the calorie carb and fat bible

The UK's Most Comprehensive Calorie Counter

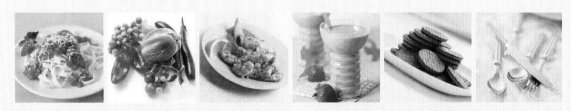

Juliette Kellow BSc RD, Lyndel Costain BSc RD & Rebecca Walton

The Calorie, Carb & Fat Bible

© Weight Loss Resources 2019
Lyndel Costain's contributions © Lyndel Costain

Published by:
Weight Loss Resources Ltd
2C Flag Business Exchange
Vicarage Farm Road
Peterborough
PE1 5TX.

Tel: 01733 345592
www.weightlossresources.co.uk

Companies and other organisations wishing to make bulk purchases of the Calorie, Carb and Fat Bible should contact their local bookstore or Weight Loss Resources direct.

Whilst every effort has been made to ensure accuracy, the publishers cannot be held responsible for any errors or omissions.

ISBN 978-1-1904512-24-0

Authors: Lyndel Costain BSc RD
Juliette Kellow BSc RD
Rebecca Walton, Weight Loss Resources

Database Editor: Sam Holt
Design and Layout: Joanne Putney

Printed and bound in the UK by Bonacia Ltd
www.bookprintinguk.com

Contents

Losing weight – the easy way

Juliette Kellow BSc RD

PIZZA, curries, chocolate, chips and the odd glass of wine! Imagine being told the best diet to help you lose weight can include all these foods and more. It sounds too good to be true, doesn't it? But the truth is, these are exactly the types of foods you can still enjoy if you opt to lose weight by counting calories.

But you'd be forgiven for not knowing you can still eat all your favourite foods *and* lose weight. In recent years, endless trendy diets have helped to make dieting a complicated business. Added to this, an increasing number of celebrities and so-called nutrition experts have helped mislead us into thinking that dieting is all about restriction and denial. Is it any wonder then that most of us have been left feeling downright confused and miserable about what we should and shouldn't be eating to shift those pounds?

Dieting doesn't have to be a complicated or unhappy experience. In fact, there's really only one word you need to remember if you want to shift those pounds healthily and still eat all your favourite foods. And that's CALORIE!

It's calories that count

When it comes to losing weight, there's no getting away from the fact that it's calories that count. Ask any qualified nutrition expert or dietitian for advice on dropping pounds and you'll receive the same reply: quite simply you need to create a calorie deficit or shortfall. In other words, you need to take in fewer calories than you use up so that your body has to draw on its fat stores to provide it with the energy it needs to function properly. The result: you start losing fat and the pounds start to drop off!

Fortunately, it couldn't be easier to create this calorie deficit. Regardless of your age, weight, sex, genetic make up, lifestyle or eating habits, losing weight is as simple as reducing your daily calorie intake slightly by modifying your diet and using up a few more calories by being slightly more active each day.

Better still, it's a complete myth that you need to change your eating and exercise habits dramatically. You'll notice I've said you need to reduce your calorie intake 'slightly' and be 'slightly' more active. It really is just LITTLE differences between the amount of calories we take in and the amount we use up that make BIG differences to our waistline over time. For example, you only need to consume one can of cola more than you need each day to gain a stone in a year. It's no wonder then that people say excess weight tends to 'creep up on them'.

10 simple food swaps you can make every day (*and won't even notice!*)

Make these simple swaps every day and in just 4 weeks you'll lose 7lb!

SWAP THIS...	FOR THIS...	SAVE...
300ml full-fat milk (*195 calories*)	300ml skimmed milk (*100 calories*)	*95 calories*
1tsp butter (*35 calories*)	1tsp low-fat spread (*20 calories*)	*15 calories*
1tbsp vegetable oil (*100 calories*)	10 sprays of a spray oil (*10 calories*)	*90 calories*
1tsp sugar (*16 calories*)	Artificial sweetener (*2 calories*)	*14 calories*
1tbsp mayonnaise (*105 calories*)	1tbsp fat-free dressing (*10 calories*)	*95 calories*
Regular sandwich (*600 calories*)	Low-fat sandwich (*350 calories*)	*250 calories*
Can of cola (*135 calories*)	Can of diet cola (*1 calorie*)	*134 calories*
Large (50g) packet of crisps (*250 calories*)	Small (25g) packet of crisps (*125 calories*)	*125 calories*
1 chocolate digestive (*85 calories*)	1 small chocolate chip cookie (*55 calories*)	*30 calories*
1 slice thick-cut wholemeal bread (*95 calories*)	1 slice medium-cut wholemeal bread (*75 calories*)	*20 calories*
	TOTAL CALORIE SAVING:	*868 calories*

The good news is the reverse is also true. You only need to swap that daily can of cola for the diet version or a glass of sparking water and you'll lose a stone in a year – it really is as easy as that!

Of course, most people don't want to wait a year to shift a stone. But there's more good news. To lose 1lb of fat each week you need to create a calorie deficit of just 500 calories a day. That might sound like a lot, but you can achieve this by simply swapping a croissant for a wholemeal fruit scone, a regular sandwich for a low-fat variety, a glass of dry white wine for a gin and slimline tonic and using low-fat spread on two slices of toast instead of butter. It is also important to become more active and increase your level of exercise; simply walking a little more will help. Losing 1lb a week, amounts to a stone in 14 weeks, or just under 4 stone in a year!

Taking control of calories

By now you've seen it really is calories that count when it comes to shifting those pounds.

A calorie-controlled diet is one of the few that allows you to include anything, whether it's pizza, wine or chocolate. A healthy diet means including a wide range of foods *(see 'Healthy Eating Made Easy' page 32).*

And that's where this book can really help. Gone are the days when it was virtually impossible to obtain information about the calorie contents of foods. This book provides calorie information for more than 22,000 different branded and unbranded UK foods so that counting calories has never been easier.

The benefits of counting calories

- *It's guaranteed to help you lose weight providing you stick to your daily calorie allowance*

- *You can include favourite foods*

- *No foods are banned*

- *It's a great way to lose weight slowly and steadily*

- *Nutrition experts agree that it's a proven way to lose weight*

Calorie counting made easy

Forget weird and wacky science, complicated diet rules and endless lists of foods to fill up on or avoid every day! Counting calories to lose weight couldn't be easier. Quite simply, you set yourself a daily calorie allowance to help you lose between ½-2lb (¼-1kg) a week and then add up the calories of everything you eat and drink each day, making sure you don't go over your limit.

To prevent hunger from kicking in, it's best to spread your daily calorie allowance evenly throughout the day, allowing a certain amount of calories for breakfast, lunch, dinner and one or two snacks. For example, if you are allowed 1,500 calories a day, you could have 300 calories for breakfast, 400 calories for lunch, 500 calories for dinner and two snacks or treats of 150 calories each. You'll find more detailed information on p26-31 (Your step-by-step guide to using this book and shifting those pounds).

QUESTION
What affects the calorie content of a food?

ANSWER:
Fat, protein, carbohydrate and alcohol all provide the body with calories, but in varying amounts:

- *1g fat provides 9 calories*

- *1g alcohol provides 7 calories*

- *1g protein provides 4 calories*

- *1g carbohydrate provides 3.75 calories*

The calorie content of a food depends on the amount of fat, protein and carbohydrate it contains. Because fat provides more than twice as many calories as an equal quantity of protein or carbohydrate, in general, foods that are high in fat tend to contain more calories. This explains why 100g of chips (189 calories) contains more than twice as many calories as 100g of boiled potato (72 calories).

DIET MYTH:
Food eaten late at night stops you losing weight

DIET FACT:
It's not eating in the evening that stops you losing weight. It's consuming too many calories throughout the day that will be your dieting downfall! Providing you stick to your daily calorie allowance you'll lose weight, regardless of when you consume those calories. Nevertheless, it's a good idea to spread your calorie allowance throughout the day to prevent hunger from kicking in, which leaves you reaching for high-calorie snack foods.

Eat for good health

While calories might be the buzz word when it comes to shifting those pounds, it's nevertheless important to make sure your diet is healthy, balanced and contains all the nutrients you need for good health. Yes, you can still lose weight by eating nothing but chocolate, crisps and biscuits providing you stick to your calorie allowance, but you'll never find a nutrition expert or dietitian recommending this. And there are plenty of good reasons why.

To start with, an unbalanced diet is likely to be lacking in essential nutrients such as protein, vitamins, minerals and fibre, in the long term putting you at risk of nutritional deficiencies. Secondly, research proves that filling up on foods that are high in saturated fat and/or salt and sugar can lead to many different health problems. But most importantly, when it comes to losing weight, it's almost impossible to stick to a daily calorie allowance if you're only eating high-calorie foods.

Filling up on lower-calorie foods also means you'll be able to eat far more with the result that you're not constantly left feeling unsatisfied. For example, six chocolates from a selection box contain around 300 calories, a lot of saturated fat and sugar, few nutrients – and are eaten in just six mouthfuls! For 300 calories, you could have a grilled skinless chicken breast (packed with protein and zinc), a large salad with fat-free dressing (a great source of fibre, vitamins and minerals), a slice of wholemeal bread with low-fat spread (rich in fibre and B vitamins) and a satsuma (an excellent source of vitamin C). That's a lot more food that will take you a lot more time to eat! Not convinced? Then put six chocolates on one plate, and the chicken, salad, bread and fruit on another!

Bottom line: while slightly reducing your calorie intake is the key to losing weight, you'll be healthier and far more likely to keep those pounds off if you do it by eating a healthy diet *(see 'Healthy Eating Made Easy' page 32).*

Eight steps to a healthy diet

1   Base your meals on starchy foods.

2   Eat lots of fruit and vegetables.

3   Eat more fish.

4   Cut down on saturated fat and sugar.

5   Try to eat less salt - no more than 6g a day.

6   Get active and try to be a healthy weight.

7   Drink plenty of water.

8   Don't skip breakfast.

SOURCE: www.nhs.uk/live-well/eat-well/eight-tips-for-healthy-eating/

Fat facts

Generally speaking, opting for foods that are low in fat can help slash your calorie intake considerably, for example, swapping full-fat milk for skimmed, switching from butter to a low-fat spread, not frying food in oil and chopping the fat off meat and poultry. But don't be fooled into believing that all foods described as 'low-fat' or 'fat-free' are automatically low in calories or calorie-free. In fact, some low-fat products may actually be higher in calories than standard products, thanks to them containing extra sugars and thickeners to boost the flavour and texture. The solution: always check the calorie content of low-fat foods, especially for things like cakes, biscuits, crisps, ice creams and ready meals. You might be surprised to find there's little difference in the calorie content when compared to the standard product.

Uncovering fat claims on food labels

Many products may lure you into believing they're a great choice if you're trying to cut fat, but you need to read between the lines on the labels if you want to be sure you're making the best choice. Here's the lowdown on what to look for:

LOW FAT	by law the food must contain less than 3g of fat per 100g for solids. These foods are generally a good choice if you're trying to lose weight.
REDUCED FAT	by law the food must contain 30 percent less fat than a similar standard product. This doesn't mean the product is low-fat (or low-calorie) though! For example, reduced-fat cheese may still contain 14g fat per 100g.
FAT FREE	the food must contain no more than 0.5g of fat per 100g or 100ml. Foods labelled as Virtually Fat Free must contain less than 0.3g fat per 100g. These foods are generally a good choice if you're trying to lose weight.
LESS THAN 8% FAT	this means the product contains less than 8g fat per 100g. It's only foods labelled 'less than 3% fat' that are a true low-fat choice.
X% FAT FREE	claims expressed as X% Fat Free shall be prohibited.
LIGHT OR LITE	claims stating a product is 'light' or 'lite' follows the same conditions as those set for the term 'reduced'.

10 easy ways to slash fat (and calories)

1   Eat fewer fried foods – grill, boil, bake, poach, steam, roast without added fat or microwave instead.

2   Don't add butter, lard, margarine or oil to food during preparation or cooking.

3   Use spreads sparingly. Butter and margarine contain the same amount of calories and fat – only low fat spreads contain less.

4   Choose boiled or jacket potatoes instead of chips or roast potatoes.

5   Cut off all visible fat from meat and remove the skin from chicken before cooking.

6   Don't eat too many fatty meat products such as sausages, burgers, pies and pastry products.

7   Use semi-skimmed or skimmed milk instead of full-fat milk.

8   Try low-fat or reduced-fat varieties of cheese such as reduced-fat Cheddar, low-fat soft cheese or cottage cheese.

9   Eat fewer high-fat foods such as crisps, chocolates, cakes, pastries and biscuits.

10 Don't add cream to puddings, sauces or coffee.

Getting Ready for Weight Loss Success

Lyndel Costain BSc RD

THIS BOOK not only provides tools to help you understand more about what you eat and how active you are, but guidance on how to use this information to develop a weight loss plan to suit your needs. Getting in the right frame of mind will also be a key part of your weight control journey, especially if you've lost weight before, only to watch the pounds pile back on.

The fact is that most people who want to lose weight know what to do. But often there is something that keeps stopping them from keeping up healthier habits. The same may be true for you. So what's going on? For many it's a lack of readiness. When the next diet comes along with its tempting promises it's so easy to just jump on board. But if you have struggled with your weight for a while, will that diet actually help you to recognise and change the thoughts and actions that have stopped you shifting the pounds for good?

Check out your attitude to weight loss programmes

Before starting any new weight loss programme, including the Weight Loss Resources approach, ask yourself:

Am I starting out thinking that I like myself as a person right now?	(YES or NO)
OR I feel I can only like myself once I lose weight?	(YES or NO)
Do I want to stop overeating, but at the same time find myself justifying it – in other words I want to be able to eat what I want, but with no consequences?	(YES or NO)
Do I believe that I need to take long-term responsibility for my weight?	(YES or NO)
OR Am I relying on 'it' (the diet) to do it for me?	(YES or NO)

Keep these questions, and your replies, in mind as you read through this chapter.

Next Steps

You may have already assessed the healthiness of your weight using the BMI guide on page 37. If not, why not do it now, remembering that the tools are a guide only. The important thing is to consider a weight at which you are healthy and comfortable – and which is realistic for the life you lead *(see opposite - What is a healthy weight?)*.

The next step is to have a long hard think about why you want to lose weight. Consider all the possible benefits, not just those related to how you look. Psychologists have found that if we focus only on appearance we are less likely to succeed in the long-term. This is because it so often reflects low self-esteem or self-worth – which can sabotage success – as it saps confidence and keeps us stuck in destructive thought patterns. Identifying key motivations other than simply how you look - such as health and other aspects of physical and emotional well being - is like saying that you're an OK person right now, and worth making changes for. Making healthy lifestyle choices also has the knock on effect of boosting self-esteem further.

Write down your reasons for wanting to lose weight in your Personal Plan *(see page 42)* – so you can refer back to them. This can be especially helpful when the going gets tough. It may help to think of it in terms of what your weight is stopping you from doing now. Here's some examples: to feel more confident; so I can play more comfortably with my kids; my healthier diet will give me more energy; to improve my fertility.

What is a Healthy Weight?

With all the mixed messages in the media it can be easy to get a distorted view about whether your weight is healthy or not. However, as the BMI charts suggest, there is no single 'ideal' weight for anybody. Research also shows that modest amounts of weight loss can be very beneficial to health and are easier to keep off. Therefore, health professionals now encourage us to aim for a weight loss of 5-10%. The ideal rate of weight loss is no more than 1-2 pounds (0.5-1kg) per week – so averaging a pound a week is great, and realistic progress.

The health benefits of modest weight loss include:

* *Reduced risk of developing heart disease, stroke and certain cancers*

* *Reduced risk of developing diabetes and helping to manage diabetes*

* *Improvements in blood pressure*

* *Improvements in mobility, back pain and joint pain*

* *Improvements with fertility problems and polycystic ovarian syndrome*

* *Less breathlessness and sleep/snoring problems*

* *Increased self esteem and control over eating*

* *Feeling fitter and have more energy*

Are You Really Ready to Lose Weight?

When you think of losing weight, it's easy just to think of what weight you'd like to get to. But weight loss only happens as a result of making changes to your usual eating and activity patterns – which allow you to consume fewer calories than you burn *(see 'It's calories that count' page 5)*.

So here comes the next big question. Are you really ready to do it? Have you thought about the implications of your decision? If you have lost weight in the past, and put it all back on - have you thought about why that was? And how confident do you feel about being successful this time?

To help you answer these questions, try these short exercises.

Where would you place yourself on the following scales?

Importance

How important is it to you, to make the changes that will allow you to lose weight?

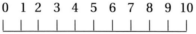

0 1 2 3 4 5 6 7 8 9 10

Not at all important   *Extremely important*

If you ranked yourself over half way along the scale then move on to the next question. If you were half way or less along the scale, you may not be mentally ready to make the required changes to lose weight. To further explore this, go to *'The Pros and Cons of Weight Loss' (page 17)*.

Confidence

How confident are you in your ability to make the changes that will allow you to lose weight?

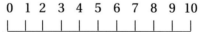

0 1 2 3 4 5 6 7 8 9 10

Not at all confident   *Extremely confident*

Now ask yourself (regarding your confidence ratings):

1. Why did I place myself here?

2. What is stopping me moving further up the scale (if anything)?

3. What things, information, support would help me move further up the scale? (if not near 10)

If you aren't sure about answers to question 3, then keep reading for some pointers.

The Pros and Cons of Weight Loss

Making lifestyle changes to lose weight is simpler if there are lots of clear benefits or pros, for example, clothes fit again, more energy, helps back pain - but there will also be associated downsides or cons. For example, some may feel it interferes with their social life, or don't have the time to plan meals or check food labels. Or overeating can help, if only temporarily, as a way of coping with unwanted feelings. Being overweight allows some people to feel strong and assertive, or to control their partner's jealousy. So in these cases there are downsides to losing weight, even if the person says they are desperate to do it.

If you are aware of the possible downsides, as well as the pros, you will be better prepared to deal with potential conflicts. Understanding what could be (or were with past weight loss efforts) barriers to success gives you the chance to address them. This boosts confidence in your ability to succeed this time, which in turn maintains your motivation.

Have a go at weighing up the pros and cons using the charts below and on page 18. Some examples are included. If you decide that the pros outweigh the cons, then great. You can also use the cons as potential barriers to plan strategies for *(see page 42)*. If you find it's the other way around, this may not be the best time to actively lose weight. Try the exercise again in a month or so.

Making Lifestyle Changes to Lose Weight Now

CONS *e.g. Must limit eating out, take aways*	PROS *e.g. Feel more energetic, slimmer*

Not Making Changes Now – how would I feel in 6 months time?

PROS *e.g. Haven't had to worry about failing;* *Still able to eat take aways a lot*	CONS *e.g. Perhaps gained more weight;* *Still don't like how I look and feel*

To change your weight, first change your mind

To lose weight you may already have a list of things to change, such as eating more fruit and veg, calculating your daily calorie intake, going for a walk each morning or buying low fat options. Others could also give you tips to try. But knowing what to do isn't the same as feeling motivated or able to do it. To be effective, you have to believe the changes are relevant, do-able and worth it.

What you think, affects how you feel, and in turn the actions you take.

Self-efficacy

In fact, research is telling us that one of the most important factors that influences weight loss success are your feelings of 'self-efficacy'. Self-efficacy is a term used in psychology to describe a person's belief that any action they take will have an effect on the outcome. It reflects our inner expectation that what we do will lead to the results we want. Not surprisingly, high levels of self-efficacy can enhance motivation, and allow us to deal better with uncertainty and conflict, and recovery from setbacks. But low levels, can reduce our motivation. We fear that whatever we do will not bring about our desired goal. This can lead self-defeating thoughts or 'self-talk', which make it hard to deal with set-backs, meaning we are more likely to give up. Here's some examples.

Examples: Low self-efficacy

'No matter how carefully I diet, I don't lose weight...'

'I have eaten that chocolate and as usual blown my diet, so I may as well give up now.'

'I had a rich dessert – I have no willpower to say no. I can't stand not being able to eat what I want.'

If you have a strong sense of self-efficacy, your mindset and 'self-talk' will be more like:

Examples: High self-efficacy

' I know from previous weight loss attempts, that if I stay focussed on what I am doing I do lose weight. I have always expected to lose too much too quickly which frustrates me. I know that I will lose weight if I keep making the right changes, and this time it is important to me.'

' The chocolate bar won't ruin my diet, but if I think it has and keep on eating, then my negative self-talk will. So I will get back on track.'

*' Losing weight is very important to me, so I **can** make better food choices. After all, the world won't stop if I say no to dessert, and I will feel great afterwards. If I think about it, I am not hungry so would just feel bloated and guilty if I ate it.'*

Willpower is a Skill

Many people feel that they just need plenty of willpower or a good telling off to lose weight. But willpower isn't something you have or you don't have. Willpower is a skill. Like the dessert example on page 19, it's a sign that you've made a conscious choice to do something, because you believe the benefits outweigh any downsides. In reality everything we do is preceded by a thought. This includes everything we eat. It just may not seem like it because our actions often feel automatic *(see 'Look out for trigger eating' page 21).*

When it comes to weight loss, developing a range of skills – including choosing lower calorie options, coping with negative self-talk and managing things that don't go to plan - will boost your sense of self-efficacy to make the changes you want. This is especially important because we live in such a weight-promoting environment.

Our weight-promoting environment

We are constantly surrounded by tempting food, stresses that can trigger comfort eating and labour-saving devices that make it easy not to be physically active. In other words, the environment we live in makes it easy to gain weight, unless we stop and think about the food choices we make and how much exercise we do. In fact, to stay a healthy weight/maintain our weight, just about all of us need to make conscious lifestyle choices everyday. This isn't 'dieting' but just part of taking care of ourselves in the environment we live in.

It is also true that some people find it more of a challenge than others to manage their weight, thanks to genetic differences in factors such as appetite control, spontaneous activity level and emotional responses to food – rather than metabolic rate, as is often believed. The good news is that with a healthy diet and active lifestyle a healthier weight can still be achieved. But do talk to your doctor if you feel you need additional support.

Coping with Common Slimming Saboteurs

Lyndel Costain BSc RD

Look out for 'trigger' eating

Much of the overeating we do or cravings we have are actually down to unconscious, habitual, responses to a variety of triggers. These triggers can be external, such as the sight or smell of food, or internal and emotion-led, such as a response to stress, anger, boredom or emptiness. Your food diary (see page 43) helps you to recognise 'trigger' or 'non-hungry' eating which gives you the chance to think twice before you eat (see below).

Get some support

A big part of your success will be having someone to support you. It could be a friend, partner, health professional, health club or website. Let them know how they can help you most.

Make lapses your ally

Don't let a lapse throw you off course. You can't be, nor need to be perfect all the time. Doing well 80-90% of the time is great progress. Lapses are a normal part of change. Rather than feel you have failed and give up, look at what you can learn from a difficult day or week and use it to find helpful solutions for the future.

Understand why you eat

When I ask people what prompts them to eat, hunger usually comes down near the bottom of their list of reasons. Some people struggle to remember or appreciate what true hunger feels like. We are lucky that we have plenty of food to eat in our society. But its constant presence makes it harder to control what we eat, especially if it brings us comfort or joy.

If you ever find yourself in the fridge even though you've recently eaten, then you know hunger isn't the reason but some other trigger. The urge to eat can be so automatic that you feel you lack willpower or are out of control. But it is in fact a learned or conditioned response. A bit like Pavlov's dogs. He rang a bell every time he fed them, and from then on, whenever they heard the bell ring they were 'conditioned' to salivate in anticipation of food.

Because this 'non-hungry' eating is learned, you can reprogramme your response to the situations or feelings that trigger it. The first step is to identify when these urges strike. When you find yourself eating when you aren't hungry ask yourself 'why do I want to eat, what am I feeling?' If you aren't sure think back to what was happening before you ate. Then ask yourself if there is another way you can feel better without food. Or you could chat to your urge to eat in a friendly way, telling it that you don't want to give into it, you have a planned meal coming soon, and it's merely a learned response. Whatever strategy you choose, the more often you break into your urges to eat, the weaker their hold becomes.

Practise positive self-talk

Self-talk may be positive and constructive (like your guardian angel) or negative and irrational (like having a destructive devil on your shoulder).

If you've had on-off battles with your weight over the years, it's highly likely that the 'devil' is there more often. 'All or nothing' self-talk for example, 'I ate a "bad food" so have broken my diet', can make you feel like a failure which, can then trigger you into the action of overeating and/or totally giving up *(see 'Diet-binge cycle' page 23)*. One of the most powerful things about it is that the last thoughts we have are what stays in our mind. So if we think 'I still look fat' or 'I will never be slim', these feelings stay with us.

To change your self-talk for the better, the trick is to first recognise it's happening (keeping a diary really helps, *see Keep a Food Diary, page 29*). Then turn it around into a positive version of the same events *(see Self-efficacy, page 18)* where the resulting action was to feel good and stay on track. Reshaping negative self-talk helps you to boost your self-esteem and feelings of self-efficacy, and with it change your self-definition - from someone who can't 'lose weight' or 'do this or that', to someone 'who can'. And when you believe you can…

The Diet – Binge Cycle

If this cycle looks familiar, use positive self-talk, and a more flexible dietary approach, to help you break free.

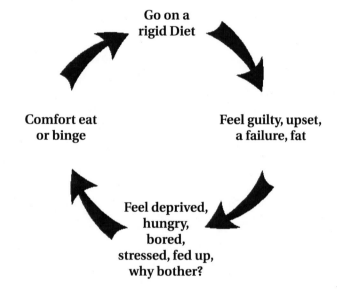

**Go on a
rigid Diet**

**Feel guilty, upset,
a failure, fat**

**Feel deprived,
hungry,
bored,
stressed, fed up,
why bother?**

**Comfort eat
or binge**

Really choose what you want to eat

This skill is like your personal brake. It also helps you to manage 'trigger/ non-hungry' eating and weaken its hold. It legalises food and stops you feeling deprived. It helps you to regularly remind yourself why you are making changes to your eating habits, which keeps motivation high. But it doesn't just happen. Like all skills it requires practise. Sometimes it will work well for you, other times it won't – but overall it will help. Basically, ask yourself if you really want to eat that food in front of you. This becomes the prompt for you to make a conscious choice, weighing up the pros and cons or consequences of making that choice, and feeling free to have it, reject it or just eat some. Remembering all the while that you can eat this food another time if you want to.

Action Planning

Successful people don't just wait for things to happen. They believe in themselves, plan ahead, take action and then refine their plan until it gets, and keeps on getting the results they want. Successful slimmers use a very similar approach. They don't rely on quick-fixes or magic formulas, but glean information from reliable sources to develop a plan or approach that suits their needs, tastes and lifestyle. Thinking of weight management as a lifelong project, which has a weight loss phase and a weight maintenance phase, is also a route to success.

When the Going Gets Tough - Staying on Track

If things start to go off track, don't panic. Learning new habits takes time. And life is never straightforward so there will be times when it all seems too much, or negative 'self- talk' creeps in to try and drag you back into old ways. So if the going gets tough:

- Value what you've achieved so far, rather than only focus on what you plan to do.

- Look back at your reasons to lose weight and refer to the list often.

- Don't expect to change too much, too quickly. Take things a step at a time.

- Accept difficulties as part of the learning and skill building process.

- Enjoy a non-food reward for achieving your goals (including maintaining your weight).

- Use recipes and meal ideas to keep things interesting.

- Talk to your supporters and get plenty of encouragement. This is really vital!

Strategies of Successful Slimmers

Thanks to research conducted by large studies such as the US National Weight Control Registry and the German Lean Habits Study, we now know more about what works best for people who have lost weight and successfully kept it off. So be inspired!

The key elements of success are to:

- Believe that you can control your weight and the changes involved are really worth it.
- Stay realistic and value what you have achieved rather than dwell on a weight you 'dream' of being.
- Be more active – plan ways to fit activity into your daily life – aim for 1 hour of walking daily.
- Plan ahead for regular meals and snacks, starting with breakfast.
- Choose a balanced, low-fat diet with plenty of fruit and vegetables *(see Healthy Eating Made Easy, page 32)*.
- Watch portion size and limit fast food.
- Sit down to eat and take time over meals, paying attention to what you are eating.
- Have a flexible approach – plan in and enjoy some favourite foods without guilt.
- Recognise and address 'all or nothing' thinking and other negative 'self-talk'.
- Keep making conscious choices.
- Learn to confront problems rather than eat, drink, sleep or wish they would go away.
- Enlist ongoing help and support from family, friends, professionals or websites.
- Regularly (at least once a week but not more than once daily) check your weight.
- Take action before your weight increases by more than 4-5lb (2kg).
- Accept that your weight management skills need to be kept up long-term.
- Take heart from successful slimmers, who say that it gets easier over time.

Your step-by-step guide to using this book and shifting those pounds

Juliette Kellow BSc RD and Rebecca Walton

1. Find your healthy weight

Use the weight charts, body mass index table and information on pages 36-43 to determine the right weight for you. Then set yourself a weight to aim for. Research shows it really helps if you make losing 10% of your weight your first overall target. It also brings important health benefits too *(see 'What is a Healthy Weight?' page 15).* You can break this down into smaller manageable steps, for example, 3kg/6.5lbs at a time. If 10% is too much, then go for a 5% loss – this has important health benefits too. In fact, just keeping your weight stable is a great achievement these days, because of our weight-promoting environment *(see page 20).*

Waist Management

In addition to BMI, another important way to assess your weight is by measuring your waist just above belly button level. It is especially useful for men as they tend to carry more excess weight around their bellies, but women should test it out too. Having excess weight around your middle (known as being 'apple-shaped') increases your risk of heart disease and type 2 diabetes. A simple way to stay aware of your waist is according to how well, or otherwise, skirts and trousers fit. Talk to your doctor about any weight and health concerns.

WAIST MEASUREMENT

	Increased Health Risk	High Risk to Health
Women	32-35in (81-88cm)	more than 35in (88cm)
Men	37-40in (94-102cm)	more than 40in (102cm)

2. Set a realistic time scale

With today's hectic lifestyles, everything tends to happen at breakneck speed, so it's no wonder that when it comes to losing weight, most of us want to shift those pounds in an instant. But it's probably taken years to accumulate that extra weight, with the result that it's unrealistic to expect to lose the excess in just a few weeks! Instead, prepare yourself to lose weight slowly and steadily. It's far healthier to lose weight like this. But better still, research shows you'll be far more likely to maintain your new, lower weight.

If you only have a small amount of weight to lose, aim for a weight loss of around 1lb (½kg) a week. But if you have more than 2 stone (28kg) to lose, you may prefer to aim for 2lb (1kg) each week. Remember though, it's better to keep going at 1lb (½kg) a week than to give up because trying to lose 2lb (1kg) a week is making you miserable! The following words may help you to keep your goal in perspective:

'Never give up on a goal because of the time it will take to achieve it – the time will pass anyway.'

Weight Fluctuations

Weight typically fluctuates on a day to day basis. You know that shock/horror feeling when you weigh yourself in the morning then later in the day, or after a meal out, and it looks like youve gained pounds in hours! But this is due to fluid not fat changes. Real changes in body fat can only happen more gradually (remember, to gain 1lb you need to eat 3500 calories more than you usually do). Don't be confused either by seemingly very rapid weight loss in the first week or so.

When calorie intake is initially cut back, the body's carbohydrate stores in the liver and muscles (known as glycogen) are used up. Glycogen is stored with three times its weight in water, meaning that rapid losses of 4.5- 6.6lb (2 -3 kg) are possible. These stores can be just as rapidly refilled if normal eating is resumed. True weight loss happens more gradually and this book helps you to lose weight at the steady and healthy rate of no more than 1-2 lbs per week.

3. Calculate your calorie allowance

Use the calorie tables on pages 39-40 to find out how many calories you need each day to maintain your current weight. Then use the table below to discover the amount of calories you need to subtract from this amount every day to lose weight at your chosen rate. For example, a 35 year-old woman who is moderately active and weighs 12 stone (76kg) needs 2,188 calories a day to keep her weight steady. If she wants to lose ½lb (¼kg) a week, she needs 250 calories less each day, giving her a daily calorie allowance of 1,938 calories. If she wants to lose 1lb (½kg) a week, she needs 500 calories less each day, giving her a daily calorie allowance of 1,688 calories, and so on.

TO LOSE...	Cut your daily calorie intake by	In three months you could lose...	In six months you could lose...	In one year you could lose...
½lb a week	250	6.5lb	13lb	1st 12lb
1lb a week	500	13lb	1st 12lb	3st 10lb
1½lb a week	750	1st 5.5lb	2st 11lb	5st 8lb
2lb a week	1,000	1st 12lb	3st 10lb	7st 6lb

TO LOSE...	Cut your daily calorie intake by	In three months you could lose...	In six months you could lose...	In one year you could lose...
¼kg a week	250	3.25kg	6.5kg	13kg
½kg a week	500	6.5kg	13kg	26kg
¾kg a week	750	9.75kg	19.5kg	39kg
1kg a week	1,000	13kg	26kg	52kg

4. Keep a food diary

Writing down what you eat and drink and any thoughts linked to that eating helps you become more aware of your eating habits. Recognising what is going on helps you feel in control and is a powerful way to start planning change. Keeping a food diary before you start to change your eating habits will also help you identify opportunities for cutting calories by substituting one food for another, cutting portion sizes of high-calorie foods or eating certain foods less often.

Simply write down every single item you eat or drink during the day and use this book to calculate the calories of each item. Then after a few days of eating normally, introduce some changes to your diet to achieve your daily calorie allowance. Remember to spread your daily calorie allowance fairly evenly throughout the day to prevent hunger. You'll find a template for a daily food and exercise diary on page 43.

Top Tip

If you only fill in your main food diary once a day, keep a pen and notepad with you to write down all those little extras you eat or drink during the day – that chocolate you ate in the office, the sliver of cheese you had while cooking dinner and the few chips you pinched from your husband's plate, for example! It's easy to forget the little things if they're not written down, but they can make the difference between success and failure.

QUESTION: Why are heavier people allowed more calories than those who have smaller amounts of weight to lose?

ANSWER: This confuses a lot of people but is easily explained. Someone who is 3 stone overweight, for example, is carrying the equivalent of 42 small packets of butter with them everywhere they go – up and down the stairs, to the local shops, into the kitchen. Obviously, it takes a lot more energy simply to move around when you're carrying that extra weight. As a consequence, the heavier you are, the more calories you need just to keep your weight steady. In turn, this means you'll lose weight on a higher calorie allowance. However, as you lose weight, you'll need to lower your calorie allowance slightly as you have less weight to carry around.

5. Control your portions

As well as making some smart food swaps to cut calories, it's likely you'll also need to reduce your serving sizes for some foods to help shift those pounds. Even 'healthy' foods such as brown rice, wholemeal bread, chicken, fish and low-fat dairy products contain calories so you may need to limit the amount you eat. When you first start out, weigh portions of foods like rice, pasta, cereal, cheese, butter, oil, meat, fish, and chicken rather than completing your food diary with a 'guesstimated' weight! That way you can calculate the calorie content accurately. Don't forget that drinks contain calories too, alcohol, milk, juices and sugary drinks all count.

6. Measure your success

Research has found that regular weight checks do help. Weighing yourself helps you assess how your eating and exercise habits affect your body weight. The important thing is to use the information in a positive way – to assess your progress - rather than as a stick to beat yourself up with. Remember that weight can fluctuate by a kilogram in a day, for example, due to fluid changes, premenstrually, after a big meal out, so weigh yourself at the same time of day and look at the trend over a week or two.

People who successfully lose weight and keep it off, also tend to continue weighing themselves at least once a week, and often daily (but not in an obsessive way), because they say it helps them stay 'on track'. Probably because they use it as an early warning system. People who weigh themselves regularly (or regularly try on a tight fitting item of clothing) will notice quickly if they have gained a few pounds - and can take action to stop gaining more. Checking your weight less often can mean that you might discover one day that you gained more than you thought. That can be pretty discouraging, and it might trigger you to just give up.

Top Tip

Don't just focus on what the bathroom scales say either – keep a record of your vital statistics, too. Many people find it doubly encouraging to see the inches dropping off, as well as the pounds!

7. Stay motivated

Each time you lose half a stone, or reach your own small goal – celebrate! Treat yourself to a little luxury – something new to wear, a little pampering or some other (non-food) treat. It also helps replace the comfort you once got from food and allows you to take care of yourself in other ways. Trying on an item of clothing that used to be tight can also help to keep you feeling motivated. Make sure you keep in touch with your supporters, and if the going gets tough take another look at the *'Coping with Common Slimming Saboteurs' section on page 21*. Once you've reviewed how well you've done, use this book to set yourself a new daily calorie allowance based on your new weight to help you lose the next half stone *(see point 3 - page 28 - Calculate your calorie allowance)*.

8. Keep it off

What you do to stay slim is just as important as what you did to get slim. Quite simply, if you return to your old ways, you are likely to return to your old weight. The great thing about calorie counting is that you will learn so much about what you eat, and make so many important changes to your eating and drinking habits, that you'll probably find it difficult to go back to your old ways – and won't want to anyway. It's still a good idea to weigh yourself at least once a week to keep a check on your weight. The key is to deal with any extra pounds immediately, rather than waiting until you have a stone to lose *(see page 30)*. Simply go back to counting calories for as long as it takes to shift those pounds and enjoy the new slim you. Page 25 has more information about how successful slimmers keep it off.

QUESTION: Do I need to stick to exactly the same number of calories each day or is it OK to have a lower calorie intake during the week and slightly more at the weekend?

ANSWER: The key to losing weight is to take in fewer calories than you need for as long as it takes to reach your target, aiming for a loss of no more than 2lb (1kg) a week. In general, most nutrition experts recommend a daily calorie allowance. However, it's just as valid to use other periods of time such as weeks. If you prefer, simply multiply your daily allowance by seven to work out a weekly calorie allowance and then allocate more calories to some days than others. For example, a daily allowance of 1,500 calories is equivalent to 10,500 calories a week. This means you could have 1,300 calories a day during the week and 2,000 calories a day on Saturday and Sunday.

Healthy Eating Made Easy

Juliette Kellow BSc RD

HEALTHY EATING doesn't just mean eating salads and smoothies. Eating healthily means we're positively encouraged to eat a wide range of foods, including some of our favourites – it's just a question of making sure we don't eat high fat, high sugar or highly processed foods too often.

Eating a healthy diet, together with taking regular exercise and not smoking, has huge benefits to our health, both in the short and long term. As well as helping us to lose or maintain our weight, a healthy diet can boost energy levels, keep our immune system strong and give us healthy skin, nails and hair. Meanwhile, eating well throughout life also means we're far less likely to suffer from health problems such as constipation, anaemia and tooth decay, or set ourselves up for serious conditions in later life such as obesity, heart disease, stroke, diabetes, cancer or osteoporosis.

Fortunately, it couldn't be easier to eat a balanced diet. To start with, no single food provides all the calories and nutrients we need to stay healthy, so it's important to eat a variety of foods. Meanwhile, most nutrition experts also agree that mealtimes should be a pleasure rather than a penance. This means it's fine to eat small amounts of our favourite treats from time to time.

To help people eat healthily, the NHS recommends eating plenty of different foods from four main groups of foods and limiting the amount we eat from a smaller fifth group. Ultimately, we should eat more fruit, vegetables, starchy, fibre-rich foods and fresh products, and fewer fatty, sugary, salty and processed foods.

The following guidelines are all based on the healthy eating guidelines recommended by health professionals.

Bread, other cereals and potatoes

Eat these foods at each meal. They also make good snacks.

Foods in this group include bread, breakfast cereals, potatoes, rice, pasta, noodles, yams, oats and grains. Go for high-fibre varieties where available, such as wholegrain cereals, wholemeal bread and brown rice. These foods should fill roughly a third of your plate at mealtimes.

TYPICAL SERVING SIZES

* *2 slices bread in a sandwich or with a meal*

* *a tennis ball sized serving of pasta, potato, rice, noodles or couscous*

* *a bowl of porridge*

* *around 40g of breakfast cereal*

Fruit and vegetables

Eat at least five portions every day.

Foods in this group include all fruits and vegetables, including fresh, frozen, canned and dried products, and unsweetened fruit juice. Choose canned fruit in juice rather than syrup and go for veg canned in water without added salt or sugar.

TYPICAL PORTION SIZES

* *a piece of fruit eg: apple, banana, pear*

* *2 small fruits eg: satsumas, plums, apricots*

* *a bowl of fruit salad, canned or stewed fruit*

* *a small glass of unsweetened fruit juice*

* *a cereal bowl of salad*

* *3tbsp vegetables*

Milk, dairy and alternatives

Eat two or three servings a day.

Foods in this group include milk, cheese, yoghurt and fromage frais. Choose low-fat varieties where available such as skimmed milk, reduced-fat cheese and fat-free yoghurt.

TYPICAL SERVING SIZES

* *200ml milk*

* *a small pot of yoghurt or fromage frais*

* *a small matchbox-sized piece of cheese*

Meat, fish and alternatives

Eat two servings a day

Foods in this group include meat, poultry, fish, eggs, beans, nuts and seeds. Choose low-fat varieties where available such as extra-lean minced beef and skinless chicken and don't add extra fat or salt.

TYPICAL SERVING SIZES

* *a piece of meat, chicken or fish the size of a deck of cards*

* *1-2 eggs*

* *3 heaped tablespoons of beans*

* *a small handful of nuts or seeds*

Healthy Eating on a plate

A simple way to serve up both balance and healthy proportions is to fill one half of your plate with salad or vegetables and divide the other half between protein-rich meat, chicken, fish, eggs or beans, and healthy carbs (potatoes, rice, pasta, pulses, bread or noodles).

Fatty and sugary foods

Eat only small amounts of these foods

Foods in this group include oils, spreading fats, cream, mayonnaise, oily salad dressings, cakes, biscuits, puddings, crisps, savoury snacks, sugar, preserves, confectionery and sugary soft drinks.

TYPICAL SERVING SIZES:

- *a small packet of sweets or a small bar of chocolate*

- *a small slice of cake*

- *a couple of small biscuits*

- *1 level tbsp mayo, salad dressing or olive oil*

- *a small packet of crisps*

Useful Tools

Body Mass Index

The Body Mass Index (BMI) is the internationally accepted way of assessing how healthy our weight is for most people. It is calculated using height and weight. Use the BMI Chart to look up your BMI, and use this table to see which range you fall into.

BMI Under 18.5	Underweight
BMI 18.5-25	Healthy
BMI 25-30	Overweight
BMI 30-40	Obese
BMI Over 40	Severely Obese

This is what different BMI ranges mean.

- **Underweight:** you probably need to gain weight for your health's sake. Talk to your doctor if you have any concerns, or if you feel frightened about gaining weight.

- **Healthy weight:** you are a healthy weight, so aim to stay in this range (note that most people in this range tend to have a BMI between 20-25).

- **Overweight:** aim to lose some weight for your health's sake, or at least prevent further weight gain.

- **Obese:** your health is at risk and losing weight will benefit your health.

- **Severely obese:** your health is definitely at risk. You should visit your doctor for a health check. Losing weight will improve your health.

Please note that BMI is not as accurate for athletes or very muscular people (muscle weighs more than fat), as it can push them into a higher BMI category despite having a healthy level of body fat. It is also not accurate for women who are pregnant or breastfeeding, or people who are frail.

Body Mass Index Table

HEIGHT IN FEET / INCHES

	4'6	4'8	4'10	5'0	5'2	5'4	5'6	5'8	5'10	6'0	6'2	6'4	6'6	6'8	6'10
6st 7	22.0	20.5	19.1	17.8	16.7	15.7	14.7	13.9	13.1	12.4	11.7	11.1	10.6	10.0	9.5
7st 0	23.7	22.1	20.6	19.2	18.0	16.9	15.9	15.0	14.1	13.3	12.6	12.0	11.4	10.8	10.3
7st 7	25.4	23.6	22.0	20.6	19.3	18.1	17.0	16.0	15.1	14.3	13.5	12.8	12.2	11.6	11.0
8st 0	27.1	25.2	23.5	22.0	20.6	19.3	18.1	17.1	16.1	15.2	14.4	13.7	13.0	12.3	11.8
8st 7	28.8	26.8	25.0	23.3	21.8	20.5	19.3	18.2	17.1	16.2	15.3	14.5	13.8	13.1	12.5
9st 0	30.5	28.4	26.4	24.7	23.1	21.7	20.4	19.2	18.1	17.2	16.2	15.4	14.6	13.9	13.2
9st 7	32.2	29.9	27.9	26.1	24.4	22.9	21.5	20.3	19.2	18.1	17.1	16.2	15.4	14.7	14.0
10st 0	33.9	31.5	29.4	27.4	25.7	24.1	22.7	21.4	20.2	19.1	18.0	17.1	16.2	15.4	14.7
10st 7	35.6	33.1	30.8	28.8	27.0	25.3	23.8	22.4	21.2	20.0	18.9	18.0	17.0	16.2	15.4
11st 0	37.3	34.7	32.3	30.2	28.3	26.5	24.9	23.5	22.2	21.0	19.8	18.8	17.9	17.0	16.2
11st 7	39.0	36.2	33.8	31.6	29.6	27.7	26.1	24.6	23.2	21.9	20.7	19.7	18.7	17.8	16.9
12st 0	40.7	37.8	35.2	32.9	30.8	28.9	27.2	25.6	24.2	22.9	21.6	20.5	19.5	18.5	17.6
12st 7	42.3	39.4	36.7	34.3	32.1	30.1	28.3	26.7	25.2	23.8	22.5	21.4	20.3	19.3	18.4
13st 0	44.0	41.0	38.2	35.7	33.4	31.4	29.5	27.8	26.2	24.8	23.5	22.2	21.1	20.1	19.1
13st 7	45.7	42.5	39.6	37.0	34.7	32.6	30.6	28.8	27.2	25.7	24.4	23.1	21.9	20.8	19.8
14st 0	47.4	44.1	41.1	38.4	36.0	33.8	31.7	29.9	28.2	26.7	25.3	23.9	22.7	21.6	20.6
14st 7	49.1	45.7	42.6	39.8	37.3	35.0	32.9	31.0	29.2	27.6	26.2	24.8	23.5	22.4	21.3
15st 0	50.8	47.3	44.0	41.2	38.5	36.2	34.0	32.0	30.2	28.6	27.1	25.7	24.4	23.2	22.0
15st 7	52.5	48.8	45.5	42.5	39.8	37.4	35.2	33.1	31.2	29.5	28.0	26.5	25.2	23.9	22.8
16st 0	54.2	50.4	47.0	43.9	41.1	38.6	36.3	34.2	32.3	30.5	28.9	27.4	26.0	24.7	23.5
16st 7	55.9	52.0	48.5	45.3	42.4	39.8	37.4	35.2	33.3	31.4	29.8	28.2	26.8	25.5	24.2
17st 0	57.6	53.6	49.9	46.6	43.7	41.0	38.6	36.3	34.3	32.4	30.7	29.1	27.6	26.2	25.0
17st 7	59.3	55.1	51.4	48.0	45.0	42.2	39.7	37.4	35.3	33.3	31.6	29.9	28.4	27.0	25.7
18st 0	61.0	56.7	52.9	49.4	46.3	43.4	40.8	38.5	36.3	34.3	32.5	30.8	29.2	27.8	26.4
18st 7	62.7	58.3	54.3	50.8	47.5	44.6	42.0	39.5	37.3	35.3	33.4	31.6	30.0	28.6	27.2
19st 0	64.4	59.9	55.8	52.1	48.8	45.8	43.1	40.6	38.3	36.2	34.3	32.5	30.8	29.3	27.9
19st 7	66.1	61.4	57.3	53.5	50.1	47.0	44.2	41.7	39.3	37.2	35.2	33.3	31.7	30.1	28.6
20st 0	67.8	63.0	58.7	54.9	51.4	48.2	45.4	42.7	40.3	38.1	36.1	34.2	32.5	30.9	29.4
20st 7	69.4	64.6	60.2	56.3	52.7	49.4	46.5	43.8	41.3	39.1	37.0	35.1	33.3	31.6	30.1
21st 0	71.1	66.2	61.7	57.6	54.0	50.6	47.6	44.9	42.3	40.0	37.9	35.9	34.1	32.4	30.9
21st 7	72.8	67.7	63.1	59.0	55.3	51.9	48.8	45.9	43.3	41.0	38.8	36.8	34.9	33.2	31.6
22st 0	74.5	69.3	64.6	60.4	56.5	53.1	49.9	47.0	44.4	41.9	39.7	37.6	35.7	34.0	32.3
22st 7	76.2	70.9	66.1	61.7	57.8	54.3	51.0	48.1	45.4	42.9	40.6	38.5	36.5	34.7	33.1
23st 0	77.9	72.5	67.5	63.1	59.1	55.5	52.2	49.1	46.4	43.8	41.5	39.3	37.3	35.5	33.8
23st 7	79.6	74.0	69.0	64.5	60.4	56.7	53.3	50.2	47.4	44.8	42.4	40.2	38.2	36.3	34.5
24st 0	81.3	75.6	70.5	65.9	61.7	57.9	54.4	51.3	48.4	45.7	43.3	41.0	39.0	37.0	35.3
24st 7	83.0	77.2	71.9	67.2	63.0	59.1	55.6	52.3	49.4	46.7	44.2	41.9	39.8	37.8	36.0
25st 0	84.7	78.8	73.4	68.6	64.2	60.3	56.7	53.4	50.4	47.6	45.1	42.8	40.6	38.6	36.7
25st 7	86.4	80.3	74.9	70.0	65.5	61.5	57.8	54.5	51.4	48.6	46.0	43.6	41.4	39.4	37.5
26st 0	88.1	81.9	76.3	71.3	66.8	62.7	59.0	55.5	52.4	49.5	46.9	44.5	42.2	40.1	38.2
26st 7	89.8	83.5	77.8	72.7	68.1	63.9	60.1	56.6	53.4	50.5	47.8	45.3	43.0	40.9	38.9
27st 0	91.5	85.1	79.3	74.1	69.4	65.1	61.2	57.7	54.4	51.5	48.7	46.2	43.8	41.7	39.7
27st 7	93.2	86.6	80.8	75.5	70.7	66.3	62.4	58.7	55.4	52.4	49.6	47.0	44.7	42.4	40.4
28st 0	94.9	88.2	82.2	76.8	72.0	67.5	63.5	59.8	56.4	53.4	50.5	47.9	45.5	43.2	41.1
28st 7	96.5	89.8	83.7	78.2	73.2	68.7	64.6	60.9	57.5	54.3	51.4	48.7	46.3	44.0	41.9
29st 0	98.2	91.4	85.2	79.6	74.5	69.9	65.8	62.0	58.5	55.3	52.3	49.6	47.1	44.8	42.6
29st 7	99.9	92.9	86.6	80.9	75.8	71.1	66.9	63.0	59.5	56.2	53.2	50.5	47.9	45.5	43.3

WEIGHT IN STONES / LBS

Weight Chart

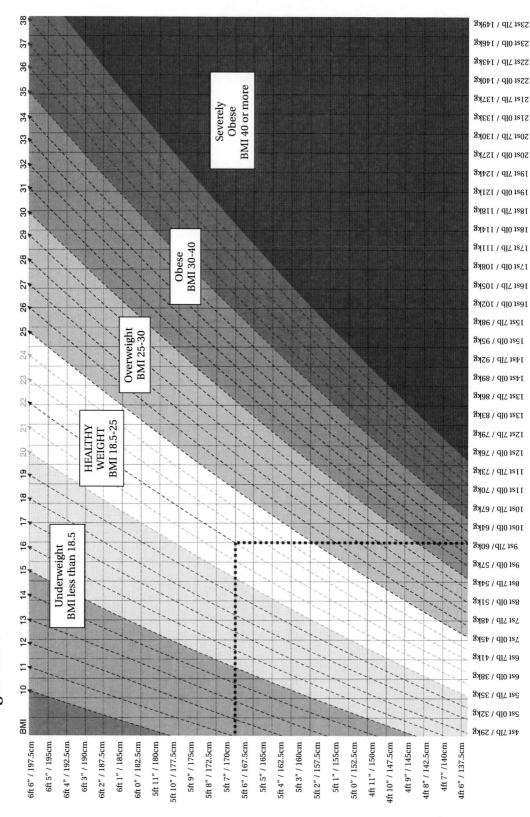

Calories Required to Maintain Weight
Adult Females

ACTIVITY LEVEL / AGE

WEIGHT IN STONES / LBS	VERY SEDENTARY			MODERATELY SEDENTARY			MODERATELY ACTIVE			VERY ACTIVE		
	<30	30-60	60+	<30	30-60	60+	<30	30-60	60+	<30	30-60	60+
7st 7	1425	1473	1304	1544	1596	1412	1781	1841	1630	2138	2210	1956
8st 0	1481	1504	1338	1605	1629	1450	1852	1880	1673	2222	2256	2008
8st 7	1537	1535	1373	1666	1663	1487	1922	1919	1716	2306	2302	2059
9st 0	1594	1566	1407	1726	1696	1524	1992	1957	1759	2391	2349	2111
9st 7	1650	1596	1442	1787	1729	1562	2062	1996	1802	2475	2395	2163
10st 0	1706	1627	1476	1848	1763	1599	2133	2034	1845	2559	2441	2214
10st 7	1762	1658	1511	1909	1796	1637	2203	2073	1888	2644	2487	2266
11st 0	1819	1689	1545	1970	1830	1674	2273	2111	1931	2728	2534	2318
11st 7	1875	1720	1580	2031	1863	1711	2344	2150	1975	2813	2580	2370
12st 0	1931	1751	1614	2092	1897	1749	2414	2188	2018	2897	2626	2421
12st 7	1987	1781	1648	2153	1930	1786	2484	2227	2061	2981	2672	2473
13st 0	2044	1812	1683	2214	1963	1823	2555	2266	2104	3066	2719	2525
13st 7	2100	1843	1717	2275	1997	1861	2625	2304	2147	3150	2765	2576
14st 0	2156	1874	1752	2336	2030	1898	2695	2343	2190	3234	2811	2628
14st 7	2212	1905	1786	2397	2064	1935	2766	2381	2233	3319	2858	2680
15st 0	2269	1936	1821	2458	2097	1973	2836	2420	2276	3403	2904	2732
15st 7	2325	1967	1855	2519	2130	2010	2906	2458	2319	3488	2950	2783
16st 0	2381	1997	1890	2580	2164	2047	2976	2497	2362	3572	2996	2835
16st 7	2437	2028	1924	2640	2197	2085	3047	2535	2405	3656	3043	2887
17st 0	2494	2059	1959	2701	2231	2122	3117	2574	2449	3741	3089	2938
17st 7	2550	2090	1993	2762	2264	2159	3187	2613	2492	3825	3135	2990
18st 0	2606	2121	2028	2823	2298	2197	3258	2651	2535	3909	3181	3042
18st 7	2662	2152	2062	2884	2331	2234	3328	2690	2578	3994	3228	3093
19st 0	2719	2182	2097	2945	2364	2271	3398	2728	2621	4078	3274	3145
19st 7	2775	2213	2131	3006	2398	2309	3469	2767	2664	4162	3320	3197
20st 0	2831	2244	2166	3067	2431	2346	3539	2805	2707	4247	3366	3249
20st 7	2887	2275	2200	3128	2465	2383	3609	2844	2750	4331	3413	3300
21st 0	2944	2306	2235	3189	2498	2421	3680	2882	2793	4416	3459	3352
21st 7	3000	2337	2269	3250	2531	2458	3750	2921	2836	4500	3505	3404
22st 0	3056	2368	2303	3311	2565	2495	3820	2960	2879	4584	3552	3455
22st 7	3112	2398	2338	3372	2598	2533	3890	2998	2923	4669	3598	3507
23st 0	3169	2429	2372	3433	2632	2570	3961	3037	2966	4753	3644	3559
23st 7	3225	2460	2407	3494	2665	2608	4031	3075	3009	4837	3690	3611
24st 0	3281	2491	2441	3554	2699	2645	4101	3114	3052	4922	3737	3662
24st 7	3337	2522	2476	3615	2732	2682	4172	3152	3095	5006	3783	3714
25st 0	3394	2553	2510	3676	2765	2720	4242	3191	3138	5091	3829	3766
25st 7	3450	2583	2545	3737	2799	2757	4312	3229	3181	5175	3875	3817
26st 0	3506	2614	2579	3798	2832	2794	4383	3268	3224	5259	3922	3869
26st 7	3562	2645	2614	3859	2866	2832	4453	3307	3267	5344	3968	3921
27st 0	3618	2676	2648	3920	2899	2869	4523	3345	3310	5428	4014	3973
27st 7	3675	2707	2683	3981	2932	2906	4594	3384	3353	5512	4060	4024
28st 0	3731	2738	2717	4042	2966	2944	4664	3422	3397	5597	4107	4076
28st 7	3787	2768	2752	4103	2999	2981	4734	3461	3440	5681	4153	4128

Calories Required to Maintain Weight
Adult Males

ACTIVITY LEVEL / AGE

WEIGHT IN STONES / LBS	VERY SEDENTARY			MODERATELY SEDENTARY			MODERATELY ACTIVE			VERY ACTIVE		
	<30	30-60	60+	<30	30-60	60+	<30	30-60	60+	<30	30-60	60+
9st 0	1856	1827	1502	2010	1979	1627	2320	2284	1878	2784	2741	2254
9st 7	1913	1871	1547	2072	2026	1676	2391	2338	1933	2870	2806	2320
10st 0	1970	1914	1591	2134	2074	1724	2463	2393	1989	2955	2871	2387
10st 7	2027	1958	1636	2196	2121	1772	2534	2447	2045	3041	2937	2454
11st 0	2084	2001	1680	2258	2168	1820	2605	2502	2100	3127	3002	2520
11st 7	2141	2045	1724	2320	2215	1868	2677	2556	2156	3212	3067	2587
12st 0	2199	2088	1769	2382	2262	1916	2748	2611	2211	3298	3133	2654
12st 7	2256	2132	1813	2444	2310	1965	2820	2665	2267	3384	3198	2720
13st 0	2313	2175	1858	2506	2357	2013	2891	2719	2322	3470	3263	2787
13st 7	2370	2219	1902	2568	2404	2061	2963	2774	2378	3555	3329	2854
14st 0	2427	2262	1947	2630	2451	2109	3034	2828	2434	3641	3394	2920
14st 7	2484	2306	1991	2691	2498	2157	3106	2883	2489	3727	3459	2987
15st 0	2542	2350	2036	2753	2545	2205	3177	2937	2545	3813	3525	3054
15st 7	2599	2393	2080	2815	2593	2253	3248	2992	2600	3898	3590	3120
16st 0	2656	2437	2125	2877	2640	2302	3320	3046	2656	3984	3655	3187
16st 7	2713	2480	2169	2939	2687	2350	3391	3100	2711	4070	3721	3254
17st 0	2770	2524	2213	3001	2734	2398	3463	3155	2767	4155	3786	3320
17st 7	2827	2567	2258	3063	2781	2446	3534	3209	2823	4241	3851	3387
18st 0	2884	2611	2302	3125	2828	2494	3606	3264	2878	4327	3917	3454
18st 7	2942	2654	2347	3187	2876	2542	3677	3318	2934	4413	3982	3520
19st 0	2999	2698	2391	3249	2923	2591	3749	3373	2989	4498	4047	3587
19st 7	3056	2741	2436	3311	2970	2639	3820	3427	3045	4584	4112	3654
20st 0	3113	2785	2480	3373	3017	2687	3891	3481	3100	4670	4178	3721
20st 7	3170	2829	2525	3434	3064	2735	3963	3536	3156	4756	4243	3787
21st 0	3227	2872	2569	3496	3112	2783	4034	3590	3211	4841	4308	3854
21st 7	3285	2916	2614	3558	3159	2831	4106	3645	3267	4927	4374	3921
22st 0	3342	2959	2658	3620	3206	2880	4177	3699	3323	5013	4439	3987
22st 7	3399	3003	2702	3682	3253	2928	4249	3754	3378	5098	4504	4054
23st 0	3456	3046	2747	3744	3300	2976	4320	3808	3434	5184	4570	4121
23st 7	3513	3090	2791	3806	3347	3024	4392	3862	3489	5270	4635	4187
24st 0	3570	3133	2836	3868	3395	3072	4463	3917	3545	5356	4700	4254
24st 7	3627	3177	2880	3930	3442	3120	4534	3971	3600	5441	4766	4321
25st 0	3685	3220	2925	3992	3489	3168	4606	4026	3656	5527	4831	4387
25st 7	3742	3264	2969	4054	3536	3217	4677	4080	3712	5613	4896	4454
26st 0	3799	3308	3014	4116	3583	3265	4749	4135	3767	5699	4962	4521
26st 7	3856	3351	3058	4177	3630	3313	4820	4189	3823	5784	5027	4587
27st 0	3913	3395	3103	4239	3678	3361	4892	4243	3878	5870	5092	4654
27st 7	3970	3438	3147	4301	3725	3409	4963	4298	3934	5956	5158	4721
28st 0	4028	3482	3191	4363	3772	3457	5035	4352	3989	6042	5223	4787
28st 7	4085	3525	3236	4425	3819	3506	5106	4407	4045	6127	5288	4854
29st 0	4142	3569	3280	4487	3866	3554	5177	4461	4101	6213	5354	4921
29st 7	4199	3612	3325	4549	3913	3602	5249	4516	4156	6299	5419	4987
30st 0	4256	3656	3369	4611	3961	3650	5320	4570	4212	6384	5484	5054

Calories Burned in Exercise

This table shows the approximate number of extra* calories that would be burned in a five minute period of exercise activity.

ACTIVITY	CALORIES BURNED IN 5 MINUTES	ACTIVITY	CALORIES BURNED IN 5 MINUTES
Aerobics, Low Impact	25	Situps, Continuous	17
Badminton, Recreational	17	Skiing, Moderate	30
Cross Trainer	30	Skipping, Moderate	30
Cycling, Recreational, 5mph	17	Squash Playing	39
Dancing, Modern, Moderate	13	Tennis Playing, Recreational	26
Fencing	24	Toning Exercises	17
Gardening, Weeding	19	Trampolining	17
Hill Walking, Up and Down, Recreational	22	Volleyball, Recreational	10
Jogging	30	Walking, Uphill, 15% Gradient, Moderate	43
Kick Boxing	30	Walking Up and Down Stairs, Moderate	34
Netball Playing	23	Walking, 4mph	24
Rebounding	18	Weight Training, Moderate	12
Roller Skating	30	Yoga	13
Rowing Machine, Moderate	30		
Running, 7.5mph	48		

*Extra calories are those in addition to your normal daily calorie needs.

My Personal Plan

Date: _____

Body Mass Index: _____

Weight: _____

Waist Measurement: _____

Height: _____

Body Fat % (if known) _____

10% Weight Loss Goal: _____

Current weight	16stone (224lb)	100kg
- 10% weight	1stone 8½lb (22½lb)	10kg
= 10% loss goal	14stone 5½lb (201½lb)	90kg

My smaller weight targets on the way to achieving my 10% goal will be:

_____ _____ _____ _____

Reasons why I want to lose weight:

_____

Changes I will make to help me lose weight:

Diet:

_____

_____

_____

Activity:

_____

_____

_____

Potential saboteurs or barriers will be:

_____

_____

_____

Ways I will overcome these:

_____

_____

_____

My supporters will be:

_____

I will monitor my progress by:

_____

_____

I will reward my progress with:

In the short term:

_____

_____

In the long term:

_____

_____

Food and Exercise Diary

Date:

/ /

Daily Calorie Allowance: **(A)**

Food/Drink Consumed	Serving Size	Calories
_____	_____	_____
_____	_____	_____
_____	_____	_____
_____	_____	_____
_____	_____	_____
_____	_____	_____
_____	_____	_____
_____	_____	_____
_____	_____	_____
_____	_____	_____
_____	_____	_____
_____	_____	_____
_____	_____	_____
_____	_____	_____
_____	_____	_____

You are aiming for your Calorie Balance (Box D) to be as close to zero as possible - ie. you consume the number of calories you need.

Your Daily Calorie Allowance (Box A) should be set to lose ½-2lb (¼-1kg) a week, or maintain weight, depending on your goals.

Total calories consumed **(B)**

Exercise/Activity	No. mins	Calories
_____	_____	_____
_____	_____	_____
_____	_____	_____
_____	_____	_____

Daily Calorie Allowance (A) *plus* Extra Calories used in Exercise (C) *minus* Total Calories Consumed (B) *equals* Calorie Balance (D)

Calories used in exercise **(C)**

$A + C - B = D$

Calorie balance **(D)**

You can also write down any comments or thoughts related to your eating if you want to.

Food Information

Nutritional Information

CALORIE AND FAT values are given per serving, plus calorie and nutrition values per 100g of product. This makes it easy to compare the proportions of fat, protein, carbohydrate and fibre in each food.

The values given are for uncooked, unprepared foods unless otherwise stated. Values are also for only the edible portion of the food unless otherwise stated. ie - weighed with bone.

Finding Foods

The Calorie, Carb & Fat Bible has an Eating Out section which is arranged alphabetically by brand. In the General Foods and Drinks A-Z most foods are grouped together by type, and then put in to alphabetical order. This makes it easy to compare different brands, and will help you to find lower calorie and/or fat alternatives where they are available.

This format also makes it easier to locate foods. Foods are categorised by their main characteristics so, for example, if it is bread, ciabatta or white sliced, you'll find it under "Bread".

Basic ingredients are highlighted to make them easier to find at a glance. You'll find all unbranded foods in bold - making the index easier to use, whether it's just an apple or all the components of a home cooked stew.

There are, however, some foods which are not so easy to categorise, especially combination foods like ready meals. The following pointers will help you to find your way around the book until you get to know it a little better.

FILLED ROLLS AND SANDWICHES - Bagels, baguettes, etc which are filled are listed as "Bagels (filled)" etc. Sandwiches are under "Sandwiches".

CURRIES - Popular types of curry, like Balti or Jalfrezi, are listed under their individual types. Unspecified or lesser known types are listed under their main ingredient.

BURGERS - All burgers from fast-food outlets are listed under "Burgers".

CHIPS & FRIES - Are listed separately, depending on the name of the particular brand. All other types of potato are listed under "Potatoes".

SWEETS & CHOCOLATES - Well-known brands, eg. Aero, Mars Bar, are listed under their brand names. Others are listed under "Chocolate" (for bars) and "Chocolates" (for individual sweets).

READY MEALS - Popular types of dishes are listed under their type, eg. "Chow Mein", "Casserole", "Hot Pot", etc. Others are listed by their main ingredient, eg. "Chicken With", "Chicken In", etc.

EATING OUT & FAST FOODS - By popular demand this edition has the major eating out and fast food brands listed separately, at the back of the book. They are alphabetised first by brand, then follow using the same format as the rest of the book, with calories provided per serving.

Serving Sizes

Many ready-meal type foods are given with calories for the full pack size, so that an individual serving can be worked out by estimating the proportion of the pack that has been consumed. For example, if you have eaten a quarter of a packaged pasta dish, divide the calorie value given for the whole pack by 4 to determine the number of calories you have consumed. Where serving sizes are not appropriate, or unknown, values are given per 100g and per 1oz/28g. Serving sizes vary greatly from person to person and, if you are trying to lose weight, it's important to be accurate – especially with high calorie foods such as those that contain a fair amount of fat, sugar, cream, cheese, alcohol etc.

Food Data

Nutrition information for basic average foods has been compiled by the Weight Loss Resources food data team using many sources of information to calculate the most accurate values possible. Some nutrition information for non-branded food records is from The Composition of Foods 6th Edition. Reproduced under licence from The Controller of Her Majesty's Stationary Office. Where basic data is present for ordinary foodstuffs such as 'raw carrots'; branded records are not included.

Nutrition information for branded goods is from details supplied by retailers and manufacturers, and researched by Weight Loss Resources staff. The Calorie Carb & Fat Bible contains data for over 1400 UK brands, including major supermarkets and fast food outlets.

The publishers gratefully acknowledge all the manufacturers and retailers who have provided information on their products. All product names, trademarks or registered trademarks belong to their respective owners and are used only for the purpose of identifying products.

Calorie & nutrition data for all food and drink items are typical values.

Caution

The information in The Calorie, Carb and Fat Bible is intended as an aid to weight loss and weight maintenance, and is not medical advice. If you suffer from, or think you may suffer from a medical condition you should consult your doctor before starting a weight loss and/or exercise regime. If you start exercising after a period of relative inactivity, you should start slowly and consult your doctor if you experience pain, distress or other symptoms.

Weights, Measures & Abbreviations

ABBREVIATIONS	
kcal	*kilocalories / calories*
prot	*protein*
carb	*carbohydrate*
sm	*small*
med	*medium*
av	*average*
reg	*regular*
lge	*large*
tsp	*teaspoon*
tbsp	*tablespoon*
dtsp	*dessertspoon*
gf	*gluten free*

BRAND ABBREVIATIONS USED	
ASDA	
Good for You	*GFY*
Chosen by You	*CBY*
Good & Counted	*G&C*
MARKS & SPENCER	*M & S*
Count on Us	*COU*
Balanced For You	*BFY*
MORRISONS	
Better For You	*BFY*
SAINSBURY'S	
Be Good to Yourself	*BGTY*
Way to Five	*WTF*
Taste the Difference	*TTD*
TESCO	
Healthy Eating	*HE*
Healthy Living	*HL*
Hearty Food Co	*HFC*
Light Choices	*LC*
WAITROSE	
Perfectly Balanced	*PB*
Cambridge Weight Plan	*CWP*

	Measure INFO/WEIGHT	per Measure KCAL	FAT	Nutrition Values per 100g / 100ml KCAL	PROT	CARB	FAT	FIBRE

ABSINTHE

	Measure INFO/WEIGHT	KCAL	FAT	KCAL	PROT	CARB	FAT	FIBRE
Average	*1 Pub Shot/35ml*	*127*	*0*	*363*	*0*	*38.8*	*0*	*0*

ACKEE

Canned, Drained, Average	*1oz/28g*	*43*	*4.3*	*151*	*2.9*	*0.8*	*15.2*	*0*

ADVOCAAT

Average	*1 Pub Shot/35ml*	*91*	*2.2*	*260*	*4.7*	*28.4*	*6.3*	*0*

AERO

Bliss, Milk Chocolate, Aero, Nestle*	1 Piece/8g	46	2.7	545	7.2	56.9	31.6	1.7
Bliss, Praline, Aero, Nestle*	1 Piece/8g	44	2.8	568	6.3	53.2	36.2	1.9
Bliss, Salted Caramel, Aero, Nestle*	1 Piece/8g	43	2.4	537	7.4	58	30.2	1.4
Creamy White Centre, Nestle*	1 Bar/46g	244	13.8	530	7.6	57.4	30	0
Honeycomb, Nestle*	1 Bar/40g	199	10	497	5.9	62.2	25	0
Milk Chocolate, Bubbles, Sharing Bag, Aero, Nestle*	1 Bag/113g	610	34.7	540	6.5	57.8	30.7	0
Milk, Giant, Bar, Nestle*	1 Bar/125g	674	38.6	539	6.6	57.7	30.9	2.2
Milk, Medium, Bar, Nestle*	1 Bar/43g	232	13.3	539	6.6	57.7	30.9	2.2
Milk, Purely Chocolate, Aero*	1 Bar/37g	197	11.2	538	6.8	57.8	30.5	1.9
Milk, Snacksize, Bar, Nestle*	1 Bar/21g	110	6.5	537	6.6	55.9	31.9	2.2
Mint, Bubbles, Aero, Nestle*	1 Bubble/3g	16	0.9	533	4.4	62.7	29.1	0.8
Mint, Nestle*	1 Bar/41g	218	11.9	531	5.4	61.6	28.9	1.1
Mint, Snack Size, Nestle*	1 Bar/21g	112	6.7	548	7.7	55.3	32.8	0.9
Mint, Standard, Aero, Nestle*	1 Bar/43g	233	13.2	542	5.2	60.5	30.8	0.9
Orange, Bubbles, Aero, Nestle*	1 Bubble/3g	16	0.9	538	5.4	60.5	30	1.4
Orange, Nestle*	6 Squares/22g	119	6.8	542	5.1	60.7	30.7	0.9

ALCOPOPS

Smirnoff Apple Bite, Frozen, Smirnoff*	1 Pint/568ml	523	0	92	0	15	0	0
Smirnoff Ice, Smirnoff*	1 Bottle/275ml	188	0	68	1.8	12	0	0

ALFALFA SPROUTS

Raw, Average	*1 Serving/33g*	*8*	*0.3*	*24*	*3*	*3*	*0.9*	*3*

ALLSPICE

Ground, Schwartz*	1 Tsp/3g	11	0.1	358	6.1	74.3	4	0
Whole, Average	*1 Tsp/2g*	*5*	*0.2*	*263*	*6.1*	*72.1*	*8.7*	*21.6*

ALMONDS

Blanched, Average	*1 Serving/100g*	*617*	*54.3*	*617*	*25.1*	*6.9*	*54.3*	*8.1*
Candied, Sugared	*1 Serving/100g*	*458*	*16.3*	*458*	*8.4*	*69.2*	*16.3*	*2.2*
Chilli , Specially Selected, Aldi*	1 Serving/30g	188	16.2	626	26	4.3	54	9.3
Chocolate Coated, Belgian, Dark, M&S*	1 Pack/60g	332	21.2	554	10.9	45.8	35.4	4.5
Flaked, Average	*1oz/28g*	*172*	*15.2*	*613*	*24.9*	*6.5*	*54.3*	*7.6*
Flaked, Toasted, Average	*1oz/28g*	*176*	*15.8*	*629*	*24.6*	*5.8*	*56.4*	*7.5*
Ground, Average	*1 Serving/10g*	*62*	*5.6*	*625*	*24*	*6.6*	*55.8*	*7.4*
Marcona, Average	*1 Serving/100g*	*608*	*53.7*	*608*	*22.1*	*13*	*53.7*	*9.7*
Milk Chocolate, Caramelised, Quibbles*	1 Pack/35g	188	10.9	536	10.4	51.7	31.1	3.8
Moroccan Spiced, Mr Filbert's*	1 Pack/110g	684	54.1	622	22.4	17.1	49.2	10.4
Rosemary, & Sea Salt, Oven Roasted, Boots*	1 Serving/25g	160	13.3	641	24.1	10.8	53.2	11.1
Toasted, Average	*1oz/28g*	*178*	*15.8*	*634*	*25*	*6.6*	*56.4*	*6.6*
Whole, Average	*1 Serving/20g*	*122*	*11*	*612*	*23.4*	*6.9*	*54.8*	*8.4*
Yoghurt Coated, Holland & Barrett*	1 Pack/100g	536	37	536	10.9	45.3	37	2.8

ALOO

Bombay, M&S*	½ Pack/114g	108	5.2	95	1.8	10.3	4.6	2.3
Gobi, Slimming World, Iceland*	1 Pack/350g	150	1.4	43	1.7	7.2	0.4	2.1
Saag, Canned, Geo Organics*	½ Can/200g	160	8.8	80	2.3	9.2	4.4	2.6
Saag, Gobi, Side, Asda*	½ Pack/148g	114	5.3	77	2.4	7.6	3.6	2.4
Saag, Gobi, Takeaway, Microwaved, Morrisons*	½ Pack/105g	88	3.6	84	2	9.5	3.4	3.9
Saag, Gobi, Waitrose*	½ Pack/150g	129	8.2	86	2	6	5.5	2.4
Saag, Indian, Serves 2, Sainsbury's*	1 Pack/300g	216	10.5	72	2	7	3.5	2.2

	Measure INFO/WEIGHT	per Measure KCAL	FAT	Nutrition Values per 100g / 100ml KCAL	PROT	CARB	FAT	FIBRE

ALOO

	Measure / INFO/WEIGHT	KCAL	FAT	KCAL	PROT	CARB	FAT	FIBRE
Saag, Inspired Cuisine, Aldi*	½ Pack/125g	116	4.8	93	2.1	11	3.8	3.3
Saag, Tesco*	1 Serving/200g	144	7	72	2.1	8	3.5	2
Tikki, Average	*1 Serving/25g*	*48*	*2*	*191*	*4.5*	*25.2*	*8*	*3.5*
AMARANTH								
Seed, Holland & Barrett*	1 Tbsp/15g	56	1	371	14	55	7	6.5
ANCHOVIES								
Fillets, in Extra Virgin Olive Oil, Drained, M&S*	¼ Jar/15g	30	1.4	210	26.4	3.7	9.9	0.1
Fillets, Tesco*	1 Serving/15g	34	2.1	226	25	0	14	0
in Oil, Canned, Drained	*1 Anchovy/4g*	*8*	*0.5*	*195*	*23.4*	*0*	*11.3*	*0*
Marinated, Sainsbury's*	¼ Pot/44g	78	4	177	22	2	9	0.1
ANGEL DELIGHT								
Butterscotch, no Added Sugar, with Semi Skimmed, Kraft*	1 Portion/89g	97	4.1	109	3.8	13	4.6	0.5
Chocolate Flavour, Kraft*	1 Sachet/67g	305	12.1	455	3.7	69.5	18	0.4
Strawberry Flavour, Kraft*	1 Sachet/59g	286	12.4	485	2.5	71	21	0
Strawberry Flavour, no Added Sugar, Kraft*	1 Sachet/47g	230	12.5	490	4.8	59	26.5	0
Vanilla Ice Cream Flavour, Kraft*	1 Sachet/59g	289	12.7	490	2.5	71.5	21.5	0
ANGEL HAIR								
Pasta, Dry	*1 Serving/50g*	*181*	*1.1*	*362*	*12.4*	*73.6*	*2.2*	*4.4*
ANTIPASTI								
in Oil, Grilled, Cucina, Aldi*	¼ Jar/43g	41	3.7	96	1.1	2.3	8.6	2.2
Mixed, in Olive Oil, Extra Virgin, Drained, M&S*	¼ Jar/40g	76	7	191	1.3	4.8	17.5	4.3
ANTIPASTO								
Artichoke, Sainsbury's*	1 Serving/50g	68	6.2	135	2	3.6	12.5	2.3
Italian, Specially Selected, Aldi*	¼ Pack/30g	97	6.9	323	28	0	23	0
Mixed Mushroom, Sainsbury's*	¼ Jar/72g	70	6.5	97	2.7	1.4	9	3.7
Mixed Pepper, Sainsbury's*	½ Jar/140g	48	1.8	34	1.3	4.2	1.3	3.5
Parma Ham, from Selection Platter, TTD, Sainsbury's*	1 Serving/100g	236	12.9	236	29.9	0.1	12.9	0
Parma, Salami Milano, Bresaola, Finest, Tesco*	¼ Pack/30g	104	7.9	345	26.4	0.5	26.3	0
Roasted Pepper, Drained, Tesco*	1 Jar /170g	128	9.4	75	0.9	5.5	5.5	4.1
APPLES								
& Cheddar, Boots*	1 Pack/70g	93	5	133	4.6	12	7.2	1.8
Bites, Average	*1 Pack/118g*	*58*	*0.1*	*49*	*0.3*	*11.6*	*0.1*	*2.2*
Braeburn, Average	*1 Apple/123g*	*58*	*0*	*47*	*0.3*	*12.9*	*0*	*2.9*
Cooking, Baked with Sugar, Flesh Only, Average	*1 Serving/140g*	*104*	*0.1*	*74*	*0.5*	*19.2*	*0.1*	*1.7*
Cooking, Raw, Peeled, Average	*1oz/28g*	*10*	*0*	*35*	*0.3*	*8.9*	*0.1*	*1.6*
Cooking, Stewed with Sugar, Average	*1 Serving/140g*	*104*	*0.1*	*74*	*0.3*	*19.1*	*0.1*	*1.2*
Cooking, Stewed without Sugar, Average	*1 Serving/140g*	*46*	*0.1*	*33*	*0.3*	*8.1*	*0.1*	*1.5*
Cox, English, Average	*1 Apple/123g*	*53*	*0.1*	*43*	*0.4*	*10.2*	*0.1*	*1.8*
Discovery, Average	*1 Apple/182g*	*82*	*0.9*	*45*	*0.4*	*10.6*	*0.5*	*1*
Dried, Average	*1 Pack/250g*	*537*	*0.7*	*215*	*0.8*	*52.8*	*0.3*	*5.9*
Empire, Average	*1 Apple/120g*	*52*	*0.1*	*44*	*0.4*	*10.7*	*0.1*	*1.8*
Fuji	*1 Apple/132g*	*64*	*0.1*	*48*	*0.4*	*11.8*	*0.1*	*1.8*
Gala, Average	*1 Apple/152g*	*66*	*0.2*	*43*	*0.3*	*10.4*	*0.1*	*1.4*
Golden Delicious, Average	*1 Med/102g*	*44*	*0.1*	*43*	*0.3*	*10.1*	*0.1*	*1.6*
Granny Smith, Average	*1 Sm/125g*	*56*	*0.1*	*45*	*0.4*	*10.7*	*0.1*	*1.8*
Green, Raw, Average	*1 Med/182g*	*86*	*0.2*	*48*	*0.4*	*11.3*	*0.1*	*1.8*
Jazz, Tesco*	1 Apple/133g	70	0.1	53	0.4	11.8	0.1	1.8
Kanzi, Tesco*	1 Apple/134g	71	0.1	53	0.4	11.8	0.1	1.8
Mackintosh, Red, Average	*1 Apple/165g*	*81*	*0.5*	*49*	*0.2*	*12.8*	*0.3*	*1.8*
Pink Lady, Average	*1 Apple/125g*	*56*	*0.1*	*45*	*0.4*	*10.6*	*0.1*	*1.9*
Pink Lady, Dried, M&S*	1 Pot/50g	101	0.1	202	2	45.3	0.2	5.3
Puree, Biona Organic*	1 Serving/100g	48	0.1	48	0.2	10.5	0.1	1.5
Red, Average	*1 Med/149g*	*71*	*0.2*	*48*	*0.3*	*11.8*	*0.1*	*2*

	Measure INFO/WEIGHT	per Measure		Nutrition Values per 100g / 100ml				
		KCAL	FAT	KCAL	PROT	CARB	FAT	FIBRE
APPLES								
Sliced, Average	*1oz/28g*	*14*	*0*	*49*	*0.4*	*11.6*	*0.1*	*1.8*
Slices, Apple, Crownfield, Lidl*	1 Slice/15g	56	0.9	389	7.2	74.5	6.1	3.5
APPLETISER*								
Juice Drink, Sparkling, Appletiser, Coca-Cola*	1 Glass/200ml	94	0	47	0	11	0	0.4
APRICOTS								
Canned, in Syrup, Average	*1oz/28g*	*18*	*0*	*63*	*0.4*	*16.1*	*0.1*	*0.9*
Dried, Average	*1 Apricot/10g*	*17*	*0.1*	*171*	*3.6*	*37.4*	*0.5*	*6.3*
Dried, Soft, Average	*1 Serving/50g*	*104*	*0.2*	*208*	*2.4*	*48.5*	*0.4*	*5.2*
Halves, in Fruit Juice, Average	*1 Can/221g*	*87*	*0.1*	*40*	*0.5*	*9.2*	*0.1*	*1*
Milk Chocolate Coated, Graze*	1 Pack/35g	158	8.6	450	6.1	55.9	24.7	5
Pitted, Dried, Soft, CBY, Asda*	1 Serving/30g	49	0.2	162	4	37	0.6	6.3
Raw, Flesh Only, Average	*1 Apricot/37g*	*19*	*0.2*	*52*	*1.5*	*12*	*0.4*	*2.2*
Raw, Weighed with Stone, Average	*1 Apricot/40g*	*19*	*0.2*	*47*	*1.4*	*10.8*	*0.4*	*1.9*
AQUAFABA								
Average	*1 Tbsp/15ml*	*3*	*0*	*18*	*1*	*2.9*	*0.2*	*0*
ARANCINI								
Aubergine, Cauldron Foods*	1 Arancini/30g	63	2.8	211	5.6	24.9	9.2	3.2
Mushroom, Vegetarian, Waitrose*	1 Arancini/50g	116	5	233	6.2	28.8	9.9	2.1
ARCHERS*								
Aqua, Peach, Archers*	1 Bottle/275ml	206	0	75	0.3	7.7	0	0
Peach (Calculated Estimate), Archers*	1 Shot/35ml	91	0	260	0	0	0	0
ARTICHOKE								
Baby, Chargrilled, Sainsbury's*	1/3 Pot/47g	72	5.6	154	2.6	7.6	12	2.6
Chargrilled, in Olive Oil, Cooks Ingredients, Waitrose*	1 Serving/30g	54	4.9	134	1.7	2.7	12.3	2.7
Chargrilled, Italian, Drained, Sainsbury's*	1/3 Tub/43g	40	2.7	92	3.1	2.8	6.1	6.5
Fresh, Raw, Average	*1oz/28g*	*13*	*0*	*47*	*3.3*	*10.5*	*0.2*	*5.4*
Hearts, Canned, Drained, Average	*½ Can/117g*	*35*	*0.1*	*30*	*1.9*	*5.4*	*0*	*2.2*
Hearts, Marinated & Grilled, Waitrose*	1 Serving/50g	57	5	114	3	3	10	3
Hearts, Sliced with Extra Virgin Olive Oil, Waitrose*	1 Serving/40g	24	1.6	59	1.3	4.4	4	7
in Oil, Tesco*	1 Piece/15g	17	1.5	115	1.9	2.4	10	4
Marinated, Roasted, M&S*	1 Pack/200g	300	26.6	150	1.9	5	13.3	2.3
ASPARAGUS								
& Green Vegetables (Steamer Pouch), Waitrose*	½ Pack/125g	28	0.6	22	2.1	2.3	0.5	2.1
Boiled, in Salted Water, Average	*5 Spears/125g*	*28*	*0.3*	*22*	*2.4*	*4.1*	*0.2*	*2*
British with Butter, Tesco*	1 Serving/50g	26	2	52	2.6	1.6	4	2
Canned, Average	*1 Can/250g*	*41*	*0.4*	*16*	*2*	*1.8*	*0.2*	*1.4*
Trimmed, Raw, Average	*1 Serving/80g*	*20*	*0.4*	*24*	*2.9*	*1.9*	*0.6*	*1.7*
White, Raw, Average	*1 Spear/17g*	*3*	*0*	*17*	*1*	*2.5*	*0.3*	*1*
AUBERGINE								
Baby, Tesco*	1 Aubergine/50g	8	0.2	15	0.9	2.2	0.4	2.3
Baked Topped, M&S*	1 Serving/150g	165	11.6	110	2.4	7.4	7.7	0.9
Fried, Average	*1oz/28g*	*85*	*8.9*	*302*	*1.2*	*2.8*	*31.9*	*2.3*
Marinated & Grilled, Waitrose*	½ Pack/100g	106	10	106	1	3	10	2
Parmigiana, M&S*	1 Pack/350g	332	18.6	95	4.6	7.6	5.3	1.1
Raw, Fresh, Average	*1 Sm/250g*	*36*	*1*	*14*	*0.9*	*2.1*	*0.4*	*1.9*
& Halloumi, Tomato Sauce, & Bulgur, Charlie Bigham's*	1 Serving/400 g	576	22.4	144	4.6	19.5	5.6	0
Sliced, Chargrilled, Frozen, Oven Cooked, Tesco*	¼ Pack/78g	35	0.2	46	1.6	6.8	0.3	4.6
AVOCADO								
Breakfast, Holy Moly*	1 Serving/30g	45	4.5	151	2	9	15	7
Flesh Only, Average	*1 Med/145g*	*276*	*28.3*	*190*	*1.9*	*1.9*	*19.5*	*3.4*
Smashed, Pure, Holy Moly*	¼ Pot/40g	64	6.4	160	2	9	16	7

	Measure INFO/WEIGHT	per Measure KCAL	per Measure FAT	Nutrition Values per 100g / 100ml KCAL	PROT	CARB	FAT	FIBRE
BACARDI*								
& Diet Cola, Bacardi*	1 Bottle/275ml	85	0	31	0	1	0	0
37.5% Volume, Bacardi*	1 Pub Shot/35ml	72	0	207	0	0	0	0
40% Volume, Bacardi*	1 Pub Shot/35ml	78	0	222	0	0	0	0
Breezer, Cranberry, Bacardi*	1 Bottle/275ml	154	0	56	0	7.1	0	0
Breezer, Lime, Bacardi*	1 Bottle/275ml	182	0	66	0	9.1	0	0
BACON								
Back, Dry Cured, Average	*1 Rasher/31g*	*77*	*4.7*	*250*	*28.1*	*0.3*	*15.1*	*0.3*
Back, Dry Fried or Grilled, Average	*1 Rasher/25g*	*72*	*5.4*	*287*	*23.2*	*0*	*21.6*	*0*
Back, Lean, Average	*1 Rasher/33g*	*57*	*4*	*174*	*16.3*	*0.1*	*12*	*0.5*
Back, Smoked, Average	*1 Rasher/25g*	*66*	*5*	*265*	*20.9*	*0*	*19.9*	*0*
Back, Smoked, Farmfoods*	1 Rasher/25g	65	3.8	260	18	0	15.4	0
Back, Smoked, Lean, Average	*1 Rasher/25g*	*41*	*1.2*	*163*	*28.2*	*1.1*	*5*	*0.2*
Back, Smoked, Rindless, Average	*1 Rasher/25g*	*60*	*4.3*	*241*	*21*	*0.1*	*17.4*	*0*
Back, Unsmoked, Average	*1 Rasher/32g*	*78*	*5.5*	*242*	*21.3*	*0.4*	*17.3*	*0*
Back, Unsmoked, Dry Cured, Deluxe, Lidl*	2 Rashers/51g	134	7.4	263	32	0.7	14.6	0.5
Back, Unsmoked, Dry Cured, Finest, Tesco*	2 Rashers/60g	156	11.8	260	19.2	1.1	19.7	0.6
Back, Unsmoked, Grilled, Freshcure, Aldi*	2 Rashers/42g	112	7.6	267	27	0.5	18	0.5
Back, Unsmoked, Rindless, Average	*1 Rasher/23g*	*56*	*3.9*	*241*	*22.5*	*0*	*16.9*	*0*
Bits, Average	*1oz/28g*	*75*	*5.9*	*268*	*18.6*	*0.7*	*21.2*	*0.1*
Chops, Average	*1oz/28g*	*62*	*4.2*	*222*	*22.3*	*0*	*14.8*	*0*
Collar Joint, Lean & Fat, Boiled	*1oz/28g*	*91*	*7.6*	*325*	*20.4*	*0*	*27*	*0*
Collar Joint, Lean & Fat, Raw	*1oz/28g*	*81*	*7.4*	*290*	*13.3*	*0*	*26.3*	*0*
Collar Joint, Lean Only, Boiled	*1oz/28g*	*53*	*2.7*	*191*	*26*	*0*	*9.7*	*0*
Fat Only, Cooked, Average	*1oz/28g*	*194*	*20.4*	*692*	*9.3*	*0*	*72.8*	*0*
Fat Only, Raw, Average	*1oz/28g*	*209*	*22.7*	*747*	*4.8*	*0*	*80.9*	*0*
Gammon Rasher, Lean Only, Grilled	*1oz/28g*	*48*	*1.5*	*172*	*31.4*	*0*	*5.2*	*0*
Lardons, Smoked, Tesco*	1 Pack/200g	518	40.6	259	17.1	2	20.3	0.8
Lean Only, Fried, Average	*1 Rasher/25g*	*83*	*5.6*	*332*	*32.8*	*0*	*22.3*	*0*
Lean Only, Grilled, Average	*1 Rasher/25g*	*73*	*4.7*	*292*	*30.5*	*0*	*18.9*	*0*
Lean, Average	*1 Rasher/33g*	*47*	*2.2*	*142*	*19.6*	*0.9*	*6.7*	*0.2*
Loin Steaks, Grilled, Average	*1 Serving/120g*	*229*	*11.6*	*191*	*25.9*	*0*	*9.7*	*0*
Medallions, Average	*1 Rasher/18g*	*27*	*0.6*	*151*	*29.4*	*0.9*	*3.3*	*0.1*
Middle, Fried	*1 Rasher/40g*	*140*	*11.4*	*350*	*23.4*	*0*	*28.5*	*0*
Middle, Grilled	*1 Rasher/40g*	*123*	*9.2*	*307*	*24.8*	*0*	*23.1*	*0*
Middle, Raw	*1 Rasher/43g*	*95*	*7.9*	*222*	*14*	*0*	*18.4*	*0*
Rashers, Lean Only, Trimmed, Average	*1 Rasher/20g*	*24*	*0.8*	*119*	*20.6*	*0*	*4*	*0*
Smoked, Crispy, Cooked, Average	*1 Serving/10g*	*46*	*2.7*	*460*	*53*	*2.1*	*26.9*	*0*
Streaky, Cooked, Average	*1 Rasher/20g*	*68*	*5.6*	*342*	*22.4*	*0.3*	*27.8*	*0*
Vegan, Pieces, Vivera*	½ Pack/88g	81	0.4	92	18	1.9	0.4	6
Vegan, Streaky, Pieces, Smoky, Waitrose*	½ Pack/55g	145	7.7	263	20.9	11.7	14	3.2
Vegetarian, Deli Style, Rashers, Quorn*	1 Rasher/15g	30	2.3	199	11.8	3	15.5	5
Vegetarian, Rashers	*1 Rasher/16g*	*33*	*1.7*	*206*	*19.5*	*8.6*	*10.4*	*2.8*
Vegetarian, Rashers, Cheatin', The Redwood Co*	1 Rasher/16g	32	1.2	196	25.9	7.3	7.3	0.5
Vegetarian, Rashers, Tesco*	1 Rasher/20g	41	2.2	203	22.5	3.3	11.1	3.9
BAGUETTE								
Beef, & Horseradish, Freshly Prepared, M&S*	1 Baguette/274g	795	31	290	12.1	37.2	11.3	2
Brie, Tomato, & Rocket, Freshly Prepared, M&S*	1 Baguette/219g	570	21.7	260	10.3	33.2	9.9	1.9
Cheese, & Pickle, Fullfillers*	1 Baguette/280g	767	31.1	274	11.9	35.5	11.1	0
Cheese, & Ham, Average	*1 Baguette/203g*	*593*	*20.8*	*292*	*14*	*35.9*	*10.3*	*1.4*
Cheese, & Onion, Asda*	¼ Loaf/42g	154	7.4	366	12	39.8	17.6	1.3
Cheese, & Tomato, Tesco*	1 Baguette/108g	243	8.3	225	9.7	29.3	7.7	1.8
Cheese, Mixed, & Spring Onion, Asda*	1 Pack/190g	629	34.8	331	9.5	32.1	18.3	1.3
Chicken, & Salad, Boots*	1 Baguette/132g	202	2.4	153	11	23	1.8	2

B

	Measure INFO/WEIGHT	per Measure KCAL	FAT	Nutrition Values per 100g / 100ml KCAL	PROT	CARB	FAT	FIBRE
BAGUETTE								
Chicken, & Stuffing, Hot, Sainsbury's*	1 Baguette/227g	543	16.3	239	13.7	29.6	7.2	0
Chicken, & Salad, Asda*	1 Serving/158g	326	9.5	206	9	29	6	2.1
Chicken, & Salad, Shapers, Boots*	1 Baguette/132g	222	2.6	168	11	27	2	1.5
Chicken, Tikka, Asda*	1 Pack/190g	439	17.9	231	10.4	32.8	9.4	1.3
Egg, Bacon, & Tomato, Freshly Prepared, M&S*	1 Baguette/182g	455	17.3	250	12.9	28	9.5	1.7
GF, Schar*	½ Baguette/88g	234	2.6	267	2.9	54	3	6.4
Ham, & Turkey, Asda*	1 Baguette/360g	774	18.4	215	11.6	30.7	5.1	1.3
Ham, & Cheese, Freshly Prepared, M&S*	1 Baguette/231g	555	11.3	240	13.4	35.9	4.9	2.4
Ham, & Salad, with Mustard Mayonnaise, Sainsbury's*	1 Baguette/100g	412	15.9	412	17.6	49.6	15.9	0.1
Mozzarella, Tomato, & Pesto, Darwins Deli*	1 Serving/210g	531	20.4	253	11.7	29.7	9.7	0
Pizza, with Mushrooms, Virtu*	1 Pack/235g	609	25.8	259	9.7	30	11	0
Prawn Mayonnaise, Asda*	1 Pack/190g	399	9.3	210	9.1	32.5	4.9	1.3
Salmon, Smoked, & Egg, Freshly Prepared	**1 Baguette/178g**	**455**	**17.3**	**255**	**13.7**	**28.4**	**9.7**	**1.6**
Steak, & Onion, Snack 'n' Go, Sainsbury's*	1 Baguette/177g	398	8.8	225	14.3	30.6	5	2.2
Tuna, Melt, Sainsbury's*	1 Serving/204g	373	8	183	11.3	25.8	3.9	0
BAILEYS*								
Almande, Dairy Free, Baileys*	1 Serving/25ml	10	0.2	38	0.6	3.1	0.8	0
Irish Cream, Original, Baileys*	1 Serving/50ml	164	6.5	327	3	25	13	0
BAKE								
Aubergine, & Grain, Moroccan Inspired, Waitrose*	½ Pack/189g	151	8.3	80	1.3	6.9	4.4	3.7
Aubergine, Tomato, & Mozzarella, Vegetarian, Tesco*	1 Pack/380g	228	9.5	60	2.7	4.8	2.5	3.6
Broccoli, & Cheese, Asda*	1 Bake/132g	269	15.4	204	5.3	19.3	11.7	2.5
Broccoli, & Cheese, M&S*	1 Pack/400g	480	31.2	120	6.5	5.4	7.8	1.6
Cheese, & Onion, Greggs, Iceland*	1 Bake/141g	434	29.6	308	6.1	23	21	0
Cheese, & Onion, Tesco*	1 Bake/110g	332	17	302	7.8	31.8	15.5	2.3
Chicken, & Stuffing, 139, Oakhouse Foods Ltd*	1 Pack/451g	383	13.5	85	6.9	6.8	3	0.8
Chicken, Creamy, Morrisons*	1 Bake/125g	367	22.2	294	9.3	23.1	17.8	2
Fruit, Strawberry, Bar, Sainsbury's*	1 Bar/35g	127	2.6	362	2.6	67.8	7.4	6.9
Haddock, Average	**1 Serving/400g**	**312**	**9.2**	**78**	**6.4**	**8**	**2.3**	**0.9**
Lentil, Spiced, Vegetarian, TTD, Sainsbury's*	1 Bake/132g	245	8.4	186	4.8	27.3	6.4	4.2
Pizza, Pepperoni, Crispy Crust, Hot Pocket, Nestle*	1 Pocket/125g	330	17	264	8	27.2	13.6	0.8
Potato, Cheese, & Onion, Roast, Asda*	½ Pack/200g	288	16	144	4.2	14	8	1.1
Potato, Cheese, & Onion, Tesco*	1 Pack/400g	376	19.6	94	2.4	10	4.9	1
Root Vegetable, with Tomato & Chilli Sauce, Morrisons*	½ Pack/152g	96	2.9	63	1.6	6.8	1.9	6.1
Sausage, with Roasted Vegetables, Musclefood*	1 Serving/619g	464	6.2	75	4.7	12	1	1.9
Vegetable, Mediterranean, Cooked, CBY, Asda*	1 Bake/120g	279	13.2	232	8.4	22.8	11	4.2
BAKING POWDER								
Average	**1 Tsp/2g**	**3**	**0**	**163**	**5.2**	**37.8**	**0**	**0**
BAKLAVA								
Average	**2 Pieces/50g**	**239**	**14.2**	**478**	**8**	**47.4**	**28.4**	**2.8**
BALTI								
Chick Pea & Spinach, Cauldron Foods*	1 Pack/400g	356	8	89	2.3	15.5	2	1
Chicken, Asda*	1 Pack/400g	400	19.6	100	11	2.5	4.9	1.7
Chicken, Garlic, Chilli, Takeaway, Iceland*	1 Pack/343g	446	24	130	11.1	4.9	7	1.5
Chicken, M&S*	½ Pack/175g	245	15.2	140	13	2	8.7	1.7
Chicken, with Pilau Rice, Asda*	1 Pack/504g	625	24.7	124	5	15	4.9	1.2
Lamb, Bhuna, Tesco*	1 Pack/400g	360	14.8	90	9.2	4.8	3.7	1.1
Prawn, Budgens*	1 Pack/350g	374	24.8	107	5.6	5.2	7.1	1.3
Vegetable, Asda*	½ Can/200g	206	12	103	2.2	10	6	2.5
Vegetable, Average	**1 Serving/200g**	**182**	**8.3**	**91**	**1.9**	**11.3**	**4.1**	**1.7**
Vegetable, Cauliflower & Chickpeas, Microwaved, Asda*	½ Pack/191g	149	7.3	78	2.5	6.4	3.8	4
Vegetable, GFY, Asda*	1 Pack/450g	324	4	72	1.9	14	0.9	1.5
Vegetable, Organic, Canned, Free & Easy*	½ Can/200g	156	4	78	3.5	13.3	2	3.7

B

	Measure INFO/WEIGHT	per Measure KCAL	FAT	Nutrition Values per 100g / 100ml KCAL	PROT	CARB	FAT	FIBRE
BAMBOO SHOOTS								
Canned, Average	*1 Sm Can/120g*	*10*	*0.1*	*8*	*1*	*0.8*	*0.1*	*0.8*
BANANA								
Chips, Average	*1oz/28g*	*143*	*8.8*	*511*	*1*	*59.9*	*31.4*	*1.7*
Green, Medium, Average	*1 Sm/101g*	*91*	*0*	*90*	*1*	*23*	*0*	*3*
Raw, Flesh Only, Average	*1 Med/118g*	*105*	*0.4*	*89*	*1.1*	*22.8*	*0.3*	*2.6*
BARLEY								
Canned, in Water, Drained, Napolina*	1 Can/240g	122	0.2	51	1.7	10	0.1	1.9
Pot, Raw, Average	*1 Serving/60g*	*212*	*1.4*	*354*	*12.5*	*73.5*	*2.3*	*17.3*
Quick Cook, Wholefoods, Tesco*	1 Portion/83g	291	1.2	351	8	70.7	1.4	11.6
BARS								
& Casahew Butter, Protein Balls, Graze*	1 Serving/30g	119	5.1	397	17	48	17	9.3
All Bran, Honey & Oat, Kellogg's*	1 Bar/27g	99	2.2	366	6	67	8	12
Almond, & Cashew, Paleo, Aldi*	1 Bar/45g	203	10.8	451	13	40	24	8.9
Almond, & Sultana, with Peanuts & Apricots, Eat Natural*	1 Bar/50g	224	11	449	13.2	47.2	22	4.6
Almond, Kale, Protein, Ball, Bounce*	1 Ball/40g	176	8.4	440	22.5	43	21	0
Almond, Madagascan Vanilla, Kind*	1 Bar/40g	203	15.6	507	16	36	39	14
Almond, Marzipan, Dark & Milk Chocolate, M&S*	1 Bar/36g	171	8.4	474	6.9	57.4	23.2	4
Almond, Nut Butter, Balls, Deliciously Ella*	1 Pack/36g	162	9.7	450	12.5	37.3	27	9.6
Almond, Spirulina, Protein, Ball, Bounce*	1 Ball/40g	70	3.5	176	9	16.8	8.8	0
Almond, Sweet & Nutty, Nature Valley*	1 Bar/30g	143	6.9	475	10	54.3	23	5.4
Apple, & Cinnamon, FattBar*	1 Bar/30g	139	11.1	464	9.1	6.8	37	33
Apple, Fruit & Oat Bakes, Go Ahead*	1 Bar/35g	127	2.7	363	2.7	72.3	7.7	4.3
Apple, Fruit Bake, Go Ahead, McVitie's*	1 Bar/35g	124	2.5	354	2.7	73.8	7.2	1.2
Apple, Fruit Bakes, Crownfield, Lidl*	1 Bar/33g	128	2.6	387	3.8	73.9	8	2
Apple, Granola, McVitie's*	1 Bar/35g	128	3.4	366	6.6	63.1	9.7	4.3
Apple, Peanut, & Almond, Goodness Knows*	1 Bar/34g	157	6.8	462	7.7	59.6	20	4.6
Apricot, & Almond, Eat Natural*	1 Bar/50g	238	13.4	476	6.6	49.7	26.7	5
Apricot, & Almond, Yoghurt Coated, Eat Natural*	1 Bar/50g	233	13.1	476	6.6	49.7	26.7	5
Apricot, & Hazelnut, Breaks, Go Ahead, McVitie's*	1 Bar/20g	89	3.5	445	8.9	61.2	17.4	4.2
Apricot, Orange, & Ginger, Juicy, Get Fruity*	1 Bar/35g	131	4.6	375	6.6	54	13	6.8
Banana, & Date, Tesco*	1 Bar/26g	88	0.9	340	14	60	3.6	5.6
Bananito, Dark Chocolate Dipped, Mighty Bee*	1 Bar/25g	86	2	344	2.9	68.5	8.2	7.5
Banoffee Pie, Nakd*	1 Bar/35g	129	4.6	368	6.9	53.1	13.2	4.6
Beetroot, & Apple, Yes!*	1 Bar/32g	123	3.7	386	4.8	62.3	11.6	6.6
Berries & Yoghurt, Protein, Alpen*	1 Bar/34g	124	2.5	364	19	47	7.3	17
Berry Delight, The Foodie Market, Aldi*	1 Bar/35g	141	5.2	402	6.4	57	15	6.8
Berry, Delight, GF, Nak'd*	1 Bar/35g	135	5.2	385	9	52	15	6
Berry, Mixed, Moist, Get Fruity*	1 Bar/35g	140	4.6	399	6	61	13	6.3
Berry, Mixed, Trek, Natural Balance Foods*	1 Bar/68g	204	1.5	300	15.6	56.5	2.2	6
Berry, Nut Free, Get Buzzing*	1 Bar/62g	173	8.7	279	3.2	50	14	2.9
Biscuit, & Choco, Milk, Choceur, Aldi*	1 Bar/33g	174	9.6	526	7.9	59	29	1.3
Biscuit, Chocolate, Chunky, Belmont Biscuit Co, Aldi*	1 Bar/24g	126	6.7	526	6.6	61	28	1.8
Biscuit, Chocolate, Mint, Penguin, McVitie's*	1 Bar/25g	133	6.9	531	5.4	65	27.7	1.5
Biscuit, Chocolate, Orange, Penguin, McVitie's*	1 Bar/25g	133	6.9	531	5.4	65	27.7	1.5
Biscuit, Chocolate, Original, Penguin, McVitie's*	1 Bar/20g	106	5.6	515	5.1	61.4	27.1	2.4
Biscuit, Groovy, Aldi*	1 Bar/27g	123	5.3	457	4.9	64.2	19.7	1.8
Biscuit, Raisin & Chocolate Hobnobs, Snack, McVitie's*	1 Bar/32g	132	3.9	420	5.5	71.1	12.5	3.6
Bliss Balls, Salted Caramel, Tom & Luke*	1 Pack/70g	272	12.7	389	12.9	47.9	18.2	5.9
Blueberry, & Yoghurt Nougat, Shapers, Boots*	1 Bar/23g	85	3	369	1.8	76	13	1.7
Blueberry, Muffin, Fibre, Asda*	1 Bar/24g	86	2.3	359	3.6	54	9.5	22
Brazil, & Sultana, GF, Deluxe, Lidl*	1 Bar/45g	218	12.8	485	13.2	41.5	28.4	5.1
Brazil, Sultanas, Almonds & Hazelnuts, Eat Natural*	1 Bar/50g	227	11.3	454	11.2	40	22.6	5
Brownie, Chocolate Orange, Weight Watchers*	1 Bar/18g	63	1.8	346	21	29.6	9.8	27.8

B

BARS

INFO/WEIGHT	Measure	per Measure		Nutrition Values per 100g / 100ml				
		KCAL	FAT	KCAL	PROT	CARB	FAT	FIBRE
Brownie, Chocolate, Fibre, Asda*	1 Bar/24g	89	2.9	369	5	49	12	23
Cacao, & Almond, Energy Ball, Deliciously Ella*	1 Ball/40g	173	11.1	433	12.5	35.3	27.8	7.2
Cacao, & Cashew, Quinoa, Perkier*	1 Bar/35g	137	6.3	391	14	39	18	14
Cacao, & Orange, Protein Balls, Alesto, Lidl*	1 Pack/45g	165	4.5	367	20.2	45.8	10	5.8
Cacao, Protein, Hike, The Foodie Market, Aldi*	1 Bar/55g	190	2.9	345	19	52	5.3	7.4
Cacao, Raw Fruit & Nut, Wild Trail*	1 Bar/30g	115	3.3	383	8.6	56	11	11
Caramel, Almond, & Sea Salt, Kind*	1 Bar/40g	200	15.6	500	14	39	39	18
Caramel, Chewy, Mini, Sainsbury's*	1 Bar/18g	80	3.3	444	3.5	66.4	18.2	0.5
Caramel, Crazy, Tesco*	1 Bar/40g	192	9.2	480	3.9	64	23	1
Caramel, Crunchy, Tesco*	1 Bar/21g	98	5.2	467	4.6	56	25	1.4
Caramel, Nougat, Soft, Shapers, Boots*	1 Bar/25g	86	2.5	343	2.9	60.4	10	0.6
Caramel, Salted, Huel*	1 Bar/49g	200	7.8	408	24	36	16	9
Caramel, Salted, Protein, Ball, Bounce*	1 Ball/40g	170	7	425	1	30	17.5	25
Caramel, Salted, Square, Fibre One*	1 Bar/24g	87	2.8	362	4	49.5	11.7	21.2
Caramel, Skinny Whip*	1 Bar/25g	96	2.3	384	3.6	64	9.2	15.2
Caramel, Wafer, Chewy, Ms Mollys*	1 Bar/18g	88	3.9	489	6.2	66.5	21.6	2
Carb Crusher, Caramel Nut, Myprotein*	1 Bar/60g	212	8.4	353	35	20	14	18
Carrot, Cake, Fibre One*	1 Bar/25g	90	3.4	361	4.2	44	13.4	23.9
Cashew, Cookie, Raw Fruit & Nut, GF, Nak'd*	1 Bar/35g	143	8	410	10	46	23	5
Cashew, Crush, The Foodie Market, Aldi*	1 Bar/35g	158	8	451	12	46	23	7.6
Cereal, & Milk, Nesquik, Nestle*	1 Bar/25g	108	3.7	433	6.2	68.5	14.9	1
Cereal, Apple & Cinnamon, Boka*	1 Bar/30g	88	0.8	293	5.7	58	2.5	19
Cereal, Apple & Cinnamon, Fruit 'n' Grain, Asda*	1 Bar/37g	131	2.6	353	4.5	68	7	2.9
Cereal, Apple & Sultana, Light, Alpen*	1 Bar/20g	63	0.7	330	4.1	59.4	3.6	21.7
Cereal, Apricot, Almond, & Yoghurt, Tesco*	1 Bar/35g	156	6.8	447	5.9	59.7	19.4	4.9
Cereal, Banana Bonanza, Tesco*	1 Bar/21g	82	1.8	390	6.6	69	8.8	4.3
Cereal, Banoffee, Light, Alpen, Weetabix*	1 Bar/19g	66	1.3	346	4.7	54	7	24
Cereal, Cherry Bakewell, Light, Alpen*	1 Bar/19g	65	1.1	341	5.1	56	5.6	23
Cereal, Choc Chip, Brunch, Cadbury*	1 Bar/32g	140	5.3	445	6.1	64.5	17	4.8
Cereal, Choco Mallow, Boka*	1 Bar/30g	93	0.9	309	5.8	53	2.9	24
Cereal, Chocolate & Fudge, Light, Alpen*	1 Bar/21g	71	1.3	342	4.9	55	6.5	22
Cereal, Chocolate Chip, Special K, Kellogg's*	1 Bar/21g	84	1.5	401	9	76	7	1.5
Cereal, Chocolate Delight, Dark, Fibre, Special K, Kellogg's	1 Bar/24g	97	3.4	404	4.5	57	14	17
Cereal, Chocolate, & Fudge, Asda*	1 Bar/19g	66	1.3	347	4.5	53	6.9	28
Cereal, Chocolate, Double, Asda*	1 Bar/19g	67	1.2	352	5.5	58	6.3	21
Cereal, Chocolate, Double, Light, Alpen*	1 Bar/19g	67	1.2	351	5.6	58	6.3	20
Cereal, Chocolate, Milk, Double, Special K, Kellogg's*	1 Bar/20g	79	1.8	396	9	66	9	10
Cereal, Chocolate, Milk, Double, Special K, Kellogg's*	1 Bar/20g	80	2	400	10	65	10	10
Cereal, Citrus Fruits, Light, Alpen*	1 Bar/21g	59	0.9	283	5.6	55.9	4.1	22.4
Cereal, Cornflake, Crunchy, Tesco*	1 Bar/21g	91	2.5	431	4.3	76	12	1
Cereal, Cranberry & Orange, Weight Watchers*	1 Bar/28g	102	1.1	365	4.5	77.6	4.1	2.3
Cereal, Cranberry & Yoghurt, Harvest Morn, Aldi*	1 Bar/29g	117	2.6	403	6.5	71.9	9	4.1
Cereal, Crunchy Granola, Apple Crunch, Nature Valley*	1 Bar/21g	92	3.2	440	7.3	69	15	5.7
Cereal, Crunchy Granola, Ginger Nut, Nature Valley*	1 Bar/42g	189	7.1	451	7.9	64.2	16.9	2.3
Cereal, Crunchy Granola, Peanut Butter, Nature Valley*	1 Bar/21g	95	4	452	9.5	64.3	19	4.8
Cereal, Dark Chocolate, & Cranberries, Special K*	1 Bar/27g	100	2.5	372	5.9	68	9.1	10
Cereal, Fruit & Fibre, Asda*	1 Bar/29g	111	2.8	390	6	69	10	4.1
Cereal, Fruit & Nut, Alpen*	1 Bar/28g	109	2.3	390	5.8	73	8.3	2.9
Cereal, Fruit & Nut, with Milk Chocolate, Alpen*	1 Bar/29g	123	3.8	425	6.4	70.5	13	2.2
Cereal, Fruit, Average	*1 Bar/34g*	*130*	*3.9*	*382*	*5.9*	*64.7*	*11.5*	*6.5*
Cereal, Frusli, Blueberry, Jordans*	1 Bar/30g	113	2.1	375	5.2	70.2	7.1	4.9
Cereal, Frusli, Cranberry & Apple, Jordans*	1 Bar/30g	113	2.1	376	5.1	75.6	7.1	5
Cereal, Frusli, Raisin & Hazelnut, Jordans*	1 Bar/30g	117	3.7	390	5.8	64.3	12.2	4.5

B

BARS

	Measure INFO/WEIGHT	per Measure KCAL	FAT	Nutrition Values per 100g / 100ml KCAL	PROT	CARB	FAT	FIBRE
Cereal, Frusli, Red Berries, Jordans*	1 Bar/30g	112	2.2	374	4.8	75.1	7.2	5.4
Cereal, Hazelnut, Brunch, Cadbury*	1 Bar/35g	160	7.4	460	7	60.5	21.4	2.2
Cereal, Milk Chocolate Chip, Chewy, Harvest Morn, Aldi*	1 Bar/22g	95	3.1	432	5.6	68	14	4.2
Cereal, Muesli, Apple, No Added Sugar, Crownfield, Lidl*	1 Bar/25g	96	2.8	386	6.3	67.9	11.2	6.7
Cereal, Nut & Seed, Organic, Green & Black's*	1 Bar/50g	258	16.3	516	8.4	47.2	32.6	10
Cereal, Oat & Raisin, Basics, Sainsbury's*	1 Bar/25g	98	2.2	391	5.1	72.8	8.8	3.8
Cereal, Oat & Raisin, Soft Oaties, Nutri-Grain, Kellogg's*	1 Bar/40g	173	6.4	432	6	66	16	3.5
Cereal, Raisin & Nut Snack Bar, Benecol*	1 Bar/25g	98	2.8	390	3.9	68.5	11.1	2
Cereal, Raisin, Raisin, Cadbury*	1 Bar/35g	150	5.4	430	5.6	66.4	15.5	1.8
Cereal, Red Fruit, Chewy & Crispy, Sainsbury's*	1 Bar/23g	82	1.2	358	6	69.4	5.2	10.5
Cereal, Rice Snaps, Asda*	1 Bar/20g	77	2.1	385	3.5	60	10.5	15.5
Cereal, Strawberry with Yoghurt, Alpen*	1 Bar/29g	120	2.9	415	4.8	75	10	2.7
Cereal, Strawberry, Fruit 'n' Grain, Asda*	1 Bar/37g	126	2.6	340	4.2	65	7	4.5
Cereal, Summer Fruits, Light, Alpen*	1 Bar/21g	70	0.9	334	4.4	58.7	4.1	22.4
Cereal, Summer Fruits, Tesco*	1 Bar/19g	66	0.8	350	4.5	65.3	4	17.4
Cereal, White Chocolate & Strawberry, Value, Tesco*	1 Bar/21g	85	1.7	405	6.2	76.2	8.1	2.4
Cereal, White Chocolate, & Strawberry, Ms Mollys*	1 Bar/21g	82	1.4	390	5.5	74.7	6.7	4.2
Chocolate Hazelnut Whip, Fulfil Nutrition*	1 Bar/55g	210	9.9	382	36	27	18	5.5
Chocolate, & Caramel, Rice Krispies Squares, Kellogg's*	1 Bar/36g	155	5	430	4.5	71	14	2
Chocolate, & Peanut, Tracker, Mars*	1 Bar/26g	112	5	432	6.6	50.6	19.1	15.5
Chocolate, Brownie, Average	*1 Bar/68g*	*240*	*4*	*353*	*14.7*	*60.3*	*5.9*	*8.8*
Chocolate, Brownie, Double, Protein, PhD Nutrition*	1 Bar/60g	199	5.2	332	33.3	31.7	8.7	0
Chocolate, Caramel, & Sea Salt, Nomo*	1 Bar/38g	212	13.7	559	1.9	55	36	0
Chocolate, Caramel, HiLo, Healthspan*	1 Bar/60g	193	6	322	33.3	23.3	10	0
Chocolate, Caramel, Nut Roll, Advantage, Atkins*	1 Bar/44g	170	12	386	18.2	43.2	27.3	18.2
Chocolate, Caramel, Protein, Battle Bites*	1 Bar/62g	227	8.7	366	32.3	25	14	0
Chocolate, Caramel, Wacko, Belmont, Aldi*	1 Bar/21g	102	4.6	485	5.3	65	22	1.7
Chocolate, Coconut, Protein, Battle Bites*	1 Bar/62g	236	10.5	381	32.3	23.1	16.9	0
Chocolate, Cosmic Whip, Tesco*	1 Bar/22g	100	3.7	452	3.6	72.4	16.6	0.8
Chocolate, Crispy Wafer, Dark, Tasty Little Numbers*	1 Bar/20g	100	5.1	499	6.4	60.4	25.6	7
Chocolate, Crispy, Free From, Tesco*	1 Bar/30g	132	4.6	440	4.1	71.2	15.4	0.5
Chocolate, Dark, & Peanut Butter, Deluxe, Lidl*	1 Bar/40g	218	14.6	545	20.2	30.5	36.5	6.8
Chocolate, Dark, & Raspberry, Tesco*	1 Bar/23g	92	2.2	401	7	69	9.8	4.5
Chocolate, Dark, Chewy Delight, Special K, Kellogg's*	1 Bar/24g	97	3.4	404	4.5	57	14	17
Chocolate, Dark, Intense, The Dark One, M&S*	1 Bar/32g	180	10.9	564	9.6	53.1	34.2	2.5
Chocolate, Dark, Mint, Hi-Fi, Slimming World*	1 Bar/20g	70	1.8	351	4	54	8.8	20
Chocolate, Dark, Nuts, & Sea Salt, Kind*	1 Bar/40g	198	14.8	495	14	23	37	17
Chocolate, DArk, Sea SAlt, & Almond, Yes!*	1 Bar/35g	188	13.3	538	20.2	21.2	37.9	15.4
Chocolate, Double, Snack, Skinny Whip*	1 Bar/25g	96	2.3	385	3.7	64	9.3	15
Chocolate, Fruit & Nut, M&S*	1 Bar/50g	235	12	470	6.5	57.1	24.1	2.5
Chocolate, Fudge Fandango, Protein, The Protein Works*	1 Bar/50g	185	7	370	30	27	14	15.8
Chocolate, Hazelnut, Weight Watchers*	1 Stick/11g	54	3	470	6.2	51	26	2.3
Chocolate, Honeycomb, Bunnycomb, Mini Moos*	1 Bar/25g	143	9.4	571	2.7	59.5	37.6	0
Chocolate, Huel*	1 Bar/49g	200	7.9	406	24	36	16	10
Chocolate, Juice Plus*	1 Bar/55g	210	6.4	382	24.8	39.4	11.6	10.2
Chocolate, Meal Replacement, Ultra Slim, Tesco*	1 Bar/60g	219	6.7	365	28.5	37.3	11.1	8.2
Chocolate, Milk, Chewy Delight, Special K, Kellogg's*	1 Bar/24g	95	3.1	397	5	57	13	17
Chocolate, Milk, Swiss, M&S*	1 Bar/50g	285	18.4	570	0.2	51	36.8	2
Chocolate, Mint, Club, Mcvitie's*	1 Bar/23g	117	6.1	510	5.7	61.2	26.4	2.3
Chocolate, Mint, Meal Replacement, Crunchy, CWP*	1 Bar/55g	215	7	391	27	42.7	12.8	5.6
Chocolate, Mint, Milk, Vitamin & Protein, Fulfil Nutrition*	1 Bar/55g	189	6.9	344	35.9	18.8	12.5	18.8
Chocolate, Mint, Polar, Sainsbury's*	1 Bar/25g	135	7.6	534	4.9	59.9	29.9	2.6
Chocolate, Mint, Protein, Shred & Burn, Musashi*	1 Bar/60g	214	6.2	356	33.6	2.2	10.3	6.1

BARS

INFO/WEIGHT	per Measure KCAL	per Measure FAT	KCAL	PROT	CARB	FAT	FIBRE
Chocolate, Mint, Whip'd, Aussie Bodies*	1 Bar/60g	652	21.2	1087	100	11	35.3	43.7
Chocolate, Orange, Huel*	1 Bar/49g	200	7.9	406	24	36	16	10
Chocolate, Peanut Butter, Smart, PhD Nutrition*	1 Bar/64g	239	10.2	373	31	38	16	1
Chocolate, Peanut, & Caramel, Shapers, Boots*	1 Bar/24g	96	4.1	401	6.6	42	17	28
Chocolate, Peanut, Almond, Sweet & Salty, Nature Valley*	1 Bar/30g	139	7.2	464	10.1	45.5	24	13
Chocolate, Polar, Sainsbury's*	1 Bar/25g	133	7.2	533	5.5	63	28.6	1.2
Chocolate, Protein, Diet Chef Ltd*	1 Bar/60g	225	7.1	375	29.3	37.5	11.9	4.2
Chocolate, Racer, Dairyfine, Aldi*	1 Bar/38g	185	9.5	486	8.6	54	25	4.2
Chocolate, Sandwich, Seal, Aldi*	1 Bar/25g	131	7	523	5.5	60.6	28.1	3.1
Chocolate, The Milk One, M&S*	1 Bar/32g	174	10.1	545	8.3	56	31.6	1.5
Chocolate, Titan, Aldi*	1 Bar/38g	169	6.8	444	3.5	66	18	0.5
Chocolate, Toffee Pecan, M&S*	1 Bar/36g	179	9.8	498	4.9	58.3	27.3	0.7
Chocolate, Viennese, Sandwich, Fox's*	1 Biscuit/14g	76	4.4	542	6.9	57.4	31.6	1.6
Chocolate, Wafer, Blue Riband, 99 Calories, Nestle*	1 Bar/19g	99	4.7	514	5.5	66.5	24.6	2
Chocolate, White, Creamy, The White One, M&S*	1 Bar/32g	184	12	574	6.6	51.6	37.5	1.7
Chocolix, Schar*	1 Bar/22g	101	3.9	463	3.6	70	18	4.2
Cinnamon, & Apple, Fruit & Peanut, Asda*	1 Bar/35g	135	5.6	386	12	40	16	16
Club, Fruit, Jacob's*	1 Bar/25g	124	6.2	496	5.6	62.2	25	2.3
Club, Milk Chocolate, Jacob's*	1 Bar/24g	123	6.3	511	5.8	62.6	26.4	2
Club, Mint, Jacob's*	1 Bar/24g	124	6.5	517	5.6	62.5	27.2	1.7
Club, Orange, Crunchies, McVitie's*	1 Bar/24g	115	6.1	481	5.1	59	25.7	1.4
Club, Orange, Jacob's*	1 Bar23g	117	6.1	509	5.7	61.8	26.5	2.3
Coco Pops, & Milk, Kellogg's*	1 Bar/20g	85	2.6	423	7	70	13	1
Cocoa, & Hazelnut, Goodness, Go Ahead!*	1 Bar/30g	111	4	369	7.4	56	13.4	7.8
Cocoa, & Hazelnut, Nut Butter, Nature Valley*	1 Bar/38g	191	10	503	7.6	56	26.3	6.1
Cocoa, Brownie, Trek, The Natural Health Company*	1 Bar/68g	223	4.1	328	17	53	6	8
Cocoa, Crunch, Nak'd*	1 Bar/30g	105	2.6	351	18.4	47.2	8.8	6.3
Cocoa, Delight, Wholefood, GF, Nak'd*	1 Bar/35g	135	5.3	386	9.4	49.4	15.1	6.8
Cocoa, Orange, GF, Nak'd*	1 Bar/35g	145	7	415	11	45.1	20	6.4
Cocoa, Twist, Nak'd*	1 Bar/30g	99	1.7	329	7	59.9	5.6	6
Coconut, & Oat, Energy Ball, Deliciously Ella*	1 Ball/40g	145	4.8	362	7.4	56.5	11.9	7.7
Coconut, Chocolate Crisp, Weight Watchers*	1 Bar/25g	89	2.6	356	3.6	71.2	10.4	3.2
Coconut, Cumin, Protein, Balls, Bounce*	1 Ball/40g	184	10	460	22.5	40	25	0
Coffee, Caramel, Huel*	1 Bar/49g	200	7.9	407	24	36	16	10
Cookie, Oaty, Maryland*	1 Bar/19g	94	4.6	493	6.8	58.5	24.2	6.1
Cranberry, & Dark Chocolate, Yes!*	1 Bar/35g	183	11.9	523	20.3	25.4	34.1	16.5
Cranberry, Crunchy, Meal Replacement, CWP*	1 Bar/55g	214	6.8	389	27.7	42.9	12.3	4.5
Fibre, Chocolate Brownie, Morrisons*	1 Bar/24g	88	3	368	5	48.1	12.6	20.7
Fibre, Lemon Drizzle, Morrisons*	1 Bar/24g	85	2.6	353	3.5	48.7	10.9	23.5
Flapjack, Buttery, Traditional, Organic, Dove's Farm*	1 Bar/40g	173	7.5	432	6.1	59.4	18.8	5.7
Flapjack, Cocoa, & Raisin, Protein, Trek*	1 Bar/50g	222	10.7	444	18	43.1	21.4	4.2
Frosties, & Milk, Kellogg's*	1 Bar/25g	102	2.8	408	7	71	11	1
Frosties, Snack Bar, Kellogg's*	1 Bar/25g	104	2.8	414	7	72	11	1
Fruit & Fibre, Coconut, Apricot, Oats, Spelt, Eat Natural*	1 Bar/40g	165	7	413	6.4	51.6	17.5	6.1
Fruit & Fibre, Plum, Peanut, Oats, Spelt, Eat Natural*	1 Bar/40g	173	7.8	432	10.1	51.1	19.4	6.4
Fruit & Nut, Salted Caramel, & Peanuts, Eat Natural*	1 Bar/45g	223	12.8	496	26	31.3	28.4	5.4
Fruit & Grain, Apple, Harvest Morn, Aldi*	1 Bar/37g	129	3	349	4.2	65	8	4.5
Fruit & Grain, Strawberry, Harvest Morn, Aldi*	1 Bar/37g	130	2.6	349	4.2	65	7	4.5
Fruit & Nut, Eat Natural*	1 Bar/50g	223	11.2	446	11.6	49.8	22.3	5.3
Fruit & Nut, with Chocolate, & Orange, Eat Natural*	1 Bar/45g	224	12.8	498	26.1	31.1	28.5	6
Fruit 'n' Fibre, Kellogg's*	1 Bar/25g	95	2.2	380	5	71	9	5
Fruit, & Nut, Apricot, Almond, & Pumpkin Seed, Benecol*	1 Bar/40g	171	8	428	7	52	20	6.8
Fruit, GF, Schar*	1 Bar/25g	99	3	396	3.2	65	12	8.2

B

BARS

	Measure INFO/WEIGHT	per Measure KCAL	FAT	KCAL	PROT	CARB	FAT	FIBRE
Fudge, Brownie, Carb Killa, Grenade*	1 Bar/60g	215	8	359	38.9	22.6	13.3	11.3
Ginger, Bread, GF, Nak'd*	1 Bar/35g	158	10.8	450	10	35	31	9.4
Ginger, Bread, Nak'd*	1 Bar/35g	157	10.7	450	10	35.4	30.8	9.4
Goji, & Coconut, Protein, Balls, Alesto, Lidl*	1 Pack/45g	173	6.3	384	12.9	49.1	14	5.3
Golden Syrup, Morning, Oat So Simple, Quaker*	1 Bar/35g	142	3.5	407	8.2	67.6	10	6.8
Granola, Chocolate & Nut, Crunchy Nut, Kellogg's*	1 Bar/32g	167	10.6	521	12	41	33	6.6
Granola, Crunchy, Oats & Chocolate, Nature Valley*	1 Bar/21g	98	4.1	464	8.3	59.8	19.8	7.1
Granola, Maple Syrup, Crunchy, Harvest Morn, Aldi*	2 Bars/42g	189	6.7	450	8.2	65	16	5.9
Granola, Oats & Honey, Crunchy, Harvest Morn, Aldi*	2 Bars/42g	191	6.7	455	8.2	66	16	6.2
Hazelnut, Dark Chocolate Coated, Vive*	1 Bar/50g	227	14	453	21	26	28	13
Hazelnut, Wafer, Princessa, Nestle*	1 Bar/34g	188	11.3	552	5.6	57.1	33.1	1.7
Hobnobs, Choc & Golden Syrup, McVitie's*	1 Bar/31g	129	4	421	6.3	68.2	13.1	4.8
Honey, & Almond, Crunchy, Original, Jordans*	1 Bar/30g	139	6.8	463	8.3	56.7	22.7	6.7
Honeycomb, Club, Jacob's*	1 Bar/23g	116	6	512	5.7	61.9	26.3	2.3
Honeycomb, Milk Chocolate, Mighty Fine*	1 Bar/30g	133	3.8	444	3.1	79.7	12.7	1
Jaffa Cake, Benefit, Harvest Morn, Aldi*	1 Bar/66g	228	3.6	346	5.2	58	5.5	22
Jive, Chocolate, Shortcake Finger, Dairyfine, Aldi*	1 Twin Bar/42g	194	9.7	463	4.6	58	23	0.9
LCMs, Choc Chip, Kellogg's*	1 Bar/22g	90	2.2	411	4.1	75.1	9.9	0.7
Lemon Drizzle, Nak'd*	1 Bar/35g	133	5.4	381	6.1	51.8	15.5	5.1
Malt Loaf, Soreen*	1 Bar/42g	124	1	295	8.2	57.8	2.3	5.1
Maple Pecan, Salted, The Yes Bar*	1 Bar/40g	220	17	550	12.5	32.5	42.5	7.5
Maple, Glazed Pecan, & Sea Salt, Kind*	1 Bar/40g	213	17.2	532	14	33	43	13
Marshmallow, Chewy, Rice Krispies Squares, Kellogg's*	1 Bar/28g	119	3.4	424	3	76	12	0.9
Marshmallow, Vanilla, Mallow & Marsh*	1 Bar/35g	134	3.7	383	7.1	68.9	10.6	0
Melto, GF, Schar*	1 Bar/30g	165	9.9	549	6.8	55	33	0
Millionaire, Salted Caramel, Hazelnut, M&S*	1 Bar/62g	285	12	459	2.2	67.1	19.4	3.4
Millionaires Shortcake, Hi-Fi, Slimming World*	1 Bar/20g	71	2	353	4.7	52	9.8	18
Mint Truffle, M&S*	1 Bar/33g	189	13.1	574	4.4	47.9	39.7	3.5
Muesli, & Seeds, Bountiful, Aldi*	1 Bar/30g	98	1.4	328	3	53	4.8	18
Muesli, Fruit, Morning, Oat So Simple, Quaker*	1 Bar/35g	139	3.2	398	7.7	68.1	9.1	6.6
Muesli, Fruit, Special, Jordans*	1 Bar/40g	140	2.4	349	5	68.8	6	5
Muesli, Peanut, No Added Sugar, Crownfield, Lidl*	1 Bar/25g	98	3.3	391	7.9	65.7	13.2	4.7
Nine Bar, Mixed Seed with Hemp, Original, Wholebake*	1 Bar/40g	222	16.2	555	18.3	29.2	40.5	5.2
Nougat, Chewy, Barratt*	1 Bar/35g	133	1.5	380	4.6	79.2	4.2	2.1
Nougat, Cool Mint, & Dark Chocolate, Shapers, Boots*	1 Bar/25g	81	3.1	324	2.4	48	12.4	1.2
Nougat, Honeycomb, Shapers, Boots*	1 Bar/22g	96	2.9	435	2.8	76	13	1.2
Nougat, Salted Caramel, Shapers, Boots*	1 Bar/23g	95	2.5	412	2.8	73	11	3.5
Nougat, Summer Strawberry, Shapers, Boots*	1 Bar/23g	83	3	361	2.7	73	13	0.6
Nut, Dark Chocolate & Apricot, Natural, Nice & Natural*	1 Bar/35g	163	10.2	465	15.2	35.2	29.1	5.4
Nut, Feast, Mixed, Eat Natural*	1 Bar/50g	278	20.5	556	18.8	28	41	0
Nutri-Grain, Apple, Kellogg's*	1 Bar/37g	131	3.3	355	4	67	9	4
Nutri-Grain, Apple, Soft & Fruity, Kellogg's*	1 Bar/37g	133	3	359	4	70.3	8.1	4
Nutri-Grain, Blackberry & Apple, Soft & Fruity, Kellogg's*	1 Bar/37g	133	3	359	4	70.3	8.1	4
Nutri-Grain, Blueberry, Kellogg's*	1 Bar/37g	133	3	359	3.5	69	8	3.5
Nutri-Grain, Elevenses, Choc Chip Bakes, Kellogg's*	1 Bar/45g	179	5.8	397	4	66	13	2
Nutri-Grain, Elevenses, Raisin Bakes, Kellogg's*	1 Bar/45g	168	4	374	4.5	68	9	2.5
Nutri-Grain, Strawberry, Kellogg's*	1 Bar/37g	133	3	359	3.5	69	8	3.5
Nutri-Grain, Strawberry, Soft & Fruity, Kellogg's*	1 Bar/37g	133	3	359	4	70.3	8.1	4
Nutty Nougat Caramel, Tesco*	1 Bar/40g	200	11.1	490	8.7	52.7	27.2	3.8
Nutty, Snack Size, Asda*	1 Bar/38g	182	9.5	479	9	54	25	0.9
Oat, Berry & Vanilla, Mini, Graze*	1 Bite/30g	136	6.3	452	12	51	21	5.3
Oat, Choc Chip & Raisin, Mini, Graze*	1 Bite/30g	140	7.6	477	11	53	26	6.2
Oat, Choc Salt Caramel, Tribe*	1 Bar/50g	206	8	412	14	49	16	8.7

BARS

INFO/WEIGHT	Measure	per Measure KCAL	per Measure FAT	Nutrition per 100g/100ml KCAL	PROT	CARB	FAT	FIBRE
Orange, & Cacao, Dark, Millionaire, Graze*	1 Bar/50g	188	7	376	21	38	14	6.6
Peach, & Apricot, Special K, Kellogg's*	1 Bar/23g	90	1.4	383	8	75	6	2.5
Peanut Butter, Breakfast, Bounce*	1 Bar/45g	168	7.2	374	22	27	16	16
Peanut Butter, Crunchy, Nature Valley*	1 Pack/42g	204	9	486	10.2	59.7	21.5	6.5
Peanut Butter, Dark Chocolate Coated, Vive*	1 Bar/50g	219	13	438	21	28	26	13
Peanut Butter, Dark Chocolate, Specially Selected, Aldi*	1 Bar/40g	213	14.8	533	23	21	37	15
Peanut Butter, Mega Nuts, Tasti*	1 Bar/40g	216	14	540	14.9	38.4	35.1	3.4
Peanut, & Choco, Mister Choc, Lidl*	1 Bar/38g	190	10.6	500	10	51	28	2.8
Peanut, & Dark Chocolate, Tesco*	1 Bar/35g	175	10.4	500	22.2	33	29.7	6
Peanut, & Date, Breakfast, M&S*	1 Bar/40g	171	9.5	428	22.8	19.5	23.8	21.8
Peanut, Caramel, Payday, Hershey*	1 Bar/19g	88	4.8	462	13.5	51.9	25	3.8
Peanut, Mr Toms*	1 Bar/40g	210	13	525	20	42.5	32.5	2.5
Peanut, Nutty Crunch, Go Ahead, McVitie's*	1 Bar/20g	94	4.8	483	11	52.8	24.6	3.6
Peanut, Sweet & Salty Nut, Nature Valley*	1 Bar/30g	143	7.8	478	12.3	43.1	26.1	11
Peanuts, Coconut, & Chocolate, Vegan, Eat Natural*	1 Bar/45g	223	13.5	496	11.9	40.4	30	7.8
Pecan, Pie, GF, Nak'd*	1 Bar/35g	156	10.3	477	7.6	36.4	31.4	8.9
Popcorn, Peanut Butter, Fibre One*	1 Bar/21g	90	4.3	427	7.6	41.4	20.3	23.9
Popcorn, Peanut, & Sunflower, Asda*	1 Bar/20g	90	4.4	448	8.6	45	22	16
Protein, Banana, Hike, Aldi*	1 Bar/55g	169	0.8	306	20	45	1.5	18
Protein, Boysenberry Ripple, Whip'd, Aussie Bodies*	1 Bar/30g	94	2.8	313	30	4	9.3	14.7
Protein, Caramel & Hazelnut, Elite, Myprotein*	1 Bar/70g	244	7.7	348	37	32	11	6.6
Protein, Caramel Cashew, Barebells*	1 Bar/55g	199	8.2	361	36	26	15	7.9
Protein, Caramel Chaos, Carb Killa, Grenade*	1 Bar/60g	214	7.9	357	38.7	22.5	13.2	11.1
Protein, Chocolate Brownie, GF, Quest*	1 Bar/60g	191	7.2	318	33	12	12	25
Protein, Chocolate Chip Cookie Dough, GF, Quest*	1 Bar/60g	206	9	344	34	12	15	23
Protein, Cinnamon Roll, GF, Quest*	1 Bar/60g	191	7.2	318	33	16	12	23
Protein, Cookies & Cream, Barebells*	1 Bar/55g	197	6.6	358	36	30	12	6.1
Protein, Cookies & Cream, Fulfil*	1 Bar/55g	208	9.3	379	36.4	14.9	16.9	20.8
Protein, Cookies & Cream, GF, Quest*	1 Bar/60g	209	9	349	35	12	15	23
Protein, Flapjack, Oat Crunch, Natural Balance Foods*	1 Bar/56g	249	12.9	444	18	43	23	3
Protein, Hazelnut, & Nougat, Barebell*	1 Bar/55g	205	9.4	373	36	26	17	7.7
Protein, Low Sugar, Chocolate, USN*	1 Bar/35g	116	4.2	332	31	30	12	13
Protein, Madagascan Vanilla, High Fibre, Bounce*	1 Bar/45g	164	6.8	364	20	28	15	15
Protein, Mint Chocolate Chunk, GF, Quest*	1 Bar/60g	209	9	348	33	11	15	24
Protein, Mint Dark Chocolate, Barebells*	1 Bar/55g	192	7.2	350	36	30	13	0
Protein, Peanut Blast, Natural Energy, Ball, Bounce*	1 Ball/49g	210	8	429	28.6	38.8	16.3	4.1
Protein, Peanut Butter, Ball, The Protein Ball Co.*	1 Pack/45g	176	7.6	390	23	32	17	13
Protein, Peanut Butter, Promax Lean, Maximuscle *	1 Bar/55g	190	6.2	346	36.7	24.8	11.2	12.7
Protein, Peanut Peak, Chunks, Trek, Natural Balance*	1 Bar/60g	232	7.9	386	20.9	42	13.2	7
Protein, Salty Peanut, Barebells*	1 Bar/55g	200	8.2	364	36	27	15	7.1
Protein, Vanilla Cheesecake, Protein 20, Science in Sport*	1 Bar/55g	212	8.2	386	37	39	15	0.9
Protein, White Chocolate Raspberry, GF, Quest*	1 Bar/60g	215	9.6	358	33	13	16	23
Pumpkin Seed, & Almond, Tesco*	1 Bar/35g	204	15.8	582	20	21	45	6.6
Quinoa, Goji, & Cranberry, Perkier*	1 Bar/35g	129	3.9	370	12.7	51.1	11.2	10.1
Raisin, Munch, Tesco*	1 Bar/32g	135	4.1	423	6.2	68	13	4.7
Raspberry Crunch, Protein, Weight Watchers*	1 Bar/23g	68	2.5	297	21.9	49.8	10.9	9.7
Red Berry, Juicy, Special K, Kellogg's*	1 Bar/27g	104	1.7	384	5.3	73	6.3	7.7
Rhubarb, & Ginger, Porridge Oat, Stoats*	1 Bar/50g	221	11.1	442	7.9	52.6	22.2	5.3
Rice Krispies, Snack, Kellogg's*	1 Bar/20g	83	2	415	7	70	10	0.5
Rice Krispies, Squares, Totally Chocolatey, Kellogg's*	1 Bar/36g	156	5.3	439	4.5	72	15	1.5
Rocky Road, M&S*	1 Bar/68g	330	18	486	4.1	56.7	26.5	1.9
Rocky Road, Rice Krispies Squares, Kellogg's*	1 Square/34g	143	3.7	420	4	76	11	1.5
Rocky Road, Romance Me, Hi-Fi, Slimming World*	1 Bar/20g	73	1.5	366	4.8	62.7	7.3	15.4

	Measure INFO/WEIGHT	per Measure KCAL	FAT	Nutrition Values per 100g / 100ml KCAL	PROT	CARB	FAT	FIBRE
BARS								
Salted Caramel, Dark Chocolate Coated, Vive*	1 Bar/50g	219	13	438	21	28	26	13
Sesame Snaps, Anglo-Dal*	1 Pack/30g	157	8.8	522	12.2	49.4	29.4	0
Sesame Snaps, in Chocolate, Anglo-Dal*	1 Pack/40g	211	11.9	527	9.3	55.6	29.7	0
Strawberry, & Vanilla, Vitamin & Protein, Fulfil Nutrition*	1 Bar/60g	185	4.9	309	33.4	10.1	8.2	33.1
Strawberry, & Chocolate, Skinny Whip*	1 Bar/25g	96	2.3	385	3.7	64	9.3	15
Strawberry, Fruit & Oat Bakes, Go Ahead*	1 Bar/35g	129	2.7	369	2.8	73.4	7.8	4.2
Strawberry, Fruit Bakes, Go Ahead, McVitie's*	1 Bar/35g	131	3	375	3.5	72	8.5	4
Strawberry, Shapers, Boots*	1 Bar/22g	75	2.4	343	2.5	77	11	0.9
Tiffin, GF, Free From, Co-Op*	1 Bar/62g	321	19.8	518	3.2	53	32	4
Toffee, & Chocolate, Snack, Skinny Whip*	1 Bar/25g	96	2.3	384	3.6	64	9.2	15.2
Toffee, Sticky, Hi-Fi, Slimming World*	1 Bar/20g	69	2	343	4	51	9.9	17
Tracker, Chocolate Chip, Mars*	1 Bar/37g	178	8.7	480	6.8	58	23.6	3.8
Tracker, Roasted Nut, Mars*	1 Bar/26g	127	6.6	489	8.1	55	25.3	4.9
Wafer, Hanuta, Ferrero*	1 Slice/44g	238	14	542	7.6	54	31.9	0
White Chocolate, Cookie Dough, Fulfil Nutrition*	1 Bar/55g	195	7.2	355	38.6	20.2	13.2	14.2
BASA								
Fillets, Lemon & Herb, Tempura Batter, Gastro, Youngs*	1 Fillet/147g	240	9.7	163	16.3	9.4	6.6	0.3
Fillets, Lightly Dusted, Parsley, Oven Baked, Asda*	1 Fillet/119g	246	11.3	206	14	16	9.5	0.5
Fillets, Lime, Chilli & Coriander, Dusted, Gastro, Youngs*	1 Fillet/152g	288	13.9	189	15.6	11	9.1	0.4
Fillets, Rocket, Basil & Parmesan Sauce, Gastro, Youngs*	1 Serving/136g	136	4.2	100	17.7	0.2	3.1	0.2
Fillets, Sea Salt & Cracked Black Pepper, Gastro, Youngs*	1 Fillet/151g	261	12.1	173	14.7	10.5	8	0.3
Fillets, Skinless & Boneless, Aldi*	1 Fillet/120g	140	2.9	117	23.7	0.1	2.4	0
Fillets, Skinless, & Boneless, Oven Cooked, Morrisons*	1 Fillet/89g	76	1.4	85	17.6	0	1.6	0
Fillets, Smoked, Skinless, Tesco*	1 Fillet/125g	112	2.8	90	17.5	0	2.2	0
BASIL								
Dried, Ground	**1 Tsp/1.4g**	**4**	**0.1**	**251**	**14.4**	**43.2**	**4**	**0**
Fresh, Average	**1 Tbsp/5g**	**2**	**0**	**40**	**3.1**	**5.1**	**0.8**	**0**
BATTER MIX								
for Yorkshire Puddings & Pancakes, Tesco*	1 Serving/17g	34	0.3	200	2.3	43.3	1.5	2.5
for Yorkshire Puddings, Baked, Aunt Bessie's*	1 Pudding/13g	48	1.1	356	9.8	34	8.1	2.3
Pancake, Buttermilk, Krusteaz*	3 Pancakes/16g	57	0.8	352	11.3	66	4.7	3.4
BAY LEAVES								
Dried, Average	**1 Tsp/0.6g**	**2**	**0.1**	**313**	**7.6**	**48.6**	**8.4**	**0**
BEAN SPROUTS								
Mung, Raw, Average	**1oz/28g**	**9**	**0.1**	**31**	**2.9**	**4**	**0.5**	**1.5**
Mung, Stir-Fried in Blended Oil, Average	**1 Serving/90g**	**65**	**5.5**	**72**	**1.9**	**2.5**	**6.1**	**0.9**
Raw, Average	**1 Serving/150g**	**55**	**2.6**	**37**	**2.2**	**3.2**	**1.8**	**1.2**
BEANS								
& Seeds, Steamer, Waitrose*	1 Bag/160g	213	7.7	133	9.4	8.1	4.8	9.9
Aduki, Cooked in Unsalted Water, Average	**1 Tbsp/30g**	**37**	**0.1**	**123**	**9.3**	**22.5**	**0.2**	**5.5**
Aduki, Dried, Raw	**1 Tbsp/30g**	**82**	**0.2**	**272**	**19.9**	**50.1**	**0.5**	**11.1**
Baked, & Sausage in Tomato Sauce, Smart Price, Asda*	½ Can/203g	256	12.2	126	5	13	6	0
Baked, & Sausage, Asda*	½ Can/203g	211	4	104	6.7	13	2	3.5
Baked, & Sausages, in Tomato Sauce, Bramwells, Aldi*	1 Can/400g	412	11.6	103	5.2	12	2.9	3.5
Baked, Barbecue, Beanz, Heinz*	1 Can/390g	343	0.8	88	4.9	14.6	0.2	3.8
Baked, Cheesy & Sausage, Meal For One, Iceland *	1 Pack/494g	721	30.6	146	6.4	14.3	6.2	3.7
Baked, Curried, Average	**½ Can/210g**	**203**	**1.9**	**96**	**4.8**	**17.2**	**0.9**	**3.6**
Baked, Curry, Beanz, Heinz*	1 Can/390g	382	1.2	98	4.8	17	0.3	4
Baked, Five, in Tomato Sauce, Heinz*	1 Can/415g	361	0.8	87	5.4	13.6	0.2	4.3
Baked, Gigantes, in Tomato Sauce, Odysea *	1 Jar/355g	593	29.1	167	5.8	14.1	8.2	0
Baked, in Tomato Sauce, Average	**1 Can/400g**	**318**	**1.6**	**80**	**4.6**	**13.9**	**0.4**	**3.7**
Baked, in Tomato Sauce, Canned, Co-Op*	1 Can/420g	370	2.1	88	4.7	14	0.5	4.1
Baked, in Tomato Sauce, Canned, Nisa Heritage*	1 Can/400g	356	2	89	4.4	14	0.5	4.8

B

BEANS

	Measure INFO/WEIGHT	per Measure KCAL	FAT	Nutrition Values per 100g / 100ml KCAL	PROT	CARB	FAT	FIBRE
Baked, in Tomato Sauce, Reduced Sugar & Salt	½ Can/210g	159	0.7	76	4.6	13.6	0.3	3.8
Baked, in Tomato Sauce, Reduced Sugar, Tesco*	1 Can/419g	302	2.5	72	4.2	10.9	0.6	3.1
Baked, in Tomato Sauce, Rich, Simply, M&S*	½ Can/205g	184	0.8	90	5.1	14.6	0.4	4
Baked, in Tomato Sauce, Stockwell & Co., Tesco*	½ Can/210g	183	1	87	3.7	14.6	0.5	4.4
Baked, Peri Peri, Beanz, Heinz*	½ Can/195g	176	1.4	90	5.2	13.7	0.7	4.2
Baked, Sweet Chilli, Mean, Beanz, Heinz*	½ Can/195g	142	0.6	73	4.5	13	0.3	3.6
Baked, with Sausages, in Tomato Sauce, Corale, Aldi*	1 Can/400g	412	11.6	103	5.2	12	2.9	3.5
Barbecue, Good Grains, Worldwide Foods, Aldi*	1 Pack/256g	264	3.1	103	5.5	15	1.2	5
Black, Cooked, Average	1 Cup/172g	227	0.9	132	8.8	23.7	0.5	8.7
Black, Refried, Ultimate, Capsicana*	½ Pack/100g	104	0.5	104	5.4	17.8	0.5	4.3
Borlotti, Canned, Average	1oz/28g	29	0.1	103	7.6	16.9	0.5	4.7
Borlotti, Dried, Raw, Average	1 Serving/100g	335	1.2	335	23	60	1.2	24.7
Broad, Canned, Drained, Average	1 Can/195g	136	1.1	70	6.9	9.2	0.6	6.8
Broad, Dried, Raw, Average	1oz/28g	69	0.6	245	26.1	32.5	2.1	27.6
Broad, Fresh, without Pod, Boiled, Average	1 Serving/80g	78	0.5	97	7.9	11.7	0.6	6.5
Broad, Fried & Salted, Captain Tiptoes*	1 Serving/30g	122	5.1	405	24.5	29.6	17	18
Broad, Frozen, Average	1 Serving/80g	63	0.6	79	7.6	10.8	0.7	5.3
Butter, Canned, Drained, Average	1oz/28g	23	0.1	81	6	12.8	0.5	4.3
Butter, Dried, Boiled, Average	1oz/28g	30	0.2	106	7.2	18.6	0.6	5.2
Butter, Dried, Raw, Average	1oz/28g	81	0.5	290	19.1	52.9	1.7	16
Cannellini, Canned, Drained, Average	1 Portion/80g	75	0.4	94	8.7	15	0.5	5.7
Cannellini, Dried, Tesco*	1 Serving/32g	83	0.3	260	24.8	37.4	0.8	20.9
Chilli, Canned, Average	1 Can/420g	381	3.1	91	5.2	15.8	0.7	4.4
Eda-Yummy, Mix, Macro*	1 Pack/30g	124	4.4	415	22.2	39.7	14.8	17.1
Edamame, Sainsbury's*	1 Serving/150g	212	9.6	141	12.3	6.8	6.4	4.2
Edamame, with Soy Sauce, On the Go, Sainsbury's*	1 Pot/100g	119	5.8	119	11.4	20	5.8	6.5
Five, Canned, in Tomato Sauce, Sainsbury's*	½ Can/200g	168	1	84	4.9	12.4	0.5	5.4
Flageolet, Canned, Average	1 Can/265g	235	1.6	89	6.8	14	0.6	3.5
French, Boiled, Average	1 Serving/150g	38	0	25	2.3	3.8	0	3.7
French, Raw	1oz/28g	6	0.1	20	1.6	2.7	0.4	1.8
Green, Cut, Average	1oz/28g	7	0.1	24	1.7	3.6	0.2	2.7
Green, Fine, Average	1 Serving/75g	18	0.3	24	1.8	3.2	0.4	2.9
Green, Sliced, Average	1oz/28g	6	0.1	23	1.9	3.5	0.2	2.1
Green, Sliced, Frozen, Average	1 Serving/50g	13	0	26	1.8	4.4	0.1	4.1
Green, Whole, Average	1oz/28g	6	0.1	22	1.6	3	0.4	1.7
Haricot, Canned, Average	1 Can/400g	307	2	77	6.2	10.7	0.5	5.9
Kidney, Red, Canned, Drained, Average	½ Can/120g	115	0.7	96	7.4	20.7	0.5	5.5
Kidney, Red, Canned, in Water, Four Seasons, Aldi	*1 Can/240g	223	1.2	93	6.8	12	0.5	7.2
Kidney, Red, Canned, in Water, Sweet Harvest, Aldi*	1 Can/240g	290	1.2	121	8.4	17	0.5	6.7
Kidney, Red, Dried, Boiled in Unsalted Water	1oz/28g	29	0.1	103	8.4	17.4	0.5	6.7
Kidney, Red, Dried, Raw	1oz/28g	74	0.4	266	22.1	44.1	1.4	15.7
Kidney, Red, in Chilli Sauce, Sainsbury's*	1 Can/420g	365	1.7	87	5.3	15.6	0.4	4.5
Mexican, Creationz, Heinz*	1 Can/390g	308	3.1	79	4	11.7	0.8	4.5
Mixed, Canned, Average	1 Can/300g	300	3.5	100	6.8	15.6	1.2	4.1
Mixed, in Mild Chilli Sauce, Sainsbury's*	1 Can/420g	328	1.3	78	4.9	13.8	0.3	3.7
Mung, Whole, Dried, Boiled in Unsalted Water	1oz/28g	25	0.1	91	7.6	15.3	0.4	3
Mung, Whole, Dried, Raw	1oz/28g	78	0.3	279	23.9	46.3	1.1	10
Pinto, Dried, Boiled in Unsalted Water	1oz/28g	38	0.2	137	8.9	23.9	0.7	0
Pinto, Dried, Raw	1oz/28g	92	0.4	327	21.1	57.1	1.6	14
Refried, Average	1 Serving/215g	162	1.5	76	4.6	12.7	0.7	1.8
Runner, Average	1 Serving/80g	15	0.3	19	1.3	2.8	0.4	2.2
Soya, Dried, Boiled in Unsalted Water	1oz/28g	39	2	141	14	5.1	7.3	6.1
Soya, Shelled, Frozen, Raw, Average	1 Serving/80g	99	4.3	124	12.2	6.9	5.3	4.4

BEEF

INFO/WEIGHT	Measure	per Measure KCAL	FAT	Nutrition Values per 100g / 100ml KCAL	PROT	CARB	FAT	FIBRE
Brisket, Boiled, Lean	1 Serving/100g	225	11	225	31.4	0	11	0
Brisket, Boiled, Lean & Fat	1 Serving/100g	268	17.4	268	27.8	0	17.4	0
Brisket, Braised, Lean	1 Serving/100g	280	17.4	280	29	0	17.4	0
Brisket, Raw, Lean	1oz/28g	39	1.7	139	21.1	0	6.1	0
Brisket, Raw, Lean & Fat	1oz/28g	60	4.4	216	18.2	0	15.8	0
Brisket, Slow Cooked, Rolled, Oven Cooked, Waitrose*	½ Pack/122g	264	13.3	216	29.3	0.2	10.9	0
Brisket, with Red Wine Sauce, Slow Cooked, M&S*	½ Pack/260g	296	12.5	114	15.6	2.1	4.8	0.5
Carpaccio Del Lago, Dry Cured, Unearthed*	½ Pack/35g	41	0.5	116	26	0.5	1.4	0.5
Cheeks, Ox, Aberdeen Angus, Waitrose*	1 Serving/100g	123	4.6	123	22	0	4.6	0
Diced, Casserole, Lean, Average	1oz/28g	35	1.1	126	23	0	3.8	0
Escalope, Healthy Range, Average	1 Serving/170g	233	6.7	137	24.2	1.2	4	0.4
Flank, Pot-Roasted, Lean	1oz/28g	71	3.9	253	31.8	0	14	0
Flank, Raw, Lean	1oz/28g	49	2.6	175	22.7	0	9.3	0
Fore Rib, Lean & Fat, Average	1oz/28g	40	1.8	144	21.7	0	6.2	0.2
Fore Rib, Raw, Lean	1oz/28g	41	1.8	145	21.5	0	6.5	0
Fore Rib, Roasted, Lean	1oz/28g	66	3.2	236	33.3	0	11.4	0
Fore Rib, Roasted, Lean & Fat	1oz/28g	84	5.7	300	29.1	0	20.4	0
Grill Steak, Average	1 Steak/170g	501	39.5	295	19.3	2.1	23.2	0.1
Grill Steak, Peppered, Average	1 Serving/172g	419	24.4	244	23.6	5.2	14.2	0.3
Joint, for Roasting, Average	1oz/28g	38	1	134	24.5	1.4	3.4	0.2
Joint, Sirloin, Roasted, Lean	1oz/28g	53	1.8	188	32.4	0	6.5	0
Joint, Sirloin, Roasted, Lean & Fat	1oz/28g	65	3.5	233	29.8	0	12.6	0
Joint, with Onion Gravy, Asda*	½ Pack/215g	316	10.1	147	24	2.2	4.7	0.5
Mince, Cooked, Average	1 Serving/75g	214	15.3	286	24	0	20.3	0
Mince, Extra Lean, Raw, Average	1 Serving/100g	124	5	124	21.2	0.1	5	0
Mince, Extra Lean, Stewed	1oz/28g	50	2.4	177	24.7	0	8.7	0
Mince, Lean, Raw, Average	1oz/28g	48	2.8	172	20.8	0	10	0.1
Mince, Raw, Average	1oz/28g	68	5.1	242	19.6	0.2	18.1	0
Mince, Raw, Frozen, Average	1 Serving/100g	176	10	176	20.4	0	10	0
Mince, Steak, Extra Lean, Average	1oz/28g	37	1.6	131	20.5	0.4	5.6	0
Mince, Steak, Raw, Average	1 Serving/125g	318	25	254	17.2	0	20	0
Mince, Stewed	1oz/28g	59	3.8	209	21.8	0	13.5	0
Peppered, Sliced, Average	1 Slice/20g	26	1.1	129	18.2	1.3	5.6	1
Potted, Binghams*	1 Serving/30g	76	6.6	254	13.8	1	22	0.6
Roast, Sliced, Average	1 Slice/35g	48	1.3	136	26.1	0.4	3.6	0.2
Roast, Sliced, Garlic & Horseradish Dressing, Waitrose*	1 Pack/100g	123	2.6	123	23.2	1.7	2.6	0.5
Salt, Average	1 Serving/70g	80	1.7	114	21.7	1	2.5	0.1
Salted, Dried, Raw	1oz/28g	70	0.4	250	55.4	0	1.5	0
Silverside, Pot-Roasted, Lean	1oz/28g	54	1.8	193	34	0	6.3	0
Silverside, Pot-Roasted, Lean & Fat	1oz/28g	69	3.8	247	31	0	13.7	0
Silverside, Raw, Lean	1oz/28g	38	1.2	134	23.8	0	4.3	0
Silverside, Raw, Lean & Fat	1oz/28g	60	4.1	213	20.2	0	14.7	0
Silverside, Salted, Boiled, Lean	1oz/28g	52	1.9	184	30.4	0	6.9	0
Silverside, Salted, Raw, Lean	1oz/28g	39	2	140	19.2	0	7	0
Silverside, Salted, Raw, Lean & Fat	1oz/28g	64	5	227	16.3	0	18	0
Sliced, Cooked, From Supermarket, Average	1 Slice/35g	47	1.2	135	23.6	2	3.5	0.5
Steak, 8oz Rump & Chips	1 Serving/466g	870	41.1	187	10.7	16.2	8.8	0
Steak, Braising, Braised, Lean	1oz/28g	63	2.7	225	34.4	0	9.7	0
Steak, Braising, Lean, Raw, Average	1oz/28g	40	1.4	144	24.8	0	5	0
Steak, Braising, Raw, Lean & Fat	1oz/28g	44	2.4	158	20.5	0	8.5	0
Steak, Economy, Average	1oz/28g	53	2.4	190	26.9	1.2	8.7	0.4
Steak, Fillet, Cooked, Average	1oz/28g	54	2.4	191	28.6	0	8.5	0
Steak, Fillet, Lean, Average	1oz/28g	42	2	150	21	0	7.3	0

B

BEEF

	Measure INFO/WEIGHT	per Measure KCAL	FAT	Nutrition Values per 100g / 100ml KCAL	PROT	CARB	FAT	FIBRE
Steak, Fillet, Lean, Cooked, Average	**1oz/28g**	**52**	**2.2**	**186**	**28.6**	**0**	**8**	**0**
Steak, Flat Iron, British, Raw, Market Street, Morrisons*	½ Pack/182g	248	9.3	136	22.5	0	5.1	0
Steak, Flat Iron, Waitrose*	1 Steak/180g	358	22.5	199	20.5	0.9	12.5	0.5
Steak, Frying, Average	**1 Steak/110g**	**128**	**2.7**	**116**	**23.7**	**0**	**2.5**	**0**
Steak, Matured, Black Garlic Butter, Sainsbury's*	1 Steak/134g	219	9	163	24.3	1.2	6.7	0.5
Steak, Medallion, Extra Lean, British, Sainsbury's*	1 Steak/166g	246	4.6	148	30.5	0.5	2.8	0.5
Steak, Ranch, with Garlic Butter, Finest, Tesco*	1 Steak/136g	199	6.9	146	24	0.9	5.1	0.5
Steak, Rib Eye, Thick Cut, British, Raw, Morrisons*	1 Steak/440g	1113	87.1	253	18.8	0	19.8	0
Steak, Ribeye, As Sold, Tesco*	1 Steak/227g	575	45	253	18.8	0	19.8	0
Steak, Rump, Cooked, Average	**1oz/28g**	**69**	**4**	**246**	**29.1**	**0.5**	**14.1**	**0**
Steak, Rump, Grilled, Rare, Lean	**1 Steak/227g**	**381**	**15.6**	**168**	**26.5**	**0**	**6.9**	**0**
Steak, Rump, Lean, Cooked, Average	**1oz/28g**	**50**	**1.7**	**179**	**31**	**0**	**6.1**	**0**
Steak, Rump, Raw, Lean & Fat	**1oz/28g**	**49**	**2.8**	**174**	**20.7**	**0**	**10.1**	**0**
Steak, Rump, Raw, Lean, Average	**1 Steak/175g**	**219**	**7.2**	**125**	**22**	**0**	**4.1**	**0**
Steak, Sirloin, British, Birchwood Farm, Lidl*	1 Steak/175g	236	7.9	135	24.5	0	4.5	0
Steak, Sirloin, Fried, Rare, Lean	**1oz/28g**	**53**	**2.3**	**189**	**28.8**	**0**	**8.2**	**0**
Steak, Sirloin, Fried, Rare, Lean & Fat	**1oz/28g**	**65**	**3.9**	**231**	**26.5**	**0**	**13.9**	**0**
Steak, Sirloin, Grilled, Medium-Rare, Lean	**1oz/28g**	**49**	**2.2**	**176**	**26.6**	**0**	**7.7**	**0**
Steak, Sirloin, Grilled, Medium-Rare, Lean & Fat	**1oz/28g**	**59**	**3.5**	**211**	**24.6**	**0**	**12.5**	**0**
Steak, Sirloin, Grilled, Rare, Lean	**1oz/28g**	**46**	**1.9**	**166**	**26.4**	**0**	**6.7**	**0**
Steak, Sirloin, Grilled, Well-Done, Lean	**1oz/28g**	**63**	**2.8**	**225**	**33.9**	**0**	**9.9**	**0**
Steak, Sirloin, Grilled, Well-Done, Lean & Fat	**1oz/28g**	**71**	**4**	**254**	**31.5**	**0**	**14.3**	**0**
Steak, Sirloin, Raw, Lean & Fat	**1oz/28g**	**56**	**3.6**	**201**	**21.6**	**0**	**12.7**	**0**
Steak, Sirloin, Raw, Lean, Average	**1 Steak/150g**	**202**	**6.8**	**135**	**23.5**	**0**	**4.5**	**0**
Steak, Stewed, in Gravy, Canned, Stockwell & Co., Tesco*	½ Can/200g	234	9.6	117	14.1	4.4	4.8	0.1
Steaks, Bavette, Chimichurri, Waitrose*	1 Steak/55g	88	3.1	161	27	0.2	5.7	0.5
Steaks, British, Louisiana Inspired, BBQ, Waitrose*	1 Steak/112g	197	6.3	176	28	3.1	5.6	0.7
Steaks, Meat Free, Quorn*	1 Fillet/95g	106	4.7	112	11.7	5	4.9	5.4
Stewed Steak, Average	**1 Serving/220g**	**258**	**10.1**	**117**	**15.8**	**3.3**	**4.6**	**0**
Stewing Steak, Lean & Fat, Raw, Average	**1 Serving/100g**	**136**	**4.3**	**136**	**24.2**	**0.1**	**4.3**	**0.1**
Stewing Steak, Raw, Lean	**1oz/28g**	**34**	**1**	**122**	**22.6**	**0**	**3.5**	**0**
Stewing Steak, Stewed, Lean	**1oz/28g**	**52**	**1.8**	**185**	**32**	**0**	**6.3**	**0**
Stewing Steak, Stewed, Lean & Fat	**1oz/28g**	**57**	**2.7**	**203**	**29.2**	**0**	**9.6**	**0**
Stir Fry Strips, Raw, Average	**1 Serving/125g**	**149**	**3.8**	**119**	**23**	**0**	**3**	**0.2**
Topside, Lean & Fat, Raw, Average	**1oz/28g**	**55**	**3.6**	**198**	**20.4**	**0**	**12.9**	**0**
Topside, Raw, Lean	**1oz/28g**	**32**	**0.8**	**116**	**23**	**0**	**2.7**	**0**
Topside, Slices, Peppered, Warren & Sons, Lidl*	1 Slice/26g	34	0.8	130	23.5	2	3	0.5
Vegetarian, Slices, Peppered Style, Quorn*	¼ Pack/25g	29	0.5	115	14.5	7.6	2.1	4
Vegetarian, Steak Strips, Frozen, Quorn*	¼ Pack/75g	75	1.8	100	14.3	4.3	2.4	6
Vegetarian, Steaks, Peppered, Quorn*	1 Steak/123g	138	6	112	11.7	5	4.9	5.4
Wafer Thin Sliced, Cooked, Average	**1 Slice/10g**	**13**	**0.3**	**129**	**24.5**	**0.5**	**3.2**	**0.2**

BEEF &

Onions, Minced, Asda*	½ Can/196g	314	19.6	160	13	4.6	10	0.1
Onions, with Gravy, Minced, Lean, Sainsbury's*	1 Sm Can/198g	285	13.9	144	17	3.1	7	0.2

BEEF BOURGUIGNON

and Dauphinoise Potatoes, Charlie Bigham's*	1 Serving/426 g	562	30.2	132	8	7.9	7.1	0
Finest, Tesco*	½ Pack/300g	247	7.8	82	9.9	4.8	2.6	0.5
Slow Cooked, British, Oven Baked, Extra Special, Asda*	½ Pack/320g	505	26.5	158	17	3.1	8.3	1.2
with Garlic Mash, The Best, Morrisons*	1 Pack/336g	363	14.1	108	8.1	8.7	4.2	1.5

BEEF BRAISED

& Mash, Mini Meal, Tesco*	1 Pack/241g	251	9.2	104	6.5	10.5	3.8	1.1
Steak & Mash, Tastes of Home, M Kitchen, Morrisons*	1 Meal/250g	209	6	87	6.4	9.1	2.5	1.1
Steak, & Mash, British, Meal for One, M&S*	1 Meal/450g	369	11.2	82	6.7	7.3	2.5	1.9

	Measure INFO/WEIGHT	per Measure KCAL	FAT	Nutrition Values per 100g / 100ml KCAL	PROT	CARB	FAT	FIBRE
BEEF BRAISED								
Steak, with Root Vegetable Crush, British, COU, M&S*	1 Pack/380g	243	3.8	64	7.1	5.9	1	1.4
Tender, Pub Specials, Birds Eye*	1 Pack/450g	243	3.6	54	5.5	6.1	0.8	1.8
BEEF CRISPY CHILLI								
Cantonese, Chilled, Sainsbury's*	1 Pack/250g	682	38.8	273	11.4	22.1	15.5	1.9
Tesco*	1 Pack/250g	472	17.2	189	10.8	21	6.9	0.5
BEEF DINNER								
British Classic, Serves 1, Sainsbury's*	1 Pack/400g	500	12.4	125	8.5	14.7	3.1	2.1
Roast with Trimmings	*1 Dinner/840g*	*1310*	*63*	*156*	*6.1*	*17.7*	*7.5*	*2.3*
Roast, Homestyle, Kershaws*	1 Pack/400g	304	8	76	3.4	10.3	2	1.5
Roast, Oven Cooked, Morrisons*	1 Pack/380g	361	8.7	95	8.5	9.4	2.3	1.4
BEEF IN								
Black Bean Sauce, CBY, Asda*	1 Pack/375g	368	12.4	98	8.5	8.2	3.3	0.8
Black Bean Sauce, Chinese Takeaway, Morrisons*	½ Pack/168g	234	11.3	139	10.3	8.3	6.7	2.3
Black Bean Sauce, Chinese, Tesco*	1 Pack/400g	396	12.4	99	9.1	8.7	3.1	0.5
Black Bean Sauce, M&S*	½ Pack/175g	210	10.2	120	10.9	5.4	5.8	1.4
Black Bean with Rice, Weight Watchers*	1 Pack/320g	288	4.2	90	5	14.6	1.3	0.1
Black Bean, Chinese Favourites Box, M&S*	½ Pack/120g	152	8.3	127	7.8	7.6	6.9	1.4
Gravy, Ale, Rich, Slow Cooked Brisket, COU, M&S*	1 Pack/350g	242	6.7	69	8.4	3.7	1.9	1.6
Gravy, Roast, Birds Eye*	1 Pack/227g	177	3.9	78	13.4	2.2	1.7	0
Gravy, Traditional, Morrisons*	1 Pack/286g	366	10	128	17.9	6	3.5	0.5
in Black Bean Sauce, Inspired Cuisine, Aldi*	1 Serving/400g	555	20	139	5	17.2	5	2.8
Steak, & Ale, with Cheesy Mash, Morrisons*	1 Pack/385g	393	13.1	102	7.4	10	3.4	0.8
BEEF RAGU								
with Rigatoni Pasta, Chianti, BFY, M&S*	1 Pack/400g	484	12.4	121	10.3	12.1	3.1	1.5
BEEF WELLINGTON								
Average	*1 Serving/200g*	*530*	*33.3*	*265*	*12.4*	*17*	*16.6*	*1*
Extra Special, Asda*	1 Serving/218g	605	37.1	277	11	20	17	0.9
Fillet, Easy to Cook, Waitrose*	1 Wellington/180g	490	26.8	272	14.5	19.3	14.9	1.4
BEEF WITH								
Black Bean Sauce, Chilli, Sainsbury's*	1 Pack/300g	336	14.4	112	8.7	8.6	4.8	1
Onion, & Gravy, Minced, Princes*	1 Serving/200g	342	24.4	171	9.9	5.5	12.2	0
Oyster Sauce, Ooodles of Noodles, Oriental Express*	1 Pack/425g	378	5.5	89	4.9	14.2	1.3	1.5
Peppercorn Sauce, Steak, Just Cook, Sainsbury's*	½ Pack/128g	174	7.3	136	17.7	3.4	5.7	1.2
Peppercorn Sauce, Steak, Rump, M&S*	½ Pack/213g	281	8.7	132	19.4	4.2	4.1	0.1
Peppercorn Sauce, Steak, Rump, Waitrose*	½ Pack/180g	189	5.9	105	17.9	0.9	3.3	0.2
Vegetables, & Gravy, Minced, Birds Eye*	1 Pack/178g	155	6.1	87	9.1	5.1	3.4	0.6
BEER								
Ale, 1698, Kentish Strong, Shepherd Neame*	1 Bottle/500ml	285	0	57	0.4	4.8	0	0
Ale, Alcohol Free, Without, St Peter's*	1 Bottle/500ml	135	0.5	27	0.2	6.4	0.1	0
Ale, American Pale, Low Tide, 0.5%, Shipyard*	1 Bottle/500ml	85	0	17	0.3	3.2	0	0
Ale, Bottled, Old Speckled Hen*	1 Bottle/330ml	124	0.3	38	0.2	1.8	0.1	0.2
Ale, Goliath, Wychwood, Marstons PLC*	1 Bottle/500ml	191	0	38	0.4	2.8	0	0
Ale, Honey Dew, Fullers*	1 Bottle/500ml	232	0	46	0	4.6	0	0
Ale, Hopped Bourbon, Cask, Innis & Gunn*	1 Bottle/330ml	201	0	61	0.3	4.9	0	0
Ale, Hopping Hare, Hall & Woodhouse Ltd*	1 Bottle/500ml	189	0	38	0.4	3	0	0
Ale, IPA, Punk AF, Alcohol Free, Brewdog *	1 Can/330ml	50	0	15	0	3	0	0
Ale, Low Alcohol, Nanny State, BrewDog*	1 Bottle/330ml	20	0.3	6	0.1	1	0.1	0
Ale, Low Alcohol, Old Speckled Hen*	1 Bottle/500ml	110	0.5	22	0.4	4.1	0.1	0
Ale, Old Peculiar, Theakstons*	1 Serving/500ml	250	0	50	0	4.6	0	0
Ale, Old Speckled Hen*	1 Pint/568ml	185	0.6	32	0.2	1.6	0.1	0.2
Ale, Pale, Alcohol Free, Innis & Gunn*	1 Can/330ml	66	0	20	0.5	4.7	0	0
Ale, Pale, Big Easy, Low Alcohol, Thornbridge*	1 Bottle/330ml	63	0.3	19	0.1	3.6	0.1	0
Ale, Pale, IPA, Greene King*	1 Pint/568ml	157	0.1	28	0.2	1.6	0	0.1

B

BEER

INFO/WEIGHT	Measure per Measure		Nutrition Values per 100g / 100ml				
	KCAL	FAT	KCAL	PROT	CARB	FAT	FIBRE
Ale, Pale, IPA, Innis & Gunn*	1 Bottle/330ml	162	0	49	0.3	4.6	0	0
Ale, Pale, IPA, TTD, Sainsbury's*	½ Bottle/250ml	128	0	51	0.5	4.4	0	0.5
Ale, Pale, Sierra Nevada*	1 Bottle/350g	175	0	50	0.4	4	0	0
Ale, Wychcraft, Wychwood, Marstons PLC*	1 Bottle/500ml	210	0	42	0.3	4.2	0	0
Argus, Lidl*	1 Bottle/250ml	200	0	80	0	0	0	0
Becks Blue Lemon, No Alcohol, Beck & Co*	1 Bottle/1196ml	275	0.1	23	0.2	6	0	0
Bitter, Average	*1 Can/440ml*	*141*	*0*	*32*	*0.3*	*2.3*	*0*	*0*
Bitter, Banks, Marstons PLC*	1 Pint/568ml	193	0.1	34	0.3	3.4	0	0
Bitter, Cask, Draught, London Pride, Fullers*	1 Pint/568ml	201	0	35	0	0	0	0
Bitter, Draught, Average	*1 Pint/568ml*	*182*	*0*	*32*	*0.3*	*2.3*	*0*	*0*
Bitter, Keg, Average	*1 Pint/568ml*	*176*	*0*	*31*	*0.3*	*2.3*	*0*	*0*
Bitter, Low Alcohol, Average	*1 Pint/568ml*	*74*	*0*	*13*	*0.2*	*2.1*	*0*	*0*
Bitter, Original, Tetley's*	1 Can/440ml	140	0	32	0.2	4.6	0	0
Bitter, Oxford Gold, Brakspear*	1 Bottle/500ml	161	0	32	0	0	0	0
Bitter, Savers, Morrisons*	1 Can/440ml	75	0	17	0	0	0	0
Bitter, Strong, Broadside, Adnams*	1 Bottle/500ml	285	0	57	0	0	0	0
Brown Ale, Bottled, Average	*1 Bottle/330ml*	*99*	*0*	*30*	*0.3*	*3*	*0*	*0*
Brune, Leffe*	1 Bottle/330ml	184	0	56	0.5	11.3	0	0
Craft, 3.5% ABV, (Calculated Estimate)	*1 Bottle/330ml*	*102*	*0*	*31*	*0*	*0*	*0*	*0*
Craft, 4% ABV, (Calculated Estimate)	*1 Bottle/330ml*	*116*	*0*	*35*	*0*	*0*	*0*	*0*
Craft, 4.5% ABV, (Calculated Estimate)	*1 Bottle/330ml*	*132*	*0*	*40*	*0*	*0*	*0*	*0*
Craft, 5% ABV, (Calculated Estimate)	*1 Bottle/330ml*	*146*	*0*	*44*	*0*	*0*	*0*	*0*
Craft, 5.5% ABV, (Calculated Estimate)	*1 Bottle/330ml*	*160*	*0*	*49*	*0*	*0*	*0*	*0*
Craft, 6% ABV, (Calculated Estimate)	*1 Bottle/330ml*	*175*	*0*	*53*	*0*	*0*	*0*	*0*
Craft, 6.5% ABV, (Calculated Estimate)	*1 Bottle/330ml*	*189*	*0*	*57*	*0*	*0*	*0*	*0*
Craft, 7% ABV, (Calculated Estimate)	*1 Bottle/330ml*	*204*	*0*	*62*	*0*	*0*	*0*	*0*
Craft, 7.5% ABV, (Calculated Estimate)	*1 Bottle/330ml*	*218*	*0*	*66*	*0*	*0*	*0*	*0*
Craft, 8% ABV, (Calculated Estimate)	*1 Bottle/330ml*	*233*	*0*	*71*	*0*	*0*	*0*	*0*
Craft, 8.5% ABV, (Calculated Estimate)	*1 Bottle/330ml*	*248*	*0*	*75*	*0*	*0*	*0*	*0*
Especial, Modelo*	1 Bottle/355ml	145	0	41	0	1.1	0	0
Guinness* Extra Stout, Bottled	1 Bottle/500ml	215	0	43	4	0	0	0
Guinness, Draught*	*1 Can/440ml*	*158*	*0.2*	*36*	*0.3*	*3*	*0*	*0*
Guinness, Stout*	*1 Pint/568ml*	*205*	*0*	*36*	*0.3*	*3*	*0*	*0*
Kilkenny, Diageo*	1 Pint/568ml	210	0	37	0.3	3	0	0
Light, Superior, Ultra, Michelob*	1 Bottle/330ml	73	0	22	0.2	0.6	0	0
Low Calorie, Low Carb, Cobra*	1 Bottle/330ml	96	0	29	0.1	1.3	0	0
Mackeson, Stout	*1 Pint/568ml*	*205*	*0*	*36*	*0.4*	*4.6*	*0*	*0*
Mild, Draught, Average	*1 Pint/568ml*	*136*	*0*	*24*	*0.2*	*1.6*	*0*	*0*
Non Alcoholic, Zero, Cobra*	1 Bottle/330ml	79	0	24	0.8	2	0	0
Oak Aged, Original, Innis & Gunn*	1 Bottle/330ml	182	0	55	0.3	4.7	0	0
Pale Ale, Dead Pony Club, Brewdog *	1 Bottle/330ml	116	0	35	0	0	0	0
Peroni, Libera, Non-Alcholic, Miller Brewing Company*	1 Bottle/330ml	73	0	22	0.2	5.3	0	0
Prohibition Brew, Alcohol Free, Budweiser *	1 Can/330ml	112	0	34	0.2	8	0	0
Raspberry, Framboise, Lindemans*	1 Serving/355ml	185	0	52	0	8.8	0	0
Rum Finish, Oak Aged, Innis & Gunn*	1 Bottle/330ml	188	0	57	0.3	4.8	0	0
Stout, Coopers*	1 Pint/375ml	191	0	51	0	2.9	0	0
Stout, Dark Matters, Aldi*	1 Bottle/328ml	128	0	39	0	0	0	0
Weissbier, Alcohol Free, Erdinger*	1 Bottle/500ml	125	0	25	0.4	5.3	0	0
Weissbier, Hefe, Franziskaner*	1 Bottle/500ml	225	0	45	0	0	0	0
Weissbier, Non Alcoholic, Franziskaner*	1 Bottle/500ml	105	0.5	21	0.6	4.4	0.1	0
Wheat, Tesco*	1 Bottle/500ml	155	0	31	0.5	0.4	0	0
Zero, Alcohol Free, Birra Moretti*	1 Bottle/330ml	66	0	20	0.5	4.4	0	0

	Measure INFO/WEIGHT	per Measure KCAL	FAT	Nutrition Values per 100g / 100ml KCAL	PROT	CARB	FAT	FIBRE
BEETROOT								
& Feta, Protein Pot, Aldi*	1 Pack/140g	151	8	108	4.3	8.7	5.7	2.6
Baby, Horseradish, & Black Pepper, Finest, Tesco*	4 Beetroot/80g	77	0.3	96	2.3	18.5	0.4	4.4
Baby, Pickled, Average	*1 Beetroot/12g*	*5*	*0*	*37*	*1.7*	*7.2*	*0.1*	*1.2*
Cooked, Boiled, Drained, Average	*1 Serving/100g*	*44*	*0.2*	*44*	*1.7*	*10*	*0.2*	*2*
Grated, Tesco*	1 Serving/80g	34	0.1	42	1.7	7.2	0.1	2.8
Grated, with Horseradish, Smak*	1 Tbsp/15g	9	0.1	59	1.6	12	0.5	0
Juniper & Black Pepper, Finest, Tesco*	1 Beetroot/20g	15	0	75	1.8	16.8	0.1	0
Pickled, in Balsamic Vinaigrette, M&S*	½ Pack/125g	89	1.5	71	1.6	12.4	1.2	2.2
Pickled, in Sweet Vinegar, Average	*1oz/28g*	*16*	*0*	*57*	*1.2*	*12.8*	*0.1*	*1.5*
Pickled, in Vinegar, Average	*1 Serving/50g*	*18*	*0*	*36*	*1.6*	*7.3*	*0.1*	*1.2*
Raw, Unprepared, Average	*1oz/28g*	*8*	*0*	*29*	*1.4*	*5.4*	*0.1*	*1.7*
Rosebud, M&S*	½ Pack/90g	45	0.3	50	1.9	8.9	0.3	3.2
Rosebud, Sweet Chilli Marinated, M&S*	1 Serving/80g	52	0.2	65	1.5	12.3	0.3	3.6
Steamed, Love Beets*	1 Beetroot/30g	12	0	41	1.5	7.2	0.1	2.9
with Balsamic Vinaigrette, Side Salad, M&S*	1 Pack/225g	146	2.9	65	0.7	12.4	1.3	2.2
BERRIES								
Medley, Grapes, Strawberry, Blueberry, Blackberry, Tesco*	1/2 Pack/120g	67	0.2	56	0.6	12.2	0.2	1
Mix, Naturally Wonky, Frozen, Morrisons*	1 Serving/80g	23	0.2	29	0.9	5.6	0.3	0.3
Mixed, Fresh, Average	*1 Serving/80g*	*29*	*0.2*	*37*	*0.9*	*8.3*	*0.2*	*3.4*
Mixed, Lidl*	1 Serving/85g	47	0.2	55	0.9	6.9	0.2	0
Mixed, Strawberries, Raspberries & Blueberries, Tesco*	½ Pack/150g	102	0.4	68	0.7	14.5	0.3	2.4
Mixed, Summer Fruits, Frozen, Tesco*	1 Serving/80g	30	0.2	37	1.1	6.2	0.2	3.2
Summer, Mixed, Frozen, Farmfoods*	1 Avg Serving/80g	37	0	46	0.9	7.6	0	0
Very Berry, Luxury, Mix, Holland & Barrett*	1 Serving20g	44	0.1	222	1.3	60	0.5	2.5
BHAJI								
Aubergine, & Potato, Fried in Vegetable Oil, Average	*1oz/28g*	*36*	*2.5*	*130*	*2*	*12*	*8.8*	*1.7*
Cabbage, & Pea, Fried in Vegetable Oil, Average	*1oz/28g*	*50*	*4.1*	*178*	*3.3*	*9.2*	*14.7*	*3.4*
Cauliflower, Fried in Vegetable Oil, Average	*1oz/28g*	*60*	*5.7*	*214*	*4*	*4*	*20.5*	*2*
Indian Snack Selection, Chef Select, Lidl*	1 Serving/50g	125	7.2	250	5.6	22.1	14.3	5.3
Mushroom, Fried in Vegetable Oil, Average	*1oz/28g*	*46*	*4.5*	*166*	*1.7*	*4.4*	*16.1*	*1.3*
Okra, Bangladeshi, Fried in Butter Ghee, Average	*1oz/28g*	*27*	*1.8*	*95*	*2.5*	*7.6*	*6.4*	*3.2*
Onion, Fried in Vegetable Oil, Takeaway, Average	*1 Bhaji/70g*	*190*	*10.3*	*270*	*9.8*	*24.6*	*14.7*	*5.6*
Onion, Frozen, Tesco*	1 Bhaji/14g	28	1.4	203	6.3	20.1	9.8	4.5
Onion, Indian Starter Selection, M&S*	1 Bhaji/22g	57	3.7	260	5.7	19.3	17	3.5
Onion, Indian, Mini, Asda*	1 Bhaji/18g	33	1.8	186	4.9	19	10	6
Onion, M&S*	1 Bhaji/42g	100	5.3	237	5.1	24	12.6	3.5
Onion, Tesco*	1 Bhaji/47g	85	4.9	181	5.7	16.2	10.4	4.3
Potato, & Onion, Fried in Vegetable Oil, Average	*1oz/28g*	*45*	*2.8*	*160*	*2.1*	*16.6*	*10.1*	*1.6*
Potato, Onion & Mushroom, Fried, Average	*1oz/28g*	*58*	*4.9*	*208*	*2*	*12*	*17.5*	*1.5*
Potato, Spinach & Cauliflower, Fried, Average	*1oz/28g*	*47*	*4.2*	*169*	*2.2*	*7.1*	*15.1*	*1.4*
Spinach, & Potato, Fried in Vegetable Oil, Average	*1oz/28g*	*53*	*3.9*	*191*	*3.7*	*13.4*	*14.1*	*2.3*
Spinach, Fried in Vegetable Oil, Average	*1oz/28g*	*23*	*1.9*	*83*	*3.3*	*2.6*	*6.8*	*2.4*
Sweet Potato, & Spinach, Indian, Waitrose*	1 Bhaji/37g	91	2.9	247	3.5	37.8	8	4.7
Vegetable, Fried in Vegetable Oil, Average	*1oz/28g*	*59*	*5.2*	*212*	*2.1*	*10.1*	*18.5*	*2.4*
BHUNA								
Chicken, Curry, Tesco*	1 Serving/300g	396	22.8	132	11.4	4.5	7.6	0.5
Chicken, Indian Takeaway, Tesco*	1 Pack/350g	438	27.6	125	8.3	4.6	7.9	2.2
Chicken, Tikka, Tesco*	1 Pack/350g	438	23.4	125	11.3	5	6.7	0.9
Chicken, with Rice, Ready Meal, Average	*1 Pack/350g*	*444*	*20.8*	*127*	*9.4*	*8.9*	*5.9*	*1.4*
Lamb, 405, Oakhouse Foods Ltd*	1 Meal/400g	412	14	103	4.8	13	3.5	0.8
Prawn, King, M&S*	1 Pack/400g	308	15.2	77	6.7	3.3	3.8	1.5
Prawn, King, Morrisons*	1 Pack/350g	301	20.6	86	6.5	1.8	5.9	0.5

	Measure INFO/WEIGHT	per Measure KCAL	per Measure FAT	Nutrition Values per 100g / 100ml KCAL	PROT	CARB	FAT	FIBRE
BILBERRIES								
Fresh, Raw	*1oz/28g*	*8*	*0.1*	*29*	*0.6*	*6.8*	*0.2*	*1.8*
BILTONG								
Average	*1 Serving/25g*	*64*	*1*	*256*	*50*	*0*	*4*	*0*
BIRYANI								
Chicken, Aromatic, BGTY, Sainsbury's*	1 Pack/385g	397	8.5	103	6.8	12.5	2.2	3.5
Chicken, Indian, Asda*	1 Pack/450g	778	22.5	173	9	23	5	0.7
Chicken, LC, Tesco*	1 Serving/450g	495	10.3	110	7	15	2.3	3.4
Chicken, Ready Meal, Average	*1 Pack/400g*	*521*	*17.1*	*130*	*7.5*	*15.2*	*4.3*	*1.6*
Chicken, Tikka, Ready Meal, Average	*1 Pack/400g*	*460*	*11.5*	*115*	*7.3*	*14.8*	*2.9*	*1.5*
Chicken, Vegetarian, Linda McCartney*	½ Pack/180g	300	11.7	167	8.6	17	6.5	3.3
Jackfruit, Vegetarian, Waitrose*	1 Pack/375g	386	14.2	103	2.1	12.8	3.8	4.6
Lamb, Average	*1 Serving/200g*	*390*	*19.4*	*195*	*7.3*	*20.9*	*9.7*	*0*
Lamb, Bangladeshi, Hello Fresh*	1 Serving/528g	554	16	105	6.2	13.1	3	0
Lamb, HL, Tesco*	1 Pack/400g	560	17.6	140	5.1	19	4.4	3.1
Vegetable, HL, Tesco*	1 Pack/450g	454	9.4	101	2.7	17.9	2.1	1.6
Vegetable, Waitrose*	1 Pack/450g	521	19.8	116	2.4	14.9	4.4	3.6
Vegetarian, Chicken Style, Lunch Pot, Quorn*	1 Pot/300g	300	13	100	3.5	10.9	4.4	1.7
BISCUITS								
Breakfast, Fruit & Seed, Weight Watchers *	2 Biscuits/36g	159	5.4	442	8	64.7	15.1	7.9
Abbey Crunch, McVitie's*	1 Biscuit/9g	43	1.6	477	6	72.8	17.9	2.5
Abernethy, Simmers*	1 Biscuit/12g	61	2.7	490	5.7	69.2	21.9	0
Ace Milk Chocolate, McVitie's*	1 Biscuit/24g	122	5.9	510	6.1	66.2	24.5	1.6
All Butter, M&S*	1 Biscuit/8g	42	2.1	505	5.8	63.1	25	2.2
Almond & Chocolate, Biscotti, TTD, Sainsbury's*	1 Biscuit/30g	132	4.8	440	8.4	65.6	16	3.1
Almond, Thins, TTD, Sainsbury's*	1 Biscuit/4g	16	0.5	450	6.7	72.8	14.7	3.1
Amaretti, Average	*1 Biscuit/5g*	*22*	*0.8*	*434*	*8.1*	*66.4*	*15.4*	*2.8*
Amaretti, Doria*	1 Biscuit/4g	17	0.3	433	6	84.8	7.8	0
Amaretti, M&S*	1 Biscuit/6g	30	1.1	480	9.6	71.3	17.2	3.8
Anzac, Bitesmart*	1 Biscuit/20g	84	4.6	420	5.1	46.8	23	0
Apple & Cinnamon Thins, Finest, Tesco*	1 Biscuit/5g	22	0.8	470	5.9	71.7	17.5	1.5
Apple Crumble, Officially Low Fat, Fox's*	1 Biscuit/23g	85	0.6	365	5.4	80.4	2.4	2.5
Arrowroot, Thin, Crawfords*	1 Biscuit/7g	35	1.2	450	6.9	71.4	15.2	2.8
Baked Bites, Cheddar, Mini, Cathedral City*	1 Pack/22g	115	6.4	521	12.2	51.4	29.2	2.6
Bars, Disco Bits, Oki Doki*	1 Bar/27g	121	5	449	4.9	65.6	18.4	0
Belgian Chocolate Chip, Walkers Shortbread Ltd*	2 Biscuits/25g	124	6.1	494	5.1	63.3	24.5	2.2
Belgian Chocolate, Selection, Finest, Tesco*	1 Biscuit/10g	52	2.7	515	6	62	27	3
Belgian Milk Chocolate, M&S*	1 Biscuit/12g	60	2.5	490	6.2	70.1	20.3	2.5
Billionaire, Salted Caramel, Squares, Moments, McVitie's*	1 Square/41g	194	10.4	473	3.8	56.6	25.4	1.3
Biscotti, Chocolate Chip, Kate's Cakes Ltd*	1 Biscotti/36g	134	4.6	372	6.5	57.9	12.7	2.7
Biscotti, Chocolate, Heinz*	1 Biscuit/20g	80	1.7	398	8.5	72	8.7	5.8
Bourbon Creams, Asda*	1 Biscuit/14g	68	2.9	487	6.3	66	21	2.8
Bourbon Creams, Sainsbury's*	1 Biscuit/13g	60	2.4	476	5.7	70.4	19.1	1.7
Bourbon Creams, Tesco*	1 Biscuit/14g	66	2.9	486	5.6	66.2	21.4	3.4
Bourbon Creams, Value, Multipack, Tesco*	1 Biscuit/13g	62	2.9	494	5.9	68	22.8	1.7
Bourbon, Average	*1 Biscuit/13g*	*63*	*2.8*	*488*	*5.7*	*68.2*	*21.3*	*2.1*
Brandy Snap, Askeys*	1 Basket/20g	98	4.3	490	1.9	72.7	21.3	0
Brandy Snaps, Average	*1 Biscuit/15g*	*69*	*2.2*	*460*	*2.7*	*79.8*	*14.4*	*0.5*
Brazil Nut, Chocolate, Ringtons*	1 Biscuit/25g	137	8.6	547	6.2	53.2	34.4	1.7
Breakfast, Blueberries, Soft Bakes, Belvita*	1 Biscuit/50g	194	6	388	5.5	63	12	7.5
Breakfast, Blueberry Flaxseeds, Seeds & Berries, Belvita*	1 Biscuit/15g	66	2.1	441	8.4	66	14	7
Breakfast, Choc Chips, Crunchy, Belvita*	1 Pack/50g	208	6	415	8	63	12	12
Breakfast, Choc Chips, Soft Bakes, Belvita*	1 Pack/50g	202	7.5	405	5.7	61	15	6.9
Breakfast, Choco Hazelnut, Tops, Belvita*	1 Pack/50g	230	8	460	7.2	69	16	4.9

BISCUITS

	Measure INFO/WEIGHT	per Measure KCAL	FAT	Nutrition Values per 100g / 100ml KCAL	PROT	CARB	FAT	FIBRE
Breakfast, Chocolate Chip, Bakes, Genius*	1 Bake/28g	142	7.9	507	5.2	56	28.3	4
Breakfast, Cocoa, Chocolate Chip, Belvita*	1 Pack/50g	220	7.5	440	7.8	66	15	7.1
Breakfast, Cranberry & Orange, High in Fibre, M&S*	2 Biscuits/30g	142	6.9	473	6.6	54.9	23	10
Breakfast, Golden Grain, Soft Bakes, Belvita*	1 Pack/50g	192	6	385	5.9	63	12	6.7
Breakfast, Golden Oats, Belvita*	1 Pack/50g	220	7.5	440	7.7	67	15	5.7
Breakfast, Hazlenuts, Crunchy, Belvita*	1 Pack/50g	210	6	420	8.7	63	12	12
Breakfast, Honey & Nuts, Belvita*	1 Pack/50g	228	7.5	455	7.6	69	15	4.4
Breakfast, Honey & Oat, Eat Well, M&S*	2 Biscuits/20g	88	3	442	9	65.6	15	4.3
Breakfast, Milk & Cereals, Belvita*	1 Pack/50g	220	7.2	440	7.9	67	14.5	6.5
Breakfast, Oat, Golden, Asda*	1 Pack/45g	210	9	467	6	64	20	5.1
Breakfast, Original, All Bran, Kellogg's*	1 Pack/40g	176	8	440	8	49	20	16
Breakfast, Porridge Oats, Raspberry & Yoghurt, Mcvities*	2 Biscuits/51g	248	10.8	487	9.1	63.5	21.1	3.2
Breakfast, Porridge Oats, Red Berries , McVitie's*	4 Biscuits/50g	226	6.9	452	9.6	71	13.8	5.1
Breakfast, Red Berries, Soft Bakes, Belvita*	1 Pack/50g	190	5.5	380	5.5	65	11	6.6
Butter, Chocolate Brownie, Farmhouse Biscuits*	1 Biscuit/17g	88	5.1	528	5.3	56.1	30.6	0
Butter, Dark Chocolate, Momento, Aldi*	1 Biscuit/14g	69	3.2	491	6.2	63.5	22.6	4.2
Butter, Dark Chocolate, Tesco*	1 Biscuit/14g	72	3.7	511	6.9	58.3	26.7	4.9
Butter, Milk Chocolate, Belmont Biscuit Co, Aldi*	1 Biscuit/14g	69	3.2	492	7.3	63	23	2.8
Butter, Milk Chocolate, Ritter Sport*	1 Biscuit/25g	139	8.5	555	6.1	55	34	0
Butter, Milk Chocolate, Tesco*	1 Biscuit/14g	71	3.6	508	7.8	61	25.4	2.2
Butter, Salted Caramel, & Choc Chip, Farmhouse Biscuits*	1 Biscuit/15g	74	3.8	495	4.4	60.7	25.6	0
Cafe Noir, with Coffee Flavour Icing, McVitie's*	1 Biscuit/6g	27	0.8	458	4.9	76	14	1.7
Cantucci, with Honey, Loyd Grossman*	1 Biscuit/7g	32	1.1	450	9.5	66.3	16.3	0.9
Cantuccini, Sainsbury's*	1 Biscotti/8g	35	1.3	440	10.4	63.1	16.2	4.4
Cantuccini, with Almonds, Average	**1 Biscotti/30g**	**130**	**5**	**433**	**10**	**60**	**16.7**	**3.3**
Caramel Squares, Thorntons*	2 Biscuits/32g	150	6.4	470	6.2	65	20	2.4
Caramelised, Biscoff, Lotus*	1 Biscuit/8g	38	1.5	484	4.9	72.7	19	1.3
Chcoolate Coated, GF, Chocoful, Prewett's*	1 Bar/20g	100	4.8	502	7.3	63.2	24	0
Chcoolate, Milk, Special Assortment, Tesco*	1 Biscuit/17g	89	4.6	521	5.6	62.9	27	1.8
Cheese Melts, Carr's*	1 Biscuit/4g	21	1	493	10.8	59.6	22.9	2.5
Cheese Sandwich, Ritz*	1 Biscuit/9g	50	2.8	530	9.5	55	30.2	2
Cheese Savouries, Sainsbury's*	1 Serving/30g	159	9.4	531	11.3	50	31.3	2.1
Cheese, & Chutney, Delicious, Boots*	1 Pack/134g	290	14.7	217	9	19	11	2.3
Cheese, Baked, Cheddars, Jacob's*	1 Cheddar/4g	20	1.2	525	10.8	47	31.8	2.9
Cherry Bakewell, Handfinished, M&S*	1 Biscuit/40g	200	9.7	495	5.9	62.1	24	0.5
Choc Chip, Paterson's*	1 Biscuit/17g	79	3.6	474	5.6	64	21.6	3.1
Choco Leibniz, Dark Chocolate, Bahlsen*	1 Biscuit/14g	69	3.6	493	6.8	59	26	5.1
Choco Leibniz, Milk, Bahlsen*	1 Biscuit/14g	71	3.5	505	7.5	61	25	2.4
Choco Leibniz, Orange Flavour, Bahlsen*	1 Biscuit/14g	70	3.7	504	7.9	58.5	26.4	0
Choco Leibniz, White, Bahlsen *	2 Biscuits/28g	142	7	508	5.1	65	25	0
Chocoful, Caramel, GF, Prewetts*	1 Bar/20g	97	4.3	485	6.5	64.5	21.5	3
Chocolate & Coconut, Duchy Originals*	1 Biscuit/13g	68	4.3	543	6.3	52.1	34.4	2.6
Chocolate Chip & Peanut, Trufree*	1 Biscuit/11g	55	2.6	496	4	66	24	2
Chocolate Chip GI, Diet Chef Ltd*	1 Pack/20g	90	3.6	450	7.4	64.4	17.9	6.4
Chocolate Fingers, Milk, Cadbury*	1 Biscuit/6g	31	1.6	515	6.8	60.8	27.1	1.7
Chocolate Fingers, Salted Peanut Crunch, Cadbury*	4 Fingers/21g	100	5.5	478	6.6	52.9	26.5	1.4
Chocolate Florentine, M&S*	1 Serving/39g	195	9.7	500	7.4	64.5	24.9	1.7
Chocolate Ginger, Organic, Duchy Originals*	1 Biscuit/12g	64	3.6	518	4.6	59.7	29	2.1
Chocolate Ginger, Thorntons*	1 Biscuit/19g	96	5.3	512	5.9	58.2	28.4	0
Chocolate Kimberley, Jacob's*	1 Biscuit/20g	86	3.4	428	3.9	64.4	17.2	1.1
Chocolate Sandwich Finger, M&S*	1 Biscuit/31g	161	8.8	520	6.2	58.2	28.4	3.2
Chocolate Viennese, Fox's*	1 Biscuit/16g	85	4.9	530	6.7	56.6	30.7	1.7
Chocolate, Breakaway, Nestle*	1 Bar/19g	99	4.9	511	6.1	63.5	25.2	3

BISCUITS

INFO/WEIGHT	Measure	per Measure KCAL	FAT	Nutrition Values per 100g / 100ml KCAL	PROT	CARB	FAT	FIBRE
Chocolate, Fingers, Average	*1 Biscuit/6g*	*31*	*1.6*	*514*	*6.7*	*61.4*	*26.8*	*1.5*
Chocolate, Golden Crunch, Free From Milk, Tesco*	1 Biscuit/17g	85	4.9	510	4.2	57.2	29.4	4.6
Chocolate, Milk, Nobbles, Schar*	1 Biscuit/13g	67	3.8	517	6	56	29	4
Chocolate, Milk, Take Away, Belmont Biscuit Co, Aldi*	1 Biscuit/28g	136	5.9	487	8	65	21	2.5
Chocolate, O's, GF, Schar*	1 Biscuit/10g	51	2.5	499	6.6	62	24	4.1
Chocolate, O's, Mini, GF, Schar*	1 Biscuit/11g	55	2.6	508	5.8	66	24	2.5
Chocolate, Stencil, Gail's*	100g	402	18	402	6.5	52	18	3.8
Classic, Milk Chocolate, Fox's*	1 Biscuit/13g	67	3.1	517	6.1	64.9	24	1.6
Cocoa Cream, Lidl*	1 Biscuit/25g	117	4.5	468	6	69	18	3
Coconut, Ring, Average	*1 Biscuit/9g*	*44*	*2*	*490*	*6.1*	*67.4*	*21.8*	*2.6*
Coffee, GF, Barkat*	2 Biscuits/15g	72	2.8	479	2	75	19	0
Cookies 'n Cream, Eat Me, Aldi*	1 Biscuit/12g	58	2.1	467	5.4	72	17	2.9
Cornish Fairings, Original, Furniss Of Cornwall*	1 Biscuit/17g	75	2.5	448	5.1	72.9	15.1	0
Cranberry & Pumpkin Seed, BGTY, Sainsbury's*	1 Biscuit/17g	68	2.8	410	7.2	56.6	17.1	13.9
Crispy Fruit Slices, Apple, Sultana, Go Ahead, McVitie's*	1 Slice/13g	50	0.9	388	5.4	74	7.1	2.9
Crispy Fruit Slices, Forest Fruit, Go Ahead, McVitie's*	1 Biscuit/13g	49	0.9	380	5.4	73.7	7	3
Crispy Slices, Raspberry, Go Ahead, McVitie's*	1 Slice/13g	50	0.9	385	5.3	74	7	2.8
Crunch Creams, Double Choc, Fox's*	1 Biscuit/15g	77	3.8	511	4.7	65	25	2.7
Crunchers, Salted, Savoury, Crackers, Sainsbury's*	1 Cracker/5g	22	1	448	6.1	59.4	20.4	1.4
Crunchie, Cadbury*	1 Biscuit/13g	64	3.1	495	4.8	65.7	23.6	0.9
Crunchy Caramel, Tesco*	1 Bar/21g	98	5.2	467	4.6	56	25	1.4
Custard Cream, Gluten & Wheat Free, Lovemore*	1 Biscuit/15g	71	2.5	475	0	33	16.8	0
Custard Creams, Asda*	1 Biscuit/12g	59	2.7	495	5	67	23	2
Custard Creams, Crawfords*	1 Biscuit/11g	57	2.7	517	5.9	69.2	24.1	1.5
Custard Creams, Everyday Value, Tesco*	1 Biscuit/13g	62	2.6	495	5.6	69.7	20.9	1.7
Custard Creams, M&S*	1 Biscuit/13g	63	2.8	494	5.5	67.2	22	2.4
Custard Creams, Sainsbury's*	1 Biscuit/13g	67	3	514	5.5	70.4	23.4	1.6
Custard Creams, Tesco*	1 Biscuit/12g	58	2.4	490	5.7	70.1	20.5	1.1
Custard Creams, Trufree*	1 Biscuit/12g	60	2.8	504	8.7	65	23	1
Dark Chocolate Ginger, M&S*	1 Biscuit/21g	105	5.7	505	5	58.8	27.6	4.2
Dark Chocolate Gingers, Border*	1 Biscuit/17g	74	3.4	445	4.4	61.4	20.1	2.9
Diet Fibre, Gullon*	2 Biscuits/16g	65	2.6	405	6.5	48.7	16.4	23
Digestive with Wheatgerm, Hovis*	1 Biscuit/12g	57	2.4	475	8.3	65	20	3.3
Digestive, Caramels, Milk Chocolate, McVitie's*	1 Biscuit/17g	81	3.7	478	5.6	65.1	21.7	2.3
Digestive, Chocolate	*1 Biscuit/17g*	*84*	*4.1*	*493*	*6.8*	*66.5*	*24.1*	*2.2*
Digestive, Chocolate Chip, Asda*	1 Biscuit/14g	68	3.2	491	6	65	23	2.9
Digestive, Chocolate, Free From, Co-Op*	1 Biscuit/11g	54	2.3	495	6.3	69	21	2.9
Digestive, Chocolate, GF, Just Free, Lidl*	1 Biscuit/13g	64	2.8	482	6.3	66	20.8	3.2
Digestive, Chocolate, Milk, Ms Mollys*	1 Biscuit/17g	83	3.7	490	7	64.6	21.9	3.2
Digestive, Cracker Selection, Tesco*	1 Biscuit/12g	56	2.3	464	7.1	65.2	19.4	4.3
Digestive, Crawfords*	1 Biscuit/12g	58	2.4	484	7.1	68.8	20	3.4
Digestive, Dark Chocolate, McVitie's*	1 Biscuit/17g	83	4.1	495	6	60.8	24.2	4.2
Digestive, Dark Chocolate, Thins, McVitie's*	1 Biscuit/6g	31	1.5	499	6	60.9	24.7	4.7
Digestive, Everyday Value, Tesco*	1 Biscuit/16g	80	3.4	490	6.7	66.5	21	3
Digestive, GF, Schar*	1 Biscuit/10g	48	2.2	483	6.1	62	22	6.2
Digestive, Gluten & Wheat Free, Lovemore*	1 Biscuit/15g	55	2.7	378	3.4	49.3	18.5	18.4
Digestive, Lemon & Ginger, McVitie's*	1 Biscuit/15g	72	3.1	480	6.7	66.7	20.7	2.7
Digestive, Light, McVitie's*	1 Biscuit/15g	66	2.1	444	7.3	69.5	14.4	3.6
Digestive, McVitie's*	1 Biscuit/15g	70	3.2	470	7.2	62.7	21.5	3.6
Digestive, Milk Chocolate, 25% Reduced Fat, McVitie's*	1 Biscuit/17g	78	2.9	459	7.2	68.6	17.3	3.2
Digestive, Milk Chocolate, Asda*	1 Biscuit/17g	82	3.7	494	7.2	65	22	2.6
Digestive, Milk Chocolate, Basics, Sainsbury's*	1 Biscuit/14g	71	3.4	496	6.5	62.9	23.7	2.9
Digestive, Milk Chocolate, Cadbury*	1 Biscuit/16g	80	3.8	490	7.4	61.3	23.3	3.9

BISCUITS

INFO/WEIGHT	Measure	per Measure		Nutrition Values per 100g / 100ml				
		KCAL	FAT	KCAL	PROT	CARB	FAT	FIBRE
Digestive, Milk Chocolate, Homewheat, McVitie's*	1 Biscuit/17g	83	4.1	486	6	61.5	24	4
Digestive, Milk Chocolate, McVitie's*	1 Biscuit/17g	84	4	488	6.7	62.7	23.4	2.9
Digestive, Milk Chocolate, Mini, McVitie's*	1 Bag/25g	124	6.2	496	6.6	61.9	24.7	2.9
Digestive, Milk Chocolate, Sainsbury's*	1 Biscuit/17g	87	6.3	511	6.9	65.9	36.8	2.5
Digestive, Milk Chocolate, Slices, McVitie's*	1 Slice/28g	140	7.4	500	4.5	60.5	26.3	2
Digestive, Milk Chocolate, Tesco*	1 Biscuit/17g	85	4.1	498	6.6	62.8	23.9	3.1
Digestive, Milk Chocolate, Thins, McVitie's*	1 Biscuit/6g	32	1.5	508	6.9	64.3	24.1	3.1
Digestive, Milk Chocolate, Trufree*	1 Biscuit/12g	63	3	521	4	70	25	2
Digestive, Oat, Weight Watchers*	1 Biscuit/11g	50	2.1	457	6	66.3	18.6	6.9
Digestive, Plain Chocolate, Tesco*	1 Biscuit/17g	85	4.1	499	6.2	63.5	24.4	2.8
Digestive, Plain, Average	**1 Biscuit/14g**	**67**	**2.9**	**480**	**7.1**	**65.6**	**20.5**	**3.5**
Digestive, Plain, M&S*	1 Biscuit/16g	80	3.9	490	6.5	62.7	23.8	3.3
Digestive, Reduced Fat, McVitie's*	1 Biscuit/15g	70	2.4	467	7.1	72.8	16.3	3.4
Digestive, Sugar Free, Gullon*	1 Biscuit/13g	57	2.1	430	6.2	68	16	6.5
Digestive, Sweetmeal, Asda*	1 Biscuit/14g	68	3.1	499	7	66	23	3.5
Digestive, Sweetmeal, Sainsbury's*	1 Biscuit/13g	61	2.5	469	7.3	64.3	19.1	5.3
Digestive, Value, Tesco*	1 Biscuit/15g	74	3.4	490	6.9	64	22.4	3.3
Digestive, Whole Wheat, Organic, Dove's Farm*	1 Biscuit/13g	56	2.4	446	5.9	61.6	19.5	7.8
Digestives, Chocolate Chip Coconut, Twists, McVitie's*	1 Biscuit/9g	47	2.4	505	6.6	57.9	26.1	5.3
Digestives, Double Chocolate, Mcvitie's*	1 Biscuit/17g	83	4.1	497	6.5	60.9	24.3	3.6
Dorset Knob, Original White, Moores*	1 Biscuit/13g	52	1	398	12	70.5	7.6	0
Double Choc Chip, Trufree*	1 Biscuit/11g	58	3	523	3	67	27	1.8
Extremely Chocolatey, Dark Chocolate Rounds, M&S*	1 Biscuit/19g	97	5.6	510	6.2	55.7	29.3	6.3
Extremely Chocolatey, Milk Chocolate, Rounds, M&S*	1 Pack/44g	227	11.7	517	6.4	61.6	26.7	2.3
Fig Roll, Tesco*	1 Biscuit/19g	70	1.6	375	4	69.3	8.8	3.1
Fior di Neve, Italiamo, Lidl*	1 Biscuit/12g	60	3.2	516	5.1	62	27	0
Florentines, Decadent Dark Chocolate, Thomas J Fudge*	1 Florentine/19g	107	7.1	565	8	46.8	37.3	0
Forest Fruit, Yoghurt, Breaks, Go Ahead, McVitie's*	2 Slices/36g	144	3.6	402	5.4	72.6	10	2.2
Freddo, Face Cakes, Cadbury*	1 Cake/30g	126	5.7	420	6	57	19	1.4
Fruit Shortcake, McVitie's*	1 Biscuit/8g	37	1.5	462	5.6	65.9	18.9	3.1
Fruit Shortcake, Morrisons*	1 Biscuit/8g	38	1.5	469	6.2	68	18.7	1.9
Fruit Shortcake, Tesco*	1 Biscuit/9g	43	1.7	473	5.8	70.1	18.8	1.9
Fruit Slices, Apple, Raisin & Currant, Belmont, Aldi*	1 Biscuit/15g	57	1	379	7	72.8	6.4	1.3
Garibaldi, Asda*	1 Biscuit/10g	39	0.9	375	4.7	68.5	9.1	2.2
Garibaldi, Sainsbury's*	1 Biscuit/9g	34	0.8	378	4.6	67.6	9.2	3.3
Garibaldi, Tesco*	1 Biscuit/10g	40	0.9	400	4.7	74	9.1	2.2
Ginger Crunch Creams, Fox's*	1 Biscuit/15g	77	3.5	501	4.1	68	23	1.6
Ginger Crunch, Hand Baked, Border*	1 Biscuit/12g	54	2.3	470	4.7	71.4	20.4	0
Ginger Nuts, CBY, Asda*	1 Biscuit/10g	46	1.5	452	5.4	73.5	14.7	2.1
Ginger Nuts, McVitie's*	1 Biscuit/10g	46	1.5	452	5.4	73.5	14.7	2.1
Ginger Nuts, Morrisons*	1 Biscuit/10g	46	1.5	456	5.7	74.6	14.6	1.9
Ginger Nuts, Tesco*	1 Biscuit/10g	46	1.4	465	5.7	74.6	14.6	1.9
Ginger Nuts, Value, Tesco*	1 Biscuit/12g	55	1.9	460	5.2	74.2	15.8	1.6
Ginger Snap, Fox's*	1 Biscuit/8g	35	1	443	4.6	77.1	12.8	1.5
Ginger Snap, Sainsbury's*	1 Biscuit/10g	46	1.5	454	5.2	75	14.4	1.8
Ginger Snaps, Hand Baked, Ringtons *	1 Biscuit/15g	69	2.4	458	5	73.9	16.2	0
Ginger Thins, Asda*	1 Biscuit/5g	23	0.8	462	6	73	16	1.9
Ginger, Belgian Dark Chocolate, Thins, Waitrose*	1 Biscuit/10g	48	2.2	481	6.2	61.2	22.5	4.6
Ginger, Snap, 35% Reduced Fat, Sainsbury's*	1 Biscuit/10g	42	0.9	421	6.8	77.1	9	2.4
Gingernut	**1 Biscuit/11g**	**50**	**1.7**	**456**	**5.6**	**79.1**	**15.2**	**1.4**
Golden Crunch Creams, Fox's*	1 Biscuit/15g	75	3.8	515	4.7	64.8	26.3	1.2
Golden Crunch, Bronte*	1 Biscuit/15g	69	3.3	474	5.1	62.5	22.6	0
Happy Faces, Jacob's*	1 Biscuit/16g	78	3.6	485	4.8	66.1	22.3	1.6

B

BISCUITS

	Measure INFO/WEIGHT	per Measure KCAL	per Measure FAT	Nutrition Values per 100g / 100ml KCAL	PROT	CARB	FAT	FIBRE
Hobnobs, Chocolate Creams, McVitie's*	1 Biscuit/12g	60	3.1	503	6.7	60.3	26.1	4
Hobnobs, McVitie's*	1 Biscuit/15g	72	3.2	473	7	61.8	20.7	5.4
Hobnobs, Milk Chocolate, McVitie's*	1 Biscuit/19g	92	4.5	479	6.8	60.7	23.3	4.5
Hobnobs, Plain Chocolate, McVitie's*	1 Biscuit/16g	81	3.9	498	6.7	63.3	24.3	4.2
Hobnobs, Vanilla Creams, McVitie's*	1 Biscuit/12g	60	3	501	6.1	62.3	25.2	3.6
Jaffa Cakes, Asda*	1 Cake/12g	43	1	368	4.7	67.5	8.8	1.9
Jaffa Cakes, Belmont Biscuit Co, Aldi*	1 Biscuit/13g	52	1.3	400	3.7	72.8	10.2	1
Jaffa Cakes, Dark Chocolate, M&S*	1 Cake/11g	45	1.5	395	3.7	64.9	13.2	2.8
Jaffa Cakes, Dark Chocolate, Mini, M&S*	1 Cake/5g	20	0.8	410	3.9	62.8	15.8	1.9
Jaffa Cakes, McVitie's*	1 Cake/12g	46	1	380	4.9	70.8	8	2.2
Jaffa Cakes, Mini Roll, McVitie's*	1 Cake/26g	99	2.7	374	3.5	67.1	10.1	2.3
Jaffa Cakes, Sainsbury's*	1 Cake/11g	41	1	373	4.3	69.3	8.8	2
Jaffa Cakes, Smart Price, Asda*	1 Cake/12g	43	1	374	4.3	69	9	2
Jaffa Cakes, Value, Tesco*	1 Cake/12g	45	1.1	388	4.7	70	9.4	2.2
Jam Creams, Jacob's*	1 Biscuit/15g	75	3.4	486	5	67.4	21.8	1.6
Jam Sandwich Creams, M&S*	1 Biscuit/17g	80	3.7	485	5.7	64.5	22.6	1.8
Jam Sandwich Creams, Sainsbury's*	1 Biscuit/15g	75	3.4	488	4.9	65.6	22.4	2.2
Jam Sandwich Creams, Tesco*	1 Biscuit/15g	72	3.2	482	4.8	67.1	21.4	1.2
Jammie Dodgers, Minis, Lunchbox, Burton's*	1 Pack/20g	89	3	445	6	70	15.1	2.3
Jammie Dodgers, Original, Burton's*	1 Biscuit/18g	78	2.5	436	5.4	71.3	13.9	1.7
Jammy Wheels, GF, Prewett's*	1 Biscuit/24g	95	5.6	394	5	60.1	23.2	4.7
Lebkuchen, Sainsbury's*	1 Biscuit/10g	39	0.8	400	5.7	76.1	8	1.3
Lemon, & Chia, Weight Watchers*	1 Biscuit/10g	42	1.5	418	15.4	49.4	15.4	10.2
Lemon, All Butter, Half Coated, Finest, Tesco*	1 Biscuit/17g	84	4.5	505	5.6	60.4	26.9	3.6
Lion, Caramel, Masterpieces, Godiva*	1 Biscuit/12g	65	3.5	540	8.6	60	29	0
Malt, Basics, Sainsbury's*	1 Biscuit/8g	36	1.2	470	7.1	73.6	15.7	0
Malted Milk, Asda*	1 Biscuit/8g	39	1.8	490	7	66	22	2
Malted Milk, Average	***1 Biscuit/9g***	***42***	***1.9***	***490***	***7***	***65.6***	***22.2***	***1.8***
Malted Milk, Chocolate, Tesco*	1 Biscuit/10g	52	2.5	500	6.7	64.4	24	1.9
Malted Milk, Milk Chocolate, Sainsbury's*	1 Biscuit/11g	56	2.7	505	6.4	64.4	24.2	2.1
Malted Milk, Sainsbury's*	1 Biscuit/8g	40	1.8	488	7.1	65.5	21.9	2
Malted Milk, Tesco*	1 Biscuit/9g	44	1.9	495	6.6	66.8	21.8	2
Maple Leaf, M&S*	1 Biscuit/13g	50	1.9	395	5.1	59.8	14.8	2
Maria, Gullon*	1 Biscuit/6g	24	0.7	408	7	75	11	4.5
Marie, Crawfords*	1 Biscuit/7g	33	1.1	475	7.5	76.3	15.5	2.3
Mikado, Jacob's*	1 Biscuit/13g	53	1.6	397	4.2	67.7	12.1	2.5
Milk Chocolate Digestive, Everyday Value, Tesco*	1 Biscuit/17g	82	3.7	494	7.2	65.4	22.3	1.7
Milk Chocolate, All Butter, M&S*	1 Biscuit/14g	70	3.6	490	7.9	57.4	25.5	1.4
Milkshake, Belmont Biscuit Co, Aldi*	1 Biscuit/25g	134	7.5	536	6.4	59	30	1.7
Mint, Viscount*	1 Biscuit/14g	73	4	525	4.5	61.6	28.5	1.8
Moments, Chocolate, Special K, Kellogg's*	1 Bar/25g	96	2.3	383	5.5	72	9.1	2.3
Morning Coffee, Tesco*	1 Biscuit/5g	22	0.7	450	7.6	72.3	14.5	2.4
Nice, Asda*	1 Biscuit/8g	38	1.7	480	6	68	21	2.4
Nice, Average	***1 Biscuit/8g***	***36***	***1.6***	***484***	***6.3***	***67.3***	***21***	***2.5***
Nice, Sainsbury's*	1 Biscuit/8g	41	2	498	5.8	63.2	23.9	3.5
Nice, Value, Multipack, Tesco*	1 Biscuit/8g	39	1.7	485	6.5	68	20.8	2.4
Oat & Wholemeal, Crawfords*	1 Biscuit/14g	67	3	482	7.7	64.2	21.6	4.8
Oat Bites, Cheese, Diet Chef Ltd*	1 Pack/23g	99	3.6	430	15	57.4	15.8	4.9
Oat Crisps, Orange, Swedish, Gille*	1 Biscuit/8g	40	2	500	4.7	63.8	25	0
Oat Crumbles, Border*	1 Biscuit/15g	66	3.1	443	5.3	58.9	20.7	1.8
Oat Crunch, M&S*	1 Biscuit/14g	65	2.7	450	7.8	62	18.7	6.1
Oat, & Chocolate Chip, GF, Breaks, Nairn's*	1 Biscuit/10g	47	2	470	7.6	61.8	20.1	5.5
Oat, & Stem Ginger, GF, Breaks, Nairn's*	1 Biscuit/10g	46	1.9	463	8.2	62.4	18.8	5.7

BISCUITS

	Measure INFO/WEIGHT	per Measure KCAL	FAT	Nutrition Values per 100g / 100ml KCAL	PROT	CARB	FAT	FIBRE
Oat, Beetroot, Nigella, & Three Seed, Waitrose*	1 Biscuit/10g	48	2.4	481	11.9	50.7	23.9	7.7
Oat, Black Sesame & Seaweed, 1, Waitrose*	1 Biscuit/5g	27	1.3	487	10.5	55.5	23.1	7.8
Oat, Dark Chocolate Chip, Nairn's*	1 Biscuit/10g	46	1.7	454	8.1	63.8	16.9	6.7
Oat, Fruit & Spice, Nairn's*	1 Biscuit/10g	43	1.5	425	7.8	65.3	14.7	7.6
Oat, Mixed Berries, Nairn's*	1 Biscuit/10g	43	1.5	427	7.5	64.8	15.3	7.1
Oatie Crumbles, CBY, Asda*	1 Biscuit/14g	68	2.9	483	6.6	65.6	20.6	4.5
Oatie Crumbles, Milk Chocolate, Asda*	1 Biscuit/19g	93	4.4	489	7	62	23	4.6
Oaties, Belmont Biscuit Co, Aldi*	1 Biscuit/20g	95	4.2	476	7.8	62	21	4.8
Oaties, Chocolate, Milk, Aldi*	1 Biscuit/20g	95	4.2	476	7.8	62	21	4.8
Oaties, Oatland, Tesco*	1 Biscuit/15g	70	3.1	470	6.5	64.9	20.5	4.5
Oaties, Tower Gate, Lidl*	1 Biscuit/15g	74	3.2	491	8.9	63	21	7
Oatmeal Crunch, Jacob's*	1 Biscuit/8g	37	1.5	458	6.8	65.9	18.6	3.6
Oatmeal, Asda*	1 Biscuit/12g	54	2.5	470	6	62	22	6
Orange Sultana, Go Ahead, McVitie's*	1 Biscuit/15g	58	1.2	400	5.1	75.7	8.1	3
Oreo, Chocolate Cream, Thins, Mondelez*	4 Biscuits/24g	117	4.8	488	5.4	69	20	3.5
Oreo, Thins, Mondelez*	4 Biscuits/24g	118	5.1	490	4.8	69	21	2.6
Oreos, Choc o Brownie, Mondelez*	1 Biscuit/11g	52	2.1	473	5.7	67	19	3.8
Parmesan Cheese, Sainsbury's*	1 Biscuit/3g	18	1	553	14.7	56.4	29.9	1.8
Parsnip, & Poppy Seed, Savoury, Biccies, Ella's Kitchen*	1 Pack/20g	87	2.8	433	6.5	67.9	13.8	5.6
Party Rings, Iced, Fox's*	1 Biscuit/6g	29	0.9	459	5.1	75.8	15	0
Peanut Butter, American Style, Sainsbury's*	1 Biscuit/13g	63	2.9	504	5.2	68.7	23.1	2.2
Petit Beurre, Stella Artois*	1 Biscuit/6g	26	0.9	440	9	73	15	0
Pink Wafers, Crawfords*	1 Biscuit/7g	36	1.9	521	2.5	68.6	26.5	1.1
Pink Wafers, Eat Me, Aldi*	1 Biscuit/8g	44	2.6	552	4.2	58.4	32.9	2.9
Pink Wafers, Sainsbury's*	1 Biscuit/8g	36	1.8	486	4.6	64.2	23.4	1.7
Raspberry & Cream Viennese, Melts, Fox's*	1 Biscuit/16g	84	4.5	521	4	62.1	28.1	1.7
Raspberry Creams, Bolands*	1 Biscuit/13g	64	3	504	4.6	67.3	23.6	2.2
Raspberry, Yoghurt Breaks, Go Ahead, McVitie's*	1 Pack/35g	143	3.6	408	5.4	73.6	10.2	2.3
Redcurrant Puffs, Eat Well, M&S*	1 Biscuit/7g	32	1.4	470	5.6	67.7	19.8	2
Rich Shorties, Asda*	1 Biscuit/10g	50	2.3	486	6	66	22	2
Rich Tea, 25% Less Fat, Tesco*	1 Biscuit/10g	44	1.1	435	7.1	77	11	1.3
Rich Tea, Average	*1 Biscuit/10g*	*45*	*1.5*	*451*	*6.8*	*72.8*	*14.5*	*2.5*
Rich Tea, Basics, Sainsbury's*	1 Biscuit/8g	35	1.2	450	7.1	71.3	15.2	2.9
Rich Tea, Belmont Biscuit Co, Aldi*	1 Biscuit/8g	37	1.2	464	7.4	74	15	3.2
Rich Tea, CBY, Asda*	1 Biscuit/8g	34	1	447	7.2	72.9	13.4	3
Rich Tea, Classic, McVitie's*	1 Biscuit/8g	39	1.3	459	7	71.3	15.5	2.9
Rich Tea, Finger, Essential, Waitrose*	1 Biscuit/5g	22	0.7	450	7.2	72.5	14.3	3
Rich Tea, Finger, Tesco*	1 Finger/5g	23	0.7	451	7.4	72.9	14.4	2.3
Rich Tea, Fingers, Morrisons*	1 Finger/4g	22	0.7	550	10	90	17.5	5
Rich Tea, Light, McVitie's*	1 Biscuit/8g	36	0.9	436	7.6	75.3	10.7	3.1
Rich Tea, Sainsbury's*	1 Biscuit/8g	35	1	454	7.5	75.2	13.2	2
Rich Tea, Tesco*	1 Biscuit/10g	43	1.4	450	7.3	71.8	14.2	3.1
Rocky, Chocolate & Caramel, Fox's*	1 Biscuit/21g	107	4.1	507	6.9	60.3	19.3	15.5
Rocky, Chocolate, Fox's*	1 Biscuit/21g	106	5.4	505	5.7	62.4	25.7	2.4
Rosemary & Thyme, Oaten, Duchy Originals, Waitrose*	1 Biscuit/12g	58	2.7	467	8.5	56.8	21.5	6
Roundie, Milk Chocolate Covered Wafer, Cadbury*	1 Biscuit/30g	161	9.3	536	6.8	56	31	2.8
Rounds, Reese's, Hershey*	1 Biscuit/18g	96	5.6	533	11	50	31	2.7
Safari Snacks, Belmont Biscuit Co, Aldi*	1 Bag/22g	108	4.8	492	6.4	65	22	2.8
Savoury, Gluten, Wheat & Dairy Free, Sainsbury's*	1 Biscuit/17g	77	2.9	467	11.7	65.1	17.7	2.4
Sea Salt & Black Pepper, for Cheese, TTD, Sainsbury's*	3 Biscuits/20g	93	4.3	484	8.8	60.1	22.4	3.8
Shortbread, All Butter, Fingers, Walkers Shortbread Ltd*	2 Fingers/48g	256	14.5	533	5.6	58.4	30.3	2.1
Shortbread, Salted Toffee, GF, Free From, Sainsbury's*	1 Biscuit/20g	100	4.8	502	4.7	65.8	24.2	0.9
Shortcake with Real Milk Chocolate, Cadbury*	1 Biscuit/15g	75	3.5	500	6.3	65.8	23.5	0

B

BISCUITS

INFO/WEIGHT	Measure	per Measure KCAL	FAT	Nutrition Values per 100g / 100ml KCAL	PROT	CARB	FAT	FIBRE
Shortcake, Average	**1 Biscuit/11g**	**55**	**3**	**501**	**6.3**	**66.1**	**27.1**	**2.1**
Shortcake, Caramel, Mini, Thorntons*	1 Biscuit/15g	71	4.6	492	4.8	46.3	31.9	0.6
Shortcake, Caramel, Squares, Tesco*	1 Square/54g	274	16.4	507	4.6	54.1	30.4	0.4
Shortcake, Dairy Milk Chocolate, Cadbury*	1 Bar/49g	252	13.5	515	7.5	59.2	27.5	0
Shortcake, Dutch, M&S*	1 Biscuit/17g	90	5.1	540	5.4	59	30.8	2.5
Shortcake, Fruit, Crawfords*	1 Biscuit/8g	34	1.5	419	5.4	55.9	19.3	2.4
Shortcake, Sainsbury's*	1 Biscuit/11g	53	5.2	479	6.1	65.3	47.2	2.5
Shortcake, Snack, Cadbury*	2 Biscuits/15g	70	3.7	475	7	54.5	25	1.7
Shortcake, Tesco*	1 Biscuit/11g	53	2.3	485	6.8	66.3	21	1.8
Shorties, Cadbury*	1 Biscuit/15g	77	3.6	511	6.5	67.3	24	0
Shorties, Fruit, Value, Tesco*	1 Serving/10g	46	1.7	457	5.7	69.3	17.4	3
Shorties, Rich Highland, Tesco*	1 Biscuit/10g	48	2.2	485	6.1	65.3	21.7	2.6
Shorties, Rich, Tesco*	1 Biscuit/10g	48	2.2	484	6.4	65.6	21.8	2
Shorties, Sainsbury's*	1 Biscuit/10g	50	2.2	500	6.4	69.8	21.8	2
Snappy, Milk Chocolate Finger, Tesco*	2 Fingers/21g	113	6.1	528	6.5	60.8	28.3	2
Speculaas, Large, Hema*	1 Biscuit/23g	106	4.8	459	5.4	61.2	20.8	2.6
Spiced, German, Christmas, Favorina, Lidl*	1 Biscuit/10g	47	1.9	472	5.8	70.2	18.7	0
Stem Ginger, Brakes*	1 Biscuit/13g	62	3.1	495	5.6	62.6	24.7	0
Stornoway, Water, Stag Bakeries Ltd*	1 Biscuit/9g	31	1.2	341	6.5	47.9	13.6	1.7
Strawberry, Biscuit Moments, Special K, Kellogg's*	2 Biscuits/25g	98	2	391	5	74	8	1.5
Sugar Wafers, Vanilla, Flavoured, Triunfo*	1 Biscuit/10g	53	2.5	511	4.1	70.1	24.3	0.6
Tasties, Jam & Cream, Sandwich, Mcvitie's*	1 Biscuit/15g	74	3.4	488	4.8	65.6	22.4	2.2
The Oaty, Wheat Free, Rude Health*	1 Biscuit/12g	55	2.2	437	9	57.2	17.5	7.9
Treacle Crunch Creams, Fox's*	1 Biscuit/13g	65	3.2	502	4.5	65.3	24.8	1.4
Triple Chocolate, Fox's*	1 Biscuit/21g	100	5.2	478	5.7	57.3	25.1	2.5
Twix, Caramel Slice, McVitie's*	1 Slice/29g	142	7.8	491	4.5	57.3	26.8	1.4
Viennese Creams, Raspberry, M&S*	1 Biscuit/17g	90	4.9	520	4.6	60.4	28.6	1.3
Viennese Finger, Belmont Biscuit Co, Aldi*	1 Biscuit/16g	84	4.7	521	4.8	61	29	1.5
Viennese Swirls, All Butter, Waitrose*	1 Biscuit/14g	76	4.7	548	4.9	55.2	33.7	2.1
Viennese Whirl, Fox's*	1 Biscuit/25g	130	7	518	6.7	60.1	27.8	0
Viennese, Chocolate, Melts, Fox's*	1 Biscuit/12g	64	3.4	526	6.1	60.5	28.3	2.4
Viennese, Milk Chocolate, Thins, Tesco*	1 Biscuit/9g	48	2.7	533	5.1	59.7	30.1	1.5
Viennese, Sandwich, Chocolate, M&S*	1 Biscuit/15g	80	4.6	535	7.2	58	30.6	1.7
Viennese, with Milk Chocolate Filling	**1 Biscuit/15g**	**81**	**4.5**	**533**	**6.5**	**59.6**	**29.4**	**2.1**
Wafer, Vanilla, Loacker*	1 Pack/45g	231	12.6	514	7.5	58	28	0
Water, Asda*	1 Biscuit/6g	25	0.5	412	10	75	8	3.3
Water, Average	**1 Biscuit/6g**	**24**	**0.7**	**440**	**10.8**	**75.8**	**12.5**	**3.1**
Water, High Bake, Jacob's*	1 Biscuit/5g	22	0.4	414	10.5	76.4	7.4	3
Water, High Bake, Sainsbury's*	1 Biscuit/5g	21	0.4	412	9.8	76.3	7.5	3.2
Water, High Baked, Tesco*	1 Biscuit/5g	21	0.3	413	9.7	77.4	6.6	2.7
Water, Table, Carr's*	1 Biscuit/3g	14	0.3	417	10.1	74.7	7.6	4.2
Water, Table, Large, Carr's*	1 Biscuit/8g	31	0.6	408	9.9	73.1	7.5	4.1
Water, Table, Small, Carr's*	1 Biscuit/3g	14	0.3	406	10.1	80	7.6	4.2
Wheat, Fig, Plum, & Cranberry, 1, Waitrose*	1 Biscuit/10g	40	1.2	399	9.3	62.6	11.8	3
Yoghurt Break, Red Cherry, Go Ahead, McVitie's*	1 Slice/18g	72	1.8	407	5.5	73.4	10.1	2.2
Yoghurt Break, Strawberry, Go Ahead, McVitie's*	1 Slice/18g	72	1.8	402	52	72.4	10.3	3.4
Yorkie, Nestle*	1 Biscuit/25g	128	6.7	510	6.7	60.4	26.8	1.3

BISON

INFO/WEIGHT	Measure	per Measure KCAL	FAT	Nutrition Values per 100g / 100ml KCAL	PROT	CARB	FAT	FIBRE
Raw	**1oz/28g**	**31**	**0.5**	**109**	**21.6**	**0**	**1.8**	**0**

BITES

INFO/WEIGHT	Measure	per Measure KCAL	FAT	Nutrition Values per 100g / 100ml KCAL	PROT	CARB	FAT	FIBRE
Blueberry, & Lemon, Oat Squares, Superfood, Graze*	1 Bite/30g	136	7.5	454	5	53	25	4.8
Brownie, Chocolate, Tesco*	1 Bite/11g	43	1.6	394	5.3	58	15	30.7
Brownies, Co-Op*	1 Bite/12g	49	2.2	412	5.1	56	18	2.2

BITES	Measure INFO/WEIGHT	per Measure KCAL	FAT	Nutrition Values per 100g / 100ml KCAL	PROT	CARB	FAT	FIBRE
Caramel Crispy, Extremely Chocolatey, Mini, M&S*	1 Bite/11g	50	2	455	4.7	68.2	17.9	2.8
Caramel Shortcake, Mini, Bakers Selection, Asda*	1 Bite/12g	60	3.1	499	5.6	60	26	1.4
Carrot, with Cannellini Bean Dip, Plant Kitchen, M&S*	1 Pack/115g	155	6.3	135	10.2	6.6	5.5	9.3
Chocolate Cornflake, Mini, M&S*	1 Bite/11.8g	55	2.4	470	6.2	66.3	20.1	3.6
Chocolate Orange, Mini, M&S*	1 Bite/22g	95	4.8	430	5.5	54.6	21.6	1.8
Chocolate, Double, Mini, M&S*	1 Bite/17g	82	4.1	469	5.8	57.2	23.6	2.1
Chocolate, Whipped, Protein, Optimum Nutrition*	1 Pack/76g	243	8.4	320	27	37	11	9.1
Coconut, Crunchy, Sesame Seed, Ape*	1 Serving/30g	149	11.4	498	7.2	31	38	20
Cornflake Clusters, Morrisons*	1 Cluster/10g	47	1.8	474	6.2	70.4	18.2	2.1
Flapjack, Co-Op*	1 Bite/16g	73	3.4	455	5.6	58	21	3.9
Flapjack, Mini, M&S*	1 Bite/14g	64	3.1	458	6.1	56.7	21.9	5
Granola, & Yoghurt, Mini, M&S*	1 Piece/10g	49	2.3	492	7.1	62.3	23.4	2
Honeycomb Clusters, Rich & Chocolatey, Mini, Waitrose*	1 Bite/11g	50	2	456	4.8	66.2	18.5	2.9
Jalapeno, Cream Cheese, Tesco*	1 Bite/20g	63	3.9	313	7.2	26.7	19.4	1.6
Millionaires, Tesco*	1 Bites/12g	60	3.4	500	5.1	55.6	28	2.5
Protein, Honey & Seed, Oat Squares, Graze*	1 Square/30g	140	8.1	465	15	42	27	4.4
Protein, Peanut Butter, & Chocolate, Oat Squares, Graze*	1 Bar/30g	149	8.7	496	16	40	29	17
Quinoa, Sour Cream & Onion, Passions, Aldi*	1 Pack/20g	85	2.9	425	10	60	14.5	5.5
Rocky Road, Mini, M&S*	1 Bite/12g	50	1.6	410	5.2	66.9	13.3	2.5
Rocky Road, Mini, Waitrose*	1 Bite/14g	71	3.8	506	5.2	59	27.1	2.4
Saag Aloo, with Potato, & Spinach, Gosh!*	4 Bites/88g	177	1.1	202	7.1	24	1.3	7.7
Salted Caramel Popcorn, Mini, Extremely Indulgent, M&S*	1 Bite/9g	42	1.7	481	5.1	69.9	19.8	1.6
Salted Caramel, CWP*	1 Serving/57g	203	5.9	356	23	43	10.4	6.3
Spinach, & Pine Nuts, Gosh!*	4 Bites/88g	207	10.5	236	8.1	27	12	6
Spinach, Oven Cooked, Strong Roots*	3 Bites/75g	202	10	269	4.3	30.5	13.3	5.1
Spinach, Strong Roots*	3 Bites/93g	202	11.2	218	3.4	20.8	12.1	6.4
Tahini, Chocolate, Gail's*	100g	432	23	432	7.9	46	23	5.6
Tiffin, Chocolate, Belgian, Free From, Lazy Day Foods*	1 Tiffin/15g	73	4.5	488	3	52	30	3.5
BITTER LEMON								
Fever-Tree*	1 Glass/200ml	77	0	38	0	9.2	0	0
Low Calorie, Tesco*	1 Glass/200ml	6	0.2	3	0.1	0.3	0.1	0.1
Schweppes*	1 Glass/250ml	85	0	34	0	8.2	0	0
BLACK PUDDING								
Average, Uncooked	*1 Serving/40g*	*101*	*6*	*252*	*10.2*	*19*	*14.9*	*0.6*
BLACKBERRIES								
Fresh, Raw, Average	*1 Blackberry/8g*	*2*	*0*	*25*	*0.9*	*5.1*	*0.2*	*5.3*
Frozen, Average	*1 Serving/80g*	*37*	*0.1*	*46*	*0.9*	*9.6*	*0.2*	*5.3*
in Fruit Juice, Average	*½ Can/145g*	*52*	*0.3*	*36*	*0.6*	*7.9*	*0.2*	*1.3*
in Light Syrup, Canned, Tesco*	½ Can/145g	70	0.1	48	0.5	10.6	0.1	1.5
BLACKCURRANTS								
Dried, Graze*	1 Pack/30g	95	0.3	317	3.3	79	1	0
Fresh, Raw, Average	*1 Serving/80g*	*22*	*0*	*27*	*0.9*	*6.5*	*0*	*3.5*
in Light Syrup, British, Canned, Tesco*	½ Can/145g	71	0.1	49	0.5	10.4	0.1	2.1
Stewed with Sugar	*1oz/28g*	*16*	*0*	*58*	*0.7*	*15*	*0*	*2.8*
Stewed without Sugar	*1oz/28g*	*7*	*0*	*24*	*0.8*	*5.6*	*0*	*3.1*
BLANCMANGE								
Chocolate Flavour, Made Up, Pearce Duff*	1 Serving/140g	137	5.6	98	3.3	12.3	4	0
Raspberry Flavour, Pearce Duff*	1 Serving/138g	123	2.5	89	3.1	15	1.8	0
Strawberry Flavour, Pearce Duff*	1 Serving/138g	123	2.5	89	3.1	15	1.8	0
Vanilla Flavour, Pearce Duff*	1 Serving/138g	123	2.5	89	3.1	15	1.8	0
BLUEBERRIES								
Dried, Love Life, Waitrose*	1 Serving/30g	107	0.2	358	1.1	80.1	0.8	3.6
Frozen, Average	*1 Serving/80g*	*41*	*0.2*	*51*	*0.6*	*13.8*	*0.2*	*4.4*

	Measure INFO/WEIGHT	per Measure KCAL	per Measure FAT	Nutrition Values per 100g / 100ml KCAL	PROT	CARB	FAT	FIBRE
BLUEBERRIES								
Raw, Average	**50 Berries/68g**	**39**	**0.2**	**57**	**0.7**	**14.5**	**0.3**	**2.4**
BOAR								
Wild, Raw, Average	**1 Serving/200g**	**244**	**6.7**	**122**	**21.5**	**0**	**3.3**	**0**
BOILED SWEETS								
Average	**1 Sweet/7g**	**21**	**0**	**327**	**0**	**87.1**	**0**	**0**
Blackcurrant & Liquorice, Co-Op*	1 Sweet/8g	32	0.4	405	0.9	91	5	0
Cherry Drops, Bassett's*	1 Sweet/5g	18	0	390	0	98.1	0	0
Clear Fruits, Sainsbury's*	1 Sweet/7g	26	0	372	0.1	92.9	0	0
Fruit Drops, Co-Op*	1 Sweet/6g	24	0	395	0.2	98	0	0
Fruit Sherbets, Assorted, M&S*	1 Sweet/9g	35	0.4	405	0.3	91.6	4.3	0.1
Lockets, Mars*	1 Pack/43g	165	0	383	0	95.8	0	0
Mentho-Lyptus, Cherry, Sugar Free, Hall's*	1 Lozenge/4g	8	0	234	0	62.4	0	0
Mentho-Lyptus, Extra Strong, Hall's*	1 Lozenge/4g	14	0	389	0	96.9	0	0
Pear Drops, Bassett's*	1 Sweet/4g	16	0	390	0	96.4	0	0
Pear Drops, Sugar Free, Sula*	1 Sweet/3g	7	0	235	0.1	97	0.1	0
Soothers, Blackcurrant, Hall's*	1 Lozenge/5g	16	0	365	0	91.4	0	0
Soothers, Cherry, Hall's*	1 Pack/45g	165	0	365	0	91.3	0	0
Soothers, Strawberry Flavour, Hall's*	1 Sweet/5g	19	0	385	0	96	0	0
BOK CHOY								
Tesco*	1 Serving/100g	11	0.2	11	1	1.4	0.2	1.2
BOLOGNESE								
Soya, Vegan, Sauce, Fresh, Waitrose*	½ Pot/175g	163	9.4	93	6.2	3.5	5.4	3
Spaghetti, Al Forno, Sainsbury's*	1 Pack/400g	460	19.6	115	7.8	10	4.9	1.1
Spaghetti, As Consumed, Savers, Morrisons*	1 Pack/300g	338	10.4	120	4.5	16.3	3.7	1.6
Spaghetti, BGTY, Sainsbury's*	1 Pack/400g	364	5.6	91	7.1	12.2	1.4	0.6
Spaghetti, CBY, Asda*	1 Pack/100g	108	2	108	6	15.6	2	2
Spaghetti, Charlie Bigham's*	1 Serving/364 g	503	20.8	138	7.1	13.2	5.7	0
Spaghetti, Cook*	1 Portion/390g	491	14.8	126	8.9	14.8	3.8	1.6
Spaghetti, Egg Pasta in Rich Beef Sauce, Waitrose*	1 Pack/400g	404	10.4	101	7.6	11.7	2.6	1
Spaghetti, HL, Tesco*	1 Pack/360g	342	7.2	95	6.4	12	2	1.6
Spaghetti, Italian, Microwaved, Morrisons*	1 Pack/400g	398	9.1	101	6.5	12.7	2.3	1.6
Spaghetti, Meal for One, M&S*	1 Pack/400g	612	31.6	153	7.4	12.3	7.9	1.6
Spaghetti, Mushroom, Plant Chef, Tesco*	1 Pack/426g	511	9.8	120	9.1	14.6	2.3	2.4
Spaghetti, Serves 1, Basics, Sainsbury's*	1 Pack/300g	276	5.4	92	4.9	12.9	1.8	2.1
Spaghetti, Slow Cooked, TTD, Sainsbury's*	1 Pack/400g	474	16.7	125	8	12	4.4	3
Spaghetti, with Cheese Alternative, Plant Kitchen, M&S*	1 Pack/370g	485	15.5	131	5.8	16.4	4.2	2.2
Tortellini, Beef, Rich, Italian, Giovanni Rana*	½ Pack/125g	222	9	178	7.6	20.6	7.2	4.1
Turkey, Microwaved, Slimzone, Asda*	1 Pack/419g	381	3.8	91	7.2	12	0.9	2.4
Vegetarian, Spaghetti, Quorn*	1 Pack/300g	255	1.8	85	4.4	14.8	0.6	1.5
BOMBAY MIX								
Average	**1oz/28g**	**141**	**9.2**	**503**	**18.8**	**35.1**	**32.9**	**6.2**
BON BONS								
Fruit, Bassett's*	1 Serving/7g	25	0	380	0.1	94.2	0	0
Lemon, Bassett's*	1 Sweet/7g	30	0.7	425	0	83.7	9.8	0
Mixed Fruit Flavour, Vimto, Tangerine Confectionery Ltd*	1 Sweet/5g	20	0.3	409	0.1	85.8	6.7	0.6
BOOST								
Duo, Cadbury*	2 Bars/68g	391	19	575	5.6	59	28	1.9
Protein, Cadbury*	1 Bar/49g	249	13.3	507	25	42	27	1.2
Standard Bar, Cadbury*	1 Bar/49g	250	13.8	515	5.8	58.6	28.5	1.5
Treat Size, Cadbury*	1 Bar/24g	130	7.4	535	5.3	59.6	30.5	0
BOUILLABAISSE								
Average	**1 Serving/400g**	**556**	**38.8**	**139**	**11.2**	**2**	**9.7**	**0.4**

	Measure INFO/WEIGHT	per Measure KCAL	FAT	Nutrition Values per 100g / 100ml KCAL	PROT	CARB	FAT	FIBRE
BOUILLON								
Powder, Miso, Marigold*	1 Tsp/5g	12	0.5	248	7	34	9.3	1.4
Powder, Swiss Vegetable, Green Tub, Marigold*	1 Tsp/5g	12	0.4	245	10.1	30.1	8.5	0
BOUNTY								
Dark, Mars*	1 Funsize/29g	141	7.9	493	3.6	55.8	27.5	0
Milk, Mars*	1 Funsize/29g	139	7.3	487	3.7	58.9	25.7	0
BOUQUET GARNI								
Handtied, Fresh, Asda*	1 Bunch/2.4g	11	0.2	455	8.3	69.4	7.9	31.6
BOVRIL*								
Beef Extract, Drink, Made Up with Water, Bovril*	1 Serving/12g	22	0.1	184	38.9	4.6	1.2	0
Chicken Savoury Drink, Bovril*	1 Serving/13g	16	0.2	129	9.7	19.4	1.4	2.1
BRANDY								
37.5% Volume, Average	*1 Pub Shot/35ml*	*72*	*0*	*207*	*0*	*0*	*0*	*0*
40% Volume, Average	*1 Pub Shot/35ml*	*78*	*0*	*224*	*0*	*0*	*0*	*0*
Cherry, Average	*1 Pub Shot/35ml*	*89*	*0*	*255*	*0*	*32.6*	*0*	*0*
BRAWN								
Average	*1 Serving/100g*	*153*	*11.5*	*153*	*12.4*	*0*	*11.5*	*0*
BRAZIL NUTS								
Average	*6 Whole/20g*	*136*	*13.7*	*682*	*15.3*	*2.8*	*68.4*	*5.4*
Milk Chocolate, Tesco*	1 Nut/8g	47	3.5	585	9.9	38	43.7	1.9
BREAD								
50/50, Wonderloaf, Med Sliced, Warburton's*	1 Slice/43g	106	1.2	244	8.8	43.4	2.8	4.3
American, Sandwich, 7 Cereal, Harrys*	2 Slices/79g	223	5.4	282	10.7	41.2	6.8	6.5
Ancient Grain, Pave, Bakery, Tesco*	1 Slice/80g	213	3.9	267	9.8	44.1	4.9	3.3
Apricot & Sesame Seed, Lifefibre*	1 Slice/43g	148	4.4	344	8.1	55	10.3	6.2
Arabic, El Amar Bakery*	1 Serving/110g	318	1.3	289	11.6	57.9	1.2	0
Bagel, Baked with Marmite, Marmite*	1 Bagel/85g	240	2.6	282	12.9	49.3	3.1	2.8
Bagel, Caramelised Onion & Poppyseed, Waitrose*	1 Bagel/86g	222	2.2	258	9.7	49.2	2.5	2.4
Bagel, Caramelised Onion & Poppy Seed, Tesco*	1 Bagel/85g	221	2.1	260	10.9	47.6	2.5	3.8
Bagel, Cinnamon & Raisin, Tesco*	1 Bagel/85g	230	1.4	270	10.4	51.3	1.7	3.8
Bagel, Cinnamon & Raisin, Warburton's*	1 Bagel/80g	212	1.2	265	10.1	51	1.5	3.6
Bagel, Fruit & Spice, Sainsbury's*	1 Bagel/85g	234	1.8	275	9.7	54.3	2.1	3.8
Bagel, Fruit & Fibre, Kingsmill*	1 Bagel/85g	225	1.2	265	9.8	50.8	1.4	5.2
Bagel, Keto, The Low Carb & Keto Bakery UK*	1 Bagel/70g	137	6.3	196	21.4	2.9	9	21.4
Bagel, Mini, Sainsbury's*	1 Bagel/25g	67	0.4	268	11.2	52.4	1.6	2.8
Bagel, Multi Seed, BFree*	1 Bagel/80g	186	2	232	4.1	51.4	2.5	6.5
Bagel, Multi Seed, New York Bagel Co*	1 Bagel/90g	244	4.3	271	12.4	41.6	4.8	5.8
Bagel, Multigrain, Sainsbury's*	1 Bagel/113g	293	3.5	259	10	49.6	3.1	2
Bagel, Onion & Poppy Seed, Average	*1 Bagel/85g*	*225*	*2.8*	*264*	*9*	*50.5*	*3.3*	*3.2*
Bagel, Onion, New York Bagel Co*	1 Bagel/85g	222	1.6	261	10.6	50.4	1.9	3.1
Bagel, Original, Organic, New York Bagel Co*	1 Bagel/85g	221	1	260	9.9	51.5	1.2	1.6
Bagel, Plain	*1 Bagel/104g*	*290*	*2*	*279*	*10.6*	*53.8*	*1.9*	*2.9*
Bagel, Plain, Asda*	1 Bagel/85g	226	2	265	15	46	2.3	2.9
Bagel, Plain, Average	*1 Bagel/78g*	*202*	*1.5*	*259*	*10.1*	*50.4*	*1.9*	*3.1*
Bagel, Plain, Free From, Tesco*	1 Bagel/80g	215	5.5	270	3.4	47.7	6.9	4.7
Bagel, Plain, GFY, Asda*	1 Bagel/84g	218	1.8	259	10	50	2.1	1.8
Bagel, Plain, New York Bakery Co*	1 Bagel/90g	232	1.1	258	10.1	50.1	1.2	3.1
Bagel, Plain, So Organic, Sainsbury's*	1 Bagel/85g	216	2.3	254	9	48.4	2.7	3.6
Bagel, Plain, Tesco*	1 Bagel/85g	225	1.3	265	9.3	52.2	1.5	2.7
Bagel, Red Onion, & Chive, New York Bakery Co*	1 Bagel/90g	235	1	261	10.6	50.5	1.1	3.1
Bagel, Sesame Seed, Essential, Waitrose*	1 Bagel/85g	243	2.7	286	9.6	54.6	3.2	3.6
Bagel, Sesame Seed, GFY, Asda*	1 Bagel/84g	227	2.1	271	11	51	2.5	2.6
Bagel, Sesame, M&S*	1 Bagel/87g	240	2.8	275	10.2	51.2	3.2	2.1
Bagel, Sesame, New York Bakery*	1 Bagel/90g	242	2.5	269	10.7	47.8	2.8	4.5

BREAD

INFO/WEIGHT	Measure	per Measure		Nutrition Values per 100g / 100ml				
		KCAL	FAT	KCAL	PROT	CARB	FAT	FIBRE
Bagel, Thins, Plain, New York Bakery Co*	1 Thin/48g	133	0.6	277	9.4	55.8	1.2	2.7
Bagel, Thins, Seeded, Sliced, New York Bakery Co*	1 Thin/45g	129	1.5	286	10	52.1	3.4	3.9
Bagel, Thins, Sesame, Warburton's*	1 Thin/50g	130	1.7	260	10.1	46.8	3.4	3.6
Bagel, Wee Soda, Genesis Crafty*	1 Bagel/65g	148	2.5	227	6.9	41.3	3.9	2.9
Bagel, White, Asda*	1 Bagel/86g	227	2.7	264	10	49	3.1	0
Bagel, White, Original, Weight Watchers*	1 Bagel/67g	158	0.5	236	9.5	42.4	0.8	10.7
Bagel, Wholemeal, & White, Mini, New York Bakery Co*	1 Bagel/45g	114	1	254	10.8	45.2	2.2	5.1
Bagel, Wholemeal, Average	*1 Bagel/90g*	*235*	*2.7*	*261*	*12.7*	*44.6*	*3*	*7.7*
Bagel, Wholemeal, Multiseed, M&S*	1 Bagel/84g	215	5.6	255	13.1	35.4	6.6	8.3
Bagel, Wholemeal, New York Bagel Co*	1 Bagel/90g	225	2	250	10.9	42.8	2.2	7.7
Baguette, Bake At Home, Tesco*	½ Baguette/75g	216	0.9	289	8.6	59.1	1.2	3.5
Baguette, Crusty Brown, M&S*	½ Loaf/71g	160	1.1	225	9.8	42.7	1.6	6.3
Baguette, French, Tesco*	1 Serving/60g	144	0.7	240	7.8	49.5	1.2	3.4
Baguette, Garlic, Slices, Frozen, CBY, Asda*	1 Slice/26g	92	4.7	355	8.2	38.3	18.1	2.8
Baguette, GF, Schnitzer*	½ Baguette/80g	186	6.2	233	4.7	30	7.8	12
Baguette, Granary, Average	*1 Serving/100g*	*250*	*2.8*	*250*	*20*	*46*	*2.8*	*6*
Baguette, Granary, Co-Op*	1 Serving/60g	150	1.5	250	20	46	2.5	6
Baguette, Homebake, Half, Tesco*	1 Serving/75g	217	0.9	289	8.6	49.1	1.2	3.5
Baguette, Malted Grain, Bake At Home, M&S*	½ Baguette/75g	187	1.7	249	9.7	43.6	2.3	7.6
Baguette, Multiseed, Mini, GF, Fria*	1 Baguette/70g	203	6	290	3.5	47	8.5	6
Baguette, Part Baked, Classique, Deli France, Delifrance*	1 Pack/250g	745	3	298	9.8	54.8	1.2	2.7
Baguette, Part Baked, H.W. Nevill's*	½ Baguette/75g	216	0.9	289	8.6	59.1	1.2	3.5
Baguette, Part Baked, Half, Tesco*	½ Baguette/75g	216	0.9	289	8.6	59.1	1.2	3.5
Baguette, Paysanne, Stonebaked, Asda*	1/6 Loaf/46g	119	1.4	259	10	48	3	3.3
Baguette, Ready to Bake, Sainsbury's*	½ Baguette/62g	150	0.8	242	7.8	49.7	1.3	2.8
Baguette, Sourdough, la Brea Bakery*	1 Serving/60g	160	0.4	266	8.8	56.1	0.7	1.8
Baguette, White, Half, Crusty, M&S*	1 Baguette/162g	420	1.8	260	8.4	53.5	1.1	2.3
Baguette, White, Homebake, Tesco*	1 Baguette/150g	434	1.8	289	8.6	59.1	1.2	3.5
Baguette, White, Ready to Bake, Asda*	1 Serving/60g	168	1.1	280	10	56	1.8	2.6
Baguette, White, Sainsbury's*	1 Serving/50g	132	0.8	263	9.3	53.1	1.5	2.7
Baguette, Wholemeal, Part Baked, Asda*	½ Baguette/75g	176	1	235	8.2	47.7	1.3	3
Baguette, Wholemeal, Part Baked, Mini, Landgut*	½ Baguette/25g	56	0.2	223	7.5	46	1	0
Banana, with Dates & Hazelnuts, Graze*	1 Slice/19g	59	2.7	309	4.8	38.7	14.4	2.7
Baps, Brown, Large, Asda*	1 Bap/58g	140	0.9	242	10	47	1.6	0
Baps, Brown, Large, G H Sheldon*	1 Bap/64g	169	4.3	264	5.3	47.5	6.7	4
Baps, Brown, Malted Grain, Large, Tesco*	1 Bap/93g	228	3.1	245	9.9	42.7	3.3	5.3
Baps, Cheese Topped, Baker's Soft, Tesco*	1 Bap/65g	176	3.3	268	10.8	43.5	5.1	2.6
Baps, Cheese Topped, G H Sheldon*	1 Roll/70g	197	5.8	282	12.4	38.6	8.3	1.4
Baps, Multigrain, Tesco*	1 Bap/98g	238	3.1	244	8.7	45.1	3.2	1.9
Baps, White Sandwich, Kingsmill*	1 Bap/80g	209	3.2	261	10.1	46.2	4	2.2
Baps, White, Average	*1 Bap/65g*	*167*	*2.3*	*257*	*9.5*	*47*	*3.5*	*1.9*
Baps, White, Floured, Waitrose*	1 Bap/60g	147	1.2	244	8	48.6	2	1.1
Baps, White, Giant, Sainsbury's*	1 Bap/86g	235	3.2	273	8.3	51.7	3.7	3.4
Baps, White, Giant, Waitrose*	1 Bap/104g	260	3.7	250	9.5	45	3.6	4.8
Baps, White, Large, Tesco*	1 Bap/100g	250	1	250	9.2	49.7	1	2.6
Baps, White, Sliced, Large, Asda*	1 Bap/58g	148	1	255	10	50	1.7	0
Baps, White, Soft, Floured, M&S*	1 Bap/61g	175	3.4	285	11.5	46.6	5.5	2.8
Baps, White, Super Soft, The Bakery, M&S*	1 Roll/60g	161	2.8	268	8.4	46.6	4.7	3
Baps, White, Warburton's*	1 Bap/57g	144	2.5	252	9.8	43.4	4.3	2.7
Baps, Wholemeal, Brace's*	1 Bap/59g	137	2.6	234	10.5	42.5	4.4	4.3
Baps, Wholemeal, Country Oven*	1 Bap/40g	92	1.3	231	9.5	41	3.3	4.1
Baps, Wholemeal, Giant, Rathbones*	1 Bap/110g	230	2.1	209	9.4	39	1.9	8
Baps, Wholemeal, Giant, Sainsbury's*	1 Bap/86g	230	3.5	268	9.7	48.1	4.1	7.7

BREAD

	Measure INFO/WEIGHT	per Measure KCAL	FAT	Nutrition Values per 100g / 100ml KCAL	PROT	CARB	FAT	FIBRE
Baps, Wholemeal, Tesco*	1 Bap/46g	104	2.4	227	9.6	41.4	5.3	5.6
Baps, Wholemeal, Waitrose*	1 Bap/80g	191	3.4	238	12	34.8	4.2	6.7
Barmbrack, Irish, Rankin Selection*	1 Slice/48g	142	1.6	295	4.5	61.5	3.4	3.2
Beau & Bon, Cereales et Graines, Harrys*	2 Slices/46g	136	3.4	298	13	41.6	7.5	6
Best of Both, Farmhouse, Hovis*	1 Slice/44g	99	1.4	226	9.5	40	3.1	4.9
Best of Both, Med Sliced, Eat Well, M&S*	1 Slice/36g	83	0.8	229	9.4	41.2	2.2	3.5
Best of Both, Medium, Hovis*	1 Slice/38g	86	0.8	230	10.2	40.4	2.2	3.9
Best of Both, Thick Sliced, Hovis*	1 Slice/47g	108	1	230	10.2	40.4	2.2	3.9
Black Olive, Finest, Tesco*	1 Serving/72g	184	4.6	255	9.7	39.7	6.4	2.9
Bloomer, Brown, Slices, GF, Made Without Wheat, M&S*	1 Slice/53g	131	2.9	247	4.3	41.4	5.4	7.8
Bloomer, COU, M&S*	1 Slice/33g	78	0.5	235	9.5	45.5	1.5	3.6
Bloomer, Honey, & Sunflower, Asda*	1 Slice/40g	110	2.5	274	9.5	42.8	6.2	4.5
Bloomer, Multi Seed, Organic, Sainsbury's*	1 Serving/60g	160	4.1	266	10.9	40.3	6.8	8.8
Bloomer, Multi Seed, Sliced, M&S*	1 Slice/54g	150	3.9	280	10.5	43.6	7.2	3.1
Bloomer, Multiseed, Average	**1 Slice/50g**	**120**	**2.4**	**240**	**11.8**	**37.2**	**4.9**	**7.7**
Bloomer, Multiseed, Finest, Tesco*	1 Slice/50g	145	3.8	290	9.8	40.2	7.6	7.4
Bloomer, Multiseed, TTD, Sainsbury's*	1 Slice/50g	119	1.8	239	12	39.7	3.6	8.8
Bloomer, Soft Grain, M&S*	1 Slice/34g	80	0.5	235	9.5	45.5	1.5	3.6
Bloomer, Sunflower Seeded, with Rye, TTD, Sainsbury's*	2 Med Slices/57g	181	6.9	317	12.6	36	12.1	6.8
Bloomer, White, Crusty, Bakery, Tesco*	1 Serving/100g	244	1.7	244	8.3	47.2	1.7	3.3
Bloomer, White, Sliced, Waitrose*	1 Slice/50g	130	0.9	259	8.5	52.1	1.8	2.6
Bloomer, Wholemeal, Organic, M&S*	1 Slice/50g	110	2.1	220	10.2	35.5	4.2	6.4
Both in One, Village Bakery, Aldi*	1 Slice/40g	95	1	237	8.5	43	2.5	4.3
Breadcakes, Big Brown, Morrisons*	1 Cake/63g	154	2.1	245	9	44.6	3.4	4.3
Brioche, Buns, Burger, Sliced, St Pierre*	1 Bun/50g	164	4.1	328	9	53.3	8.2	2.5
Brioche, Burger Bun, Deluxe, Lidl*	1 Bun/50g	170	4.9	339	10.1	51.8	9.8	1.6
Brioche, Burger Buns, Luxury, Specially Selected, Aldi*	1 Bun/50g	159	3.7	317	9.5	52	7.3	3.1
Brioche, Burger Buns, Signature, Morrisons*	1 Bun/55g	156	2.3	284	9.4	51	4.2	2.2
Brioche, Burger Buns, Warburton's*	1 Roll/54g	159	3.2	294	10.2	49.1	6	1.2
Brioche, Chocolate & Custard, Rolls, Mini, Lidl*	1 Roll/50g	152	4.5	305	7	48	9	2
Brioche, Chocolate Chip, Brioche Pasquier*	1 Brioche/35g	132	5.6	376	7.7	49	16	2.8
Brioche, Chocolate, Marbled, Waitrose*	¼ Loaf/100g	305	9.6	305	6.8	46.7	9.6	2.3
Brioche, French Marble, with Vanilla, Bon Appetit, Aldi*	1 Serving/50g	132	3.4	264	6.6	42.6	6.7	1.8
Brioche, Loaf, Butter, Sainsbury's*	1/8 Loaf/50g	174	5.2	347	8	55	10.5	2.2
Brioche, Loaf, Finest, Tesco*	1 Serving/66g	242	9	367	7.4	52.9	13.6	1.9
Brioche, Loaf, Hand Plaited, Aldi*	1 Slice/50g	178	5.5	355	8.1	50	11	1.7
Brioche, Loaf, Sliced, Tesco*	2 Slices/42g	151	5	360	7.3	54.8	11.9	2
Brioche, Milk, Rolls, Brioche Pasquier*	1 Brioche/35g	127	4.4	364	8.8	53	12.6	1.5
Brioche, Raisin, Swirls, Sainsbury's*	1 Swirl/45g	130	3.4	288	6.9	47.3	7.5	2
Brioche, Rolls, Chocolate Chip, Morrisons*	1 Roll/35g	130	4.8	372	8.1	52.6	13.8	2.3
Brioche, Rolls, Chocolate Chip, Tesco*	1 Serving/35g	131	4.4	374	7.6	56.3	12.7	2.1
Brioche, Rolls, Sweet, GF, Schar*	1 Roll/50g	146	3.6	293	3.4	52	7.3	3
Brown, Baps, Henllan Bakery*	1 Bap/69g	171	1.9	248	10	47.7	2.8	0
Brown, Bloomer, Half, Jackson's Bakery*	1 Slice/45g	113	1.3	252	10	44.6	2.8	4.4
Brown, Bloomer, Organic, Bakery, Tesco*	1 Slice/80g	193	1.8	241	9	42.8	2.3	6.5
Brown, Ciabatta, Rolls, GF, Dietary Specials*	1 Roll/50g	137	4	274	5.8	36.9	8.1	8.9
Brown, Danish, Weight Watchers, Warburton's*	1 Slice/20g	48	0.4	233	10.3	40.7	1.8	6.2
Brown, Deli Sub, Roll, Asda*	1 Roll/60g	142	1.9	236	0	35	3.2	0
Brown, Farmhouse, GF, Newburn, Warburton's*	1 Slice/35g	82	1.9	234	7.8	35.8	5.4	5.7
Brown, Farmhouse, Linwoods*	1 Slice/25g	56	0.4	225	7.3	44.4	1.7	5.8
Brown, Farmhouse, Soft, Sliced, GF, Genius *	1 Slice/36g	92	2.1	256	2.2	44	5.8	9.1
Brown, GF, 300g Loaf, Warburton's*	1 Slice/27g	70	1.8	259	4.5	42.4	6.7	5.6
Brown, GF, Genius *	1 Slice/35g	97	4.7	277	6.7	42.2	13.3	9.5

B

BREAD

INFO/WEIGHT	Measure	per Measure KCAL	FAT	Nutrition Values per 100g / 100ml KCAL	PROT	CARB	FAT	FIBRE
Brown, Gluten & Wheat Free, Sliced	1 Slice/25g	56	1.3	224	3.4	41	5.2	9.4
Brown, Granary Malted, thick Sliced, Waitrose*	1 Slice/40g	95	0.9	238	9.4	44.8	2.3	5.1
Brown, Kingsmill Gold, Seeds & Oats, Kingsmill*	1 Slice/45g	126	4.4	280	12.2	35.6	9.8	4.9
Brown, Malted Grain, Medium, Roberts*	1 Slice/30g	70	0.4	233	8.3	46.6	1.4	3.2
Brown, Malted, Average	*1 Thin Slice/25g*	*60*	*0.6*	*242*	*9.4*	*45.5*	*2.4*	*4.2*
Brown, Malted, Farmhouse Gold, Morrisons*	1 Slice/38g	94	0.5	248	8.2	49.6	1.4	3
Brown, Med Slice, Smart Price, Asda*	1 Slice/37g	77	0.6	210	8	41	1.6	6
Brown, Med Sliced	*1 Slice/34g*	*74*	*0.7*	*218*	*8.5*	*44.3*	*2*	*3.5*
Brown, Med Sliced, Asda*	1 Slice/36g	78	0.6	216	8	42	1.8	4.1
Brown, Med Sliced, Bettabuy, Morrisons*	1 Slice/31g	66	0.4	212	8.6	42	1.3	3.6
Brown, Med Sliced, Sainsbury's*	2 Slices/80g	187	2.3	234	11.9	36.7	2.9	6.6
Brown, Med Sliced, Savers, Morrisons*	1 Slice/30g	78	0.4	260	9.7	50.7	1.3	4
Brown, Mixed Grain, Original, Vogel*	1 Slice/45g	102	0.6	227	9.8	47.1	1.2	6.4
Brown, Multi Grain, Wheat Free, GF	1 Slice/33g	76	1.7	229	5.1	40.8	5.1	5.6
Brown, Multigrain, Sliced, Half Pan, Pat The Baker*	1 Slice/40g	94	1.3	234	10.4	41.6	3.3	7.8
Brown, Oaty, Super, Sliced, Roberts*	1 Slice/33g	76	0.7	229	8.6	43.6	2.2	3.9
Brown, Premium, Med Sliced, Warburton's*	1 Slice/24g	61	0.9	258	10.6	43.2	3.7	4.3
Brown, Sainsbury's*	1 Slice/34g	81	0.7	239	8.4	46.8	2.1	4.2
Brown, Sandwich Bread, GF, Udi's*	1 Slice/37g	79	1.1	216	5.2	39.2	2.9	6.3
Brown, Seeded, Dumpy, Low GI, Sasko*	1 Slice/55g	128	2.3	232	9.4	35	4.2	8
Brown, Seeded, GF, Loaf, Made Without Wheat, M&S*	1 Slice/33g	89	3.2	268	4.8	34.5	9.7	11.9
Brown, Seeded, Rolls, Free From, Tesco*	1 Roll/75g	167	5.5	222	6.7	28.8	7.3	7.4
Brown, Sliced, By Brennans, Weight Watchers*	1 Slice/20g	51	0.4	257	9.5	45.4	2.1	6.8
Brown, Sliced, Free From, Tesco*	1 Slice/42g	81	1.7	193	5.3	29.3	4	9.3
Brown, Soda, M&S*	1 Slice/40g	92	1.4	229	9.2	43.6	3.6	4.9
Brown, Soft, Farmhouse , Warburton's*	1 Slice/42g	104	1.1	246	9.9	42.8	2.7	5.3
Brown, Sunflower & Barley, Vogel*	1 Slice/42g	100	1.9	239	9.4	40.3	4.5	6.7
Brown, Super Seeded, Sliced, Loaf, Extra Special, Asda*	1 Slice/44g	131	4.3	298	12	39	9.7	5.5
Brown, Thick Slice, Tesco*	1 Serving/50g	110	1.2	219	10.3	38.9	2.5	5.3
Brown, Thin Sliced, Sainsbury's*	1 Slice/29g	65	0.5	225	8.2	43.8	1.9	3.9
Brown, Toasted, Average	*1 Med Slice/24g*	*65*	*0.5*	*272*	*10.4*	*56.5*	*2.1*	*4.5*
Brown, Toastie, Thick Sliced, Kingsmill*	1 Slice/44g	101	1.4	230	9.5	40.5	3.3	4.7
Brown, Very Dark, Albert Heijn*	1 Slice/35g	84	1.4	240	12	35	4	7.4
Buckwheat, Artisan*	1 Loaf/400g	736	7	184	6.1	38.1	1.8	4.3
Buns, Burger Seeded, Sliced, Warburton's*	1 Roll/60g	158	3.2	264	9	43.6	5.3	2.7
Buns, Burger, American Style, Sainsbury's*	1 Bun/50g	131	2.1	261	10.5	45.6	4.1	3.6
Buns, Burger, Brioche, TTD, Sainsbury's*	1 Bun/80g	257	8.2	322	7.8	48.1	10.3	2.6
Buns, Burger, Cheese & Onion Topped, Finest, Tesco*	1 Serving/105g	309	10	294	10.2	41.9	9.5	2.8
Buns, Burger, GF, Made Without Wheat, M&S*	1 Bun/80g	201	5	251	4.8	38.9	6.2	10.4
Buns, Burger, Giant, Sainsbury's*	1 Bun/95g	249	4.9	262	8.7	45.2	5.2	2.9
Buns, Burger, M&S*	1 Bun/58g	162	3.3	280	10.1	45.7	5.7	2.5
Buns, Burger, Sainsbury's*	1 Bun/56g	154	2.9	275	9.2	47.8	5.2	4.1
Buns, Burger, Seeded, Large, Tesco*	1 Bun/90g	240	3.2	267	9.5	47.7	3.6	2.9
Buns, Burger, Sesame, American Style, Sainsbury's*	1 Bun/60g	162	3.8	270	7.3	46.2	6.3	2.2
Buns, Burger, Sesame, Sliced, Tesco*	1 Bun/60g	168	4	280	7.9	47.3	6.6	2.1
Buns, White, Burger, Waitrose*	1 Serving/64g	169	2.5	264	10	47.2	3.9	2.7
Buns, White, Stay Fresh, Tesco*	1 Bun/56g	152	3.7	271	7.5	45.5	6.6	0
Butterbread, Nature's Own*	1 Slice/30g	70	0.6	231	11.5	46.2	1.9	0
Challah, Average	*1 Slice/50g*	*143*	*3.6*	*286*	*8.9*	*53.6*	*7.1*	*3.6*
Cheese, & Garlic, Pizza Style, Sainsbury's*	¼ Bread/63g	199	8.1	318	10.7	39.7	13	2.2
Cheese, & Garlic, Stonebaked, Morrisons*	¼ Bread/69g	228	9.9	331	10.9	39.5	14.4	1.9
Cheese, & Onion, Tear & Share, Sainsbury's*	¼ Bread/71g	202	6.6	285	9.8	40.6	9.3	1.9
Cheese, & Onion, Toastie, Warburton's*	1 Slice/42g	120	5.8	286	7.5	33.1	13.7	0

BREAD

INFO/WEIGHT		per Measure KCAL	FAT	Nutrition Values per 100g / 100ml KCAL	PROT	CARB	FAT	FIBRE
Cheese, & Tomato, Tear & Share, Sainsbury's*	¼ Bread/72g	211	9.5	293	8	35.7	13.2	1.5
Cheese, Morrisons*	1 Serving/96g	297	13.6	311	9.9	35.9	14.2	3
Cheese, Onion & Garlic, Tear & Share, Waitrose*	¼ Bread/112g	326	14.6	290	9.4	33.9	13	2.1
Cheese, Tear & Share, Tesco*	¼ Loaf/73g	225	7.8	310	8.8	44	10.7	0.8
Cheese, Three, Bloomer, Bakery, Tesco*	1 Slice/82g	214	5.3	261	13.1	36.7	6.4	2
Cheese, Topped, Baton, Bakery, Tesco*	½ Baton/100g	292	4.5	292	10.7	51.2	4.5	2
Cholla, Average	*1/10 Loaf/154g*	*421*	*14.3*	*274*	*6.9*	*40.8*	*9.3*	*1*
Ciabatta, Black Olive, Bake At Home, Aldi*	¼ Baguette/75g	220	3.1	294	8.9	54	4.1	3.3
Ciabatta, Black Olive, Part Baked, Sainsbury's*	¼ Ciabatta/67g	172	2.5	257	8.8	46.8	3.8	2.4
Ciabatta, Finest, Tesco*	1/6 Ciabatta/45g	124	2.7	275	10.4	44.8	5.9	2.7
Ciabatta, Gail's*	100g	223	0.7	223	6.6	46	0.7	2.2
Ciabatta, Green Olive, Tesco*	¼ Ciabatta/70g	155	3.1	222	7.4	38.2	4.4	1.9
Ciabatta, Half, M&S*	1 Ciabatta/135g	354	5.5	262	10.3	48.1	4.1	2.1
Ciabatta, Half, Organic, Sainsbury's*	½ Ciabatta/63g	152	0.6	241	9.1	48.7	1	2.3
Ciabatta, Half, Part Baked, TTD, Sainsbury's*	¼ Pack/67g	173	3.3	257	8.6	44.6	4.9	3.5
Ciabatta, Half, Tesco*	1 Ciabatta/135g	351	4.7	260	8.9	47.7	3.5	2.2
Ciabatta, Italian Style, Waitrose*	1 Ciabatta/89g	231	1.2	260	10.7	51.2	1.4	2.2
Ciabatta, Loaf, Finest, Tesco*	1 Serving/45g	115	2.1	257	10.1	41.8	4.7	3.3
Ciabatta, Olive & Rosemary, Mini, Tesco*	1 Pack/75g	319	8.2	425	17.8	63	10.9	3.6
Ciabatta, Organic, Tesco*	1/3 Ciabatta/100g	240	3.6	240	8.7	43.2	3.6	2.4
Ciabatta, Part Baked, Half, Sainsbury's*	½ Ciabbatta/67g	174	2.5	260	8.9	47.7	3.7	2.2
Ciabatta, Plain, Half, Two, Waitrose*	1 Roll/80g	248	5.8	310	10	51.3	7.2	2.2
Ciabatta, Plain, Tesco*	1 Serving/60g	166	3.1	277	9	47.4	5.1	2.5
Ciabatta, Ready to Bake, Sainsbury's*	½ Ciabatta/66g	172	2.4	260	8.9	47.7	3.7	2.2
Ciabatta, Square, Bake at Home, Part Baked, Asda*	1 Roll/60g	157	2.1	262	8.4	49.1	3.5	2.1
Ciabatta, Stick, Organic, M&S*	1 Stick/140g	315	2	225	8.9	48.5	1.4	4.2
Ciabatta, Sun Dried Tomato & Basil, Tesco*	¼ Ciabatta/75g	193	4.3	257	8.9	42.4	5.7	2.4
Ciabatta, Tomato & Basil, GFY, Asda*	1 Serving/55g	143	1.2	260	9	51	2.2	0
Ciabatta, TTD, Sainsbury's*	¼ Pack/68g	185	4	274	10.4	44.8	5.9	2.7
Cinnamon, & Raisin, Toasty Loaf, Rankin*	1 Slice/40g	113	2	283	6.6	54.2	5	2.5
Cinnamon, Swirl, Asda*	1 Serving/25g	87	3.2	349	6	52	13	1.6
Cob, Cheese & Chutney, Bakery, Tesco*	1 Slice/50g	124	2.2	249	11.3	39.7	4.4	2.5
Corn, Soft, Mexican, Discovery*	1 Tortilla/40g	119	2.8	297	7.4	51	7.1	2.3
Corn, Soft, Old El Paso*	1 Tortilla/42g	121	2	289	8.5	51.8	4.8	2.4
Corn, with Sunflower Seed & Mixed Spice, Bakery, Tesco*	1 Slice/50g	131	2	262	9.9	45	4.1	2.6
Cottage Loaf, Stonebaked, Asda*	1 Serving/67g	155	0.9	232	10	45	1.3	3.2
Crostini, Olive Oil, TTD, Sainsbury's*	1 Roll/4g	16	0.3	409	11.4	72.2	8.3	3.3
Farl, Irish Soda, Irwin's Bakery*	1 Farl/150g	334	5.1	223	4	44	3.4	2.3
Farmhouse, Batch, Multiseed, Love Life, Waitrose*	1 Slice/50g	130	3.5	259	9.9	39.2	7	7.2
Farmhouse, Poppy Seed, Crusty, Loaf, M&S*	1 Slice/40g	104	1.3	260	9.4	47.6	3.3	2.3
Farmhouse, Wholemeal, Average	*1 Slice/43g*	*94*	*1.4*	*219*	*10.7*	*36.2*	*3.3*	*7.3*
Farmhouse, with Oatmeal, Batch, Finest, Tesco*	1 Slice/44g	110	1.4	240	9.8	43.2	3.1	5.2
Ficelle, Mixed Olive, Waitrose*	1/5 Stick/50g	133	1.4	267	7.5	51.1	2.8	3.4
Fig, & Almond, BrÃƒÆ'Ã‚'derna Cartwright*	4 Slices/100g	267	7.5	267	9.2	39.7	7.5	0
Fig, & Hazelnut, Loaf, M&S*	1 Serving/100g	285	8.2	285	11	38.9	8.2	5.4
Five Seed, Fully Loaded, Aldi*	1 Slice/50g	135	3.3	270	10.9	36.4	6.7	7.9
Flat, Italian, Piada Sfogliata, Italiamo, Lidl*	1 Piece/130g	402	12.5	309	7.9	45.9	9.6	2
Flatbread, Folded, Lge Plain, by, Sainsbury's*	1 Flatbread/65g	192	3.4	295	8.5	51.4	5.3	4.1
Flatbread, Folded, Plain, Sainsbury's*	1 Flatbread/33g	97	1.7	295	8.5	51.4	5.3	4.1
Flatbread, Garlic & Herb, Tear & Share, Sainsbury's*	¼ Bread/68g	201	6.3	297	10.9	42.5	9.3	3.7
Flatbread, Garlic, & Cheese, Handcrafted, Tesco*	¼ Bread/58g	176	5.1	305	10.5	44.6	8.9	2.4
Flatbread, Garlic, BGTY, Sainsbury's*	¼ Bread/56g	177	5.7	316	9.6	46.6	10.1	2.7
Flatbread, Khobez, White, Dina Foods Ltd*	1 Bread/56g	158	0.6	282	10.5	57.5	1.1	3

B

BREAD

INFO/WEIGHT	Measure	per Measure KCAL	FAT	Nutrition Values per 100g / 100ml KCAL	PROT	CARB	FAT	FIBRE
Flatbread, Multi Seed, Tower Gate, Lidl*	1 Bread/8g	34	1.1	430	13.1	57.4	13.9	11.2
Flatbread, Multiseed, Folded, Tesco*	1 Flatbread/35g	107	2.4	305	10.4	47.8	6.8	5.3
Flatbread, Piadina, Durum Wheat, Crosta & Mollica*	1 Flatbread/75g	234	6.5	312	8.4	48.8	8.7	2.5
Flatbread, Plain, Folded, Asda*	1 Flatbread/35g	109	2.4	313	9.6	52	6.8	3.1
Flatbread, Plain, Folded, Luxury, Iceland*	1 Flatbread/35g	113	2.7	323	9.1	53	7.7	2.5
Flatbread, Seeded, Morrisons*	1 Serving/35g	114	3.8	325	9.9	44.1	10.8	5.7
Flatbread, Super Seeded, Folded, Village Bakery, Aldi*	1 Flatbread/35g	123	4.6	352	9.7	47	13	5.5
Flatbread, Tomato, & Garlic, Sainsbury's*	1/3 Bread/73g	191	4.9	261	8.4	41.7	6.7	3.4
Flatbread, White, Folded, Village Bakery, Aldi*	1 Flatbread/35g	106	2.1	303	9.1	51.4	6	2.6
Flatbread, Wholemeal, Folded, Sainsbury's*	1 Flatbread/35g	102	2.4	292	9.5	44	7	7.4
Flour, From Dinner Kit, Old El Paso*	1 Tortilla/42g	144	4.9	344	8.7	51.1	11.7	0
Flour, Soft, Discovery*	1 Tortilla/40g	119	2.8	298	8	49.6	7.1	2.4
Focaccia, Balsamic Onion, & Thyme, Co-Op*	1 Focaccia/60g	155	3.6	258	7.3	41	6	4.9
Focaccia, Harissa Peperonata, Bake at Home, M&S*	1 Bun/114g	282	8.3	247	7.9	35.8	7.3	3.2
Focaccia, Onion & Herb, Tesco*	½ Pack/190g	547	23.8	288	8.7	35.2	12.5	3.7
Focaccia, Roast Cherry Tomato & Olive, GFY, Asda*	½ Pack/148g	350	6	237	9	41	4.1	2.8
Focaccia, Roasted Onion & Cheese, M&S*	1 Serving/89g	240	4.1	270	10.4	45.7	4.6	2.8
Focaccia, Rosemary & Sea Salt, TTD, Sainsbury's*	1 Serving/50g	130	3.5	261	7.4	40.7	7	2.8
Focaccia, Rosemary, & Sea Salt, Tesco*	1 Focaccia/50g	151	4.2	301	9.4	45.5	8.3	3.4
Focaccia, Sliced, Deli Kitchen*	1 Slice/90g	219	5	243	8.7	38.5	5.5	2.3
Focaccia, Sun Dried Tomato, & Olive, Chef Select, Lidl*	1/3 Focaccia/50g	128	3.9	257	7	38.3	7.8	2.6
Focaccia, Tomato, & Mozzarella, Chef Select, Lidl*	1 Serving/50g	133	3.4	266	8.8	41.2	6.8	2.2
Focaccia, Tomato, & Rosemary, TTD, Sainsbury's*	1 Serving/50g	118	3	236	6.9	37.1	6.1	2.7
French, Sliced, Parisian*	2 Slices/39g	100	1	256	5.1	48.7	2.6	0
French, Stick, Average	*1 Serving/60g*	*147*	*0.2*	*245*	*8.7*	*52.2*	*0.4*	*2.1*
Fried, Average	*1 Slice/28g*	*141*	*9*	*503*	*7.9*	*48.5*	*32.2*	*1.6*
Fruit Loaf, & Cinnamon, Finest, Tesco*	1 Slice/37g	134	4.9	363	6.4	54.6	13.2	1.5
Fruit Loaf, Apple & Cinnamon, Soreen*	1 Serving/10g	31	0.4	307	6.9	60.5	4.2	0
Fruit Loaf, Apple, M&S*	1 Slice/39g	100	0.6	255	8.5	51.9	1.5	3.3
Fruit Loaf, Banana, Soreen*	1 Slice/25g	76	1.2	305	7.2	55.6	5	4.4
Fruit Loaf, Cinnamon & Raisin, Soreen*	1/8 Loaf/25g	77	1	308	7.7	54.1	4	4.1
Fruit Loaf, Fruity Five, Snack Pack, Soreen*	1 Pack/45g	148	4	329	7.1	54.9	9	2.7
Fruit Loaf, Luxury, Christmas, Soreen*	1 Serving/28g	85	0.6	303	4.5	66.6	2.1	0
Fruit Loaf, Mixed Berry, Weight Watchers*	1 Slice/34g	79	0.9	231	7.6	44.3	2.6	7.7
Fruit Loaf, Plum, Lincolnshire, Soreen*	1 Slice/25g	65	0.8	261	8.4	49.3	3.4	2.1
Fruit Loaf, Sliced, Bakers Selection, Asda*	1 Serving/36g	100	1.5	278	8.2	50	4.2	3.6
Fruit Loaf, Sliced, Sainsbury's*	1 Slice/40g	104	1.4	260	8.9	47.9	3.6	2.4
Fruit Loaf, Sliced, Tesco*	1 Slice/36g	101	1.3	281	7.9	52.6	3.6	3.2
Fruit Loaf, Sultana & Cherry, Sainsbury's*	1 Slice/50g	178	6.1	357	2.7	59	12.2	1.7
Fruit Loaf, Toffee Apple, Soreen*	1 Bar/30g	98	1.5	326	8	59.8	5.1	4.5
Fruit Loaf, Winter Spice, Soreen*	1 Slice/52g	155	1.5	299	7.3	63.8	2.8	5.2
Fruit, & Spice, Extra Thick, Sliced, Vogel*	2 Slices/120g	290	4.1	241	8.3	41.7	3.4	4.9
Fruit, Loaf, Banana, Lunchbox, Soreen*	1 Bar/30g	98	1.7	326	8.1	59.5	5.5	4.6
Fruit, Loaf, Toasted, Cafe Instore, Asda*	1 Slice/33g	89	1.2	269	8	51	3.7	2.9
Fruit, Raisin Swirl, Sun-Maid*	1 Slice/33g	95	1.9	287	8.3	50.4	5.8	2.6
Garlic, & Cheese, Slices, Tesco*	1 Slice/30g	114	5	380	11.7	43.9	16.8	2
Garlic, & Tomato, Pizza, Italiano, Tesco*	½ Bread/140g	405	15.1	289	7.5	40.5	10.8	2.5
Garlic, & Herb, Slices, Reduced Fat, Asda*	1 Slice/33g	91	1.6	277	8.5	49	4.9	1.8
Garlic, 30% Less Fat, Morrisons*	1 Serving/80g	231	7.4	289	7.9	43.8	9.2	2.7
Garlic, Average	*1 Serving/100g*	*327*	*13.8*	*327*	*8.1*	*43.7*	*13.8*	*1.4*
Garlic, Baguette, Average	*1 Slice/20g*	*66*	*2.8*	*330*	*7.8*	*43.1*	*14.2*	*1.8*
Garlic, Baguette, Everyday Essentials, Aldi*	¼ Baguette/43g	148	6.4	349	8.1	45	15	1.4
Garlic, Baguette, Extra Strong, Italiano, Tesco*	¼ Baguette/53g	178	8.7	340	7.9	39.8	16.6	2.8

BREAD

INFO/WEIGHT	Measure	per Measure		Nutrition Values per 100g / 100ml				
		KCAL	FAT	KCAL	PROT	CARB	FAT	FIBRE
Garlic, Baguette, Extra Strong, Sainsbury's*	½ Baguette/85g	278	12.6	327	8.4	40	14.8	3.4
Garlic, Baguette, Free From, Tesco*	¼ Baguette/39g	137	6.2	352	1.2	49.1	15.8	4.4
Garlic, Baguette, HFC, Tesco*	1 Serving/85g	325	18.9	383	6.7	38.2	22.2	1.7
Garlic, Baguette, Italian, Asda*	¼ Baguette/48g	173	9.5	364	7	39	20	3.4
Garlic, Baguette, Italiano, Tesco*	¼ Baguette/53g	186	9.9	355	6.9	39.2	18.8	2.4
Garlic, Baguette, LC, Tesco*	¼ Baguette/52g	130	2.9	250	7	42.2	5.5	2.4
Garlic, Baguette, M&S*	¼ Baguette/52g	172	8.2	330	6.8	38.6	15.8	2.9
Garlic, Baguette, Morrisons*	½ Baguette/95g	316	12.1	333	8	45.9	12.7	1.5
Garlic, Baguette, Sainsbury's*	½ Baguette/85g	342	16.3	403	8.9	48.6	19.2	2.3
Garlic, Baguette, Slices, Tesco*	1 Serving/60g	187	9.2	312	9.8	33.8	15.3	1.7
Garlic, Baguette, Value, Tesco*	½ Baguette/85g	270	11.1	318	8.1	42	13.1	2.3
Garlic, Baguette, Waitrose*	½ Baguette/85g	290	15.2	341	7.1	37.8	17.9	0
Garlic, Cheesy, Slices, M&S*	1 Slice/28g	103	5	368	10.1	40.8	17.7	2.5
Garlic, Ciabatta, & Herb Butter, Sainsbury's*	½ Ciabatta/105g	345	16.3	329	8.5	38.8	15.5	0
Garlic, Ciabatta, Finest, Tesco*	1 Serving/65g	205	8.9	316	8.1	40.1	13.7	2.4
Garlic, Ciabatta, Italiano, Tesco*	1 Ciabatta/65g	211	9.4	324	7.7	40.9	14.4	2.2
Garlic, Ciabatta, Morrisons*	¼ Pack/73g	241	9.6	330	9.6	42.1	13.1	2.7
Garlic, Focaccia, & Rosemary, Sainsbury's*	¼ Focaccia/75g	219	7.4	292	8	43	9.8	2.8
Garlic, Focaccia, & Herb, Italian Style, Morrisons*	1/6 Focaccia/76g	259	10.9	341	8.5	44.7	14.3	2.5
Garlic, Homebake, Tesco*	1 Serving/60g	209	12.3	348	7.1	33.7	20.5	1.5
Garlic, Italian Style Stone Baked, Morrisons*	½ Pack/115g	420	22	365	7.9	40.4	19.1	1.9
Garlic, Pizza Bread, Co-Op*	1 Pizza/240g	756	31.2	315	8	41	13	2
Garlic, Slices, 50 % Less Fat, Asda*	1 Slice/29g	75	1.1	262	7.9	47.1	3.9	3.2
Garlic, Slices, Asda*	1 Slice/27g	88	3.3	328	8	46.2	12.4	2.8
Garlic, Slices, BGTY, Sainsbury's*	1 Slice/32g	96	2.1	304	8.9	51	6.6	2.7
Garlic, Slices, Chilled, Sainsbury's*	1 Pack/368g	1369	60	372	9.1	47.3	16.3	3.2
Garlic, Slices, LC, Tesco*	1 Slice/30g	75	1.7	250	7.3	42.3	5.7	2.9
Garlic, Slices, Morrisons*	1 Slice/32g	109	4.1	341	8.5	46.9	12.9	1.7
Garlic, Stonebaked, M&S*	1 Loaf/85g	314	14.4	369	8.6	44.4	16.9	2.4
Garlic, with Cheese, Asda*	1 Slice/34g	130	6.1	382	11	44	18	0
Giraffe, Sainsbury's*	1 Serving/50g	119	0.2	238	8.9	48.1	0.5	2.7
Grained, Soft, Farmhouse, Warburton's*	1 Slice/42g	109	1.7	258	10.2	44.6	4	5
Grains, & Seeds, Tasty, Warburton's*	1 Slice/38g	100	1.6	264	10.6	45.6	4.3	5.2
Granary, Average	**1 Med Slice/35g**	**85**	**1**	**242**	**9.8**	**44**	**2.8**	**4.8**
Granary, Baps, Large, Asda*	1 Bap/64g	143	1.4	224	10	41	2.2	4.3
Granary, M&S*	1 Slice/30g	75	0.9	250	9.5	46.4	3.1	3.2
Granary, Malted, Med Brown, Asda*	1 Slice/35g	81	0.9	231	9	43	2.6	3.3
Granary, Med Sliced, 800g, Hovis*	1 Slice/38g	97	0.9	256	10.3	46.4	2.4	3.7
Granary, Sliced, Sm Loaf, Hovis*	1 Slice/33g	84	0.8	256	10.3	46.4	2.4	3.7
Granary, Thick Slice, COU, M&S*	1 Slice/25g	60	0.6	240	10.5	44.1	2.2	6
Granary, Thick, Sliced, 800g, Hovis*	1 Slice/44g	112	1	256	10.3	46.4	2.4	3.7
Granary, Waitrose*	1 Slice/40g	88	1	220	9.4	39.9	2.5	4.3
Granary, Wholemeal, Average	**1 Slice/35g**	**80**	**0.9**	**228**	**10.8**	**38.4**	**2.6**	**6.6**
Half & Half, Medium, Warburton's*	1 Slice/40g	95	0.8	240	8.8	44.2	2	5
Half & Half, Toastie, Warburton's*	1 Slice/47g	112	0.9	240	8.8	44.2	2	5
Hardo, Sliced, National bran*	1 Slice/41g	138	0.9	336	11.1	66	2.2	4.4
Herby, Basket, Snack, Graze*	1 Punnet/20g	101	5	503	8	61	25	3
Herby, Basket, Snack, Retail, Graze*	1 Punnet/18g	90	4.3	500	8.1	61	24	3.5
High Bran, Loaf, M&S*	2 Slices/62g	143	2.4	230	13.1	31.7	3.9	7.7
Irish, Barm Brack, Tesco*	1 Serving/75g	232	5.2	310	16	47.6	6.9	3
Irish, Brown Soda, Tesco*	1 Serving/50g	110	1.9	219	9.2	36.2	3.8	6.4
Irish, Cottage Wheaten, Loaf, Tesco*	1 Serving/50g	116	1.3	231	8.6	41.4	2.6	4.2
Jalapeno Chilli, & Three Cheese, Bloomer, Bakery, Tesco*	1 Serving/82g	217	3.3	265	12	43.5	4.1	3

BREAD

INFO/WEIGHT	Measure	per Measure		Nutrition Values per 100g / 100ml				
		KCAL	FAT	KCAL	PROT	CARB	FAT	FIBRE
Juvela*	1 Slice/25g	60	0.8	240	3.3	50	3	1.7
Linseed & Wheat, Healthy Grain, Irish Pride*	1 Slice/38g	96	0.5	253	10.8	41	1.3	7
Low Carb, Protein Rich, Carbzone*	1 Slice/50g	132	6.5	264	22	7.5	13	14
Low GI, Multiseed, Percy Ingle*	1 Med Slice/35g	99	3.1	283	0	0	8.9	6
Malt Loaf, Buttered, 2 Slices, Soreen*	1 Pack/45g	150	3.9	333	7.5	54.2	8.6	4.4
Malt Loaf, Apple, Lunchbox, Soreen*	1 Slice/30g	92	1.3	307	7.7	57	4.5	4.4
Malt Loaf, Family, Asda*	1 Serving/20g	54	0.3	270	8	56	1.5	5
Malt Loaf, Fruited, Sliced, Weight Watchers*	1 Slice/23g	68	0.4	294	8.9	60.2	1.9	3.6
Malt Loaf, Fruity, Sliced, Soreen*	2 Slices/43g	129	1.3	300	8.2	58.2	3	3.9
Malt Loaf, Original, Low Fat, Soreen*	1 Slice/22g	63	0.4	288	7.5	60	1.6	2
Malt Loaf, Seeds & More, Soreen*	1 Serving/52g	174	3.8	336	10.1	54.3	7.4	5.9
Malt Loaf, Tesco*	1 Slice/50g	146	1.4	291	8.6	58	2.7	4.8
Malted Grain, Thick Cut, Loaf, Morrisons*	1 Slice/42g	106	1.1	251	10.1	44.5	2.5	5
Malted, & Seeded, Batch, Organic, Waitrose*	1 Slice/50g	118	2	236	10.9	39.5	3.9	6.2
Malted, Bloomer, Thick Sliced, Iceland*	1 Slice/51g	136	1.9	269	8.9	48	3.8	3.9
Malted, Brown, Slice, BGTY, Sainsbury's*	1 Slice/22g	53	0.6	239	12.1	41.4	2.8	5.8
Malted, Brown, Thick Sliced, Organic, Tesco*	1 Slice/44g	111	0.9	249	8.9	48.8	2	3.5
Malted, Crusty, Sainsbury's*	1 Slice/42g	109	1.4	259	8.6	48.6	3.3	4.4
Malted, Danish, Weight Watchers, Warburton's*	1 Slice/20g	51	0.3	249	11.8	45.1	1.5	4.2
Malted, Farmhouse, Morrisons*	1 Serving/40g	94	0.7	235	9.1	45.6	1.8	4.7
Malted, Grain, Baton, Tesco*	¼ Baton/57g	143	0.5	251	10.5	47.6	0.9	5
Malted, Grain, Co-Op*	1 Slice/43g	99	0.9	230	8	46	2	3
Malted, Grain, Good As Gold, Kingsmill*	1 Slice/47g	114	1.2	243	9.5	45.4	2.6	4.2
Malted, Grain, Loaf, Bakery, Tesco*	1 Slice/40g	100	0.4	250	10.5	47.6	0.9	5
Malted, Grain, Loaf, Sliced, Bakery, Tesco*	1 Slice/50g	122	0.7	244	9.1	46.6	1.4	4.3
Malted, Wheat Loaf, Crusty, Finest, Tesco*	1 Slice/50g	115	0.8	230	9.8	44.2	1.5	4.4
Malted, Wheatgrain, Roberts Bakery*	1 Slice/30g	80	1	265	11	48	3.3	3.6
Mediterranean, Olive, Waitrose*	1 Slice/30g	82	2.8	273	7.4	40.1	9.2	4.9
Mediterranean, Style, Stonebaked Tomato Batard, Tesco*	¼ Loaf/100g	256	3.1	256	9.8	45.5	3.1	3.5
Mixed Grain, Original, Sandwich, Vogel*	2 Slices/72g	144	1	201	9.7	34.7	1.4	4.5
Mixed Seed, Organic, Duchy Originals*	1 Slice/43g	114	3.4	269	10.9	39.1	8.1	5.3
Multi-Seed, Protein Punch, GF, Cob, Genius *	1 Slice/77g	189	7.7	246	14	19	10	11
Multi-Seeded, Farmhouse, Sliced, Loaf, Waitrose*	1 Slice/33g	96	2.9	291	11.2	38.5	8.8	6.7
Multicereal, Toast, Thins, Carrefour*	1 Serving/20g	77	1.2	383	16	62	5.9	8.5
Multigrain, Batch, Sliced, Tesco*	1 Slice/50g	120	0.9	241	9.3	43.7	1.8	6.2
Multigrain, Brown, Farmhouse Baker's, M&S*	1 Slice/51g	115	2.8	225	13	31.2	5.4	5.1
Multigrain, Crusty, Finest, Tesco*	1 Slice/40g	98	1.4	245	9	44.7	3.4	5
Multigrain, Farmhouse, Deluxe, Lidl*	1 Slice/40g	101	1.2	253	10.1	44.3	2.9	4.6
Multigrain, GF, Just Free, Lidl*	1 Slice/34g	23	0.4	69	1.6	10.1	1.3	4.6
Multigrain, GF, Sainsbury's*	1 Slice/17g	39	0.8	229	5.1	40.8	5	5.6
Multigrain, Med Sliced, Batch, Tesco*	1 Slice/50g	120	0.9	241	9.3	43.7	1.8	6.2
Multigrain, Sliced, Fresh And Easy*	1 Slice/40g	110	1	275	10	52.5	2.5	5
Multigrain, Sliced, Weight Watchers*	1 Slice/21g	50	0.5	238	9.5	42.9	2.4	9.5
Multigrain, Soft Batch, Sainsbury's*	1 Slice/44g	106	2.9	242	11.3	34.5	6.5	5.6
Multigrain, Thick Sliced, Tesco*	1 Slice/50g	112	1.2	225	8.4	42.2	2.5	3.9
Multiseed, Farmhouse Batch, Finest, Tesco*	1 Slice/44g	108	1.9	245	9.9	40.4	4.4	7.5
Multiseed, Farmhouse, Finest, Tesco*	1 Slice /50g	135	3.8	270	12.5	37	7.7	5.8
Multiseed, Sandwich, Thins, GF, Warburton's*	1 Thin/50g	142	4	284	6.5	43.1	8.1	6.5
Multiseed, Sliced, Free From, Tesco*	1 Slice/29g	85	3.4	294	6.7	34.8	11.8	10.7
Multiseeded, Bloomer, TTD, Sainsbury's*	1 Slice/50g	128	1.8	256	12	39.7	3.6	8.8
Naan, Asda*	1 Naan/130g	308	2.3	237	7.7	47.4	1.8	2.2
Naan, Average	**1 Naan/130g**	**344**	**5.6**	**264**	**8.3**	**48.5**	**4.3**	**2**
Naan, Bombay Brassiere, Sainsbury's*	1 Naan/140g	372	4.3	266	9.8	49.6	3.1	2.9

BREAD

	Measure INFO/WEIGHT	per Measure KCAL	FAT	Nutrition Values per 100g / 100ml KCAL	PROT	CARB	FAT	FIBRE
Naan, Chicken Tikka, Tandoori, Naanzza*	½ Naan/150g	337	9.6	225	10.9	30.7	6.4	1.3
Naan, Chilli & Mango, Finest, Tesco*	½ Naan/90g	230	5.1	255	8.4	41.9	5.7	3.2
Naan, Fresh, BGTY, Sainsbury's*	1 Serving/150g	368	4.6	245	9.4	44.9	3.1	2.2
Naan, Garlic & Coriander, Free From, Tesco*	1 Naan/90g	215	6	240	5.1	38.7	6.7	4.9
Naan, Garlic & Coriander, Tesco*	½ Naan/65g	184	3	283	7.5	51.2	4.6	3.3
Naan, Garlic & Coriander, TTD, Sainsbury's*	1 Naan/70g	219	8.4	313	7	44	12	2.9
Naan, Garlic & Coriander, Asda*	1 Naan/165g	473	10.1	287	7.9	48	6.1	5
Naan, Garlic & Coriander, Heritage*	1 Naan/130g	344	4.7	265	7.5	49	3.6	2.7
Naan, Garlic & Coriander, Mini, Asda*	1 Naan/110g	320	12.5	291	6.9	40.2	11.4	2.5
Naan, Garlic & Coriander, Mini, Sainsbury's*	1 Naan/48g	147	3.4	307	8.3	51.2	7	3
Naan, Garlic & Coriander, Mini, Sharwood's*	1 Naan/65g	196	4.2	302	8	51.5	6.5	2.8
Naan, Garlic & Coriander, Mini, Tesco*	1 Naan/50g	130	2.3	261	7.6	45.9	4.6	3
Naan, Garlic & Coriander, Mini, Weight Watchers*	1 Naan/40g	100	1	250	9.3	47.6	2.5	4.2
Naan, Garlic & Coriander, Patak's*	1 Naan/127g	373	7.7	294	7.9	50.9	6.1	2.4
Naan, Garlic & Coriander, Sainsbury's*	½ Naan/63g	167	2.5	264	8.1	47.3	4	3.4
Naan, Garlic & Coriander, The Spice Tailor*	1 Naan/110g	366	12.1	333	8.5	49	11	2.2
Naan, Garlic & Coriander, Weight Watchers*	1 Naan/60g	155	2.6	259	8.9	46	4.3	3.4
Naan, Garlic, & Coriander, Pana*	1 Naan/137g	372	11.4	271	7.1	42.1	8.3	2.1
Naan, Indian Meal for One, BGTY, Sainsbury's*	1 Serving/45g	115	1.9	257	10.3	44.2	4.3	2.1
Naan, Meal For Two, Korma/Tikka Masala, Tesco*	1 Naan/97g	291	6.8	300	8.6	49.1	7	3.3
Naan, Ocado*	½ Naan/75g	194	1.7	258	8.4	48.3	2.3	5.3
Naan, Onion & Mint, M&S*	½ Naan/135g	351	11.7	260	8.9	35.8	8.7	2.5
Naan, Onion Bhaji, Sharwood's*	1 Pack/130g	378	9.9	291	7.3	48.4	7.6	2.2
Naan, Peshwari, Apple & Coconut, Mini, Sharwood's*	1 Naan/65g	179	3.1	275	7.5	47.1	4.8	6.7
Naan, Peshwari, Flame Baked, Finest, Tesco*	½ Naan/75g	221	6.2	295	7.2	46.6	8.3	2.5
Naan, Peshwari, M&S*	1 Serving/127g	394	12.8	310	9.2	45.8	10.1	1.9
Naan, Peshwari, Mini, Bilash, Aldi*	1 Naan/58g	212	9.5	366	7	45.1	16.4	4.9
Naan, Peshwari, Sainsbury's*	1 Naan/166g	511	18.3	308	7.1	45.1	11	4.7
Naan, Peshwari, Sharwood's*	1 Naan/130g	334	6.9	257	7.2	45.1	5.3	2.5
Naan, Peshwari, Tesco*	1 Naan/215g	684	26.7	318	7.5	48.9	12.4	4.8
Naan, Plain, Average	*1 Naan/160g*	*437*	*10.5*	*273*	*8*	*45.7*	*6.5*	*2.1*
Naan, Plain, Finest, Tesco*	½ Naan/80g	206	4.1	257	8	43.2	5.1	3.1
Naan, Plain, Indian, Mini, Asda*	1 Naan/110g	329	12.6	299	6.6	42.2	11.5	2.1
Naan, Plain, Large, Sainsbury's*	½ Naan/70g	191	4.6	273	7.1	46.2	6.6	3
Naan, Plain, Mega, Indian Takeaway, Asda*	1 Naan/222g	572	8.4	258	7	49	3.8	2.5
Naan, Plain, Mini, Asda*	1 Naan/58g	156	2.7	269	8	49	4.6	2.3
Naan, Plain, Mini, BGTY, Sainsbury's*	1 Naan/50g	124	0.6	248	7.6	49.8	1.3	3.3
Naan, Plain, Mini, Weight Watchers*	1 Naan/44g	108	1.1	245	9.1	46.5	2.5	4.9
Naan, Plain, Sharwood's*	1 Naan/120g	326	8.9	272	8.5	42.9	7.4	2.4
Naan, Plain, Tesco*	1 Naan/150g	392	6.9	261	8.4	46.4	4.6	2.3
Naan, Plain, Value, Tesco*	1 Naan/135g	363	9.7	269	8.1	42.9	7.2	1.6
Naan, Santosh*	½ Naan/50g	150	3	300	8	48	6	2
Naan, Smart Price, Asda*	1 Naan/100g	233	1.9	233	8.7	45.3	1.9	2.8
Naan, Take Away, Tesco*	1 Naan/39g	97	1.3	248	8.7	45.6	3.4	1.7
Naan, Tandoori Baked, Waitrose*	1 Naan/140g	372	4.3	266	9.8	49.6	3.1	2.9
Naan, Tandoori, Sharwood's*	1 Naan/130g	330	6.5	254	7.3	45	5	2
Oatmeal, Farmhouse, Soft, M&S*	1 Slice/45g	110	2	245	11.1	39.5	4.4	5.2
Oatmeal, Sliced Loaf, Tesco*	1 Slice/50g	111	1.7	222	7.4	40.5	3.4	2.8
Olive, Mixed, Gail's*	100g	230	8.1	230	6.7	32.6	8.1	3
Olive, Waitrose*	1 Slice/28g	86	3	306	9	43.6	10.6	2
Onion, Roasted, M&S*	1 Slice/50g	125	1.6	250	9	46.7	3.3	2.1
Pain De Mie, 7 Cereales, Carrefour*	1 Slice/39g	108	2.3	277	9	44	6	4
Pain De Mie, Cereales, et Graines, Harrys*	2 Slices/46g	150	4.4	323	13	44.4	9.5	4

B

BREAD

	Measure INFO/WEIGHT	per Measure KCAL	FAT	Nutrition Values per 100g / 100ml KCAL	PROT	CARB	FAT	FIBRE
Paleo, Almond, GF, Non GMO, Julian Bakery*	1 Slice/43g	60	3	140	16.3	14	7	11.6
Pane Pugliese, Italian, Toasting, Crosta & Mollica*	1 Slice/69g	184	0.8	267	8.6	55.5	1.2	0.2
Pave, Walnut, Sainsbury's*	1 Serving/50g	140	4.8	280	9	40	9.5	3.5
Pave, Walnut, TTD, Sainsbury's*	1 Serving/50g	138	3.6	277	9.5	41.5	7.3	3.7
Petit Pain, Homebake, Mini, Tesco*	1 Roll/50g	144	0.6	289	8.6	59.1	1.2	3.5
Petit Pain, Mini, Homebake, Tesco*	1 Roll/45g	110	0.6	245	7.8	49.7	1.3	2.5
Petit Pain, Organic, Tesco*	1 Roll/100g	235	0.8	235	7.8	49.1	0.8	1.2
Petit Pain, Part Bake, Weight Watchers*	1 Roll/50g	111	0.4	223	6.8	43.5	0.9	6.8
Pitta, 159, Pride Valley*	1 Pitta/63g	159	1.2	252	10.1	51.2	1.9	2.6
Pitta, Brown, Organic, Waitrose*	1 Pitta/53g	124	0.5	234	8.5	43.9	1	7.4
Pitta, Free From, Sainsbury's*	1 Pitta/65g	164	2.5	252	4.1	50	3.9	2.9
Pitta, Garlic, Morrisons*	1 Pitta/60g	149	1.1	249	9.7	51.1	1.8	0
Pitta, Mediterranean Style, The Bakery, M&S*	1 Pitta/85g	247	3.7	291	6.7	54.9	4.3	2.8
Pitta, Pockets, Sainsbury's*	1 Pitta/75g	188	0.8	250	8.5	52	1	3.5
Pitta, Sd Tomato, Olive & Oregano, Extra Special, Asda*	1 Pitta/75g	194	0.8	259	7.1	55.2	1.1	1.6
Pitta, Seeded, HL, Tesco*	1 Pitta/60g	153	3.6	255	10.8	39.4	6	12.8
Pitta, Spelt, Albert Heijn*	1 Pitta/80g	196	0.8	245	2.5	48	1	0
Pitta, White, Average	*1 Pitta/75g*	*191*	*1.1*	*255*	*9.2*	*50.8*	*1.5*	*2.7*
Pitta, White, Essential, Waitrose*	1 Pitta/60g	157	0.5	262	9	53.4	0.9	2.3
Pitta, White, Free From, Tesco*	1 Pitta/55g	140	1.2	255	6.5	52.6	2.1	5.5
Pitta, White, Greek Style, Asda*	1 Pitta/50g	126	1	253	8	51	1.9	0
Pitta, White, Large, Tesco*	1 Pitta/80g	220	0.8	275	9.4	54.9	1	4.5
Pitta, White, Mini, Asda*	1 Pitta/18g	44	0.1	245	8.9	49	0.8	3.2
Pitta, White, Mini, Sainsbury's*	1 Pitta/20g	54	0.2	268	8.8	54.6	1.2	2
Pitta, White, Mini, Tesco*	1 Pitta/30g	84	0.6	280	9.8	55.1	2.1	3.4
Pitta, White, Sainsbury's*	1 Pitta/58g	160	0.7	275	9.8	54.7	1.2	3.1
Pitta, White, Soft, Sandwich, Warburton's*	½ Pitta/36g	81	0.9	228	9.8	41.4	2.6	1.8
Pitta, White, Speciality Breads, Waitrose*	1 Pitta/60g	149	0.7	249	10.3	49.3	1.2	3.5
Pitta, White, Tesco*	1 Pitta/58g	160	0.6	275	9.4	54.9	1	4.5
Pitta, White, Weight Watchers*	1 Pitta/45g	106	0.3	238	8.7	45.9	0.7	6.7
Pitta, Wholegrain, GF, BFree*	1 Pitta/55g	118	1.6	215	5.5	37.7	2.9	8.2
Pitta, Wholemeal with Extra Virgin Olive Oil, Tesco*	1 Pitta/60g	135	1.6	225	8.3	41.5	2.6	5.5
Pitta, Wholemeal, Acropolis, Lidl*	1 Pitta/57g	136	0.9	238	12	44	1.6	6
Pitta, Wholemeal, Asda*	1 Pitta/56g	133	0.9	238	12	44	1.6	6
Pitta, Wholemeal, Average	*1 Pitta/64g*	*154*	*1.1*	*241*	*11*	*45.8*	*1.7*	*6.4*
Pitta, Wholemeal, Dina*	1 Pitta/75g	182	1.1	243	10.6	46.7	1.5	4.9
Pitta, Wholemeal, Essential, Waitrose*	1 Pitta/60g	159	0.7	264	9.7	50.1	1.2	7.2
Pitta, Wholemeal, Healthy Eating, Co-Op*	1 Pitta/63g	135	1.3	215	12	37	2	9
Pitta, Wholemeal, Hollyland Bakery*	1 Pitta/20g	48	0.3	242	13.1	43.7	1.6	6
Pitta, Wholemeal, M&S*	1 Pitta/60g	155	1.6	255	10	45	2.6	5.5
Pitta, Wholemeal, Mini, M&S*	1 Pitta/18g	44	0.4	247	10.3	45.8	2.5	5.6
Pitta, Wholemeal, Mini, Sainsbury's*	1 Pitta/30g	69	0.5	231	10	43.8	1.7	6.2
Pitta, Wholemeal, Mini, Tesco*	1 Pitta/30g	76	0.5	255	11.8	48.2	1.7	4.2
Pitta, Wholemeal, Sainsbury's*	1 Pitta/57g	154	0.9	271	10.9	49.7	1.5	7.4
Pitta, Wholemeal, Simple & Versatile, As Sold, Tesco*	1 Pitta/58g	145	0.7	250	9.6	46.2	1.2	7.8
Pitta, Wholemeal, So Organic, Sainsbury's*	1 Pitta/60g	140	1	233	9.8	44.8	1.6	8.1
Pitta, Wholemeal, Tesco*	1 Pitta/58g	145	0.7	250	9.6	46.2	1.2	7.8
Pitta, Wholemeal, Waitrose*	1 Pitta/60g	145	0.5	242	12.4	46	0.9	3.1
Potato, & Rosemary, M&S*	1 Serving/40g	108	2.7	270	9.4	42.2	6.8	2.3
Potato, Farls, Irish, Rankin Selection, Irwin's Bakery*	1 Farl/60g	110	2.2	184	2.3	34.4	3.6	2.5
Potato, Farls, M&S*	1 Farl/55g	79	0.2	144	4.2	33.8	0.4	4.7
Potato, Farls, Sunblest*	1 Farl/100g	156	0.9	156	3.8	33.2	0.9	1.9
Pumpernickel, Average	*1 Slice/50g*	*96*	*0.6*	*191*	*5.5*	*37.9*	*1.1*	*7.8*

BREAD

	Measure INFO/WEIGHT	per Measure KCAL	FAT	Nutrition Values per 100g / 100ml KCAL	PROT	CARB	FAT	FIBRE
Pumpernickel, Organic, Bavarian Pumpernickel*	1 Slice/50g	90	0.5	180	6	38	1	10
Pumpernickel, Organic, Biona*	1 Slice/80g	158	1.4	197	4.6	36	1.7	9.6
Pumpernickel, Rye, Kelderman*	1 Slice/50g	92	0.5	185	6	38	1	0
Pumpkin Seed, Chleb Dyniowy, The Polish Bakery*	1 Slice/40g	100	2	250	7.1	45.5	5.1	6.4
Pumpkin Seed, Raisin & Sunflower Seed, Sainsbury's*	1 Slice/30g	76	0.8	255	11.6	45.9	2.8	3.4
Pure Grain, Heart of Nature, Pure Nature*	1 Slice/55g	172	9.1	313	9.7	24.8	16.6	7.9
Pure Grain, with Prunes, Pure Nature*	1 Slice/50g	169	10.4	338	8	28.3	20.8	9
Raisin, & Pumpkin Seed, Organic, Tesco*	1 Slice/30g	76	1.7	253	9.7	40.6	5.8	3.8
Raisin, with Cinnamon, Warburton's*	1 Slice/36g	96	1.3	267	7.2	51.1	3.7	3.2
Richly Fruited, Loaf, Waitrose*	1 Slice/34g	99	1.5	292	7.5	54.2	4.4	2.8
Roll, Malted Wheat, Bakery, Waitrose*	1 Roll/85g	222	1	262	7.9	52.2	1.2	5.5
Roll, Oatmeal, Deli, M&S*	1 Roll/75g	202	2.8	270	10.9	46.3	3.7	3.7
Roll, Scotch, Sainsbury's*	1 Roll/79g	200	1.9	253	9.2	47	2.4	3.4
Roll, Sourdough, Seeded, Gail's*	1 Roll/70g	196	5.5	280	10.2	39.8	7.9	4.6
Roll, Super Seeded, GF, Made Without Wheat, M&S*	1 Roll/75g	170	6.2	227	8	24	8.3	12
Roll, Wholemeal, Deli, Iceland*	1 Roll/59g	143	1.5	242	9.3	42.4	2.6	5.8
Rolls, American Style Deli, Tesco*	1 Roll/65g	162	2.2	249	7.8	46.8	3.4	1.6
Rolls, Ancient Grain, Tesco*	1 Roll/80g	231	6.7	289	14.7	34.4	8.4	8.6
Rolls, Best of Both, Hovis*	1 Roll/62g	148	2.9	239	9.8	39.7	4.6	5
Rolls, Brioche, Average	*1 Roll/49g*	*177*	*6.9*	*361*	*8.8*	*50.1*	*14.1*	*1.5*
Rolls, Brioche, Butter, Tesco*	1 Serving/35g	120	3.7	344	8.5	52.9	10.5	2.2
Rolls, Brioche, Continental Classics*	1 Roll/35g	122	3.3	349	8.2	58.3	9.3	0
Rolls, Brioche, Finest, Tesco*	1 Roll/52g	207	11.6	398	10.8	38.3	22.4	2
Rolls, Brioche, French Milk, Bon Appetit, Aldi*	1 Roll/35g	116	2.7	330	8.3	56	7.8	2.2
Rolls, Brioche, Hot Dog, Specially Selected, Aldi*	1 Roll/45g	142	3.4	316	9.4	52	7.5	2
Rolls, Brioche, Hot Dog, TTD, Sainsbury's*	1 Roll/70g	229	7.3	327	8.3	48.6	10.4	2.8
Rolls, Brioche, La Boulangere, Lidl*	1 Roll/35g	122	3.6	350	8.2	55.5	10.2	1.8
Rolls, Brioche, Plain Chocolate Chip, Sainsbury's*	1 Roll/35g	126	4.5	361	8	52.1	12.9	2.1
Rolls, Brioche, Sainsbury's*	1 Roll/35g	123	3.9	352	8.1	53.5	11.3	1.8
Rolls, Brioche, Tesco*	1 Roll/26g	92	2.9	349	8.5	54	11	0
Rolls, Brown, bake at Home, Aldi*	1 Roll/45g	131	1.5	291	10	52	3.3	5.8
Rolls, Brown, Ciabatta, Schar*	1 Roll/50g	138	4.1	274	5.8	40	8.1	8.9
Rolls, Brown, Crusty	*1 Roll/50g*	*128*	*1.4*	*255*	*10.3*	*50.4*	*2.8*	*3.5*
Rolls, Brown, Free From, Tesco*	1 Roll/65g	174	5.3	268	5.4	43.2	8.2	3.6
Rolls, Brown, Large, Asda*	1 Roll/57g	138	0.9	242	10	47	1.6	0
Rolls, Brown, M&S*	1 Roll/105g	242	6.4	230	9.2	37.3	6.1	4.4
Rolls, Brown, Malted Grain, Tesco*	1 Roll/58g	144	1.9	248	8.7	46.2	3.2	1.9
Rolls, Brown, Mini, M&S*	1 Roll/33g	80	2.5	245	9.8	35.5	7.6	3.8
Rolls, Brown, Morning, Farmfoods*	1 Roll/50g	134	1.8	269	12	47	3.7	4.2
Rolls, Brown, Old Fashioned, Waitrose*	1 Roll/63g	152	2.6	241	9.6	41.3	4.1	4.7
Rolls, Brown, Part Baked, Sunnyhills, Aldi*	1 Roll/50g	129	1.5	258	9.3	45.3	3	6.3
Rolls, Brown, Seeded, Organic, Sainsbury's*	1 Roll/70g	166	3.2	237	9.9	39.1	4.6	6.5
Rolls, Brown, Snack, Allinsons*	1 Roll/47g	128	2.5	272	10.2	43.5	5.3	4.9
Rolls, Brown, Soft, Average	*1 Roll/50g*	*134*	*1.9*	*268*	*10*	*51.8*	*3.8*	*3.5*
Rolls, Brown, Soft, Organic, Sainsbury's*	1 Roll/70g	166	3.2	237	9.9	39.1	4.6	6.6
Rolls, Brown, Soft, Tesco*	1 Roll/50g	125	0.5	250	9.2	49.7	1	2.6
Rolls, Cheese Topped, Sandwich, Warburton's*	1 Roll/62g	168	4	270	12.1	40.7	6.5	2.6
Rolls, Cheese Topped, Village Green*	1 Roll/56g	159	4.1	284	13.1	41.2	7.4	4.8
Rolls, Cheese, Rustique, Waitrose*	1 Roll/90g	255	3.4	283	11.3	49.7	3.8	2.6
Rolls, Cheesy Topped, Village Bakery, Aldi*	1 Serving/100g	206	4.4	206	8	0	4.4	1.4
Rolls, Chunky Cheese, Tesco*	1 Roll/80g	219	4.8	274	12.8	41.1	6	2
Rolls, Ciabatta, Cheese Topped, Mini, Finest, Tesco*	1 Roll/30g	85	2.4	282	11.5	40.9	8.1	3.8
Rolls, Ciabatta, Garlic, Asda*	1 Roll/93g	333	16.7	358	9	40	18	2.3

BREAD

	Measure INFO/WEIGHT	per Measure KCAL	FAT	Nutrition Values per 100g / 100ml KCAL	PROT	CARB	FAT	FIBRE
Rolls, Ciabatta, GF, Schar*	1 Roll/50g	112	1.3	219	3.7	41	2.6	8.7
Rolls, Ciabatta, Mini, Finest, Tesco*	1 Roll/30g	89	2	297	9.9	49.1	6.8	4.1
Rolls, Ciabatta, Sun Dried Tomato, Mini, Finest, Tesco*	1 Roll/30g	79	1.9	262	8.7	42.3	6.4	2.6
Rolls, Ciabatta, Tesco*	1 Roll/100g	295	5.6	295	9.2	50.5	5.6	3
Rolls, Country Grain, Mini, M&S*	1 Roll/31g	85	3	275	10.2	38.9	9.7	3.8
Rolls, Crisp, Original, Organic, Kallo*	1 Roll/9g	34	0.5	390	11	74	5.6	3
Rolls, Crusty, French, M&S*	1 Roll/65g	159	0.8	245	8.1	50.5	1.2	3.3
Rolls, Crusty, Part-Baked, Budgens*	1 Roll/50g	148	0.7	296	9.4	61.4	1.4	2.5
Rolls, Finger, Morrisons*	1 Roll/46g	119	0.8	259	10.7	50	1.8	2.3
Rolls, Finger, White, Sainsbury's*	1 Roll/40g	96	1	240	9	45.2	2.6	3.2
Rolls, Focaccia, Tesco*	1 Roll/75g	226	7	302	8.7	45.6	9.4	3.8
Rolls, Granary Malted Wheatgrain, Soft, M&S*	1 Roll/80g	208	3.1	260	9.3	47.2	3.9	2.3
Rolls, Granary, Average	**1 Roll/70g**	**176**	**2.7**	**251**	**9.6**	**45.2**	**3.9**	**3.3**
Rolls, Granary, Bakers Premium, Tesco*	1 Roll/65g	158	0.8	243	9.9	47.8	1.3	2.3
Rolls, Granary, Mini, Tesco*	1 Roll/34g	92	2.2	271	10	43.5	6.5	3.8
Rolls, Granary, Waitrose*	1 Roll/59g	160	3.8	271	10	47.2	6.4	3.8
Rolls, Green Olive, M&S*	1 Roll/75g	210	4.5	280	11.2	44	6	1.8
Rolls, Half & Half, Warburton's*	1 Roll/55g	144	2.5	261	10.4	42.7	4.5	4
Rolls, Heyford Wholemeal, Soft & Grainy, Waitrose*	1 Roll/75g	164	1.3	219	11.2	36.7	1.7	5.8
Rolls, Hot Dog, Tesco*	1 Roll/85g	200	2.8	235	7.3	44	3.3	1.9
Rolls, Hot Dog, Value, Tesco*	1 Roll/40g	93	0.8	232	8.7	45	1.9	2.2
Rolls, Hot Dog, White, Warburton's*	1 Roll/55g	142	2.1	259	8.8	46.4	3.9	1.6
Rolls, Low GI, Lidl*	1 Roll/60g	177	5.1	295	14	44.9	8.5	8.4
Rolls, Malted Grain, Sainsbury's*	1 Roll/68g	190	2.9	280	8.7	51.6	4.3	4.2
Rolls, Malted Grain, Submarine, M&S*	1 Roll/109g	300	4.7	275	8.9	53.6	4.3	3
Rolls, Malted, Whole Grain Rolls, Batched, Soft, M&S*	1 Roll/80g	180	3.6	225	7.8	38.5	4.5	3.1
Rolls, Mini Submarine, M&S*	1 Roll/23g	63	1.1	275	11.4	47.7	4.9	1.1
Rolls, Morning, Scottish, Warburton's*	1 Roll/50g	138	0.4	276	10.9	56.2	0.8	2.1
Rolls, Morning, Tesco*	1 Roll/48g	117	1.2	243	10.4	44.8	2.5	4.7
Rolls, Multi Seed, Free From, Free From, Tesco*	1 Roll/70g	214	8.3	305	5.4	44.2	11.8	6.3
Rolls, Multigrain, Sourdough, Paul Hollywood*	1 Roll/75g	192	2.5	256	8.4	46.1	3.3	4.2
Rolls, Multigrain, Torpedo, Sainsbury's*	1 Roll/112g	328	7.5	293	10.5	47.7	6.7	6.3
Rolls, Multiseed, Deli, Tesco*	1 Roll/65g	188	4.6	289	10.5	40.7	7.1	10.3
Rolls, Multiseed, Genius*	1 Roll/70g	209	7.8	299	3.9	40.6	11.2	10
Rolls, Nut & Raisin, Bakery, Tesco*	1 Serving/120g	426	11.2	355	9	56.8	9.3	4
Rolls, Oatmeal, Soft, M&S*	1 Roll/83g	224	3.9	270	12.3	43.4	4.7	3.4
Rolls, Olive, Mixed, Waitrose*	1 Roll/90g	240	2.5	267	8.8	50	2.8	3
Rolls, Panini, Sainsbury's*	1 Roll/90g	249	5.6	276	11	44.1	6.2	3
Rolls, Panini, White, Tesco*	1 Roll/85g	232	4.1	273	10.7	44.9	4.8	3.4
Rolls, Part Baked, Mini, Tesco*	1 Roll/50g	120	0.6	240	7.8	49.5	1.2	3.4
Rolls, Poppy Seeded Knot, Waitrose*	1 Roll/60g	169	3.2	282	10.3	48.3	5.3	2.2
Rolls, Posh Dog, The Grill, M&S*	1 Roll/64g	195	5.6	305	8.7	45.4	8.8	4.5
Rolls, Pumpkin Seed, Lidl*	1 Roll/80g	271	9	339	15	42.5	11.2	3.8
Rolls, Rustic, Ready to Bake, Paul Hollywood*	1 Roll/75g	199	0.8	265	8.5	54.7	1	1.7
Rolls, Rye, Toasting, Good & Hot*	1 Roll/65g	143	0.7	220	7.3	44.6	1.1	7.1
Rolls, Scotch, Morning, Tesco*	1 Roll/50g	136	0.6	273	11.8	52	1.3	3.2
Rolls, Scottish Morning, Morrisons*	1 Roll/60g	157	1.3	261	11.3	51.4	2.2	2.4
Rolls, Seeded, Deli, Rowan Hill Bakery, Lidl*	1 Roll/75g	243	8.2	324	11.4	42.2	11	5.4
Rolls, Seeded, Mixed Mini Loaf Pack, M&S*	1 Roll/76g	220	7.3	290	10.6	39.7	9.6	4
Rolls, Seeded, Soft, GF, Newburn, Warburton's*	1 Roll/65g	176	6.2	270	9	33.8	9.5	6.7
Rolls, Snack, Mini, Tesco*	1 Roll/35g	95	2.1	271	19	43	6	4
Rolls, Soft, White, Rowan Hill Bakery, Lidl*	1 Roll/66g	157	1.6	238	8.5	44	2.5	2.8
Rolls, Soft, Wholemeal, Finger, M&S*	1 Roll/66g	145	1.3	220	12.6	38	2	5.8

B

BREAD

	Measure INFO/WEIGHT	per Measure KCAL	FAT	Nutrition Values per 100g / 100ml KCAL	PROT	CARB	FAT	FIBRE
Rolls, Stone Baked, Bakery Instore, Lidl*	1 Roll/100g	292	1.5	292	9.5	58.4	1.5	3.5
Rolls, Sub, White, Batch, Warburton's*	1 Roll/80g	215	3.5	269	11	45	4.4	2.4
Rolls, Sub, Wholemeal, Warburton's*	1 Roll/94g	231	4.1	246	10.9	40.6	4.4	6.3
Rolls, Submarine, Sainsbury's*	1 Roll/117g	305	4.6	261	9.1	47.4	3.9	2.4
Rolls, Sun Dried Tomato, Homebake, Tesco*	1 Roll/50g	123	1.5	246	11.3	44	3	0
Rolls, Sunflower Seed, Toasting, Good & Hot*	1 Roll/65g	162	3.2	250	8.5	41	5	8
Rolls, Tiger, Crusty, Baked by Us, Morrisons*	1 Roll/63g	143	1.8	227	6.3	46	2.9	2.5
Rolls, Triple Seeded, Genius *	1 Roll/70g	209	7.8	299	3.9	40.6	11.2	10
Rolls, White with Mixed Seeds & Bran, Wheatfield Bakery*	1 Roll/76g	190	3.9	250	8.5	41.6	5.1	6.1
Rolls, White, 4 Pack, Warburton's*	1 Roll/58g	145	2.5	253	9.7	42.6	4.3	2.4
Rolls, White, 50/50, Soft, Kingsmill*	1 Roll/63g	154	2.4	245	9.3	41.2	3.8	4.4
Rolls, White, BGTY, Sainsbury's*	1 Roll/50g	114	0.5	227	9.1	45.3	1	3
Rolls, White, Cheese Topped, Asda*	1 Roll/46g	121	2	264	10	46	4.4	2
Rolls, White, Cheese Topped, Sainsbury's*	1 Roll/75g	218	6.4	291	12.1	41.6	8.5	2
Rolls, White, Crusty, Average	*1 Roll/50g*	*140*	*1.2*	*280*	*10.9*	*57.6*	*2.3*	*1.5*
Rolls, White, Crusty, Bakery, Tesco*	1 Roll/70g	193	0.6	276	9.3	56.7	0.8	2.6
Rolls, White, Crusty, Home Bake, Tesco*	1 Roll/69g	185	1	270	9.3	54.2	1.4	2.9
Rolls, White, Crusty, Morning, M&S*	1 Roll/65g	176	0.8	270	8.8	53.8	1.3	2.7
Rolls, White, Dinner, Village Bakery, Aldi*	1 Roll/70g	183	0.9	262	8.8	52	1.3	3
Rolls, White, Finest, Tesco*	1 Roll/80g	198	2	247	9.3	45.3	2.5	3
Rolls, White, Finger, Smart Price, Asda*	1 Roll/50g	121	0.8	242	9	48	1.6	2.1
Rolls, White, Finger, Tesco*	1 Roll/45g	112	0.4	250	9.2	49.7	1	2.6
Rolls, White, Finger, Value, Tesco*	1 Roll/50g	116	1	232	8.7	45	1.9	2.2
Rolls, White, Floured, Batch, Tesco*	1 Roll/76g	193	2.5	254	8.8	47.3	3.3	2.2
Rolls, White, Floury Batch, Sainsbury's*	1 Roll/68g	168	1.9	247	8.3	47.2	2.8	2.2
Rolls, White, Floury, Roberts Bakery*	1 Roll/63g	160	1.6	254	8.4	49.5	2.5	2
Rolls, White, Free From, Co-Op*	1 Roll/65g	80	1.4	123	3.5	19	2.1	6
Rolls, White, Hot Dog, Jumbo, Sainsbury's*	1 Roll/85g	239	5.2	281	7.5	49.1	6.1	2.9
Rolls, White, Hot Dog, Tesco*	1 Roll/65g	162	0.6	250	9.2	49.7	1	2.6
Rolls, White, Hot Dog, Tesco*	1 Roll/70g	177	2.5	254	9	45.5	3.6	1.9
Rolls, White, Large, Warburton's*	1 Roll/88g	229	3.1	259	10.2	44.3	3.5	2.5
Rolls, White, Low Price, Sainsbury's*	1 Roll/44g	107	0.7	243	8.9	48.2	1.6	2.1
Rolls, White, Mini, Submarine, M&S*	1 Roll/30g	86	1.5	285	11.4	47.7	4.9	1.1
Rolls, White, Morning, Co-Op*	1 Roll/47g	134	1.4	285	12	53	3	2
Rolls, White, Old Fashioned, Waitrose*	1 Roll/64g	176	2.9	275	8.8	49.8	4.5	2.8
Rolls, White, Organic, Sainsbury's*	1 Roll/65g	170	2	262	8.7	49.9	3	1
Rolls, White, Part Baked, Morrisons*	1 Roll/75g	227	1	303	9.6	63	1.4	2.6
Rolls, White, Sandwich, Sliced, Warburton's*	1 Roll/55g	146	2.1	265	9.7	46.6	3.9	2.4
Rolls, White, Scottish, Tesco*	1 Roll/48g	117	1.2	243	10.4	44.8	2.5	4.7
Rolls, White, Seeded, Sainsbury's*	1 Roll/80g	217	4.7	271	10.9	43.4	5.9	4.8
Rolls, White, Seeded, Soft, M&S*	1 Roll/75g	214	4.3	285	11.7	46.2	5.7	2.8
Rolls, White, Sliced, Morrisons*	1 Roll/59g	157	2.1	266	8.4	48.7	3.5	2.8
Rolls, White, Sliced, Warburton's*	1 Roll/55g	146	2.2	265	9.7	46.6	3.9	2.4
Rolls, White, Snack, Sainsbury's*	1 Roll/67g	159	0.7	237	7.9	49.2	1	2.3
Rolls, White, Soft, Average	*1 Sm Roll/45g*	*114*	*1.5*	*253*	*9.2*	*46.5*	*3.3*	*2.2*
Rolls, White, Soft, Dietary Specials*	1 Roll/75g	130	2.9	172	2.2	29.8	3.8	4.7
Rolls, White, Soft, Farmhouse, TTD, Sainsbury's*	1 Slice/47g	111	0.8	235	8.1	45.4	1.7	2.9
Rolls, White, Soft, GF, Newburn Bakehouse, Warburton's*	1 Roll/65g	159	4	244	7.3	37.1	6.2	5.4
Rolls, White, Soft, Hovis*	1 Roll/70g	180	3.1	257	9.5	44.8	4.4	3
Rolls, White, Soft, M&S*	1 Roll/60g	150	1.9	250	10.3	45.2	3.1	2.7
Rolls, White, Soft, Morrisons*	1 Roll/42g	100	0.8	238	9.1	46.4	1.9	2.4
Rolls, White, Soft, Tesco*	1 Roll/55g	137	0.6	250	9.2	49.7	1	2.6
Rolls, White, Softgrain, GFY, Asda*	1 Roll/54g	128	1	237	9	46	1.9	2.9

B

BREAD

INFO/WEIGHT	Measure	per Measure KCAL	FAT	Nutrition Values per 100g / 100ml KCAL	PROT	CARB	FAT	FIBRE
Rolls, White, Split, Asda*	1 Roll/45g	113	1.5	251	10	45	3.4	2.8
Rolls, White, Submarine, M&S*	1 Roll/109g	300	5.4	275	11	47	5	1
Rolls, White, Super Soft, Bakers Selection, Asda*	1 Roll/64g	173	2.9	272	7.5	49	4.6	2.5
Rolls, White, Tesco*	1 Roll/65g	180	2.5	277	8.7	52	3.8	2.7
Rolls, White, Tesco*	1 Roll/30g	79	0.7	262	9.7	50.5	2.3	2.9
Rolls, Wholemeal	*1 Roll/45g*	*108*	*1.3*	*241*	*9*	*48.3*	*2.9*	*5.9*
Rolls, Wholemeal & White, Kingsmill*	1 Roll/60g	151	2.5	251	9.5	43.7	4.2	3.5
Rolls, Wholemeal, & Oat, Warburton's*	1 Roll/70g	167	2.5	239	10.5	38	3.6	6
Rolls, Wholemeal, Asda*	1 Roll/58g	130	1.6	225	11	39	2.8	6
Rolls, Wholemeal, Deli, Tesco*	1 Serving/65g	156	3.1	240	9	40.2	4.8	5.7
Rolls, Wholemeal, Finest, Tesco*	1 Roll/75g	182	2.6	243	11.3	39	3.4	5.9
Rolls, Wholemeal, Finger, Six, Bakers Selection, Asda*	1 Roll/49g	112	0.7	228	9.5	41	1.4	6.6
Rolls, Wholemeal, Floury Batch, Sainsbury's*	1 Roll/68g	152	2.3	223	9.9	37.8	3.4	6.5
Rolls, Wholemeal, Mini, Assorted, Waitrose*	1 Roll/35g	86	2.1	244	9.7	37.9	6	7.3
Rolls, Wholemeal, Morrisons*	1 Roll/67g	155	2.7	231	10.2	38.6	4	6.3
Rolls, Wholemeal, Oat Topped, Deli, Tesco*	1 Roll/65g	170	3.5	260	10.9	38.3	5.3	6.7
Rolls, Wholemeal, Oat Topped, Tesco*	1 Roll/65g	166	2.9	255	11.3	42.2	4.5	5.1
Rolls, Wholemeal, Oaty, Deli Rolls, Morrisons*	1 Roll/65g	153	2	235	10.4	41.3	3.1	6.6
Rolls, Wholemeal, Old Fashioned, Waitrose*	1 Roll/57g	135	2.7	236	11.1	37.2	4.8	6.6
Rolls, Wholemeal, Organic, Sainsbury's*	1 Roll/66g	152	1.8	230	10.7	41	2.7	6.6
Rolls, Wholemeal, Plaited, Morrisons*	1 Roll/100g	195	1	195	6	30	1	6
Rolls, Wholemeal, Sainsbury's*	1 Roll/65g	153	2.1	236	10.7	40.8	3.3	7.4
Rolls, Wholemeal, Seeded, The Country Miller, Waitrose*	1 Roll/75g	190	7.7	255	13.6	26.9	10.3	7.6
Rolls, Wholemeal, Sliced, Sandwich, Warburton's*	1 Roll/56g	130	2.2	233	10.5	35.8	3.9	6.6
Rolls, Wholemeal, Soft, Average	*1 Roll/65g*	*151*	*2.7*	*233*	*10.8*	*37.3*	*4.1*	*6.3*
Rolls, Wholemeal, Soft, Batch Baked, Warburton's*	1 Roll/65g	158	2.1	245	10.7	37.3	3.2	6.1
Rolls, Wholemeal, Soft, Sainsbury's*	1 Roll/60g	133	2	221	9.9	37.8	3.4	6.5
Rolls, Wholemeal, Soft, Seeded, Sainsbury's*	1 Roll/75g	193	5.6	257	11.8	35.6	7.4	6.2
Rolls, Wholemeal, Sunflower & Honey, Sainsbury's*	1 Roll/100g	311	8.1	311	10.8	45.9	8.1	5.4
Rolls, Wholemeal, Super Soft, Bakers Selection, Asda*	1 Roll/65g	181	2.5	280	9.8	48	3.9	6.9
Rolls, Wholemeal, Tasty, Kingsmill*	1 Roll/68g	171	2.5	251	10.7	39.1	3.7	6.5
Rolls, Wholemeal, Tesco*	1 Roll/46g	115	1.8	250	10.9	41.8	4	7.5
Rolls, Wholemeal, The Best, Morrisons*	1 Roll/72g	174	2.1	242	10.5	39.7	2.9	7.6
Rolls, Wholemeal, Village Bakery, Aldi*	1 Roll/63g	144	0.9	228	10	40	1.5	5.3
Rolls, Wholmeal, Deli, Tesco*	1 Roll/65g	156	3.1	240	9	40.2	4.8	5.7
Rolls, York Baps, Adkins Bakery*	1 Roll/100g	264	2.2	264	10.7	53.7	2.2	2.4
Roti, Tesco*	1 Bread/95g	256	5.2	269	8.4	46.4	5.5	3.2
Rye, & Flax, Organic, Profusion*	1 Slice/50g	120	4.4	241	20.1	14.4	8.9	11.4
Rye, & Mixed Seed, Dark, Boule, Finest, Tesco*	1 Slice/35g	86	1.2	248	12.1	39.2	3.4	5.9
Rye, Average	*1 Slice/25g*	*55*	*0.4*	*219*	*8.3*	*45.8*	*1.7*	*4.4*
Rye, Dark, Sliced, Trianon*	1 Slice/41g	74	0.6	180	6.5	35	1.5	0
Rye, German Style, Bolletje*	1 Slice/60g	114	1.2	190	6	35	2	9.5
Rye, German Style, Kelderman*	1 Slice/64g	113	0.6	177	6.1	34.4	1	8.3
Rye, German Style, Loaf, Bakery in Store, M&S*	2 Slices/50g	112	0.6	225	9.5	40.8	1.1	6.3
Rye, Half Wheat, The Polish Bakery, Tesco*	1 Slice/40g	93	0.6	233	5.7	51.1	1.5	6.6
Rye, Light, Boule, Bakery, Waitrose*	1 Slice/50g	132	2.1	264	8.5	45.6	4.2	5.2
Rye, Light, Finest, Tesco*	1 Slice/20g	47	0.4	237	10.4	44.3	2	3.7
Rye, Russian, Gail's*	1 Loaf/800g	1704	8.8	213	6.2	41.3	1.1	5.2
Rye, Seeded, Organic, The Village Bakery*	1 Slice/50g	107	1.6	214	5	37.8	3.2	7.2
Rye, Sourdough, Part Baked, TTD, Sainsbury's*	1 Slice/30g	70	0.4	233	6.5	45	1.3	7.8
Rye, Stone Baked, Dutch Style , Kelderman*	1 Slice/55g	128	0.5	233	8.1	46	0.9	5.1
Rye, Swedish Style, Kelderman*	1 Slice/50g	92	1.6	185	7.2	31.5	3.2	4.3
Rye, Vitality, Organic, Biona*	1 Slice/71g	147	1.4	207	5.3	37	2	9.9

BREAD

	Measure INFO/WEIGHT	per Measure KCAL	FAT	Nutrition Values per 100g / 100ml KCAL	PROT	CARB	FAT	FIBRE
Rye, Whole Grain, Schneiderbrot*	1 Slice/50g	100	0.5	201	5.2	38.9	1	7.7
Rye, Wholegrain , Sliced, Rowan Hill Bakery, Lidl*	1 Slice/56g	118	1	210	5.8	38	1.8	9.3
Rye, Wholegrain, with Sunflower Seeds, Rowan Hill*	1 Slice/56g	126	2.6	225	6.3	35	4.6	9.3
Rye, Wholemeal with Sunflower Seeds, Organic, Biona*	1 Slice/72g	150	2.9	210	7	36	4	6
Rye, Wholemeal, Mestemacher*	1 Slice/72g	165	0.6	229	4.9	44.6	0.9	11.5
Rye, Wholemeal, Organic, House Of Westphalia*	1 Slice/71g	131	0.9	184	4.5	34.2	1.2	9.2
Rye, with Pumpkin Seed, Organic, Lindale*	1 Slice/71g	150	2.9	211	6.1	32.1	4.1	10.6
Rye, with Sprouted Seeds, Yeast Free, Biona Organic*	1 Slice/35g	71	0.7	204	5.3	36.6	2	9.9
Rye, with Sunflower Seeds, Organic, Schneider Brot*	1 Slice/72g	138	2.6	191	6.2	33.4	3.6	7.9
Sandwich Thins, 50/50, Kingsmill*	1 Thin/40g	99	1.1	245	10	43	2.7	4.3
Sandwich Thins, Brown, Warburton's*	1 Thin/40g	100	1.1	252	9.9	45.2	2.8	3.5
Sandwich Thins, Half & Half, Warburtons *	1 Thin/40g	100	1.2	251	10	44.5	2.9	3.6
Sandwich Thins, Seeded, Free From, Tesco*	1 Thin/50g	125	3.8	250	7.8	32.3	7.6	10.8
Sandwich Thins, Seeded, GF, Warburton's*	1 Thin/43g	122	3.5	284	6.5	43.1	8.1	6.5
Sandwich Thins, Seeded, Kingsmill*	1 Thin/40g	106	1.8	264	9.6	43.6	4.6	4.8
Sandwich Thins, White, CBY, Asda*	1 Thin/42g	105	1.1	250	8	47	2.7	2.3
Sandwich Thins, White, GF, Warburton's*	1 Thin/50g	124	3.2	247	6	38.7	6.3	5.7
Sandwich Thins, White, Kingsmill*	1 Thin/40g	99	1	248	9.4	45.6	2.5	2.9
Sandwich Thins, White, Warburton's*	1 Thin/40g	100	1.1	251	9	46.2	2.8	2.5
Sandwich Thins, Wholemeal, Kingsmill*	1 Thin/41g	98	1.2	240	10.3	39.8	3	6.1
Sandwich Thins, Wholemeal, Protein & Fibre, Warburton's*	1 Thin/50g	121	2.8	241	14.7	29.6	5.5	7.3
Seeded, Batch, Finest, Tesco*	1 Slice/65g	168	4	259	9.3	41.8	6.1	6.1
Seeded, Batch, Hovis*	1 Slice/50g	134	3.4	267	10.9	38.1	6.7	5.6
Seeded, Deliciously, Lower Carb, Hovis*	1 Slice/36g	100	3	277	15.7	27.2	8.3	15.1
Seeded, Farmhouse, GF, Warburton's*	1 Slice/35g	92	3.2	262	8.7	33	9.1	6.5
Seeded, Farmhouse, Loaf, Extra Special, Asda*	1 Slice/44g	92	0.5	207	11	38	1.2	8
Seeded, Farmhouse, Organic, Cranks*	2 Slices/94g	232	3.5	247	10.1	39.9	3.7	6.9
Seeded, Free From, Gluten, Wheat, & Milk, Tesco*	1 Slice/42g	95	3.7	227	7	25.7	8.8	8.7
Seeded, GF, Sandwich Thins, Free From, Waitrose*	1 Thin/50g	132	5.1	263	9.3	24.5	10.2	18
Seeded, GF, Sliced, Cob, Waitrose*	2 Slices/67g	186	4.9	278	5.8	42.7	7.3	9.2
Seeded, Med Sliced, Average	*1 Slice/44g*	*116*	*2.9*	*262*	*11.3*	*38.6*	*6.5*	*5.6*
Seeded, Mighty, GF, Mini Loaf, Warburton's*	1 Slice/27g	75	2.9	277	7.7	33.5	10.9	7
Seeded, Rye, Loaf, la Brea Bakery*	1 Slice/55g	120	0.6	218	7	42.5	1	5.7
Seeded, Seriously, Gold, Kingsmill*	1 Slice/50g	136	3.4	272	10.9	41.6	6.9	6.4
Seeded, The Really Seeded One, Kingsmill*	1 Slice/44g	118	3.2	268	10.4	37.3	7.3	5.5
Seeded, Triple, Farmhouse, Loaf, GF, Genius*	1 Slice/36g	100	2.9	277	3.5	43.8	8	8
Seeded, with Sunflower, & Linseed, Sliced, Baker Street*	1 Slice/39g	98	2.2	251	8.3	36.4	5.6	10.7
Sesame Seed, la Brea Bakery*	1 Slice/35g	85	0.8	244	8.8	47.1	2.3	2
Skinni Wrap, Tortilla, Plain, Deli Kitchen*	1 Wrap/31g	94	1.1	302	9	57	3.5	3
Soda	*1oz/28g*	*72*	*0.7*	*258*	*7.7*	*54.6*	*2.5*	*2.1*
Soda, Farls, M&S*	1 Farl/110g	267	3	243	9.6	50.1	2.7	2.3
Soda, Farls, Tesco*	1 Farl/142g	325	4.5	229	7.1	42.2	3.2	2.6
Soda, Fruit, M&S*	1 Slice/40g	105	1.9	260	5.9	51.3	4.6	2.5
Soda, M&S*	1 Slice/40g	82	0.6	205	8.7	39.2	1.6	4.2
Softgrain, Mighty White*	1 Slice/36g	81	0.5	224	7.2	45.5	1.5	3.7
Sourdough, 7 Seed, Bake at Home, Promise*	1 Slice/67g	121	1.3	181	7.1	26.6	1.9	14.6
Sourdough, Average	*1 Slice/50g*	*144*	*0.9*	*289*	*11.8*	*56.4*	*1.8*	*2.4*
Sourdough, Dark, French, Seasonal, Gail's*	1 Loaf/2kg	4280	18.4	214	7.5	43	0.9	2.4
Sourdough, Dark, with Seeds, GF, No.23, Gradz Bakery*	1 Slice/40g	102	4	255	6.8	41	10	13
Sourdough, Highlander, Premium, The Polish Bakery*	1 Slice/40g	94	0.6	235	5.8	51.3	1.6	6.6
Sourdough, Honey, Walnut, & Almond, Gail's*	1 Loaf/500g	1425	46	285	9.5	41.2	9.2	3.1
Sourdough, Loaf, Finest, Tesco*	1 Slice/33g	86	1.8	262	9.6	41.9	5.5	3.3
Sourdough, Malted Wheat, Sliced, Bertinet Bakery*	1 Slice/80g	189	1	236	8.9	45.7	1.2	3.6

BREAD

INFO/WEIGHT	per Measure		Nutrition Values per 100g / 100ml				
Measure	KCAL	FAT	KCAL	PROT	CARB	FAT	FIBRE
Sourdough, Multi Seeded, Sliced, Warburtons *	1 Slice/60g	152	3.7	253	10.2	37.4	6.1	4
Sourdough, Potato, & Rosemary, Gail's*	1 Loaf/500g	1190	14.5	238	7.6	44	2.9	2.4
Sourdough, Quinoa, Gail's*	1 Loaf/500g	1155	7	231	9.2	45.3	1.4	2.4
Sourdough, Rye, Banneton, Sainsbury's*	1 Serving/50g	115	0.6	230	6.6	46.1	1.1	4.7
Sourdough, Rye, Bloomer, Tesco*	1 Slice/40g	97	0.5	243	8.3	47.2	1.2	4.9
Sourdough, San Francisco, Gail's*	1 Loaf/500g	850	3.5	170	6.4	34.6	0.7	1.2
Sourdough, Sandwich Thins, Made Without Wheat, M&S*	2 Thins/100g	210	4.2	210	6.7	32	4.2	8.8
Sourdough, Seeded, Gail's*	1 Loaf/500g	1400	39.5	280	10.2	39.8	7.9	4.6
Sourdough, Sour Cherry, Gail's*	1 Loaf/500g	1190	4.5	238	6.9	50.6	0.9	4.4
Sourdough, Sultana, & Fennel, Gail's*	100g	205	0.7	205	5.9	42	0.7	2.4
Sourdough, White, Cob, Free From, Tesco*	1 Slice/50g	92	1.4	184	5.1	31	2.7	7.4
Sourdough, Whole Grain, Malted, Gail's*	1 Loaf/900g	2214	53.1	246	9.3	8.7	5.9	5.6
Soya, & Linseed, Vogel*	1 Slice/42g	95	2.1	227	11.7	34.1	4.9	6.8
Soya, & Linseed, Sliced, Burgen *	1 Slice/44g	126	4.8	287	15.2	26.9	11	9.8
Soya, & Linseed, The Best, Morrisons*	1 Slice/44g	116	2.7	264	11.2	37.9	6.1	6.3
Spelt, Soul bakery*	1 Slice/45g	116	0.8	258	10.4	50	1.7	7.6
Spinach, & Goats Cheese, Twist, Waitrose*	1 Twist/45g	114	2.9	253	11.8	34.7	6.5	4.3
Sprouted Grain, Ezekiel *	1 Slice/34g	80	0.5	235	11.8	44.1	1.5	0.9
Sprouted Grain, Rolls, Finest, Tesco*	1 Roll/80g	209	3.3	262	8.4	45.5	4.1	4.5
Sprouted Spelt, with Raisins, Everfresh Bakery*	¼ Loaf/100g	230	1.9	230	9.2	43.9	1.9	6.6
Stoneground, Sm Loaf, Organic, Sainsbury's*	1 Slice/24g	50	0.5	208	10	37.9	2.1	7.9
Stoneground, Wholemeal, Thick, Love Life, Waitrose*	1 Slice/40g	86	1.1	214	10.1	36.5	2.8	7.9
Sundried Tomato, & Pepper, Bloomer, Bakery, Tesco*	1 Slice/50g	132	1.5	266	9.9	47.3	3.1	4.5
Sunflower, & Pumpkin Seed, So Organic, Sainsbury's*	1 Slice/30g	76	1.6	254	11.4	40	5.4	12.9
Sunflower, & Pumpkin, Cob, Sliced, Finest, Tesco*	1 Slice/40g	120	4.4	299	12.3	34.7	10.9	6.6
Sunflower, & Honey, Bloomer, Co-Op*	1 Serving/80g	221	4.7	276	9.9	43	5.9	5.3
Sunflower, Bakers Selection, Asda*	1 Slice/60g	162	5.9	270	11.3	50	9.8	8.3
Sunflower, Multi-Grain, Allinson*	1 Slice/47g	113	2.2	240	9.8	39.6	4.7	3.9
Sunflower, Seed, Organic, Natural, Mestemacher*	1 Slice/75g	162	3	216	5.6	34.7	4	9.4
Sunflower, Spelt, Gail's*	1 Loaf/400g	980	25.2	245	10.3	36.7	6.3	6.2
Super Grained, Med Sliced, Loaf, Finest, Tesco*	2 Slices/84g	266	6.5	317	12.8	43.9	7.7	10.4
Super Seeded, Farmhouse, Batch, Specially Selected, Aldi*	1 Slice/50g	138	3.9	276	11	38	7.8	6.4
Superseeded, Sliced Loaf, Extra Special, Asda*	1 Slice/44g	135	4.4	306	12	38	10	6.3
Sweet Potato, with Pumpkin & Sunflower Seeds, BFree*	1 Slice/40g	93	2.5	232	3.5	30.6	6.3	9.2
Tiger, Artisan, Bloomer, GF, Warburton's*	2 Slices/100g	241	5.3	241	7.1	38.5	5.3	5.5
Tiger, Baton, Bakery, Tesco*	½ Baton/100g	288	2	288	9.1	57.4	2	2.2
Tiger, Bloomer, The Great, Village Bakery, Aldi*	1 Slice/58g	159	2.6	274	8.8	49	4.4	2.1
Tiger, Bloomer, Thick Sliced, Iceland*	1 Slice/57g	168	4	295	8	48.2	7.1	3.2
Tiger, Loaf, Bloomer, Bakery, Tesco*	1 Slice/50g	133	1.6	266	8.4	49.2	3.2	3.2
Tiger, White, Warburton's*	1 Slice/40g	106	1.3	266	8.4	49.2	3.2	3.2
Toaster, White, Rathbones*	1 Slice/38g	92	0.5	243	9.1	48.6	1.3	2.3
Toastie Pockets, Brown, Easy Fill, Warburtons*	1 Pocket/55g	134	1.6	243	9.8	42.2	3	4.2
Tomato, & Chilli, BGTY, Sainsbury's*	¼ Bread/65g	155	3.1	238	11.9	36.9	4.7	2.8
Tomato, & Herb, Tear & Share, Tesco*	¼ Pack/73g	164	3.2	226	6.3	40.2	4.4	2.1
Tortilla, Plain, GF, Free From, Sainsbury's*	1 Wrap/40g	84	1.8	211	4.3	31	4.4	15.3
Tortilla, Wheat & Corn, Asda*	1 Tortilla/40g	125	1.9	314	9.4	58	4.8	0.6
Walnut, Waitrose*	1/8 Loaf/50g	170	7.6	339	10	40.6	15.2	5.9
Wheat, & Wholemeal Spelt, & Seeds, Love Life, Waitrose*	1 Slice/34g	88	2.6	267	10.5	33.5	7.9	9.9
Wheat, & Rye, Bloomer, Half, Waitrose*	1 Slice/44g	110	1.4	250	8.2	44.4	3.2	5.2
Wheat, Spelt, & Rye, Loaf, Baked by Us, Morrisons*	1 Serving/70g	165	1.4	236	11.3	39.9	2	6.6
Wheaten, Big Slice	**1 Slice/65g**	**139**	**1.7**	**214**	**7.5**	**40.2**	**2.6**	**3.6**
Wheaten, Loaf, Sliced, Genesis*	1 Slice/40g	86	1	214	7.5	40.2	2.6	3.6
Wheaten, Loaf, Sliced, No Added Sugar, Genesis Crafty*	1 Slice/40g	86	1	214	7.5	40.2	2.6	3.6

BREAD

	Measure INFO/WEIGHT	per Measure KCAL	FAT	Nutrition Values per 100g / 100ml KCAL	PROT	CARB	FAT	FIBRE
Wheaten, M&S*	1 Slice/33g	74	1.2	225	9.3	42.9	3.5	3.9
Wheaten, Sliced, Healthy, Irwin's Bakery*	1 Slice/40g	76	0.8	190	9	40.5	1.9	6.2
Wheatgerm, Hovis, Soft, Sliced, M&S*	1 Slice/23g	50	0.7	220	10.1	38.5	3	4.6
White, & Wholemeal, Slimsters Squares, Irish Pride*	1 Square/41g	100	0.4	245	11.6	44	1	7
White, Average	*1 Slice/40g*	*94*	*0.8*	*235*	*8.4*	*49.3*	*1.9*	*1.5*
White, Batch Loaf, Extra Special, Asda*	1 Slice/47g	109	0.9	233	9	45	1.9	2.2
White, Batch, Warburton's*	1 Slice/42g	98	0.9	233	9.8	43.6	2.1	2.7
White, Baton, Part-Baked, TTD, Sainsbury's*	1 Serving/50g	125	0.4	250	7.5	51.4	0.9	3
White, Baton, Sesame Seed, Bakery, Sainsbury's*	1 Serving/50g	139	2	278	11.1	47.9	3.9	3.5
White, Ciabatta, Roll, GF, Dietary Specials*	1 Roll/50g	106	0.9	213	4.1	40.9	1.8	8.3
White, Classic, Med Sliced, Hovis*	1 Slice/38g	91	0.9	240	11.4	40.3	2.3	2.5
White, Commercially Prepared, Average	*1oz/28g*	*74*	*0.9*	*266*	*7.6*	*50.6*	*3.3*	*2.4*
White, Commercially Prepared, Toasted, Average	*1oz/28g*	*82*	*1.1*	*293*	*9*	*54.4*	*4*	*2.5*
White, Country Maid*	1 Slice/33g	76	0.7	229	8.5	44.1	2.1	3
White, Country, Sliced, Warburtons*	1 Slice/31g	72	0.7	233	9.1	43.1	2.2	2.2
White, Crusty, Farmhouse, Sliced, Bakery, Tesco*	1 Slice/40g	103	0.5	259	9.4	51.1	1.2	3.3
White, Crusty, Fresh, Finest, Tesco*	1 Slice/52g	130	1	250	8.6	48.5	1.9	2.4
White, Crusty, Hovis*	1 Slice/44g	103	1	233	8.8	44.3	2.2	2.1
White, Crusty, Premium, Warburton's*	1 Slice/31g	77	0.7	254	10.6	46.5	2.3	2.6
White, Crusty, Sliced Loaf, Tesco*	1 Slice/50g	127	0.6	254	9.2	50.1	1.2	3.2
White, Crusty, Split Tin, Bakery, Tesco*	1 Slice/50g	134	0.8	268	9.4	52.6	1.5	3.3
White, Danish Style, Thick Sliced, Light, Tesco*	1 Slice/22g	55	0.6	255	9.4	47.3	2.9	2.7
White, Danish, Lighter, Warburton's*	1 Slice/26g	63	0.3	243	10.5	45.8	1.2	2.6
White, Danish, Med Sliced, Tesco*	1 Slice/20g	50	0.5	249	9.9	45.3	2.4	3.3
White, Danish, Soft & Light, Thick Cut, Asda*	1 Slice/26g	60	0.4	230	9	45	1.6	2.1
White, Danish, Soft, Weight Watchers, Warburton's*	1 Slice/21g	50	0.3	243	9.8	46.5	1.3	2.9
White, Danish, Thick Sliced, Tesco*	1 Slice/24g	60	0.6	250	9.7	47.4	2.3	2.9
White, Extra Thick Sliced, Kingsmill*	1 Slice/58g	135	1.4	232	8.8	43.8	2.4	2.8
White, Farmhouse Crusty, M&S*	1 Slice/34g	82	0.7	240	8.9	46.6	2.2	3
White, Farmhouse Gold Premium, Morrisons*	1 Slice/38g	90	0.5	236	8.9	47.4	1.2	2.2
White, Farmhouse, GF, Newburn, Warburton's*	1 Slice/35g	83	2.1	236	6.8	35.6	6.1	5.5
White, Farmhouse, Hovis*	1 Slice/44g	103	1	234	8.7	44.6	2.3	2.4
White, Farmhouse, Seeded, Waitrose*	1 Serving/75g	192	4.1	256	10.8	40.9	5.5	5.6
White, Farmhouse, Sliced, Bakery, Tesco*	1 Slice/44g	106	1	240	7.9	46	2.3	2
White, Farmhouse, Sliced, Rowan Hill Bakery, Lidl*	1 Slice/44g	101	0.7	229	8.3	44.4	1.5	2.4
White, Farmhouse, Soft, 400g Loaf, Warburton's*	1 Slice/27g	66	0.7	245	10.1	43.7	2.6	2.8
White, Farmhouse, Soft, 800g Loaf, Warburton's*	1 Slice/43g	104	1.1	243	9	45	2.5	2.3
White, Fibre, Morrisons*	1 Slice/40g	96	0.7	240	8	48.4	1.7	0.3
White, Fried in Blended Oil	*1 Slice/28g*	*141*	*9*	*503*	*7.9*	*48.5*	*32.2*	*1.6*
White, Gluten & Wheat Free, Free From, Sainsbury's*	1 Slice/89g	189	4.5	212	3.4	32.1	5.1	12.5
White, Gold Seeded, Kingsmill*	1 Slice/44g	108	2.5	245	9.7	38.8	5.7	3.5
White, Harvest Crust Premium, Ormo*	1 Slice/40g	92	0.6	229	9.4	47.4	1.5	2.7
White, Loaf, Danish, Asda*	1 Serving/23g	53	0.5	236	9	45	2.2	2
White, Loaf, Gluten & Wheat Free, Lovemore*	1 Serving/35g	111	3.8	316	0	3.4	10.9	0
White, Loaf, Sliced, Finest, Tesco*	1 Slice/44g	103	0.6	236	8.6	45.5	1.3	4.1
White, Med Sliced, Average	*1 Slice/39g*	*93*	*0.6*	*238*	*7.5*	*48.5*	*1.6*	*1.8*
White, Med Sliced, Basics, Sainsbury's*	1 Slice/36g	83	0.5	231	8	46.4	1.5	2.1
White, Med Sliced, Brace's*	1 Slice/32g	75	0.4	235	9.5	46.6	1.2	2.6
White, Med Sliced, Great Everyday, Kingsmill*	1 Slice/40g	93	0.8	232	9	44.6	2	2.7
White, Med Sliced, Mother's Pride*	1 Slice/36g	82	0.6	229	8	45.6	1.6	3
White, Med Sliced, Stay Fresh, Tesco*	2 Slices/72g	172	1.6	240	8.3	45.8	2.2	2
White, Med Sliced, Tesco*	1 Slice/40g	96	0.9	239	8.1	45.6	2.2	2.3
White, Med Sliced, Value, Tesco*	1 Slice/36g	81	0.4	225	7.9	46.1	1	2.1

BREAD

INFO/WEIGHT	Measure	per Measure		Nutrition Values per 100g / 100ml				
		KCAL	FAT	KCAL	PROT	CARB	FAT	FIBRE
White, Medium, 400g Loaf, Warburton's*	1 Slice/24g	58	0.5	244	10.3	45.1	1.9	2.4
White, Medium, Warburton's*	1 Slice/40g	98	0.8	244	9.1	46.4	2	2.3
White, Mega Bite, Pan, Thick Sliced, Pat The Baker*	1 Slice/45g	105	0.6	233	9.4	44.6	1.4	2.8
White, Mega Thick, Roberts Bakery*	1 Slice/66g	154	1.2	233	8.3	46.2	1.8	2.2
White, Mighty, GF, Mini Loaf, Warburton's*	1 Slice/27g	67	1.8	249	6.7	37.9	6.5	5.8
White, Milk Roll, Warburton's*	1 Slice/18g	46	0.5	248	9.4	45	2.8	2.4
White, Multiseed, Farmhouse, Sliced, 400g, Waitrose*	1 Slice/33g	96	2.9	291	11.2	38.5	8.8	6.7
White, Multiseed, Med Sliced, Batch, Tesco*	1 Slice/33g	88	2	267	9.9	40.3	6.1	5.5
White, Old English, Warburton's*	1 Slice/40g	99	1.2	248	9.8	44.3	2.9	2.8
White, Organic, Bloomer, Bakery, Tesco*	1 Slice/40g	98	0.9	247	9.8	44.8	2.2	4.2
White, Organic, Sainsbury's*	1 Slice/36g	84	0.6	234	8.9	45.5	1.8	2.3
White, Plain, Scottish, Sunblest*	1 Slice/57g	133	1.5	233	10.1	42.3	2.6	2.8
White, Premium, M&S*	1 Slice/40g	95	0.8	235	8.5	45.8	1.9	2.7
White, Rolls, GF, Promise*	1 Roll/60g	118	1.3	197	5	33.1	2.2	12.6
White, Sandwich Thins, Rowan Hill Bakery, Lidl*	1 Thin/42g	115	1	274	9.6	51.9	2.4	3
White, Sandwich, Bakery, Sainsbury's*	1 Slice/50g	121	0.3	242	10.3	49	0.6	2.9
White, Sandwich, Irish Pride*	1 Slice/38g	89	0.5	233	9.4	44.6	1.4	2.8
White, Scottish Plain, Medium, Mother's Pride*	1 Slice/50g	114	0.8	227	8.7	44.6	1.5	3
White, Sea Salt & Black Pepper, Bloomer, Bakery, Tesco*	1 Slice/50g	131	0.8	262	10.1	50.4	1.6	3
White, Seeded, Batch, Loaf, Truly Irresistible, Co-Op*	1 Slice/47g	129	3.4	275	11.6	41.1	7.2	4.3
White, Seeds, Oats, & Honey, TTD, Sainsbury's*	1 Slice/50g	154	5.4	308	12.1	36.7	10.9	7.1
White, Sliced, Brennans*	1 Slice/40g	88	0.6	219	8.7	43	1.4	2.8
White, Sliced, GF, Free From, Tesco*	1 Slice/42g	80	1.7	190	5.2	29.7	4	7.3
White, Sliced, Roberts Bakery*	1 Slice/35g	87	0.7	249	10	48	2.1	2.5
White, Sm Loaf, Classic, Hovis*	1 Slice/33g	75	0.8	228	11.4	40.3	2.3	6.5
White, Soft Batch, Sliced, Sainsbury's*	1 Slice/44g	102	0.8	232	8.2	45.4	1.9	2.3
White, Soft Crusty, M&S*	1 Slice/25g	64	0.6	256	9.3	49	2.5	2.4
White, Soft, Batch Loaf, Sliced, Tesco*	1 Slice/50g	116	1	233	7.5	46.1	2.1	2.1
White, Soft, Extra Thick, Hovis*	1 Slice/67g	156	1.1	233	8.7	44.6	1.7	2.4
White, Soft, GF, Sliced, Promise*	2 Slices/80g	147	2.1	184	1.7	28.6	2.6	19.8
White, Soft, Gold, Kingsmill*	1 Slice/47g	112	1.5	239	8.2	44.5	3.1	2.7
White, Soft, M&S*	1 Slice/47g	105	0.8	225	7.3	46.1	1.7	2.4
White, Soft, Pain De Mie, EpidÃƒÂ¢Ã¢â šÂ¬Ã¢ žÂ¢Or*	1 Slice/36g	96	1.6	270	10.4	44.5	4.6	4.4
White, Soft, Rolls, Genius*	1 Roll/70g	196	4.9	280	2	49.2	7	5.9
White, Soft, Sliced, Hovis*	1 Slice/25g	58	0.6	234	8.7	44.6	2.3	2.4
White, Soft, Thick Sliced, Kingsmill*	1 Slice/44g	105	0.9	238	8	45.6	2	2.7
White, Soft, Toastie, Thick Sliced, Asda*	1 Slice/50g	120	1.1	239	8.1	46	2.2	2.3
White, Sourdough, Country, Oval, la Brea Bakery*	1 Slice/60g	143	0.4	239	8.8	49.4	0.6	1.6
White, Sourdough, Free From, Waitrose*	2 Slices/67g	185	3.6	277	5.4	48.2	5.4	6.9
White, Sourdough, Specially Selected, Aldi*	1 Slice/58g	136	0.5	234	8.4	47	0.8	2.1
White, Sourdough, The Rustik Bakery*	1 Slice/35g	79	0.4	225	9.1	43	1.2	3.9
White, Sourdough, Waitrose*	1 Slice/50g	119	0.6	237	9	45.9	1.2	3.3
White, Square, Extra Thick Sliced, Hovis*	1 Slice/67g	155	1.3	231	8.5	44.7	2	2.6
White, Square, Med Sliced, Hovis*	1 Slice/40g	92	0.8	231	8.5	44.7	2	2.6
White, Square, Thick Sliced, Hovis*	1 Slice/50g	116	1	231	8.5	44.7	2	2.6
White, Sunflower, & Pumpkin, Cob, Waitrose*	1 Slice/33g	89	2.1	270	11.1	39.3	6.3	5.9
White, Super Grained, Farmhouse, Medium, Finest, Tesco*	1 Slice/44g	106	0.8	241	10.4	43.4	1.8	4.9
White, Super Seeds, Farmhouse, Sainsbury*	1 Slice/50g	152	5.2	303	11.9	37.9	10.3	5.6
White, Thick Sliced, Brace's*	1 Slice/38g	90	0.5	235	9.5	46.6	1.2	2.6
White, Thick Sliced, Fine Lady*	1 Slice/44g	113	0.5	254	7.8	53.1	1.2	2.3
White, Thick Sliced, Healthy, Warburton's*	1 Slice/38g	84	0.7	222	10.3	41.2	1.8	4.1
White, Thick Sliced, M&S*	1 Slice/42g	96	0.5	228	7.3	46.7	1.3	2.8
White, Thick Sliced, Organic, Tesco*	1 Slice/44g	108	0.9	245	8.5	46.8	2.1	3.1

BREAD

INFO/WEIGHT	Measure	per Measure KCAL	FAT	Nutrition Values per 100g / 100ml KCAL	PROT	CARB	FAT	FIBRE
White, Thick Sliced, Sainsbury's*	1 Slice/44g	95	0.8	216	8.7	41.1	1.9	7.1
White, Thick Sliced, Square Cut, Asda*	1 Slice/44g	101	0.7	230	8	46	1.5	2.1
White, Thick Sliced, Sunblest*	1 Slice/40g	91	0.6	228	8	45.7	1.5	2.8
White, Thick Sliced, Super Toastie, Morrisons*	1 Slice/50g	128	1.5	257	8.7	48.9	3	2.1
White, Thick Sliced, Tesco*	1 Slice/44g	106	0.7	240	8.2	47.8	1.5	3
White, Thick, So Organic, Sainsbury's*	1 Slice/44g	102	1	231	8.2	44.6	2.2	3.1
White, Thick, Super Soft, M&S*	1 Slice/48g	120	1.3	249	9	45.3	2.7	3.6
White, Thickest, Warburton's*	1 Slice/58g	137	1.2	239	9.9	43.8	2	2.6
White, Thin Sliced, Sainsbury's*	1 Slice/29g	66	0.4	228	7.1	46.4	1.5	2.8
White, Thin Sliced, Tesco*	1 Slice/30g	68	0.4	228	9.5	44.5	1.3	3.4
White, Toasted, Average	*1 Slice/33g*	*87*	*0.5*	*265*	*9.3*	*57.1*	*1.6*	*1.8*
White, Toastie, 400g Loaf, Warburton's*	1 Slice/29g	70	0.5	244	10.3	45.1	1.9	2.4
White, Toastie, GF, Genius*	1 Slice/33g	90	2	272	2.4	47	6.1	9.3
White, Toastie, Loved by Us, Co-Op*	1 Slice/50g	120	1.2	240	7.9	45.4	2.4	2.6
White, Toastie, Thick Cut, Hovis*	1 Slice/50g	115	1	230	8.5	44.8	2	2.5
White, Toastie, Thick, Love to Toast, Kingsmill*	1 Slice/50g	116	1	232	9	44.6	2	2.7
White, Toastie, Warburton's*	1 Slice/47g	116	0.9	244	9.1	46.4	2	2.3
White, Trio of Olive, Bloomer, Bakery, Tesco*	1 Serving/82g	199	4	243	6.8	41.3	4.9	3
White, Wholesome, Loaf, Sainsbury's*	1 Serving/36g	81	0.7	224	9.4	42.5	1.8	4.4
Whole Seed, Cob, Crusty, Bakery, Tesco*	1 Slice/50g	179	6.1	359	13.7	45.7	12.3	5.2
Whole Seed, Loaf, Sliced, Tesco*	1 Slice/40g	109	2.9	272	10.9	38.4	7.2	5.3
Wholegrain, & Rye, Schneider Brot*	1 Slice/50g	98	0.6	197	5.9	36.6	1.2	8.2
Wholegrain, & Oats, Warburton's*	1 Slice/40g	98	1.4	245	11.7	38.8	3.5	5.9
Wholegrain, Average	*1 Slice/44g*	*117*	*1.9*	*265*	*13.4*	*43.3*	*4.2*	*7.4*
Wholegrain, Batch, Finest, Tesco*	1 Slice/44g	112	1.2	254	9.8	47.7	2.7	4.2
Wholegrain, Brennans*	1 Slice/39g	79	0.6	203	9	40	1.5	4.9
Wholegrain, Med Sliced, Irish Pride*	1 Slice/38g	90	0.8	237	9.2	46.6	2.1	7.6
Wholegrain, Soft, M&S*	1 Slice/51g	115	2.8	225	13	31.2	5.4	8.2
Wholegrain, Toasted, Average	*1 Slice/40g*	*117*	*1.9*	*288*	*14.5*	*47.1*	*4.6*	*8.1*
Wholemeal & Oat, Loaf, Vogel*	1 Slice/42g	86	0.6	205	8.7	34.3	1.5	9.7
Wholemeal & Tasty Spelt, Sliced, Hovis*	1 Slice/47g	108	1	230	11.1	38.4	2.1	6.7
Wholemeal Loaf, British Farmers, Hovis*	1 Slice/47g	108	1.3	229	10	37.9	2.8	6.8
Wholemeal Oatbran, Sliced, Tesco*	1 Slice/45g	90	0.7	200	10.1	35.3	1.6	7.4
Wholemeal, & Oat Flakes, Gold, Kingsmill*	1 Slice/47g	103	1.6	220	10	37.3	3.4	7
Wholemeal, & Rye, Cob, Waitrose*	1 Slice/33g	80	0.7	242	11.7	40.5	2.1	6.9
Wholemeal, & Rye, Farmhouse,, Extra Special, Asda*	1 Slice/50g	112	1.2	225	11	36	2.5	7.3
Wholemeal, 7 Seeded, Irwin's Bakery*	1 Slice/38g	90	2	237	9.5	33.4	5.2	9.4
Wholemeal, American Sandwich, Harry's*	1 Slice/43g	110	2.1	259	9	45	5	5
Wholemeal, Ancient Grains, The Best, Morrisons*	2 Slices/80g	222	2.2	277	11.8	48.3	2.7	5.9
Wholemeal, Average	*1 Slice/40g*	*88*	*1*	*215*	*9.2*	*41.6*	*2.5*	*5.8*
Wholemeal, Baker`s Soft, Medium, Tesco*	1 Slice/40g	94	1.1	235	10.8	37.8	2.8	6.9
Wholemeal, Batch, Sliced, Organic, Duchy, Waitrose*	1 Slice/50g	121	1.2	242	10.2	41.8	2.3	6.8
Wholemeal, Bloomer, Heroic, Sliced, Roberts*	1 Slice/37g	87	0.6	236	10.7	41	1.7	6.7
Wholemeal, Brennans*	1 Slice/33g	78	1.4	236	11.2	38.4	4.2	7.7
Wholemeal, Brown, Med Sliced, 400g, Hovis*	1 Slice/29g	64	0.5	221	10	37.8	1.8	6.8
Wholemeal, COU, M&S*	1 Slice/21g	45	0.5	213	13.6	33.7	2.6	7
Wholemeal, Crusty, Finest, Tesco*	1 Slice/50g	103	0.8	206	10.8	37	1.7	6.9
Wholemeal, Crusty, Kingsmill*	1 Slice/42g	104	1.8	247	11.2	41.1	4.2	7
Wholemeal, Danish, BFY, Morrisons*	1 Slice/17g	39	0.3	228	11.2	47.9	1.8	6.2
Wholemeal, Farmhouse, Bakery in Store, M&S*	1 Slice/35g	80	1	229	11.4	35.3	3	7.9
Wholemeal, Farmhouse, Hovis*	1 Slice/44g	91	1	207	11	36	2.2	7.1
Wholemeal, Farmhouse, Med Sliced, Waitrose*	1 Slice/36g	84	0.7	232	10.8	39.1	1.9	7.5
Wholemeal, Farmhouse, Rowan Hill Bakery, Lidl*	1 Slice/47g	102	0.7	218	10.3	37.8	1.4	6.3

B

BREAD

INFO/WEIGHT	Measure	per Measure KCAL	FAT	Nutrition Values per 100g / 100ml KCAL	PROT	CARB	FAT	FIBRE
Wholemeal, Farmhouse, Soft, Tesco*	1 Slice/44g	103	1.1	234	11.3	28.1	2.6	6.3
Wholemeal, Farmhouse, Thick Sliced, 400g, Waitrose*	1 Slice/33g	77	0.6	232	10.8	39.1	1.9	7.5
Wholemeal, Farmhouse, Thick Sliced, Waitrose*	1 Slice/44g	103	0.8	232	10.8	39.1	1.9	7.5
Wholemeal, Fh, Stoneground, Batch, Finest, Tesco*	1 Slice/50g	108	1.4	215	10.3	36.1	2.8	6.9
Wholemeal, Granary, Med Sliced, Hovis*	1 Slice/47g	111	1.1	236	10.6	39.8	2.4	6.8
Wholemeal, Healthy Range, Pat The Baker*	1 Slice/27g	58	0.5	215	10	36.4	1.8	6.6
Wholemeal, High Protein, High Fibre, Warburton's*	1 Slice/29g	66	1	227	13.5	32	3.3	7.8
Wholemeal, Light, Irish Pride*	1 Slice/28g	68	0.4	241	13.3	44.1	1.3	4.5
Wholemeal, Little Brown Loaf, Unsliced, Hovis*	1 Slice/40g	86	1.1	216	10	37.8	2.7	6.8
Wholemeal, Live Good, Hovis*	1 Slice/26g	67	0.4	258	10	46.9	1.5	6.9
Wholemeal, Loaf, 400g, Kingsmill*	1 Slice/29g	68	0.8	234	10.2	39	2.8	6.2
Wholemeal, Loaf, Sliced, Thick, 800g, Hovis*	1 Slice/47g	104	0.8	221	10	37.8	1.8	6.8
Wholemeal, Longer Life, Thick Slice, Sainsbury's*	1 Slice/45g	101	1.6	224	10.6	37.4	3.6	5.9
Wholemeal, Lower Carb , Hovis*	1 Slice/36g	84	1.3	234	16	27	3.7	14.4
Wholemeal, Med Sliced, Great Everyday, Kingsmill*	1 Slice/40g	91	1.5	227	10.5	37.7	3.8	6.2
Wholemeal, Med Sliced, Little Big Loaf, Kingsmill*	1 Slice/39g	93	1.5	239	10.5	37.7	3.8	6.2
Wholemeal, Med Sliced, Loaf, 800g, Village Bakery, Aldi*	1 Slice/40g	90	0.9	225	11	37	2.3	6.2
Wholemeal, Med Sliced, M&S*	1 Slice/40g	80	1.2	200	10.5	32.7	3.1	6.7
Wholemeal, Med Sliced, Morrisons*	1 Slice/33g	72	0.5	216	9.6	38	1.4	6.5
Wholemeal, Med Sliced, Premium, Tesco*	1 Slice/36g	71	0.2	196	9.8	37.8	0.6	7.2
Wholemeal, Med Sliced, Roberts Bakery*	1 Slice/37g	86	0.6	233	10.9	38.1	1.5	6.6
Wholemeal, Med Sliced, Sainsbury's*	1 Slice/36g	77	0.9	214	10.3	37.8	2.4	7.4
Wholemeal, Med Sliced, The Village Bakery*	1 Slice/33g	69	0.7	209	9.8	38	2	6
Wholemeal, Med Sliced, Waitrose*	1 Slice/36g	76	0.9	213	10.1	37.6	2.4	7
Wholemeal, Medium, 400g Loaf, Warburton's*	1 Slice/24g	55	0.7	231	10.6	37.8	2.8	6.4
Wholemeal, Medium, 800g Loaf, Warburton's*	1 Slice/45g	103	1.3	231	10.6	37.8	2.8	6.4
Wholemeal, Medium, Sliced, Everyday Essentials, Aldi*	1 Slice/40g	85	0.7	213	10	36	1.7	6.3
Wholemeal, Medium, Sliced, H.W. Nevill's*	1 Slice/36g	83	0.9	231	9.6	39	2.5	7
Wholemeal, Multi Seeded, TTD, Sainsbury's*	1 Slice/47g	110	3.4	234	11.7	30.7	7.2	8.1
Wholemeal, Multigrain, Soft Batch, Sainsbury's*	1 Slice/44g	106	2.9	242	11.3	34.5	6.5	5.6
Wholemeal, Multiseed, Batch, So Organic, Sainsbury's*	1 Slice/30g	79	2.2	263	11.8	30.9	7.4	12.9
Wholemeal, Nimble, Hovis*	1 Slice/22g	51	0.6	233	12.3	37	2.5	6.8
Wholemeal, Oat Topped, TTD, Sainsbury's*	1 Slice/47g	109	1.3	232	10	38.5	2.8	0.3
Wholemeal, Organic, 400g Loaf, Bakery, Sainsbury's*	1 Slice/50g	137	1.2	274	11.3	46.9	2.4	9.7
Wholemeal, Premium, Thick Slice, M&S*	1 Slice/50g	95	1.5	190	9.8	30.8	3	6.4
Wholemeal, Rustic, Tin, Tesco*	1 Slice/37g	92	1.3	249	12.2	44	3.5	3.1
Wholemeal, Seed Sensations, Hovis*	1 Slice/44g	109	2.5	249	11.9	31.4	5.6	12.4
Wholemeal, Seeded Batch, Truly Irresistible, Co-Op*	1 Slice/47g	115	1.9	245	11.5	36.2	4	6.6
Wholemeal, Seeded, Farmhouse, Rowan Hill Bakery, Lidl*	1 Slice/33g	84	2.1	256	12.4	32.7	6.3	9.4
Wholemeal, Seeded, Roll, Love Life, Waitrose*	1 Roll/72g	192	6.3	266	12.6	34.1	8.8	6.4
Wholemeal, Seeded, Rowan Hill Bakery, Lidl*	1 Slice/33g	86	1.9	261	12.7	34.9	5.8	9
Wholemeal, Seeded, Signature, Allinson*	1 Slice/46g	118	4	256	11.1	28.9	8.7	8.9
Wholemeal, Sliced, Loaf, Average	**1 Slice/40g**	**90**	**0.9**	**224**	**9.9**	**38.8**	**2.4**	**6.9**
Wholemeal, Sliced, McCambridge*	1 Slice/38g	90	0.7	237	7.9	44.7	1.8	0
Wholemeal, Sliced, Medium, Tesco*	1 Slice/40g	93	1.2	234	11.9	36.7	2.9	6.6
Wholemeal, Sliced, Ramsey Bakery*	1 Slice/28g	81	0.8	291	8.5	36	2.9	8.2
Wholemeal, Soft, Multiseed, Farmhouse, TTD, Sainsbury's*	1 Slice/50g	140	4.4	280	12.1	33.4	8.8	9.3
Wholemeal, Soft, Thick Sliced, Rowan Hill Bakery, Lidl*	1 Slice/44g	97	0.8	221	10	37.8	1.8	6.8
Wholemeal, Square Cut, Thick Sliced, Asda*	1 Slice/44g	91	1	208	10	37	2.2	6
Wholemeal, Stoneground, Batch Baked, Warburton's*	1 Slice/45g	101	1.2	224	10.3	35.7	2.6	6.9
Wholemeal, Stoneground, Organic, Waitrose*	1 Sm Slice/25g	57	0.9	228	10.8	38.2	3.6	7.1
Wholemeal, Stoneground, Thick Sliced, Sainsbury's*	1 Slice/44g	92	0.8	210	10.2	37.9	1.9	7.8
Wholemeal, Super Soft, Thick Sliced, 800g, M&S*	2 Slices/100g	234	2.3	234	11	39.2	2.3	6.2

BREAD

	Measure INFO/WEIGHT	per Measure KCAL	FAT	Nutrition Values per 100g / 100ml KCAL	PROT	CARB	FAT	FIBRE
Wholemeal, Supersoft, Eat Well, M&S*	1 Slice/33g	81	1.1	245	10.9	40	3.3	6.7
Wholemeal, Tasty, Medium, Kingsmill*	1 Slice/40g	93	1.1	233	10.2	38.6	2.8	6.3
Wholemeal, Tasty, Thick, Kingsmill*	1 Slice/44g	105	1.7	239	10.5	37.7	3.8	6.2
Wholemeal, The Champion, Batch, Allinson*	1 Slice/46g	108	1.3	234	11	37.8	2.9	6.1
Wholemeal, Thick Slice, Brennans*	1 Slice/27g	69	0.6	257	9.2	45.4	2.1	6.8
Wholemeal, Thick Sliced, Bakers Gold, Asda*	1 Slice/44g	99	1.4	225	12	37	3.2	6
Wholemeal, Thick Sliced, Great Everyday, Kingsmill*	1 Slice/44g	100	1.7	227	10.5	37.7	3.8	6.2
Wholemeal, Thick Sliced, Rathbones*	1 Slice/42g	106	0.9	253	9.5	45.7	2.2	6
Wholemeal, Thick Sliced, Sainsbury's*	1 Slice/44g	103	1.3	234	11.9	36.7	2.9	6.6
Wholemeal, Thick Sliced, So Organic, Sainsbury's*	1 Slice/50g	120	1.6	239	9.6	39.3	3.2	7.2
Wholemeal, Thick Sliced, Tesco*	1 Slice/40g	96	1.1	240	9.5	40.9	2.7	6.8
Wholemeal, Thick Sliced, Waitrose*	1 Slice/44g	94	1.1	213	10.1	37.6	2.4	7
Wholemeal, Thick, Weight Watchers, Warburton's*	1 Slice/28g	64	0.6	225	10	38.4	2.2	6
Wholemeal, Toasted, Average	**1 Med Slice/26g**	**58**	**0.6**	**224**	**8.6**	**42.3**	**2.2**	**5.8**
Wholemeal, Toastie, Sliced, Tesco*	1 Slice/50g	116	1.4	234	11.9	36.7	2.9	6.6
Wholemeal, Unsliced, Organic, Dove's Farm*	1 Med Slice/35g	77	0.9	221	11.4	37.9	2.6	8.3
Wholemeal, with Rye, Rich & Tasty, Warburton's*	1 Slice/45g	109	1.1	246	9.9	40.6	2.4	7.5
Wholemeal. Medium, Brace's*	1 Med Slice/32g	72	0.7	226	10.2	44.3	2.2	6
Wholesome, Five Seeded, GF, Genius*	1 Slice/36g	102	3.4	285	3.7	42.3	9.4	7.8
Wholesome, Vitality, GF, Schar*	1 Slice/32g	84	2.9	262	4.5	36	9.2	8.8
Wholewheat, Harvest	1 Serving/42g	90	1	214	7.1	45.2	2.4	7.1
Wholewheat, Nature's Own*	1 Slice/28g	66	1	236	14.3	39.3	3.6	10.7
Wholewheat, No Crusts, Harry's*	1 Slice/25g	58	1.1	233	8	40	4.5	5.5
Wholewheat, Soft, Trader Joe's*	1 Slice/37g	70	1	189	10.8	37.8	2.7	5.4
Whtie, 50/50, Vitamin Boost, Sliced, Kingsmill*	1 Slice/38g	89	0.8	234	9.4	41.9	2.2	4.7
Wrap, Brown, Soft, Easy Roll, Warburton's*	1 Wrap/65g	190	2.9	292	12	49.3	4.5	3.2
Wrap, Half & Half, Warburton's*	1 Wrap/41g	121	1.8	296	12.8	49.6	4.4	3.8
Wrap, Mediterranean Herb, Soft, Village Bakery, Aldi*	1 Wrap/64g	188	2.6	294	8	54.7	4.1	2
Wrap, Original, Super Soft, Village Bakery, Aldi*	1 Wrap/64g	202	4	316	7.9	56	6.3	2.3
Wrap, Seeded, GF, Newburn Bakehouse, Warburton's*	1 Wrap/60g	178	4.5	297	5.5	48.1	7.5	7.4
Wrap, Tortilla, 8 Pack, Asda*	1 Tortilla/50g	143	3	286	8	50	6	1.9
Wrap, Tortilla, 8 Pack, LC, Tesco*	1 Tortilla/50g	135	1	270	7.1	53.2	2.1	3.5
Wrap, Tortilla, Beetroot, Fibre Fest, Genius*	1 Wrap/40g	83	1.4	208	5.3	32	3.6	13
Wrap, Tortilla, Beetroot, GF, Warburton's*	1 Wrap/45g	131	2.6	292	4.6	52.2	5.8	6.4
Wrap, Tortilla, BGTY, Sainsbury's*	1 Wrap/50g	131	0.8	263	7.3	52.4	1.7	4.3
Wrap, Tortilla, Both in One, Sunnyhills, Aldi*	1 Wrap/64g	184	2.9	287	8.1	52	4.5	3
Wrap, Tortilla, Corn, & Wheat, Santa Maria*	1 Tortilla/40g	118	2.2	294	7.7	50	5.6	0
Wrap, Tortilla, Corn, Soft, Sainsbury's*	1 Wrap/40g	126	1.9	314	9.4	58	4.8	0
Wrap, Tortilla, Deli, Multigrain, Mission Deli*	1 Tortilla/61g	202	6.1	330	7.9	50.5	10	3
Wrap, Tortilla, Flour, Soft, Mini, Stand n Stuff, Old El Paso*	1 Tortilla/12g	36	0.6	296	8.5	52.5	5.2	2.7
Wrap, Tortilla, Flour, Soft, Old El Paso*	1 Tortilla/41g	123	2.1	299	8.5	53.7	5.2	1.9
Wrap, Tortilla, Flour, Stand n Stuff, Old El Paso*	1 Tortilla/24g	71	1.2	296	8.5	52.5	5.2	2.7
Wrap, Tortilla, Garlic, & Parsley, Sainsbury's*	1 Tortilla/60g	166	3.7	277	7.2	48	6.2	1.8
Wrap, Tortilla, GF, Lovemore*	1 Wrap/50g	150	4.2	299	1.8	48.1	8.3	4.1
Wrap, Tortilla, Healthy 'n' White, Wrap 'n' Roll, Discovery*	1 Tortilla/40g	161	3.5	288	8	49.7	6.3	2.6
Wrap, Tortilla, Large, Essential, Waitrose*	1 Tortilla/64g	190	3.7	297	7.2	52.5	5.8	3.1
Wrap, Tortilla, LC, Tesco*	1 Tortilla/64g	166	1.3	260	7.1	53.2	2.1	3.5
Wrap, Tortilla, Less Than 3% Fat, BGTY, Sainsbury's*	1 Tortilla/51g	128	1.1	250	7.8	50.1	2.2	2.9
Wrap, Tortilla, Low Carb, Carbzone*	1 Wrap/65g	182	8.4	280	18	10	13	26
Wrap, Tortilla, Low Carb, Gerry's Wraps*	1 Wrap/43g	142	3.7	330	6.9	30.3	8.6	31.9
Wrap, Tortilla, Low Fat, M&S*	1 Serving/180g	225	4	125	6.3	20.6	2.2	1.9
Wrap, Tortilla, Mediterranean Herb, Rowan Hill, Lidl*	1 Wrap/64g	178	2.2	278	7.3	53	3.5	2.5
Wrap, Tortilla, Mediterranean Style, Morrisons*	1 Wrap/64g	177	2.4	277	7.7	51.8	3.7	3

B

BREAD

INFO/WEIGHT	Measure	per Measure KCAL	FAT	Nutrition Values per 100g / 100ml KCAL	PROT	CARB	FAT	FIBRE
Wrap, Tortilla, Mexican, Asda*	1 Tortilla/34g	100	2.8	295	7.9	47.2	8.3	3.9
Wrap, Tortilla, Morrisons*	1 Serving/60g	132	2.1	220	6.2	42	3.5	1.7
Wrap, Tortilla, Multiseed, Discovery*	1 Tortilla/57g	160	2.8	280	8.7	50.1	5	3.6
Wrap, Tortilla, Multiseed, Tesco*	1 Wrap/64g	186	4	290	8.6	47.6	6.3	4.4
Wrap, Tortilla, Original, Mini, Mission Deli*	1 Wrap/31g	93	2	299	7.6	50.9	6.6	2.7
Wrap, Tortilla, Plain , Ocado*	1 Wrap/53g	154	4.4	291	6.7	45.7	8.4	3.1
Wrap, Tortilla, Plain, Atkins*	1 Tortilla/40g	123	5.2	308	22.5	11	13	25
Wrap, Tortilla, Plain, HL, Tesco*	1 Wrap/64g	182	3.2	284	8.2	49.7	5	3.7
Wrap, Tortilla, Plain, Mini, Morrisons*	1 Tortilla/34g	91	1.4	267	8.1	48.9	4	2.8
Wrap, Tortilla, Plain, Ready to Eat, Sunnyhills, Aldi*	1 Wrap/64g	181	2.2	283	7.1	54.5	3.4	3
Wrap, Tortilla, Plain, Sainsbury's*	1 Wrap/64g	185	2.9	290	7.4	53.4	4.6	2.7
Wrap, Tortilla, Plain, Tesco*	1 Tortilla/64g	182	3.2	284	8.1	49.7	5	3.8
Wrap, Tortilla, Plain, Village Bakery, Aldi*	1 Wrap/65g	194	4.9	298	7.8	49.6	7.6	2.7
Wrap, Tortilla, Quinoa, & Chia Seed, BFree*	1 Wrap/42g	105	2.4	250	7.6	36	5.7	11.4
Wrap, Tortilla, Rice, Mountain Bread*	1 Wrap/25g	68	0.3	272	10	53	1.3	2.6
Wrap, Tortilla, Seeded, Love Life, Waitrose*	1 Tortilla/64g	185	3.6	290	8.8	46.6	5.7	4.3
Wrap, Tortilla, Small, Rapiditas, Bimbo*	1 Wrap/18g	55	1.5	306	8.1	50	8.2	0
Wrap, Tortilla, Soft Flour, Sainsbury's*	1 Wrap/40g	123	2.6	307	8.5	52.5	6.5	0
Wrap, Tortilla, Soft, M&S*	1 Wrap/64g	186	3.8	290	8	49.7	6	2.5
Wrap, Tortilla, Spicy Tomato, Morrisons*	1 Tortilla/55g	158	3.1	288	8.6	50.5	5.7	0.7
Wrap, Tortilla, Spicy Tomato, Tesco*	1 Tortilla/63g	175	3.5	278	7.8	49.2	5.6	2.4
Wrap, Tortilla, Super Seed, Protein, GF, Warburton's*	1 Wrap/45g	133	3	295	17	39	6.7	5.5
Wrap, Tortilla, Sweet Chilli, Tesco*	1 Wrap/64g	184	2.9	288	7.4	53.1	4.5	2.7
Wrap, Tortilla, Sweet Potato, GF, BFree*	1 Wrap/42g	91	0.8	217	5.4	33	1.9	15.2
Wrap, Tortilla, Tomato, & Herb, Tesco*	1 Serving/63g	165	3.5	262	7.9	45.1	5.5	2.1
Wrap, Tortilla, Tomato, Low Carb, High Protein, Carbzone*	1 Wrap/40g	112	4.8	280	20	11	12	23
Wrap, Tortilla, Value, Tesco*	1 Wrap/47g	129	2.4	275	8.5	49.1	5	4.3
Wrap, Tortilla, Wheat & White, Mini, Mission Deli*	1 Wrap/31g	93	2.1	299	7.5	50	6.9	3.6
Wrap, Tortilla, White, Bakers Selection, Asda*	1 Tortilla/62g	181	2.9	290	7.9	53	4.6	2.5
Wrap, Tortilla, White, GF, Free From, Tesco*	1 Wrap/40g	84	1.8	211	4.3	31	4.4	15.3
Wrap, Tortilla, White, GF, Warburton's*	1 Wrap/45g	138	2.6	306	3.9	57	5.8	5.3
Wrap, Tortilla, White, M&S*	1 Tortilla/64g	170	2.4	265	7.9	49	3.8	1.6
Wrap, Tortilla, White, Weight Watchers*	1 Wrap/50g	118	0.6	236	6.9	46.5	1.3	8.8
Wrap, Tortilla, Whole & White, HL, Tesco*	1 Wrap/64g	182	1.7	284	8.5	54.1	2.7	4.5
Wrap, Tortilla, Whole 'n' White, Goodness, Kids, Tesco*	1 Wrap/27g	72	1.2	265	8.3	47.6	4.5	5.8
Wrap, Tortilla, Whole Wheat, Stand n Stuff, Old El Paso*	1 Tortilla/24g	71	1.2	294	8.9	50.3	5.2	6
Wrap, Tortilla, Whole, & White, Mini, Kids, Sainsbury's*	1 Tortilla/26g	67	1.4	258	9.2	42.9	5.5	6.2
Wrap, Tortilla, Wholemeal , M&S*	1 Wrap/64g	160	2.4	250	11.2	42.5	3.8	6.5
Wrap, Tortilla, Wholemeal, Bakers Selection, Asda*	1 Wraps/63g	177	4.1	283	8	46	6.5	4
Wrap, Tortilla, Wholemeal, Discovery*	1 Wrap/40g	109	3.3	273	9.2	40.4	8.3	6.4
Wrap, Tortilla, Wholemeal, Essential, Waitrose*	1 Wrap/64g	181	4.1	283	9.2	43.4	6.4	7.3
Wrap, Tortilla, Wholemeal, Mission Deli*	1 Wrap/60g	175	5	292	8.4	41.6	8.3	8.8
Wrap, Tortilla, Wholemeal, Weight Watchers*	1 Wrap/50g	118	0.8	236	8.1	52.8	1.5	11
Wrap, Tortillas, GF, Old El Paso*	1 Tortilla/36g	96	0.8	268	1.9	58	2.2	3.8
Wrap, White, Soft, Easy Roll, Warburton's*	1 Wrap/65g	192	2.8	296	11.7	51.6	4.3	2
Wrap, Wholegrain, GF, Mini, Warburton's*	1 Wrap/35g	101	2.3	288	9.2	44.7	6.6	6.7
Wrap, Wholemeal, High Protein & Fibre, Warburton's*	1 Wrap/68g	184	3.3	271	15	38.4	4.8	7.3
Wrap. Tortilla, Plain, GF, Genius*	1 Wrap/40g	84	1.8	211	4.3	31	4.4	15.3
Wraps, Tortilla, Sweet Potato, Free From, Sainsbury's*	1 Wrap/40g	73	1.3	182	4.4	26.2	3.2	15.3
Wraps, Tortilla, Wholemeal, Asda*	1 Wrap/63g	191	4.7	304	7.6	48	7.5	8

BREAD & BUTTER PUDDING

INFO/WEIGHT	Measure	per Measure KCAL	FAT	Nutrition Values per 100g / 100ml KCAL	PROT	CARB	FAT	FIBRE
Average	*1 Serving/250g*	*400*	*19.5*	*160*	*6.2*	*17.5*	*7.8*	*0.3*
BGTY, Sainsbury's*	1 Serving/125g	126	2.9	101	6.3	13.4	2.3	5.4

	Measure INFO/WEIGHT	per Measure KCAL	FAT	Nutrition Values per 100g / 100ml KCAL	PROT	CARB	FAT	FIBRE
BREAD & BUTTER PUDDING								
Individual, M&S*	1 Pudding/130g	280	16.4	215	4.4	21.4	12.6	0.5
Tesco*	½ Pack/198g	494	31.8	250	5	20.8	16.1	0.4
BREAD MIX								
Ciabatta, Made Up with Water & Olive Oil, Wrights*	1 Slice/45g	113	1.8	251	10	43.6	4	1.8
Crusty White, Made Up, Tesco*	1 Slice/126g	316	2.3	251	9.4	49.3	1.8	2.5
Focaccia, Garlic & Herb, Asda*	1 Serving/125g	385	10	308	11	48	8	3.3
Mixed Grain, Sainsbury's*	1 Serving/45g	103	0.7	228	7.7	46	1.5	4.4
Multiseed, Baked, Sainsbury's*	1 Slice/44g	112	4.3	252	10.8	30.5	9.6	6.8
Multiseed, Crunchy Four Seed, Tesco*	1 Pack/500g	1370	37	274	11.3	38.1	7.4	4.9
Pain De Compagne, Made Up, Francine*	2 Slices/100g	237	2.5	237	9.7	42.3	2.5	0
Parmesan & Sun Dried Tomato, Made Up, Wrights*	1 Slice/45g	103	0.6	229	9.3	46	1.3	2.4
White Loaf, Asda*	1 Slice/60g	128	0.2	213	7.9	43	0.3	3.5
White, Premium, Dry Mix, Made Up, Wright's*	1 Avg Slice/45g	112	0.8	248	10.4	46.3	1.7	3
Wholemeal, CBY, Asda*	1 Slice/45g	93	0.3	207	9.6	37.5	0.6	6.5
Wholemeal, Hovis*	1 Serving/65g	148	3.1	227	10	35.8	4.8	6.8
Wholemeal, Made Up, M&S*	1 Loaf/600g	1410	14.4	235	11	42	2.4	5.3
BREADCRUMBS								
Average	**1oz/28g**	**98**	**0.5**	**350**	**10.8**	**74.8**	**1.9**	**2.6**
BREADFRUIT								
Raw	**1oz/28g**	**19**	**0.1**	**67**	**0.9**	**16.4**	**0.2**	**0**
BREADSTICKS								
Asda*	1 Serving/5g	21	0.4	412	12	73	8	2.9
Bruschetta, Olive & Rosemary, Graze*	1 Punnet/29g	138	7.5	480	13.4	53	26	4.1
Chive & Onion Twists, Tesco*	3 Twists/24g	115	5.3	480	11.6	57.6	22.1	2.2
Ciabatta, Basil & Parsley, Specially Selected, Aldi*	1 Serving/55g	208	8.8	378	9.6	46	16	2.9
Ciabatta, Garlic, Sainsbury's*	1 Breadstick/36g	147	7.2	412	10.5	45.8	20.1	3.3
Grissini, Black Olive, Crosta & Mollica*	1 Grissini/10g	41	0.9	410	10	69.7	9.4	3.2
Grissini, Italian, Sainsbury's*	1 Breadstick/5g	20	0.4	408	11.6	72.9	7.8	2.9
Grissini, Thin with Olive Oil, Forno Bianco*	1 Stick/5g	21	0.4	420	11	77	7.5	0
Grissini, Waitrose*	1 Breadstick/6g	25	0.4	397	12	72.5	6.2	3.1
Grissini, with Wholemeal Flour, Faidon*	1 Stick/14g	63	2.3	447	12.8	62.6	16.2	4.5
Italian Original, Tesco*	1 Stick/5.5g	23	0.4	414	11.2	73.1	7.9	2.8
Mini, Sainsbury's*	4 Breadsticks/5g	20	0.4	404	15.6	68.7	7.4	4.8
Mini, Tesco*	1 Stick/2g	7	0.1	412	11.1	73.2	7.7	2.9
Olive Oil & Rosemary, Finest, Tesco*	2 Sticks/10g	42	1.2	427	13.9	64.4	12.6	4.1
Plain, You Count, Love Life, Waitrose*	1 Breadstick/5g	17	0.1	349	13.4	70.1	1.7	5.6
Sesame Seed Grissini, Sainsbury's*	1 Breadstick/6g	27	0.7	424	13.5	66.2	11	3.1
Sesame, Tesco*	3 Sticks/24g	113	4.6	469	15.3	57.2	19.3	2.6
BREAKFAST CEREAL								
Advantage, Weetabix*	1 Serving/30g	105	0.7	350	10.2	72	2.4	9
All Bran, All Bran, Fibre Crunch, Berry Burst, Kellogg's*	1 Serving/45g	176	5	391	7.6	59	11	13
All Bran, Asda*	1 Serving/40g	110	1.4	276	15	46	3.5	27
All Bran, Bran Flakes, & Fruit, Kellogg's*	1 Serving/40g	143	2.4	358	8	68	6	9
All Bran, Bran Flakes, Chocolate, Kellogg's*	1 Serving/30g	106	1.8	354	10	65	6	13
All Bran, Fibre Crunch, Kellogg's*	1 Serving/45g	184	5	409	7.6	63	11	13
All Bran, Fruit 'n' Fibre, Kellogg's*	1 Serving/30g	114	1.8	380	8	69	6	9
All Bran, Golden Crunch, Kellogg's*	1 Serving/45g	182	5	405	8	62	11	13
All Bran, High Fibre, Morrisons*	1 Serving/40g	109	1.4	272	14.8	45.5	3.5	27
All Bran, Muesli, Cranberry & Sultana, Kellogg's*	1 Serving/45g	158	2.5	350	10	58	5.5	14
All Bran, Original, High Fibre, Kellogg's*	1 Serving/40g	134	1.4	334	14	48	3.5	27
Almond, Oats & More, Nestle*	1 Serving/40g	162	3.5	404	11	67	8.8	7
Almond, Pecan & Cashew Muesli, Kellogg's*	1 Serving/45g	188	6.3	418	11	62	14	8
Alpen*, Crunchy Bran*	1 Serving/40g	120	1.9	299	11.8	52.3	4.7	24.8

BREAKFAST CEREAL

	Measure INFO/WEIGHT	per Measure KCAL	FAT	Nutrition Values per 100g / 100ml KCAL	PROT	CARB	FAT	FIBRE
Apple & Cinnamon, Crisp, Sainsbury's*	1 Serving/50g	216	7.4	433	6.2	69.1	14.7	3.4
Apple & Cinnamon Crisp, Tesco*	1 Serving/50g	217	6.6	433	8.7	67.1	13.1	6.1
Apple & Cinnamon, Oat & Fruit Breakfast, Quaker*	1 Sachet/200g	172	3.6	86	2.3	14	1.8	2.3
Apple & Raisin, Additions, Weetabix*	2 Biscuits/43g	149	0.8	344	9.5	66	1.8	13
Apple, & Cinnamon, Crisp, Crownfield, Lidl*	1 Serving/30g	129	3.6	429	8.2	68.5	12	6.9
Apricot Wheats, Harvest Morn, Aldi*	1 Serving/30g	101	0.4	337	7.6	72.3	1.4	8
Apricot Wheats, Whole Grain, Tesco*	1 Serving/40g	130	0.6	326	7.6	70.6	1.4	8
Apricot Wheats, Wholegrain, Essential, Waitrose*	1 Serving/45g	151	0.6	335	8	71.3	1.4	8.3
Balance, Sainsbury's*	1 Serving/30g	111	0.4	370	11.4	77.7	1.5	3.2
Banana, Papaya & Honey Oat, Crunchy, Waitrose*	1 Serving/40g	170	4.8	426	9.6	69.8	12	5.5
Benefit Flakes, Original, Harvest Morn, Aldi*	1 Serving/40g	154	0.5	384	12	80	1.3	2.2
Berries, Clusters, & Seeds, Protein, Special K, Kellogg's*	1 Serving/40g	148	1.3	371	12	69	3.2	8.9
Berry Granola, Rude Health*	1 Serving/40g	178	6.4	446	10	61	16	7
Bircher Mix, Almonds, & Honey, Dorset Cereals*	1 Serving/30g	117	3.3	389	10	55	11	8.5
Bircher Muesli, Love Life, Waitrose*	1 Serving/45g	153	3.5	341	8.8	57.7	7.7	6.8
Biscuit, with Coconut & Raisin, Additions, Weetabix*	2 Biscuits/43g	157	2.5	363	9.5	62	5.7	13
Bitesize Wheats, Crownfield, Lidl*	1 Serving/40g	142	0.8	356	10.6	67	1.9	14
Bitesize, Weetabix*	1 Serving/40g	135	0.8	338	11.5	68.4	2	10
Bixies, Wheat Biscuits, Wholegrain, Crownfield, Lidl*	2 Biscuits/40g	145	0.8	362	10.8	70.3	1.9	10
Blueberry Wheaties, Asda*	1 Bowl/45g	150	0.6	333	7.9	71	1.4	8.2
Blueberry Wheats, Tesco*	1 Serving/50g	168	0.8	336	7.5	71.6	1.5	8.5
Blueberry Wheats, Wholegrain, Essential, Waitrose*	1 Serving/45g	150	0.6	333	7.9	70.8	1.4	8.2
Blueberry, & Banana, with Live Cultures, GoodBelly, Nestle*	1 Serving/40g	162	4	404	12	61	10	9.8
Bran Crunch, Raisin, Kellogg's*	1 Pack/80g	280	1.5	350	6.2	83.8	1.9	7.5
Bran Flakes, Asda*	1 Serving/47g	157	1.5	333	11	65	3.2	14
Bran Flakes, Free From, Tesco*	1 Serving/30g	107	0.7	358	7.5	69.3	2.3	15
Bran Flakes, Kellogg's*	1 Serving/30g	108	1	359	12	63	3.2	15
Bran Flakes, Sultana Bran, Kellogg's*	1 Serving/40g	138	0.8	344	8	67	2	13
Bran Flakes, Sultana, Dry, Sainsbury's*	1 Serving/30g	98	0.6	325	8.3	68.6	1.9	12.1
Bran Flakes, Tesco*	1 Serving/30g	107	0.7	356	10.8	64.3	2.4	16.8
Bran Flakes, Wholegrain, Essential, Waitrose*	1 Serving/30g	107	0.7	356	10.8	64.7	2.4	16
Bran Flakes, Wholegrain, Sainsbury's*	1 Serving/30g	109	0.9	363	10.1	67.1	3	13.6
Cheerios, Honey Nut, Nestle*	1 Serving/30g	112	1.1	374	7	78.3	3.7	5.2
Cheerios, Honey, Nestle*	1 Serving/50g	184	1.4	369	6.6	79.2	2.8	5.8
Cheerios, Low Sugar, As Sold, Nestle*	1 Serving/30g	120	2.3	399	11.1	67.4	7.6	8.5
Cheerios, Multigrain, Nestle*	1 Serving/30g	114	1.3	380	9.4	72	4.2	8.9
Cheerios, Nestle*	1 Serving/30g	114	1.1	381	8.6	74.5	3.8	7.1
Cheerios, Oat Crisp, Nestle*	1 Portion/40g	154	2.1	385	11	70	5.2	8.5
Choc & Nut Crisp, Tesco*	1 Serving/40g	185	8	462	8.3	62.5	19.9	4.8
Choco Crackles, Morrisons*	1 Serving/30g	115	0.7	383	5.5	84.8	2.4	1.9
Choco Hoops, Aldi*	1 Serving/30g	116	1.4	385	7	79.1	4.5	0
Choco Hoops, Asda*	1 Serving/40g	154	1.8	385	7	79	4.5	4
Choco Squares, Asda*	1 Serving/30g	130	4.2	434	10	67	14	4
Chocolate Crisp, Minis, Weetabix*	1 Serving/36g	134	1.9	371	9	71.7	5.3	8.5
Chocolate Hoops, Average	***1 Serving/30g***	***116***	***1.3***	***386***	***7.2***	***79.3***	***4.4***	***3.4***
Chocolate Rice, Puffed, Average	***1 Serving/30g***	***117***	***1.2***	***389***	***5.7***	***81***	***4.1***	***3.2***
Chocolatey Squares, Mornflake*	1 Serving/30g	140	5.6	466	6.4	66.7	18.7	2.8
Cinnamon Chips, Harvest Morn, Aldi*	1 Serving/40g	166	4.4	416	6.8	70	11	0
Cinnamon Grahams, Nestle*	1 Serving/40g	164	3.9	411	4.7	76.1	9.8	4.2
Clusters, Honey, & Nut, Harvest Morn, Aldi*	1 Serving/45g	200	6.3	445	9.6	68	14	5.6
Clusters, Nestle*	1 Serving/30g	113	1	377	9	74	3.4	7.9
Coco Pops, Kellogg's*	1 Serving/30g	115	0.6	382	6.3	84	1.9	3
Coco Rice, GF, Nestle*	1 Serving/30g	115	0.7	382	6.2	82	2.4	3.1

BREAKFAST CEREAL

INFO/WEIGHT	Measure	per Measure KCAL	per Measure FAT	Nutrition Values per 100g / 100ml KCAL	PROT	CARB	FAT	FIBRE
Coco Shreddies with 125ml Semi Skimmed Milk, Nestle*	1 Serving/40g	210	2.7	525	18	90.2	6.7	8.7
Coco Snaps, Value, Tesco*	1 Serving/30g	117	0.7	390	7	84.1	2.4	2.4
Cookie Crunch, Nestle*	1 Serving/40g	154	1.1	385	4.6	85.3	2.8	1.8
Corn Flakes, Asda*	1 Serving/30g	111	0.2	370	7	84	0.7	3
Corn Flakes, Golden, Organic, Whole Earth*	1 Serving/30g	111	0.2	369	8	80	0.8	5
Corn Flakes, Honey Nut, Average	*1 Serving/30g*	*118*	*1.3*	*393*	*7*	*81.4*	*4.3*	*2.4*
Corn Flakes, Honey Nut, Harvest Home, Nestle*	1 Serving/30g	118	1.3	392	7.4	81.1	4.2	2.5
Corn Flakes, Kellogg's*	1 Serving/30g	113	0.3	378	7	84	0.9	3
Corn Flakes, Organic, Lima*	1 Serving/50g	178	0.5	355	8.3	77.7	1	6.4
Corn Flakes, Sainsbury's*	1 Serving/25g	93	0.2	371	7.3	83.8	0.7	3
Corn Flakes, Tesco*	1 Serving/30g	116	0.3	386	7.6	85.2	1.1	2.5
Corn Flakes, Value, Tesco*	1 Serving/30g	116	0.3	386	7.6	85.2	1.1	2.5
Cornflakes, Co-Op*	1 Serving/30g	116	0.3	386	7.6	85	1.1	2.5
Cornflakes, Essential, Waitrose*	1 Serving/30g	116	0.3	385	7.4	84.8	1.1	3.1
Cornflakes, GF, Nestle*	1 Serving/30g	115	0.3	384	7.4	84.6	1.1	3.1
Cornflakes, Honey, GF, Nestle*	1 Serving/30g	114	0.2	381	5.6	86.2	0.8	3.5
Country Crisp with Real Raspberries, Jordans*	1 Serving/50g	214	7.9	429	7.5	64.1	15.8	7.1
Country Crisp with Real Strawberries, Jordans*	1 Serving/50g	214	7.8	428	7.5	64.1	15.7	7.1
Country Crisp, Four Nut Combo, Jordans*	1 Serving/50g	240	12.4	480	8.9	55.4	24.7	6.9
Craze, Chocolate Hazelnut, Harvest Morn, Aldi*	1 Serving/40g	167	4.4	418	7.9	70	11	3.2
Crispy Minis, Banana, Weetabix*	1 Serving/40g	156	2	389	9.3	72	4.9	9.7
Crunchy Bran, Weetabix*	1 Serving/40g	140	1.4	350	11.9	57.6	3.6	20
Crunchy Choco, Crisp & Square, Tesco*	1 Serving/50g	212	7	423	8	66.3	14	6
Crunchy Nut, Clusters, Honey & Nut, Kellogg's*	1 Serving/40g	161	2	402	6	82	5	2.5
Crunchy Nut, Clusters, Milk Chocolate Curls, Kellogg's*	1 Serving/40g	183	7.2	458	8	66	18	4
Crunchy Nut, Clusters, Peanut Butter, Kellogg's *	1 Serving/30g	146	7.5	488	14	49	25	5.5
Crunchy Nut, Clusters, Summer Berries, Kellogg's*	1 Serving/40g	176	6	439	8	68	15	5
Crunchy Nut, Corn Flakes, Kellogg's*	1 Serving/30g	118	1.2	392	6	83	4	2.5
Crunchy Nut, Oat Granola, with Chocolate, Kellogg's*	1 Serving/45g	224	11.2	497	8	57	25	6
Curiously Cinnamon, Nestle*	1 Serving/30g	124	3	412	4.9	75.9	9.9	4.1
Fibre Flakes, GF, Organic, Dove's Farm*	1 Serving/30g	105	0.4	351	7.1	69.7	1.5	15
Flakes & Grains, Exotic Fruit, BGTY, Sainsbury's*	1 Serving/30g	113	1.5	377	6.8	76.4	4.9	5.9
Flakes & Clusters, Tesco*	1 Serving/50g	220	8.5	440	11.2	55.4	17	10.5
Frosted Flakes, Tesco*	1 Serving/30g	112	0.1	374	4.9	87.8	0.4	2.4
Frosted Wheats, Kellogg's*	1 Serving/30g	104	0.6	346	10	72	2	9
Frosties, Caramel, Kellogg's*	1 Serving/30g	113	0.2	377	5	88	0.6	2
Frosties, Kellogg's*	1 Serving/30g	112	0.2	375	4.5	87	0.6	2
Fruit & Fibre, Flakes, Waitrose*	1 Serving/40g	143	2.5	357	8.2	67.2	6.2	9.9
Fruit & Fibre, Morrisons*	1 Serving/30g	110	2.2	366	8.8	66.5	7.2	8.5
Fruit & Fibre, Value, Tesco*	1 Serving/40g	144	2.2	359	11.4	65.7	5.6	8
Fruit & Nut Crisp, Minis, Weetabix*	1 Serving/40g	148	1.6	371	9.9	69	4.1	9.3
Fruit & Fibre, Asda*	1 Serving/40g	155	2.6	387	8.8	69	6.5	8.8
Fruit & Fibre, Harvest Morn, Aldi*	1 Serving/30g	114	1.8	380	8.4	69	6.1	8
Fruit 'n' Fibre, Kellogg's*	1 Serving/40g	152	2.4	380	8	69	6	9
Fruit Wheats, Raspberry, Morrisons*	1 Serving/45g	150	0.6	333	8	70.8	1.4	8.4
Fruit, Nuts & Flakes, M&S*	1 Serving/30g	117	2.6	391	9.1	69.6	8.5	3.5
GoFree, Honey Flakes, GF, Nestle*	1 Serving/30g	115	0.2	384	5.6	87	0.8	2.3
Golden Grahams, Nestle*	1 Serving/30g	112	0.9	375	6	81	3	3.4
Golden Honey Puffs, Tesco*	1 Serving/30g	115	0.4	382	6.6	86.3	1.2	3
Golden Nuggets, Nestle*	1 Serving/40g	152	0.3	381	6.2	87.4	0.7	1.5
Granola	*1 Serving/45g*	*194*	*8.7*	*430*	*17.5*	*48.8*	*19.4*	*16.8*
Granola, & Strawberries with Bio Yoghurt, Rumblers*	1 Pot/168g	267	9.7	159	4.3	22.4	5.8	1.1
Granola, 3 Seed, & Oat, Wholegrain, M&S*	1 Serving/45g	217	9	483	16.1	50.8	20	7.7

B

BREAKFAST CEREAL

INFO/WEIGHT	Measure	per Measure		Nutrition Values per 100g / 100ml				
		KCAL	FAT	KCAL	PROT	CARB	FAT	FIBRE
Granola, 4 Nut, & Flame Raisin, Wholegrain, M&S*	1 Serving/45g	206	8.3	458	10	59.5	18.5	6.5
Granola, 5 Ways, Honey, Almonds & Seeds, Nutri Brex*	1 Serving/40g	165	5.9	413	12.4	54.1	14.7	7
Granola, Berry & Orange, Wholegrain, M&S*	1 Serving/45g	178	4.3	396	8.5	65.5	9.6	6.7
Granola, Cherry Bakewell, 1, Waitrose*	1 Serving/40g	181	4.8	452	12	70	12	8
Granola, Chocolate with Orange, Troo*	1 Serving/45g	207	10.1	461	15.7	44.6	22.5	19.7
Granola, Chocolate, Dorset Cereals*	1 Serving/40g	206	12	515	8.8	47.2	30	10.5
Granola, Crunchy Nut Glorious Oat, Kellogg's*	1 Serving/45g	212	9.4	470	7	61	21	4.5
Granola, Crunchy Oat, Raisin, Almond, Harvest Morn, Aldi*	1 Serving/40g	166	4.6	416	8.2	66.9	11.4	6.4
Granola, Crunchy Oat, Tropical Fruits, Harvest Morn, Aldi*	1 Serving/40g	174	5.2	436	9.4	66	13	7.4
Granola, Dark Choc Zing, Spoon*	1 Serving/30g	140	6.4	468	9.7	54.4	21.5	8.7
Granola, Fruit, Simply Sumptuous, Lidl*	1 Bowl/45g	198	8.1	440	10	56	18	7.1
Granola, Hazelnuts, & Pecans, Super Goodness, Quaker*	1 Serving/45g	187	5	416	9.6	67	11	8
Granola, High Protein, Lizi's*	1 Serving/40g	180	6.8	450	27	44	17	6.7
Granola, High Protein, Well & Good, Co-Op*	1 Serving/45g	193	4.9	429	28	52	11	6.4
Granola, Honey, & Maple Syrup, Scrumshus*	1 Serving/25g	111	4.4	444	9.2	58.8	17.6	7.6
Granola, Honey, Dorset Cereals*	1 Serving/40g	204	12	511	13	44	30	7.4
Granola, Mango, & Coconut, Wholegrain, M&S*	1 Serving/45g	196	6.7	435	10.5	61.3	14.8	7.4
Granola, Muesli, Fruit & Nut, The Best, Morrisons*	1 Serving/45g	174	4.4	387	8.5	63.2	9.8	6
Granola, Multigrain Nutty, G&B, Asda*	1 Serving/40g	178	7.6	444	12	52	19	7.6
Granola, Nut, Simply Nut, Dorset Cereals*	1 Serving/40g	200	10.8	500	11	48	27	8.3
Granola, Nuts, Pumpkin Seeds, & Fruit, Aldi*	1 Serving/45g	210	8.6	466	27	45	19	5
Granola, Nutty Fruit, Result Plan*	1 Serving/45g	194	6	431	9.8	62.2	13.3	6.9
Granola, Oat Clusters, Apple & Cinnamon, Quaker*	1 Pack/48g	193	3.8	403	8	70.2	8	9.4
Granola, Oat, Golden Crunch, 30% Less Fat, Quaker*	1 Serving/45g	193	4.6	429	8.7	71.5	10.3	7.2
Granola, Oat, Simply Oat, Dorset Cereals*	1 Serving/40g	177	6.8	443	8.8	60	17	7.4
Granola, Organic, Lizi's, The GoodCarb Food Company*	1 Serving/50g	246	14	493	11.3	48.6	28.1	7.4
Granola, Original, Lizi's, The GoodCarb Food Company*	1 Serving/50g	248	14.6	496	10.9	46.2	29.3	10.6
Granola, Pink Apple & Cinnamon, Diet Chef Ltd*	1 Pack/40g	193	10.7	483	10.1	49.3	26.8	11.2
Granola, Pumpkin & Sunflower, Super Goodness, Quaker*	1 Serving/45g	185	4.5	411	10	67	10	7.6
Granola, Quaker*	1 Serving/48g	210	7	438	10.4	72.9	14.6	6.2
Granola, Raisin, & Almond, Crownfield, Lidl*	1 Serving/50g	209	5.7	418	9.5	66.9	11.4	5.1
Granola, Raspberry, Apple, Carrot, W.K. Kellogg's*	1 Serving/45g	191	6.3	425	8.1	62	14	9.4
Granola, Salted Caramel, & Popcorn, Finest, Tesco*	1 Serving/50g	230	8	460	8.7	68.3	16	4.1
Granola, Strawberry, Apple, & Raspberry, Asda*	1 Serving/50g	220	7.5	439	9.4	64	15	7.6
Granola, Strawberry, Crunchy, Weight Watchers*	1 Serving/50g	150	1.4	300	9	57	2.8	24
Granola, Summer Fruits, Pomegranate Infused, M&S*	1 Serving/50g	200	6.4	400	8.6	63.2	12.7	5.8
Granola, Super Berry, Tesco*	1 Serving/45g	195	6	434	9.2	66	13.3	6.5
Granola, Super Fruity, Jordan's*	1 Serving/45g	194	5.6	431	9.5	66.6	12.4	7.5
Granola, Super Nutty, Aldi*	1 Serving/45g	217	9.9	483	11	56	22	7.2
Granola, Super Nutty, Finest, Tesco*	1 Serving/50g	229	8.7	457	12.2	59.3	17.4	7
Granola, Super Seedy, with Calming Ginger, Troo*	1 Serving/45g	206	9.6	457	15.7	46.7	21.3	22
Granola, Super, Cocoa, Cashew, Almond, Spelt, Kellogg's*	1 Serving/45g	204	8.6	454	11	55	19	9.4
Granola, Tropical Twist, Paleo, Planet Organic*	1 Serving/35g	197	14.3	536	16	36	39	7.8
Granola, Very Berry, Aldi*	1 Serving/45g	191	5.4	424	11	64	12	8.1
Granola, Very Berry, Asda*	1 Serving/45g	187	4.9	417	10	66	11	8
Grape Nuts, Kraft*	1 Serving/45g	158	0.9	350	10.9	81.9	2	11.9
Harvest Crunch, Nut, Quaker*	1 Serving/40g	184	7.8	459	8	62.5	19.5	6
Harvest Crunch, Real Red Berries, Quaker*	1 Serving/50g	224	8.5	447	7	66	17	4.5
High Bran, CBY, Asda*	1 Serving/40g	136	1.5	341	13.6	49.5	3.8	27.1
High Fibre Bran, Co-Op*	1 Serving/40g	110	1.6	275	15	46	4	27
High Fibre Bran, Sainsbury's*	1 Serving/40g	140	1.6	350	13.7	54	3.9	22.1
High Fruit Muesli, BGTY, Sainsbury's*	1 Serving/50g	164	1	328	6.7	71	1.9	6.6
Honey & Nut Crisp, Mini, Weetabix*	1 Serving/40g	150	0.8	375	9.4	75.1	2	9.3

BREAKFAST CEREAL

	Measure INFO/WEIGHT	per Measure KCAL	FAT	Nutrition Values per 100g / 100ml KCAL	PROT	CARB	FAT	FIBRE
Honey Cheerios with 125ml Semi Skimmed Milk, Nestle*	1 Serving/30g	174	2.9	580	21	99.7	9.7	5.7
Honey Hoops, Harvest Morn, Aldi*	1 Serving/30g	117	1	389	6.5	81	3.4	4
Honey Loops, Kellogg's*	1 Serving/30g	110	0.9	367	8	77	3	6
Honey Nut Clusters, Tesco*	1 Bowl/50g	220	7.2	441	9.2	65.7	14.4	6
Honey Nut Crunch , Asda*	1 Serving/40g	176	5.2	441	10	68	13	5.3
Honey Raisin & Almond, Crunchy, Waitrose*	1 Serving/40g	170	4.8	425	10.5	68.8	12	5.7
Hoops, Multigrain, Asda*	1 Serving/30g	113	1.2	376	6.5	78.4	4	4.6
Hoops, Multigrain, Tesco*	1 Serving/30g	112	1.1	375	6.5	78.6	3.8	4.6
Hoops, Mutigrain, Harvest Morn, Aldi*	1 Serving/30g	114	1	380	9	75	3.4	7.4
Hot Oat, Aldi*	1 Serving/40g	142	3.3	356	11.6	58.8	8.3	8.9
Hot Oats, Instant, Tesco*	1 Serving/30g	108	2.6	360	11.8	58.4	8.7	7.9
Instant Oats, Dry Weight	*1 Sachet/36g*	*129*	*3.1*	*359*	*11.5*	*59.1*	*8.5*	*8.3*
Jungle Bites, Asda*	1 Serving/30g	112	0.6	375	8	78	2	6.5
Just Right, Kellogg's*	1 Serving/40g	148	0.8	371	7	79	2	4.5
Krave, Chocolate & Hazelnut, Kellogg's*	1 Serving/30g	136	4.8	452	7.2	68	16	3.4
Krave, Milk Chocolate, Kellogg's*	1 Serving/30g	134	4.5	445	7.1	69	15	3
Lion, Nestle*	1 Serving/40g	166	3.1	415	7.2	76.9	7.7	4.3
Luxury Muesli, Diet Chef Ltd*	1 Pack/40g	166	4.7	414	10.6	61	11.8	10.9
Malted Wheaties, CBY, Asda*	1 Serving/40g	146	0.8	366	10.3	72.7	1.9	8.2
Malted Wheats, Waitrose*	1 Serving/30g	110	0.6	365	10	72.7	1.9	8.5
Malties, Sainsbury's*	1 Serving/40g	146	0.8	366	10.1	71.8	1.9	10.8
Malties, Wholegrain, Aldi*	1 Serving/40g	146	0.8	366	10.1	71.8	1.9	10.8
Malty Flakes with Red Berries, Tesco*	1 Serving/30g	111	0.6	369	9.9	78.1	1.9	3.1
Malty Flakes, Tesco*	1 Serving/40g	148	0.6	371	11	78.4	1.5	4.3
Maple & Pecan Crisp, Sainsbury's*	1 Serving/50g	226	9.8	452	7.9	61.3	19.5	5.4
Maple & Pecan Crisp, Tesco*	1 Serving/50g	215	7.6	430	10.5	62.5	15.2	10.2
Maple & Pecan, Crisp, Asda*	1 Serving/30g	135	5.7	451	8	62	19	6
Millet Rice Oatbran Flakes, Nature's Path*	1 Serving/56g	204	3.2	365	11.3	67	5.8	10
Milo Duo, Nestle*	1 Serving/30g	116	1.7	386	8.2	75.6	5.6	4.9
Mini Bites, Cinnamon, Wholegrain, Be Natural *	1 Serving/30g	106	0.4	354	9.2	69.6	1.3	11.1
Mini Wheats, Original, Frosted, Kellogg's*	1 Serving/30g	106	0.6	352	9.3	83.3	1.8	11.1
Minibix, Weetabix*	1 Serving/40g	134	1.5	335	8.8	71.2	3.8	8.1
Muesli Base, Wholesome, Waitrose*	1 Portion/50g	125	4.2	250	11.5	31.8	8.4	5
Muesli, 4 Fruit, Almond & Hazelnut, M&S*	1 Serving/45g	162	3.3	360	8.5	61.6	7.3	7.1
Muesli, 8 Fruit, Nut, & Seed, Luxury, M&S*	1 Serving/45g	177	6.3	393	10.2	51.8	14	9.7
Muesli, Almonds & Apricot, Toasted, Crisp, Eat Natural*	1 Serving/50g	206	7.5	412	9.2	44.6	15	6.6
Muesli, Basics, Sainsbury's*	1 Serving/50g	178	2.6	355	11.2	61.5	5.1	9.2
Muesli, Berry, & Cherry, Luscious, Dorset Cereals*	1 Serving/45g	149	0.9	332	7	67	2.1	8.3
Muesli, Bircher, Fruity, The Best, Morrisons*	1 Serving/40g	158	3.6	396	8.8	66.5	9	6.9
Muesli, COU, M&S*	1 Serving/60g	201	1.5	335	7.6	70.2	2.5	8.1
Muesli, Creamy Tropical Fruit, Finest, Tesco*	1 Serving/80g	283	4.5	354	7.2	68.8	5.6	6.9
Muesli, Crunchy, Organic, Sainsbury's*	1 Serving/40g	168	5.8	420	10.6	62	14.4	9.2
Muesli, De Luxe, No Added Salt or Sugar, Sainsbury's*	1 Serving/40g	161	5.6	403	11.9	57.6	13.9	8.4
Muesli, Fruit & Nut, 55%, Asda*	1 Serving/40g	151	5.6	378	9	54	14	7
Muesli, Fruit & Nut, Luxury, Co-Op*	1 Serving/40g	150	4	375	8	64	10	6
Muesli, Fruit & Nut, Luxury, Lidl*	1 Serving/57g	205	5.6	360	8	60	9.8	7.5
Muesli, Fruit & Nut, Luxury, Simply Sumptuous, Lidl*	1 Serving/45g	179	6.2	398	8	57.6	13.8	5.8
Muesli, Fruit & Nut, Luxury, Waitrose*	1 Serving/40g	145	3.8	363	9	60.3	9.5	6.5
Muesli, Fruit & Nut, M&S*	1 Serving/40g	128	1.1	320	7.4	74.5	2.8	7.4
Muesli, Fruit & Nut, Organic, M&S*	1 Serving/50g	166	3	333	8.2	61.6	6	7.6
Muesli, Fruit & Nut, Tesco*	1 Serving/50g	190	5.6	380	8.4	60.3	11.3	5.3
Muesli, Fruit & Nut, Whole Wheat, Organic, Asda*	1 Serving/50g	172	3.5	343	10	60	7	7
Muesli, Fruit & Fibre, M&S*	1 Serving/45g	171	4.7	380	8.7	59	10.4	7.6

BREAKFAST CEREAL

	Measure INFO/WEIGHT	per Measure KCAL	FAT	Nutrition Values per 100g / 100ml KCAL	PROT	CARB	FAT	FIBRE
Muesli, Fruit & Nut, Essential, Waitrose*	1 Serving/45g	173	6.1	384	8.6	51.5	13.5	11
Muesli, Fruit & Nut, Jordans*	1 Serving/50g	180	4.7	361	8	61.2	9.4	7.5
Muesli, Fruit & Nut, Luxury, Sainsbury's*	1 Serving/50g	178	4.6	355	10.3	57.9	9.1	11.3
Muesli, Fruit & Nut, Sainsbury's*	1 Serving/30g	114	3.1	379	9.5	58.7	10.3	6.9
Muesli, Fruit & nut, TTD, Sainsbury's*	1 Serving/45g	188	6.3	418	10.8	58.5	13.9	7.9
Muesli, Fruit & Nut, Wholegrain, M&S*	1 Serving/30g	105	1.6	349	9.5	60	5.5	10.8
Muesli, Fruit Nut & Seed, Organic, Dorset Cereals*	1 Serving/70g	251	6.9	358	10.8	56.6	9.8	8.4
Muesli, Fruit Sensation, M&S*	1 Serving/50g	158	1.5	315	6	66	3	7.4
Muesli, Fruit, Nuts & Seeds, Dorset Cereals*	1 Serving/45g	172	4	383	10	58	8.9	8.6
Muesli, Fruit, Sainsbury's*	1 Serving/40g	132	1.8	330	8.1	64.3	4.5	9.6
Muesli, Fruit, Waitrose*	1 Serving/30g	101	1.4	338	7.2	66.8	4.7	6.8
Muesli, GF, Nature's Harvest, Holland & Barrett*	1 Serving/60g	234	7.8	390	14.1	54.1	13	3.3
Muesli, Golden Sun, Lidl*	1 Serving/40g	144	3.9	360	8	60	9.8	7.5
Muesli, High Fruit & Fibre, BuyWholeFoodsOnline*	1 Serving/30g	119	4.8	397	11	53.1	16.1	9.9
Muesli, Light & Crispy, Jordans*	1 Serving/50g	172	2.5	343	7.7	66.7	5	9.5
Muesli, Luxury Fruit, Harvest Morn, Aldi*	1 Serving/50g	179	2.3	358	7.2	69	4.6	5.6
Muesli, Luxury, Finest, Tesco*	1 Serving/50g	197	6.6	394	8.3	60.8	13.1	5.4
Muesli, Natural, No Added Sugar or Salt, Jordans*	1 Serving/45g	161	2.2	357	9.5	63.7	5	9.7
Muesli, No Added Sugar Or Salt, Organic, Jordans*	1 Serving/50g	175	4.4	350	9.2	58.4	8.8	9.3
Muesli, No Added Sugar, Mornflake*	1 Serving/40g	147	2.4	367	10.2	63.9	6	8.2
Muesli, No Added Sugar, Morrisons*	1 Serving/50g	166	2.6	331	11.2	64.7	5.1	6.3
Muesli, No Added Sugar, Waitrose*	1 Serving/40g	146	2.5	364	12	64.9	6.3	6.7
Muesli, Nuts & Seeds , Tesco*	1 Serving/50g	195	5.5	390	10.9	57.2	11	9.2
Muesli, Original, Holland & Barrett*	1 Serving/30g	105	2.5	351	11.1	61.2	8.4	7.1
Muesli, Original, Raisins, Hazelnuts, & Almonds, Alpen*	1 Serving/40g	144	2.3	359	10.5	66.6	5.8	7.3
Muesli, Original, Simply, Hubbards*	1 Serving/50g	212	6.7	424	11.8	59.4	13.4	9.2
Muesli, Really Nutty, Dorset Cereals*	1 Serving/70g	253	6.1	362	9.8	61.1	8.7	6.3
Muesli, Really Nutty, Simply Sumptuous, Lidl*	1 Serving/45g	167	3.9	371	9.5	59.2	8.7	8.9
Muesli, Roasted Nut, Gloriously, Dorset Cereals*	1 Serving/45g	189	7.2	419	14.5	49	16	8.7
Muesli, Seriously Nutty, Mornflake*	1 Bowl/45g	202	10.1	449	14.5	43.4	22.5	7.6
Muesli, Simply Delicious, Dorset Cereals*	1 Serving/45g	160	3.3	356	9.9	58.1	7.4	8.9
Muesli, Simply Fruity, As Sold, Dorset Cereals*	1 Serving/45g	152	1.1	337	7.3	68	2.4	6.8
Muesli, Simply Sumptuous, Luxury Fruit, Lidl*	1 Serving/45g	154	1.5	343	6.5	68.7	3.3	6.2
Muesli, Six Nut, Finest, Tesco*	1 Serving/50g	224	9.6	448	14.2	50.2	19.3	8.4
Muesli, Special, Fruit, Jordans*	1 Serving/50g	162	1.4	323	6.6	68	2.7	8.4
Muesli, Super Berry, Jordans*	1 Serving/50g	174	3.8	348	9	60.8	7.6	8.1
Muesli, Super High Fibre, Dorset Cereals*	1 Serving/70g	250	6.6	357	8	60.1	9.4	8.4
Muesli, Swiss Style with Fruit, Tesco*	1 Serving/40g	144	2.1	360	10.4	67.4	5.3	7.4
Muesli, Swiss Style, Co-Op*	1 Serving/40g	148	2.4	370	11	67	6	6
Muesli, Swiss Style, No Added Salt or Sugar, Sainsbury's*	1 Serving/50g	178	3	357	10.9	64.9	6	6
Muesli, Swiss Style, No Added Salt or Sugar, Tesco*	1 Serving/50g	182	3.2	364	11	61	6.4	9.6
Muesli, Swiss Style, No Added Sugar or Salt, Asda*	1 Serving/50g	182	3.5	363	11	64	7	8
Muesli, Swiss Style, No Added Sugar, CBY, Asda*	1 Serving/45g	166	2.5	369	11	65	5.6	7.6
Muesli, Swiss Style, No Added Sugar, Lidl*	1 Serving/30g	111	1.8	371	10.9	64.5	6	7.8
Muesli, Swiss Style, Smart Price, Asda*	1 Serving/60g	222	3.6	370	9	70	6	10
Muesli, Swiss Style, Tesco*	1 Serving/50g	189	3.1	378	10.4	67	6.2	6.4
Muesli, Swiss, Original, Harvest Morn, Aldi*	1 Serving/45g	164	2.1	365	10	65	4.7	10
Muesli, The Ultimate, Organic, Rude Health*	1 Serving/50g	163	4.5	326	10.8	50.5	9	12.3
Muesli, Toasted Spelt, Barley, Oat Flakes, Dorset Cereals*	1 Serving/40g	148	4.5	371	9.5	57.9	11.3	7.4
Muesli, Toasted, GF with Buckwheat, Eat Natural*	1 Serving/50g	230	11.4	461	11.7	53.2	22.8	2
Muesli, Tropical, Sainsbury's*	1 Serving/50g	182	3.4	365	6.5	69.4	6.8	6.4
Muesli, Whole Wheat, No Added Sugar & Salt, Tesco*	1 Serving/40g	154	5	386	9.5	59.1	12.4	7.4
Muesli, with Berries, Swiss, Dry, Love Life, Waitrose*	1 Serving/45g	172	4.3	383	13.5	55.7	9.6	9.8

BREAKFAST CEREAL

	Measure INFO/WEIGHT	per Measure KCAL	FAT	Nutrition Values per 100g / 100ml KCAL	PROT	CARB	FAT	FIBRE
Muesli, with Toasted Nuts & Seeds, Eat Natural*	1 Portion/50g	219	11.1	438	11.5	38.9	22.2	7.9
Multigrain Boulders, Tesco*	1 Serving/30g	112	0.4	375	8.2	82.3	1.3	3.6
Multigrain Flakes with Fruit & Nuts, Aldi*	1 Serving/30g	108	0.7	360	7.5	77.1	2.4	4.5
Multigrain Flakes, with Fruit, Tesco*	1 Serving/40g	147	0.9	367	7.2	77.3	2.2	4.7
Multigrain Hoops, Free From, Tesco*	1 Serving/30g	113	1	376	7.4	77.3	3.2	4.2
Multigrain Hoops, Harvest Morn, Aldi*	1 Serving/30g	109	0.9	364	9.3	69	2.9	12
Multigrain, Fitnesse, Nestle*	1 Serving/30g	109	0.4	363	8	79.8	1.3	5.1
Multigrain, Hoops, Average	***1 Serving/30g***	***112***	***1.1***	***374***	***6.6***	***77.4***	***3.6***	***6.1***
Nesquik, Chocolatey Corn & Rice, Nestle*	1 Serving/30g	111	0.5	369	8.4	76	1.7	8.7
Nutri Brex, Biscuits, GF, Nutri Brex*	3 Biscuits/46g	174	1.7	378	12.3	70	3.6	6.8
Nuts & Seeds, with Honey, Eat Natural*	1 Serving/30g	138	6.7	461	12.5	48.3	22.3	8.9
Nuts, Clusters, & Seeds, Protein, Special K, Kellogg's*	1 Serving/40g	157	2.8	392	13	65	7	8.3
Nutty Crunch, Alpen*	1 Serving/40g	159	4.5	398	10.7	63.6	11.2	6.5
Nutty Crunch, Deliciously, M&S*	1 Serving/45g	220	10.5	488	9.9	57.4	23.3	4.6
Oat & Bran Flakes, Sainsbury's*	1 Serving/30g	97	1.7	324	12.2	56	5.7	17.7
Oat Bran, Hodgson Mill*	1 Serving/40g	48	1.2	120	6	23	3	6
Oat Clusters, Triple Chocolate Crunch, M&S*	1 Serving/45g	212	8.9	471	8.5	61.9	19.8	5.6
Oat Granola, Quaker*	1 Serving/50g	206	4.4	411	8.6	73	8.8	5.2
Oat Granola, Raisin, Quaker*	1 Serving/45g	188	4.1	418	8	70.9	9.1	6.9
Oat Meal, Medium, Heart's Content, Mornflake*	1 Serving/30g	108	2.4	359	11	60.4	8.1	8.5
Oatbran 100%, Pure & Simple, Mornflake*	1 Serving/40g	146	3.8	364	13.4	47.3	9.4	18.2
Oatbran Flakes, Nature's Path*	1 Serving/30g	124	1.4	414	8.7	83	4.7	6.7
Oatbran Sprinkles, Mornflake*	1 Serving/40g	146	3.8	364	13.4	47.3	9.4	18.2
Oatbran, Original Pure, Mornflake*	1 Serving/30g	104	2.9	345	14.8	49.7	9.7	15.2
Oatibix Flakes, Red Berries, Oatibix*	1 Serving/30g	121	2.5	403	11	67	8.3	8.1
Oatibix, Flakes, Weetabix*	1 Serving/50g	190	2.8	381	9.5	73.2	5.6	3.5
Oatibix, Original, Bitesize, Weetabix*	1 Serving/36g	133	2.4	370	10.6	66.5	6.8	10.1
Oatibix, Weetabix*	2 Biscuits/48g	189	3.8	394	12.5	64.3	8	7.3
Oatmeal, Coarse, Prewett's*	1 Serving/40g	137	4.2	343	14.3	47.6	10.6	16
Oatmeal, Quick Oats, Dry, Quaker*	1 Serving/30g	114	2	380	14	66.7	6.7	10
Oatmeal, Raw	***1oz/28g***	***112***	***2.4***	***401***	***12.4***	***72.8***	***8.7***	***6.8***
Oats, Ginger Bread, Bench Press, Instant, Oomf*	1 Pot/75g	296	3.4	395	28.3	57.1	4.5	6.7
Oats, Golden Syrup Flavour, Instant, Hot, Waitrose*	1 Serving/39g	153	2.3	393	7.8	77.4	5.8	6
Oats, Instant, Protein, Ironmaxx *	1 Hp Tbsp/20g	79	1.4	396	14.1	67.9	7.2	5
Oats, Jumbo, Asda*	1 Serving/40g	148	2.4	369	12	61	6.1	9.4
Oats, Jumbo, Organic, Waitrose*	1 Serving/50g	180	4	361	11	61.1	8.1	7.8
Oats, Original, Instant, Hot, Waitrose*	1 Sachet/27g	97	2.2	359	11	60.4	8.1	8.5
Oats, Pure, Free From, Sainsbury's*	1 Serving/40g	164	3.2	410	14.9	64	8	11
Oats, Superfast, Mornflake*	1 Serving/40g	147	3.4	367	12.1	56.1	8.4	9.1
Oats, Tesco*	1 Serving/40g	142	3.2	356	11	60	8	8
Oats, Wholegrain, Organic, Quaker*	1 Serving/25g	89	2	356	11	60	8	9
Organic, Weetabix*	2 Biscuits/38g	134	0.7	358	11.5	68.6	2	10
Physalis, Almond, & Fig, Supermix Powder, Germline*	1 Serving/35g	141	3.8	403	13	61	11	6.3
Pillows, Choco Nut, Free From, Tesco*	1 Serving/30g	136	4.7	453	6.4	70.8	15.6	2.1
Porage Oats, Old Fashioned, Dry, Scotts*	1 Serving/40g	142	3.2	355	11	60	8	9
Porage Oats, Original, Dry, Scotts*	1 Serving/40g	149	3.2	372	11	60	8	9
Porage Oats, Original, So-Easy, Dry, Scotts*	1 Serving/30g	109	2.6	364	11	60	8.5	9
Porage Oats, Syrup Swirl, So-Easy, Dry, Scotts*	1 Sachet/37g	135	2.2	366	8	70	6	6.5
Porridge 5 Grain, 5 Seed, Rude Health*	1 Serving/50g	176	4.1	351	12.2	57.1	8.2	12.4
Porridge Oats, & Bran, Co-Op*	1 Serving/40g	141	2.8	353	12.5	60	7	12
Porridge Oats, Co-Op*	1 Serving/40g	144	3.2	360	12	61	8	9
Porridge Oats, Dry Weight, Value, Tesco*	1 Serving/50g	180	4	359	11	60.4	8.1	8.5
Porridge Oats, Everyday Essentials, Aldi*	1 Serving/40g	162	2.6	405	12	70	6.4	8.9

BREAKFAST CEREAL

	Measure INFO/WEIGHT	per Measure KCAL	FAT	Nutrition Values per 100g / 100ml KCAL	PROT	CARB	FAT	FIBRE
Porridge Oats, Golden Syrup, Asda*	1 Sachet/36g	137	2.1	381	9.3	70	5.7	6.8
Porridge Oats, Honey Flavour, Paw Ridge, Quaker*	1 Sachet/29g	103	2	361	9.6	64.7	7	7.9
Porridge Oats, Mornflake*	1 Serving/40g	147	3.4	367	12.1	56.1	8.4	9.1
Porridge Oats, Organic, Kavanagh's, Aldi*	1 Serving/40g	148	2.1	370	12	64	5.3	8.6
Porridge Oats, Organic, Tesco*	1 Serving/50g	184	4.2	368	12.1	56.1	8.4	10
Porridge Oats, Original, Asda*	1 Sachet/27g	101	2	375	12	61	7.4	8.4
Porridge Oats, Original, Dry, Quaker*	1 Serving/45g	160	3.6	356	11	60	8	4
Porridge Oats, Plain, Jumbo, Moma Foods*	1 Pot/40g	144	2.4	361	11.7	60.3	6	9.3
Porridge Oats, Rolled, Tesco*	1 Serving/50g	180	4	359	11	60.4	8.1	8.5
Porridge Oats, Scottish, Organic, Sainsbury's*	1 Serving/45g	172	2.2	383	10	74.4	5	7.9
Porridge Oats, Scottish, Tesco*	1 Serving/50g	180	4	359	11	60.4	8.1	8.5
Porridge Oats, Sprouted, Organic, Rude Health*	1 Serving/10g	38	0.6	375	16	64	6.5	10
Porridge Oats, with Oatbran & Wheatbran, Tesco*	1 Portion/50g	187	4.1	375	11	58.3	8.3	11.4
Porridge Oats, with Wheatbran, Essential, Waitrose*	1 Serving/50g	168	3.8	336	11.2	55.8	7.6	13
Porridge To Go, Cinnamon, Quaker*	1 Square/55g	217	4.5	394	6.3	68	8.2	10.8
Porridge, 5 Grain, & Seed, Organic, Harvest Morn, Aldi*	1 Serving/50g	190	5	380	12	55	10	11
Porridge, Apple & Cinnamon, Express, Dry, Sainsbury's*	1 Sachet/36g	138	2.1	383	8.6	70.3	5.9	7.2
Porridge, Apple & Cinnamon, Variety Box, Graze*	1 Bag/67g	240	3.4	356	8	68	5	10
Porridge, Apple, Cinnamon, & Raisin, Nutri Boost, Quaker*	1 Sachet/38g	149	2.5	391	12	66	6.5	9.3
Porridge, Apple, Sultana & Cinnamon, M&S*	1 Sachet/40g	144	3	360	10.3	62.3	7.5	8.6
Porridge, Berry Burst, Oat So Simple, Quaker*	1 Serving/39g	144	2.3	370	8	70	6	6.5
Porridge, Berry Burst, Wholegrain, Instant , M&S*	1 Pot/70g	252	3.3	360	12.6	62.7	4.7	8.4
Porridge, Blueberry, Cranberry, Guava, Made Up, Quaker*	1 Serving/35g	128	2.3	365	9	63	6.7	9.1
Porridge, Blueberry, Frozen, Tesco*	1 Pack/250g	202	4.4	81	3.5	12	1.8	1.7
Porridge, Brochan*	1 Serving/30g	112	1.7	374	15.4	61.5	5.7	7.8
Porridge, Caramel, Instant, Pot, Oat So Simple, Quaker*	1 Pot/57g	208	3.2	365	10.5	67.7	5.6	6.3
Porridge, Chocolate, Free From, Ocado*	1 Serving/45g	174	2.7	384	11	66	6	11
Porridge, Chocolate, High Protein, Pot, Fuel 10K*	1 Pot/70g	263	4.7	376	19.4	55.9	6.7	6.3
Porridge, Chocolate, Ready Brek, Weetabix*	1 Serving/30g	114	2.4	380	10	63.6	8	7
Porridge, Coconut, & Chia, Moma Foods*	1 Serving/55g	233	9.5	423	10.8	53.2	17.3	9.4
Porridge, Complete Protein, Bulk Powders*	1 Serving/50g	188	3.1	377	29.9	47	6.2	6.5
Porridge, Cranberry & Raisin, Sachets, Dry, Moma Foods*	1 Sachet/70g	248	2.7	354	13.9	63.6	3.9	6.4
Porridge, Cranberry & Raspberry, Fruity, Dorset Cereals*	1 Sachet/30g	99	1.8	330	10.2	58.7	6	12.3
Porridge, Fresh, Double Cream, & Demerara Sugar, M&S*	1 Pot/200g	254	15.2	127	4.3	9.7	7.6	1.3
Porridge, GF, Oat So Simple, Quaker*	1 Sachet/35g	130	2.5	370	13.2	58.5	7.2	9.2
Porridge, Golden Honey, Oatibix, Weetabix*	1 Serving/40g	145	2.6	363	9.2	66.7	6.6	7
Porridge, Golden Syrup, Dry, Oat So Simple, Quaker*	1 Sachet/36g	137	2.2	380	8.4	68.7	6.2	6.8
Porridge, Golden Syrup, Instant, As Consumed, Slim Fast*	1 Sachet/29g	99	1.3	340	17.4	53.2	4.6	7.9
Porridge, Golden Syrup, Prepared, Oatilicious, Lidl*	1 Sachet/39g	140	1.5	358	8.8	69	3.9	6
Porridge, Honey & Vanilla, Express Pot, Quaker*	1 Pot/57g	213	2.9	374	15.1	64.1	5.1	5.5
Porridge, Instant, Sweet Cinnamon, Harvest Morn, Aldi*	1 Pot/57g	211	2.6	371	15	64	4.5	7.8
Porridge, Made with Semi Skimmed Milk, Waitrose*	1 Serving/50g	277	7.5	554	24.6	80.4	15	8.6
Porridge, Maple & Pecan, Oat So Simple, Quaker*	1 Pack/35g	132	2.3	376	8.4	66.6	6.5	8.8
Porridge, Maple Syrup Flavour, Pot, As Sold, M&S*	1 Pot/70g	260	2.6	371	11.6	70.7	3.7	4.3
Porridge, Morning Glory, Rude Health*	1 Bowl/50g	176	4.1	351	12.2	57.1	8.2	12.4
Porridge, Multigrain, Jordans*	1 Serving/40g	134	2.2	335	10.4	60.9	5.5	10
Porridge, Nutty, Pot, As Sold, Wolfys*	1 Pot/90g	385	11.9	428	12.6	56.6	13.2	6.9
Porridge, Oat, & Barley, Instant, M&S*	1 Pot/70g	257	4.3	367	11.4	62.2	6.1	9.4
Porridge, Oatmeal, Rude Health*	1 Serving/40g	152	2.6	380	10.2	66	6.4	7.6
Porridge, Oats, 100% Whole Grain, Rolled, Jumbo, Quaker*	1 Serving/40g	150	3.2	374	11	60	8	9
Porridge, Oats, 100% Whole Grain, Rolled, Quaker*	1 Portion/40g	150	3.2	374	11	60	8	9
Porridge, Oats, Apple & Blueberry, Instant, Pot, Tesco*	1 Pot/205g	210	2.9	102	3.6	18.1	1.4	1.5
Porridge, Oats, Berry & Cherry, Instant, Pot, Tesco*	1 Pot/225g	207	2.9	92	3.2	16.2	1.3	1.4

BREAKFAST CEREAL

	Measure INFO/WEIGHT	per Measure KCAL	FAT	Nutrition Values per 100g / 100ml KCAL	PROT	CARB	FAT	FIBRE
Porridge, Oats, Berry, Instant, Free From, Asda*	1 Sachet/27g	98	1.1	364	10	68	4.1	7.6
Porridge, Oats, Cinnamon, Instant, Pot, Tesco*	1 Pot/225g	212	3.2	94	3.3	16.4	1.4	1.4
Porridge, Oats, Dry, Smart Price, Asda*	1 Serving/50g	186	4	372	11	60	8	8
Porridge, Oats, GF, Organic, Scottish, Alara *	1 Serving/40g	148	2.2	369	11.8	67.9	5.5	7.5
Porridge, Oats, Golden Syrup, Instant, Pot, Tesco*	1 Pot/55g	210	2.7	380	11.4	70	4.9	5.5
Porridge, Oats, Golden Syrup, Sainsbury's*	1 Sachet/39g	143	2.1	367	6.3	73.6	5.3	6.7
Porridge, Oats, Irish, Multi Seed, Flahavans*	1 Serving/40g	166	5.3	415	14	55.4	13.3	9
Porridge, Oats, No Added Sugar, Love Life, Waitrose*	1 Pot/60g	224	3.8	373	17.5	57.8	6.4	7.2
Porridge, Oats, Original, Instant, Pot, Tesco*	1 Pot/256g	208	3.3	81	3.1	13.5	1.3	1.6
Porridge, Oats, Twice the Fibre, M&S*	1 Portion/60g	230	3.5	384	10.4	62.6	5.9	19.5
Porridge, Oats, Whole, Chunky, Traditional, Jordans*	1 Serving/40g	143	2.7	358	6.7	63.6	6.8	7.9
Porridge, Original, Diet Chef Ltd*	1 Sachet/40g	157	2.5	392	12	67	6.3	9.8
Porridge, Original, Dry, Oat So Simple, Quaker*	1 Sachet/27g	100	2.1	370	11	58.9	7.7	10.5
Porridge, Original, Express, Sachet, Sainsbury's*	1 Pack/27g	100	2.2	370	11	58	8	10.8
Porridge, Original, Pot, Made Up, Asda*	1 Pot/221g	199	2.7	90	3.3	16	1.2	2.1
Porridge, Original, Pot, Made Up, Morrisons*	1 Pot/225g	205	2.7	91	3.5	16	1.2	1.1
Porridge, Original, Ready Brek, Weetabix*	1 Serving/40g	149	3.5	373	11.7	57.9	8.7	7.9
Porridge, Original, Simply, Sachet, Asda*	1 Sachet/27g	96	2.2	356	11	60	8	8
Porridge, Original, Super Goodness, Quaker*	1 Serving/31g	114	2.8	372	14.1	56.7	9.1	9.9
Porridge, Plain, Instant, Quaker*	1 Serving/34g	124	2.9	364	11	60	8.5	9
Porridge, Raspberry & Cranberry, Made Up, Quaker*	1 Sachet/39g	217	5.6	564	26	81.6	14.6	9.4
Porridge, Ready Oats, CBY, Asda*	1 Serving/40g	149	3.5	374	12	58	8.7	7.9
Porridge, Red Berry, Instant, As Consumed, Slim Fast*	1 Sachet/29g	99	1.3	341	17.2	53.1	4.5	7.9
Porridge, Rice & Buckwheat, Free From, Sainsbury's*	1 Serving/50g	179	0.4	358	6.8	81.1	0.7	1.4
Porridge, Spiced Sultana, Diet Chef Ltd*	1 Pack/37g	148	2.5	400	9.6	70.8	6.7	8.8
Porridge, Super Seeds, Instant, Dry, Moma Foods*	1 Sachet/70g	258	4.8	368	18.5	55.6	6.9	7.7
Porridge, Vanilla & Banana, Diet Chef Ltd*	1 Pack/40g	151	2.2	378	10.7	70.6	5.6	9.8
Porridge, with Cocao Nib, Diet Chef Ltd*	1 Pack/40g	164	3.5	410	10.9	67.3	8.8	9.5
Protein Crunch, Chocolate, Weetabix*	1 Serving/30g	114	1	379	20	64	3.2	7
Protein Crunch, Weetabix*	1 Serving/30g	114	0.8	379	20	66	2.5	6.1
Puffed Rice, Average	**1 Serving/30g**	**115**	**0.8**	**382**	**7.1**	**82.2**	**2.8**	**3**
Puffed Rice, Organic, Natural, Kallo*	1 Bowl/25g	92	0.5	370	7	81	2	3
Puffed Rice, Wholegrain, Brown, Original, Organic, Kallo*	1 Serving/25g	95	0.8	380	8	80	3	9
Puffed Wheat, Quaker*	1 Serving/15g	49	0.2	328	15.3	62.4	1.3	5.6
Puffed Wheat, Tesco*	1 Serving/28g	104	0.9	373	13.9	72.2	3.2	5.7
Raisin & Almond, Crunchy, Jordans*	1 Serving/45g	186	5.7	412	9.9	61.6	12.6	6.6
Raisin Oats & More, & 125ml Semi Skimmed Milk, Nestle*	1 Serving/40g	207	3.9	518	19.8	88	9.8	6.2
Raisin Wheats, Kellogg's*	1 Serving/45g	104	0.6	345	9	69	2	9
Raisin, Bran Flakes, Asda*	1 Serving/50g	166	1.5	331	7	69	3	10
Raisin, Oats & More, Nestle*	1 Serving/30g	112	1.4	373	8.9	73.7	4.7	5.8
Red Berries, Additions, Weetabix*	2 Biscuits/43g	152	0.8	350	9.8	67	1.9	13
Red Berries, Special K, Kellogg's*	1 Serving/30g	112	0.4	374	14	76	1.5	3
Red Berry, & Almond, Luxury Crunch, Jordans*	1 Serving/40g	176	7.4	441	8.2	60.5	18.5	6.6
Rice & Wheat Flakes, Toasted, Love Life, Waitrose*	1 Serving/30g	115	0.4	382	11.7	79.7	1.3	2.2
Rice Krispies, Kellogg's*	1 Serving/30g	116	0.4	387	7	86	1.2	2
Rice Krispies, Multi-Grain, Shapes, Kellogg's*	1 Serving/30g	111	0.8	370	8	77	2.5	8
Rice Pops, GF, Nestle*	1 Serving/30g	116	0.4	385	7.5	85	1.2	1.5
Rice Pops, Organic, Dove's Farm*	1 Serving/30g	107	0.2	357	6.8	86.1	0.8	2
Rice Snaps, Asda*	1 Serving/28g	105	0.4	376	7	84	1.3	1.5
Rice Snaps, Everyday Value, Tesco*	1 Serving/30g	115	0.3	380	7.5	84.5	0.9	1.4
Right Balance, Morrisons*	1 Serving/50g	181	1.1	362	6.9	78.6	2.2	5.3
Shredded Wheat, Average	**2 Biscuits/45g**	**157**	**0.8**	**348**	**9**	**77**	**1.8**	**10**
Shredded Wheat, Bitesize, Nestle*	1 Serving/40g	148	0.9	369	11.8	69.6	2.2	11.8

BREAKFAST CEREAL

INFO/WEIGHT	Measure	per Measure		Nutrition Values per 100g / 100ml				
		KCAL	FAT	KCAL	PROT	CARB	FAT	FIBRE
Shredded Wheat, Honey Nut, Nestle*	1 Serving/40g	151	2.6	378	11.2	68.8	6.5	9.4
Shreddies, Apple & Cinnamon, Limited Edition, Nestle*	1 Serving/40g	148	0.6	370	9.3	75	1.5	9.2
Shreddies, Coco Orange Flavoured, Nestle*	1 Serving/40g	150	0.8	374	8.5	76.2	2	8.6
Shreddies, Coco, Nestle*	1 Serving/45g	161	0.9	358	8.4	76.5	2	8.6
Shreddies, Crunchy Cranberry & Oat Granola, Nestle*	1 Serving/45g	181	3.1	403	13	68	7	7.2
Shreddies, Frosted, Nestle*	1 Serving/45g	166	0.7	370	9.2	76	1.5	9
Shreddies, Frosted, Variety Pack, Nestle*	1 Pack/45g	163	0.6	363	6.7	81.1	1.3	6.8
Shreddies, Honey, Nestle*	1 Serving/45g	169	0.7	375	8.2	78.1	1.5	8.1
Shreddies, Malt Wheats, Tesco*	1 Serving/45g	169	0.9	375	10.3	73.8	2	8.2
Shreddies, Nestle*	1 Serving/45g	186	1	371	10	73.7	1.9	9.9
Special Flakes, Gluten, Wheat, & Milk, Free From, Tesco*	1 Serving/30g	115	0.6	382	6.5	83	2	3
Special Flakes, Honey, Oats, & Almonds, Tesco*	1 Serving/30g	116	0.7	385	7.2	82.5	2.2	3.1
Special Flakes, Red Fruits, Asda*	1 Serving/30g	115	0.4	382	7.1	84	1.3	2.7
Special Flakes, Tesco*	1 Serving/20g	74	0.3	371	11	78.4	1.5	4.3
Special Flakes, with Red Berries, Crownfield, Lidl*	1 Serving/30g	113	0.5	377	6.5	81	1.6	6.4
Special K, Bliss, Strawberry & Chocolate, Kellogg's*	1 Serving/30g	115	0.9	383	13	76	3	2.5
Special K, Kellogg's*	1 Serving/30g	114	0.4	379	14	76	1.5	2.5
Special K, Oats & Honey, Kellogg's*	1 Serving/30g	114	0.9	381	9	77	3	5
Special K, Peach & Apricot, Kellogg's*	1 Serving/30g	112	0.3	373	14	77	1	2.5
Special K, Protein Plus, Kellogg's*	1 Serving/29g	100	3	345	34.5	31	10.3	17.2
Special K, Purple Berries, Kellogg's*	1 Serving/30g	112	0.3	374	13	77	1	3.5
Start, Kellogg's*	1 Serving/30g	117	1	390	8	79	3.5	5
Strawberry Crisp, Asda*	1 Serving/45g	194	7	431	8.1	64.7	15.5	5.9
Strawberry, Alpen*	1 Serving/40g	144	1.9	359	9.4	69.5	4.8	7.9
Sugar Puffs, Quaker*	1 Serving/30g	114	0.5	379	5.3	85.8	1.6	3.7
Sultana Bran, Co-Op*	1 Serving/40g	130	1.2	325	9	66	3	11
Sultana Bran, HL, Tesco*	1 Serving/30g	98	0.6	325	8.2	68	1.9	12
Sultana Bran, Morrisons*	1 Serving/30g	98	0.9	325	8.8	65.8	3	11.4
Sultana Bran, Waitrose*	1 Serving/30g	97	0.6	324	8.2	68.6	1.9	11.6
Weet Bix, Sanitarium*	2 Biscuits/30g	106	0.4	352	12	67	1.4	10.5
Weet-Bix, Blends, Multi-Grain, Sanitarium*	2 Biscuits/48g	185	2.1	385	10.7	70.2	4.4	8.9
Weetabix, Banana, Weetabix*	1 Serving/44g	157	0.9	357	10	70.4	2	9.8
Weetabix, Chocolate, Weetabix*	2 Biscuits/45g	166	1.8	368	10.1	67.9	4	10
Weetaflakes, Weetabix*	1 Serving/30g	102	0.4	340	8.9	72.9	1.4	11
Weetos, Chocolate, Weetabix*	1 Serving/30g	113	1.5	378	8.4	75.1	4.9	5.8
Wheat Biscuits, As Sold, Savers, Morrisons*	2 Biscuits/36g	127	0.6	353	10.8	67.6	1.8	11.6
Wheat Biscuits, Average	*2 Biscuits/38g*	*130*	*0.8*	*347*	*11.7*	*68.4*	*2.2*	*9.9*
Wheat Biscuits, Stockwell & Co., Tesco*	2 Biscuits/36g	127	0.6	352	11.4	67.4	1.6	11.1
Wheat Bisks, Chocolate, Asda*	2 Biscuits/43g	158	1.5	367	10	69	3.4	10
Wheat Bisks, Harvest Morn, Aldi*	2 Biscuits/38g	136	0.8	358	11.5	68.6	2	10
Wheat Bisks, Wholegrain, M&S*	2 Biscuits/40g	141	0.7	353	10.9	68.1	1.7	10.7
Wheat Shreds, Bitesize, Crownfield, Lidl*	1 Serving/40g	142	0.8	356	10.6	67	1.9	14
Wheat Shreds, Harvest Morn, Aldi*	2 Biscuits/45g	156	0.8	346	13	64	1.8	13
Wholegrain Hoops, Goldenvale, Aldi*	1 Serving/30g	111	0.8	371	6.9	74	2.6	10.7
Wholegrain Wheats, Classic, Organic, Kellogg's*	1 Serving/40g	148	1	371	14	68	2.5	10
Wholegrain Wheats, Raisin, Organic, Kellogg's*	1 Bowl/45g	155	0.9	345	9	69	2	9
Wholegrain, Apricot, Wheats, Sainsbury's*	1 Serving/45g	151	0.6	335	8	71.3	1.4	8.3
Wholegrain, Fruit & Fibre, Sainsbury's*	1 Serving/40g	149	2.3	372	9.3	66.1	5.7	9.4
Wholegrain, Mini Wheats, Sainsbury's*	1 Serving/40g	144	0.7	359	11.8	68.2	1.8	11.2
Wholegrain, Minis, Weetabix*	1 Serving/40g	149	0.8	372	10.2	73.2	2	10
Wholesome Crunch, Granola, Pecan & Brazil Nut, Quaker*	1 Serving/45g	189	5	420	11.1	61.8	11.1	13.2
Wholesome Crunch, Granola, Goji & Blueberry, Quaker*	1 Serving/45g	181	3.6	402	11	64.5	7.9	13.5
Yoghurt & Raspberry, Crisp, Sainsbury's*	1 Serving/45g	191	6.7	424	7.5	65.2	14.8	6.4

INFO/WEIGHT	Measure	per Measure KCAL	FAT	Nutrition Values per 100g / 100ml KCAL	PROT	CARB	FAT	FIBRE
BRESAOLA								
Average	*1 Serving/28g*	*51*	*1*	*181*	*33.6*	*0.4*	*3.7*	*0.2*
Finest, Tesco*	1 Serving/35g	64	1.4	182	36	0.5	4	0
Waitrose*	2 Slices/14g	21	0.2	150	33.9	0.5	1.3	0.5
BROCCOLI								
& Cauliflower, Floret Mix, Fresh, Tesco*	1 Serving/80g	27	0.7	34	3.9	2.5	0.9	2.7
Florets, Frozen, Four Seasons, Aldi*	1 Avg Serving/80g	32	0.4	40	4.1	3.5	0.5	2.6
Green, Boiled, Average	*1 Serving/80g*	*19*	*0.6*	*24*	*3.1*	*1.1*	*0.8*	*2.3*
Green, Raw, Average	*1 Serving/80g*	*24*	*0.7*	*30*	*3.7*	*1.6*	*0.8*	*2.5*
Purple Sprouting, Boiled, Average	*1 Serving/80g*	*15*	*0.5*	*19*	*2.1*	*1.3*	*0.6*	*2.3*
Purple Sprouting, Raw	*1oz/28g*	*10*	*0.3*	*35*	*3.9*	*2.6*	*1.1*	*3.5*
Steamed, Average	*1 Serving/100g*	*24*	*0.8*	*24*	*3.1*	*1.1*	*0.8*	*2.3*
Tenderstem, Average	*1 Serving/80g*	*28*	*0.4*	*35*	*4.1*	*2.9*	*0.6*	*2.3*
BROWNIES								
Chocolate, Almonds, & White Chocolate Drizzle, GF, M&S*	1 Piece/46g	211	12.4	458	7.2	43.9	27	5.2
Average	*1 Brownie/60g*	*243*	*10.1*	*405*	*4.6*	*0*	*16.8*	*0*
Chocolate Chip, Cadbury*	1 Brownie/25g	116	7.2	465	4.8	46	29	3
Chocolate Chip, Free From, Morrisons*	1 Slice/30g	143	8	478	6	52.5	26.5	2.9
Chocolate, & Orange, Bites, Amaze, Cadbury*	1 Bite/14g	65	3.3	470	5.3	56.4	24.1	3.1
Chocolate, Average	*1 Serving/100g*	*446*	*22.3*	*446*	*5.9*	*55.6*	*22.3*	*2.2*
Chocolate, Chewy, M&S*	1 Brownie/29g	130	6	455	6.5	59.8	21.1	2
Chocolate, Chunky, Belgian, M&S*	1 Brownie/55g	242	11.2	440	6.2	57.7	20.3	2.5
Chocolate, Double, Bites, Amaze, Cadbury*	1 Bite/14g	65	3.3	470	5.3	56.7	24.1	3.1
Chocolate, Double, Mini Bites, Sainsbury's*	1 Serving/18g	73	3.1	406	5.5	55.9	17.2	2.6
Chocolate, Fudge, Mini, Thorntons*	1 Bite/14g	61	2.8	435	5.6	57.4	20	0
Chocolate, Fudgy, M&S*	1 Brownie/87g	400	21.9	460	4.8	56.9	25.2	3
Chocolate, Mini Bites, Asda*	1 Brownie/15g	62	3	420	5	55	20	1.4
Chocolate, Mix, Made Up, Lo Dough*	1 Brownie/53g	65	2.3	123	6.8	29.9	4.3	13.3
Chocolate, Orange, Organic, The Village Bakery*	1 Brownie/30g	126	6.7	421	5	50.5	22.2	0.9
Chocolate, Sainsbury's*	1 Brownie/60g	265	13.6	442	4.6	55	22.6	1.6
Chocolate, Slices, M&S*	1 Brownie/36g	158	8.7	440	5.3	51.1	24.1	1.3
Chocolate, Tray Bake, Tesco*	1 Brownie/37g	155	6.8	420	5.5	57.1	18.4	5.7
Chocolate, Waitrose*	1 Brownie/45g	192	8.9	426	6.3	55.6	19.8	2.7
Chocolate, Wheat & GF, Mrs Crimble's*	1 Slice/48g	180	9.6	379	4.2	47.9	20.3	1.5
The Graze Brownie, Graze*	1 Portion/30g	110	5.4	368	7.1	50.5	17.9	3.8
BRUSCHETTA								
Cheese & Tomato, Asda*	1 Bruschetta/38g	68	1.7	180	8.6	26	4.6	2.9
Garlic, & Parsley, Valentina*	1 Bruschetta/10g	55	3.1	538	8.4	56.9	30.4	0
Pane Italia*	1 Serving/75g	367	18.8	489	12.4	53.6	25.1	1.4
Red Pepper & Onion, Brunchetta, Golden Vale*	1 Pack/90g	266	17.1	296	14.6	17	19	1.3
Soft Cheese & Cranberry, Brunchetta, Golden Vale*	1 Pack/95g	200	8.6	211	8.2	24.8	9	1.3
Toasted, Olive Oil & Sea Salt, Tesco*	1 Serving/30g	126	4.6	420	11.5	58.7	15.5	4.5
Topping, Tomato & Basil, Spirit of Summer, M&S*	½ Jar/140g	99	4.9	71	1.6	6.6	3.5	3.2
BRUSSELS SPROUTS								
& Sweet Chestnuts, Asda*	1 Serving/100g	73	1.7	73	3.1	11	1.7	4.2
Boiled, Average	*1 Serving/80g*	*27*	*1*	*33*	*3*	*3*	*1.2*	*3.3*
Button, Raw, Average	*1 Serving/80g*	*28*	*1*	*36*	*3.3*	*2.8*	*1.3*	*3*
Canned, Drained	*1oz/28g*	*5*	*0.2*	*17*	*1.6*	*1.5*	*0.6*	*1.6*
Raw, Average	*1 Serving/80g*	*28*	*0.8*	*35*	*3.3*	*3.1*	*1*	*2.9*
Steamed, Average	*1 Serving/100g*	*35*	*1.3*	*35*	*3.1*	*3.2*	*1.3*	*3.5*
with Chestnuts, & Bacon, Tesco*	1 Serving/100g	151	6.6	151	4.7	14.4	6.6	7.7
BUBBLE & SQUEAK								
Fried in Vegetable Oil	*1oz/28g*	*35*	*2.5*	*124*	*1.4*	*9.8*	*9.1*	*1.5*
Tesco*	½ Pack/325g	256	3.7	79	1.5	14.7	1.1	1.9

	Measure INFO/WEIGHT	per Measure KCAL	FAT	Nutrition Values per 100g / 100ml KCAL	PROT	CARB	FAT	FIBRE
BUCKWHEAT								
Average	*1oz/28g*	**102**	**0.4**	**364**	**8.1**	**84.9**	**1.5**	**2.1**
Tatrapallid Hommikuks, Balsnack*	1 Serving/40g	130	1.2	326	11	70	2.9	11
BUFFALO								
Steak, Rump, Extra Lean, Pan Fried, Iceland*	1 Steak/125g	214	3.3	171	36.9	0.1	2.6	0.1
BULGUR WHEAT								
Dry Weight, Average	*1oz/28g*	**99**	**0.5**	**353**	**9.7**	**76.3**	**1.7**	**8**
Quinoa & Rainbow Vegetables, As Prepared, Waitrose*	1 Pack/300g	372	11.4	124	3.1	17.6	3.8	3.6
with Chick Peas, & Quinoa, Ready to Eat, Sainsbury's*	½ Pack/125g	239	4.1	191	7.7	30	3.3	4.7
BUNS								
Bath, Tesco*	1 Bun/80g	262	8.9	328	8	48.9	11.1	5.8
Belgian, Asda*	1 Bun/133g	464	19.9	350	4.8	49	15	2.2
Belgian, Co-Op*	1 Bun/118g	413	15.3	350	5	54	13	2
Belgian, Sainsbury's*	1 Bun/110g	398	11.3	362	6.1	61.3	10.3	1.9
Belgian, Tesco*	1 Bun/123g	438	15.7	356	5.2	54.9	12.8	2.2
Butterfly, GF, Free From, Asda*	1 Bun/37g	159	7.7	434	3.2	58	21	0.5
Chelsea	*1 Bun/78g*	**285**	**10.8**	**366**	**7.8**	**56.1**	**13.8**	**1.7**
Chelsea, Gail's*	100g	374	11.3	374	7.5	59.1	11.3	3
Chelsea, Sainsbury's*	1 Bun/85g	239	4.4	281	6.9	51.6	5.2	2.9
Chelsea, Tesco*	1 Bun/85g	269	6.5	316	7.9	53.9	7.6	2.3
Choux, Caramel, Asda*	1 Bun/189g	745	51	394	4.3	33.5	27	1.3
Choux, Chocolate, Tesco*	1 Choux Bun/74g	259	18.1	350	7.3	24.4	24.5	1.2
Choux, Fresh Cream, Tesco*	1 Bun/95g	340	23.7	358	4.9	28.5	24.9	0.9
Choux, M&S*	1 Bun/78g	247	17.3	317	5.4	25.6	22.2	0.3
Cinnamon, Tear & Share, Bakery, Tesco*	¼ Bun/108g	363	10.7	334	6.9	52.9	9.8	3.3
Currant	*1 Bun/60g*	**178**	**4.5**	**296**	**7.6**	**52.7**	**7.5**	**0**
Finger, Iced, Essential, Waitrose*	1 Bun/40g	139	3.5	347	6.7	59.2	8.7	2.6
Fruit, Waitrose*	1 Bun/54g	155	2.3	287	8.1	54	4.3	1.6
Hot Cross	*1 Bun/50g*	**156**	**3.5**	**312**	**7.4**	**58.5**	**7**	**1.7**
Hot Cross, Asda*	1 Bun/60g	190	3.8	317	10	55	6.3	3.3
Hot Cross, BGTY, Sainsbury's*	1 Bun/70g	189	1.8	270	6.7	53.7	2.6	2.4
Hot Cross, Bramley Apple & Cinnamon, Waitrose*	1 Bun/70g	194	2.7	277	7.7	52.2	3.8	1.5
Hot Cross, Bramley Apple, & Cinnamon, Finest, Tesco*	1 Bun/70g	190	3.8	271	7.4	46.2	5.5	3.5
Hot Cross, Chocolate, Free From, Sainsbury's*	1 Bun/70g	202	8.4	288	3.7	36.4	12	9.6
Hot Cross, Co-Op*	1 Bun/60g	165	3.6	275	8	47	6	3
Hot Cross, Extra Fruit, Finest, Tesco*	1 Bun/80g	218	3.4	272	8.4	48.6	4.2	3.1
Hot Cross, Fruity, Free From, Sainsbury's*	1 Bun/70g	195	6.2	279	3.3	41.4	8.8	10.2
Hot Cross, GF, M&S*	1 Bun/70g	206	4.1	294	2.9	54.1	5.9	6.1
Hot Cross, Luxury, Rowan Hill Bakery, Lidl*	1 Bun/75g	204	3.5	272	8.3	47	4.7	4
Hot Cross, Mini, M&S*	1 Bun/41g	110	1.4	265	7.8	51.4	3.4	3.7
Hot Cross, Morrisons*	1 Bun/72g	178	1.4	247	7.4	49.9	2	3.3
Hot Cross, Richly Fruited, Tesco*	1 Bun/70g	180	2.2	257	8.8	56.7	3.1	3.3
Hot Cross, Salted Caramel, & Chocolate Chip, Tesco*	1 Bun/72g	205	4.5	284	8.1	47.1	6.2	3.8
Hot Cross, Sticky Toffee, The Best, Morrisons*	1 Bun/77g	222	3.5	288	6.8	52.8	4.6	4
Hot Cross, White, Sainsbury's*	1 Bun/70g	199	3.4	284	7.9	50.6	4.8	3.4
Hot Cross, Wholemeal, Asda*	1 Bun/70g	182	4.2	262	9	43	6	6
Hot Cross, Wholemeal, Waitrose*	1 Bun/66g	176	3.2	267	9.6	43.2	4.9	5.7
Iced Finger, Average	*1 Bun/40g*	**130**	**3.1**	**325**	**7.2**	**57**	**7.7**	**2.3**
Iced Finger, Coconut, Genesis Crafty*	1 Bun/64g	210	6.9	328	7.7	52.4	10.8	2.4
Iced Finger, Sainsbury's*	1 Bun/40g	130	3.3	326	7	55.4	8.2	1.4
Iced Finger, Tesco*	1 Bun/40g	135	3.6	338	6.2	57.2	9	1.9
Iced, Filled with Raspberry Jam, M&S*	1 Bun/48g	155	3.2	320	6.4	58.9	6.6	1.9
Vanilla Iced, Soft, M&S*	1 Bun/39g	125	3.1	320	7.6	54.9	8	2.9

B

BURGERS

INFO/WEIGHT	Measure	per Measure KCAL	FAT	Nutrition Values per 100g / 100ml KCAL	PROT	CARB	FAT	FIBRE
American Style, Tesco*	1 Burger/125g	250	9.1	200	13	20.4	7.3	3.9
Aubergine, & Feta, Aromatic & Minty, Waitrose*	1 Burger/101g	238	12.9	235	5.2	22.3	12.7	5.3
BBQ, Gourmet, Flame Grilled, Rustlers*	1 Burger/215g	593	27.7	276	14.6	24.7	12.9	0
Bean, Chilli, Crisp & Spicy, Frozen, Cooked, Waitrose*	1 Burger/95g	226	8.3	238	5.8	31	8.7	6.1
Bean, Green, Vegan, My Best Veggie, Lidl*	1 Serving/100g	144	7.9	144	7.1	7.3	7.9	7.8
Bean, Mexican Style, Meat Free, Tesco*	1 Burger/106g	214	9.6	202	4.8	22	9.1	6.4
Bean, Mexican, Tomato Salsa, Love Life, Waitrose*	1 Burger/93g	255	14.3	274	6.5	24.3	15.4	6.1
Bean, Nacho, Spicy, Iceland*	1 Burger/140g	326	16.5	233	6.9	20.1	11.8	4.4
Bean, Spicy Veg, with Chipotle Chilli, Good Life*	1 Burger/109g	219	9.6	201	5.2	22	8.8	6.4
Bean, Spicy, BGTY, Sainsbury's*	1 Burger/113g	223	11.2	197	4.5	19.6	9.9	5.7
Bean, Spicy, Cauldron Foods*	1 Burger/88g	203	9.8	232	5.4	27.4	11.2	6.2
Bean, Spicy, in Herby Nacho Crumb, Morrisons*	1 Burger/102g	185	8.1	181	5.2	19.5	7.9	5.5
Bean, Spicy, Quarter Pounder, Mae's Kitchen, Aldi*	1 Burger/105g	287	13.6	274	5.4	30	13	9.7
Bean, Spicy, Vegetarian, Tesco*	1 Burger/106g	214	9.6	202	4.8	22	9.1	6.4
Beef, & Caramelised Red Onion, Steak, TTD, Sainsbury's*	1 Burger/133g	287	15.3	216	20.2	7.8	11.5	0.5
Beef, 100%, Average	*1 Burger/52g*	*148*	*11.6*	*286*	*20.5*	*0.6*	*22.3*	*0.1*
Beef, 100%, Birds Eye*	1 Burger/41g	120	10.2	292	17.3	0	24.8	0
Beef, 100%, Half Pounders, Sainsbury's*	1 Burger/148g	462	33.1	313	26	1.7	22.4	0.2
Beef, 100%, Organic, Waitrose*	1 Burger/57g	140	9.6	247	23.6	0	16.9	0
Beef, 100%, Quarter Pounders, Aldi*	1 Burger/114g	320	23.3	282	24.3	0.1	20.5	1.3
Beef, 100%, Sainsbury's*	1 Burger/44g	133	10.4	302	21.4	0.9	23.6	0.9
Beef, 97%, Grilled, Heck*	1 Burger/113g	246	12.5	217	26.9	3.4	11	0
Beef, Aberdeen Angus, Asda*	1 Burger/112g	249	13.3	222	22.2	6.7	11.8	0.9
Beef, Aberdeen Angus, Fresh, Waitrose*	1 Burger/113g	269	21	238	16.4	1.2	18.6	0
Beef, Aberdeen Angus, Gourmet, Finest, Tesco*	1 Burger/106g	258	15.8	243	25.2	2	14.9	0
Beef, Aberdeen Angus, M&S*	1 Burger/142g	298	18.9	210	18.3	4.1	13.3	0.1
Beef, Aberdeen Angus, Quarter Pounder, TTD, Sainsbury's*	1 Burger/69g	208	14.9	301	25.8	0.5	21.6	0.5
Beef, Aberdeen Angus, Scotch, Deluxe, Lidl*	1 Burger /170g	430	30.4	253	21.9	0.7	17.9	0.6
Beef, Barbecue, Tesco*	1 Burger/114g	295	22.7	260	15.6	3.5	20	0.5
Beef, Best, Cheese, Gherkin, Tomato, & Mustard, M&S*	1 Burger/167g	414	32.2	248	15.4	3.2	19.3	0.1
Beef, BGTY, Sainsbury's*	1 Burger/110g	177	6	161	20.8	7.1	5.5	1.1
Beef, Black Pepper, Smokey, Sainsbury's*	1 Burger/84g	205	13.2	245	22.7	2.6	15.8	0.5
Beef, British, Grilled, Finest, Tesco*	1 Burger/95g	185	11.8	195	17.2	3.3	12.4	0.9
Beef, British, Organic, Duchy, Waitrose*	1 Burger/65g	152	9.4	234	22.8	2.9	14.4	0.9
Beef, British, Organic, Waitrose*	1 Burger/85g	226	16.6	266	19	3.5	19.5	1
Beef, British, Waitrose*	1 Burger/113g	279	21	247	18.6	1.2	18.6	0
Beef, Caramelised Onion, Grilled, Finest, Tesco*	1 Burger/88g	196	11.4	223	19.1	7.4	12.9	0.5
Beef, Chargrill, Tesco*	1 Burger/114g	246	18.4	217	17	0.8	16.2	2.5
Beef, Cheddar Cheese, Hereford, Waitrose*	1 Burger/85g	199	12.3	234	23.2	2.3	14.5	0.6
Beef, Classic, Flame Grilled, Rustlers*	1 Burger/216g	613	31.9	284	16.1	20.6	14.8	0
Beef, Flame Grilled, Feasters*	1 Burger/58g	164	13.5	282	19.3	2.6	23.2	0
Beef, Frozen, Tesco*	1 Burger/44g	117	8.4	266	14.8	4.6	19.1	0
Beef, Morrisons*	1 Burger/57g	169	14.3	298	12.3	5.5	25.2	0.6
Beef, Original, & Best, Birds Eye*	1 Burger/46g	115	8.9	252	14.1	5.1	19.5	0.4
Beef, Original, with Onion, Grilled, Birds Eye*	1 Burger/38g	110	9.5	287	13.4	2.6	24.8	0.3
Beef, Our Best Ever, M&S*	1 Burger/170g	450	36.4	265	16.5	1.7	21.4	0
Beef, Quarter Pounder, 5% Fat, Grilled, Ashfield Farm, Aldi*	1 Burger/89g	128	3.7	144	23	4	4.2	0.5
Beef, Quarter Pounder, Reduced Fat, Grilled, Asda*	1 Burger/94g	178	8	189	20	6.9	8.5	1.6
Beef, Quarter Pounders, Chilled, Morrisons*	1 Burger/115g	228	13.9	198	17.2	4.4	12.1	0.2
Beef, Quarter Pounders, Farmfoods*	1 Burger/113g	289	22.1	256	14.4	5.4	19.6	0.1
Beef, Quarter Pounders, GF, Butchers Selection, Asda*	1 Burger/93g	210	13.1	225	16	8.5	14	0.5
Beef, Quarter Pounders, Morrisons*	1 Burger/114g	338	28.6	298	12.3	5.5	25.2	0.6
Beef, Quarter Pounders, Original, Birds Eye*	1 Burger/85g	251	21.2	296	15	2.7	25	0.5

B

BURGERS

	Measure INFO/WEIGHT	per Measure KCAL	per Measure FAT	Nutrition Values per 100g / 100ml KCAL	PROT	CARB	FAT	FIBRE
Beef, Quarter Pounders, Red Fat, Birchwood Farm, Lidl*	1 Burger/113g	205	9.4	181	18	3.2	8.3	0.5
Beef, Quarter Pounders, Red Fat, Tesco*	1 Burger/95g	171	12.4	180	14	1.8	13	0.8
Beef, Quarter Pounders, Scotch, Sainsbury's*	1 Burger/114g	255	15.4	225	22.2	3.5	13.6	0.5
Beef, Quarter Pounders, Scotch, The Best, Morrisons*	1 Burger/97g	223	13.9	230	21	4	14.3	0.5
Beef, Quarter Pounders, Steak Country, Lidl*	1 Burger/68g	188	15.1	276	16.3	2.4	22.2	0.1
Beef, Quarter Pounders, with Onion, BGTY, Sainsbury's*	1 Burger/83g	171	7.8	205	26.6	3.8	9.3	0.9
Beef, Red Onion & Cheese, Butchers Selection, Asda*	1 Burger/114g	243	13.7	213	21	5	12	0.5
Beef, Scotch, Ultimate, TTD, Sainsbury's*	1 Burger/119g	265	15.8	223	25.3	0.5	13.3	1
Beef, Steak, 5oz, As Sold, Birds Eye*	1 Burger/142g	476	41.2	335	17	1.4	29	0.5
Beef, Steak, British, Cooked, TTD, Sainsbury's*	1 Burger/110g	276	19.2	250	21.6	1.8	17.4	0.5
Beef, Steak, Extra Lean, Musclefood*	1 Burger/113g	160	5.4	142	19.6	5.7	4.8	1.3
Beef, Steak, Fillet, Donald Russell*	1 Burger/200g	362	16	181	20	0	8	0
Beef, Steak, Full of Flavour, Finest, Tesco*	1 Burger/88g	265	18.7	302	26.4	0.5	21.3	1
Beef, with Onion, Sainsbury's*	1 Burger/42g	102	6.2	243	20.7	6.9	14.8	1
Beef, with West Country Cheddar, TTD, Sainsbury's*	1 Burger/112g	252	13.7	225	26.4	2.3	12.2	0
Beet, Plant Kitchen, M&S*	1 Burger/120g	144	1.7	120	0	19.9	1.4	5.1
Beetroot, & Root Vegetable, Vegetarian, Asda*	½ Pack/107g	158	8.8	148	3.7	11	8.2	7.2
Beetroot, & Feta, Morrisons*	1 Burger/106g	159	6.7	150	5.3	15.9	6.3	4.3
Beetroot, BBQ, Tesco*	1 Burger/96g	137	1	143	5	26.3	1	4.6
Beetroot, with Mint, Gosh!*	1 Burger/125g	196	7	157	5.1	24.4	5.6	5.9
Black Bean, Beetroot, Bean Supreme*	1 Burger/85g	108	3.6	127	5.7	13.8	4.2	5.7
Cauliflower, What's Cooking, Lidl*	1 Burger/96g	211	11	220	5.5	22.3	11.5	2.5
Cheeseburger	**1 Serving/275g**	**706**	**29**	**257**	**13.7**	**25.6**	**10.6**	**1.8**
Cheeseburger, Bacon with Bun, Chargrilled, Tesco*	1 Burger/265g	726	42.1	274	13	19.6	15.9	1
Cheeseburger, Quarter Pounder, Rustlers*	1 Burger/190g	505	25.1	266	13.6	22.4	13.2	0
Cheeseburger, with Sesame Seed Bun, Tesco*	1 Burger/275g	644	32.2	234	12.2	20.1	11.7	2
Chicken, Average	**1 Burger/46g**	**111**	**5.6**	**242**	**14.9**	**18.7**	**12.1**	**1**
Chicken, Breaded, Ovenbaked, Iceland*	1 Burger/49g	122	6	251	15.7	18.6	12.4	1.2
Chicken, Breaded, Value, Tesco*	1 Burger/57g	165	10.8	290	10.5	19.2	19	1.4
Chicken, Cajun Spiced, Tesco*	1 Burger/90g	207	8.9	230	19.5	15.7	9.9	0
Chicken, Cajun, Fillets, Birds Eye*	1 Pack/180g	275	8.8	153	21.5	5.8	4.9	0.3
Chicken, Fresh, Non Coated, Waitrose*	1 Burger/100g	141	4	141	16	10.4	4	0.9
Chicken, GF, Made Without Wheat, M&S*	1 Burger/114g	209	10.3	184	15.2	8.9	9.1	2.8
Chicken, Golden Breadcrumbs, Frozen, Birds Eye*	1 Burger/56g	130	6.9	232	13.8	16.4	12.4	0.3
Chicken, Italia, Grilled, Heck*	1 Burger/114g	121	2.6	106	18.7	1.5	2.3	0
Chicken, Quarter Pounders, Birds Eye*	1 Burger/117g	280	16.1	239	13.5	15.2	13.8	0.6
Chicken, Southern Fried, Snax On The Go*	1 Burger/132g	318	11.1	241	11.9	28.8	8.4	1.3
Chicken, Style, Vegetarian, Quorn*	1 Burger/60g	122	5.1	205	12.1	16.5	8.6	6.6
Chicken, Thigh, Oakhurst, Aldi*	1 Burger/138g	324	15.2	235	17	16	11	0.7
Cod, Fish Fillet, Breaded, Birds Eye*	1 Burger/118g	241	8.6	204	13	21	7.3	1
Hemp, Vegetarian, Bean Supreme*	1 Burger/85g	148	5.8	174	9.3	15.2	6.8	7.3
Hot & Spicy, Vegan, Quorn*	1 Burger/66g	139	5.7	211	11.1	20.3	8.7	3.4
Kale, & Quinoa, Vegetarian, Strong Roots*	1 Burger/75g	151	8.5	201	4.2	19.5	11.3	2.4
Lamb, Minted, Average	**1 Burger/56g**	**125**	**7.4**	**223**	**20.6**	**5.5**	**13.2**	**0.2**
Lamb, Minted, Grilled, Specially Selected, Aldi*	1 Burger/92g	223	14.7	242	17	6.4	16	0.5
Lamb, Minted, Quarter Pounder, Grilled, Iceland*	1 Burger/85g	231	17	271	18	3	19.9	1.9
Lamb, Moroccan Spiced, Waitrose*	1 Burger/88g	215	13.2	245	16.9	10.5	15	0.1
Lamb, Waitrose*	1 Burger/67g	99	4.7	148	15.7	5.4	7	0.9
Lentil, & Spinach, Quarter Pounder, Indian, Sainsbury's*	1 Burger/114g	222	11.9	196	4.2	18.9	10.5	4.5
Manhattan, Amy's Kitchen*	1 Burger/68g	88	2.9	129	3.8	18	4.2	1.8
Mc2, No Beef, The Vegetarian Butcher*	1 Burger/80g	135	6.5	169	15.2	8	8.1	1.5
Meat Free, Average	**¼ Pounder/113g**	**195**	**8.8**	**172**	**17.5**	**7.9**	**7.8**	**3**
Meat Free, Sainsbury's*	1 Burger/45g	67	1.8	149	19.1	6.4	4	5.6

B

	Measure INFO/WEIGHT	per Measure KCAL	FAT	Nutrition Values per 100g / 100ml KCAL	PROT	CARB	FAT	FIBRE
BURGERS								
Meat Free, Spicy, Bean & Nacho, Cooked, Asda*	1 Burger/113g	247	9.6	218	5.3	27.7	8.5	4.7
Meat Free, Traditional, Fry's*	1 Burger/80g	119	4.5	148	14	7.4	5.6	6.2
Mix, Vegetarian, Slim & Save*	1 Serving/38g	140	4.5	371	30.8	31.9	12	6.1
Mushroom, with Lentil, & Butter Bean, Gosh!*	1 Burger/125g	174	3.9	139	6	25	3.1	6.6
Ostrich, Quarter Pounder, Oslinc*	1 Burger/113g	132	1.5	117	22.9	3.5	1.3	1.1
Plant Based, Beyond Burger, Vegan, Beyond Meat*	1 Patty/114g	318	21.1	280	21.5	6.6	18.6	0.5
Pork, Free Range, Waitrose*	1 Burger/115g	306	19.9	266	19.3	7.7	17.3	1
Pork, & Apple, Quarter Pounder, Grilled, Asda*	1 Burger/80g	147	6.4	184	23.9	4.1	8	0.5
Pork, & Chorizo, Quarter Pounders, Tesco*	1 Burger/88g	240	15.8	273	21.1	5.9	18	1.3
Pork, Pulled, Quarter Pounder, Grilled, Linda McCartney*	1 Burger/97g	150	4.5	154	16.1	11.1	4.6	2
Pumpkin, & Spinach, Vegetarian, Strong Roots*	1 Burger/80g	162	7.5	202	3.9	24.6	9.3	2.3
Pumpkin, & Sweet Potato, Vegetarian, Vivera*	1 Burger/99g	98	3	99	5.1	10.3	3	5.4
Quarter Pounder, Loved by Us, Co-Op*	1 Burger/114g	301	23.9	265	19	0.5	21	0
Quarter Pounder, Mozzarella, Vegetarian, Linda McCartney*	1 Burger/98g	238	13.5	243	18.2	10.3	13.8	2.3
Quarter Pounder, Quorn*	1 Burger/114g	170	6.8	150	14.4	7.7	6	4
Quarter Pounder, Steak, Deluxe, Lidl*	1 Burger/98g	237	17.6	242	18	2.1	18	0
Quarter Pounder, Vegan, Vivera*	1 Burger/113g	251	15.8	222	15	5.7	14	5.2
Quinoa, Sweet Potato, & Lentil, Vegetarian, Sainsbury's*	1 Burger/88g	168	8.2	192	4.7	19.3	9.4	5.8
Salmon, Quarter Pounders, Tesco*	1 Burger/114g	145	2.7	128	15.9	10.6	2.4	1.2
Salmon, Smoky BBQ, The Grill, M&S*	1 Burger/90g	175	8.4	194	16.4	10.3	9.3	1.7
Soya, Quarter Pounders, Meat Free Butcher, Aldi*	1 Burger/108g	297	18.4	275	13	16	17	3.6
Steak, Peppered, M&S*	1 Burger/114g	310	24.4	272	18.8	0.8	21.4	0.7
Sweet Potato, & Edamame, Meat Free, Morrisons*	1 Burger/88g	144	8	164	6.4	10.6	9.1	7.2
Sweet Potato, & Black Bean, Tesco*	1 Burger/97g	145	1.5	150	5.3	25.6	1.6	5.8
Sweet Potato, & Quinoa, Vegetarian, Waitrose*	1 Burger/91g	222	11.8	244	5.1	23.8	13	5.4
Sweet Potato, Chickpea, Carrot, Red Pepper, Aldi*	1 Burger/115g	172	2.6	150	4.2	25	2.3	6.1
Sweetcorn, & Chickpea, M&S*	1 Burger/120g	200	5.2	167	5.7	21.8	4.3	9.1
Turkey, British, Grilled, Sainsbury's*	1 Burger/97g	171	6.5	176	24.6	4.1	6.7	0.5
Turkey, Sea Salt & Pepper, Butchers Selection, Asda*	1 Burger/96g	141	4.4	147	23	3.2	4.6	0.5
Vegan, Onion Bhaji, Frozen, As Consumed, Tesco*	1 Burger/117g	167	8.5	143	3.5	12.3	7.3	7.1
Vegan, Vivera*	1 Burger/100g	169	7.3	169	18.5	4.8	7.3	5
Vegetable, Average	*1 Burger/56g*	*100*	*4.5*	*179*	*4.4*	*22.4*	*8*	*2.3*
Vegetable, Frozen, Oven Baked, Asda*	1 Burger/106g	204	8.4	192	3.9	25	7.9	3.6
Vegetable, Organic, Tesco*	1 Burger/90g	108	3.9	120	2.6	17.6	4.3	2.1
Vegetable, Quarter Pounders, Crisp & Golden, Waitrose*	1 Burger/113g	236	8.8	209	4.8	28.2	7.8	3.4
Vegetable, Quarter Pounders, Meat Free, Vegan, Tesco*	1 Burger/106g	229	10.6	216	3.7	25.8	10	3.9
Vegetable, Quarter Pounders, Sainsbury's*	1 Burger/102g	225	10.1	221	4.8	26	9.9	4.4
Vegetable, Spicy, Asda*	1 Burger/56g	108	6.2	193	3.4	20	11	0
Vegetable, Tesco*	2 Burgers/108g	178	5.9	165	2.9	23.7	5.5	4.9
Vegetarian, Average	*1 Patty/60g*	*112*	*5.3*	*187*	*17.2*	*2.9*	*8.8*	*3.3*
Vegetarian, Frozen, Grilled, Quorn*	1 Burger/50g	87	4	174	15.7	7.4	8.1	4.7
Vegetarian, Quarter Pounders, Grilled, Linda McCartney*	1 Burger/105g	232	12.5	220	17.3	9.8	11.9	2.4
Veggie, Frozen, Birds Eye*	1 Burger/125g	222	5.5	181	4.2	23	4.5	2.1
Venison, Finnebrougue Estate*	1 Burger/142g	170	7	120	19.9	4.2	4.9	0.5
Zebra, Cooked, Kezie*	1 Burger/110g	160	3.8	145	25.3	2.2	3.5	0
BURRITO								
Bean, & Rice, Mexican, GF, Amy's Kitchen*	1 Burrito/158g	234	6	148	4.5	24	3.8	3.2
Beef	*1 Serving/225g*	*536*	*20.2*	*238*	*12*	*27*	*9*	*2.2*
Beef, Chilli, As Consumed, Morrisons*	½ Pack/200g	368	16	184	8.9	17.7	8	2.7
Beef, Chilli, Inspired Cuisine, Aldi*	1 Pack/400g	748	26.4	187	6.8	24	6.6	2.6
Beef, Spicy, Tex Mex, Tesco*	1 Burrito/192g	326	8.4	170	6.5	24.8	4.4	2.6
Beef, with Rice, Beans, Sweet Potato, & Sour Cream, M&S*	1 Pack/217g	432	11.1	199	9.1	27.9	5.1	2.3
Black Bean, Chilli, Everdine*	1 Serving/450g	594	14.4	132	4.2	19.4	3.2	4.5

B

	Measure INFO/WEIGHT	per Measure KCAL	FAT	Nutrition Values per 100g / 100ml KCAL	PROT	CARB	FAT	FIBRE
BURRITO								
Pork, Pulled, BBQ, Scratch, Waitrose*	½ Pack/404g	654	18.6	162	10.1	18.2	4.6	0
Veg Medley, Bowl, Musclefood*	1 Serving/435g	344	7.8	79	5.6	8.4	1.8	3.6
BUTTER								
Almond, 100%, Sainsbury's*	1 Tbsp/20g	128	10.9	639	29.3	4.3	54.4	7.6
Almond, Cherry Bakewell, Pip & Nut*	1 Tbsp/15g	88	7.1	584	17.9	22.3	47.6	4.5
Brandy, Average	***1 Serving/10g***	***56***	***3.8***	***556***	***0.2***	***46.2***	***38.4***	***0.1***
Cashew, Pip & Nut*	1 Serving/15g	87	6.6	580	18	27	44	0
Creamery, Average	***1 Serving/10g***	***74***	***8.1***	***736***	***0.5***	***0.4***	***81.4***	***0***
Fresh, Average	***1 Thin Spread/7g***	***51***	***5.7***	***735***	***0.6***	***0.4***	***81.3***	***0***
Garlic, Crushed, Lurpak*	1 Serving/10g	69	7.5	692	1.3	3.7	75	0
Goat's, St Helen's Farm*	1 Thin Spread/7g	56	6.2	794	0.5	0	88	0
Granules, Butter Buds*	1 Tsp/1.4g	5	0.1	368	1.8	77.9	6.5	2.3
Reduced Fat, Fresh, Average	***1 Thin Spread/7g***	***26***	***2.8***	***368***	***2.3***	***1.2***	***39.4***	***0.2***
Salted, Average	***1 Thin Spread/7g***	***51***	***5.7***	***729***	***0.4***	***0.3***	***81.1***	***0***
Slightly Salted, Spreadable, Danpak*	1 Thin Spread/7g	49	5.5	707	0.5	0.6	78	0
Spreadable, Fresh, Average	***1 Thin Spread/7g***	***51***	***5.7***	***730***	***0.4***	***0.3***	***80.8***	***0***
Spreadable, Lighter, Norpak, Aldi*	1 Thin Spread/7g	36	4	519	0.6	0.7	57	0.5
Spreadable, Reduced Fat, Average	***1 Thin Spread/7g***	***38***	***4.2***	***540***	***0.5***	***0.5***	***60***	***0***
with Olive Oil, Lighter, Spreadable, Lurpak*	1 Thin Spread/7g	38	4.2	543	0.3	0.4	60	0
BUTTERMILK								
Average	***1 Mug/400ml***	***177***	***1.3***	***44***	***4.2***	***5.9***	***0.3***	***0***
BUTTERNUT SQUASH								
& Red Onion, Quick Roast, M&S*	1 Pack/340g	109	0.3	32	1	6	0.1	1.5
& Mixed Vegetable, Selection, M&S*	1 Pack/100g	170	0.3	170	3	5.1	0.3	2.7
Chips, Crinkle Cut, Cooked, Sainsbury's*	½ Pack/95g	66	0.9	70	2.2	11.7	0.9	3.1
Chunks, Frozen, Four Seasons, Aldi*	1 Serving/80g	30	0.4	37	0.9	7.4	0.5	1.4
Frozen, Tesco*	1 Serving/80g	29	0.2	36	1	6.1	0.2	2.7
Noodles, Ready Prepared, Sainsbury's*	½ Pack/152g	50	0.8	33	1.1	5.8	0.5	1.4
Squaffles, Cooked, Sainsbury's*	½ Pack/150g	102	2.6	68	1.7	10.4	1.7	2
Winter, Boiled, Flesh Only	***1 Serving/80g***	***27***	***0.1***	***34***	***0.7***	***8.8***	***0.1***	***2.6***
Winter, Butternut, Baked, Average	***1 Serving/100g***	***32***	***0.1***	***32***	***0.9***	***7.4***	***0.1***	***1.4***
Winter, Butternut, Raw, Prepared, Average	***1 Serving/80g***	***29***	***0.1***	***36***	***1.1***	***8.3***	***0.1***	***1.6***
Winter, Butternut, Raw, Unprepared, Average	***1 Serving/80g***	***24***	***0.1***	***30***	***0.9***	***6.8***	***0.1***	***1.3***
BUTTONS								
Chocolate, Orange, Free From, Asda*	1 Bag/25g	140	8.8	562	2.4	58	35	2.6
Milk Chocolate, Asda*	1 Bag/70g	368	21	526	7	57	30	1.5
Milk Chocolate, Giant, Dairy Milk, Cadbury*	1 Button/2g	11	0.6	530	7.6	56.5	30.5	0.7
Milk Chocolate, M&S*	1 Pack/75g	375	19	500	8.6	59.8	25.3	1.9
Milk Chocolate, Tesco*	1 Bag/70g	359	19.3	513	7.1	59.1	27.6	2.1
Mixed, White & Milk, Dairy Milk, Cadbury*	¼ Bag/28g	150	8.4	536	3.6	60.7	30	1.1
White Chocolate, Co-Op*	½ Pack/35g	186	9.8	530	7	64	28	0
White Chocolate, Dairy Milk, Cadbury*	1 Pack/32g	174	9.5	540	4.7	63	29.5	0
White Chocolate, Milkybar, Nestle*	1 Bag/30g	164	9.5	546	7.5	58.1	31.6	0
White Chocolate, Tesco*	1 Bag/70g	388	23.4	554	5.1	58	33.5	0

	Measure INFO/WEIGHT	per Measure KCAL	FAT	Nutrition Values per 100g / 100ml KCAL	PROT	CARB	FAT	FIBRE
CABBAGE								
& Leek, Crunchy Mix, Ready to Cook, Sainsbury's*	1 Serving/125g	34	0.6	27	1.9	3.7	0.5	2.6
& Leek, Ready for Use, Cooked, Sainsbury's*	1 Bag/200g	68	1	34	1.5	4.9	0.5	3.2
& Leek, Ready Sliced, Sainsbury's*	1 Pack/240g	53	1.2	22	1.1	2.2	0.5	2.1
& Leek, Sliced, Tesco*	1/3 Pack/100g	32	0.6	32	2.1	3.4	0.6	2.6
Boiled, Average	*1 Serving/90g*	*14*	*0.3*	*15*	*1*	*2.2*	*0.3*	*1.7*
Creamed, Cooked, Sainsbury's*	½ Pack/150g	95	6.8	67	2	2.6	4.8	2.5
Greens, Trimmed, Average	*1oz/28g*	*8*	*0.1*	*28*	*2.9*	*3*	*0.5*	*3.4*
Raw, Average	*1 Serving/100g*	*21*	*0.4*	*21*	*1.3*	*3.2*	*0.4*	*1.8*
Red, Average	*1 Serving/90g*	*19*	*0.2*	*21*	*1*	*3.7*	*0.3*	*2.2*
Red, Braised with Red Wine, M&S*	½ Pack/150g	180	7.2	120	1.4	17.1	4.8	1
Red, Braised, with Bramley Apples, M&S*	½ Pack/150g	126	3	84	1	14	2	2.8
Red, Pickled, Average	*1 Serving/50g*	*13*	*0.1*	*26*	*0.9*	*4.6*	*0.2*	*1.6*
Red, Spiced, Steamer, Sainsbury's*	½ Pack/150g	105	3.3	70	1	10.5	2.2	2.9
Red, with Apple, Bramley, British, Sainsbury's*	1 Pack/300g	213	1.5	71	1.2	14.9	0.5	2.3
Red, with Apple, Finest, Tesco*	½ Pack/150g	177	8.8	118	1.6	14.7	5.9	4.6
Red, with Apple, Red Wine & Cranberries, Waitrose*	1/3 Pack/97g	116	5.7	120	1.4	14.2	5.9	2.6
Savoy, Boiled in Salted Water, Average	*1 Serving/90g*	*15*	*0.4*	*17*	*1.1*	*2.2*	*0.5*	*2*
Savoy, Raw, Average	*1 Serving/90g*	*24*	*0.4*	*27*	*2.1*	*3.9*	*0.5*	*3.1*
Spring Greens, Boiled, Average	*1 Serving/80g*	*16*	*0.6*	*20*	*1.9*	*1.6*	*0.7*	*2.6*
Spring Greens, Raw, Average	*1 Serving/80g*	*22*	*0.7*	*28*	*2.5*	*2.6*	*0.8*	*2.9*
Steamed, Average	*1 Serving/100g*	*15*	*0.3*	*15*	*1*	*2.2*	*0.3*	*1.7*
Sweetheart, Raw	*1 Serving/100g*	*26*	*0.6*	*26*	*2.1*	*3.2*	*0.6*	*2.8*
Trio, with Pancetta, Finest, Tesco*	½ Pack/91g	79	5	87	4.4	3.4	5.5	3.4
White, Raw, Average	*1oz/28g*	*8*	*0.1*	*27*	*1.4*	*5*	*0.2*	*2.1*
CACAO								
Powder, Green Origins*	1 Tsp/5g	18	0.6	353	25	21	11	35
Powder, Natural, 100%, Food Thoughts*	1 Tsp/5g	21	1	418	28.1	14.5	21	31
CAKE								
Almond, Slices, Mr Kipling*	1 Slice/35g	144	6.5	411	6	54.2	18.5	1.8
Almond, Slices, Sainsbury's*	1 Serving/27g	120	7.1	444	5.9	45.9	26.3	1.5
Almond, Slices, Weight Watchers*	1 Slice/26g	95	2.6	365	5.2	63.8	9.9	2.4
Almond, Square, Regal Cake*	1 Slice/42g	185	10.5	440	5.2	49.8	25	0
Angel, Average	*1 Slice/44g*	*175*	*7.9*	*397*	*4.2*	*54.9*	*17.9*	*0.8*
Angel, Layer, Tesco*	1 Serving/34g	130	5	387	5	57.8	14.8	1.1
Angel, Sainsbury's*	1/8 Cake/41g	171	8.1	417	4.1	55.7	19.8	0.8
Angel, Slices, Mr Kipling*	1 Slice/33g	139	6.1	413	2.9	59	18.2	0.7
Angel, Slices, Snap Packs, Mr Kipling*	1 Slice/34g	148	6.6	417	2.7	60.1	18.5	0.6
Angel, Slices, Tesco*	1 Slice/29g	117	5	407	3.8	57.9	17.4	1.6
Apple, & Blackcurrant, Crumble, Graze*	1 Punnet/33g	121	7.5	365	6.1	34.5	22.7	3.1
Apple, Bramley, & Blackberry Crumble, M&S*	1/8 Cake/56g	221	10	395	4.4	54.1	17.9	1.5
Apple, Crumble, Slices, Weight Watchers*	1 Slice/26g	90	2	346	4.5	64.8	7.7	2.3
Apple, Home Style, M&S*	1 Cake/54g	189	7.9	350	5.3	49.4	14.7	1.5
Apple, Slices, Delightful, Mr Kipling*	1 Slice/29g	92	1.1	317	4.4	66.2	3.9	1.3
Apple, Sticky Toffee, Finest, Tesco*	1 Slice/51g	247	9.2	487	3	52.7	18.1	0.6
Bakewell, Cherry, Co-Op*	1 Cake/47g	205	8	435	3.7	67.2	16.9	1.8
Bakewell, Cherry, Delightful, Mr Kipling*	1 Cake/45g	176	5.8	390	3.9	66.4	12.9	1.2
Bakewell, Cherry, M&S*	1 Cake/44g	185	7.8	420	4.5	61.7	17.7	1
Bakewell, Cherry, Mini, Sainsbury's*	1 Cake/27g	101	3.3	370	3.4	62.2	12	0.4
Bakewell, Cherry, Mr Kipling*	1 Cake/45g	193	8.3	428	3.9	61.3	18.5	1.4
Bakewell, Cherry, Slices, GFY, Asda*	1 Slice/29g	98	0.7	337	3.4	75.4	2.4	0.7
Bakewell, Cherry, Waitrose*	1 Cake/44g	184	8.5	419	3.8	57.4	19.3	2.1
Bakewell, Lemon, Average	*1 Cake/42g*	*173*	*6.4*	*411*	*3.7*	*64.6*	*15.2*	*1.3*
Bakewell, Lemon, CBY, Asda*	1 Cake/42g	181	7.3	432	3.8	64.4	17.4	1.4

CAKE

	Measure INFO/WEIGHT	per Measure KCAL	FAT	Nutrition Values per 100g / 100ml KCAL	PROT	CARB	FAT	FIBRE
Bakewell, Lemon, Mr Kipling*	1 Cake/43g	185	7.4	430	3.6	64.4	17.3	1
Bakewell, Slices, Mr Kipling*	1 Slice/35g	146	6.2	414	4.1	59.2	17.6	1
Bakewell, Slices, Weight Watchers*	1 Slice/26g	84	0.6	324	3.7	71	2.4	2
Bakewell, The Handmade Flapjack Company*	1 Cake/75g	311	17.1	415	4.5	47.4	22.8	0
Banana, Bread, Brilliant, Graze*	1 Cake/23g	72	3.6	312	5.2	40.4	15.6	3
Banana, Iced, Waitrose*	1/6 Cake/55g	190	5.9	345	4.2	58	10.7	2.7
Banana, Loaf, Tesco*	1 Slice/40g	152	6.9	380	5.3	50.3	17.2	1.6
Banana, Loaf, The Best, Morrisons*	1 Serving/75g	273	13.4	364	5.7	44.1	17.9	2
Banana, Loaf, Waitrose*	1 Slice/70g	236	7.5	337	5	55.2	10.7	1.7
Banana, with An Afternoon Tea Infusion, Graze*	1 Punnet/18g	55	2.5	307	5	39	14	3
Bara Brith, Tan Y Castell*	1 Serving/100g	261	1	261	4	58.8	1	1.5
Battenberg, Mini, Mr Kipling*	1 Cake/32g	128	3.2	399	3.8	72.9	10	1.2
Battenberg, Mr Kipling*	1 Serving/38g	161	4.6	421	5	73.3	12	1.6
Battenberg, Tesco*	1 Serving/43g	161	4.4	377	4.9	65.2	10.4	1.3
Berry, & Polenta, Gail's*	100g	300	17	300	5.7	30	17	3.1
Birthday, M&S*	1 Serving/60g	240	7.1	400	2.3	70.9	11.9	0.8
Birthday, Piece of Cake, M&S*	1 Serving/85g	395	24.4	465	4.3	39.7	28.7	0.9
Birthday, Present, Tesco*	1 Serving/79g	347	13.9	439	3.5	66.6	17.6	0.4
Butterfly, Mr Kipling*	1 Cake/29g	114	6.4	392	4.4	43.4	22.2	0.6
Caramel, Crunchy, Devondale*	1 Cake/80g	359	19.2	449	2.9	56.3	24	1.3
Caramel, Salted, The Best, Morrisons*	1/6 Cake/63g	262	12.2	416	3.9	56.2	19.4	0.5
Caramel, Shortcake, Slices, McVitie's*	1 Slice /32g	146	7.7	463	4.3	56.5	24.4	1.6
Caramel, Slices, M&S*	1 Slice/64g	304	16.1	475	4.9	60.4	25.2	2.6
Carrot, & Orange, Extra Special, Asda*	1/6 Cake/65g	240	11.7	369	4.7	47	18	0.9
Carrot, & Orange, Finest, Tesco*	1/8 Cake/50g	205	10.2	410	4.6	51.2	20.5	2.1
Carrot, & Orange, Waitrose*	1/6 Cake/47g	164	7.4	350	5.3	46.8	15.7	1.8
Carrot, & Walnut, Aldi*	1/4 Cake/100g	409	23	409	5.1	44	23	2.2
Carrot, & Walnut, Layered, Asda*	1 Serving/42g	172	8	409	4.6	55	19	1
Carrot, & Walnut, Mini Classics, Mr Kipling*	1 Cake/39g	172	9.8	440	4.5	48.6	25.2	1
Carrot, Average	*1 Slice/56g*	*211*	*10.4*	*377*	*4.6*	*47.6*	*18.6*	*1.4*
Carrot, Free From, Finest, Tesco*	1 Slice/67g	288	17.7	429	3	43.3	26.3	3.5
Carrot, GF , Finest, Tesco*	1 Serving/50g	204	10.4	407	3.4	50.4	20.9	1.9
Carrot, Handmade, Delicious, Boots*	1 Slice/75g	292	13.5	389	4.1	53	18	1.4
Carrot, Iced, Tesco*	1 Serving/61g	246	12	404	3.1	53.7	19.6	1.6
Carrot, Lidl*	1/6 Cake/71g	280	13.7	394	4.7	48.9	19.3	3
Carrot, Mini, Weight Watchers*	1 Cake/31g	120	3.3	388	3.7	68.9	10.8	2.7
Carrot, Organic, Respect Organics*	1 Slice/45g	179	10.1	398	3.1	47.4	22.4	1.5
Carrot, Slices, Asda*	1 Slice/80g	302	13.2	377	3.4	53.8	16.5	1.7
Carrot, Slices, Less Than 3% Fat, BGTY, Sainsbury's*	1 Slice/30g	94	0.8	313	3.4	68.7	2.7	2.4
Carrot, Slices, Weight Watchers*	1 Slice/27g	84	0.2	311	2.8	73	0.8	0.9
Carrot, The Best, Morrisons*	1/6 Cake/64g	255	12.5	398	4.3	50	19.5	2.5
Carrot, TTD, Sainsbury's*	1 Slice/72g	287	13.7	398	4.5	51.1	19	2.5
Carrot, with Cream Cheese Icing, On the Go, Sainsbury's*	1 Cake/64g	251	11.9	392	4.3	51.5	18.6	1
Cherry & Almond Slices, GF, Free From, Sainsbury's*	1 Slice/33g	144	7.9	442	6.5	48.7	24.3	1
Cherry Crumble, Rowan Hill Bakery, Lidl*	1 Slice/50g	196	7	392	3.4	62.6	13.9	1.6
Chocolate	*1oz/28g*	*128*	*7.4*	*456*	*7.4*	*50.4*	*26.4*	*1.7*
Chocolate Chip, Co-Op*	1/6 Cake/63g	275	16.9	440	5	44	27	0.5
Chocolate Chip, Slices, Mr Kipling*	1 Slice/25g	109	5.1	442	6.2	57.4	20.5	1.6
Chocolate Slices, Mr Kipling*	1 Slice/32g	132	6	411	3.4	56.3	18.7	1.7
Chocolate, & Blood Orange, Bars, Lunchbox, Soreen*	1 Bar/30g	105	2.5	349	8.9	57.5	8.2	5.2
Chocolate, & Madeira, Marble Loaf, M&S*	1/6 Cake/88g	380	20.4	430	5	50	23.1	1
Chocolate, & Orange, Rolls, M&S*	1 Cake/60g	228	17	380	3.6	27	28.4	1.3
Chocolate, & Salted Caramel, Delice, TTD, Sainsbury's*	1 Serving/65g	207	12.3	319	3.6	32.5	19	1.9

CAKE

Measure INFO/WEIGHT		per Measure		Nutrition Values per 100g / 100ml				
		KCAL	FAT	KCAL	PROT	CARB	FAT	FIBRE
Chocolate, Belgian, Waitrose*	1 Slice/55g	244	12.7	447	5.2	53.1	23.3	2
Chocolate, Birthday, Tesco*	1 Serving/54g	229	13.2	425	5.9	45.5	24.4	2.1
Chocolate, Box, Asda*	1 Serving/60g	263	13.8	439	5	53	23	0.7
Chocolate, Brownie, Devondale*	1 Cake/60g	246	12.9	410	4.4	51	21.5	2.1
Chocolate, Brownie, Fudge, Entenmann's*	1/8 Cake/55g	168	2.4	306	4	62.7	4.4	1.5
Chocolate, Caterpillar, Tesco*	1 Serving/54g	221	9.2	410	4.8	57.8	17.1	2.6
Chocolate, Celebration, Tesco *	1 Slice/61g	281	15.5	462	5.2	51.9	25.5	2.1
Chocolate, Crispy Clusters, Mini, Tesco*	1 Cluster/8g	37	1.5	470	7	67.8	18.7	2.5
Chocolate, Cubes, Easter, Tesco*	1 Cube/47g	205	8.8	437	4.9	60.6	18.7	3.6
Chocolate, Double, Ganache, M&S*	1/12 Cake/61g	281	16.8	460	5.9	46.1	27.6	2.5
Chocolate, Flourless, Gail's*	100g	465	33	465	8.9	31	33	5
Chocolate, Free From, Finest, Tesco*	1 Slice/64g	279	16.1	438	4.1	46.9	25.3	3.2
Chocolate, Fudge	*1 Serving/110g*	*415*	*19.1*	*377*	*4.4*	*50.4*	*17.4*	*1.4*
Chocolate, Fudge Slice, Waitrose*	1 Slice/60g	230	9.7	383	4.7	54.6	16.2	1.5
Chocolate, Fudge, & Vanilla Cream, M&S*	1/6 Cake/69g	310	17.9	450	5.2	49.8	26	1.3
Chocolate, Fudge, Alabama, Morrisons*	1/6 Cake/58g	195	6.4	337	4.5	55.1	11	2.3
Chocolate, Fudge, Belgian, TTD, Sainsbury's*	1 Avg Slice/66g	282	14.3	428	4.4	52.5	21.7	2.5
Chocolate, Fudge, Classics, M&S*	1 Serving/71g	195	7.5	275	2.8	42.8	10.6	1.1
Chocolate, Fudge, Hot, Frozen, Tesco*	1 Slice/75g	255	10.7	341	5.7	46	14.3	2.9
Chocolate, Happy Birthday, Tesco*	1 Serving/58g	241	13.2	415	4.7	46.9	22.7	2.9
Chocolate, Heaven, Extra Special, Asda*	1/6 Cake/66g	255	13.1	388	4	48	20	1
Chocolate, Iced, Tesco*	1 Serving/40g	158	6.3	395	4.7	58.5	15.8	1.8
Chocolate, Individual with Mini Eggs, Cadbury*	1 Cake/26g	119	6.1	455	4.6	57.5	23.1	1.3
Chocolate, Indulgence, Finest, Tesco*	1 Slice/51g	207	9.1	405	4.8	55.9	17.9	1.2
Chocolate, Large, Happy Birthday, Tesco*	1/14 Cake/63g	291	16	462	4.2	53.4	25.4	1.7
Chocolate, Log, Mini, Free From, Sainsbury's*	1 Slice/45g	202	10.8	450	5.6	51	24	3
Chocolate, Mini Roll, Bites, Tesco*	1 Bite/18g	78	3.6	435	6	58	19.8	1.9
Chocolate, Mousse, Galaxy, Mars*	1 Serving/71g	250	15.5	354	5.3	33	22	0
Chocolate, Orange, Sponge, Asda*	1 Serving/70g	298	18.2	425	4.9	42.9	26	3
Chocolate, Party, M&S*	1 Serving/61g	240	12.6	395	4.6	46.9	20.8	1.1
Chocolate, Party, Sainsbury's*	1 Slice/58g	225	9.5	388	5.4	53.5	16.4	2.5
Chocolate, Party, Tesco*	1 Slice/62g	244	13.1	394	4.6	46.3	21.2	0.9
Chocolate, Rice Crispy, Knightsbridge, Lidl*	1 Cake/24g	88	4.2	368	3.9	48.7	17.5	0.1
Chocolate, Rich, Christmas, Tesco*	1 Slice/82g	300	13.5	367	7	47.5	16.5	1.6
Chocolate, Roll, Triple, Cadbury*	1 Serving/40g	165	6.7	410	4.3	60.1	16.6	1.5
Chocolate, Sainsbury's*	1 Serving/30g	118	5.6	395	4.1	52.6	18.5	1.3
Chocolate, Sensation, Sainsbury's*	1 Serving/92g	320	17.7	348	3.7	40	19.2	2.3
Chocolate, Slice, Asda*	1 Slice/100g	405	20	405	5.2	50	20	2.3
Chocolate, Sponge, Morrisons*	1 Serving/59g	179	7.6	303	4.4	42.5	12.8	0.7
Chocolate, Sponge, Tesco*	1 Serving/37g	129	3.6	358	5.1	60.8	10.1	1.7
Chocolate, Sponge, Victoria, Co-Op*	1 Slice/61g	201	9.8	330	5	42	16	1
Chocolate, The Best, Morrisons*	1/6 Cake/69g	294	15	426	4.3	52.5	21.7	1.5
Chocolate, The Handmade Flapjack Company*	1 Cake/75g	303	16.2	404	12.5	39.8	21.6	0
Chocolate, Thorntons*	1 Serving/87g	408	25.1	469	5.2	47.1	28.8	0.6
Chocolate, Triple Layer, Celebration, Tesco*	1/24 of cake/79g	345	18.8	430	5	47.7	23.4	2.8
Chocolate, Truffle, Mini, Finest, Tesco*	1 Cake/28g	125	6.6	448	5.9	52.9	23.7	0.3
Chocolate, White, Triple Layer, Party Cake, Asda*	1 Slice/68g	306	15.6	450	2.9	57	23	1.1
Chocolate, Wiggles The Caterpillar, Mini, Sainsbury's*	1 Cake/30g	139	6.7	462	4.8	59.9	22.2	1.8
Chocolate, Wiggles The Caterpillar, Sainsbury's*	1 Slice/40g	170	7.6	425	5.2	57.3	19	1.9
Chocolate, with Butter Icing, Average	*1oz/28g*	*135*	*8.3*	*481*	*5.7*	*50.9*	*29.7*	*0*
Chorley, Asda*	1 Cake/60g	269	12.6	449	6	59	21	2.2
Christmas, Bites, M&S*	1 Bite/21g	75	1.7	359	4	66.5	8.3	1.1
Christmas, Connoisseur, M&S*	1 Slice/60g	216	5.5	360	4.1	64.7	9.2	3.3

CAKE

INFO/WEIGHT	Measure	per Measure KCAL	FAT	Nutrition Values per 100g / 100ml KCAL	PROT	CARB	FAT	FIBRE
Christmas, Fruit, Iced, Bar, Bakers Selection, Asda*	1 Serving/67g	233	5.3	349	3.8	64	7.9	2.5
Christmas, Iced Rich Fruit, Finest, Tesco*	1/8 Cake/50g	183	4.3	366	4.3	66.4	8.6	3.3
Christmas, Iced, Slices, Tesco*	1 Slice/45g	168	4.4	369	2.9	67.6	9.6	1.2
Christmas, Rich Fruit, Free From, Tesco*	1/12 Cake/75g	284	6.4	376	3	71	8.5	1.6
Christmas, Rich Fruit, Organic, Tesco*	1 Serving/76g	282	7.6	374	3.9	67.1	10	2
Christmas, Rich Fruit, Tesco*	1 Serving/75g	261	7.2	348	3.8	60.6	9.6	2.1
Christmas, Slices, Mr Kipling*	1 Slice/43g	159	3.8	368	3	68.4	8.8	1.4
Christmas, Top Iced, Rich Fruit , Essential, Waitrose*	1 Slice/75g	278	5.8	368	3.6	69.6	7.7	2.9
Coconut	*1 Slice/70g*	*304*	*16.7*	*434*	*6.7*	*51.2*	*23.8*	*2.5*
Coconut, & Raspberry, M&S*	1 Serving/52g	231	13.9	445	5	45.5	26.8	2.3
Coconut, Snowball, Bobby's*	1 Cake/18g	80	4	436	2.2	57.3	22.1	0
Coconut, Snowball, Tunnock's*	1 Cake/30g	134	6.2	446	4.2	56.7	20.8	3.6
Coconut, Sponge, Mini Classics, Mr Kipling*	1 Cake/38g	155	8.7	409	3.7	47	22.9	0.9
Coffee, & Walnut Slices, HE, Tesco*	1 Slice/23g	69	0.5	301	4.4	65.7	2.3	2.8
Coffee, & Walnut, Slices, Free From, Tesco*	1 Slice/38g	158	7.3	418	3.5	57.1	19.2	1.2
Coffee, Iced, M&S*	1 Slice/33g	135	6.5	410	4.4	54.5	19.6	1.6
Coffee, Sponge Roll, M&S*	1/6 Roll/42g	160	7.4	385	3.1	53.1	17.8	1.4
Coffee, The Best, Morrisons*	1/6 Cake/69g	296	13.5	429	3.8	59.1	19.5	0.8
Colin the Caterpillar, M&S*	1 Slice/60g	234	12.8	390	5.3	57.2	21.3	1.3
Cookies & Cream, Fitbakes*	1 Cake/78g	173	7	221	12	40	9	0
Cornflake, Average	*1 Cake/18g*	*83*	*3.7*	*464*	*5.2*	*64.6*	*20.4*	*2*
Cornflake, Chocolate Clusters, Asda*	1 Cake/14g	64	2.6	460	8.2	65.2	18.5	2.7
Cornflake, Chocolate, Mini Bites, Tesco*	1 Bite/14g	62	2.5	446	7.1	64.1	17.9	5.9
Cream Sponge, Morrisons*	1 Serving/46g	138	6.4	302	3.8	39.8	13.9	1.2
Cream, Oysters, M&S*	1 Cake/72g	227	15.3	315	3.6	27.5	21.2	3
Cream, Slices, M&S*	1 Slice/80g	310	18.3	387	2.3	45.7	22.9	0.6
Date, & Walnut Loaf, Sainsbury's*	1/10 Slice/40g	148	8.2	371	6.7	40.1	20.4	1
Date, Chocolate, & Halva, Baby, Tin, Mini, Gail's*	100g	487	30	487	6.4	45	30	4.6
Eccles, All Butter, M&S*	1 Cake/86g	345	14.8	400	4.5	57.4	17.2	3.2
Eccles, Fresh Baked	*1 Cake/45g*	*171*	*7.6*	*381*	*4.3*	*56.3*	*17*	*1.5*
Fairy, Average	*1 Cake/23g*	*96*	*4.6*	*416*	*5.1*	*53*	*20.2*	*1.5*
Fairy, Chocolate, Ms Mollys*	1 Cake/23g	95	4.9	413	4.2	49.7	21.4	2.5
Fairy, Iced, Average	*1 Cake/23g*	*91*	*3.4*	*394*	*4.2*	*60.8*	*14.8*	*0.9*
Fairy, Iced, Ms Mollys*	1 Cake/23g	96	4.6	416	4.3	54.3	19.8	1.8
Fairy, Lemon Iced, Average	*1 Cake/23g*	*90*	*3.1*	*393*	*4.4*	*63.2*	*13.6*	*1.1*
Fairy, Plain, Average	*1 Cake/23g*	*95*	*4.6*	*413*	*5.5*	*51.1*	*20.2*	*1.5*
Fairy, Plain, Sainsbury's*	1 Cake/20g	84	4.3	422	4.9	46.4	21.5	1.2
Fairy, Plain, Value, Tesco*	1 Cake/15g	52	1.3	348	5.3	62.4	8.6	0.9
Fairy, Strawberry Iced, Tesco*	1 Cake/24g	94	3.2	392	4.9	62.9	13.4	1.4
Fairy, Vanilla Iced, Average, Tesco*	1 Cake/23g	89	2.8	388	4.4	65.1	12.2	1.2
Fairy, Victoria, Sainsbury's*	1 Cake/50g	218	10.8	436	3.7	56.1	21.5	1.3
Flake, Cadbury*	1 Cake/20g	90	4.6	445	6.3	54.5	22.3	0
Flamingo Slices, Mr Kipling*	1 Slice/27g	112	5	415	3.7	57.8	18.5	1.8
Fondant Fancies, Lemon, Waitrose*	1 Cake/40g	176	7.1	441	2.5	67.9	17.7	0.6
Fondant Fancies, Sainsbury's*	1 Cake/28g	103	2.5	373	2.7	69.7	9.1	0.7
Fondant, Dark Chocolate, Graze*	1 Pack/40g	157	5.8	393	3.5	66.2	14.5	0
Fondant, with Chocolate, Mini, Delhaize*	1 Cake Mini/20g	88	6.2	440	4.6	36.3	30.8	3.8
French Fancies, Average	*1 Cake/27g*	*100*	*2.5*	*371*	*2.7*	*69.6*	*9.1*	*0.8*
French Fancies, Lemon, Average	*1 Cake/28g*	*106*	*2.7*	*378*	*2.5*	*69.9*	*9.8*	*0.5*
French Fancies, Lemon, Mr Kipling*	1 Cake/28g	106	2.7	378	2.5	69.9	9.8	0.5
French Fancies, Mr Kipling*	1 Cake/28g	106	2.8	378	2.6	69.7	9.9	0.6
French Fancies, Strawberry, Mr Kipling*	1 Cake/28g	106	2.7	379	2.5	70.6	9.6	0.4
Fruit, Iced, Slices, Tesco*	1 Slice/50g	171	2.9	342	2.8	68	5.8	3.3

CAKE	Measure INFO/WEIGHT	per Measure KCAL	FAT	Nutrition Values per 100g / 100ml KCAL	PROT	CARB	FAT	FIBRE
Fruit, Luxury, Fully Iced Slice, The Best, Morrisons*	1 Serving/50g	178	3.8	356	3.7	66.6	7.6	3.1
Fruit, Petit Cakes Aux Fruits, Bonne Maman*	1 Cake/30g	122	6.3	407	5.4	48	21	0
Fruit, Plain, Average	*1 Slice/90g*	*319*	*11.6*	*354*	*5.1*	*57.9*	*12.9*	*0*
Fruit, Rich, Average	*1 Slice/70g*	*225*	*8.8*	*322*	*4.9*	*50.7*	*12.5*	*1.7*
Fruit, Rich, Golden Bow, TTD, Sainsbury's*	1 Slice/85g	324	7.7	381	3.3	70.3	9	2.7
Fruit, Rich, Iced	*1 Slice/70g*	*249*	*8*	*356*	*4.1*	*62.7*	*11.4*	*1.7*
Fruit, Rich, Iced, Bar, Finest, Tesco*	1 Serving/100g	360	10.7	360	3.8	61.3	10.7	4.2
Fruit, Rich, Iced, Finest, Tesco*	1 Slice/57g	191	4.7	335	3.6	61.2	8.3	4.4
Fruit, Rich, Iced, Top, Sainsbury's*	1 Slice/75g	268	5.3	357	3	69.3	7.1	2.2
Fruit, Rich, M&S*	1 Serving/50g	158	3.2	315	3.1	60.9	6.5	4.3
Fruit, Rich, Slices, Free From, Sainsbury's*	1 Slice/40g	144	5	361	4.5	57.4	12.6	3.7
Fruit, Slices, Value, Tesco*	1 Slice/23g	84	4	372	4	48.7	17.7	1.3
Fudge, Brownie, The Handmade Flapjack Company*	1 Cake/75g	286	9.2	381	4.9	62.8	12.3	0
Genoa, Tesco*	1 Serving/44g	150	3.9	340	3.7	59.1	8.8	3.1
Ginger, & Syrup, Tesco*	1 Serving/32g	134	7	420	4.5	51.4	21.8	0.7
Ginger, Drizzle, Iced, Co-Op*	1/6 Cake/64g	226	7.7	350	3	58	12	1
Ginger, Jamaica, McVitie's*	1/9 Cake/26g	92	2.6	362	3.7	63.1	10.4	1.6
Ginger, Loaf , Stem, Waitrose*	1 Slice/35g	134	4.8	384	3.7	60.1	13.7	2.6
Ginger, Stem, Mrs Crimble's*	1 Slice/48g	153	1	319	2.5	71	2.1	3.2
Granola, Square, All Butter, Finest, Tesco*	1 Square/72g	322	16.1	447	7.8	50.7	22.4	5.9
Granola, Square, M&S*	1 Square/72g	330	18.1	464	7.9	49.3	25.5	5
Honey, Mini, Gail's*	100g	413	22.5	413	4.9	45.9	22.5	3.8
Jaffa Chocolate, Fitbakes*	1 Cake/65g	169	5.2	259	13	43	8	0
Lemon Drizzle, Fitbakes*	1 Cake/77g	154	4.6	199	10	48	6	0
Lemon, & Orange, Finest, Tesco*	1 Serving/53g	216	10.7	410	4.5	52.4	20.3	1.1
Lemon, & Poppy Seed, Slices, Weight Watcher*	1 Slice/19g	69	2.1	364	3.7	60.9	11.3	1.9
Lemon, Average	*1 Slice/81g*	*320*	*14.5*	*396*	*4.1*	*54.8*	*18*	*0.6*
Lemon, Buttercream & Lemon Curd, The Cake Shop*	1 Cake/28g	124	7.8	444	3.5	43.4	27.8	0.6
Lemon, Drizzle Cake, Asda*	1 Serving/50g	150	6	299	2.8	45	12	0.4
Lemon, Drizzle, Classic, M&S*	1 Serving/100g	333	13.6	333	4	47.5	13.6	2.2
Lemon, Drizzle, Finest, Tesco*	1 Slice/68g	266	11.2	391	3.6	56.3	16.5	1.6
Lemon, Drizzle, The Best, Morrisons*	1/6 Cake/72g	287	11.8	398	3.2	59.1	16.3	1.1
Lemon, Loaf, M&S*	1 Slice/47g	190	8.8	400	2.1	55.8	18.6	0.6
Lemon, Madeira, Half Moon, Dan Cake*	1 Slice/50g	215	10	430	3.5	59	20	0
Lemon, Slice, GF, Free From, Sainsbury's*	1 Slice/35g	169	10.1	477	6.5	47.6	28.6	1.8
Lemon, Slices, Free From, Tesco*	1 Slice/38g	156	6.6	410	3	59.5	17.5	1
Lemon, Slices, Iced, Tesco*	1 Slice/29g	114	4.9	394	3	56.1	17.1	2
Lemon, Slices, Low Fat, Weight Watchers*	1 Slice/26g	79	0.5	303	3.1	68.1	2	2.2
Lemon, Slices, Mr Kipling*	1 Slice/33g	135	5.1	409	2.7	64.2	15.5	0.7
Lemon, Slices, Sainsbury's*	1 Slice/30g	130	6.3	432	4.1	56	20.9	1.7
Leo the Lion, Birthday, Asda*	1 Slice/81g	325	12.9	402	2.6	62	16	0.5
Madeira	*1 Slice/40g*	*157*	*6.8*	*393*	*5.4*	*58.4*	*16.9*	*0.9*
Madeira, All Butter, Sainsbury's*	1 Serving/30g	116	5.9	388	5.2	47.4	19.7	0.8
Madeira, Cherry, Sainsbury's*	1 Slice/34g	117	2.6	349	4	64.8	7.9	1.3
Madeira, Cherry, Tesco*	1 Serving/38g	135	4.2	357	4.6	58.9	11	1.8
Madeira, Iced, Sainsbury's*	1/8 Cake/47g	182	6.6	388	3.6	61.6	14.1	0.7
Madeira, Iced, Tesco*	1 Slice/40g	157	5.8	393	3.8	60.7	14.6	1.7
Madeira, Lemon Iced, Co-Op*	1 Cake/290g	1131	52.2	390	4	53	18	0.6
Madeira, Lemon Iced, Tesco*	1 Slice/40g	169	7.4	418	4.9	58.1	18.2	1.1
Madeira, Morrisons*	1 Slice/35g	139	5.5	395	5	58.2	15.6	0.7
Madeira, Ms Mollys*	1 Slice/56g	237	10.4	423	4.3	59.2	18.5	1.3
Madeira, Party, Sainsbury's*	1 Slice/75g	321	15.2	427	4.1	56.8	20.2	1.1

C

C

	Measure INFO/WEIGHT	per Measure KCAL	FAT	Nutrition Values per 100g / 100ml KCAL	PROT	CARB	FAT	FIBRE
CAKE								
Madeira, Tesco*	1 Serving/37g	141	5.4	382	5.7	56.5	14.6	0.9
Madeleine, La, Bonne Maman*	1 Cake/25g	112	6.8	449	6.4	44	27	2.3
Madeleines, Classic, French, GF, Mrs Crimbles*	1 Cake/30g	136	7.8	453	4.7	49	26	0
Madeleines, Tesco*	1 Cake/25g	122	7.3	486	4.8	50.5	29.1	1.5
Manor House, Mr Kipling*	1 Serving/69g	277	13.8	400	5.3	49.7	20	1.4
Marble, Tesco*	1/8 Cake/45g	184	8.4	410	4.4	55.9	18.7	1.5
Mini Rolls, Cadbury*	1 Roll/27g	117	6.2	435	4.8	50.5	23	2.3
Mini Rolls, Chocolate, Average	*1 Cake/27g*	*122*	*6.2*	*453*	*4.8*	*56.9*	*22.9*	*0.9*
Mini Rolls, Chocolate, Tesco*	1 Roll/26g	117	5.6	450	5.6	57	21.5	3.3
Mini Rolls, Cola, Chocolate, Cadbury*	1 Roll/27g	115	6.1	435	4.8	50.4	23.1	2.3
Mini Rolls, Double Chocolate, Tesco*	1 Mini Roll/26g	117	5.6	451	5.6	57	21.5	3.3
Mini Rolls, Jaffa, Average	*1 Cake/29g*	*111*	*3.3*	*382*	*3.5*	*67.2*	*11.2*	*1.4*
Mini Rolls, Jam, Average	*1 Cake/29g*	*115*	*4.5*	*395*	*3.8*	*59.8*	*15.6*	*1.8*
Mini Rolls, Jammy Strawberry, Cadbury*	1 Cake/29g	119	4.8	411	4.9	59.8	16.5	0.5
Mini Rolls, Raspberry Ripple , Cadbury*	1 Roll/27g	120	5.5	440	4.5	58.7	20.1	2
Mint Aero, Celebration, Nestle*	1 Slice/58g	232	11.8	400	4	49.7	20.3	1.7
Orange, Marmalade, M&S*	1 Slice/50g	195	9.2	390	3.6	53.2	18.3	1.8
Pandoro, Italian	*1/8 Cake/87g*	*357*	*18.2*	*408*	*7.1*	*47.2*	*20.8*	*1.6*
Panettone, Average	*1 Portion/90g*	*345*	*15.3*	*383*	*8*	*52*	*17*	*0*
Panettone, Classic, Sainsbury's*	1 Slice/63g	227	8.2	363	7.4	53.3	13.1	1.2
Panettone, Finest, Tesco*	1/8 Cake/93g	318	11.8	339	6.1	49.1	12.6	2.5
Panettone, Prosecco Maron Glace, TTD, Sainsbury's*	1 Slice/85g	328	14.6	386	6.6	50.1	17.2	2.2
Passionfruit, & Coconut, Gail's*	100g	357	18	357	4.8	42	18	1.4
Pecan, Cinnamon, Crumb, Gail's*	100g	500	32.9	500	6.4	44.6	32.9	2.7
Plum, & Ginger, Crumble, Graze*	1 Punnet/33g	119	9.1	361	6.2	35.1	27.6	3.3
Polenta, & Almond, Mini, Gail's*	100g	388	22	388	8.4	38	22	2.4
Pumpkin, Patch, Cadbury*	1 Cake/31g	149	7.1	480	5.3	61.7	22.9	2.4
Punschrulle Punsch Roll, Delicato*	1 Roll/40g	173	8	433	5	59	20	0
Raisin, Fruit Slab, Basics, Sainsbury's*	1 Slice/50g	183	6.2	367	5.3	57.3	12.5	1.9
Raspberry, Rockin' Raspberry, Slices, Mr Kipling*	1 Slice/21g	85	4.2	397	4.3	50.6	19.5	1
Raspberry, Slice, Dairy Milk, Cadbury*	1 Slice/29g	122	5.7	420	4.6	55	19.6	1.8
Raspberry, Sponge, Value, Tesco*	1 Slice/39g	130	4.6	334	3.4	53.4	11.9	0.7
Red Velvet, The Best, Morrisons*	1/6 Cake/63g	277	13.2	440	3.7	58.8	20.9	0.8
Red Velvet, TTD, Sainsbury's*	1 Slice/71g	302	16	428	2.8	52.8	22.7	0.8
Rock	*1 Sm Cake/40g*	*158*	*6.6*	*396*	*5.4*	*60.5*	*16.4*	*1.5*
Rock, Tesco*	1 Serving/87g	311	8.4	357	7.4	60.1	9.7	1.6
Sea Salt Caramel, Banana, & Pecan, Gail's*	100g	617	49.7	617	4	37.1	49.7	2.5
Shrek Birthday, Tesco*	1/16 Cake/72g	248	8.8	344	3.3	64	12.2	0.5
Simnel Slices, Mr Kipling*	1 Slice/47g	177	5.9	379	2.9	63.4	12.6	1.2
Snowballs, Sainsbury's*	1 Snowball/18g	80	4.1	445	2.5	55.6	23	3.6
Snowballs, Tesco*	1 Snowball/18g	79	4	432	2.5	55.8	22.1	5.4
Sponge	*1 Slice/53g*	*243*	*13.9*	*459*	*6.4*	*52.4*	*26.3*	*0.9*
Sponge, Fatless	*1 Slice/53g*	*156*	*3.2*	*294*	*10.1*	*53*	*6.1*	*0.9*
Sponge, Fresh Cream & Strawberry, Asda*	1/12 Cake/60g	170	6	284	4.6	44	10	1.1
Sponge, Jam Filled	*1 Slice/65g*	*196*	*3.2*	*302*	*4.2*	*64.2*	*4.9*	*1.8*
Sponge, Raspberry, Sandwich, Sainsbury's*	1 Slice/42g	159	6.3	383	3.8	57.4	15.1	0.9
Sponge, Roll, Chocolate, M&S*	¼ Cake/66g	251	12.1	380	3.9	50.5	18.4	1.8
Sponge, with Butter Icing	*1 Slice/65g*	*318*	*19.9*	*490*	*4.5*	*52.4*	*30.6*	*0.6*
Stollen, Bites, Finest, Tesco*	1 Bite/17g	68	3.2	398	5	50.9	18.8	4.4
Stollen, Bites, Waitrose*	1 Bite/18g	71	3.1	395	4.6	54.5	17.1	2.2
Stollen, Chocolate & Rum, Finest, Tesco*	1/8 Cake/68g	262	9.5	381	5.3	57	13.8	3.9
Stollen, Kuchenmeister*	1 Serving/80g	357	16	446	5	61.2	20	2.5
Stollen, Marzipan Butter, Mini, Favorina, Lidl*	1 Stollen/18g	81	4.2	452	9.5	49.2	23.3	0

CAKE

INFO/WEIGHT	Measure	per Measure KCAL	FAT	Nutrition Values per 100g / 100ml KCAL	PROT	CARB	FAT	FIBRE
Stollen, Marzipan, Marzipan, Finest, Favorina, Lidl*	1 Slice/50g	206	9.3	412	6.2	53.4	18.6	0
Stollen, Slices, Average	*1 Slice/42g*	*160*	*6.3*	*381*	*5.5*	*55.8*	*15*	*3.1*
Stollen, Slices, Finest, Tesco*	1 Slice/33g	130	5.8	394	5.2	52.5	17.6	2.5
Stollen, Slices, Waitrose*	1 Slices/35g	143	5.8	402	4.7	57.3	16.3	3.8
Strawberry, Milkshake, Slices, Mr Kipling*	1 Slice/34g	139	5.5	402	3.3	61.1	16	0.6
Strawberry, Sponge Roll, M&S*	1/6 Cake/49g	160	4.6	330	2.8	58	9.5	0.8
Sultana, Fair Trade, Co-Op*	1/8 Cake/45g	155	4	345	5	60	9	1
Sultana, Fingerellas, Mrs Crimble's*	2 Cakes/25g	102	4	410	5.7	80	16	1.8
Swiss Roll, Average	*1oz/28g*	*77*	*1.2*	*276*	*7.2*	*55.5*	*4.4*	*0.8*
Swiss Roll, Butter Cream, M&S*	1/6 Roll/46g	162	4.3	354	2.9	63.9	9.5	0.5
Swiss Roll, Chocolate Flavour, Value, Tesco*	1 Slice/20g	79	3.9	394	5.5	49.2	19.5	1.4
Swiss Roll, Chocolate, Double, Tesco*	1 Slice/29g	104	2.3	361	2.5	69	8	1.3
Swiss Roll, Chocolate, Individual	*1 Roll/26g*	*88*	*2.9*	*337*	*4.3*	*58.1*	*11.3*	*0*
Swiss Roll, Chocolate, Lyons*	1 Serving/50g	190	9.6	379	4.3	47	19.3	0.9
Swiss Roll, Chocolate, M&S*	1 Serving/46g	168	11.1	365	4.6	32.6	24.2	1.2
Swiss Roll, Chocolate, Morrisons*	1/6 Roll/26g	103	4.9	401	4.4	56.4	18.9	3.1
Swiss Roll, Chocolate, Triple, Specially Selected, Aldi*	1 Serving/34g	153	7.4	453	5.4	58	22	1.1
Swiss Roll, Chocolate, Value, Tesco*	1 Serving/20g	81	3.7	404	5	54.1	18.7	2.1
Swiss Roll, Lemon, Tesco*	1 Slice/32g	118	3	371	3.7	67.4	9.4	1
Swiss Roll, Raspberry & Vanilla, Morrisons*	1 Serving/28g	98	2.7	350	4.2	61.8	9.5	0
Swiss Roll, Raspberry Jam, Mr Kipling*	1/6 Cake/52g	184	5.3	355	2.8	63	10.2	1
Swiss Roll, Raspberry, Average	*1 Slice/35g*	*107*	*1.2*	*305*	*3.8*	*64.8*	*3.5*	*0.6*
Swiss Roll, Strawberry & Cream, Tesco*	1 Slice/32g	113	2.5	353	3.5	66.6	7.8	1.4
Tea Loaf, Rowan Hill Bakery, Lidl*	1 Slice/50g	135	0.4	270	3.8	63.3	0.9	3.4
Tiffin, Chocolate, Sainsbury's*	1 Cake/61g	184	11.6	301	2.7	29.8	19	1.3
Toffee, & Pecan Slices, M&S*	1 Slice/36g	160	8.5	445	4.7	54	23.7	1.3
Toffee, Apple, McVitie's*	1 Slice/26g	95	2.9	363	3.8	61.5	11	1.6
Toffee, Iced, Tesco*	1 Serving/35g	132	5.2	376	3.3	57.2	14.9	1.6
Toffee, Temptation, Tesco*	1 Slice/67g	228	12.8	340	2.9	39.1	19.1	0.3
Toffee, Terror Whirls, Mr Kipling*	1 Whirl/28g	141	7.9	509	3.9	58.3	28.7	1.2
Toffee, The Handmade Flapjack Company*	1 Cake/75g	346	18.8	462	5.1	54	25.1	0
Toffee, Thorntons*	1/6 Cake/70g	302	16.8	431	4.6	49.2	24	0.8
Triple Chocolate , Fitbakes*	1 Cake/15g	46	2.2	298	15	35	14	0
Twinkie, Hostess*	1 Serving/77g	270	8.1	351	2.3	62.8	10.5	0
Vanilla, Sponge, Fresh Cream, Sainsbury's*	1 Slice/50g	152	5.1	304	7.5	45.6	10.2	0.4
Victoria Sandwich, Average	*1 Slice/68g*	*267*	*12.9*	*392*	*4.4*	*50.9*	*19*	*1*
Victoria Sandwich, Individual, M&S*	1 Pack/75g	299	13.1	399	3.6	55.8	17.5	1.8
Victoria Sponge, Free From, Finest, Tesco*	1 Slice/61g	238	11.8	393	2.9	51.3	19.4	0.8
Victoria Sponge, Fresh Cream, Value, Tesco*	1 Slice/60g	224	12.8	374	3.8	41.4	21.3	0.7
Victoria Sponge, Hand Finished, Deluxe, Lidl*	1 Slice/57g	223	9.6	389	4.4	54.3	16.8	1.5
Victoria Sponge, Lemon, Co-Op*	1 Slice/42g	151	8	360	4	44	19	0.7
Victoria Sponge, Mini, Bobby's*	1 Cake/35g	164	9.6	469	4	51.3	27.5	0.2
Victoria Sponge, Mini, Mr Kipling*	1 Cake/36g	152	6.9	420	3.9	58.5	19	0.8
Victoria Sponge, Mini, Weight Watchers*	1 Cake/30g	103	2.5	343	5.7	57.2	8.3	8.4
Victoria Sponge, Tesco*	1 Pack/68g	280	12.1	412	3.5	59	17.8	0.9
Victoria Sponge, TTD, Sainsbury's*	1 Slice/57g	229	11	401	5	51.8	19.3	1.4
Victoria Sponge, Waitrose*	1 Serving/45g	183	8.5	405	3.8	54.4	18.8	1.8
Victoria, Individual, On the Go, Sainsbury's*	1 Cake/57g	228	9.7	400	3.9	56.9	17.1	0
Viennese, M&S*	1 Cake/51g	250	14.1	495	4.1	58.9	28	2.8
Viennese, Whirl, Average	*1 Cake/28g*	*131*	*6.9*	*467*	*4.1*	*56.7*	*24.8*	*1.1*
Viennese, Whirl, Chocolate, Mr Kipling*	1 Whirl/28g	134	7.8	484	4.6	53.1	28	2.1
Viennese, Whirl, Lemon, Mr Kipling*	1 Cake/28g	115	4.5	409	4.2	62.2	15.9	0.7
Viennese, Whirl, Mr Kipling*	1 Whirl/28g	140	8	498	3.8	55.4	28.5	2.2

	Measure INFO/WEIGHT	per Measure KCAL	FAT	Nutrition Values per 100g / 100ml KCAL	PROT	CARB	FAT	FIBRE
CAKE								
Walnut, Sandwich, Sainsbury's*	1/8 Cake/48g	182	8.3	379	5.4	53.8	17.3	1.3
Walnut, Tesco*	1 Slice/40g	161	6.9	403	5.5	55.8	17.3	1.1
Wedding, Rich Fruit, with Cognac, Iced, Sainsbury's*	1 Slice/55g	212	5.5	385	3.8	68.9	10	2
Welsh, All Butter, Waitrose*	1 Cake/35g	138	5.2	393	6.2	57.4	14.9	2.2
Welsh, Average	**1oz/28g**	**121**	**5.5**	**431**	**5.6**	**61.8**	**19.6**	**1.5**
Yorkshire Parkin, Bakers Delight*	1oz/28g	111	4.1	395	5.1	60.3	14.8	1.5
CAKE BAR								
Blueberry, Trimlyne*	1 Cake/50g	142	1.1	283	3.9	64	2.2	2.2
Caramel, Tesco*	1 Cake/26g	103	4.9	395	5.1	50.8	19	8.2
Carrot, Tesco*	1 Bar/68g	239	12.6	351	4.7	41.4	18.5	2.4
Chocolate & Orange, Go Ahead, McVitie's*	1 Cake/33g	109	2	330	4.3	64.9	6	1
Chocolate Chip, Average	**1 Cake/28g**	**428**	**21.6**	**428**	**6.3**	**51.9**	**21.6**	**1.6**
Chocolate Chip, Sainsbury's*	1 Cake/25g	108	5.6	430	6.1	51.2	22.3	0.6
Chocolate Chip, Tesco*	1 Cake/30g	124	5.9	415	7	51.4	19.7	2.3
Chocolate Dream, Go Ahead, McVitie's*	1 Bar/36g	141	4.8	391	4.6	63.2	13.4	0.9
Chocolate, Average	**1 Cake/28g**	**125**	**6.2**	**446**	**5.6**	**56.3**	**22.1**	**1.9**
Chocolate, Snack Cakes, Penguin, McVitie's*	1 Bar/24g	122	7.2	510	4.8	54.6	30.2	1.6
Chocolate, Squidgy, Minis, Soreen*	1 Cake/30g	99	1.8	330	9.2	59.5	6	3.4
Chocolate, Tesco*	1 Cake/30g	130	5.8	433	5.5	58.6	19.2	1.7
Double Chocolate, Free From, Sainsbury's*	1 Cake/50g	196	7.9	391	4.2	58.2	15.7	1
Double Chocolate, Free From, Tesco*	1 Serving/45g	190	9.1	425	4.2	55.6	20.3	4.1
Flake, Cadbury*	1 Cake/25g	120	6.2	470	4.8	56.5	24.4	1.9
Galaxy, Salted Caramel, Festive, Galaxy, Mars*	1 Bar/26g	113	5.3	438	5.6	58.7	20.4	0
Golden Syrup, McVitie's*	1 Cake/33g	127	4.8	385	3.6	60.2	14.4	1.2
Jaffa Cakes, Spooky, McVitie's*	1 Bar/25g	96	3.5	390	3.2	62.1	14.2	2.7
Jaffa, McVitie's*	1 Bar/25g	96	3.5	395	3.1	62.9	14.5	2.5
Jamaica Ginger, McVitie's*	1 Cake/33g	128	4.9	388	3.5	60.2	14.7	1.2
Lemon Meringue, Indulgence, Weight Watchers*	1 Bar/24g	21	0.3	86	1.1	7.1	1.3	0
Milk Chocolate, Cadbury*	1 Bar/25g	110	5.6	445	4.9	53.8	22.8	2.9
Milky Way, McVitie's*	1 Cake/26g	124	6.2	476	5.1	58.5	23.6	1.2
Peanut, High Fibre, Squares, Tesco*	1 Square/24g	92	3.1	383	6	49	13	23
Toffee, Squidgy, Minis, Soreen*	1 Bar/30g	95	1.3	317	7.7	59.7	4.2	5.9
Vanilla, & Raspberry, Mini Rolls, Ms Mollys*	1 Roll/20g	74	2.2	368	4.7	62	11	1.2
CAKE MIX								
Carrot Cake, Betty Crocker*	¼ Pack/125g	504	8.4	403	5.8	78.9	6.7	1.4
Cheesecake, Original, Made Up, Asda*	1/6 Cake/85g	228	10.2	268	4.1	36	12	1.4
Cheesecake, Tesco*	1 Serving/76g	199	7.9	262	4.1	38	10.4	1.6
Sponge, Value, Tesco*	1 Slice/55g	181	4.8	329	4.6	57.9	8.8	1.4
Yellow, Super Moist, Betty Crocker*	1 Cake/128g	517	9.5	404	3.3	81.6	7.4	1.1
CALLALOO								
Leaves, Raw, Unprepared	**1 Cup/28g**	**6**	**0.1**	**23**	**2.5**	**4**	**0.3**	**0**
CALZONE								
Cream Cheese & Pepperonata, Waitrose*	½ Pizza/165g	383	15.8	232	7	29.4	9.6	1.5
Ham & Mushroom, Waitrose*	½ Pizza/145g	362	13.5	250	10	31.6	9.3	1.6
Speciale, Ristorante, Dr Oetker*	½ Pizza/145g	381	20.3	263	11	23	14	0
Three Cheese, Waitrose*	1 Pizza/265g	747	31.8	282	10.4	33	12	1.4
CANAPES								
Aegean Tomato, Finest, Tesco*	1 Canape/15g	45	2.2	300	7.2	34.3	14.7	2.1
Salmon & Dill, Finest, Tesco*	1 Canape/15g	47	2.4	315	9.2	32.7	16.1	1.9
Salmon, Smoked, Tesco*	3 Canapes/25g	60	4.6	241	14.7	4.1	18.3	0.5
Smoked Salmon, Youngs*	1 Canape/10g	21	1.5	210	15.9	2	15.2	0.7
CANNELLONI								
Beef, As Prepared, Waitrose*	1 Pack/360g	501	26.7	139	6.2	11.5	7.4	1

INFO/WEIGHT	Measure	per Measure		Nutrition Values per 100g / 100ml				
		KCAL	FAT	KCAL	PROT	CARB	FAT	FIBRE
CANNELLONI								
Beef, Meal for One, M&S*	1 Pack/400g	572	30.8	143	6.7	10.7	7.7	2.1
Butternut Squash, with Spinach & Goats' Cheese, Tesco*	1 Pack/350g	490	29.4	140	5.1	10.7	8.4	1.9
Mushroom, Italian, Sainsbury's*	1 Pack/450g	598	31	133	5.2	12.5	6.9	0.5
Spinach & Rocotta, Microwaved, Vegetarian, Asda*	1 Pack/377g	433	18.8	115	5.6	11	5	1.2
Spinach & Ricotta, Meal for One, M&S*	1 Pack/400g	412	17.2	103	4.8	10.2	4.3	2.2
Spinach & Ricotta, Serves 1, BGTY, Sainsbury's*	1 Pack/400g	364	9.2	91	4.5	11.8	2.3	2.6
Spinach, & Ricotta, Charlie Bigham's*	1 Serving/329 g	481	31.6	146	4.4	9.9	9.6	0
Spinach, & Ricotta, Fresh, Ready Meal, Average	**1 Serving/300g**	**393**	**22**	**131**	**5**	**10.8**	**7.4**	**1.2**
Spinach, & Ricotta, Low Fat, COU, M&S*	1 Pack/400g	340	7.6	85	4.8	11.4	1.9	1.7
Spinach, & Ricotta, Ready Meal, Average	**1 Serving/300g**	**426**	**22**	**142**	**5.6**	**13.3**	**7.3**	**1.4**
Spinach, & Ricotta, Sainsbury's*	1 Pack/400g	520	27.2	130	4.9	11.6	6.8	1.4
Spinach, & Ricotta, Italian Cuisine, Aldi*	1 Pack/385g	443	20.4	115	5.4	10	5.3	1.9
Spinach, & Ricotta, Low Fat, Well & Good, Co-Op*	1 Pack/380g	309	8.7	81	3.7	11	2.3	1
Tubes, Dry, Average	**1oz/28g**	**101**	**1**	**361**	**12.5**	**69.1**	**3.6**	**1.2**
Vegetarian, Tesco*	1 Pack/400g	552	34.4	138	5.3	9.8	8.6	1.5
CAPERS								
Capucine, in Brine, Sainsbury's*	1 Serving/15g	4	0.1	28	2	1.7	0.7	3.4
in Vinegar, Average	**1 Tsp/5g**	**2**	**0**	**34**	**1.7**	**3**	**0.6**	**0**
CAPPELLETTI								
Ham, & Cheese, Cooked, Tesco*	½ Pack/150g	288	7.5	192	8.8	27.2	5	1.6
Parma Ham, Fresh, Waitrose*	½ Pack/125g	368	11.5	294	14.1	38.6	9.2	2.2
Prosciutto, & Ricotta, Made Without Wheat, M&S*	½ Pack/125g	326	8.9	261	9.1	37.5	7.1	5.2
Tomato, & Mozzarella, GF, Free From, Morrisons*	½ Pack/151g	231	3.3	153	4.3	25.6	2.2	6.7
with Parma Ham, M&S*	½ Pack/125g	342	9.1	274	15.7	35.4	7.3	1.8
CAPRI SUN								
Blackcurrant, No Added Sugar, Capri-Sun*	1 Capri Sun/200ml	10	0	5	0	0.9	0	0
Orange	**1 Pouch/200ml**	**90**	**0**	**45**	**0**	**11**	**0**	**0**
Orange, 100%, Juice	**1 Pouch/200ml**	**75**	**0**	**38**	**0.5**	**9.2**	**0**	**0.1**
CARAMAC								
Nestle*	1 Bar/30g	174	11	571	5.9	55.5	36.1	0
CARAWAY								
Seeds, Schwartz*	1 Pack/38g	170	8.1	448	23.3	40.9	21.2	0
CARBONARA								
Chicken, & Bacon, BFY, M&S*	1 Pack/375g	476	11.2	127	10.1	14.4	3	0.8
Chicken, & Bacon, Calorie Counted, Asda*	1 Pack/342g	328	6.5	96	9	10	1.9	0.7
Chicken, Mushroom, & Ham, Spaghetti, Asda*	1 Pack/700g	686	14	98	10	10	2	1.5
Creamy, As Prepared, Pot Pasta*	1 Pot/260g	275	11.5	105	2.9	13	4.4	0.5
Mushroom, Vegan, Waitrose*	1 Pack/380g	437	19.4	115	2.3	14	5.1	2
	1 serving/450 g	864	40.5	192	7.6	19.3	9	1.8
Penne, Taste of Italy, Tesco*	½ Pack/400g	604	18.5	151	7.9	19	4.6	0.9
Spaghetti, BGTY, Sainsbury's*	1 Pack/400g	392	7.6	98	5.9	14	1.9	0.7
Spaghetti, Charlie Bigham's*	1 Serving/337 g	607	33	180	7.6	14.7	9.8	0
Spaghetti, COU, M&S*	1 Pack/330g	346	7.2	105	6.1	15.7	2.2	0.8
Spaghetti, Heated, HL, Tesco*	1 Pack/365g	372	5.1	102	6	16	1.4	0.8
Spaghetti, Italian Quisine, Microwaved, Aldi*	1 Pack/400g	669	33.4	174	7.1	16	8.7	1.5
Spaghetti, M&S*	1 Pack/400g	660	36	165	6.5	14.2	9	0.6
Spaghetti, M&S*	1 Pack/400g	560	27.2	140	5.2	14	6.8	0.9
Spaghetti, Ready Meal, Average	**1 Pack/400g**	**524**	**21.5**	**131**	**5.9**	**14.4**	**5.4**	**1.1**
Spaghetti, Tesco*	1 Pack/380g	338	4.9	89	5.4	13.4	1.3	1
Spaghetti, Waitrose*	1 Pack/383g	658	31.8	172	7	16.9	8.3	0.8
Tagliatelle, PB, Waitrose*	1 Pack/350g	357	12.6	102	5.3	12.1	3.6	0.7
Tagliatelle, Ready Meal, Average	**1 Serving/400g**	**460**	**13.4**	**115**	**5.5**	**15.8**	**3.3**	**1**
Tagliatelle, TTD, Sainsbury's*	1 Pack/400g	658	31.1	167	7.3	15.7	7.9	1.9

C

	Measure INFO/WEIGHT	per Measure KCAL	FAT	Nutrition Values per 100g / 100ml KCAL	PROT	CARB	FAT	FIBRE
CARDAMOM								
Black, Ground, Average	*1 Tsp/2g*	*6*	*0.1*	*311*	*10.8*	*68.5*	*6.7*	*28*
CAROB POWDER								
Average	*1 Tsp/2g*	*3*	*0*	*159*	*4.9*	*37*	*0.1*	*0*
CARP								
Fillet, Raw, Average	*1 Fillet/218g*	*244*	*10.2*	*112*	*17.5*	*0*	*4.7*	*0*
CARROT & SWEDE								
Carrot, & Swede, Hilltop farm*	1 Pack/400g	288	17.6	72	0.6	6.4	4.4	2.1
Carrot, & Swede, Inspired Cuisine, Aldi*	1 Pack/450g	266	8.6	59	1.1	8.3	1.9	2.4
Diced, for Mashing, Average	*½ Pack/250g*	*58*	*0.7*	*23*	*0.6*	*4.7*	*0.3*	*1.9*
Fresh, Co-Op*	1 Serving/100g	26	0.5	26	0.5	4.1	0.5	2.4
Mash, From Supermarket, Average	*1 Serving/150g*	*138*	*7.5*	*92*	*1.3*	*10.4*	*5*	*1.3*
Mash, Healthy Range, Average	*1 Serving/150g*	*98*	*4.2*	*66*	*1.3*	*8.6*	*2.8*	*2.1*
CARROTS								
& Peas, Sainsbury's*	1 Serving/200g	100	1	50	3.3	8.3	0.5	3.8
& Houmous Dip, Tesco*	1 Pack/120g	96	4.9	80	1.9	7.1	4.1	3.6
Baby, Canned, Average	*1 Can/195g*	*40*	*0.5*	*21*	*0.5*	*4.2*	*0.3*	*2.1*
Baby, Fresh, Average	*1 Serving/80g*	*28*	*0.1*	*35*	*0.6*	*8.2*	*0.1*	*2.9*
Batons, Fresh, Average	*½ Pack/150g*	*41*	*0.4*	*28*	*0.6*	*5.7*	*0.3*	*2.6*
Boiled, Average	*1oz/28g*	*6*	*0.1*	*22*	*0.6*	*4.4*	*0.4*	*2.3*
Canned, Average	*1oz/28g*	*6*	*0.1*	*20*	*0.5*	*4*	*0.2*	*1.9*
Carrot, & Parsnip, Mash Direct*	½ Pack/200g	106	1.2	53	1	8.6	0.6	4.8
Chantenay, Cut, Frozen, Tesco*	1 Serving/80g	24	0.3	29	0.6	4.3	0.4	3.1
Chantenay, Wood Farm, Raw, Aldi*	1 Serving/80g	34	0.4	42	0.6	7.9	0.5	2.4
Raw, Average	*1 Med/61g*	*25*	*0.1*	*41*	*0.9*	*9.6*	*0.2*	*2.8*
Raw, Scrubbed, Average	*1 Serving/80g*	*24*	*0.4*	*30*	*0.7*	*6*	*0.5*	*2.4*
Sliced, Canned, Average	*1 Serving/180g*	*36*	*0.2*	*20*	*0.7*	*4.1*	*0.1*	*1.5*
Sliced, Fresh, Average	*1 Serving/60g*	*17*	*0.2*	*28*	*0.7*	*5.7*	*0.3*	*2*
Whole, Raw, Peeled, Average	*1 Carrot/75g*	*21*	*0.2*	*29*	*0.6*	*6.4*	*0.3*	*2.2*
CASHEW NUTS								
Cheese Flavour, Graze*	1 Pack/26g	140	10.8	540	15.3	35.7	41.5	0
Cracking Black Pepper, Graze*	1 Punnet/36g	216	16.6	600	19	26	46	4
Plain, Average	*½ Pack/25g*	*146*	*12.2*	*584*	*15.7*	*18.8*	*48.9*	*3.4*
Roasted & Salted, Average	*1 Serving/50g*	*306*	*25.6*	*612*	*18.8*	*19.6*	*51.1*	*3.1*
Wasabi, Roasted, Vitasia, Lidl*	1 Serving/30g	185	14.6	616	17.5	25.6	48.6	0
Whole, Fancy, Kirkland Signature, Costco*	1 Serving/'30g	183	14.4	610	17	26	48	3.2
CASSAVA								
Baked, Average	*1oz/28g*	*43*	*0.1*	*155*	*0.7*	*40.1*	*0.2*	*1.7*
Boiled in Unsalted Water, Average	*1oz/28g*	*36*	*0.1*	*130*	*0.5*	*33.5*	*0.2*	*1.4*
Gari, Average	*1oz/28g*	*100*	*0.1*	*358*	*1.3*	*92.9*	*0.5*	*0*
CASSEROLE								
Beef	*1 Serving/336g*	*490*	*23*	*146*	*16.3*	*4.6*	*6.8*	*0.6*
Beef, & Ale with Dumplings, Sainsbury's*	1 Pack/450g	711	32.8	158	7.7	15.4	7.3	0.6
Beef, & Ale with Mashed Potato, HL, Tesco*	1 Pack/450g	364	11.2	81	5.1	10.9	2.5	0.6
Beef, & Ale, Average	*1 Serving/300g*	*251*	*6.8*	*84*	*9.4*	*6.5*	*2.2*	*1.3*
Beef, & Dumplings, Parsley Box*	1 Pack/270g	275	10.5	102	5.4	11	3.9	0.9
Beef, & Red Wine, Average	*1 Serving/350g*	*290*	*7.3*	*83*	*7.2*	*8.2*	*2.1*	*1.5*
Beef, & Red Wine, Inspired Cuisine, Aldi*	1 Pack/420g	344	9.7	82	6.3	7.8	2.3	1.5
Beef, Low & Slow, Slimming World, Iceland*	1 Serving/175g	88	1.2	50	6.6	3.7	0.7	0.9
Beef, Meal for One, Tesco*	1 Pack/450g	425	18.9	94	3.6	10.6	4.2	1.7
Beef, with Dumplings, Classic, Waitrose*	1 Pack/442g	583	18.6	132	7.7	15.3	4.2	1.6
Beef, with Dumplings, Ready Meal, Average	*1 Serving/350g*	*464*	*21.1*	*132*	*9.5*	*10.1*	*6*	*1.5*
Beef, with Herb Potatoes, Ready Meal, Average	*1 Serving/475g*	*504*	*17.1*	*106*	*6.8*	*11.5*	*3.6*	*1.6*
Chicken, & Asparagus, HL, Tesco*	1 Serving/450g	342	10.3	76	6.3	8.3	2.3	0.5

	Measure INFO/WEIGHT	per Measure KCAL	FAT	Nutrition Values per 100g / 100ml KCAL	PROT	CARB	FAT	FIBRE
CASEROLE								
Chicken, & Dumpling, 548, Wiltshire Farm Foods*	1 Serving/440g	485	22.5	110	5.2	11	5.1	0.8
Chicken, & Dumplings, Sainsbury's*	1 Serving/450g	612	24.8	136	9.1	12	5.5	1.2
Chicken, & Vegetable, Ready Meal, Healthy Range	*1 Serving/330g*	*265*	*11.9*	*80*	*4.7*	*7.6*	*3.6*	*1.1*
Chicken, & Dumplings, Keep in the Cupboard, Tesco*	1 Pack/300g	207	4.5	69	3.8	9.7	1.5	0.8
Chicken, & Dumplings, Parsley Box*	1 Pack/270g	254	4.6	94	8.3	11	1.7	1
Chicken, & Mushroom, Slim Cook, Tesco*	1 Pack/495g	193	2	39	5.6	2.6	0.4	1.6
Chicken, & Vegetable, Tesco*	¼ Pack/240g	192	5	80	9.6	4.7	2.1	2.2
Chicken, Leek & Mushroom, Tesco*	1 Pack/350g	382	22	109	4.5	8.6	6.3	1
Chicken, with Dumpling, 252, Oakhouse Foods Ltd*	1 Meal/400g	464	24.4	116	6.7	7.5	6.1	1
Chicken, with Dumplings, M&S*	½ Pack/227g	261	10	115	9.7	9	4.4	0.9
Lamb, & Rosemary, Eat Well, M&S*	1 Pack/380g	325	11	86	7.6	7	2.9	2.2
Pork, Normandy Style, Finest, Tesco*	1 Pack/450g	405	21.6	90	7.6	4.1	4.8	2.3
Rabbit, Average	*1oz/28g*	*29*	*1.4*	*102*	*11.6*	*2.6*	*5.1*	*0.4*
Red Lentil, & Mixed Bean, Cook*	1 Serving/290g	218	4.4	75	4.5	14.2	1.5	6.6
Sausage, & Potato, M&S*	1 Serving/200g	190	11.8	95	3.3	7.5	5.9	0.9
Sausage, CBY, Asda*	1 Pot/400g	240	15.2	60	3.6	1.9	3.8	2.1
Sausage, Pork, & Leek, 248, Oakhouse Foods Ltd*	1 Serving/400g	520	30	130	6.9	8.8	7.5	0.6
Sausage, Pork, Diet Chef Ltd*	1 Pack/300g	303	18.3	101	6.6	4.9	6.1	1.4
Sausage, with Root Vegetables, Mini's, Kirstys*	1 Pack/250g	210	9.8	84	4.4	6.1	3.9	3.7
Steak, & Mushroom, 214, Wiltshire Farm Foods*	1 Pack/360g	322	16.2	89	5	7.2	4.5	1.3
Steak, & Mushroom, Asda*	½ Pack/304g	411	30.4	135	7	4.2	10	0.3
Steak, & Ale, Average	*1 Serving/275g*	*324*	*14.4*	*118*	*9*	*8.8*	*5.2*	*1*
Steak, & Mushroom, Average	*1 Serving/275g*	*274*	*15.5*	*100*	*6.2*	*6*	*5.6*	*1*
Vegetable, Root, & Kale, Waitrose*	1 Pack/357g	343	15	96	1.9	11.6	4.2	2.1
Vegetables, Mix, Frozen, Boiled, Iceland*	1 Serving/80g	20	0.2	25	0.7	4.1	0.3	1.7
Zuppa Di Pesce, Fish, & Seafood, Stir Fried, Iceland*	½ Pack/250g	320	20.5	128	11.3	2.3	8.2	0
CASEROLE MIX								
Beef & Ale, Colman's*	1 Pack/45g	144	0.9	320	9.2	66.3	2	2.3
Beef, Colman's*	1 Pack/40g	123	0.6	308	7.5	66	1.5	2.5
Beef, Recipe, Colman's*	1 Pack/42g	142	0.5	338	9.1	13.1	1.1	4
Beef, Recipe, Schwartz*	1 Pack/43g	123	0.9	287	7	56.6	2.1	6.6
Chicken Chasseur, Asda*	1 Pack/80g	273	0.8	341	9	74	1	1.4
Chicken, Authentic, Schwartz*	1 Serving/66g	210	0.7	318	14	62.1	1	2.1
Chicken, Recipe, As Sold, Colman's*	1 Pack/40g	131	1	328	6.2	68.2	2.6	3.1
Lamb, Authentic, Schwartz*	1 Pack/35g	116	1.2	332	7.7	68	3.3	1.3
Peppered Beef, Schwartz*	1 Pack/40g	129	2	323	7	62.9	4.9	7.3
Sausage, As Sold, Colman's*	1 Pack/39g	136	1	350	10	70	2.5	6
Sausage, As Sole, Morrisons*	½ Pack/250g	120	1	48	2.2	7.3	0.4	3.2
Sausage, Classic, Schwartz*	1 Pack/35g	96	0.9	275	12.4	50.1	2.7	14.9
CASSOULET								
Duck, & Wild Boar, Cook*	1 Serving/280g	347	17.6	124	8.4	9.4	6.3	2.2
Lamb, & Spinach, High in Protein, Asda*	1 Pack/400g	340	10.4	85	7.2	4	2.6	4.5
Toulouse, Hearty, with a Kick of Chilli, Hello Fresh*	1 Serving/604g	459	20	76	5.3	5.6	3.3	0
CATFISH								
Cooked, Steamed, Weighed with Bone, Average	*1 Serving/100g*	*101*	*3.1*	*101*	*18.2*	*0*	*3.1*	*0.7*
CAULIFLOWER								
BBQ, Bites, Tesco*	½ Pack/128g	83	1.1	65	2.3	10.9	0.9	2.2
Bites, Buffalo, Tesco*	½ Pack/115g	163	7.5	142	2.6	16.5	6.5	3.7
Boiled, Average	*1 Serving/80g*	*22*	*0.7*	*28*	*2.9*	*2.1*	*0.9*	*1.6*
Cauliflower, with Reduced Fat Sour Cream, M&S*	1 Pack/280g	112	7.3	40	1.2	1.8	2.6	2.3
Cous Cous, Ready to Cook, As Sold, Morrisons*	1 Pack/330g	129	3	39	3.6	2.8	0.9	2.6
Grills, Tesco*	1 Grill/96g	236	13.7	246	5.6	22	14.3	3.2
Indian Spiced, Yoghurt & Mint Dressing, Sainsbury's*	1 Pack/270g	226	5.4	84	2.6	13.3	2	1.1

C

	Measure INFO/WEIGHT	per Measure KCAL	FAT	Nutrition Values per 100g / 100ml KCAL	PROT	CARB	FAT	FIBRE
CAULIFLOWER								
Popcorn, with Spicy Buffalo Dip, Plant Kitchen, M&S*	½ Pack/113g	213	12.7	189	2.3	18.7	11.3	1.6
Raw, Average	*1 Serving/80g*	*25*	*0.7*	*31*	*3.2*	*2.7*	*0.8*	*1.6*
Rice, Nature's Pick, Aldi*	1 Pot/250g	85	2.2	34	2.9	2.1	0.9	2.7
Spiced, Roasted, Tesco*	½ Pack/70g	59	4.4	84	2.2	3.9	6.2	1.8
Steamed, Average	*1 Serving/100g*	*28*	*0.9*	*28*	*2.9*	*2.1*	*0.9*	*1.6*
CAULIFLOWER CHEESE								
& Bacon, Gastropub, M&S*	1 Pack/300g	318	21	106	6.3	4.5	7	1
& Broccoli, Average	*1 Serving/200g*	*127*	*6.4*	*64*	*3.8*	*4.6*	*3.2*	*2*
Asda*	1 Pack/450g	486	36	108	4.6	4.3	8	1.5
Average	*1 Meal/400g*	*362*	*23.3*	*90*	*4.5*	*4.6*	*5.8*	*1.3*
BFY, Morrisons*	1 Pack/300g	231	12.3	77	4.5	5.4	4.1	1.2
Florets in a Cheese Sauce, As Prepared, Sainsbury's*	½ Pack/194g	149	7.7	77	4.8	4.3	4	2.2
Fresh, Oven Heated, Tesco*	½ Pack/161g	129	7.1	80	4.4	4.7	4.4	2.1
Frozen, Iceland*	1 Serving/200g	190	12	95	4	5.5	6	1.6
Frozen, Oven Baked, Asda*	½ Pack/150g	187	10.6	125	5.9	8.3	7.1	1.9
Heated, Finest, Tesco*	½ Pack/168g	209	13.8	124	5.7	6.4	8.2	1.4
M&S*	½ Pack/225g	263	17.5	117	6.7	4.3	7.8	1.3
Made with Semi-Skimmed Milk	*1oz/28g*	*28*	*1.8*	*100*	*6*	*5.2*	*6.4*	*1.3*
Made with Skimmed Milk	*1oz/28g*	*27*	*1.7*	*97*	*6*	*5.2*	*6*	*1.3*
Made with Whole Milk	*1oz/28g*	*29*	*1.9*	*105*	*6*	*5.2*	*6.9*	*1.3*
Morrisons*	1 Pack/400g	384	20.8	96	4.2	7.6	5.2	0.9
Rich, & Creamy, Co-Op*	½ Pack/165g	206	13.7	125	5.4	6.5	8.3	1.1
TTD, Sainsbury's*	¼ Pack/148g	169	11.1	114	5.1	5.8	7.5	1.3
with Wexford Mature Cheddar, M&S*	½ Pack/225g	263	17.6	117	6.7	4.3	7.8	1.3
CAVIAR								
Average	*1oz/28g*	*25*	*1.3*	*89*	*11.6*	*0.5*	*4.6*	*0*
CELERIAC								
Boiled in Salted Water, Average	*1oz/28g*	*5*	*0.1*	*18*	*0.9*	*1.9*	*0.4*	*3.2*
Raw, Average	*1 Serving/80g*	*17*	*0.3*	*21*	*1*	*1.9*	*0.4*	*3.2*
CELERY								
Boiled in Salted Water	*1 Serving/50g*	*4*	*0.2*	*8*	*0.5*	*0.8*	*0.3*	*1.2*
Raw, Trimmed, Average	*1 Stalk/40g*	*3*	*0.1*	*7*	*0.5*	*0.9*	*0.2*	*1.1*
CHAMPAGNE								
Average	*1 Glass/125ml*	*95*	*0*	*76*	*0.3*	*1.4*	*0*	*0*
CHANNA MASALA								
M&S*	1 Pack/225g	360	23.7	160	5.6	11.2	10.5	8.2
Waitrose*	1 Pack/300g	300	18.3	100	3.7	7.4	6.1	7.9
CHAPATIS								
Brown Wheat Flour, Waitrose*	1 Chapati/42g	128	3.4	305	8.6	49.4	8	4.6
Elephant Atta*	1 Chapati/45g	129	2.9	287	7.5	53.1	6.4	3.2
Indian Style, Asda*	1 Chapati/43g	95	0.4	221	8	45	1	2.9
Loyd Grossman*	1 Chapatti/60g	179	2.8	298	9	52.4	4.7	5
Made with Fat	*1 Chapati/60g*	*197*	*7.7*	*328*	*8.1*	*48.3*	*12.8*	*0*
Made without Fat	*1 Chapati/55g*	*111*	*0.6*	*202*	*7.3*	*43.7*	*1*	*0*
Morrisons*	1 Chapati/40g	108	2.8	269	8.6	49.8	6.9	0
Plain, Original, Wrap, Patak's*	1 Chapati/42g	115	3.2	273	9.4	48.8	7.5	0
Sainsbury's*	1 Chapatti/95g	306	7	322	8.9	52.8	7.4	4.1
Wholemeal, Patak's*	1 Chapati/42g	130	4	310	11.2	44.9	9.5	9
CHARD								
Average	*1 Serving/80g*	*15*	*0.2*	*19*	*1.4*	*3.3*	*0.2*	*0.8*
Silverbeet, Fresh, Steamed	*1 Serving/100g*	*15*	*0*	*15*	*1.9*	*1.3*	*0*	*3.3*
Swiss, Boiled in Unsalted Water	*1oz/28g*	*6*	*0*	*20*	*1.9*	*4.1*	*0.1*	*2.1*
Swiss, Raw	*1oz/28g*	*5*	*0.1*	*17*	*1.7*	*3.4*	*0.2*	*1.5*

	Measure INFO/WEIGHT	per Measure KCAL	FAT	Nutrition Values per 100g / 100ml KCAL	PROT	CARB	FAT	FIBRE
CHEDDARS								
Baked, Mini, Blue Cheese, Jacob's*	1 Pack/25g	132	7.9	530	8.8	50.3	31.8	2.5
Cheese & Ham, Baked, Mini, McVitie's*	1 Bag/30g	160	8.9	534	11	55.5	29.8	2
Cheese, Baked, Mini, Original, Jacobs*	1 Bag/25g	128	7.3	512	10.6	50.1	29.2	2.5
Chilli Beef, Baked, Mini, Jacob's*	1 Pack/50g	262	15	522	9	52.2	29.9	2.7
Mini, Average	**1 Bag/26g**	**134**	**7.8**	**516**	**11.2**	**50.8**	**29.9**	**2.4**
Mini, BBQ, Jacob's*	1 Pack/25g	131	7.6	525	9.3	51.6	30.3	2.6
Red Leicester, Baked, Mini, Jacob's*	1 Pack/25g	132	7.9	530	8.7	50.2	31.8	2.5
Stilton, Baked, Mini, Jacob's*	1 Pack/25g	132	7.9	530	8.8	50.3	31.8	2.5
CHEESE								
& Nuts, Salt & Pepper, Fridge Raiders, Mattessons*	1 Pack/40g	163	10.4	407	25	17	26	0
Babybel, Cheddar Variety, Mini, Fromageries Bel*	1 Cheese/20g	75	6.2	375	24	0	31	0
Babybel, Cheddar, Light, Mini, Fromageries Bel*	1 Mini/20g	59	4.4	296	24	0.5	22	0
Babybel, Emmental, Fromageries Bel*	1 Serving/20g	63	4.9	316	23	1	24.5	0
Babybel, Goat's Variety, Mini, Fromageries Bel*	1 Cheese/20g	65	5.4	327	21	0	27	0
Babybel, Gouda Variety, Mini, Fromageries Bel*	1 Cheese/20g	68	5.6	340	22	0	28	0
Babybel, Light, Mini, Fromageries Bel*	1 Babybel/20g	42	2.4	208	25	0	12	0
Babybel, Original, Mini, Fromageries Bel*	1 Cheese/20g	61	4.8	304	22	0.1	24	0
Beechwood, Smoked, Slices, Tesco*	1 Slice/25g	75	6	299	20.7	0	24	0
Bites, Mini, Sainsbury's*	1 Serving/20g	65	4.7	323	25.3	3.1	23.3	0
Blue, Castello, Soft, Castello*	¼ Pack/37g	162	15.6	432	14	0.5	41.5	0
Blue, French, CBY, Asda*	1 Serving/30g	90	7.4	301	20	0	24.5	0
Blue, Saint Agur*	1 Serving /30g	109	9.9	363	16	0.2	33	0
Blue, Shropshire, The Delicatessen, Tesco*	1 Serving/30g	123	10.5	410	23.7	0.1	35	0
Blue, Sliced for Burger, Castello*	1 Slice/25g	100	9.2	400	17	0.5	37	0
Brie, Average	**1 Serving/25g**	**74**	**6**	**296**	**19.7**	**0.3**	**24**	**0**
Brie, Breaded, Bites, Frozen, Tesco*	1 Bite/17g	54	3.4	319	8.6	24.2	20.2	2.8
Brie, Cornish, Lactofree, Arla*	1 Serving/30g	105	9.3	351	17	1.7	31	0
Brie, Reduced Fat, Average	**1 Serving/50g**	**99**	**5.7**	**198**	**23**	**0.8**	**11.4**	**0**
Burrata, 1, Waitrose*	1 Serving/30g	67	5.6	222	13.4	0.2	18.6	0
Caerphilly, Average	**1 Serving/50g**	**187**	**15.6**	**374**	**23**	**0.1**	**31.3**	**0**
Cambazola, Tesco*	1 Serving/30g	128	12.3	425	13.5	0.5	41	0
Camembert, Average	**1 Serving/50g**	**141**	**11.1**	**283**	**20.5**	**0.1**	**22.2**	**0**
Camembert, Breaded, Average	**1 Serving/90g**	**307**	**20.9**	**342**	**16.6**	**14.2**	**23.2**	**0.4**
Cantal, French, Sainsbury's*	1 Serving/30g	106	8.7	353	23	0.1	29	0
Cheddar, Average	**1 Serving/30g**	**123**	**10.3**	**410**	**25**	**0.1**	**34.4**	**0**
Cheddar, Canadian, Average	**1 Serving/30g**	**123**	**10.3**	**409**	**25**	**0.1**	**34.3**	**0**
Cheddar, Davidstow, Mature, Average	**1 Serving/28g**	**115**	**9.6**	**410**	**25**	**0.1**	**34.4**	**0**
Cheddar, Extra Mature, Average	**1 Serving/30g**	**123**	**10.3**	**410**	**25.1**	**0.1**	**34.4**	**0**
Cheddar, Extra Mature, Spreadable, Cathedral City*	1 Serving/30g	76	5.8	254	15.9	4.5	19.2	0
Cheddar, Grated, Average	**1 Serving/50g**	**206**	**17.2**	**413**	**24.4**	**1.5**	**34.3**	**0**
Cheddar, Mature, Average	**1 Serving/30g**	**123**	**10.3**	**410**	**25**	**0.1**	**34.4**	**0**
Cheddar, Mature, Grated, Average	**1 Serving/28g**	**113**	**9.3**	**404**	**24.7**	**1.6**	**33.2**	**0**
Cheddar, Mature, Lactose Free, Cathedral City*	1 Serving/30g	125	10.5	416	25.4	0.1	34.9	0
Cheddar, Mature, Reduced Fat, Average	**1 Serving/25g**	**68**	**4.2**	**271**	**30**	**0.1**	**16.7**	**0**
Cheddar, Mature, Spreadable, Cathedral City*	1 Serving/30g	77	5.9	256	15.8	3.9	19.7	0
Cheddar, Mature, Spreadable, Lighter, Cathedral City*	1 Serving/30g	61	3.7	203	16.8	6.3	12.3	0
Cheddar, Medium, Average	**1 Serving/30g**	**123**	**10.4**	**411**	**24.9**	**0.2**	**34.5**	**0**
Cheddar, Mild, Average	**1 Serving/30g**	**123**	**10.3**	**409**	**25**	**0.1**	**34.3**	**0**
Cheddar, Reduced Fat, Average	**1 Serving/30g**	**76**	**4.2**	**255**	**32.2**	**0.1**	**14**	**0**
Cheddar, Smoked, Average	**1 Serving/30g**	**123**	**10.3**	**411**	**25.2**	**0.1**	**34.4**	**0**
Cheddar, with Caramelised Onion, Tesco*	1 Serving/50g	183	14	366	21.4	7.1	28	0.4
Cheddar, with Onion & Chives, Davidson*	1 Serving/25g	100	8.3	400	24.3	0.6	33.3	0
Chedds, Bricks, Cathedral City, Dairy Crest Ltd*	1 Brick/18g	75	6.3	416	25.4	0.1	34.9	0

CHEESE

INFO/WEIGHT	Measure	per Measure		Nutrition Values per 100g / 100ml				
		KCAL	FAT	KCAL	PROT	CARB	FAT	FIBRE
Cheshire	*1oz/28g*	*106*	*8.8*	*379*	*24*	*0.1*	*31.4*	*0*
Cottage, Low Fat, 2% Fat, Natural, Average	*1 Serving/75g*	*68*	*1.4*	*90*	*13.7*	*3.6*	*1.9*	*0*
Cottage, Plain, Average	*1 Tbsp/20g*	*19*	*0.7*	*93*	*12*	*3.3*	*3.5*	*0.1*
Cottage, Plain, Reduced Fat, Average	*100g*	*85*	*1.9*	*85*	*12.3*	*4.4*	*1.9*	*0.1*
Cottage, Virtually Fat Free, Average	*1 Tbsp/20g*	*16*	*0.2*	*79*	*13*	*4.5*	*1*	*0*
Cottage, Whole Milk, Natural, Average	*1 Serving/75g*	*77*	*3.4*	*103*	*12.5*	*2.7*	*4.5*	*0*
Cottage, with Black Pepper, HE, Tesco*	1 Pot/125g	101	2.2	81	12.1	4	1.8	0
Cottage, with Chives, Low Fat, Westacre*	1 Pot/100g	81	1.4	81	13.7	3.5	1.4	1.2
Cottage, with Chives, Virtually Fat free, Longley Farm*	½ Pot/125g	88	0.1	70	14.3	2.9	0.1	0
Cottage, with Onion & Chive, GFY, Asda*	¼ Tub/75g	50	1	66	9.3	3.8	1.4	0.5
Cottage, with Pineapple, 70% Less fat, CBY, Asda*	¼ Tub/75g	70	1	93	8.4	11.9	1.3	0
Cottage, with Pineapple, Fat Free, Tesco*	1 Serving/30g	22	0.1	73	8.8	8.6	0.4	0
Cottage, with Sweet Chilli, & Red Pepper, CBY, Asda*	½ Tub/150g	118	2	79	9.9	7.1	1.3	0.3
Cream, Average	*1 Portion/30g*	*132*	*14.2*	*439*	*3.1*	*0*	*47.4*	*0*
Cream, Garlic & Herbs, Light, Boursin*	1 Portion/20g	26	1.8	131	8	4.5	9	0
Cream, Reduced Fat, Average	*1 Serving/20g*	*23*	*1.1*	*117*	*13*	*4*	*5.3*	*0.1*
Cream, Roll, Chives & Garlic, Jermi *	1 Serving/30g	111	11.1	369	6.4	2	37.1	0.5
Cream, Roll, Salmon, Jermi *	1 Serving/30g	100	9.7	332	7.8	2.2	32.4	0.5
Cream, with Onion & Chives, Morrisons*	1 Serving/20g	38	3	190	11	3	15	0
Creme de Saint Agur, Saint Agur*	1 Serving/10g	28	2.5	285	13.5	2.3	24.7	0
Dairylea, Light, Slices, Kraft*	1 Slice/25g	44	1.9	177	16	8.2	7.6	1.6
Danish Blue, Average	*1 Serving/30g*	*106*	*8.7*	*352*	*20.8*	*0*	*29.1*	*0*
Demi Pont L'eveque, Finest, Tesco*	1 Serving/46g	138	10.6	301	21.1	0.4	23	0
Dolcelatte, Average	*1 Serving/30g*	*110*	*9.7*	*366*	*17.8*	*0.4*	*32.3*	*0.4*
Double Gloucester, Average	*1 Serving/30g*	*121*	*10.2*	*404*	*24.5*	*0.1*	*34*	*0*
Doux De Montagne, Average	*1 Serving/25g*	*88*	*7.1*	*352*	*22.9*	*1.5*	*28.3*	*0*
Edam, Average	*1 Serving/10g*	*33*	*2.5*	*326*	*25.3*	*0*	*24.9*	*0*
Edam, Dutch, Garlic & Herb Wedge, Asda*	1 Serving/60g	197	15	329	26	0	25	0
Edam, Slices, Average	*1 Slice/30g*	*96*	*7.2*	*320*	*25*	*0.4*	*24.1*	*0*
Edam, Slices, V Taste, Morrisons*	1 Slice/22g	67	5.2	305	1.1	21.4	23.8	0.5
Emmental, Average	*1 Serving/10g*	*37*	*2.8*	*368*	*28.4*	*0*	*28.4*	*0*
Emmental, Light, Slices, President*	1 Slice/20g	60	3.6	298	34	0	18	0
Emmental, Spreadable, Low Low, Kerry*	1 Serving/20g	40	2.7	200	13	6.7	13.5	0
Feta, Apetina, Light, 10 % Fat, Arla*	1 Serving/30g	52	3	173	18.4	0.6	10.1	0
Feta, Average	*1 Serving/30g*	*79*	*6.4*	*262*	*16.3*	*1*	*21.5*	*0*
Feta, Light, Greek, Salad, 40% Reduced Fat, Attis*	1 Portion/30g	51	3.6	170	20	0.6	12	0
Fondue, Swiss, Easy Cook, Tesco*	¼ Pack/100g	235	17	235	15.5	4	17	0
Fontina, Average	*1 Serving/28g*	*109*	*9*	*389*	*25*	*0*	*32.1*	*0*
for Pizza, Grated	*1 Serving/50g*	*163*	*12.2*	*326*	*25*	*1.6*	*24.4*	*0*
German, Smoked, with Jalapeno, Milbona, Lidl*	1 Slice/20g	66	5.3	332	19.5	3.5	26.6	0.5
Goats, Average	*1 Tsp/10g*	*26*	*2.1*	*262*	*13.8*	*3.8*	*21.2*	*0*
Goats, Breaded, Bites, Sainsbury's*	1 Bite/25g	84	6.2	337	13	15.1	25	0.8
Goats, French, Mild, Average	*1 Serving/30g*	*49*	*3.5*	*163*	*11.2*	*3*	*11.8*	*0*
Goats, Premium, Average	*1 Serving/30g*	*98*	*7.8*	*327*	*20.5*	*0.6*	*26.1*	*0*
Goats, Soft, Average	*1 Serving/30g*	*79*	*6.3*	*262*	*16.7*	*1.8*	*20.8*	*0.5*
Gorgonzola, Average	*1 Serving/30g*	*100*	*8.1*	*334*	*20*	*0*	*27*	*0*
Gouda, Average	*1 Serving/30g*	*113*	*9.4*	*376*	*24*	*0*	*31.5*	*0*
Gran Padano, Reserva, Deluxe, Lidl*	1 Serving/10g	39	2.8	388	33	0	28.4	0
Grana Padano, Italian Cheese, Waitrose*	1 Serving/14g	54	4	388	33	0	28.4	0
Greek Style, Salad Cheese, Everyday Value, Tesco*	1 Serving/30g	80	6.2	270	17.2	1.9	21	0
Greek Style, Salad, Light, Essential, Waitrose*	1 Serving/30g	57	3.6	190	20	0.6	12	0
Gruyere	*1oz/28g*	*115*	*9.3*	*409*	*27.2*	*0*	*33.3*	*0*
Halloumi, Average	*1 Serving/80g*	*253*	*19.7*	*316*	*20.8*	*1.6*	*24.7*	*0*

CHEESE

INFO/WEIGHT	Measure	per Measure		Nutrition Values per 100g / 100ml				
		KCAL	FAT	KCAL	PROT	CARB	FAT	FIBRE
Halloumi, Light Average	**1 Serving/100g**	**245**	**15.3**	**245**	**24.7**	**1.7**	**15.3**	**0**
Halloumi, Pesto, The Grill, M&S*	½ Pack/113g	318	23.6	283	19.8	3.2	21	1.1
Halloumi, with Chilli, Burger Slices, Aldi*	1 Slice/50g	168	13.5	335	23	1.2	27	0.5
Healthy Range, Average	**1 Slice/20g**	**39**	**2.1**	**197**	**20.6**	**5.2**	**10.4**	**0**
Healthy Range, Slices, Average	**1 Slice/25g**	**45**	**2.2**	**180**	**19.5**	**5.4**	**9**	**0**
Iberico, TTD, Sainsbury's*	1 Serving/30g	117	9.6	390	23.8	1	32.1	1
Italian, Hard, Dairy Free, Shredded, Follow Your Heart*	1 Tbsp/10g	34	2.6	344	0	29	26	0
Jarlsberg, Slices, Average	**1 Slice/15g**	**54**	**4**	**360**	**27**	**0**	**27**	**0**
Kvarg, Coconut, Lindahls, Nestle*	1 Serving/30g	18	0.1	60	11	3.4	0.2	0
Kvarg, Raspberry, Lindahls, Nestle*	1 Pot/150g	90	0.3	60	11.3	3.4	0.2	0
Kvarg, Stracciatella, Lindahls, Nestle*	1 Pot/150g	94	0.9	63	11	3.4	0.6	0
Labneh, Fresh, Lite, Almarai*	1 Serving/30ml	238	9.8	119	9	8.5	4.9	0
Labneh, Turkish, President*	1 Serving/30g	52	3.8	173	8.2	7	12.5	0
Lactose Free, Arla*	1 Serving/30g	103	8.1	344	25.3	1	27	0
Lactose Free, Semi Hard, Lactofree, Arla*	1 Portion/30g	103	8.1	344	25.3	1	27	0
Lancashire	**1oz/28g**	**104**	**8.7**	**373**	**23.3**	**0.1**	**31**	**0**
Leerdammer, Lighter, Sliced, M&S*	1 Slice/23g	62	3.9	271	29.5	0.1	17	0
Leerdammer, Original, Sliced, Leerdammer*	1 Slice/20g	71	5.5	356	27	0.1	27.5	0
Manchego	**1 Serving/70g**	**340**	**30.8**	**485**	**22.2**	**0.1**	**44**	**0**
Mascarpone, Average	**1 Serving/30g**	**131**	**13.1**	**437**	**5.6**	**4.1**	**43.6**	**0**
Mature, Half Fat, Average	**1 Serving/25g**	**66**	**3.9**	**265**	**29.9**	**0.4**	**15.6**	**0.1**
Mild, Reduced Fat, Grated, Average	**1 Serving/30g**	**70**	**3.3**	**235**	**31.5**	**2.2**	**11.1**	**0**
Monteray Jack, Slices, Morrisons*	1 Slice/25g	99	7.9	396	24	3.2	31.6	0
Monterey Jack, Iga*	1 Serving/28g	110	9	393	25	0	32.1	0
Mozzarella, Average	**½ Ball/63g**	**172**	**12.9**	**275**	**21.2**	**1.2**	**20.6**	**0**
Mozzarella, Reduced Fat, Average	**½ Ball/63g**	**115**	**6.4**	**184**	**21.2**	**1**	**10.2**	**0**
Mozzarella, Sticks, Free From, Tesco*	2 Sticks/25g	75	4.5	301	15.3	18.6	18	1.7
Mozzarella, Sticks, Melting, Crispy Golden Crumb, M&S*	½ Pack/75g	269	18.1	359	18.2	16.4	24.1	1.8
Mozzarella, Sticks, Sainsbury's*	1 Stick/15g	53	3.2	356	15.5	23.2	21.8	2.4
NeufchÃƒÂ¢tel, Soft, Average	**1 Serving/30g**	**76**	**6.9**	**253**	**9**	**3.6**	**23**	**0**
Norvegia, Sliced Light, Tine*	1 Slice/10g	27	1.6	272	32	0	16	0
Ossau-Iraty, Average	**1 Serving/30g**	**120**	**10.2**	**400**	**22.3**	**0.2**	**34**	**0**
Parmesan, Average	**1 Tbsp/10g**	**42**	**2.8**	**422**	**40**	**2**	**28.5**	**0**
Pecorino, Italian, Tesco*	1 Serving/30g	119	9.9	397	22	0	33	0
Pepper Jack, Sliced, Sargento*	1 Slice/21g	80	7	381	19	0	33.3	0
Quark, Average	**1 Serving/20g**	**13**	**0**	**66**	**11.9**	**4**	**0.2**	**0**
Quark, Strawberry, Graham's The Family Dairy *	1 Serving/30g	23	0.1	78	11.4	7.2	0.4	0
Raclette, Richsmonts*	1 Slice/28g	100	8	357	25	0	28.6	0
Reblochon, Average	**1 Serving/30g**	**95**	**8**	**318**	**19.7**	**0**	**26.6**	**0**
Red Leicester, Average	**1 Serving/30g**	**120**	**10.1**	**400**	**23.8**	**0.1**	**33.7**	**0**
Red Leicester, Reduced Fat, Average	**1 Serving/30g**	**78**	**4.6**	**261**	**30.2**	**0.1**	**15.4**	**0**
Red Leicester, Slices, V Taste, Morrisons*	1 Slice/22g	72	5.2	329	2.1	24.5	23.8	4
Ricotta, Average	**1 Serving/50g**	**67**	**4.8**	**134**	**9.3**	**2.9**	**9.5**	**0**
Roquefort, Average	**1oz/28g**	**105**	**9.2**	**375**	**19.7**	**0**	**32.9**	**0**
Roule, French, Sainsbury's*	1 Serving/30g	96	9.2	321	8.5	3	30.5	0
Roule, Garlic, & Herb, Lidl*	1 Serving/30g	90	8.4	301	7.3	5	28	0
Sage Derby	**1oz/28g**	**113**	**9.5**	**402**	**24.2**	**0.1**	**33.9**	**0**
Salami, Slices, Mlekpol*	1 Slice/13g	45	3.5	343	25	0	27	0
Shropshire, Blue, Average	**1 Serving/50g**	**196**	**17.1**	**391**	**21**	**0**	**34.2**	**0**
Slices, Average	**1 Slice/23g**	**82**	**6.6**	**358**	**24**	**0.8**	**28.6**	**0**
Slices, Caractere, Intense & Nutty, Fol Epi*	1 Slice/22g	79	6.3	365	26	0.5	29	0
Slices, Lighter, Emporium Kids, Aldi*	1 Slice/25g	48	2.8	194	17	7.4	11	0.5
Slices, Red Leicester, Tesco*	1 Slice/30g	120	10.1	400	23.7	0	33.7	0

CHEESE

INFO/WEIGHT	Measure	per Measure KCAL	FAT	Nutrition Values per 100g / 100ml KCAL	PROT	CARB	FAT	FIBRE
Slices, Smoked with Ham, Aldi*	1 Slice/21g	66	5.2	313	21	1	25	0.1
Soft, 50% Lighter, NUME, Morrisons*	1 Serving/30g	51	3.8	169	9.7	4.2	12.5	0.5
Soft, Creamfields*	1 Serving/30g	72	6.7	239	4.3	4.7	22.4	0.5
Soft, Extra Light, Average	*1 Serving/20g*	*25*	*1.2*	*125*	*14.3*	*3.6*	*5.9*	*0.1*
Soft, Full Fat, Aldi*	1 Serving/30g	73	6.9	243	5	3.3	23	1.3
Soft, Full Fat, Average	*1 Serving/50g*	*156*	*15.2*	*312*	*8.2*	*1.7*	*30.3*	*0*
Soft, Full Fat, Original, Lactose Free, Kraft*	1 Serving/30g	84	8.2	280	4.5	2.7	27.5	0.3
Soft, Garlic & Herb, Roulade, M&S*	1 Portion/100g	295	27.3	295	7.8	4.1	27.3	1.3
Soft, Garlic & Herbs, Light, Med Fat, Philadelphia*	1 Serving/20g	30	2.1	149	7.3	5.4	10.5	0.5
Soft, Garlic, & Herb, Lighter, Sainsbury's*	1 Serving/30g	49	3.3	163	9.6	6.4	11	0
Soft, Light, Average	*1 Tbsp/30g*	*54*	*3.9*	*179*	*12.1*	*3.2*	*13.1*	*0*
Soft, Med Fat, Average	*1 Serving/30g*	*62*	*5.4*	*207*	*8.4*	*3*	*17.9*	*0*
Soft, Mediterranean Herbs, Full Fat, Philadelphia*	1 Serving/30g	64	5.7	213	5	4.1	19	0.3
Soft, Salmon & Dill, Light, Med Fat, Philadelphia*	1 Serving/20g	28	2	142	7.3	5.1	10	0.5
Soft, Sweet Chilli, Light, Med Fat, Philadelphia*	1 Serving/20g	30	2	148	6.8	7.3	10	0.5
Soft, White, Lactofree, Arla*	1 Serving/30g	59	5	197	8.6	3	16.5	0
Soft, with Black Pepper, Light, Sainsbury's*	½ Pack/100g	205	16.5	205	11	3	16.5	0
Soft, with Chives, Light, Med Fat, Philadelphia*	1 Serving/20g	30	2.2	151	7.4	5.2	11	0.6
Soft, with Garlic & Herbs, Full Fat, Deli, Boursin*	1 Serving/28g	84	8.3	299	3.5	5	29.5	0
Spreadable, Lighter, Squares, Mclelland*	1 Square/17g	33	2.4	192	14	2.5	14	0
Spreadable, Original, Squares, Mclelland*	1 Square/17g	41	3.4	244	13.4	2.6	20	0
Spreadable, Protein, Eat Lean, Kavli*	1 Serving/30g	42	1.8	140	17.2	4	6	0
Stilton, Average	*1 Serving/30g*	*123*	*10.6*	*410*	*22.4*	*0.1*	*35.5*	*0*
Stilton, Blue, Average	*1 Serving/30g*	*124*	*10.7*	*412*	*22.8*	*0.1*	*35.7*	*0*
Stilton, White & Apricot, M&S*	1oz/28g	94	6.5	337	13.8	18.5	23.1	0
Stilton, White with Cranberries, Tesco*	1 Serving/50g	184	14.8	368	15.8	9.5	29.7	0.7
Stilton, White, Average	*1oz/28g*	*101*	*8.8*	*362*	*19.9*	*0.1*	*31.3*	*0*
Taleggio D.o.p., Finest, Tesco*	1 Serving/30g	89	7.5	297	18	0	25	0
Tetilla Queso, Sol & Mar, Lidl*	1 Serving/30g	98	8.1	328	21	0.1	27	0.5
Twisted, Cheestrings*	1 String/20g	61	4.5	305	23	2.5	22.5	0
Vacherin Badoz, Waitrose*	1 Serving/30g	87	7.2	289	17.6	0.7	24	0
Wedge, Leerdammer*	1 Serving/30g	107	8.2	356	27	0	27.5	0
Wensleydale, & Ginger, Truckle, Morrisons*	1 Truckle/90g	330	23.7	367	18	14	26.3	1.1
Wensleydale, Average	*1 Serving/25g*	*92*	*7.8*	*369*	*22.4*	*0.1*	*31*	*0*
Wensleydale, with Blueberries, M&S*	1 Portion/30g	111	7.9	370	18.7	13.4	26.4	0.9
Wensleydale, with Cranberries, Sainsbury's*	1 Serving/50g	180	13.9	359	20.7	6.4	27.8	0

CHEESE ALTERNATIVE

INFO/WEIGHT	Measure	per Measure KCAL	FAT	Nutrition Values per 100g / 100ml KCAL	PROT	CARB	FAT	FIBRE
Cheddar Style, Coconut Based, Sainsbury's*	1 Serving/30g	91	6.9	304	0.7	21.7	22.9	4
Cheddar Style, Coconut Based, Slices, Sainsbury's*	1 Slice/20g	61	4.6	304	0.7	21.7	22.9	4
Cheddar, Coconut Base, Free From, Morrisons*	1 Serving/30g	97	7	323	1.7	26	23.2	1.5
Cheddar, Mature, Free From, Asda*	1 Serving/30g	86	6.3	285	0.5	21	21	5.1
Cheezly, Feta Style in Oil, The Redwood Co*	1 Serving/25g	119	11.8	475	2.5	10.6	47	0
Greek Style, Coconut Based, Free From, Sainsbury's*	1 Serving/30g	91	7.3	303	0.5	19.5	24.4	1.5
Greek, White, Block, Violife*	1 Serving/30g	92	8.7	305	0	11	29	0
Hard, Italian Style, Free From, Tesco*	1 Serving/30g	92	5.9	306	1.2	29.5	19.6	3.6
Mozzarella, Grated, Free From, Asda*	1 Serving/30g	94	7.8	313	0.5	18	26	3.2
Mozzarella, Grated, Free From, Tesco*	1 Serving/30g	94	7.8	313	0	18.3	26	3.2
Mozzarella, Slices, Dairy Free	*1 Slice/19g*	*80*	*6*	*420*	*10.5*	*10.5*	*31.5*	*0*
Smoked, Gouda Style, Slices, Follow Your Heart*	1 Slice/20g	57	4.6	285	0	20	23	0
Soft, Coconut Based, Garlic & Herb, Sainsbury's*	1 Serving/30g	83	7.9	277	6.6	2.2	26.3	2.5
Soft, Coconut Based, Original, Free From, Sainsbury's*	1 Serving/30g	85	8	285	6.5	3.4	26.8	2
Soft, Cream Cheese, Koko*	1 Serving/30g	60	5.6	199	0.4	7.6	18.7	0.9
Soft, Garlic & Herb, Free From, Asda*	1 Serving/15g	40	3.8	266	5.8	2.4	25	2.2

	Measure INFO/WEIGHT	per Measure KCAL	FAT	Nutrition Values per 100g / 100ml KCAL	PROT	CARB	FAT	FIBRE
CHEESE ALTERNATIVE								
Treenut, Organic, Nutcrafter Creamery*	1 Serving/30g	163	16.3	543	27.7	7.4	54.3	6.7
Vegetarian, Average	*1 Serving/30g*	*110*	*8.4*	*368*	*28.2*	*0*	*28.1*	*0*
CHEESE PUFFS								
Average	*1 Bag/25g*	*129*	*7.4*	*517*	*7.8*	*54.8*	*29.5*	*1.5*
Cheeky, Tesco*	1 Bag/20g	108	7	542	6.7	50.2	34.9	0
Morrisons*	1 Bag/25g	136	8.7	542	6.7	50.2	34.9	1.1
Sainsbury's*	1 Pack/100g	530	32	530	9.1	51.4	32	1.9
Shapers, Boots*	1 Bag/16g	80	3.8	500	7.1	64	24	0.9
Value, Tesco*	1 Pack/16g	84	4.6	525	6.2	60	28.8	0.6
CHEESE SINGLES								
Maasdamer, Hochland*	1 Slice/17g	58	4.7	345	28	1.8	28	0
Slices, Creamfields*	1 Slice/17g	47	3.7	278	12	7.6	22	0.6
CHEESE SPREAD								
Average	*1 Serving/30g*	*76*	*6.4*	*254*	*9.4*	*5.9*	*21.4*	*0.1*
Cheese & Ham, Primula*	1 Serving/20g	43	2.9	214	12.8	7.8	14.6	0
Dairylea, Light, Tub, Kraft*	1 Serving/30g	47	2.2	158	16.5	5.2	7.2	0
Dairylea, Tub, Kraft*	1 Serving/25g	60	4.9	240	11	5.3	19.5	0
with Chives, Primula*	1 Serving/30g	65	4.5	217	12.5	8.2	15	4.5
with Prawn, Primula*	1 Squeeze/25g	48	3.6	190	12.5	3.3	14.4	3.6
CHEESE STRAWS								
All Butter, Finest, Tesco*	1 Straw/13g	73	5.2	587	17.9	33.7	41.8	2.1
Cheddar, M&S*	1 Straw/11g	59	3.8	535	14.9	40.1	34.9	2.4
Cheese Twists, Tesco*	1 Twist/8g	40	2.1	507	13.8	52.1	26.4	2.8
Finest, Tesco*	1 Straw/7g	39	2.6	558	13.3	41.5	37.6	1.5
Homemade or Bakery, Average	*1 Straw/41g*	*173*	*12.6*	*422*	*12*	*24.2*	*30.7*	*0.7*
Selection, Sainsbury's*	1 Straw/7g	41	2.9	558	16.6	34.5	39.3	2.8
CHEESE TRIANGLES								
Average	*1 Triangle/14g*	*33*	*2.2*	*238*	*10.3*	*14.2*	*15.6*	*0.2*
Dairylea, Light, Kraft*	1 Triangle/16g	26	1.4	167	15	6.3	9	0.4
Light, Extra, The Laughing Cow, Fromageries Bel*	1 Triangle/18g	19	0.4	108	17	5.5	2	0
Light, with Blue Cheese, The Laughing Cow*	1 Triangle/16g	24	1.4	151	13	5.5	8.5	0
Lighter, Valley Spire, Lidl*	1 Triangle/17g	24	1.3	141	12	6	7.5	0.5
Reduced Fat, Average	*1 Triangle/18g*	*27*	*1.2*	*154*	*15.4*	*7*	*7*	*0*
Valley Spire, Lidl*	1 Triangle/17g	42	3.6	246	9	5	21	0.5
CHEESE TWISTS								
All Butter, M&S*	1 Pack/125g	625	33.4	500	14.2	50.2	26.7	3.2
Asda*	1 Twist/8g	42	2.4	500	14	48	28	5
Cheddar, Sainsbury's*	1 Twist/8g	43	2.3	513	12.9	51.6	27.8	2.6
Gruyere & Poppy Seed, Truly Irresistible, Co-Op*	1 Twist/8g	42	2.4	520	13.2	48.8	30.1	2.5
Gruyere & Poppy Seed, TTD, Sainsbury's*	1 Serving/8g	41	2.3	509	13.7	50.5	28	2.6
Gruyere, & Poppy Seed, All Butter, Waitrose*	1 Twist/8g	40	2.2	505	12.7	48.2	28	4.8
Parmesan, All Butter, TTD, Sainsbury's*	1 Serving/8g	38	2	487	13.8	51	25.3	2.8
Pre Packed, Average	*1 Twist/8g*	*41*	*2.2*	*515*	*13.7*	*47.9*	*27.7*	*2.3*
CHEESECAKE								
After Noon, Mango & Passionfruit, 3 Pack, Gu*	1 Portion/45g	155	11.3	345	3.4	26.5	25.2	0.4
American Red White & Blueberry, Sainsbury's*	1/6 Cake/83g	264	15.4	318	3.8	35.1	18.5	0.4
Apple, & Cinnamon, Baked, M&S*	1 Serving/116g	390	22	335	3.7	39.7	18.9	2.1
Average	*1 Slice/115g*	*490*	*40.8*	*426*	*3.7*	*24.6*	*35.5*	*0.4*
Berry, Autumn, Waitrose*	1 Slice/92g	316	20.3	343	4.4	31.5	22.1	2
Berry, Red, Waitrose*	1 Slice/101g	350	22.5	346	4.6	31.3	22.2	1.4
Blackcurrant, Average	*1 Serving/90g*	*237*	*11.9*	*263*	*3.6*	*32.3*	*13.2*	*2.4*
Blackcurrant, Healthy Range, Average	*1 Serving/90g*	*182*	*4.7*	*203*	*4.7*	*33.6*	*5.3*	*2.1*
Blackcurrant, Value, Tesco*	1 Serving/70g	174	8.6	248	2.8	31.4	12.3	1

CHEESECAKE

INFO/WEIGHT	Measure	per Measure		Nutrition Values per 100g / 100ml				
		KCAL	FAT	KCAL	PROT	CARB	FAT	FIBRE
Blackcurrant, Weight Watchers*	1 Cake/103g	191	2.9	185	4.6	35.4	2.8	3.5
Blueberry, & Lemon Flavour Wedges, Sainsbury's*	1 Serving/80g	262	16.9	327	5.1	29.2	21.1	1.2
Blueberry, & Vanilla, TTD, Sainsbury's*	1 Serving/95g	353	24.8	372	5.4	28.9	26.1	2.1
Blueberry, Gorgeous, Cooked, Aunt Bessie's*	1 Portion/75g	225	6.1	300	3.9	33.5	8.2	0.9
Caramel, Salted, Frozen, Tesco*	1 Serving/75g	241	10.6	321	6.5	41.5	14.1	0.9
Caramel, Salted, Mini, Iceland*	1 Cake/22g	85	4.7	380	3.2	44.5	20.9	0.6
Caramel, Swirl, Cadbury*	1 Slice/91g	373	23.5	410	6	40.1	25.8	0
Cherry, Healthy Range, Average	*1 Serving/90g*	*172*	*3*	*191*	*3.7*	*36.4*	*3.3*	*1.1*
Chocolate, & Hazlenut, Gold, Sara Lee*	1 Slice/65g	205	12.8	316	5.9	28.7	19.7	1.1
Chocolate, & Honeycomb, Slice, Sainsbury's*	1 Slice/98g	333	20.3	340	3.7	33.7	20.7	2.4
Chocolate, & Irish Cream Liqueur, Tesco*	1 Serving/93g	385	28	414	5	30.7	30.1	0.8
Chocolate, & Vanilla, Gu*	1 Pot/90g	379	27.1	421	4.1	34.6	30.1	1.6
Chocolate, & Vanilla, Reduced Fat, M&S*	1 Serving/114g	319	13.7	280	7	37.9	12	1.5
Chocolate, & Vanilla, Tesco*	1 Serving/90g	330	19.4	365	5.2	37.1	21.5	1.6
Chocolate, Average	*1 Serving/75g*	*265*	*15.7*	*353*	*5.7*	*35.6*	*20.9*	*1.9*
Chocolate, Belgian, M&S*	1 Slice/100g	385	23.9	385	5.3	39.2	23.9	2.5
Chocolate, Belgian, Milk, Specially Selected, Aldi*	1/6 Cake/93g	386	25.1	415	5.8	37	27	1.6
Chocolate, Belgian, Tesco*	1/6 Cake/90g	392	25.8	436	5.1	37.9	28.7	2.8
Chocolate, Double, Wedge, Sainsbury's*	1 Serving/75g	327	24.8	436	5.7	29	33	1.7
Chocolate, Orange, Aldi*	1/6 Pack/83g	262	16.6	316	4.4	29	20	1.1
Chocolate, Orange, Gu*	1 Pot/85g	295	21.4	347	3.7	25.7	25.2	1.3
Chocolate, Pure Indulgence, Thorntons*	1 Serving/75g	308	17.6	410	5.6	44.3	23.4	0.6
Chocolate, Slice, M&S*	1 Pack/100g	409	25.6	409	4.5	39.2	25.6	2.1
Citrus, Good Choice, Mini, Iceland*	1 Cake/111g	198	4.7	178	3.5	31.6	4.2	0.4
Dark Muscovado, Gail's*	1 Cheesecake	367	27	367	5.8	25	27	0.7
Fruit, Average	*1 Serving/75g*	*207*	*10.9*	*276*	*5.3*	*32.3*	*14.5*	*1.6*
Irish Cream, McVitie's*	¼ Slice/190g	616	36.9	324	4.4	33	19.4	0.4
Lemon, Asda*	1 Slice/90g	319	21.2	354	4.3	31.2	23.5	1.1
Lemon, Average	*1 Serving/90g*	*307*	*19.5*	*341*	*4.1*	*33*	*21.6*	*1.8*
Lemon, BGTY, Sainsbury's*	1/6 Cake/71g	142	2.7	200	4.4	37	3.8	0.5
Lemon, Creamy & Light, M&S*	1/6 Cake/68g	236	13.8	350	3.5	32.3	20.4	0.4
Lemon, Dessert, GF, Made Without Wheat, M&S*	1 Pot/100g	319	17.2	319	3.2	37.1	17.2	1.3
Lemon, Meringue, Tesco*	1 Slice/94g	352	25	375	3.8	30.1	26.6	0.3
Lemon, Sicilian, Slices, Finest, Tesco*	1 Slice/100g	351	21	351	3	36.8	21	1.2
Lemon, Sicillian, Oppo*	1 Cheesecake/75g	159	5.6	212	6.4	25	7.5	9.9
Lemon, Swirl, Asda*	1 Pack/125g	445	29.9	356	3.1	32.1	23.9	1.8
Lemon, Swirl, Individual, Sainsbury's*	1 Pot/125g	380	23	304	3	31.1	18.4	0.9
Lemon, Swirl, Ms Mollys*	1 Serving/75g	243	11.5	324	5.2	40.9	15.3	0.7
Lemon, Swirl, Sainsbury's*	1/6 Cake/95g	350	21	369	4.8	37.2	22.1	1
Lemon, Tesco*	1 Slice/93g	315	21	339	5.2	28.6	22.6	0.3
Lemon, Value, Tesco*	1 Serving/79g	221	11.8	281	4.3	32.2	15	4.2
Lemon, Zesty, M&S*	1/6 Cake/97g	325	18.9	335	4	38.7	19.5	2.6
Madagascan Vanilla, Slices, Finest, Tesco*	1 Slice/90g	367	23.4	408	5.4	37.9	26	0.3
Mandarin, Co-Op*	1 Slice/99g	297	16.8	300	4	32	17	0.3
Mandarin, Morrisons*	1 Serving/135g	335	16.9	248	3.8	32.2	12.5	0.8
Mango, & Passion Fruit, Baked, Weight Watchers, Heinz*	1 Dessert/85g	159	1.9	187	4.2	36.9	2.2	1
Millionaires, Pot, Tesco*	1 Pot/100g	274	14	274	3.8	32.9	14	0.6
Millionaires, Toffee & Chocolate, Thorntons*	1 Serving/94g	351	20.1	373	4.7	40	21.4	1
Mulled Wine, 428, Oakhouse Foods Ltd*	1 Cake/95g	316	16.6	333	4.3	39.4	17.5	1
New York, Baked, Waitrose*	1/12 Cake/83g	317	22.6	380	5.1	28.3	27.1	1.2
New York, Mini, Iceland*	1 Cake/22g	86	5.1	385	3.6	40.7	23	0.5
Raspberry, & Mascarpone, Best, Morrisons*	1 Cake/84g	257	14	306	3.9	34.8	16.7	1
Raspberry, & Strawberry, M&S*	1 Slice/105g	340	21.1	325	3.9	33.4	20.2	1.2

	Measure INFO/WEIGHT	per Measure KCAL	FAT	Nutrition Values per 100g / 100ml KCAL	PROT	CARB	FAT	FIBRE
CHEESECAKE								
Raspberry, & Vanilla, Slices, M&S*	1 Slice/100g	300	17.5	300	4.4	30.4	17.5	1.7
Raspberry, BGTY, Sainsbury's*	1 Pot/95g	154	2.5	163	6.6	28.2	2.6	2.8
Raspberry, Rapture, Slices, Tesco*	1 Slice/110g	341	20.4	310	4.2	30.8	18.5	1.8
Raspberry, Ripple, Sainsbury's*	1 Portion/95g	355	21.8	373	4.5	37	22.9	0.9
Rhubarb, Crumble, Sainsbury's*	1 Serving/114g	268	10.6	235	3.1	34.8	9.3	2.4
Rocky Road, Aldi*	1 Serving/75g	240	9.8	320	6.6	44	13	0.7
Rocky Road, CBY, Asda*	1 Serving/75g	302	17.3	402	4.5	43.4	23.1	1.4
Strawberry, & Cream, Finest, Tesco*	1 Serving/104g	325	22.4	312	4.3	25.3	21.5	0.5
Strawberry, & Rhubarb, Slice, M&S*	1 Pack/100g	377	23.8	377	4.3	35.7	23.8	1.3
Strawberry, Devonshire, McVitie's*	1/6 Cake/66g	192	10.7	291	4.4	31.8	16.2	3.6
Strawberry, Finest, Tesco*	1 Slice/113g	383	25.1	339	4.8	30.1	22.2	0.9
Strawberry, Free From, Tesco*	1 Serving/77g	228	12.1	296	1.6	36.4	15.7	1.3
Strawberry, Frozen, Sainsbury's*	1/6 Cake/84g	277	14.2	332	4.3	40.4	17	2.3
Strawberry, Shortcake, Sara Lee*	1/6 Slice/68g	230	15.7	337	4.9	27.6	23	0.5
Toffee, & Pecan, Wedge, Sainsbury's*	1 Serving/75g	296	21.8	395	5.4	28.1	29	3.1
Toffee, Lidl*	1 Pot/100g	275	12.3	275	3	37.6	12.3	1
Toffee, M&S*	1 Serving/105g	357	22.6	340	5.2	37.2	21.5	0.9
Toffee, Mini, Asda*	1 Cake/20g	57	2.4	286	4.6	40	12	2.1
Toffee, Tesco*	1 Serving/100g	265	12.9	265	4.3	33.1	12.9	0.8
Vanilla	*1 Serving/100g*	*395*	*26.2*	*395*	*5.3*	*42.8*	*26.2*	*1.1*
Vanilla, & Berry, Weight Watchers*	1 Dessert/85g	156	3	184	3.6	34	3.5	1.8
Vanilla, Creamy, New York, Slices, Tesco*	1 Slice/90g	314	21.4	349	5.1	28.3	23.7	0.8
Vanilla, Madagascan, Finest, Tesco*	1 Serving/90g	319	19	354	5.7	35.1	21.1	0.7
Vanilla, Madagascan, Oppo*	1 Pot/75g	159	5.6	212	6.4	24	7.5	0
Vanilla, New York, Slices, M&S*	1 Slice/105g	361	23.6	344	4.5	30.1	22.5	1.5
Vanilla, Tesco*	1 Serving/115g	417	28.4	363	5.7	29.4	24.7	0.6
White Chocolate, & Mixed Berry, Finest, Tesco*	1 Serving/70g	246	13.7	353	4.5	38.9	19.6	1.3
Zillionaires, Gu*	1 Pot/92g	362	22	396	3.6	42	24	1.3
CHERRIES								
Black in Syrup, Average	*1 Serving/242g*	*160*	*0*	*66*	*0.6*	*16*	*0*	*0.7*
Black, Fresh, Average	*1 Serving/80g*	*41*	*0.1*	*51*	*0.9*	*11.5*	*0.1*	*1.6*
Black, in Kirsch, Drained, Opies*	1 Jar/250g	155	0.5	62	0.5	15	0.2	1.1
Dark, Sweet, Frozen, Aldi*	1 Serving/80g	53	0.4	66	1.1	14	0.5	2.1
Dark, Sweet, Pitted, Frozen, Essential, Waitrose*	1 Serving/80g	44	0.1	55	0.9	11.5	0.1	2.1
Dried, Wholefoods, Tesco*	1 Serving/25g	86	0.2	345	1.9	81.6	0.8	4.6
Glace, Average	*1oz/28g*	*79*	*0*	*280*	*0.4*	*71.2*	*0.2*	*1.1*
Picota, Average	*1 Serving/80g*	*42*	*0.1*	*52*	*0.9*	*11.4*	*0.1*	*1.2*
Pitted, Dark, Sweet, Frozen, Tesco*	1 Serving/80g	53	0.2	66	1.1	13.9	0.2	2.1
Raw, Average	*1oz/28g*	*14*	*0*	*49*	*0.9*	*11.2*	*0.1*	*1.4*
Stewed without Sugar, Average	*1oz/28g*	*12*	*0*	*42*	*0.8*	*10.1*	*0.1*	*0.8*
Sweet & Juicy, Good Health, Waitrose*	½ Pack/90g	43	0.1	48	0.5	11.5	0.1	0.9
CHERRYADE								
Barr's*	1 Serving/200ml	32	0	16	0	4	0	0
Sugar Free, Tesco*	1 Glass/200ml	2	0	1	0	0	0	0
CHESTNUTS								
Average	*1 Serving/100g*	*174*	*2.3*	*174*	*2.9*	*31*	*2.3*	*8.9*
Candied, Marrons Glace, Wholefoods Online*	1 Piece/20g	65	0.2	325	0.8	76.4	0.8	4.8
Roasted, Peeled, Average	*1 Nut/10g*	*17*	*0.3*	*170*	*2*	*36.6*	*2.7*	*4.1*
CHEWING GUM								
Airwaves, Sugar Free, Wrigleys*	1 Pack/15g	23	0	155	0	62	0	0
Doublemint, Wrigleys*	1 Stick/3g	10	0	370	0	74.1	0	0
Extra, Cool Breeze, Wrigleys*	1 Piece/2g	3	0	153	0	64	0	0
Extra, Peppermint, Sugar Free, Wrigleys*	1 Piece/2g	3	0	155	0	39	0	0

	INFO/WEIGHT	KCAL	FAT	KCAL	PROT	CARB	FAT	FIBRE
CHEWING GUM								
Peppermint, Sugar Free, Active, Aldi*	2 Pieces/3g	4	0	146	0	61	0	0
Spearmint, Extra, Wrigleys*	1 Piece/1g	1	0	143	0	64.3	0	0
Spearmint, Wrigleys*	1 Piece/3g	9	0	295	0	73	0	0
CHICK PEAS								
Canned, Drained, Average	*1 Can/240g*	*276*	*6*	*115*	*7.4*	*15.2*	*2.5*	*4.6*
Canned, in Salted Water, Drained, East End*	½ Can/120g	86	1.6	72	4.3	8.6	1.3	4.5
Canned, in Water, Drained, Four Seasons, Aldi*	½ Can/120g	131	2.4	109	6.2	14	2	5
Canned, in Water, Drained, Morrisons*	1 Can/180g	218	4.9	121	6.4	13.6	2.7	8.1
Chocolate, Mix, Super Snacks, The Food Doctor*	1 Serving/30g	148	9.5	494	17.3	35.5	31.7	14.7
Curried, Worldwide Foods, Aldi*	½ Pack/125g	172	4.8	138	7.3	15	3.8	6.5
Dried, Average	*1 Serving/100g*	*319*	*5.4*	*319*	*21.7*	*47.4*	*5.4*	*8*
Dried, Boiled, Average	*1 Serving/75g*	*85*	*1.7*	*114*	*7.3*	*16.4*	*2.2*	*2.6*
in Salted Water, Canned, Average	*1 Can/179g*	*204*	*5.2*	*114*	*7.2*	*14.9*	*2.9*	*4.1*
in Water, Canned, Average	*1 Can/250g*	*282*	*6.6*	*113*	*7.2*	*15.3*	*2.6*	*4.8*
in Water, Drained, So Organic, Sainsbury's*	½ Pack/115g	130	2.6	113	6.7	12.2	2.3	8.6
Organic, Lidl*	1 Serving/130g	110	1.3	85	5.2	11.7	1	0
Spiced, & Houmous, Tesco*	1 Pack/140g	202	8	144	6.3	14	5.7	5.6
CHICKEN								
Bites, Breaded, Sainsbury's*	1 Bite/22g	63	3.6	288	15.5	18.9	16.4	1.1
Bites, Finest Quality, Delicatessen*	3 Bites/50g	114	8	227	13	7.3	16	0
Bites, Flame Seared, with Sweetcorn Salsa, Waitrose*	½ Pack/70g	118	4.8	169	13.5	12.4	6.8	2.2
Bites, Hot & Spicy, Tesco*	1 Pack/110g	143	1.8	130	18.9	9.6	1.6	2.5
Bites, Slow Roasted, Mini, Fridge Raiders, Mattessons*	1 Mini Bag/23g	43	2.2	190	21	3.2	10	0
Bites, Southern Fried, Fridge Raiders, Mattessons*	1 Bag/60g	133	8.4	221	19	4.2	14	0.8
Bites, Southern Fried, Tesco*	4 Bites/38g	93	5.2	247	17.8	11.9	13.8	1.9
Bites, Southern Style, Mini, Fridge Raiders, Mattessons*	1 Pack/23g	37	2.1	166	17	4.2	9.2	0
Bites, Tikka, Average	*1 Serving/50g*	*96*	*5.3*	*193*	*20.7*	*3.8*	*10.5*	*1.9*
Breast, BBQ, Slices, Iceland*	1 Serving/50g	78	1.4	156	28.3	4.3	2.8	0.3
Breast, Cajun Spiced, Slices, Deluxe, Lidl*	1 Slice/24g	28	0.5	117	24	0.5	2	0.5
Breast, Chargrilled, Premium, Average	*1 Piece/10g*	*13*	*0.3*	*134*	*25.9*	*0.6*	*2.6*	*0.3*
Breast, Chargrilled, Sliced, Average	*1 Slice/19g*	*24*	*0.5*	*124*	*24.4*	*0.5*	*2.7*	*0.4*
Breast, Cheese & Bacon Wrapped, Iceland*	½ Pack/158g	291	19.4	184	16.6	1.2	12.3	0.9
Breast, Coconut, Mango, & Chilli, Sizzlers, Sainsbury's*	½ Pack/121g	181	5	149	25.9	1.8	4.1	0.5
Breast, Cooked, Classic, Slices, Asda*	1 Serving/50g	64	0.7	127	27	1	1.4	0.6
Breast, Cooked, Sliced, Ready to Eat, Asda*	½ Pack/70g	85	1	122	27	0	1.4	0
Breast, Diced, Average	*1 Serving/188g*	*242*	*4.4*	*129*	*26.9*	*0.1*	*2.4*	*0.1*
Breast, Fillet, Lean, Large, Raw, Musclefood*	1 Breast/200g	194	0.8	97	22	0	0.4	0
Breast, Fillet, Mozzarella, & Prosciutto, Tesco*	1 Pack/196g	259	10	132	20	1.6	5.1	0.1
Breast, Fillet, Pesto Breaded, Finest, Tesco*	½ Pack/151g	293	10.9	194	21.5	10.5	7.2	0.5
Breast, Fillet, Wiltshire Ham & Leek Crumb, Morrisons*	½ Pack/178g	289	11.8	162	21.3	4.1	6.6	0.7
Breast, Fillets, Breaded, Average	*1 Fillet/112g*	*246*	*11.6*	*220*	*17.6*	*14*	*10.4*	*1.3*
Breast, Fillets, Cajun, Average	*1 Fillet/93g*	*124*	*2.6*	*134*	*23.6*	*3.5*	*2.8*	*0.3*
Breast, Fillets, Chargrilled, Average	*1 Serving/100g*	*120*	*1.1*	*120*	*27.3*	*0.3*	*1.1*	*0.3*
Breast, Fillets, Korma Style, Average	*1 Serving/100g*	*132*	*2.8*	*132*	*27.4*	*0.8*	*2.8*	*0.6*
Breast, Fillets, Mini, Raw, Average	*1oz/28g*	*34*	*0.4*	*121*	*26.9*	*0.2*	*1.5*	*0.1*
Breast, Fillets, Organic, Average	*1 Serving/150g*	*153*	*1.1*	*102*	*24*	*0*	*0.8*	*0*
Breast, Fillets, Skinless & Boneless, Raw, Average	*1 Breast/100g*	*129*	*2*	*129*	*27.7*	*0*	*2*	*0*
Breast, Fillets, Southern Fried, Ovenbaked, Asda*	1 Fillet/87g	206	8.3	236	20	17	9.5	1.6
Breast, Fillets, Sweet Chilli, Tesco*	½ Pack/144g	219	3.7	152	22	10.1	2.6	0.4
Breast, Fillets, with Cheese, & Bacon, Morrisons*	½ Pack/166g	335	17.1	202	24.9	2.4	10.3	0
Breast, Flame Grilled, Slices, Iceland*	1 Pack/200g	258	2.6	129	29.2	0.1	1.3	0.1
Breast, Grilled, Average	*1 Breast/130g*	*174*	*2.8*	*134*	*29*	*0.1*	*2.2*	*0*
Breast, in Breadcrumbs, GF, Sainsbury's*	1 Fillet/150g	294	12.6	196	18	11.5	8.4	1.3

C

CHICKEN

	Measure INFO/WEIGHT	per Measure KCAL	FAT	Nutrition Values per 100g / 100ml KCAL	PROT	CARB	FAT	FIBRE
Breast, Joint, & Stuffing, Tesco*	1 Serving/128g	197	11.4	154	13.1	5	8.9	0.7
Breast, Meat & Skin, Raw, Average	*1 Serving/145g*	*249*	*13.4*	*172*	*20.8*	*0*	*9.2*	*0*
Breast, Meat & Skin, Weighed with Bone, Raw, Average	*1oz/28g*	*39*	*2.1*	*138*	*16.7*	*0*	*7.4*	*0*
Breast, Meat Only, Fried	*1 Serving/50g*	*68*	*1.7*	*137*	*24.4*	*0.4*	*3.4*	*0*
Breast, Mexican Nacho Crumb, Birds Eye*	1 Grill/90g	198	9.9	221	13	17	11	0.9
Breast, Nacho Toppers, Iceland*	1 Topper/96g	199	9.9	208	12.8	15.1	10.3	1.7
Breast, on a Stick, Chinese Marinated, Musclefood*	1 Pack/75g	93	1	124	21.9	5.9	1.3	0.5
Breast, On a Stick, Spicy Marinated, Musclefood*	1 Stick/75g	80	7.3	107	21.5	2.7	9.8	7.5
Breast, Pieces, BBQ, Sainsbury's*	½ Pack/70g	93	0.8	132	23.8	6.3	1.2	0.5
Breast, Pieces, Tikka, Average	*1 Serving/100g*	*154*	*3.4*	*154*	*28.2*	*2.8*	*3.4*	*0.4*
Breast, Piri Piri, Fillets, Cooked as per Instructions, Tesco*	1 Breast/141g	251	9.4	178	28.8	0.5	6.7	0.1
Breast, Piri Piri, Pieces, Cooked, Ready to Eat, Tesco*	1 Serving/90g	117	2.2	130	24	2.8	2.4	0.6
Breast, Roast, Sliced, From Supermarket, Average	*1 Slice/13g*	*17*	*0.4*	*139*	*25*	*1.8*	*3.5*	*0.2*
Breast, Roast, without Skin, Average	*1oz/28g*	*41*	*1.3*	*146*	*24.8*	*1*	*4.6*	*0.2*
Breast, Smoked, Sliced, Average	*1 Slice/20g*	*22*	*0.5*	*110*	*20.7*	*0.9*	*2.6*	*0.1*
Breast, Strips, Raw, Average	*1 Serving/280g*	*358*	*5.7*	*128*	*27.1*	*0.4*	*2*	*0.3*
Breast, Sweet Chilli, & Lime, Slices, Warren & Sons, Lidl*	1 Serving/90g	130	3.2	144	25.6	2	3.6	0.5
Breast, Tandoori Style, Average	*1 Serving/180g*	*237*	*6.8*	*132*	*22.3*	*2.3*	*3.8*	*1*
Breast, Tenderloins, Air Chilled, Harvestland, Perdue*	1 Tenderloin/28g	27	0.2	98	22.3	0	0.9	0
Breast, Tikka, Chunks, Ready to Eat, Sainsbury's*	½ Pack/125g	171	2.7	137	26.7	2.4	2.2	0.5
Breast, Tikka, Sliced, Average	*1oz/28g*	*34*	*0.5*	*120*	*24.9*	*2*	*1.7*	*0.6*
Breast, with Pork, & Sage Stuffing, Slices, Finest, Tesco*	1 Slice/31g	43	1	138	25	1.9	3.2	0.6
Breton, for Two, Charlie Bigham's*	1 Serving/300 g	465	32.7	155	12.9	1.4	10.9	0
Butter Basted, TTD, Sainsbury's*	1 Slice/30g	44	1.9	147	22.8	0	6.2	0.6
Cajun Style, Slices, Co-Op*	½ Pack/85g	116	2	137	28	0.6	2.4	0.5
Chargrill, Sweet & Sticky, As Sold, Birds Eye*	1 Grill/88g	148	7.2	168	17	6.6	8.2	0.5
Chunks, No Chic'n, Plant Kitchen, M&S*	½ Pack/90g	86	0.6	95	18.9	1	0.7	6.4
Curried, Coconut, & Lime, Slices, Ashfield Farm, Aldi*	1 Pack/180g	202	4.3	112	21	0.8	2.4	1.3
Dippers, Battered, Aldi*	6 Dippers/99g	264	15.8	267	12	17	16	1.9
Dippers, Battered, Tesco*	4 Dippers/78g	222	14	285	13.1	17.4	17.9	0.8
Dippers, Crispy, Average	*5 Dippers/93g*	*231*	*14.3*	*249*	*13.2*	*14.4*	*15.4*	*0.6*
Dippers, Crispy, Iceland*	5 Dippers/75g	160	7.9	214	16.8	12.4	10.5	1
Drums, & Thighs, Southern Fried, Sainsbury's*	1/5 Pack/138g	322	17	233	18.8	11.2	12.3	1.2
Drumsticks, BBQ Flavour, Average	*1 Serving/200g*	*348*	*16*	*174*	*22.6*	*3.1*	*8*	*0.4*
Drumsticks, Breaded, Fried, Average	*1oz/28g*	*66*	*3.9*	*237*	*18.7*	*9.4*	*13.9*	*0.6*
Drumsticks, Chinese Style, Average	*1 Serving/100g*	*178*	*8.1*	*178*	*22.6*	*3.6*	*8.1*	*0.7*
Drumsticks, Meat & Skin, Weighed with Bone, Raw	*1 Serving/133g*	*188*	*11*	*141*	*15.7*	*0.1*	*8.3*	*0*
Drumsticks, Meat Only, Boneless, Raw, Average	*1 Serving/100g*	*106*	*3.3*	*106*	*19.2*	*0*	*3.3*	*0*
Drumsticks, Meat Only, Weighed with Bone, Raw	*1 Serving/122g*	*159*	*9.3*	*130*	*14.4*	*0.1*	*7.6*	*0*
Drumsticks, Meat Only, Weighed with Bone, Roast	*1 Serving/100g*	*116*	*5.5*	*116*	*16*	*0.3*	*5.5*	*0.1*
Drumsticks, Pulled, Tandoori, Sainsbury's*	½ Pack/115g	202	8.4	175	22.3	4.9	7.3	0.5
Drumsticks, with Skin, Average	*1 Piece/125g*	*268*	*16.6*	*215*	*22.1*	*1.8*	*13.3*	*0.3*
Escalope, Breaded, Average	*1 Escalope/128g*	*361*	*21.6*	*282*	*13.4*	*19.1*	*16.9*	*0.7*
Escalope, Plain, Breast, Average	*1 Serving/100g*	*110*	*2.2*	*110*	*22.3*	*0.7*	*2.2*	*0.5*
Fillets, Battered, Average	*1 Fillet/90g*	*199*	*10.4*	*221*	*16.1*	*13.3*	*11.5*	*0.5*
Fillets, Breaded, Average	*1 Piece/98g*	*214*	*10.5*	*219*	*14.2*	*15.9*	*10.7*	*1.9*
Fillets, Cajun, Ashfield Farm, Aldi*	1 Fillet/122g	161	3.3	132	26	0.7	2.7	0.5
Fillets, Chargrilled, Spicy, 5 Pack, Fridge Filler, Taste Inc*	1 Fillet/35g	51	1.4	147	24.6	3	4	0
Fillets, Chinese Style, Average	*1oz/28g*	*37*	*0.5*	*132*	*24.4*	*4.6*	*1.8*	*0.5*
Fillets, Crispy, Mini, SFC*	1 Serving/100g	179	7.6	179	15	13	7.6	0
Fillets, Hickory Smoked, in Sweet Smoky Marinade, M&S*	1 Pack/120g	140	0.5	117	25.5	2.9	0.4	0
Fillets, Honey & Mustard, Average	*1 Serving/100g*	*138*	*3.7*	*138*	*18.4*	*7.5*	*3.7*	*0.8*
Fillets, Hot & Spicy, Average	*1oz/28g*	*58*	*3.1*	*206*	*16.4*	*10.5*	*11*	*1.1*

C

CHICKEN

	Measure INFO/WEIGHT	KCAL	FAT	KCAL	PROT	CARB	FAT	FIBRE
Fillets, in Tempura Batter, Crispy, Birds Eye*	1 Fillet/89g	229	12.5	257	13	19	14	1.4
Fillets, Mini, Mango, Coconut, & Lime, Tesco*	½ Pack/150g	230	2.8	153	26	7.9	1.9	0
Fillets, Mini, Sweet & Smokey, Eat Well, M&S*	½ Pack/60g	70	0.2	117	25.5	2.9	0.4	0.1
Fillets, No Chick, Crispy, Iceland*	1 Fillet/80g	158	7.5	198	17	10	9.4	3.1
Fillets, Red Thai, Mini, Average	*1oz/28g*	*36*	*0.6*	*128*	*21.7*	*5.4*	*2*	*0.6*
Fillets, Southern Fried, Meat Only, Average	*1 Piece/100g*	*222*	*12*	*222*	*16.4*	*12.2*	*12*	*1.1*
Fillets, Tandoori Style, Mini, Average	*1 Serving/100g*	*128*	*2*	*128*	*24.7*	*2.6*	*2*	*0.4*
Fillets, Tikka, Average	*1 Serving/100g*	*141*	*5*	*141*	*22.4*	*1.7*	*5*	*1.1*
Fillets, Tikka, Mini, Average	*1oz/28g*	*35*	*0.6*	*124*	*25.1*	*1.3*	*2.2*	*1.2*
Fingers, Average	*1 Serving/75g*	*188*	*9.9*	*250*	*13.7*	*18.8*	*13.2*	*1.2*
Firecracker, & Fragrant Rice, G&B, Asda*	1 Pack/353g	364	4.2	103	6.1	16	1.2	1
Garlic & Herb, Flatties, The Grill, M&S*	1 Flattie/90g	106	2.2	118	20.8	2.4	2.5	1.1
Goujons, Breaded, Average	*1 Serving/114g*	*293*	*17.1*	*258*	*15.8*	*15.2*	*15*	*1*
Goujons, Breast, Fresh, Average	*1oz/28g*	*36*	*0.5*	*127*	*28*	*0*	*1.6*	*0*
Goujons, Chipotle, Meat Free, Quorn*	1 Serving/83g	156	3.6	188	12.2	20.7	4.3	8.9
Goujons, Southern Fried, Coopers, Lidl*	3 Pieces/68g	187	9.5	275	18	19	14	0.7
Half, Mexican, Co-Op*	½ Pack/280g	350	14.8	125	16	3	5.3	0.4
Hunters, & Potato Wedges, COU, M&S*	1 Pack/360g	299	3.6	83	9.3	8.3	1	1.6
Hunters, Classic, with Potato Wedges, Iceland*	1 Pack/401g	570	14.9	142	8.4	17.6	3.7	2.3
Leg or Thigh, Hot & Spicy, Average	*1oz/28g*	*50*	*3*	*179*	*19.4*	*1*	*10.8*	*0.4*
Leg Portion, Roast, weighed with Bone, without Skin	*1 Portion/114g*	*175*	*11*	*153*	*30.9*	*0*	*9.6*	*0*
Leg Portion, Roasted Dry, with Skin, without Bone	*1 Portion/120g*	*188*	*11.8*	*156*	*16.7*	*0.2*	*9.8*	*0.2*
Leg, Meat Only, Cooked, Stewed, Average	*1 Serving/60g*	*111*	*4.8*	*185*	*26*	*0*	*8*	*0*
Leg, Meat Only, Raw, Average	*1oz/28g*	*34*	*1.1*	*120*	*20.1*	*0*	*3.8*	*0*
Leg, Meat Only, Raw, Weighed with Skin & Bone	*1oz/28g*	*21*	*0.7*	*76*	*12.8*	*0*	*2.4*	*0*
Leg, Meat Only, Stewed with Bone & Skin, Average	*1oz/28g*	*31*	*1.4*	*111*	*15.8*	*0*	*4.8*	*0*
Leg, with Skin, Raw, Average	*1 Serving/250g*	*430*	*26*	*172*	*19.1*	*0*	*10.4*	*0*
Leg, with Skin, Roasted, Weighed with Bone, Average	*1oz/28g*	*47*	*3.3*	*166*	*15.3*	*0.1*	*11.6*	*0*
Lemon, & Cumin, M&S*	1 Serving/320g	426	25.6	133	7.6	6.9	8	1.7
Light Meat, Roasted	*1oz/28g*	*43*	*1*	*153*	*30.2*	*0*	*3.6*	*0*
Meat & Skin Portions, Deep Fried, Average	*1oz/28g*	*73*	*4.7*	*259*	*26.9*	*0*	*16.8*	*0*
Meat & Skin, Roasted, Average	*1oz/28g*	*60*	*3.9*	*216*	*22.6*	*0*	*14*	*0*
Meat, Roasted, Average	*1oz/28g*	*47*	*1.9*	*167*	*25*	*0*	*6.6*	*0*
Mexican Chilli, Sliced, Eat Well, M&S*	1 Pack/130g	169	3.4	130	25.9	0.8	2.6	0.5
Mexican, Tray Bake, Tesco*	½ Pack/179g	315	14	176	16.7	9.1	7.8	1.2
Mince, Average	*1oz/28g*	*39*	*1.7*	*140*	*20.9*	*0.1*	*6*	*0.2*
Moroccan, with Jewelled Bulgur Wheat, Charlie Bigham's*	1 Serving/400 g	592	17.2	148	8.3	20.9	4.3	0
Nuggets, Battered, Average	*1 Nugget/20g*	*50*	*2.9*	*251*	*13.5*	*16.9*	*14.4*	*0.9*
Nuggets, Breaded, Average	*1 Nugget/14g*	*37*	*2*	*263*	*14.8*	*19.8*	*13.8*	*1.9*
Nuggets, Free From Gluten & Wheat, Sainsbury's*	1 Nugget/19g	47	2.5	251	13.4	19.7	13.2	0.8
Nuggets, Meat Free, Crispy, Quorn*	4 Nuggets/80g	129	3.4	161	10.3	15.8	4.2	9.6
Parmigiana, Finest, Tesco*	½ Pack/225g	326	14.8	145	17	3.7	6.6	1.3
Parmigiana, Tomato & Basil Sauce, Waitrose*	½ Pack/177g	257	11.9	145	16.2	4.6	6.7	0.8
Pieces, Boneless, Breaded, Fried, From Restaurant	*1 Piece/17g*	*51*	*3.3*	*301*	*17*	*14.4*	*19.4*	*0*
Poppers, Ready to Eat, Tesco*	1 Popper/10g	27	1.6	273	11.5	19.9	16.2	0.7
Poppets, Boneless Bucket, SFC*	1 Box/190g	426	21.8	224	15.4	16.2	11.5	1.6
Pops, Breaded, Oven Baked, Sainsbury's*	½ Pack/133g	352	17.2	265	18.4	18	12.9	1.4
Pulled, Vegetarian, Linda McCartney*	1 Pack/300g	534	22.2	178	22.6	3.8	7.4	2.8
Roll, Breast, Average	*1 Slice/10g*	*17*	*1*	*167*	*16.1*	*3.2*	*10*	*0.2*
Schnitzel, As Prepared, Easy to Cook, Waitrose*	½ Pack/99g	168	5.4	170	27	2.4	5.5	1.3
Schnitzel, Breaded, GF, Rosie & Jim *	1 Schnitzel/104g	235	11	226	16.8	15.8	10.6	0
Shredded, in Lite Mayo, Canned, Chop Chop*	1 Can/85g	138	6.6	162	19.5	3.3	7.8	0
Shredded, in Mustard Mayonnaise, Canned, Chop Chop*	1 Can/85g	130	6.4	153	16.7	4.3	7.5	0

CHICKEN

Measure INFO/WEIGHT		per Measure		Nutrition Values per 100g / 100ml				
		KCAL	FAT	KCAL	PROT	CARB	FAT	FIBRE
Shredded, Sweet Chilli, Canned, Chop Chop*	1 Can/85g	128	3.4	151	16.4	11.9	4	0
Shredded, Teriyaki, Canned, Chop Chop*	1 Can/85g	104	2	122	16.3	8.6	2.3	0
Sizzlers, Mediterranean, Ashfield Farm, Aldi*	1 Pack/300g	501	19.2	167	27	0.6	6.4	0.5
Sizzlers, Sweet Chilli, Ashfield Farm, Aldi*	¼ Pack/59g	94	2.8	159	27	2.4	4.7	0.5
Skewers, Marinated, Asda*	1 Skewer/35g	50	0.4	142	24.9	8	1.2	0.9
Skewers, Mini, Morrisons*	2 Skewers/20g	51	3.3	255	18.5	7	16.7	1.1
Skewers, Satay, Iceland*	1 Skewer/16g	30	1.2	187	20.3	8.9	7.7	0.3
Skewers, Satay, Waitrose*	½ Pack/80g	138	6.4	172	19.3	5.2	8	1.2
Skewers, Smoky BBQ, Fridge Raiders, Mattessons*	1 Pack/50g	58	0.7	116	23	2.3	1.4	0
Skewers, Sticky, with Sesame Seeds, Iceland*	1 Skewer/22g	33	0.1	152	21.7	14.4	0.5	1.4
Skewers, Yakitori, M&S*	1 Box/65g	125	4.5	192	20.9	11.2	6.9	0.6
Skin, Dry, Roasted or Grilled, Average	*1 Serving/100g*	*501*	*46.1*	*501*	*21.5*	*0*	*46.1*	*0*
Skin, Moist, Roasted or Grilled, Average	*1 Serving/100g*	*452*	*42.6*	*452*	*17*	*0*	*42.6*	*0*
Sliced, Cooked, Average	*1 Slice/15g*	*18*	*0.4*	*118*	*22.4*	*1.6*	*2.4*	*0.1*
Slices, Lemon, Garlic, & Herb, Morrisons*	¼ Pack/50g	66	0.6	132	25.1	4.4	1.3	1
Southern Fried, Popstars, Birds Eye*	¼ Pack/100g	272	14	272	17	19	14	1.1
Spatchcock, Garlic & Herb, No Bone, Raw, Co-Op*	¼ Pack/204g	336	18.5	165	18	2.3	9.1	0.7
Spatchcock, Piri Piri, Cooked as per Instructions, Tesco*	¼ Pack/178g	329	17.4	185	23.1	1	9.8	0.1
Spatchcock, Poussin, Sainsbury's*	1 Serving/122g	168	6.6	138	21.1	0.1	5.4	0.2
Steak, Breast, Cajun, The Butchers , Morrisons*	½ Pack/176g	260	3.9	148	30.4	0.9	2.2	1.3
Steaks, Average	*1 Serving/100g*	*205*	*9.4*	*205*	*21.1*	*9*	*9.4*	*0.7*
Steaks, Breaded, Co-Op*	1 Steak/125g	309	20	247	16	9.6	16	1.5
Steaks, Breaded, Garlic, Tesco*	1 Steak/84g	234	14.5	278	14.4	15.3	17.3	1.5
Steaks, Breaded, Morrisons*	1 Steak/112g	318	18.7	284	15.6	16.9	16.7	1.7
Steaks, Mango, & Coconut, Waitrose*	1 Steak/47g	81	1.6	172	31	4.1	3.5	0.5
Strips, Mexican, Sliced, M&S*	½ Pack/70g	77	0.4	110	24.3	2.3	0.6	0.5
Strips, No Chick, Iceland*	½ Pack/160g	200	5	125	19	0.8	3.1	7.4
Stuffing, TTD, Sainsbury's*	1 Slice/34g	41	1	122	22.3	1.3	3	0.5
Style, Nuggets, No Chic'n, Plant Kitchen, M&S*	½ Pack/80g	176	9.3	220	12.5	12.1	11.6	8.4
Sweet & Sour, with Egg Fried Rice, Charlie Bigham's*	1 Serving/404 g	573	16.5	142	8.1	19	4.1	0
Sweet & Sour, with Rice, Lean Cuisine*	1 Serving	300	3	300	16	51	3	2
Tenders, Southern Style, Vegan, Fry's*	1 Tender/19g	36	2.1	186	11.3	5.2	11	10.5
Thigh, Meat & Skin, Casseroled, Average	*1oz/28g*	*65*	*4.6*	*233*	*21.5*	*0*	*16.3*	*0*
Thigh, Meat & Skin, Raw, Average	*1 Serving/100g*	*218*	*14.7*	*218*	*21.4*	*0*	*14.7*	*0*
Thigh, Meat & Skin, Weighed with Bone, Raw, Average	*1 Serving/100g*	*186*	*14.1*	*186*	*13.8*	*0.2*	*14.1*	*0*
Thigh, Meat Only, Diced, Casseroled	*1oz/28g*	*50*	*2.4*	*180*	*25.6*	*0*	*8.6*	*0*
Thigh, Meat Only, Raw, Average	*1 Thigh/90g*	*113*	*4.9*	*126*	*19.4*	*0*	*5.4*	*0*
Thigh, Roast, Average	*1 Serving/100g*	*238*	*15.6*	*238*	*23.8*	*0.4*	*15.6*	*0*
Thighs, & Drumsticks, BBQ, Roast in Bag, Sainsbury's*	½ Pack/140g	299	14.3	214	26.8	3.6	10.2	0.5
Thighs, & Drumsticks, Southern Fried, M&S*	1 Serving.100g	220	12.7	220	13.7	11.8	12.7	1.9
Tikka, & Mint Raita Dip, Tesco*	1 Pack/90g	171	9.4	190	19.8	3.9	10.4	0.9
Tray Bake, Italian Inspired, Tesco*	½ Pack/168g	220	5.2	131	21.3	4.3	3.1	0.2
Vegan, Slices, Deli Style, Quorn*	½ Pack/50g	47	1.2	94	11	4.1	2.3	6.2
Vegetarian, Chicken Style Pieces, Vivera*	1 Pack/175g	208	0.9	119	19.4	6.4	0.5	0
Vegetarian, Chicken Style, Strips, Meat Free, Fry's*	1 Serving/95g	226	12.3	238	20.4	10	13	5.6
Vegetarian, Dippers, Quorn*	4 Dippers/92g	195	8	212	11.1	21.2	8.7	2.4
Vegetarian, Fillets, Breaded, Mini, Quorn*	1 Fillet/30g	59	2.9	196	10.2	15	9.6	4.5
Vegetarian, Fillets, Crispy, Quorn*	1 Fillet/100g	192	8.5	192	12.5	14.2	8.5	4
Vegetarian, Fillets, Garlic & Herb, Quorn*	1 Fillet/100g	208	9.8	208	13.9	16.1	9.8	4.1
Vegetarian, Nuggets, Crispy, Chicken Style, Quorn*	1 Nugget/17g	33	2	198	12	8	12	4.8
Vegetarian, Pieces, Chicken Style, Chilled, Quorn*	½ Pack/175g	173	4.6	99	13.8	1.7	2.6	7.1
Vegetarian, Pieces, Chicken Style, Frozen/Chilled, Quorn*	1 Serving/100g	113	2.8	113	15.3	3.9	2.8	5.3
Vegetarian, Roast Style, Quorn*	1/5 Roast/91g	96	1.8	106	15	4.5	2	4.9

CHICKEN

	Measure INFO/WEIGHT	per Measure KCAL	FAT	KCAL	PROT	CARB	FAT	FIBRE
Vegetarian, Roast, Family, Frozen, Cooked, Quorn*	1 Serving/80g	91	2.2	114	16.7	3	2.7	5
Wafer Thin, Average	*1 Slice/10g*	*12*	*0.4*	*120*	*19*	*2.8*	*3.6*	*0.2*
Whole, Roast, Average	*½ Chicken/685g*	*910*	*57.7*	*133*	*13.4*	*0.9*	*8.4*	*0.1*
Wing Quarter, Meat Only, Casseroled	*1oz/28g*	*46*	*1.8*	*164*	*26.9*	*0*	*6.3*	*0*
Wing, Breaded, Fried, Average	*1oz/28g*	*77*	*4.8*	*273*	*17.1*	*13*	*17.2*	*0.4*
Wing, Meat & Skin, Cooked, Average	*1 Wing/85g*	*216*	*14.3*	*254*	*23.8*	*0*	*16.9*	*0*
Wing, Meat Only, Cooked, Average	*1 Wing/21g*	*43*	*1.7*	*203*	*30.5*	*0*	*8.1*	*0*
Wing, Meat Only, Raw, Average	*1 Wing/29g*	*37*	*1*	*126*	*22*	*0*	*3.5*	*0*
Wings, BBQ Flavour, Average	*3 Wings/150g*	*330*	*18.7*	*220*	*20.3*	*6.6*	*12.4*	*0.6*
Wings, BBQ, Beer Bourbon, Sainsbury's*	½ Pack/127g	258	15	203	20.3	3.2	11.8	1.4
Wings, Carolina, & Memphis BBQ, Asda*	1/5 Pack/165g	369	23.2	223	23	2.6	14	0.5
Wings, Chinese Style, Average	*1oz/28g*	*72*	*4.3*	*256*	*24.2*	*5.1*	*15.5*	*0.6*
Wings, Hot & Spicy, Average	*1oz/28g*	*65*	*3.8*	*231*	*21.8*	*5.2*	*13.6*	*0.8*
Wings, Meat & Skin, Raw, Average	*1 Wing/150g*	*286*	*19.3*	*191*	*17.5*	*0*	*12.8*	*0*
Wings, Sweet Chilli, Sainsbury's*	½ Pack/127g	272	14.5	214	18.4	9.3	11.4	0.5
with Potatoes, Spanish Style, Inspired Cuisine, Aldi*	1 Pack/360g	353	10.4	98	5	12	2.9	2.3

CHICKEN &

& Cashew Nuts, Waitrose*	½ Pack/176g	209	10.4	119	9.6	5.9	5.9	2.1
BBQ, & Rice, Korean, G&B, Asda*	1 Pack/353g	399	8.8	113	7	15	2.5	1.1
Paprika, & Tenderstem Broccoli, Truly Irresistible, Co-Op*	1 Pack/245g	296	12.7	121	8.5	9.2	5.2	1.7
Black Bean Noodles, Sainsbury's*	1 Serving/130g	155	0.9	119	4.3	23.9	0.7	0.8
Black Bean Sauce, with Egg Fried Rice, Ready Meal	*1 Serving/400g*	*390*	*6.1*	*97*	*6.5*	*14.5*	*1.5*	*0.8*
Black Bean with Noodles, Tesco*	1 Pack/475g	470	7.6	99	7.6	13.6	1.6	0.2
Black Bean, Chinese Takeaway, Tesco*	1 Serving/200g	190	6.6	95	8.3	8	3.3	0.5
Cashew Nuts, Chinese, Ready Meal, Average	*1 Serving/400g*	*497*	*24*	*124*	*9.2*	*7.5*	*6*	*1.2*
Chorizo Paella, Go Cook, Asda*	½ Pack/475g	591	10.5	124	10.2	15.9	2.2	2.6
Fries, Southern Fried Style, Tesco*	1 Pack/500g	930	40	186	11.5	16	8	1.4
Gravy, COU, M&S*	1 Pack/300g	216	3.9	72	7.2	7.8	1.3	1.6
King Prawn Special Fried Rice, Finest, Tesco*	1 Pack/450g	734	32	163	7.7	17	7.1	0.7
Mushroom with Rice, Egg Fried, Average	*1 Serving/400g*	*421*	*10.1*	*105*	*6.3*	*14.4*	*2.5*	*0.8*
Pineapple, Chilled, Tesco*	1 Pack/350g	364	8.4	104	9.6	11.1	2.4	5.5
Roasted Potatoes, Spanish, Charlie Bigham's*	½ Pack/387g	479	25.9	124	7.2	9.8	6.7	0

CHICKEN ARRABIATA

Arrabbiata, COU, M&S*	1 Pack/360g	396	6.7	110	8.5	14.5	1.9	1.3
Arrabiata, Calorie Controlled, Counted, Morrisons*	1 Pack/323g	294	2.3	91	8.3	12	0.7	1.5
COU, M&S*	1 Meal/360g	396	6.5	110	8.4	14.5	1.8	1.3
Italian Kitchen, Tesco*	1 Pack/414g	492	11.6	119	8.3	14.2	2.8	1.8
Meal for One, M&S*	1 Pack/400g	528	20.8	132	7.9	12.5	5.2	1.9

CHICKEN BANG BANG

Waitrose*	1 Pack/350g	368	17.2	105	9.4	5.9	4.9	1.2

CHICKEN CANTONESE

& Rice, Sizzler, Tesco*	1 Serving/450g	639	25.6	142	7.7	14.9	5.7	0.9
Breast, Fillets, Sainsbury's*	1 Serving/154g	168	2.3	109	20.3	3.6	1.5	0.6
Chinese, Tesco*	½ Pack/175g	196	6.5	112	10.3	9.4	3.7	0.4
Honey, Sesame, Sainsbury's*	1/3 Pack/135g	116	3.6	86	9.8	5.5	2.7	0.8

CHICKEN CHASSEUR

Average	*1 Serving/400g*	*363*	*9.2*	*91*	*12.2*	*4.9*	*2.3*	*0.9*
Breast Fillets, Morrisons*	1 Pack/380g	384	11.4	101	15.7	2.9	3	0.8
Finest, Tesco*	½ Pack/200g	200	6.4	100	14.3	2.4	3.2	1.1
Parsley Box*	1 Pack/270g	227	5.7	84	11	5	2.1	0.4

CHICKEN CHILLI

Sweet, Battered, Chinese Favourites Box, M&S*	½ Pack/120g	220	4.9	183	11	24.9	4.1	1.1

	Measure INFO/WEIGHT	per Measure		Nutrition Values per 100g / 100ml				
		KCAL	FAT	KCAL	PROT	CARB	FAT	FIBRE
CHICKEN CHILLI								
Sweet, Just Cook, Sainsbury's*	½ Pack/191g	200	1.3	105	15.2	9.4	0.7	0.5
Sweet, Pieces, Morrisons*	1 Pack/200g	282	5	141	25.5	4.1	2.5	0.5
Sweet, With Noodles, Ready Meal, Average	**1 Serving/400g**	**404**	**5.8**	**101**	**6.5**	**15.5**	**1.4**	**1.4**
CHICKEN CHINESE								
Balls, M&S*	1 Ball/16g	45	2.2	280	10.8	29.2	13.6	2.1
Stir Fry, Morrisons*	1 Serving/319g	341	5.4	107	5.7	17	1.7	1.5
with Ginger & Spring Onion, Tesco*	1 Serving/350g	299	10.1	85	7.6	7.3	2.9	0.6
CHICKEN DINNER								
Baby Potatoes, Carrots, Peas, Stuffing, Gravy, Morrisons*	1 Serving/355g	245	4.3	69	8.2	4.4	1.2	4.1
Cooked, Eat Smart, Morrisons*	1 Pack/355g	245	4.3	69	8.2	4.4	1.2	4.1
Roast Potatoes, Peas, Carrots, & Stuffing, HFC, Tesco*	1 Pack/382g	368	9.1	96	9	8.8	2.4	2
Roast, 104, Oakhouse Foods Ltd*	1 Meal/400g	368	8.4	92	8.2	9.4	2.1	1.5
Roast, Calorie Controlled, Tesco*	1 Pack/381g	274	3	72	8.1	7.2	0.8	1.8
Roast, Mini Meals, Tesco*	1 Pack/218g	234	7	108	6.9	12	3.2	1.7
Roast, Mini, As Consumed, Fresh Ideas, Morrisons*	½ Pack/209g	310	13.6	148	18.7	3.3	6.5	1
Roast, Serves 1, Sainsbury's*	1 Pack/373g	466	13.4	125	9.4	12.3	3.6	2.6
Roast, What's Cooking, Lidl*	1 Pack/400g	360	7.2	90	7.7	10.4	1.8	0.6
Roast, with New Potatoes, Garden Veg, Gravy, G&B, Asda*	1 Pack/378g	238	3.4	63	6.5	6.5	0.9	1.9
CHICKEN EN CROUTE								
Chef Select, Lidl*	½ Pack/206g	558	34.8	271	12.8	16.1	16.9	1.7
Just Cook, Sainsbury's*	1 Serving/180g	481	27.2	267	16.8	15.9	15.1	0.4
CHICKEN IN								
Barbeque Sauce, Breasts, COU, M&S*	1 Pack/350g	420	6.7	120	8.5	20.6	1.9	0.6
BBQ Sauce, Breast, Sainsbury's*	1 Serving/170g	199	1.2	117	14.5	13.1	0.7	1.3
BBQ, Smoky, SlimWell, Aldi*	1 Pack/500g	331	4.3	70	10	3.2	0.9	3.4
Black Bean Sauce, Sainsbury's*	1 Pack/465g	484	7.9	104	5	17.3	1.7	0.3
Black Bean Sauce, Slimming World*	1 Pack/500g	330	3.5	66	10.1	4.2	0.7	1.2
Black Bean Sauce, Takeaway, Iceland*	1 Pack/375g	345	11.2	92	8.6	7	3	1.5
Black Bean Sauce, with Egg Fried Rice, Frozen, Tesco*	1 Pack/369g	464	14.1	126	8.3	13.9	3.8	1.3
Black Bean, Rice, & Veg, Balanced 2 Go, Oh So Lean*	1 Pack/400g	424	4	106	9.9	15.3	1	0
Dijon, with Rice, TTD, Sainsbury's*	1 Pack/368g	552	11.4	150	8	21.9	3.1	0.9
Gravy, Breast, Sainsbury's*	1 Box/200g	124	1	62	11.8	2.9	0.5	0.2
Hunter's BBQ Sauce, Asda*	½ Pack /190g	348	14.1	183	19.1	10.3	7.4	0
Lemon & Garlic Marinade, Thighs, Go Cook, Asda*	½ Pack/265g	493	30.2	186	19.7	1.2	11.4	0.8
Madeira Sauce with Mushrooms, Finest, Tesco*	½ Pack/200g	210	8.3	105	13.8	3	4.2	1
Mushroom, Sauce, Tesco*	1 Pack/370g	289	8	78	7.8	6.2	2.2	1.3
Oyster Sauce & Mushrooms, Tesco*	1 Pack/350g	252	5.6	72	8	6.3	1.6	0.7
Prosecco Sauce, Finest, Tesco*	½ Pack/167g	231	10.2	139	18	2.7	6.1	0.7
Reggae Reggae Sauce, Drumsticks, Levi Roots*	1 Serving/100g	165	7.3	165	21.5	3.4	7.3	0
Smoky BBQ Marinade, Breast, Fillets, Mini, CBY, Asda*	3 Fillets/150g	144	1.5	96	18.5	3.3	1	0
Sweet Chilli Sauce, Breast, Fresh Tastes, Asda*	½ Pack/180g	288	9	160	18.4	10.3	5	0.5
Tomato & Basil Sauce, Breast Fillets, Morrisons*	½ Pack/171g	231	7.5	135	21.3	2.5	4.4	1.4
Tomato & Basil Sauce, Breast, GFY, Asda*	1 Pack/392g	447	13.3	114	12	9	3.4	1.5
Tomato & Herb Sauce, Breasts, Tesco*	½ Pack/173g	155	2.4	90	15	3.6	1.4	0.5
White Wine & Tarragon Sauce, Breasts, Finest, Tesco*	½ Pack/200g	326	20.2	163	16.8	1.3	10.1	0
White Wine Sauce, & Mash, for Two, Charlie Bigham's*	1 Serving/412 g	532	30.1	129	7.4	8.9	7.3	0
CHICKEN LEMON								
Battered, Cantonese, Sainsbury's*	1 Pack/350g	560	19.6	160	10.7	16.6	5.6	0.9
Battered, Chinese Meal for Two, Tesco*	½ Serving/175g	294	13	168	6.6	18.8	7.4	2
Cantonese, Sainsbury's*	½ Pack/140g	218	8.8	156	11	13.9	6.3	0.6
COU, M&S*	1 Pack/150g	150	1.4	100	17.9	5.6	0.9	0.8

C

	Measure INFO/WEIGHT	per Measure KCAL	FAT	Nutrition Values per 100g / 100ml KCAL	PROT	CARB	FAT	FIBRE
CHICKEN MOROCCAN								
Harissa Spiced, Cook*	1 Pack/315g	350	12.9	111	11.5	7.8	4.1	1.6
Style, Sainsbury's*	½ Pack/269g	334	7	124	14.7	10.4	2.6	3.1
CHICKEN PASANDA								
Sainsbury's*	1 Serving/200g	368	24.8	184	14.7	3.4	12.4	2.3
with Pilau Rice, HL, Tesco*	1 Pack/440g	466	11	106	5.7	15.2	2.5	0.9
CHICKEN PIRI PIRI								
Peri Peri, Chips, & Apple Slaw, Gousto*	1 Portion/571g	662	33.7	116	8.3	8.4	5.9	0.8
Piri Piri, & Potato Wedges, BFY, M&S*	1 Pack/370g	340	5.2	92	9.1	9.9	1.4	1.9
Piri Piri, & Sunshine Rice, Portuguese, Asda*	1 Pack/368g	449	7.4	122	7.1	17	2	3
CHICKEN SUPREME								
Breast, Sainsbury's*	1 Serving/187g	421	29.5	225	20.6	0.3	15.8	0.6
with Rice, Asda*	1 Pack/450g	616	31.5	137	15	3.4	7	1.1
with Rice, HE, Tesco*	1 Pack/400g	384	6.4	96	4.9	15.6	1.6	1.5
CHICKEN SZECHUAN								
Tesco*	1 Pack/350g	385	10.5	110	7.2	13.6	3	0.3
with Noodles, Sainsbury's*	1 Pack/450g	423	14	94	6	10.4	3.1	0.9
CHICKEN TANDOORI								
& Basmati Rice, Aromatic, Asda*	1 Pack/380g	399	8	105	7.5	12	2.1	3.7
& Spiced Rice, As Consumed, Eat Smart, Morrisons*	1 Pack/380g	416	4.8	113	7.8	16.1	1.3	2.8
Fresh Tastes, Asda*	1 Pack/400g	356	5.6	89	6.4	12.7	1.4	2.1
Oven Baked, Asda*	½ Pack/141g	186	5.9	132	20	3.6	4.2	0.6
Sizzler, Sainsbury's*	1 Pack/400g	536	29.2	134	12.8	4.3	7.3	1.7
Sizzler, Tesco*	1 Serving/175g	243	11.6	139	10	10	6.6	1
with Cauliflower Rice, G&B, Asda*	1 Pack/380g	365	9.9	96	8.9	7.3	2.6	3.9
with Rice, City Kitchen, Tesco*	1 Pack/385g	597	21.2	155	6.7	19.6	5.5	1.8
with Vegetable Pilau Rice, HL, Tesco*	1 Pack/348g	400	9	115	8.4	14.1	2.6	1.9
CHICKEN TERIYAKI								
& Noodles, Asda*	½ Pack/340g	445	8.8	131	9	18	2.6	0.9
Japanese with Ramen Noodles, Sainsbury's*	1 Pack/450g	482	9.4	107	6.5	15.5	2.1	0.8
Noodles, HL, Tesco*	1 Pack/367g	282	1.8	77	6.4	10.5	0.5	2.3
Teriyaki, Japanese, Sainsbury's*	1 Pack/380g	486	11.4	128	7.4	16.8	3	2.1
Teriyaki, Japanese, Street Kitchen*	1 Pack/255g	398	4.1	156	1.6	31	1.6	0
CHICKEN TIKKA								
& Lemon Rice, Deli Meal, M&S*	1 Pack/360g	342	7.2	95	9.8	10.2	2	0.7
& Basmati Rice, Aromatic, Weight Watchers*	1 Pack/382g	359	7.6	94	6.4	12.1	2	1.2
& Rice, Toddler Meal, Annabel Karmel*	1 Pack/200g	204	3	102	6.1	15.6	1.5	1.4
Chargrilled, & Spiced Cauliflower Rice, BFY, M&S*	1 Pack/400g	284	8.8	71	7.2	5	2.2	1.3
Cheeky, with Brown Rice, Gousto*	1 Serving/476g	476	8.1	100	10.1	11.8	1.7	1.3
Less Than 3% Fat, BGTY, Sainsbury's*	1 Pack/303g	373	3.6	123	6	21.3	1.2	1
Masala, & Pilau Rice, Charlie Bigham's*	½ Pack/403g	737	43.9	183	6.9	15.3	10.9	0
Masala, 874, Oakhouse Foods Ltd*	1 Serving/400g	604	26	151	8	14.3	6.5	1.8
Masala, with Rice, Weight Watchers, Heinz*	1 Pack/310g	333	7.4	108	5.4	15.8	2.4	0.7
Takeaway	**1 Serving/350g**	**421**	**15**	**120**	**20.3**	**0**	**4.3**	**0.3**
with Pilau Rice, GFY, Asda*	1 Pack/450g	382	2.7	85	7	13	0.6	1.8
CHICKEN WITH								
& Ham, with Mushrooms, The Main Event, Asda*	½ Pack/169g	209	6.6	124	21	1.1	3.9	0.5
a Sea Salt & Black Pepper Crust, Breasts, Asda*	1 Serving/154g	186	4.3	121	19	5	2.8	0
a Sticky Honey & Chilli Sauce, Breast, Asda*	1 Serving/175g	247	5.6	141	20	8	3.2	0
Bacon, & Leek, with Potatoes, Classic, Iceland*	1 Pack/405g	478	16.2	118	9.5	9.6	4	3
Broccoli & Pesto Pasta, BGTY, Sainsbury's*	1 Pack/301g	328	5.1	109	10.3	13.2	1.7	2.5
Caesar Melt & Prosciutto, Breast, M&S*	1 Pack/375g	488	18.8	130	19.6	1.3	5	1
Cous Cous, Lemon & Herb, Finest, Tesco*	1 Pack/370g	492	18.5	133	10.5	11.5	5	0.9
Garlic & Chilli Balti, Tesco*	1 Pack/400g	320	7.6	80	11	4.4	1.9	0.8

	Measure INFO/WEIGHT	per Measure KCAL	FAT	Nutrition Values per 100g / 100ml KCAL	PROT	CARB	FAT	FIBRE
CHICKEN WITH								
Honey & Ginger Sauce, 125, Oakhouse Foods Ltd*	1 Dinner/365g	339	8	93	8.7	9.8	2.2	1.2
Leek & Bacon, M&S*	½ Pack/183g	239	12.8	131	15.3	1.2	7	0.9
Leeks, & White Wine Sauce, Finest, Tesco*	½ Pack/180g	258	10.3	143	20.9	1.5	5.7	1.2
Lime & Coriander, Easy, Waitrose*	½ Pack/168g	203	7.9	121	18.9	0.7	4.7	0.5
Lyonnaise Potatoes, M&S*	½ Pack/260g	286	8.1	110	12.6	8	3.1	0.9
Mediterranean Style, with Couscous, Iceland*	1 Serving/373g	328	6	88	7.6	9.9	1.6	1.4
Mediterranean, 992, Oakhouse Foods Ltd*	1 Meal/480g	480	20.6	100	7.4	8.1	4.3	1.5
Mushroom & Bacon, Fillets, M&S*	½ Pack/188g	225	11.2	120	15.5	0.5	6	1.7
Pan-Fried, with Spiced Creamy Lentils, Hello Fresh*	1 Serving/481g	500	30.9	104	8.5	4.2	6.4	0
Peppered, Rice, & Veg, Balanced 2 Go, Oh So Lean*	1 Pack/400g	328	4.4	82	9.4	9.5	1.1	0
Pork Stuffing, Breast, Roast, M&S*	1 Serving/100g	165	6.5	165	24.1	3	6.5	0
Rice, Jamaican Jerk, Healthier Choice, Co-Op*	1 Pack/406g	365	9.3	90	7.8	9.8	2.3	3.4
Sage & Onion Stuffing, Breast, Roast, Sliced, M&S*	1 Slice/17g	27	1.1	165	24.1	3	6.5	0
Sundried Tomato, with Cavatappi Pasta, BFY, M&S*	1 Pack/360g	428	9.4	119	10.5	12.7	2.6	1.4
CHICORY								
Fresh, Raw, Average	**1 Head/150g**	**30**	**0.9**	**20**	**0.6**	**2.8**	**0.6**	**0.9**
CHILLI								
3 Bean, Chipotle, Hi Five*	1 Pack/467g	355	8.4	76	3.2	12.8	1.8	2.7
Bean, 3, Mexican, with Rice, Weight Watchers, Heinz*	1 Meal/400g	328	3.6	82	3	13.8	0.9	3.6
Bean, Mixed, Chipotle, with Wild Rice, Eat Well, M&S*	1 Pack/300g	312	5.7	104	3.9	15.9	1.9	3.9
Bean, Three, & Rice, As Consumed, Counted, Morrisons*	1 Pack/390g	386	4.7	99	3.5	17	1.2	3.1
Bean, Three, Slim Choice, Sainsbury's*	1 Pack/465g	437	2.8	94	3.7	16.1	0.6	4.9
Beef with Rice, GFY, Asda*	1 Serving/402g	354	6	88	4.7	14	1.5	0.9
Beef, & Rice, HL, Tesco*	1 Pack/370g	370	5.9	100	5	13.7	1.6	5.5
Beef, & Rice, Tex Mex, Tesco*	1 Pack/450g	604	13	134	5.4	20.4	2.9	2.5
Beef, Asda*	½ Pack/200g	190	7.8	95	7	8	3.9	1.2
Beef, Chunky, Slimming World*	1 Pack/550g	418	6.6	76	8.8	5.9	1.2	3.1
Beef, Chunky, Slow Cooked, M&S*	½ Pack/268g	289	8.3	108	15.3	3.6	3.1	2.1
Beef, Pulled, Cook*	1 Pack/320g	365	11.5	114	10.3	7.6	3.6	1.3
Con Carne & Rice, Everyday, Value, Tesco*	1 Pack/400g	455	11.1	115	5	15.5	2.8	3.3
Con Carne & Rice, Tex Mex, M Kitchen, Morrisons*	1 Pack/450g	580	22.9	129	0.5	14.9	5.1	0.5
Con Carne & Sweetcorn Mash, Fuller Longer, M&S*	1 Pack/400g	380	13.2	95	8.5	7.4	3.3	3.9
Con Carne with Rice, GFY, Asda*	1 Serving/400g	456	6.4	114	6	19	1.6	0.9
Con Carne with Rice, Healthy Choice, Asda*	1 Pack/400g	412	8.4	103	6	15	2.1	0.9
Con Carne with Rice, Morrisons*	1 Pack/400g	328	5.2	82	5.3	12.2	1.3	1.4
Con Carne with Rice, Organic, Sainsbury's*	1 Pack/400g	472	10.8	118	5	18.5	2.7	1.8
Con Carne, & Mexican Rice, Charlie Bigham's*	1 Serving/421 g	589	25.2	140	7.2	14.1	6	0
Con Carne, & Mexican Rice, Charlie Bigham's*	½ Pack/421g	589	25.2	140	7.2	14.1	6	0
Con Carne, & Rice, Fiesta, Aldi*	1 Pack/450g	648	24.3	144	6.7	16	5.4	2.3
Con Carne, 175, Oakhouse Foods Ltd*	1 Meal/380g	464	14.4	122	7.3	15.4	3.8	2.1
Con Carne, Asda*	1 Can/392g	376	13.7	96	7	9	3.5	0
Con Carne, Beef, Look What We Found*	1 Pack/250g	243	9.5	97	7.5	6.2	3.8	4.1
Con Carne, Beef, Slim Cook, Tesco*	1 Pack/476g	376	7.1	79	5.4	9.6	1.5	3.1
Con Carne, Canned, Morrisons*	1 Can/392g	368	11.8	94	8.8	8	3	2.4
Con Carne, Canned, Sainsbury's*	½ Can/200g	162	4.2	81	6.6	8.9	2.1	2.5
Con Carne, Canned, Tesco*	½ Can/200g	220	11.4	110	7.8	6.4	5.7	4.7
Con Carne, Classic, Canned, Stagg*	½ Can/200g	260	10	130	7	13	5	4.5
Con Carne, Diet Chef Ltd*	1 Pack/300g	333	13.5	111	7.3	10.4	4.5	2.1
Con Carne, Dynamite Hot, Stagg*	1 Serving/250g	310	15.5	124	7.6	9.6	6.2	2.5
Con Carne, From Restaurant, Average	**1 Serving/253g**	**256**	**8.3**	**101**	**9.7**	**8.7**	**3.3**	**0**
Con Carne, Frozen, Co-Op*	1 Pack/340g	306	3.4	90	6	15	1	1
Con Carne, Heston from Waitrose, Waitrose*	½ Pack/300g	429	27	143	8.4	5.9	9	2.3
Con Carne, Homepride*	1 Can/390g	234	2.3	60	2.5	11.2	0.6	0

C

	Measure INFO/WEIGHT	per Measure KCAL	FAT	Nutrition Values per 100g / 100ml KCAL	PROT	CARB	FAT	FIBRE
CHILLI								
Con Carne, M&S*	1 Pack/285g	285	10.5	100	8.7	7.4	3.7	2
Con Carne, Recipe Mix, Colman's*	1 Pack/27g	84	2.1	312	12.3	37.8	7.7	22.9
Con Carne, with Long Grain Rice, COU, M&S*	1 Pack/390g	394	6.6	101	5.4	15	1.7	2.2
Con Carne, with Rice, BGTY, Sainsbury's*	1 Pack/400g	392	8.3	99	6.3	12.5	2.1	2.2
Con Carne, with Rice, Classic, Co-Op*	1 Pack/400g	464	13.6	116	5.9	14	3.4	2.7
Con Carne, with Rice, Counted, Morrisons*	½ Pack/158g	150	2.4	95	5.9	13.5	1.5	1.6
Con Carne, with Rice, Meal for One, M&S*	1 Pack/450g	536	12.2	119	5.5	18	2.7	0.5
Con Carne, with Rice, PB, Waitrose*	1 Pack/400g	404	7.2	101	5.8	15.3	1.8	1.7
Con Veggie, Cook*	1 Portion/285g	194	4.3	68	5.9	7.8	1.5	0
Five Bean, Deliciously Ella*	½ Pack/200g	140	2	70	3.9	8.8	1	3.6
Five Bean, Mexican, Bol*	1 Pot/343g	340	7.9	99	3.7	14.3	2.3	2.9
Jackfruit, Aldi*	1 Pack/400g	436	6.8	109	2.6	19	1.7	4.3
Jackfruit, Pulled, Smoky BBQ, Corn, & Beans, Soulful*	1 Pot/380g	304	11	80	2.5	11.5	2.9	2
Medium, Uncle Ben's*	1 Jar/500g	305	4	61	1.8	11.1	0.8	0
Mexican Bean, & Sweet Potato, with Quinoa, Soulful*	1 Pot/380g	247	3.4	65	3.2	13	0.9	4.4
Mixed Bean, Chipotle, with Wild Rice, Plant Kitchen, M&S*	1 Pack/300g	312	5.7	104	3.9	15.9	1.9	3.9
Mixed Vegetable, Tesco*	1 Pack/400g	352	11.6	88	3.9	11	2.9	3.2
Non Carne, with Chickpeas, & Rice, Mexican, Bol*	1 Jar/500g	295	6.5	59	3.1	6.1	1.3	5
Pork, with Apple Salsa, Mexican, Gousto*	1 Portion/376g	688	30.5	183	10.6	18	8.1	4
Quorn, Full of Beans, Microwaved, Quorn*	1 Pack/385g	366	4.2	95	4.7	15.2	1.1	2.6
Red, Raw, Sainsbury's*	1 Avg Chilli/45g	14	0.2	30	1.8	4.2	0.5	1.5
Speckled Lentil, with Parisienne Potatoes, Everdine*	1 Serving/450g	450	14.4	100	2.9	12.7	3.2	4.5
Sweet Potato, & Bean, Mexican Rice, Charlie Bigham's*	1 Serving/420 g	433	11.8	103	3.4	16.2	2.8	0
Three Bean, & Cauliflower Rice, Goodlife*	1 Pack/400g	276	8	69	3.8	5.8	2	6.5
Three Bean, & Cous Cous, Vegan, Good Health, Waitrose*	1 Pack/400g	440	9.2	110	4	16.2	2.3	3.7
Three Bean, & Vegetable, Slimfree, Aldi*	1 Pack/500g	295	2.5	59	3.4	8.5	0.5	3.1
Three Bean, Diet Chef Ltd*	1 Pack/300g	195	2.7	65	4	10.3	0.9	3.6
Vegetable	**1oz/28g**	**16**	**0.2**	**57**	**3**	**10.8**	**0.6**	**2.6**
Vegetable & Rice, BGTY, Sainsbury's*	1 Pack/450g	410	5	91	3.5	16.7	1.1	3.5
Vegetable Garden, Stagg*	1 Can/400g	280	2	70	3.5	14	0.5	3
Vegetable, Canned, Heated, Asda*	½ Can/200g	158	1	79	3.2	14.1	0.5	2.5
Vegetable, Canned, Sainsbury's*	1 Can/400g	230	1.6	58	3.1	10.4	0.4	3.2
Vegetable, Canned, Tesco*	½ Can/200g	136	4.2	68	2.8	8.2	2.1	2.6
Vegetable, Diet Chef Ltd*	1 Pack/300g	258	4.8	86	3.4	14.5	1.6	4.4
Vegetable, Retail	**1oz/28g**	**20**	**0.6**	**70**	**4**	**9.4**	**2.1**	**0**
Vegetable, Spicy, Jane Plan*	1 Serving/300g	150	1.2	50	2.1	9.5	0.4	2
Vegetarian with Rice, Tesco*	1 Pack/500g	575	13	115	4	19	2.6	1.8
Vegetarian, Mexican, Chef's Selection, Quorn*	½ Pack/170g	143	4.3	84	6.6	6.5	2.5	4.5
Vegetarian, Soya Mince, & Rice, Waitrose*	1 Pack/402g	442	8.4	110	5.4	14.9	2.1	5.4
Vegetarian, Tesco*	1 Pack/400g	340	3.2	85	4.4	15	0.8	2.1
Vegetarian, with Rice, Chef Select, Lidl*	1 Pack/426g	403	5.8	95	2.9	16.8	1.4	1.9
Vegetarian, with Rice, Ready Meal, Average	**1 Serving/400g**	**434**	**6**	**108**	**3.8**	**20**	**1.5**	**1.3**
Veggie, Smoky, Jamie Oliver*	1 Serving/125g	111	2.6	89	4.6	10	2.1	5.1
CHILLI POWDER								
Average	**1 Tsp/4g**	**16**	**0.7**	**405**	**12.3**	**54.7**	**16.8**	**34.2**
Hot, Asda*	1 Tsp/5g	17	0.6	331	13	30	13	21
CHIPS								
American Style, Oven, Co-Op*	1 Serving/150g	255	9	170	2	26	6	3
American Style, Thin, Oven, Tesco*	1 Serving/125g	210	8.1	168	2.7	24.6	6.5	2.1
Chip Shop, Fishnchickn*	1 Portion/311g	734	38.6	236	3.2	27.9	12.4	0
Chunky Oven, Harry Ramsden's*	1 Serving/150g	184	5.4	123	2.8	19.9	3.6	1.6
Chunky, Chilled, Waitrose*	1/3 Pack/150g	237	5.6	158	2.8	26.5	3.7	3.8
Chunky, COU, M&S*	1 Serving/150g	158	2.4	105	2.1	20.5	1.6	2.3

CHIPS

INFO/WEIGHT	Measure	per Measure KCAL	FAT	Nutrition Values per 100g / 100ml KCAL	PROT	CARB	FAT	FIBRE
Chunky, Gastropub, M&S*	1 Pack/400g	520	12.4	130	2.6	22.4	3.1	2.3
Chunky, M&S*	½ Pack/200g	292	7.6	146	2	24.7	3.8	2.6
Chunky, Ready to Bake, M&S*	1 Serving/200g	310	8.4	155	2.2	26.8	4.2	2
Chunky, Slimming World*	1 Serving/200g	208	0.6	104	3.3	20.9	0.3	2.6
Chunky, with Cornish Sea Salt, Finest, Tesco*	½ Pack/176g	294	6.2	167	2.7	29.6	3.5	2.8
Crinkle Cut, Frozen, Fried in Corn Oil	*1oz/28g*	*81*	*4.7*	*290*	*3.6*	*33.4*	*16.7*	*2.2*
Crinkle Cut, Homestyle, Tesco*	1 Serving/95g	168	4	177	2.5	30.5	4.2	3.5
Crinkle Cut, Oven Baked, Aunt Bessie's*	1 Serving/100g	206	9.2	206	2.9	28	9.2	3.2
Crinkle Cut, Oven, Asda*	1 Serving/100g	134	3.8	134	2	23	3.8	8
Family Fries, Oven, Tesco*	1 Serving/125g	164	4.6	131	2	22.4	3.7	1.8
Fine Cut, Frozen, Fried in Blended Oil	*1oz/28g*	*102*	*6*	*364*	*4.5*	*41.2*	*21.3*	*2.4*
French Fries, Crispy, Oven Baked, McCain*	1 Serving/100g	231	7.7	231	3.1	35.5	7.7	3.3
Fried, Average	*1 Serving/130g*	*266*	*10.9*	*204*	*3.2*	*29.6*	*8.4*	*1.2*
Fried, Chip Shop, Average	*1 Sm/100g*	*239*	*12.4*	*239*	*3.2*	*30.5*	*12.4*	*2.2*
Frites, M&S*	1 Pack/100g	185	7.1	185	2.2	26.5	7.1	3
Frozen, Crinkle Cut, Aunt Bessie's*	1 Serving/100g	163	7.3	163	3.1	21.3	7.3	2.2
Fry or Oven, Oven Cooked, Smart Price, Asda*	1 Serving/125g	192	4.3	153	2.1	26.9	3.4	3.3
Frying, Cooked in Sunflower Oil, Value, Tesco*	1 Portion/125g	172	4.9	138	2.5	23.1	3.9	1.6
Frying, Crinkle Cut, Tesco*	1 Serving/125g	161	4.1	129	2.6	22.2	3.3	1.9
Gourmet, Cornish Sea Salt, Oven Baked, McCain*	¼ Pack/100g	206	9.9	206	2	25.6	9.9	3
Home Chips, Straight Cut, Baked, McCain*	1 Serving/150g	312	10.8	208	3.3	31	7.2	2.9
Home Chips, Straight Cut, Frozen, As Sold, McCain*	1 Serving/100g	144	4.1	144	2.3	23	4.1	2.3
Home Chips, Straight, GF, Frozen, McCain*	1 Serving/100g	138	4.3	138	2	21.8	4.3	1.9
Home, Straight Cut, Lighter, Reduced Fat, Baked, McCain*	1 Serving/100g	181	3.4	181	3.2	33	3.4	3.3
Home, Straight Cut, Lighter, Reduced Fat, Frozen, McCain*	1 Serving/125g	178	3.5	142	2.3	26	2.8	2.2
Homefries, Chunky, Weighed Baked, McCain*	1 Serving/100g	153	3.1	153	3.2	28	3.1	2.3
Homefries, Chunky, Weighed Frozen, McCain*	1 Serving/100g	123	2.5	123	2.5	22.6	2.5	1.6
Homefries, Crinkle Cut, Weighed Baked, McCain*	1 Serving/100g	176	5	176	2.6	30.1	5	2.3
Homefries, Crinkle Cut, Weighed Frozen, McCain*	1 Serving/100g	142	5.1	142	1.9	22.2	5.1	1.3
Homefries, Straight Cut, Weighed Baked, McCain*	1 Serving/100g	181	6.2	181	3.1	28.1	6.2	2.4
Homefries, Straight Cut, Weighed Frozen, McCain*	1 Serving/100g	134	4.6	134	2.2	21	4.6	1.7
Homemade, Fried in Blended Oil, Average	*1oz/28g*	*53*	*1.9*	*189*	*3.9*	*30.1*	*6.7*	*2.2*
Homemade, Fried in Corn Oil, Average	*1oz/28g*	*53*	*1.9*	*189*	*3.9*	*30.1*	*6.7*	*2.2*
Homemade, Fried in Dripping, Average	*1oz/28g*	*53*	*1.9*	*189*	*3.9*	*30.1*	*6.7*	*2.2*
Homestyle Oven, Sainsbury's*	1 Serving/125g	206	5.4	165	2.4	29.2	4.3	2.1
Homestyle, Crispy, Ovenbaked, Asda*	1 Serving/125g	249	7.4	199	2.8	32	5.9	3.6
Homestyle, Frozen, Aunt Bessie's*	1 Serving/100g	124	3.5	124	2.4	20	3.5	1.9
Homestyle, Harvest Basket, Lidl*	1 Serving/150g	202	5.8	135	2.4	21.5	3.9	2.3
Homestyle, Oven Cooked, Aunt Bessie's*	1 Serving/100g	191	7.8	191	3.1	27	7.8	2.9
Homestyle, Oven, Straight Cut , Tesco*	1 Serving/125g	218	5.1	174	2.1	30.9	4.1	2.5
Maris Piper, Oven, Chunky, Extra Special, Asda*	1 Serving/125g	211	4.4	169	2	31	3.5	2.7
Micro Chips, Crinkle Cut, Cooked, McCain*	1 Pack/100g	146	4	158	2.4	26	4.3	2.8
Micro Chips, Straight Cut, Cooked, McCain*	1 Pack/100g	163	4.8	163	2.3	27.7	4.8	2
Microwave, Cooked	*1oz/28g*	*62*	*2.7*	*221*	*3.6*	*32.1*	*9.6*	*2.9*
Oven, 5% Fat, Frozen, McCain*	1 Serving/200g	238	6	119	1.9	21	3	1.6
Oven, American Style, Champion*	1 Serving/200g	372	14.4	186	2.2	28.2	7.2	2
Oven, Best in the World, Iceland*	1 Serving/175g	332	11.7	190	3.4	28.9	6.7	3.5
Oven, Champion*	1 Pack/133g	210	6	158	2.5	27	4.5	0
Oven, Chunky & Crispy, Tesco*	½ Pack/178g	304	10.5	171	2.9	24.9	5.9	3.5
Oven, Chunky, Extra Special, Asda*	1 Serving/125g	238	7	190	3.4	31.5	5.6	3.2
Oven, Cooked, Value, Tesco*	1 Serving/125g	308	9.8	246	4.5	39.5	7.8	2.9
Oven, Crinkle Cut, Frozen, Essential, Waitrose*	1 Serving/165g	225	6.4	136	2.7	22.6	3.9	1.7
Oven, Crinkle Cut, Sainsbury's*	1 Serving/165g	297	9.1	180	3.3	29.5	5.5	2.4

C

	Measure INFO/WEIGHT	per Measure KCAL	FAT	Nutrition Values per 100g / 100ml KCAL	PROT	CARB	FAT	FIBRE
CHIPS								
Oven, Frozen, Baked	**1 Portion/80g**	**130**	**3.4**	**162**	**3.2**	**29.8**	**4.2**	**2**
Oven, Frozen, Basics, Sainsbury's*	1 Serving/165g	249	8.1	151	3	23.6	4.9	2.9
Oven, Frozen, BGTY, Sainsbury's*	1 Serving/165g	226	4.6	137	2.9	25	2.8	2.7
Oven, Frozen, Value, Tesco*	1 Serving/125g	189	5.7	151	2.8	24.7	4.6	1.9
Oven, Homefries, McCain*	1 Serving/100g	134	4.6	134	2.2	21	4.6	1.7
Oven, Morrisons*	1 Serving/100g	134	3.9	134	2.4	22.2	3.9	0
Oven, Original, McCain*	1 Serving/100g	158	3.8	158	2.5	28.5	3.8	2.3
Oven, Steak Cut, Asda*	1 Serving/100g	153	4.1	153	2	27	4.1	2.5
Oven, Steak Cut, Sainsbury's*	1 Serving/165g	266	7.8	161	2.6	27.1	4.7	2.8
Oven, Steak Cut, Waitrose*	1 Serving/165g	218	5.6	132	2.7	22.7	3.4	1.7
Oven, Steakhouse, Frozen, Tesco*	1 Serving/125g	165	4.2	132	2.7	22.7	3.4	1.7
Oven, Straight Cut, 5% Fat, Sainsbury's*	1 Serving/165g	280	8.1	170	3.4	28	4.9	2.5
Oven, Straight Cut, Asda*	1 Serving/100g	199	5	199	3.5	35	5	3
Oven, Straight Cut, BFY, Morrisons*	1 Serving/165g	249	5.8	151	2.8	27.1	3.5	2.1
Oven, Straight Cut, Reduced Fat, Tesco*	1 Serving/100g	127	3	127	2.3	22.7	3	2.1
Oven, Straight Cut, Waitrose*	1 Serving/165g	219	6.1	133	2	23	3.7	1.7
Oven, Sweet Potato, Cooked, Tesco*	¼ Pack/87g	153	4.8	175	3	26.2	5.5	4.5
Oven, Thick Cut, Frozen, Baked	**1oz/28g**	**44**	**1.2**	**157**	**3.2**	**27.9**	**4.4**	**1.8**
Oven, Thin Cut, American Style, Asda*	1 Serving/100g	240	10	240	3.4	34	10	3
Oven, Thin Fries, Morrisons*	1 Serving/100g	161	6.1	161	2.9	23.6	6.1	1.2
Potato, Lights, Reduced Fat, Lay's*	1 Serving/25g	118	5.5	470	7.5	60	22	5
Salt & Pepper, Crinkle, Tesco*	1 Serving/112g	179	5.7	160	2.3	24.6	5.1	3.4
Steak Cut, Frying, Asda*	1 Serving/97g	181	6.8	187	2.9	28	7	2.8
Steak Cut, Harvest Basket, Lidl*	1 Serving/100g	155	4	155	2.7	26.6	4	1.2
Steak Cut, Iceland*	1 Serving/100g	156	4.1	156	3.3	24.6	4.1	3.6
Steak Cut, Morrisons*	1 Serving/125g	171	3.9	137	2.1	23.7	3.1	3.1
Steak Cut, Oven, Tesco*	1 Serving/165g	233	6.4	141	2	24.4	3.9	2
Steak, Cut, Oven, Frozen, Essential, Waitrose*	1 Serving/180g	241	6.5	134	2.4	22.1	3.6	1.7
Steakhouse, Fry, Tesco*	1 Serving/125g	278	15.1	222	3.1	25.2	12.1	2
Straight Cut, Frozen, Fried in Blended Oil	**1oz/28g**	**76**	**3.8**	**273**	**4.1**	**36**	**13.5**	**2.4**
Straight Cut, Frozen, Fried in Corn Oil	**1oz/28g**	**76**	**3.8**	**273**	**4.1**	**36**	**13.5**	**2.4**
Thick Cut, Frozen, Fried in Corn Oil, Average	**1oz/28g**	**66**	**2.9**	**234**	**3.6**	**34**	**10.2**	**2.4**
Tortilla, Lightly Salted, Everyday Value, Tesco*	1 Serving/25g	125	5.9	499	5.5	64.8	23.5	2.9
Triple Cooked, Finest, Tesco*	½ Pack/178g	262	6.8	147	2.6	24.1	3.8	3
Triple Cooked, Gastro, Frozen, McCain*	1 Serving/187g	379	22.2	203	1.9	21	11.9	2.2
Triple Cooked, Gastro, Oven Baked, McCain*	1 Serving/135g	379	20.5	281	2.9	31.6	15.2	3
Vegetable, Fries, Aldi*	1 Serving/100g	192	11	192	2.5	18	11	6.7
Vegetable, Root, Ready to Roast, Tesco*	¼ Pack/125g	99	3.8	79	1.1	10.3	3	3.1
with Gravy, Mayflower*	1 Box/330g	403	19.2	122	1.8	15.8	5.8	1.4
CHIVES								
Fresh, Average	**1 Tsp/2g**	**0**	**0**	**23**	**2.8**	**1.7**	**0.6**	**1.9**
Garden, Fresh, Cooks' Ingredients, Waitrose*	1 Pack/25g	10	0.2	42	3.3	4.4	0.7	2.5
CHOC ICES								
Chocolate, Dark, Seriously Creamy, Waitrose*	1 Ice/82g	195	12.9	238	2.6	21.6	15.7	1.7
Chocolate, Real Milk, Sainsbury's*	1 Choc Ice/41g	126	8	311	3	29.9	19.8	0.6
Dark, Sainsbury's*	1 Choc Ice/41g	115	7.2	283	2.7	27.2	17.8	1.5
Dark, Sainsbury's*	1 Choc Ice/41g	115	7.2	283	2.7	27.2	17.8	1.5
Dark, Tesco*	1 Choc Ice/43g	132	8.7	305	3.5	28	20	0.1
Everyday, Value, Tesco*	1 Choc Ice/31g	95	6.3	300	2.3	26.7	19.9	1
Neapolitan Chocolate, Co-Op*	1 Ice/62g	120	8.2	194	2	16.9	13.2	0.4
Plain, Co-Op*	1 Choc Ice/42g	123	8	293	3.1	26	19	0
CHOCOLATE								
Advent Calendar, Dairy Milk, Cadbury*	1 Chocolate/4g	22	1.3	525	7.5	56.6	30.1	0.7

CHOCOLATE

	Measure INFO/WEIGHT	per Measure KCAL	FAT	Nutrition Values per 100g / 100ml KCAL	PROT	CARB	FAT	FIBRE
Advent Calendar, Maltesers, Mars*	1 Chocolate/4g	21	1.2	537	6.8	57.9	30.9	0
Alpine Milk , Milka*	1 Serving/25g	132	7.4	530	6.6	58.5	29.5	1.8
Baking, Belgian, Milk for Cakes, Luxury, Sainsbury's*	1 Chunk/8g	44	2.7	556	7.6	56.5	33.3	1.5
Bar, Animal, Nestle*	1 Bar/19g	97	5	513	5.8	63.6	26.1	0
Bar, Bliss Truffle, Cadbury*	1 Bar/40g	226	14.9	565	6.6	48.8	37.3	2.8
Bar, Bliss, Hazelnut Truffle, Cadbury*	1 Serving/100g	565	37.9	565	7.2	47.7	37.9	2.6
Bar, Cappuccino, Thorntons*	1 Bar/38g	201	13.2	529	5.2	49.7	34.7	0.5
Bar, Chocolate Cream, Fry's*	1 Piece/10g	42	1.3	415	2.8	70.8	13.2	1.2
Bar, Chopped Nuts, Dairy Milk, Cadbury*	6 Chunks/24g	130	7.8	547	7.9	52	33	2.5
Bar, Cookies & Cream, Hello, Lindt*	1 Square/10g	56	3.7	565	7	52	37	0
Bar, Dark Chocolate, Diabetic, Thorntons*	1 Bar/75g	345	26.8	460	5.4	28.5	35.8	8.1
Bar, Dark with Ginger, Thorntons*	1 Bar/90g	495	35.1	550	8	39	39	0
Bar, Dark, 60% Cocoa with Macadamia, Thorntons*	1 Bar/70g	183	12.8	523	6.5	42.3	36.5	12.6
Bar, Dark, Thorntons*	1 Sm Bar/48g	250	17.7	521	7.3	39.9	36.9	10.9
Bar, Deliciously, Free From, Sainsbury's*	1 Bar/35g	190	12.2	543	2.5	48.2	35	12.4
Bar, Duplo, Ferrero*	1 Bar18g	101	6.1	555	6.1	56	33.5	5
Bar, Extra Dark, 60% Cocoa, Lindor, Lindt*	1 Bar/150g	900	73.5	600	5	35	49	2
Bar, Free From, Asda*	1 Bar/35g	194	12.1	563	2.5	58	35	2.8
Bar, Hazel Nut & Cashew, Dairy Milk, Cadbury*	3 Chunks/18g	96	6	540	8.8	50.6	33.5	1.8
Bar, Jazz Orange, Thorntons*	1 Bar/56g	304	18.1	543	6.8	55.7	32.3	1.2
Bar, Mandolin, Cadbury*	1 Bar/28g	139	4.6	495	3.5	66.5	16.5	0.6
Bar, Milk, Thorntons*	1 Sm Bar/50g	269	16	538	7.5	54.8	32	1
Bar, Truffle, M&S*	1 Bar/35g	168	11.4	480	5.9	41.7	32.5	8.3
Bar, Viennese, Continental, Thorntons*	1 Bar/38g	206	13	542	4.2	54	34.2	0.8
Bar, White, Thorntons*	1 Bar/50g	274	15.6	547	6.5	59.5	31.3	0
Bars, Alpini, Continental, Thorntons*	1 Bar/36g	192	11.4	538	6.9	55.3	32	2.7
Bars, Baby Ruth, Candy, NestlÃƒÂ©*	1 Bar/60g	296	14.1	494	6.7	63.9	23.5	1.7
Bars, Bubbles, Galaxy, Mars*	1 Bar/31g	172	10.6	555	6.5	54.7	34.2	1.5
Bars, Chocolate, Pistacho, Lindt*	1 Bar/100g	585	40.6	585	7.1	48.2	40.6	0
Bars, Chocolate, Strawberry, Lindt*	1 Bar/100g	470	22.8	470	4.5	61.6	22.8	0
Bars, Milk Chocolate, Galaxy, Mars*	1 Bar/42g	229	13.6	546	6.7	56	32.4	1.5
Bars, Milk Chocolate, Gold, Lindt*	1 Bar/300g	1605	92.9	535	6.6	58.7	31	0
Bars, Milk Chocolate, Hazelnut, Gold, Lindt*	1 Bar/300g	1665	108.2	555	7.9	50.7	36.1	0
Bars, Milk Chocolate, Hazelnut, Lindt*	1 Bar/100g	570	38.8	570	8.5	47	38.8	0
Bars, Milk Chocolate, Lindt*	1 Bar/100g	622	47	622	4.6	44	47	0
Bars, Milk Chocolate, Raisin & Hazelnut, Lindt*	1 Bar/100g	530	31.6	530	3.1	54.7	31.6	0
Beans, Coffee, Dark, Solid, M&S*	1 Serving/10g	53	3.8	532	4.7	42.4	37.6	11.6
Bear, Lindt*	1 Bear/11g	60	3.6	572	7.5	57.7	34.6	0
Belgian Milk, TTD, Sainsbury's*	1 Piece/10g	55	3.5	549	9.6	48.3	35.3	2
Belgian, Kschocolat*	4 Pieces/40g	212	12.2	530	6	57.5	30.5	2.3
Belgian, Milk, Mini Eggs, M&S*	1 Egg/8g	43	2.5	535	7	55.8	31.7	2.7
Bloc, Hazelnut, Green & Black's*	1 Bloc/20g	116	8	578	6.8	43	40	7.4
Blueberry Intense, Excellence, Lindt*	1 Serving/40g	200	12.4	500	6	50	31	0
Bubbly Santa, M&S*	1 Santa/23g	124	7.3	540	7	55.8	31.7	2.7
Bubbly, Dairy Milk, Cadbury*	1 Bar/35g	185	10.5	525	7.7	56.9	29.7	0.7
Bunny, Easter, Mars*	1 Bunny/29g	155	9.2	535	6.2	56.2	31.7	0
Bunny, Lindt*	1 Bunny/11g	60	3.6	572	7.5	57.5	34.6	0
Buttons, Dairy Milk, Cadbury*	1 Pack/32g	170	9.7	525	7.7	56.7	29.9	0.7
Buttons, Dark, Giant, 58%, Organic, Montezuma's*	5 Buttons/15g	82	5.7	547	5	45	38	7
Buttons, Free From, Tesco*	1 Bag/25g	136	8.8	544	2.5	48.4	35	12.5
Buttons, Maltesers, Mars*	1 Bag/32g	166	8.6	518	7.4	60	27	0
Buttons, Salted Caramel, Waitrose*	¼ Pack30g	155	9.2	517	5.4	54.1	30.5	2.2
Caramel, Chunk, Dairy Milk, Cadbury*	1 Chunk/33g	158	7.6	480	5	63	23	0

CHOCOLATE

	Measure INFO/WEIGHT	per Measure KCAL	FAT	Nutrition Values per 100g / 100ml KCAL	PROT	CARB	FAT	FIBRE
Caramel, Dairy Milk, Cadbury*	1 Bar/45g	215	10.4	480	4.9	62.8	23.2	0.4
Caramel, Irresistibly Smooth, Lindor, Lindt*	1 Bar/100g	625	48	625	4.7	43	48	0
Caramelles, Mister Choc, Lidl*	1/5 Pack/25g	120	5.1	482	4.2	69	20.5	2.2
Chips, Dark, The Pantry, Aldi*	1 Serving/25g	126	6.5	505	3.8	60	26	6.1
Chips, Extra Dark, 63%, Guittard*	1/3 Cup/60g	280	19.8	467	6.7	53	33	13.3
Chips, Milk, Tesco*	¼ Pack/25g	141	8.8	563	5.9	55.1	35	1.9
Choco Roll, Biscolata*	1 Bar/28g	155	9.2	553	6	58	33	0
Chocolat Noir, Lindt*	1/6 Bar/17g	87	5.4	510	6	50	32	0
Chocolate Favourites, Tesco*	½ Box/227g	1015	43.6	447	4.2	64.3	19.2	0.3
Chomp, Cadbury*	1 Bar/24g	112	4.8	465	3.3	67.9	20	0.2
Christmas Tree Decoration, Average	**1 Chocolate/12g**	**63**	**3.6**	**522**	**7.6**	**56.4**	**29.9**	**0.4**
Christmas Tree Decoration, Cadbury*	1 Piece/12g	60	3.4	525	7.6	56.2	29.9	0
Chunk Bar, Dairy Milk, Cadbury*	1 Chunk/7g	35	2	525	7.5	57	29.8	0.1
Clusters, White, Coconut, Free From, Sainsbury's*	1 Pack/55g	302	18.3	549	2.4	57.6	33.3	4.6
Coco Mylk, Raw, Bar, Ombar*	1 Bar/35g	208	15.9	594	6.8	43.9	45.5	8
Cocoa Fudge, Hotel Chocolat*	1 Bar/45g	170	6.3	378	1.8	62.1	13.9	2.1
Coconut, White, Excellence, Lindt*	1 Square/10g	61	4.4	610	6	48	44	0
Coins, Marzipan, & Cherry , Favorina, Lidl*	1 Serving/30g	132	5.7	439	5.3	58	19	3.3
Coins, Marzipan, Plum, & Madeira, Favorina, Lidl*	1 Serving/30g	131	6	437	5.4	53	20	4.9
Coins, Milk, Sainsbury's*	1 Coin/5g	26	1.4	502	5.5	58.8	27.1	2.5
Creme Egg, Twisted, Cadbury*	2 Chocolates/21g	96	3.8	458	3.5	70	18	1.3
Crispies, Chunk, Dairy Milk, Cadbury*	1 Chunk/31g	158	8.5	510	7.6	58.6	27.4	0
Crispies, Dairy Milk, Cadbury*	1 Bar/49g	250	13.4	510	7.6	58.6	27.4	0
Crispy, Sainsbury's*	4 Squares/19g	99	5.4	521	9.1	56.9	28.5	2.1
Dairy Milk with Oreo, Dairy Milk, Cadbury*	3 Chunks/15g	85	5.4	560	6.1	53.5	35.5	0.7
Dairy Milk, 30% Less Sugar, Dairy Milk, Cadbury*	1 Sm Bar/35g	176	10.8	503	5.8	42	31	18
Dairy Milk, Cadbury*	1 Bar/45g	242	13.6	534	7.3	57	30	2.1
Dairy Milk, Oreo, Mint, Dairy Milk, Cadbury*	3 Chunks/15g	84	5.2	557	5.9	54	35	1.5
Dairy Milk, Toffee Popcorn, Dairy Milk, Cadbury*	1 Bar/150g	765	39.8	510	7	59.5	26.5	1.7
Dark + Nibs, Artisan, Raw, Raw Halo Ltd*	1 Bar/35g	212	17.6	606	8.3	29.4	50.4	0
Dark with Chilli, Thorntons*	4 Squares/20g	107	7.9	533	7.2	36.3	39.5	10.4
Dark, Finest, 85% Cocoa, Moser Roth, Aldi*	1 Bar/25g	152	12.8	608	11	18	51	15
Dark, 60%, Amazonas, Lidl*	1 Square/13g	75	5.2	574	5.7	44	40	7.5
Dark, 64%, Almonds, Popped Quinoa, Moser Roth, Aldi*	1 Square /10g	57	4.1	573	8.7	39	41	8.4
Dark, 70% Cocoa Solids, Extra Fine, Lindt*	1 Square/10g	54	4.1	537	8	33	41	12.2
Dark, 70% Cocoa Solids, Organic, Green & Black's*	1 Lge Bar/90g	496	37	551	9.3	36	41.1	11.5
Dark, 70% Cocoa Solids, Organic, Morrisons*	½ Bar/50g	266	20.6	531	7.9	31.6	41.1	11
Dark, 70%, with Raspberries, Divine Chocolate*	1 Square/5g	29	2.2	584	6.7	32.2	45	11.3
Dark, 70%, Velvet, Green & Black's*	1 Lrg Bar/90g	557	44.1	619	6.1	33	49	9.7
Dark, 70%, with Almonds, Valor Chocolates*	2 Pieces/15g	84	6.3	562	14	26	42	0
Dark, 75% Cacao, Rausch*	1 Row/31g	163	12.9	522	8.8	28.5	41.1	15
Dark, 85% Cocoa, Excellence, Lindt*	1 Serving/40g	212	18.4	530	11	19	46	16.3
Dark, 85% Cocoa, TTD, Sainsbury's*	1 Serving/25g	149	12.8	596	9.6	16.8	51.4	14.1
Dark, 95% Cocoa, Arriba, J D Gross, Lidl*	1 Square/13g	75	6.5	594	12.5	12.7	51.1	16.7
Dark, 99% Cocoa, Excellence, Lindt*	1 Serving/25g	142	12.5	567	13	8	50	20
Dark, Almond, & Sea Salt, Tony's Chocolonely*	1 Bar/180g	970	63	539	7.4	44	35	0
Dark, Assorted Collection, Velvet, Green & Black's*	1 Piece/10g	61	4.8	612	5.8	35	48	9.2
Dark, Basics, Sainsbury's*	3 Pieces/20g	103	5.8	516	4.4	56.1	29	6.3
Dark, Baton, 100%, Hotel Chocolat*	1 Baton/8g	47	4.2	586	11.9	0	52.9	29.3
Dark, Belgian, Dairy Free, Bitesize Organics*	1 Serving/30g	136	10.5	452	0	36.6	35	0
Dark, Belgian, Extra Special, Asda*	2 Squares/20g	102	8	508	11	26	40	16
Dark, Belgian, Luxury Continental, Sainsbury's*	1 Bar/100g	490	38.7	490	11.1	24.2	38.7	7.4
Dark, Belgian, No Added Sugar, Chocologic*	4 Pieces/13g	58	4.7	432	5.3	18.7	34.8	34.8

CHOCOLATE

	Measure INFO/WEIGHT	per Measure KCAL	FAT	Nutrition Values per 100g / 100ml KCAL	PROT	CARB	FAT	FIBRE
Dark, Bournville, Classic, Cadbury*	1 Bar/45g	238	13.5	530	3.8	59.5	29.9	5.5
Dark, Buttons, Giant, Bourneville, Cadbury*	1 Serving/25g	128	6.8	510	3.9	60	27	6.2
Dark, Chilli, Excellence, Lindt*	1 Serving/40g	202	12.8	506	5.4	49	32	0
Dark, Classic, Bourneville, Cadbury*	4 Squares/25g	125	6.8	505	4.7	58.8	27.3	2
Dark, Co-Op*	1 Bar/50g	252	14.5	505	4	57	29	6
Dark, Discs, Extra Fine, M&S*	1 Disc/5g	29	2.3	589	7.7	31.3	45.6	11.2
Dark, Dominican Republic, 90%, 1, Waitrose*	1 Piece/10g	63	5.5	627	11	15	55	14
Dark, Fair Trade, Co-Op*	1 Bar/45g	214	13	475	4	49	29	6
Dark, Ganache, Belgian, Godiva*	1 Piece/8g	48	3.1	582	6.7	53	37	0
Dark, Goji, Cranberry & Linseed, M&S*	1 Bar/28g	172	11.7	614	12	41.4	41.7	12.6
Dark, Hazelnut Crisp, Mini Bar, Mister Choc, Lidl*	1 Mini Bar/18g	102	6.8	566	7.7	46.2	37.9	4.4
Dark, Ikea*	1 Square/14g	78	5.5	559	8	37	39	0
Dark, Intense, 85% Cocoa, Tesco*	1 Square/10g	58	4.7	585	11.2	22	47	14.7
Dark, Madagascan, 70%, J D Gross, Lidl*	1 Square/10g	56	4.1	562	8.5	33.5	41.2	11.5
Dark, Mint, Intense, Lindt*	1 Square/10g	53	3.2	529	5	51	32	0
Dark, Orange & Almond, Moser Roth, Aldi*	1 Serving/25g	133	8	532	5.9	51	32	7.9
Dark, Orange, Velvet Fruit, Green & Black's*	8 Pieces/26g	127	7.3	490	4.1	52	28	7.9
Dark, Orange, Zesty, Tesco*	2 Squares/20g	111	7.1	554	5.7	50	35.3	6.9
Dark, Plain, 90% Cocoa, Hotel Chocolat*	1 Serving/50g	296	25.6	592	10.2	13.8	51.3	16.2
Dark, Plain, Average	**1oz/28g**	**143**	**7.8**	**510**	**5**	**63.5**	**28**	**2.5**
Dark, Plain, Rich, Co-Op*	1 Bar/200g	1010	58	505	4	57	29	6
Dark, Pure, Artisan, Raw, Raw Halo Ltd*	1 Bar/33g	201	16.9	610	7.7	30.1	51.1	0
Dark, Raspberry, Lost Gardens of Heligan*	1 Pack/37g	204	13.5	550	5.1	45.5	36.6	0
Dark, Raw Organic, Loving Earth*	1 Serving/20g	99	7.9	495	9.3	46.4	39.5	0
Dark, Rich, Tesco*	1 Serving/20g	98	6.1	491	5.8	60	30.4	11.5
Dark, Roasted Almond, Velvet Edition, Green & Black's*	1 Lrg Bar/90g	560	45	622	9.2	29	50	9.4
Dark, Rum & Raisin, Old Jamaica, Bourneville, Cadbury*	4 Chunks/23g	105	5.3	465	4.2	59.6	23.4	2
Dark, Salted Caramel, Les Recettes de L'Atelier, Nestle*	1 Piece/25g	137	8.6	547	7.8	47.2	34.5	7.4
Dark, Seriously Rich, 65%, Waitrose*	1 Sm Bar/30g	169	11.6	562	8.2	40.3	38.6	10.4
Dark, Simply, Lidl*	3 Squares/20g	98	5.6	491	4.6	51	28	8.1
Dark, Smooth, Bar, Galaxy, Mars*	1 Bar/125g	651	42	521	6.2	48	33.6	9.3
Dark, Smooth, No Added Sugar, Sainsbury's*	1 Piece/10g	53	4.2	529	8.2	34.3	42.2	11
Dark, Special, Hershey*	1 Pack/41g	180	12	439	4.9	61	29.3	7.3
Dark, Swiss, Triple Nut, Chunky, M&S*	2 Squares/33g	185	12.2	562	7.1	46.2	37.1	7.2
Dark, Tiddly Pot, Hotel Chocolat*	1 Serving/58g	311	22.4	537	13.9	30.5	38.7	8.7
Dark, Whole Nut, Tesco*	1 Serving/13g	67	4.5	539	6.1	48.3	35.7	6.5
Dark, with Almonds, Green & Black's*	1 Lrg Bar/90g	560	45	622	9.2	29	50	9.4
Dark, with Blood Orange, Godiva*	2 Pieces/15g	76	4.4	509	5.4	60	29	0
Dark, with Coconut, Indian Ocean, 1, Waitrose*	1 Square/10g	60	4.5	599	6	39	45	7
Dark, with Hazelnuts, Waitrose*	2 Squares/12g	70	4.7	561	7.4	43.4	37.6	8.9
Dark, with Mint, Velvet, Green & Black's*	1 Lrg Bar/90g	557	44.1	619	6.1	33	49	9.7
Dark, with Orange, 70% , Ecuador *	1 Square/13g	70	4.9	537	7.3	36	38	11
Dark, with Orange, Co-Op*	2 Squares/20g	108	6.8	540	6.6	47	34	7.3
Dark, with Orange, Lidl*	1 Square/13g	67	4.7	537	7.3	36	38	11
Dark, with Salted Almonds, Benugo*	1 Bar/25g	138	9.2	550	6.1	43.7	37	7
Dark, with Salted Caramel, Velvet, Green & Black's*	1 Lrg Bar/90g	540	40.5	600	5.2	39	45	8.2
Dark, with Scottish Mint, Mackies*	1 Square/6g	31	2	540	7.5	42.7	35	10.5
Dark, with Sea Salt, Velvet, Green & Black's*	1 Lrg Bar/90g	554	44.1	616	6.1	33	49	9.7
Dark, with Strawberry, & Pink Pepper, Godiva*	1 Square/8g	40	2.2	531	7.6	54	30	0
Darker Milk, Galaxy, Mars*	1 Serving/22g	119	7	542	6.1	55	32	0
Darkmilk, Cadbury*	1 Bar/35g	197	13	562	5.8	49	37	4.8
Darkmilk, Salted Caramel, Cadbury*	3 Chunks/14g	77	4.9	551	5.2	52	35	4.3
Darkmilk, with Roasted Almonds, Cadbury*	3 Chunks/14g	79	5.3	567	7.2	45	38	5.3

CHOCOLATE

	Measure INFO/WEIGHT	per Measure KCAL	per Measure FAT	Nutrition Values per 100g / 100ml KCAL	PROT	CARB	FAT	FIBRE
Desserts, Collection, Lily O'briens*	1 Chocolate/12g	61	3.8	505	5.3	57.9	31.6	2.6
Diet, Ritter Sport*	1 Square/6g	25	1.8	412	6	44	30	0
Discovery Collection, Box, Lir Chocolates Ltd*	1 Chocolate/10g	52	3.2	517	5.7	50.2	31.6	4.6
Drops, Plain, Asda*	1 Serving/100g	489	29	489	7	50	29	10
Drops, White for Cooking & Decorating, Sainsbury's*	1oz/28g	152	8.6	544	6.5	60.3	30.8	0
Easter Animals, Smarties, Smarties, Nestle*	1 Serving/21g	112	6.2	534	5	61	29.6	1.3
Egg n Spoon, Mousse Centre, Oreo Pieces, Cadbury*	1 Egg/34g	191	11.9	561	7.1	53	35	1.2
Egg, Caramel, Cadbury*	1 Egg/39g	189	9.7	485	3.9	60	25	1.1
Egg, Charlie Chick, Lindt*	1 Egg/18g	108	7.6	599	5.9	49	42	0
Eggs, M&M's, Mars*	1 Pack/80g	386	16	483	5.2	69	20	0
Eggs, Milk, Mini, Tesco*	1 Serving/14g	73	3.6	520	5.7	65	25.9	1.8
Eggs, Milk, Raspberry, Favorina, Lidl*	1 Egg/19g	86	3.6	453	4.1	64.3	19.1	0
Eggs, Vanilla, Hotel Chocolat*	1 Egg/13g	69	4.7	531	6	45.4	36.1	1.7
Espresso Coffee Kick, 5 Bars, M&S*	1 Bar/12g	77	5.5	644	5.5	46	46.2	11.3
Extra Dark, 70%, Chunks, Dr Oetker*	1 Avg Serving/10g	51	3.9	514	8.5	30	39	3.8
Ferrero Rocher, Ferrero*	1 Chocolate/13g	75	5.3	603	8.2	44.4	42.7	0
Ferrero Rocher, Heart, Ferrero*	1 Chocolate/13g	75	5.3	603	8.2	44.4	42.7	0
Fingers, Milk, Mister Choc, Lidl*	1 Finger/18g	104	6.9	579	6.2	51.7	38.4	0.9
Freddo, Caramel, Dairy Milk, Cadbury*	1 Freddo/19g	93	4.7	490	5.5	60.5	24.8	0.5
Freddo, Dairy Milk, Cadbury*	1 Freddo/18g	95	5.4	530	7.5	57	29.8	0.7
Freddo, Rice Crisps, Dairy Milk, Cadbury*	3 Squares/25g	131	7.1	523	7.4	58.6	28.3	0
Fruit & Nut, Dark, Tesco*	4 Squares/25g	124	7	494	5.8	54.8	27.9	6.5
Fruit & Nut, Dairyfine, Aldi*	4 Squares/25g	131	8	525	8.1	50	32	4.2
Galaxy, Crispy, Galaxy, Mars*	1 Portion/20g	111	6.6	546	6.4	56.7	32.2	0
Ginger, Traidcraft*	1 Bar/50g	212	7.4	424	3.9	68.2	14.8	0
Golden Biscuit Crunch, Dairy Milk, Cadbury*	4 Chunks /25g	135	8.2	545	6.2	55.5	33	0.8
Golf Balls, Milk Chocolate, Lindt*	1 Pack/110g	619	39.5	563	6.5	53.6	35.9	0
Hazelnut Crunch, Choceur, Aldi*	1 Serving/40g	226	14.4	564	9.2	49.7	36	2.4
Hazelnut, Buttercup, LoveRaw*	1 Cup/17g	110	9.5	649	9.4	25	56	0
Jazzies, Mini, Asda*	1 Jazzie/1g	4	0.1	449	3.4	81	12	0.6
Kinder Maxi, Ferrero*	1 Bar/21g	116	7.1	550	10	51	34	0
Kinder Surprise, Ferrero*	1 Egg/20g	110	6.8	552	8.1	52.3	34.2	0
Kinder, Bar, Small, Ferrero*	1 Bar/13g	71	4.4	566	8.7	53.5	35	0
Kinder, Bueno Bar, Milk, Ferrero*	1 Bar/22g	123	8	575	9.2	49.5	37.3	2
Kinder, Bueno, Bar, White, Ferrero*	1 Piece/20g	111	7	572	8.8	53	35.9	0
Kinder, Riegel, Ferrero*	1 Bar/21g	117	7.1	558	10	53	34	0
Lait Intense, Experiences, Cote D'or*	3 Squares/100g	575	40	575	7.2	44.5	40	5
Light & Whippy, Bite Sized, Sainsbury's*	1 Bar/15g	66	2.4	439	3.3	69.7	16.3	0.1
Little Bars, Dairy Milk, Cadbury*	1 Bar/18g	96	5.4	534	7.3	57	30	2.1
Macadamia Nut, Excellence, Lindt*	1 Bar/100g	560	37	560	7	51	37	0
Mandarin & Gubinge, Mylk, Loving Earth*	2 Squares/8g	55	4.4	621	4.6	42.7	50	0
Mars, Bites, Mars*	4 Bites/20g	90	3.3	449	4.1	70.2	16.6	0
Matchmakers, Mint, Cool, Quality Street, Nestle*	4 Sticks/17g	84	3.6	495	3.7	70.6	21.3	2.4
Matchmakers, Mint, Nestle*	1 Stick/4g	20	0.8	477	4.3	69.7	20.1	0.9
Matchmakers, Orange, Nestle*	4 Sticks/17g	84	3.6	492	3.7	70	21.3	2.4
Matchmakers, Yummy Honeycomb, Nestle*	4 Sticks/15g	72	3.1	495	3.7	70.6	21.3	2.4
Medley, Dark, Biscuit & Fudge, Dairy Milk, Cadbury*	1 Piece/9g	52	3.2	555	5.9	54.5	34	2
Milk for Baking, Value, Tesco*	½ Bar/50g	265	14.5	530	6.7	60	29	2.2
Milk with Crisped Rice, Dubble*	1 Bar/40g	211	11.8	528	6.4	59.6	29.4	0
Milk with Honey & Almond Nougat, Swiss, Toblerone*	1 Piece/8g	42	2.4	525	5.4	59	29.5	2.2
Milk with Peanut Butter Filling, Ghirardelli*	1 Serving/45g	250	17	556	8.9	48.9	37.8	2.2
Milk with Raisins & Hazelnuts, Green & Black's*	1 Lrg Bar/90g	500	33.2	556	9.2	46.8	36.9	3.2
Milk with Whole Almonds, Organic, Green & Black's*	1 Lrg Bar/90g	520	38	578	11.8	37.7	42.2	5.2

CHOCOLATE

	Measure INFO/WEIGHT	per Measure KCAL	FAT	Nutrition Values per 100g / 100ml KCAL	PROT	CARB	FAT	FIBRE
Milk, & White, Alpine, Sweet Winter, Milka*	¼ Bar/25g	133	7.4	531	6.2	59.5	29.5	1.6
Milk, 65%, Cocoa Excellence, Lindt*	1 Square/8g	51	4.3	635	8.9	24	54	0
Milk, Almond, Choceur, Aldi*	1 Square/29g	171	12.2	589	13	38	42	3.5
Milk, Average	*1oz/28g*	*146*	*8.6*	*520*	*7.7*	*56.9*	*30.7*	*0.8*
Milk, Bakewell Tart, Kernow*	2 Squares/17g	90	5.4	543	6.5	54	32.8	0
Milk, Bars, M&S*	1 Bar/40g	214	12.8	535	7.8	54	32	1.9
Milk, Belgian, No Added Sugar, Chocologic*	4 Squares/13g	64	4.8	484	7.9	33.7	36.2	17
Milk, Belgian, with Hazelnut, Oyster, Masterpieces, Godiva*	1 Piece/8g	48	3	576	8.2	53	36	0
Milk, Biscuit Sticks, Mikado, Kraft*	1 Stick/2.3g	11	0.5	475	7.8	67	19.8	3.1
Milk, Bubbly, Mister Choc, Lidl*	4 Squares/17g	89	5.3	538	7.9	53.5	32	2.4
Milk, Bubbly, Swiss, M&S*	1 Serving/40g	218	13.7	545	8	52	34.3	2.5
MIlk, Caramel, Sea Salt, Thins, Charbonnel Et Walker*	1 Thin/11g	61	3.6	554	6.4	58.3	32.8	0
Milk, Creamy, 33%, Mini, Whittaker's*	1 Chocolate/15g	84	5.3	562	9.2	51.8	35.6	0
Milk, Creamy, Organic, Green & Black's*	1 Bar/90g	504	32	560	9.1	50.3	35.5	1.6
Milk, Elite*	1/3 Bar/33g	170	10	515	6.1	54.6	30.3	0
Milk, Extra Au Lait, Milch Extra, Lindt*	½ Bar/50g	268	15.5	535	6.5	57	31	0
Milk, Extra Creamy, Excellence, Lindt*	1 Bar/100g	560	37.1	560	6	51.1	37.1	0
Milk, Extra Fine, Swiss, M&S*	1 Serving/25g	141	9.2	565	7.2	50.9	36.7	2.3
Milk, Fair Trade, Tesco*	1 Serving/45g	236	13.3	524	7.6	56.7	29.6	2
Milk, Figures, Hollow, Dairyfine, Aldi*	1 Serving/11g	58	3.2	523	5.5	59.9	29	3.1
Milk, Fin Carre, Lidl*	1 Pack/40g	227	14.6	568	6.2	52.7	36.5	1.9
Milk, Fruit & Nut, Fin Carre, Lidl*	4 Pieces/17g	83	4.5	499	6.4	56.7	26.7	3.4
Milk, Giant Buttons, M&S*	1 Button/8g	44	2.7	550	7.1	52.3	34.2	0.4
Milk, Latte Macchiato, Mini Bar, Mister Choc, Lidl*	1 Mini Bar/18g	106	7.4	588	7.7	46.2	41.2	2.8
Milk, Lindor, Lindt*	1 Square/11g	68	5.2	615	4.7	43	47	0
Milk, Mini Bar, Mister Choc, Lidl*	1 Mini Bar/18g	103	6.6	571	7.1	51.1	36.8	2.8
Milk, No Added Sugar, Choco Logic*	4 Segments/13g	64	4.8	484	7.9	33.7	36.2	17
Milk, Organic, Tesco*	1 Serving/25g	140	9.1	558	6.3	51.4	36.3	2.3
Milk, Rich Coffee, Bar, Tesco*	2 Squares/20g	109	6.4	547	6.6	56.6	32.3	1.7
Milk, Sainsbury's*	4 Squares/25g	133	7.7	533	9.2	54.6	30.8	2.2
Milk, Salted Caramel, Godiva*	1 Square/10g	53	3	524	7.1	57	30	0
Milk, Salted Caramel, Thin, Organic, Green & Black's*	1 Square/12g	67	4.1	550	8.4	51.5	33.5	2.6
Milk, Santas, Tesco*	1 Bag/90g	433	21.8	481	4.5	61.4	24.2	1.4
Milk, Smart Price, Asda*	1 Square/6g	32	1.9	536	8	54	32	1.8
Milk, Strawberry Yogurt, Mini Bar, Mister Choc, Lidl*	1 Mini Bar/18g	102	6.5	566	6	52.8	36.3	2.8
Milk, Swiss, Diabetic with Fruit & Nuts, Boots*	½ Bar/21g	97	6.7	462	7	55	32	2.7
Milk, Swiss, Finest, Tesco*	2 Squares/20g	112	7	558	8.5	50.6	35.2	2.3
Milk, Tesco*	1 Serving/25g	133	7.7	533	9.5	54.7	30.7	2.2
Milk, Tony's Chocolonely*	1 Sm Bar/50g	272	16.6	545	7.7	51.9	33.2	0
Milk, Value, Tesco*	1/6 Bar/16g	83	4.5	520	6.8	60	28	2.3
Milk, Whole Nut, Tesco*	1 Serving/25g	129	8.4	517	8.7	53.4	33.8	9
Milk, Wholenut, with Hazelnuts, Dairyfine, Aldi*	4 Squares/25g	144	9.5	574	8.3	47	38	4.2
Milk, Winnie the Pooh, Solid Shapes, M&S*	1 Chocolate/6g	32	1.9	540	8.1	54.1	32.4	1.3
Milk, with Orange, Divine Chocolate*	1 Sm Bar/35g	189	11	541	6.2	57.3	31.4	1.7
Milk, with Praline Filling, Ritter Sport*	½ Pack/50g	277	17	554	7.3	54	34	0
Milk, with Strawberry Cream, Elite*	1/3 Bar/33g	190	13	576	6.1	51.5	39.4	0
Milk, with Whole Almonds, Ion*	1 Piece/30g	164	10.4	545	11	51	34.5	0
Milky Bar, Giant Buttons, Mars*	1 Sweet/2g	11	0.6	546	7.5	57.7	31.6	0
Mini Eggs, Belgian, Doubly Divine, Moser Roth, Aldi*	1 Egg/11g	57	3.2	516	6.2	55	29	4.5
Mini Eggs, Cadbury*	1 Egg/3g	16	0.7	495	4.6	69.5	21.5	1.3
Mini Eggs, Caramel, Cadbury*	1 Mini Egg/11g	55	2.9	485	5.7	59	25.7	0.4
Mini Eggs, Daim, Cadbury*	1 Egg/11g	60	3.4	535	6.9	56.5	30.5	1.8
Mini Eggs, Golden, Galaxy *	½ Bag/40g	207	10.8	518	6.6	61.3	27	0

C

CHOCOLATE

	Measure INFO/WEIGHT	per Measure KCAL	FAT	Nutrition Values per 100g / 100ml KCAL	PROT	CARB	FAT	FIBRE
Mini Eggs, Lindor, Lindt*	3 Eggs/15g	92	6.8	611	5.4	45	45	0
Mini Eggs, Oreo, Cadbury*	1 Egg/10g	58	3.7	565	5.9	53.5	36	1.3
Mini, Toblerone*	1 Serving/6g	32	1.8	525	5.6	57.5	30	3.5
Mint Chips, Dairy Milk, Cadbury*	1 Bar/49g	247	12.8	505	6.6	61.6	26.1	0.6
Mint Creme, Sainsbury's*	1 Serving/20g	93	4.9	467	2.8	62.7	24.5	2.1
Mint Crisps, M&S*	1 Mint/8g	40	2.4	494	5.4	54.8	29.6	3.1
Mint, Bar, Lindor, Lindt*	1 Bar/38g	232	17.1	611	5.3	45	45	0
Mint, Bubbly, Dairyfine, Aldi*	6 Squares/25g	137	7.8	547	5.7	60	31	0.5
Mint, Fondant Thins, Dark Chocolate, Sainsbury's*	1 Thin/10g	48	2	478	4.9	67.5	19.9	4.6
Mint, Selection, Finest, After Eight, Nestle*	2 Chocolates/14g	65	3	473	4.8	63	22	2.1
Mint, Waves, Choceur, Aldi*	7 Waves/25g	129	7	516	6.4	56	28	6
Mistletoe Kisses, Mars*	1 Pack /42g	209	11.5	498	5.3	57	27.3	0
Mix Mps, Milkybar, Nestle*	1 Pack/33g	175	10.2	538	10	53.2	31.3	1.2
Mountain Bar, Dark, M&S*	1 Bar/100g	572	41.9	572	7.4	36.2	41.9	10.3
Mountain Bar, Fruit & Nut, M&S*	1 Bar/100g	551	34.3	551	7	52.4	34.3	2.5
Mountain Bar, Milk, M&S*	1 Bar/100g	552	33.9	552	6.9	53.8	33.9	2.1
Mountain Bar, White, M&S*	1 Bar/100g	574	36.9	574	6.3	54.1	36.9	0.2
Mylk, Mint Crisp, Artisan, Raw, Raw Halo Ltd*	1 Bar/33g	187	13.9	567	7	41.5	42	0
Mylk, Salted Caramel, Artisan, Raw, Raw Halo Ltd*	1 Bar/32g	198	17.2	618	6.4	28.8	53.6	0
Natural Orange, Excellence, Lindt*	1 Bar/100g	560	37	560	7	50	37	0
Natural Vanilla, Excellence, Lindt*	1 Bar/100g	590	40	590	6	51	40	0
Nibs, Raw, Cacao, Organic, Navitas Naturals*	1 Serving/28g	130	12	464	14.3	35.7	42.9	32.1
NutRageous, Reese's, Hershey*	1 Bar/51g	260	16	510	11.8	54.9	31.4	3.9
Nuts About Caramel, Cadbury*	1 Bar/55g	272	15.1	495	5.8	56.6	27.4	0
Nutty Nougat, Bite Sized, Sainsbury's*	1 Bar/23g	111	5.5	481	7.6	59	23.8	0.6
Orange Cream, Fry's*	1 Bar/50g	210	6.8	420	2.8	72.3	13.7	0
Orange, Bar, Terry's*	1 Bar/40g	210	11.7	530	7.3	58	29.5	2.1
Orange, Dark, Terry's*	1 Segment/9g	45	2.6	511	4.3	57	29.3	6.2
Orange, Milk, Mini Segments, Minis, Terry's*	1 Segment/4g	21	1.1	520	5.8	59.5	28	2.4
Orange, Milk, Terry's*	1 Orange/157g	816	44	520	5.8	59.5	28	2.4
Orange, Plain, Terry's*	1 Orange/157g	801	43.2	510	5.2	55.5	27.5	7.6
Orange, Segsations, Terry's*	1 Segsation/8g	43	2.3	520	6.9	58.5	28.5	2.8
Orange, Tuile, Lindt*	1 Tuile/3g	18	1	513	5	54	29	9.6
Oreo, Bar, Dairy Milk, Cadbury*	1 Bar/41g	226	13.7	550	6	55	33.5	1.6
Oreo, Bites, Dairy Milk, Cadbury*	1 Serving/25g	138	8.2	551	5	57	33	1.5
Oreo, Peanut Butter, Dairy Milk, Cadbury*	1 Chunk/5g	28	1.8	558	5.9	54	35	1.5
Panna Cotta & Raspberry, M&S*	1 Bar/36g	190	12.1	528	4.7	51.4	33.6	0.3
Peanut Butter Cup, Big Cup, Reese's, Hershey*	1 Cup/39g	210	12	538	10.3	53.8	30.8	2.6
Peanut Butter Cup, Mini, Reeses, Hershey*	2 Mini Cups/7g	38	2.1	542	8.8	58.3	30.5	0
Peanut Butter Cup, Miniature, Reese's, Hershey*	1 Cup/9g	44	2.6	500	9.1	59.1	29.6	2.3
Peanut Butter Cup, Reese's, Hershey*	1 Cup/21g	105	6.5	500	11.9	57.1	31	5.9
Peanut Butter Cups, Sugar Free, Reese's, Hershey*	1 Cup/11g	45	3.3	409	6.8	61.4	29.6	13.6
Peanut Butter, Buttercup, LoveRaw*	1 Cup/17g	100	7.3	590	15	32	43	0
Peanut Caramel Crisp, Big Taste, Dairy Milk, Cadbury*	1 Chunk/12g	63	3.9	547	9.8	49	34	2.5
Pen Pals, Hotel Chocolat*	1 Animal/40g	235	16.4	588	7.5	46.2	40.9	1.5
Peppermint Cream, Fry's*	1 Bar/51g	217	7.9	425	2.6	68.8	15.4	0
Peppermint, Fondant, Strong, Fortnum & Mason*	1 Chocolate/14g	58	1.8	413	2.6	71	12.9	0
Peppermint, Ritter Sport*	1 Bar/100g	483	26	483	3	60	26	0
Plain with Hazelnuts, Tesco*	4 Squares/25g	135	8.9	539	6.1	48.3	35.7	6.5
Plain, 72% Cocoa Solids, Finest, Tesco*	1 Square/10g	60	4.4	603	7.7	44	44	3.7
Plain, Belgian, Organic, Waitrose*	1 Bar/100g	505	37.6	505	9.6	32	37.6	5.6
Plain, Dark, Fruit & Nut, Rich, Sainsbury's*	4 Squares/25g	122	7	489	5.2	53.9	27.9	5.7
Plain, Ms Mollys*	1 Bar/100g	520	31	520	5.7	51	31	7

CHOCOLATE

	Measure INFO/WEIGHT	per Measure KCAL	FAT	Nutrition Values per 100g / 100ml KCAL	PROT	CARB	FAT	FIBRE
Plain, Whole Nut, Belgian, Waitrose*	4 Squares/25g	135	9.5	540	6.3	45.4	38	7.8
Plain, with Mint, Tesco*	2 Squares/20g	111	7	557	6.7	50.2	35.2	6.7
Praline, Dizzy, Hotel Chocolat*	1 Chocolate/13g	74	5.4	589	8.3	42.2	43.2	3.9
Praline, M&S*	1 Bar/34g	185	12	545	7.3	49.6	35.2	3.1
Probiotic, Bar, Ohso*	1 Bar/14g	72	5	514	5	47	36	15.5
Puddles, Hazelnut Flavour Filling, Dairy Milk, Cadbury*	¼ Bar/23g	114	6.2	505	6.3	57	27.5	0.9
Rafaello, Roche, Ferrero*	1 Sweet/10g	60	4.7	600	9.7	35.4	46.6	0
Raspberry, & Coconut Ruffles, Jamesons*	1 Serving/26g	120	5	460	2.6	67.3	19.3	3.6
Reese's Pieces, Bite Size, Minis, Hershey*	11 Pieces/39g	200	12	513	7.7	59	30.8	2.6
Reese's, Fast Break, Candy Bar, Hershey*	1 Bar/56g	260	12	464	8.9	62.5	21.4	3.6
Reindeer, Lindt*	1 Reindeer/107g	588	35.3	550	7.2	55	33	0
Rocher Noir, Carrefour*	1 Sweet/35g	195	12.6	557	5.2	51	36	4.3
Rocky Road, Clusters, Tesco*	1 Bite/11g	52	2.2	470	5.6	65.2	20.3	2.1
Salted Butterscotch, Milk, The Best, Morrisons*	2 Squares/20g	112	7.1	558	6.2	53.1	35.3	1.6
Salted Caramel, Buttercup, LoveRaw*	1 Cup/17g	108	8.9	632	6.1	33	52	0
Sharing Block, Smarties, Nestle*	3 Pieces/17g	88	4.8	529	6.6	59.6	28.9	1.8
Smooth Praline, Choceur, Aldi*	1 Square/5g	27	1.6	544	7.8	52	33	3.9
Snack Bar, Kinder*	1 Bar/21g	116	7.1	554	10	52	34	0
Snack Size, Dairy Milk, Cadbury*	1 Bar/30g	159	9	530	7.8	57.1	29.9	0
Snickers, More Nuts, Snickers*	1 Bar/58g	299	17.3	515	10.1	52.8	29.8	0
Snowman, Mousse, Dairy Milk, Cadbury*	1 Snowman/29g	162	10.2	560	6.7	54.5	35	0.4
Tasters, Dairy Milk, Cadbury*	1 Bag/45g	238	13.7	530	7.6	56.4	30.5	0
Tasting Selection, Green & Black's*	1 Piece/15g	85	5.8	567	9	41	39	6.7
Teddy Bear, Milk Chocolate, Thorntons*	1 Teddy/250g	1358	83.8	543	7.6	52.6	33.5	1
Tempties, GF, Schar*	1 Tempties/14g	80	5.2	569	8.2	48	37	3.6
Tiffin, Honeycomb, Hare-Brained, McVitie's*	1 Slice/41g	197	9.3	480	4.2	64	22.6	2
Tiffin, Limited Edition, Dairy Milk, Cadbury*	6 Chunks/24g	120	6	502	6.7	60	25	2.1
Toffee Wholenut, Moments, Milka*	1 Moment/9g	49	3.1	555	6	52	35	2
Toffee, Wholenut, Big Taste, Dairy Milk, Cadbury*	4 Chunks/33g	184	11.9	557	6.3	51	36	1.8
Toffifee, Storck*	1 Sweet/8g	43	2.4	516	5.9	58.5	28.7	0
Treatsize, Dairy Milk, Cadbury*	1 Bar/14g	73	4.2	525	7.5	57	29.8	0.7
Truffles, Belgian, Flying Tiger*	1 Truffle/10g	56	3.8	562	3.8	49	38	0
Truffles, Dark, Peppermint, Super Thin, Hotel Chocolat*	1 Truffle/9g	49	3.6	537	6.5	35	39.4	8
Turkish Delight, Dairyfine, Aldi*	3 Squares/25g	119	6	475	3.4	62	24	0.5
Turkish Delight, Lge Bar, Dairy Milk, Cadbury*	1 Square/8g	35	1.6	470	5.6	63.2	21.4	0.5
Twirl, Bites, Cadbury*	1 Bite/2g	11	0.6	530	7.7	56.5	30.3	0.8
Vanilla, Madagascan, Moser Roth, Aldi*	1 Bar/25g	148	10.2	590	8.3	48	41	0.5
Vanilla, Nestle*	1 Whip/28g	137	6.6	493	5.4	63.2	23.9	1.3
Wafer, Bar, Time Out, Cadbury*	1 Bar/21g	111	6.1	527	6.7	60	29	2.1
Whips, Double Chocolate, M&S*	1 Whip/29g	140	7.3	485	6.6	57.8	25.3	1
White with Honey & Almond Nougat, Toblerone*	1 Serving/25g	132	7.2	530	6.2	60.5	29	0.2
White with Strawberries, Divine*	1 Piece/3g	16	0.9	534	7.6	59.9	29.3	0.1
White, Average	**1oz/28g**	**148**	**8.7**	**529**	**8**	**58.3**	**30.9**	**0**
White, Creamy Vanilla, Green & Black's*	1 Lge Bar/90g	516	32.9	573	7.4	53.5	36.6	0.1
White, Creamy, Aldi*	1 Bar/40g	220	13.2	551	5.5	58	33	0
White, Creamy, Tesco*	1 Serving/25g	139	8.7	557	5.1	55.7	34.9	3.3
White, Crispy, Fair Trade, Co-Op*	½ Bar/50g	278	17.5	555	9	51	35	0.1
White, Nestle*	4 Pieces/40g	220	13	550	7.5	55	32.5	0
White, Protein Crunchers, Yumm*	1 Bag/23g	96	4.6	417	23	43	20	0
White, Value, Tesco*	1 Serving/10g	55	3.1	548	4.7	62	31.2	0
Whole Nut, Dairy Milk, Cadbury*	1 Bar/49g	270	17.4	550	8.9	49.5	35.4	1.7
Whole Nut, Sainsbury's*	4 Chunks/25g	142	9.4	566	8.5	48.5	37.6	2.6
Wildlife Bar, Cadbury*	1 Bar/21g	109	6.2	520	7.8	56.8	29.3	0

C

	Measure INFO/WEIGHT	per Measure KCAL	per Measure FAT	Nutrition Values per 100g / 100ml KCAL	PROT	CARB	FAT	FIBRE
CHOCOLATE								
Wispa, Bitsa Wispa, Cadbury*	¼ Bag/43g	238	14.7	550	7.3	53	34	0.9
with Creme Egg, Dairy Milk, Cadbury*	1 Bar/45g	210	9.3	470	5.2	64.8	20.9	0.5
with Crunchie Bits, Dairy Milk, Cadbury*	1 Bar/200g	1000	48.8	500	6.2	63.3	24.4	0
with Hazelnuts, Whole, Milka*	2 Squares/15g	83	5.3	554	8.1	50	35.5	2
with Shortcake Biscuit, Dairy Milk, Cadbury*	1 Square/6g	31	1.7	520	7.5	59	28	0
CHOCOLATE NUTS								
Peanuts, Assorted, Thorntons*	1 Bag/140g	785	57.1	561	13.8	34.8	40.8	3.6
Peanuts, Belgian Coated, M&S*	1 Serving/20g	109	7.6	545	14.7	35.6	38	5.8
Peanuts, Milk, Tesco*	1 Bag/227g	1221	86	538	17.5	31.8	37.9	4.4
CHOCOLATE RAISINS								
Californian, Tesco*	½ Bag/57g	268	11.7	472	5.2	66.2	20.7	1.3
Co-Op*	½ Pack/50g	205	7.5	410	4	64	15	1
Milk Chocolate Coated, Average	***1 Serving/50g***	***207***	***7.7***	***415***	***4.4***	***64.6***	***15.4***	***2***
Milk, Asda*	1 Serving/28g	120	4.2	430	5.1	66.4	15.1	4.2
Milk, Tesco*	1 Lge Bag/227g	933	35	411	4.8	63.3	15.4	0.9
CHOCOLATE SPREAD								
& Caramel, Gu*	1 Serving/25g	153	11.5	613	4.2	45	46	2
Average	***1 Tsp/12g***	***68***	***4.5***	***569***	***4.1***	***57.1***	***37.6***	***0***
Hazelnut, Jim Jams*	1 Tbsp/15g	74	5.5	494	6.4	49.4	36.6	0
Hazelnut, Nutella, Ferrero*	1oz/28g	149	8.7	533	6.6	56.4	31	3.5
Hazelnut, Sainsbury's*	1 Serving/12g	67	4.2	555	6	53.5	34.5	3
Hazelnut, Weight Watchers*	1 Serving/15g	50	1.8	333	4.7	45.3	12	12
La Crema, Vegan, Valsoia*	1 Serving/15g	77	4.2	514	5.2	57	28	6.8
Luxury, Atkins & Potts*	1 Tbsp/25g	115	7.1	459	6.3	46.6	28.3	2
with Nuts	***1 Tsp/12g***	***66***	***4***	***549***	***6.2***	***60.5***	***33***	***0.8***
CHOCOLATES								
All Gold, Dark, Terry's*	1 Serving/30g	152	8.7	505	4	57.5	29	4.3
All Gold, Milk, Terry's*	1 Serving/30g	158	9.2	525	4.8	58	30.5	1.5
Almond Marzipan, Milk Chocolate, Thorntons*	1 Chocolate/13g	60	2.9	464	6.6	59.4	22.6	5.6
Almond Mocca Mousse, Thorntons*	1 Chocolate/14g	76	5.3	543	8.5	40.7	37.9	2.9
Alpini, Thorntons*	1 Chocolate/13g	70	4.2	538	7	54.6	32.3	2.3
Bittermint, Bendicks*	1 Mint/18g	80	3	440	4.3	68.9	16.3	2.4
Cafe Au Lait, from Continental Selection, Thorntons*	1 Chocolate/16g	77	4	481	5.3	58.1	25	0.6
Cappuccino, from Continental Selection, Thorntons*	1 Chocolate/13g	70	4.7	538	5.9	48.5	36.2	0.8
Caramels, Sainsbury's*	1 Sweet/12g	57	2.6	490	3.5	69	22.2	0.2
Celebrations, Mars*	1 Sweet/8g	40	2	497	5.6	61.7	25	1.7
Champagne Truffles, Milk, The Best, Morrisons*	1 Truffle/12g	57	2.9	479	5.2	57.9	24.8	1.4
Coconut, Lindor, Lindt*	1 Ball/13g	79	6	632	5.4	42	48	0
Coffee Cream, Average	***1 Chocolate/12g***	***54***	***2***	***446***	***3.3***	***70.4***	***17***	***2.4***
Coffee Creme, Dark, Thorntons*	1 Chocolate/13g	52	1.4	400	3	71.5	10.8	0.8
Coffee Creme, Milk, Thorntons*	1 Chocolate/13g	52	1.3	400	2.8	74.6	10	0.8
Continental, Belgian, Thorntons*	1 Chocolate/13g	67	3.9	514	5.8	53.5	30.3	2.9
Continental, Thorntons*	1 Chocolate/15g	76	4.4	506	5.6	54.5	29.3	2.7
Country Caramel, Milk, Thorntons*	1 Chocolate/9g	45	2.4	500	4.6	62.2	26.7	0
Dairy Box, Milk, Nestle*	1 Piece/11g	50	2.1	456	4.4	65.9	19.4	0.7
Dark, Rose & Violet Creams	***1 Chocolate/13g***	***55***	***1.6***	***422***	***2.2***	***76.1***	***12.5***	***1.7***
Dark, Swiss Thins, Lindt*	1 Pack/125g	681	46.2	545	4.8	49.2	37	0
Eclipse, Truffle, Plain, Dark, Montezuma*	1 Truffle/16g	93	8.5	581	0.6	21.9	53.1	0
Filled, Average	***1 Chocolate/13g***	***58***	***2.8***	***447***	***4.9***	***62.9***	***21.3***	***1.3***
Heroes, Cadbury*	1 Sweet/8g	38	1.8	480	4.8	65.1	22.4	0.4
Italian Collection, Amaretto, M&S*	1 Chocolate/13g	60	3.1	480	4.4	59.7	25.1	2.3
Italian Collection, Favourites, M&S*	1 Chocolate/14g	74	4.7	530	5.7	50.4	33.7	1.6
Italian Collection, Panna Cotta, M&S*	1 Chocolate/13g	70	4.7	545	5.3	49.4	36.4	0.1

CHOCOLATES

INFO/WEIGHT	Measure KCAL	FAT	KCAL	PROT	CARB	FAT	FIBRE
Lemon Selector In White Chocolate, Hotel Chocolat*	1 Sphere /5g	26	1.8	525	6	47.2	35.5	0
Liqueurs, Brandy, Asda*	1 Chocolate/8g	34	1.4	409	4	60	17	0.8
Liqueurs, Brandy, Favorina, Lidl*	1 Keg/12g	53	2.6	444	1.7	54.3	21.4	0
Liqueurs, Cherry, Mon Cheri, Ferrero*	1 Chocolate/11g	50	2.2	455	3	52.8	20.3	0
Liqueurs, Cognac Truffle, Thorntons*	1 Chocolate/14g	65	3.8	464	7.3	40	27.1	2.9
Liqueurs, Cointreau, Plain, Barrels	*1 Chocolate/10g*	*44*	*1.8*	*435*	*3.5*	*57*	*18*	*0*
Milk & White, Penguins, Cocoa Loco*	1 Chocolate/11g	63	4.1	572	6.5	52.3	37.2	0
Milk Tray, Cadbury*	1 Chocolate/9g	47	2.4	495	4.7	61.5	25.8	0.7
Milk, Mini Eggs, Green & Black's*	1 Mini Egg/8g	42	2.7	562	8.6	48.3	35.5	3.8
Milk, Swiss Thins, Lindt*	1 Pack/125g	688	43.3	550	5.8	53.6	34.6	0
Mini Eggs, Godiva*	1 Egg/11g	58	3.4	519	5.5	56	30	0
Mini Eggs, Mix, Cadbury*	1 Pack/276g	1419	74.5	514	1.6	60	27	1.6
Mini Eggs, with Soft White Truffle Centre, M&S*	1 Egg/6g	33	2	550	6.5	56.3	33.9	1.4
Mint Creams, Dark, Smooth & Fragrant, Waitrose*	1 Sweet/10g	42	0.9	410	3	77.9	9.1	2.4
Mint Crisp, Bendicks*	1 Mint/8g	38	2.3	494	5.2	55	29.9	0
Mint Crisp, Dark, Elizabeth Shaw*	1 Chocolate/6g	27	1.2	458	1.9	68	20.7	0
Mint Crisp, Milk, Elizabeth Shaw*	1 Chocolate/6g	30	1.3	493	4	70.9	21.4	0
Mint Crisp, Thorntons*	1 Chocolate/7g	34	2.2	486	7.7	40	31.4	4.3
Mint, Collection, Thorntons*	¼ Sm Box16g	83	4.8	516	4.9	54	30	0
Mints, After Eight, Dark, Nestle*	1 Sweet/7g	32	0.9	461	5	63	12.9	2
Mints, After Eight, Straws, Nestle*	1 Sweet/5g	24	1.4	526	5.1	56.6	31	4
Misshapes, Assorted, Cadbury*	1 Chocolate/8g	41	2.3	515	5.2	57.5	29.1	0
Moments, Thorntons*	1 Chocolate/7g	37	2	511	5.4	59.9	27.8	1.9
Neapolitans, No Added Sugar , Chocologic*	3 Chocolates/14g	66	5.1	472	8.8	27.8	36.2	22
Orange Cream, Average	*1 Chocolate/12g*	*53*	*2*	*440*	*3.2*	*69.3*	*16.7*	*0*
Orange Crisp, Elizabeth Shaw*	1 Chocolate/6g	29	1.3	478	2.9	68.2	21.5	0
Peppermint Cream, Average	*1 Chocolate/12g*	*50*	*1.4*	*418*	*1.9*	*76.4*	*11.4*	*1.6*
Praline, Coffee, Thorntons*	1 Chocolate/7g	37	2.4	529	7	47.1	34.3	2.9
Praline, Hazelnut, Thorntons*	1 Chocolate/5g	27	1.8	540	7	48	36	4
Praline, Marzipan, Thorntons*	1 Chocolate/14g	63	3	450	5.9	58.6	21.4	2.1
Praline, Roast Hazelnut, Thorntons*	1 Chocolate/13g	70	4.4	538	6	51.5	33.8	3.1
Quality Street, Nestle*	1 Sweet/9g	44	1.9	470	3.5	67.3	20.5	1.5
Roses, Cadbury*	1 Chocolate/9g	41	1.9	480	3.3	66	22.5	1.3
Sea Shells, Belgian, Guylian*	1 Shell/11g	62	3.8	550	7.6	52	34	0
Seashells, Milk & White, Belgian, Waitrose*	1 Serving/15g	77	4.6	511	5	53.1	31	2.8
Stars, Mini Wishes, Truffle Centre, Cadbury*	1 Star/13g	70	4.1	540	6.9	55.6	31.8	1.3
Strawberries & Cream, Thorntons*	1 Chocolate/12g	64	3.9	533	5.1	54.2	32.5	0.8
Swiss Tradition, De Luxe, Lindt*	1 Pack/250g	1388	90.7	555	6.3	51.9	36.3	0
Swiss Tradition, Mixed, Lindt*	1 Pack/392g	2215	149.4	565	6.1	49.8	38.1	0
Truffle, Amaretto, Thorntons*	1 Chocolate/14g	66	3.6	471	5.5	55	25.7	2.9
Truffle, Balls, Swiss Milk Chocolate, Waitrose*	1 Chocolate/13g	78	5.8	621	4.1	47	46	1.4
Truffle, Belgian Milk, Waitrose*	1 Truffle/14g	74	4.8	525	5.8	52.9	34.1	1.2
Truffle, Belgian, Flaked, Tesco*	1 Truffle/14g	80	5.4	575	4.4	52.7	38.5	2.3
Truffle, Brandy, Thorntons*	1 Chocolate/14g	68	3.8	486	6.1	52.1	27.1	0.7
Truffle, Caramel Milk Chocolate, Aldi*	1 Truffle/12g	76	5.8	633	5.8	42.5	48.3	4.2
Truffle, Caramel, Thorntons*	1 Chocolate/14g	67	3.6	479	4.2	57.9	25.7	2.1
Truffle, Champagne, Premier, Thorntons*	1 Chocolate/17g	88	5.6	518	6.9	45.3	32.9	2.4
Truffle, Cherry, Thorntons*	1 Chocolate/14g	58	3	414	4.2	50.7	21.4	1.4
Truffle, Continental Champagne, Thorntons*	1 Chocolate/16g	78	4.5	488	6.1	51.3	28	0.6
Truffle, Dark, Balls, Lindor, Lindt*	1 Ball/12g	76	6.2	630	3.4	38.5	51.4	0
Truffle, Filled, Swiss, Balls, Finest, Tesco*	3 Balls/37g	240	19	640	5	40.7	50.8	1.5
Truffle, French Cocoa Dusted, Sainsbury's*	1 Truffle/10g	57	4.5	570	4	37	45	0
Truffle, Hazelnut, Balls, Lindor, Lindt*	1 Ball/12g	76	6.1	632	5	39.1	50.6	0

	Measure INFO/WEIGHT	per Measure KCAL	per Measure FAT	KCAL	PROT	CARB	FAT	FIBRE
CHOCOLATES								
Truffle, Hearts, Baileys*	1 Chocolate/15g	76	4.3	506	5.2	52.6	28.9	1.3
Truffle, Lemon, White, Thorntons*	1 Chocolate/14g	63	3.5	450	4.6	64.3	25	0.7
Truffle, Milk Chocolate, Balls, Lindor, Lindt*	1 Ball/12g	75	5.6	623	4.9	44	47	2.8
Truffle, Mini Milk Chocolate Balls, Lindor, Lindt*	3 Balls/15g	90	7	600	6.7	40	46.7	0
Truffle, Rum, Average	**1 Truffle/11g**	**57**	**3.7**	**521**	**6.1**	**49.7**	**33.7**	**1.9**
Truffle, Rum, Thorntons*	1 Chocolate/13g	63	3.2	485	4.8	58.5	24.6	4.8
Truffle, Selection, Tesco*	1 Chocolate/14g	75	4.2	539	5.1	62	29.8	0.5
Truffle, Seville, Thorntons*	1 Chocolate/14g	76	4.7	543	7.1	53.6	33.6	1.4
Truffle, Thorntons*	1 Chocolate/7g	33	1.9	471	6	48.6	27.1	1.4
Truffle, Vanilla, Thorntons*	1 Chocolate/13g	64	3.5	492	4.8	57.7	26.9	1.5
Truffle, Viennese, Dark, Thorntons*	1 Chocolate/10g	53	3.6	530	5.9	47	36	3
Truffle, Viennese, Milk, Thorntons*	1 Chocolate/10g	56	3.6	560	4.9	54	36	0
Truffle, White Chocolate, Balls, Lindor, Lindt*	1 Ball/12g	76	5.9	636	3.7	45	49	0
Twilight, Dark with Mint, Terry's*	1 Chocolate/6g	33	1.9	530	3.1	59.5	30.5	4.2
Winter Selection, Thorntons*	1 Chocolate/10g	51	3.1	506	6.2	51.3	30.6	3.8
CHOP SUEY								
Chicken with Noodles, Sainsbury's*	1 Pack/300g	300	7.5	100	5.7	13.6	2.5	1.2
Vegetable, M&S*	½ Pack/150g	90	6.1	60	2	3.1	4.1	2.9
CHOW MEIN								
Beef, Aldi*	1 Pack/391g	430	12.9	110	13	7.3	3.3	0.5
Beef, Ready Meal, Average	**1 Serving/400g**	**422**	**12.2**	**106**	**6**	**13.4**	**3**	**1**
Beef, Sainsbury's*	1 Pack/450g	500	11.2	111	6.6	15.5	2.5	0.8
Chicken, & Vegetable, Fuller Longer, M&S*	1 Pack/380g	266	4.9	70	6.3	8.7	1.3	2.1
Chicken, & Vegetable, COU, M&S*	1 Pack/380g	262	3.8	69	6.6	7.4	1	1.9
Chicken, & Vegetable, Slim Cook, Tesco*	1 Pack/490g	304	2.5	62	5.9	7.6	0.5	1.9
Chicken, Chinese Takeaway, Tesco*	1 Serving/350g	294	8.4	84	8.1	7.5	2.4	1.1
Chicken, Co-Op*	1 Pack/300g	270	9	90	8	9	3	0.9
Chicken, COU, M&S*	1 Pack/200g	170	5.4	85	5.9	9.5	2.7	1.4
Chicken, High Protein, Musclefood*	1 Pot/308g	293	5.9	95	9.8	9.4	1.9	0.7
Chicken, Less Than 3% Fat, BGTY, Sainsbury's*	1 Pack/400g	292	6.2	75	5.9	7.8	1.6	2.7
Chicken, Meal for Two, Meal Box, Tesco*	½ Pack/183g	221	4.8	120	9.4	13.7	2.6	2.2
Chicken, Microwaved, Slimzone, Asda*	1 Pack/475g	342	3.3	72	7.4	8.4	0.7	1.5
Chicken, Morrisons*	1 Pack/400g	368	9.2	92	5.8	13	2.3	1.1
Chicken, Noodle, G&B, Asda*	1 Pack/371g	356	10	96	5.8	11	2.7	1.9
Chicken, Noodle, Pot, Tesco*	1 Pack/262g	280	8.1	107	6.4	12.4	3.1	2
Chicken, Ready Meal, Average	**1 Serving/400g**	**375**	**9.4**	**94**	**6.5**	**11.5**	**2.4**	**1.2**
Chicken, Serves 1, Sainsbury's*	1 Pack/450g	432	11.2	96	7.8	9.5	2.5	2.6
Chicken, Taste of China, Frozen, Tesco*	1 Pack/355g	361	4.3	102	7.5	14.6	1.2	1.2
Chicken, Taste of China, Tesco*	1 Pack/372g	398	11.5	107	8.7	10.3	3.1	1.6
Pork, PB, Waitrose*	½ Pack/310g	332	2.8	107	7.6	17.2	0.9	1.6
Prawn, Takeaway, Chinese	**1 Portion/550g**	**792**	**60**	**144**	**5.6**	**6.1**	**10.9**	**2.8**
Special, COU, M&S*	1 Pack/400g	400	15.2	100	6.6	10.3	3.8	1.4
Special, Ready Meal, Average	**1 Serving/400g**	**383**	**9.7**	**96**	**6.5**	**12.1**	**2.4**	**1**
Special, Takeaway, Morrisons*	1 Pack/350g	399	11.2	114	7.4	12.7	3.2	2.4
Vegetable, Asda*	½ Pack/200g	174	5	87	2.5	13	2.5	2.1
Vegetable, Cantonese, Stir Fry, Sainsbury's*	¼ Pack/100g	85	3.8	85	2.2	10.6	3.8	1.2
Vegetable, Chinese Favourites Box, M&S*	½ Pack/100g	93	1.5	93	3.3	15.7	1.5	1.9
Vegetable, Ready Meal, Average	**1 Serving/400g**	**337**	**6.7**	**84**	**4.2**	**12.8**	**1.7**	**2**
Vegetable, Taste of China, Tesco*	½ Pack/120g	132	4.8	110	2.7	14.8	4	2
CHRISTMAS PUDDING								
Alcohol Free, 450g, Sainsbury's*	1 Serving/114g	330	3.5	290	2.7	61.3	3.1	3.2
Average	**1oz/28g**	**81**	**2.7**	**291**	**4.6**	**49.5**	**9.7**	**1.3**
BGTY, Sainsbury's*	1 Serving/114g	302	2.8	266	2.8	58.2	2.5	4.6

	Measure INFO/WEIGHT	per Measure KCAL	FAT	Nutrition Values per 100g / 100ml KCAL	PROT	CARB	FAT	FIBRE
CHRISTMAS PUDDING								
Connoisseur, Holly Lane, Aldi*	1 Pudding/100g	303	4.9	303	2.3	61	4.9	3.6
Gluten & Wheat Free, Finest, Tesco*	1 Pudding/100g	305	7.1	305	3.3	55.1	7.1	3.7
Hidden Clementine, Heston, Waitrose*	1 Serving/114g	352	7.7	310	2.9	57.8	6.8	3.1
Individual, 6 Month Matured, Sainsbury's*	1 Pudding/100g	309	5.3	309	2.4	60.8	5.3	4
Light & Fruity, 450g, Sainsbury's*	¼ Pudding/113g	331	5.3	293	1.8	59.3	4.7	3.4
Luxury	*1 Serving/114g*	*416*	*18.8*	*365*	*2.5*	*48.6*	*16.4*	*1*
Luxury, Tesco*	¼ Pudding/114g	346	11	305	3.7	50.8	9.7	1.3
Matured, Finest, Tesco*	1 Serving/113g	340	8.3	300	3.2	54.1	7.3	2.5
Nut Free & Alcohol Free, Tesco*	1 Serving/114g	395	7.6	347	2.2	68.2	6.7	2.6
Rich Fruit, Tesco*	1 Serving/114g	331	6.7	290	2.4	55	5.9	0
Sticky Toffee, Tesco*	¼ Pudding/114g	372	7.3	326	2.5	64.5	6.4	0.8
Vintage, M&S*	1/8 Pudding/113g	335	6.4	295	2.6	59.8	5.6	1.4
CHUTNEY								
Albert's Victorian, Baxters*	1 Serving/25g	40	0.1	159	1.1	37.9	0.3	1.5
Apple & Pear, TTD, Sainsbury's*	1 Serving/20g	39	0.2	193	0.6	45	0.8	1.7
Apple & Walnut, Waitrose*	1 Serving/20g	49	0.5	243	12	53.8	2.6	3.8
Apple, & Pear, Spiced, M&S*	1 Tbsp/15g	34	0	230	0.8	55.5	0.2	1.6
Apricot, Sharwood's*	1 Tsp/16g	21	0	131	0.6	32	0.1	2.3
Beetroot, & Orange, Extra Special, Asda*	1 Tbsp/15g	20	0.1	136	0.5	32	0.5	1.6
Bengal Spice Mango, Sharwood's*	1 Tsp/5g	12	0	236	0.5	58	0.2	1.2
Caramelised Onion, Sainsbury's*	1 Serving/25g	28	0.4	111	1.1	23.5	1.4	1.1
Caramelised Red Onion, Loyd Grossman*	1 Serving/10g	11	0	111	0.5	27.2	0	0.5
Caramelised Red Onion, Specially Selected, Aldi*	1 Serving/15g	31	0.1	208	1.1	50	0.5	1
Cheese Board, Cottage Delight Ltd*	1 Tbsp/15g	42	0.5	277	1	46.6	3.1	0
Chilli, Wilkin & Sons*	1 Tbsp/15g	39	0	261	0	63	0	0
Cranberry & Caramelised Red Onion, Baxters*	1 Serving/20g	31	0	154	0.3	38	0.1	0.3
Fruit, Spiced, Baxters*	1 Tsp/16g	23	0	143	6	34.8	0.1	0
Fruit, Traditional, M&S*	1oz/28g	43	0.1	155	0.9	37.2	0.3	1.7
Indian Appetisers, Pot, Waitrose*	1 Pot/158g	330	2.2	209	1.8	47.3	1.4	1.8
Lime & Chilli, Geeta's*	1 Serving/25g	69	0.4	277	2	64	1.4	1.9
Mango & Apple, Sharwood's*	1oz/28g	65	0	233	0.4	57.6	0.1	1.1
Mango & Ginger, Baxters*	1 Jar/320g	598	0.6	187	5	45.7	0.2	0.9
Mango & Chilli, Geeta's*	1 Serving/30g	74	0	246	0.5	60.7	0.1	0.2
Mango & Mint, Cofresh*	1 Tbsp/20g	31	0.1	155	1.7	36.4	0.3	2
Mango with Hint of Chilli & Ginger, Waitrose*	1 Serving/20g	52	0	259	0.5	64.2	0	0.7
Mango, Green Label, Sharwood's*	1 Tsp/10g	24	0	241	0.3	59.7	0.1	0.9
Mango, Hot & Spicy, Waitrose*	1 Serving/20g	46	0.1	230	0.6	51.6	0.3	1.8
Mango, Premium, Geeta's*	1 Serving/50g	126	0.1	253	0.8	62	0.2	0.8
Mango, Spicy, Mild, M&S*	1 Tsp/5g	11	0.1	217	0.4	49.3	1.7	1.6
Mango, Spicy, Sainsbury's*	1 Tbsp/15g	33	0.1	222	0.5	53.8	0.5	1.9
Mango, Sweet	*1 Tsp/16g*	*30*	*0*	*189*	*0.7*	*48.3*	*0.1*	*0*
Mango, Tesco*	1 Serving/20g	45	0	224	0.4	55.5	0.1	1.3
Mango, Waitrose*	1 Serving/20g	43	0.3	215	1	49	1.5	2
Mixed Fruit	*1 Tsp/16g*	*25*	*0*	*155*	*0.6*	*39.7*	*0*	*0*
Onion, Vitasia, Lidl*	1 Tbsp/15g	40	0.1	266	0.9	63.1	0.9	0
Peach, Spicy, Waitrose*	1 Serving/20g	43	0.3	215	1	49	1.5	1.5
Peanut, Kit's*	1 Tsp/10g	36	2.1	360	15	31	21	0
Pear, & Cardamom, Harvey Nichols*	1 Tsp/5g	7	0.1	147	0.8	33.6	1.1	0
Pineapple, Coconut, & Lime, Baxters*	1 Tbsp/15g	20	0.4	131	0.5	26.4	2.4	1.3
Ploughman's Plum, The English Provender Co.*	1 Tsp/10g	16	0	160	1.3	38.1	0.2	1.6
Ploughman's, M&S*	1 Tbsp/15g	22	0	150	0.8	34.6	0.3	2.9
Plum & Apple, Classic, Specially Selected, Aldi*	1 Tbsp/15g	25	0.1	166	1	39	0.5	3
Plum, Ploughman's, Tesco*	1 Tsp/5g	8	0	154	1	34.1	0.4	5.3

C

	Measure INFO/WEIGHT	per Measure KCAL	FAT	Nutrition Values per 100g / 100ml KCAL	PROT	CARB	FAT	FIBRE
CHUTNEY								
Spicy Fruit, Baxters*	1 Serving/15g	22	0	146	0.6	35.4	0.2	0
Sticky Fig & Balsamic Chutney, M&S*	1 Servin/25g	57	0.3	228	1.6	49.8	1.3	5.4
Sweet Mango, Patak's*	1 Tbsp/15g	39	0	259	0.3	67.4	0.1	0.7
Sweet Tomato & Chilli, The English Provender Co.*	1 Tsp/10g	19	0	189	0.9	46	0.2	1.7
Tomato	*1 Tsp/16g*	*20*	*0*	*128*	*1.2*	*31*	*0.2*	*1.3*
Tomato & Chilli, Specially Selected, Aldi*	1 Tbsp/15g	21	0.1	138	12	32	0.5	1.3
Tomato & Red Pepper, Baxters*	1 Jar/312g	512	1.2	164	2	38	0.4	1.5
Tomato, Baxters*	1 Tsp/12g	18	0	152	1.1	35.9	0.4	1
Tomato, Mediterranean, Branston*	1 Tbsp/15g	23	0.1	155	1.5	34.6	0.6	1.8
Tomato, Rich, & Sweet, Asda*	1 Serving/15g	18	0.1	123	1.3	25	0.5	6.4
Tomato, Waitrose*	1 Pot/100g	195	0.3	195	1.3	46.8	0.3	0
CIDER								
Apple, Low Alcohol, Sainsbury's*	1 Glass/250ml	75	0.4	30	0.5	5.4	0.2	0
Basics, Sainsbury's*	1 Glass/250ml	200	0	80	0	0	0	0
Berry, Irish, Magner's*	1 Bottle/500ml	215	0	43	0	4.3	0	0
Classic, Low Alcohol, Sheppy's*	1 Serving/200ml	56	0	28	0	0	0	0
Cyder, Organic, Aspall*	1 Serving/200ml	120	0.2	60	0.1	3.1	0.1	0
Cyder, Perronelle's Blush, Aspall*	1 Serving/200ml	122	0.2	61	0.1	5.4	0.1	0.5
Cyder, Premier Cru, Aspall*	1 Serving/200ml	120	0	60	0	3.1	0	0
Cyder, Suffolk, Medium, Aspall*	1 Serving/200ml	134	0	67	0.1	4.4	0	0
Diamond White*	1fl oz/30ml	11	0	36	0	2.6	0	0
Dry, Average	*1 Pint/568ml*	*205*	*0*	*36*	*0*	*2.6*	*0*	*0*
Dry, Strongbow*	1 Bottle/375ml	161	0	43	0	3.4	0	0
Fruit, Mixed, Alcohol Free, Kopparberg*	1 Bottle/500ml	190	2.5	38	0.5	9.2	0.5	0
Gold, Thatchers*	1 Bottle/500ml	230	0	46	0	4.5	0	0
Laid Back, 2.5%, M&S*	1 Can/330ml	125	0	38	0	0	0	0
Light, Bulmers*	1 Can/500ml	140	0	28	0	0.8	0	0
Low Alcohol	*1 Pint/568ml*	*97*	*0*	*17*	*0*	*3.6*	*0*	*0*
Low Alcohol, M&S*	1 Serving/200ml	50	0	25	0	6.5	0	0
Low Alcohol, Sainsbury's*	1 Serving/200ml	62	0	31	0	6.4	0	0
Low Carb, Stowford*	1 Bottle/500ml	140	0	28	0	0.2	0	0
Magner's*	½ Pint/284ml	105	0	37	0	2	0	0
Nordic Berries, Alska*	1 Bottle/500ml	195	0	39	0	1.1	0	0
Organic, Westons*	1 Serving/200ml	96	0	48	0	3.1	0	0
Original, Bulmers*	1 Serving/250ml	105	0	42	0	4	0	0
Original, Gaymers*	1 Bottle/330ml	148	0	45	0	4.7	0	0
Pear, Bulmers*	1 Serving/200ml	86	0	43	0	3.6	0	0
Pear, Magner's*	1 Bottle/568ml	179	0	32	0	0	0	0
Pear, Non Alcoholic, Kopparberg*	1 Bottle/500ml	170	0.5	34	0	8.4	0.1	0
Raspberry, Light, Kopparberg*	1 Can/250ml	85	1.2	34	0.5	2.6	0.5	0
Scrumpy, Average	*1 Serving/200ml*	*93*	*0*	*46*	*0*	*2.3*	*0*	*0*
Scrumpy, Westons*	1 Serving/200ml	94	0	47	0	1.8	0	0
Strawberry & Lime, Non Alcoholic, Kopparberg*	1 Bottle/500ml	205	2.5	41	0.5	10.1	0.5	0
Sweet, Average	*1 Pint/568ml*	*239*	*0*	*42*	*0*	*4.3*	*0*	*0*
Vintage	*1 Pint/568ml*	*574*	*0*	*101*	*0*	*7.3*	*0*	*0*
CINNAMON								
Ground, Average	*1 Tsp/3g*	*8*	*0.1*	*261*	*3.9*	*55.5*	*3.2*	*0*
Stick, Average	*1 Stick/1g*	*3*	*0*	*246*	*3.9*	*77*	*1.5*	*53.1*
CLAMS								
in Brine, Average	*1oz/28g*	*22*	*0.2*	*79*	*16*	*2.4*	*0.6*	*0*
Raw, Average	*20 Sm/180g*	*133*	*1.7*	*74*	*12.8*	*2.6*	*1*	*0*
CLEMENTINES								
Raw, Weighed with Peel, Average	*1 Med/61g*	*22*	*0.1*	*35*	*0.6*	*9*	*0.1*	*1.3*

	Measure INFO/WEIGHT	per Measure KCAL	FAT	Nutrition Values per 100g / 100ml KCAL	PROT	CARB	FAT	FIBRE
CLEMENTINES								
Raw, Weighed without Peel, Average	1 Med/46g	22	0.1	47	0.8	12	0.2	1.7
COCKLES								
Boiled	1 Cockle/4g	2	0	53	12	0	0.6	0
Bottled in Vinegar, Drained	1oz/28g	8	0.1	28	6.3	0	0.3	0
COCKTAIL								
Alcoholic, Juice Based, Average	1 Glass/200ml	464	29.2	232	6.4	18.7	14.6	1.4
Bloody Mary, Average	1 Glass/250ml	86	0	42	0	2.3	0	0.6
Bucks Fizz, Premixed, M&S*	1 Glass/250ml	152	0	61	0	9	0	0
Cosmo, Skinny Brands*	1 Can/250ml	90	0.2	36	0	1.3	0.1	0
Cosmopolitan, Canned, M&S*	1 Serving/200ml	456	0	228	0	22	0	0
Daiquiri, Strawberry, Frozen, Average	1 Glass/250ml	132	0	53	0	14.1	0	0
Grenadine, Orange Juice, Pineapple Juice	1 Serving/200ml	158	0.3	79	0.5	19.2	0.1	0.2
Long Island Iced Tea, Average	1 Glass/250ml	282	0	113	0	13.6	0	0
Mai Tai, Average	1 Serving/200ml	209	0.1	105	0.2	13.9	0.1	0.1
Mojito, Canned, M&S*	1 Can/250ml	208	0	83	0	8.9	0	0
Mojito, Canned, My Cocktail, Manchester Drinks Co.*	1 Can/250ml	150	0	60	0	9.1	0	0
Pina Colada	1 Glass/250ml	592	20	237	1	28	8	0
COCOA								
Nibs, Naturya*	1 Serving/10g	58	5	578	13	18.2	50.3	13.4
COCOA POWDER								
Cadbury*	1 Tbsp/16g	52	3.3	322	23.1	10.5	20.8	0
Dark, Fine, Dr Oetker*	3 Tbsp/25g	89	5.2	357	20	8.9	21	28
Dry, Unsweetened, Average	1 Tbsp/5g	11	0.7	229	19.6	54.3	13.7	33.2
Fairtrade, Co-Op*	1 Tbsp/15g	58	3.3	390	19	12	22	37
Hazelnut, Hotel Chocolat*	1 Pack/35g	37	2	105	4.8	8.7	5.6	0.5
Organic, Green & Black's*	1 Tsp/4g	16	0.8	405	22	19	21	27
Organic, Naturya*	1 Tbsp/15g	56	1.8	370	27	26	12	26
COCONUT								
Chips, Triple Toasted, Straight Up, Urban Fruit*	1 Pack/18g	85	7.5	472	5	14.8	41.6	25
Creamed, Average	1oz/28g	186	19.2	666	6	6.7	68.4	7
Curls, Lightly Salted, Crispy, Ape*	1 Pack/20g	108	7.8	540	6.9	28	39	22
Desiccated, Average	1oz/28g	169	17.4	604	5.6	6.4	62	13.7
Flaked, Neal's Yard*	1 Serving/30g	181	18.6	604	5.3	44.4	62	13.7
Flakes, Unsweetened, Dr Goerg*	1 Serving/100g	686	67	686	7	6	67	15.6
Fresh, Flesh Only, Average	1oz/28g	69	7.1	246	2.2	2.6	25.2	5.1
Ice, Average	1oz/28g	104	3.6	371	1.7	66.7	12.7	2.6
Squares, Tesco*	1 Pack/80g	371	36	464	4.8	4.4	45	11.2
COD								
Baked, Average	1oz/28g	27	0.3	96	21.4	0	1.2	0
Beer Battered, Crispy, Finest, Tesco*	1 Portion/250g	575	35	230	12	13.4	14	1.3
Dried, Salted, Average	1oz/28g	82	0.7	290	62.8	0	2.4	0
Fillet, Battered, Market St, Morrisons*	1 Fillet/137g	313	15	229	10.7	21.3	11	0.8
Fillet, in Batter, Large, Birds Eye*	1 Fillet/120g	276	15.6	230	11	17	13	0.5
Fillet, Lightly Dusted, Salt & Pepper, Sainsbury's*	1 Serving/116g	189	8.3	163	14.3	10	7.2	0.5
Fillet, Pieces, Battered, Morrisons*	½ Pack/92g	171	5.2	186	12.2	20.3	5.7	2.1
Fillets, Battered, Average	1 Fillet/125g	219	10.2	176	12.6	13	8.2	1
Fillets, Battered, Chunky, Frozen, Tesco*	1 Fillet/116g	239	12.1	206	13.6	13.8	10.4	1.5
Fillets, Battered, Extra Large, Tesco*	½ Pack/178g	464	25.3	261	12.2	20.3	14.2	1.4
Fillets, Beer Battered, Jumbo, Frozen, Chip Shop, Youngs*	1 Fillet/136g	307	17.5	226	11.8	15.2	12.9	0.8
Fillets, Breaded, Average	1 Fillet/125g	258	12.2	206	13	16.7	9.8	1
Fillets, Breaded, Chunky, Average	1 Piece/135g	204	8	151	13.7	10.9	5.9	1.4
Fillets, Breaded, Chunky, Seachill*	1 Fish/175g	320	10.5	183	14.2	17	6	0.9
Fillets, Breaded, Large, Oven Baked, Youngs*	1 Fillet/117g	254	12.1	218	11.9	18.8	10.4	1

C

C

COD	Measure INFO/WEIGHT	per Measure KCAL	FAT	Nutrition Values per 100g / 100ml KCAL	PROT	CARB	FAT	FIBRE
Fillets, Breaded, Light, Healthy Range, Average	*1 Fillet/135g*	*209*	*6.9*	*154*	*13.6*	*13.3*	*5.1*	*1.2*
Fillets, Broccoli Mornay, Cooked, Ocean Trader*	½ Pack/155g	142	5.4	92	12	2.4	3.5	1.2
Fillets, Cajun, Lemon, with Roasted Veggies, Hello Fresh*	1 Serving/605g	472	7.9	78	4.9	9.4	1.3	0
Fillets, Chunky, Average	*1 Fillet/198g*	*267*	*7.3*	*135*	*17.1*	*8.2*	*3.7*	*0.8*
Fillets, Chunky, Breaded, Waitrose*	1 Fillet/175g	320	10.5	183	14.2	17	6	0.9
Fillets, in Batter, Chunky, Inspirations, Birds Eye*	1 Fillet/142g	293	15	206	12	15.5	10.6	0.6
Fillets, Skin On, Frozen, Tesco*	1 Fillet/124g	97	0.9	78	18	0	0.7	0
Fillets, Skinless & Boneless, Raw, Average	*1 Fillet/140g*	*137*	*2.4*	*98*	*17.8*	*0*	*1.8*	*0.4*
Fillets, Smoked, Average	*1 Serving/150g*	*152*	*2.4*	*101*	*21.6*	*0*	*1.6*	*0*
Fillets, Tempura, Battered, Crispy, Gastro, Youngs*	1 Fillet/131g	252	12.1	192	12.9	14.1	9.2	0.8
Fillets, with Tomato & Basil Sauce, Simply Bake, Tesco*	1 Fillet/142g	170	8.1	120	15.2	1.8	5.7	0.1
Fillets,Beer Battered, Gastro, Youngs*	1 Fillet/119g	232	10.7	195	13.6	14.4	9	1.1
Filltes, Breaded, GF, Free From, Tesco*	1 Fillet/135g	263	10.4	195	12.7	18	7.7	1.5
in Parsley Sauce, with Mash, & Veg, Morrisons*	1 Pack/394g	272	5.1	69	5.7	7.7	1.3	1.9
Loins, Average	*1 Serving/145g*	*116*	*1.2*	*80*	*17.9*	*0.1*	*0.8*	*0.2*
Mornay, Gratin, Cooked, Just Cook, Sainsbury's*	1 Pack/320g	518	32.2	185	13.3	6.9	11.5	0.5
Mornay, Nutritionally Balanced, M&S*	1 Pack/400g	320	10.4	80	6.8	7.2	2.6	1.6
Mornay, Sainsbury's*	1 Serving/180g	277	16.9	154	15.2	2.2	9.4	0.9
Mornay, with Mash & Peas, HL, Tesco*	1 Pack/367g	337	9.2	92	7.7	8.6	2.5	2
Poached, Average	*1oz/28g*	*26*	*0.3*	*94*	*20.9*	*0*	*1.1*	*0*
Salt, Fritters, Delices dÃƒÂ¢Ã¢ šÂ¬Ã¢ žÂ¢Orient*	6 Fritters/160g	419	19.2	262	9.9	28	12	1.1
Smoked, Raw, Average	*1oz/28g*	*22*	*0.2*	*78*	*18.1*	*0*	*0.6*	*0*
Southern Fried, Chunks, M&S*	½ Pack/115g	178	7.2	155	13.7	10.5	6.3	0.9
Steaks, Battered, Chip Shop Style, Average	*1 Serving/150g*	*321*	*18*	*214*	*12.5*	*14.3*	*12*	*1.1*
Steaks, in Butter Sauce, Youngs*	1 Serving/137g	111	3.2	81	9.8	5.1	2.3	0.2
Steamed, Average	*1oz/28g*	*23*	*0.3*	*83*	*18.6*	*0*	*0.9*	*0*
Thai Green, Steamer, Cook In, Co-Op*	½ Pack/169g	149	4.7	88	13	2.4	2.8	0.9
COD & CHIPS								
& Peas, 240, Oakhouse Foods Ltd*	1 Meal/300g	510	18.6	170	6.4	22.3	6.2	2.2
Asda*	1 Serving/280g	450	14	161	8	21	5	1.1
COD IN								
Butter Sauce, Ross*	1 Serving/150g	126	5.8	84	9.1	3.2	3.9	0.1
Butter Sauce, Sainsbury's*	1 Serving/150g	198	13.5	132	10.6	2	9	0.1
Butter Sauce, Steaks, Birds Eye*	1 Pack/170g	185	9.4	109	9.8	5	5.5	0.1
Butter Sauce, Steaks, Frozen, Asda*	1 Pouch/152g	163	4	107	16	5	2.6	0.8
Butter Sauce, Tesco*	1 Pack/150g	123	5.4	82	9.4	2.9	3.6	0.5
Cheese Sauce, BGTY, Sainsbury's*	1 Serving/170g	144	4.1	85	12.8	3.1	2.4	0
Cheese Sauce, with Broccoli, Lidl*	½ Pack/155g	143	5.4	92	12	2.4	3.5	1.2
Mushroom Sauce, BGTY, Sainsbury's*	1 Serving/170g	112	2.9	66	9.9	2.8	1.7	0.1
Parsley Sauce, COU, M&S*	1 Pack/185g	130	4.6	70	10.6	1.4	2.5	0.6
Parsley Sauce, Frozen, M&S*	1 Pack/184g	156	7.2	85	11.1	1.9	3.9	1
Parsley Sauce, Meal For One, M&S*	1 Paack/400g	292	72	73	6	7.5	18	1.6
Parsley Sauce, Portions, Ocean Trader*	1 Serving/120g	112	4.7	93	9.4	4	3.9	0.1
Parsley Sauce, Pre Packed, Average	*1 Serving/150g*	*123*	*4.7*	*82*	*10.1*	*3.3*	*3.1*	*0.5*
Parsley Sauce, Skinless & Boneless, Sainsbury's*	1 Portion/150g	162	9	108	11.3	2.2	6	0.5
Parsley Sauce, Steaks, Birds Eye*	1 Steak/172g	155	4.8	90	10.5	5.6	2.8	0.1
Parsley Sauce, with Mash, Morrisons*	1 Pack/384g	319	8.5	83	7.1	7.5	2.2	2.2
Parsley Sauce, with Mash, Peas, & Carrots, Sainsbury's*	1 Serving/375g	311	71.2	83	6.9	8.8	19	1.6
Red Pepper Sauce, Sweet, Fillets, GFY, Asda*	½ Pack/170g	143	2.7	84	15	2.3	1.6	0.1
COD WITH								
a Mediterranean Pepper Sauce, Fillets, Waitrose*	1 Pack/370g	240	4.8	65	12.2	1.1	1.3	0.9
a Thai Crust, PB, Waitrose*	1 Pack/280g	249	7	89	15.1	1.6	2.5	0.6
Fish Pesto, Fillets, COOK!, M&S*	½ Pack/165g	210	5.1	127	16.4	8.4	3.1	4.2

	Measure INFO/WEIGHT	per Measure KCAL	FAT	Nutrition Values per 100g / 100ml KCAL	PROT	CARB	FAT	FIBRE
COD WITH								
Parma Ham & Sardinian Chick Peas, M&S*	½ Pack/255g	268	12.5	105	9.8	5.3	4.9	0.5
Roasted Vegetables, M&S*	1 Serving/280g	238	10.6	85	8	4.9	3.8	1.7
Sweet Chilli, COU, M&S*	1 Pack/400g	360	2	90	7.7	13.1	0.5	1.6
COFFEE								
& Chicory, Breakfast Drink, Ricore, Nestle*	1 Tsp/5g	7	0	141	2.7	9.1	0	45.3
Azera, Barista Style Instant, Nescafe*	1 Serving/200ml	2	0	1	0.1	0	0	0
Azera, Latte, To Go, Nescafe*	1 Serving/307ml	89	2.5	29	1	4.4	0.8	0.3
Baileys, Pod, Made Up, Tassimo*	1 Mug/256g	82	3.8	32	0.3	3.8	1.5	0.1
Black, Average	***1 Mug/270ml***	***5***	***0***	***2***	***0.2***	***0.3***	***0***	***0***
Cafe Caramel, Cafe Range, Nescafe*	1 Sachet/17g	72	2.4	423	9.2	64.6	14.1	1.3
Cafe Hazelnut, Nescafe*	1 Sachet/17g	73	2.4	428	9.3	66	14.1	0
Cafe Irish Cream, Cafe Range, Nescafe*	1 Sachet/23g	98	3.2	425	8.2	65.2	14.1	1.2
Cafe Latte, Dry, Douwe Egberts*	1 Serving/12g	58	2.6	480	10	60	22	0
Cafe Latte, Instant, Made Up, Maxwell House*	1 Serving/13g	53	1.7	424	6.4	68	13.6	0
Cafe Latte, Vita Coco*	1 Carton/330g	132	3.3	40	1.7	6	1	0
Cafe Mocha, Cafe Range, Nescafe*	1 Sachet/22g	92	2.9	418	8.5	66.6	13.1	0
Cafe Vanilla, Latte, Cafe Range, Nescafe*	1 Sachet/19g	73	1.6	395	9.2	68.3	8.5	4.1
Cappuccino, Cafe Mocha, Dry, Maxwell House*	1 Serving/23g	100	2.5	434	4.3	78.2	10.8	0
Cappuccino, Cafe Specials, Dry, M&S*	1 Serving/14g	55	1.6	395	14	59	11.5	0.7
Cappuccino, Cappio, Iced, Kenco*	1 Can/200ml	138	6	69	3	7	3	0
Cappuccino, Cappio, Kenco*	1 Sachet/18g	79	1.9	439	11.7	73.9	10.6	0.6
Cappuccino, Classic Roast, Sachets, Maxwell House*	1 Sachet/14g	59	1.5	420	4.5	76.5	10.5	0
Cappuccino, Co-Op*	1 Serving/13g	55	2	440	16	64	16	8
Cappuccino, Decaff, Instant, Made Up, Nescafe*	1 Mug/200ml	68	2.3	34	1	5	1.2	0
Cappuccino, Decaff, Nescafe*	1 Sachet/16g	68	2.3	428	11.6	62.6	14.6	0
Cappuccino, Decaff, Unsweetened, Nescafe*	1 Sachet/16g	70	3.1	437	14.5	51.2	19.4	4.3
Cappuccino, Dry, Maxwell House*	1 Mug/15g	52	1.4	350	12	64	9.6	0.4
Cappuccino, Dry, Waitrose*	1 Sachet/13g	58	2.3	439	15.1	56	17.2	4.4
Cappuccino, for Filter Systems, Kenco*	1 Sachet/6g	22	0.8	375	19	44	13.5	0
Cappuccino, Iced, Cowbelle, Aldi*	1 Serving/250ml	169	4.5	68	3.3	9.6	1.8	0.3
Cappuccino, Instant, Aldi*	1 Sachet/13g	49	1.7	393	12.5	55.1	13.6	0
Cappuccino, Instant, Asda*	1 Sachet/15g	60	2.3	399	13	53	15.2	0.9
Cappuccino, Instant, Made Up, Maxwell House*	1 Serving/280g	123	5.3	44	0.6	5.8	1.9	0
Cappuccino, Instant, Sachet , Kenco*	1 Sachet/19g	72	15.9	383	6.9	70	85	0
Cappuccino, Instant, Unsweetened, Douwe Egberts*	1 Serving/12g	48	1.9	400	11	53	16	0
Cappuccino, Light, Alcafe, Aldi*	1 Serving/200ml	54	1	27	1.6	4.5	0.5	0.5
Cappuccino, M&S*	1 Serving/164g	66	2.6	40	1.5	4.4	1.6	0
Cappuccino, Made Up, Dolce Gusto, Nescafe*	1 Serving/240ml	84	3.7	35	1.6	4	1.5	0.3
Cappuccino, Original, Sachets, Nescafe*	1 Sachet/18g	80	3.1	444	11.7	60.3	17.4	0
Cappuccino, Sainsbury's*	1 Serving/12g	49	1.9	411	14.9	52.9	15.5	0.4
Cappuccino, Semi Skimmed Milk, Average	***1 Serving/200ml***	***63***	***2.3***	***31***	***2.2***	***3.2***	***1.2***	***0***
Cappuccino, Sweetened, Instant, Alcafe, Aldi*	1 Sachet/135ml	61	1.6	45	0.5	8.2	1.2	0.4
Cappuccino, to Go, Original, Nescafe*	1 Serving/19g	84	3.3	444	11.7	60.3	17.4	0
Cappuccino, Unsweetened, Cappio, Kenco*	1 Sachet/14g	57	2	407	9.9	60	14	0.6
Cappuccino, Unsweetened, Gold, Nescafe*	1 Sachet/14g	55	1.8	392	12.9	52.5	13	5.7
Capuccino, Alcafe, Aldi*	1 Sachet/135ml	61	1.6	45	0.5	8.2	1.2	0.4
Chococino, Made up, Dolce Gusto, Nescafe*	1 Serving/210g	147	5.4	70	2.3	9.4	2.6	0.7
Coconut, Caffe, Alpro*	1 Carton/250ml	88	2.8	35	0.2	5.2	1.1	0.9
Columbian, Nescafe*	1 Serving/2g	2	0	111	16.7	11.1	0	5.6
Compliment*	1 Serving/14ml	20	1.8	143	1.4	6.4	12.9	0
Espresso, Instant, Nescafe*	1 Tsp/2g	2	0	118	7.8	3.1	0.2	34.1
Espresso, Made Up, Dolce Gusto, Nescafe*	1 Serving/60ml	1	0.1	2	0.1	0	0.2	0.3
Frappe Iced, Nestle*	1 Sachet/24g	92	1	384	15	72	4	0.5

COFFEE

INFO/WEIGHT	Measure	per Measure KCAL	FAT	Nutrition Values per 100g / 100ml KCAL	PROT	CARB	FAT	FIBRE
Gold Blend, Decafefinated, Nescafe*	1 Tsp/5g	3	0	63	7	9	0.2	27
Gold Blend, Nescafe*	1 Cup 200ml/5g	3	0	63	7	9	0.2	27
Ground, Made Up with Water, Average	*1 Serving/200ml*	*2*	*0*	*1*	*0*	*0*	*0*	*0*
Hazlenut, Caffe, Alpro*	1 Serving/250ml	78	2.2	31	0.2	5.2	0.9	1
Ice Mocha Drink, Nescafe, Nestle*	1 Bottle/280ml	160	3.4	57	1.1	10.5	1.2	0
Iced, Mocha, Jimmys Iced Coffee*	1 Carton/300g	138	3.6	46	2.3	6.6	1.2	0
Iced, Original, Jimmys Iced Coffee*	1 Carton/330ml	129	3.6	39	2.4	4.9	1.1	0
Iced, Skinny, Jimmys Iced Coffee*	1 Carton/330ml	99	0	30	2.6	4.8	0	0
Infusion, Avg with Semi-Skimmed Milk	*1 Cup/220ml*	*15*	*0.4*	*7*	*0.6*	*0.7*	*0.2*	*0*
Infusion, Avg with Single Cream	*1 Cup/220ml*	*31*	*2.6*	*14*	*0.4*	*0.3*	*1.2*	*0*
Instant Edition, Skinny Coffee Club*	1 Serving/2g	6	0	309	19	48.4	0.3	18
Instant, Alta Rica, Nescafe*	1 Tsp/2g	2	0	98	13.8	10	0.3	21
Instant, Decaffeinated, Nescafe*	1 Tsp/2g	2	0	101	14.9	10	0.2	8.4
Instant, Fine Blend, Nescafe*	1 Tsp/2g	1	0	63	7	9	0.2	27
Instant, Made with Skimmed Milk	*1 Serving/270ml*	*15*	*0*	*6*	*0.6*	*0.8*	*0*	*0*
Instant, Made with Water & Semi Skimmed Milk	*1 Serving/350ml*	*24*	*0.7*	*7*	*0.4*	*0.5*	*0.2*	*0*
Instant, Made with Water, & Whole Milk	*1 Cup/220ml*	*18*	*0.9*	*8*	*0.5*	*0.6*	*0.4*	*0*
Instant, Original, Nescafe*	1 Tsp/2g	2	0	118	7.8	3.1	0.2	34.1
Instant, with Skimmed Milk, Costa Rican, Kenco*	1 Mug/300ml	17	0.1	6	0.6	0.8	0	0
Irish Latte, Gold, Nescafe*	1 Mug/22g	90	2.2	411	8.3	70.6	9.9	2.6
Latte Macchiato, Made Up, Dolce Gusto, Nescafe*	1 Serving/220g	89	4.2	40	2	4.1	1.9	0.3
Latte, Cafe, M&S*	1 Serving/190g	142	5.3	75	4.3	8.3	2.8	0
Latte, Caramel, Instant, Sachets, Sainsbury's*	1 Sachet/17g	70	1.7	412	8.2	71.2	10	0
Latte, Honest, Honest Organic Coffee*	1 Bottle/250ml	112	4.5	45	0	4.9	1.8	0
Latte, Iced, M&S*	1 Bottle/300ml	186	3.6	62	2.9	9.8	1.2	0.5
Latte, Instant, Sachet, Sainsbury's*	1 Sachet/18g	75	1.9	417	16.1	63.3	10.6	2.8
Latte, Instant, Sachets, Kenko*	1 Sachet/20g	85	2.2	430	9.3	73	11	2
Latte, Macchiato, Tassimo*	1 Cup/275ml	135	7.7	49	2.3	3.6	2.8	0
Latte, Nescafe*	1 Sachet/22g	110	6.3	498	14.5	45.7	28.5	0
Latte, Nitro, Canned, Nescafe*	1 Can/192ml	100	2.3	52	2.7	7	1.2	0.8
Latte, No Sugar, In Cup, From Machine, Kenco*	1 Cup/4g	17	0.9	400	7.6	44	22	0
Latte, Skinny, Nescafe*	1 Sachet/20g	72	1.1	359	24.1	54.3	5.3	1.1
Latte, Skinny, Sachets, Made Up, Tesco*	1 Serving/219g	72	1.3	33	1.7	5.2	0.6	0.2
Latte, Soya, Caramel, Chilled, Alpro*	1 Serving/200ml	84	24	42	2.1	5.2	12	1.3
Latte, Vanilla, Iced, Sachets, Kenco*	1 Sachet/21g	83	1.5	395	7.4	75	7	0.3
Macchiato, Caramel, Iced, Pre-made, Starbucks*	1 Cup/220ml	136	3.5	62	2.8	9.1	1.6	0
Macchiato, Latte, Classic, Tassimo*	1 Serving/295ml	90	6.1	31	0.3	2.4	2.1	0.2
Made with 1% Milk, Average	*1 Mug/250ml*	*15*	*0.2*	*6*	*0.5*	*0.8*	*0.1*	*0*
Mocha, Double Chocolate, Gold, Nescafe*	1 Sachet/23g	93	2.3	403	9.4	66.3	9.8	5.1
Mocha, Made Up, Dolce Gusto, Nescafe*	1 Serving/210g	117	5.1	56	2.4	6.1	2.4	0.6
Mocha, Sainsbury's*	1 Serving/22g	84	3	383	14	51	13.7	1.3
Mocha, Skinny, Nescafe*	1 Sachet/21g	77	0.7	367	13.6	70.3	3.5	4.3
Skinny Cappuccino, Made Up, Dolce Gusto, Nescafe*	1 Mug/15g	49	0.1	337	33.3	48.8	0.9	2.3

COFFEE CREAMER

	Measure	per Measure KCAL	FAT	Nutrition KCAL	PROT	CARB	FAT	FIBRE
Mocha, Walden Farms*	1 Tsp/5g	1	0	15	0.1	0.4	0.3	0

COFFEE WHITENER

	Measure	per Measure KCAL	FAT	Nutrition KCAL	PROT	CARB	FAT	FIBRE
Light, Tesco*	1 Tsp/3g	12	0.2	406	1	85.5	6.7	0
Original, Coffee Mate, Nestle*	1 Tsp/3.5g	19	1.2	547	2.4	56.7	34.4	0
Tesco*	1 Tsp/3g	16	0.9	533	1.2	61.3	31.4	0
Virtually Fat Free, Coffee Mate, Nestle*	1 Tsp/5g	10	0.2	200	1	42	3	0

COGNAC

	Measure	per Measure KCAL	FAT	Nutrition KCAL	PROT	CARB	FAT	FIBRE
40% Volume	*1 Pub Shot/35ml*	*78*	*0*	*222*	*0*	*0*	*0*	*0*

	Measure INFO/WEIGHT	per Measure KCAL	FAT	Nutrition Values per 100g / 100ml KCAL	PROT	CARB	FAT	FIBRE
COLA								
Average	*1 Can/330ml*	*135*	*0*	*41*	*0*	*10.9*	*0*	*0*
Coke, Cherry, Coca-Cola*	1 Bottle/500ml	225	0	45	0	11.2	0	0
Coke, Cherry, Zero, Coca-Cola*	1 Can/330ml	1	0	0	0	0	0	0
Coke, Diet with Cherry, Coca-Cola*	1 Bottle/500ml	5	0	1	0	0	0	0
Coke, Diet, Caffeine Free, Coca-Cola*	1 Can/330ml	1	0	0	0	0.1	0	0
Coke, Mango, Exotic, Diet, Coca-Cola*	1 Bottle/500ml	2	0	0	0	0	0	0
Coke, Vanilla, Coca-Cola*	1 Bottle/500ml	215	0	43	0	10.6	0	0
Coke, with Vanilla, Diet, Coca-Cola*	1 Glass/200ml	1	0	0	0	0.1	0	0
Curiosity, Fentiman's*	1 Bottle/275ml	129	0	47	0.1	11.6	0	0
Diet, Average	*1 Serving/200ml*	*1*	*0*	*1*	*0*	*0*	*0*	*0*
Light, 0% Sugar, Harboe*	1 Serving/200ml	2	1	1	0.5	0.5	0.5	0
Pepsi Max, Ginger, Pepsi*	1 Can/250ml	1	0	0	0	0	0	0
Pepsi Max, Raspberry, Pepsi*	1 Serving/250ml	1	0	0	0.1	0.1	0	0
Xero, Tesco*	1 Glass/250ml	1	0	0	0	0.1	0	0
Zero, Caffeine Free, Coca-Cola*	1 Glass/200ml	0	0	0	0	0	0	0
Zero, Coca-Cola*	1 Can/330ml	1	0	0	0	0	0	0
COLESLAW								
& Potato Salad, Baby, Finest, Tesco*	1 Serving/50g	105	9.6	210	1.4	7.2	19.2	1.4
Apple, Raisin & Walnut, TTD, Sainsbury's*	1 Serving/75g	212	19.6	283	2.3	8	26.2	2.8
Basics, Sainsbury's*	1 Serving/25g	27	2.4	107	1	3.7	9.8	1.6
Beetroot, & Pomegranate, Sainsbury's*	½ Pot/60g	48	2.6	80	2	7.3	4.3	0
Beetroot, Apple, & Pink Cabbage, Skinny Slaw, M&S*	1 Pack/225g	220	11.2	98	1.5	10.8	5	2
Cheese, Deli Style, Waitrose*	¼ Tub/75g	247	24.3	330	3.8	5.1	32.5	0.9
Cheese, M&S*	1 Serving/57g	185	19.1	325	4.2	2	33.5	1.7
Cheese, Sainsbury's*	1 Serving/75g	184	16.8	246	3.8	6.5	22.4	1.4
Coronation, Sainsbury's*	¼ Pot/75g	145	11.6	193	1	11.4	15.5	1.9
COU, M&S*	½ Pack/125g	75	3.4	60	1.3	7.4	2.7	1.7
Creamy, Asda*	1 Serving/25g	62	6	248	0.9	7	24	1.8
Creamy, Co-Op*	1 Serving/30g	68	6.6	228	0.9	5.7	22	1.3
Creamy, LC, Tesco*	1/3 Pot/100g	105	8.8	105	1.2	4.9	8.8	1.6
Creamy, Morrisons*	1 Serving/50g	112	10.9	224	0.7	5.4	21.8	1.5
Creamy, Tesco*	1 Serving/75g	142	13.4	190	1	5.5	17.8	1.5
Crunchy, with Mayonnaise, Tesco*	¼ Pack/75g	75	5.5	100	1.2	6.4	7.3	1.7
Deli Salad, Tesco*	1 Serving/50g	91	8.5	183	0.9	5.5	17.1	1.6
Deli Style, M&S*	1 Serving/50g	103	9.6	206	1.6	5.5	19.1	2.7
Eastmans, Tesco*	1 Serving/50g	67	5.8	134	1.2	5.2	11.7	1.5
Essential, Waitrose*	1 Tbsp/20g	50	4.9	248	0.8	5.4	24.6	1.2
From Restaurant, Average	*3/4 Cup/99g*	*147*	*11*	*148*	*1.5*	*12.9*	*11.1*	*0*
Fruit, Celery, & Nut, Sainsbury's*	1 Serving/75g	143	11.6	191	2.1	96	15.5	2.4
Half Fat, Waitrose*	1 Serving/100g	38	2.7	38	0.6	2.9	2.7	1.2
Jalapeno, Sainsbury's*	1 Serving/75g	142	13.4	190	0.9	5.6	17.9	1.6
Luxury, Asda*	1 Serving/50g	108	10.5	217	0.9	6	21	0
Luxury, Lidl*	1 Serving/50g	102	9.7	203	0.9	5.9	19.4	0
Luxury, Rich & Creamy, TTD, Sainsbury's*	1 Serving/50g	123	11.8	246	1.8	5.9	23.6	1.5
Premium, Co-Op*	1 Serving/50g	160	17	320	1	3	34	2
Rainbow, Finest, Tesco*	¼ Pack/84g	192	18.7	229	1.3	4.9	22.3	1.7
Red Cabbage, & Vegetable, Lightly Pickled, M&S*	1 Pack/140g	126	3.6	90	2.2	12.7	2.6	3.3
Red, Tesco*	½ Pack/70g	53	1	76	1	13.5	1.5	2.4
Reduced Fat, Average	*1 Tbsp/20g*	*23*	*1.9*	*113*	*1*	*6.4*	*9.3*	*2*
Reduced Fat, Co-Op*	1 Serving/50g	69	6	138	0.9	6.7	12	1.6
Reduced Fat, Essential, Waitrose*	1/6 Tub/50g	65	5.1	130	1.2	8.3	10.2	1.6
Reduced Fat, Luxury, Iceland*	1 Serving/20g	25	2.2	126	0.7	4.8	11	0
Reduced Fat, M&S*	½ Tub/112g	230	22.4	205	1.1	5.4	20	2.8

C

	Measure INFO/WEIGHT	per Measure KCAL	FAT	Nutrition Values per 100g / 100ml KCAL	PROT	CARB	FAT	FIBRE
COLESLAW								
Reduced Fat, Tesco*	1 Serving/30g	37	3.1	123	0.2	7	10.4	0.6
TTD, Sainsbury's*	¼ Med Pot/75g	185	17.7	246	1.8	5.9	23.6	1.5
with Reduced Calorie Dressing, Retail	*1 Serving/40g*	*27*	*1.8*	*67*	*0.9*	*6.1*	*4.5*	*1.4*
COLESLAW MIX								
Ranch, Asda*	½ Pack/149g	167	12.8	112	1.4	6.1	8.6	2.1
COLEY								
Portions, Raw, Average	*1 Serving/92g*	*65*	*0.6*	*71*	*15.9*	*0*	*0.6*	*0*
Steamed, Average	*1oz/28g*	*29*	*0.4*	*105*	*23.3*	*0*	*1.3*	*0*
CONCHIGLIE								
Cooked, Average	*1 Serving/185g*	*247*	*1.6*	*134*	*4.8*	*26.6*	*0.8*	*0.6*
Dry Weight, Average	*1 Serving/100g*	*352*	*1.7*	*352*	*12.5*	*71.6*	*1.7*	*2.6*
Shells, Dry, Average	*1 Serving/100g*	*346*	*1.5*	*346*	*12.3*	*70.4*	*1.5*	*3*
Whole Wheat, Dry Weight, Average	*1 Serving/75g*	*237*	*1.5*	*316*	*12.6*	*62*	*2*	*10.7*
CONCHIGLIONI								
Dry, Waitrose*	1 Serving/75g	256	1	341	12.5	69.8	1.3	3.7
CONSERVE								
Apricot, Average	*1 Tbsp/15g*	*37*	*0*	*244*	*0.5*	*59.3*	*0.2*	*1.5*
Blackberry, Bramble, & Gin, M&S*	1 Tsp/5g	12	0.1	233	0.8	54.2	1.1	1.4
Blackcurrant, Average	*1 Tbsp/15g*	*37*	*0*	*245*	*0.6*	*60*	*0.1*	*1.9*
Blackcurrant, Bonne Maman*	1 Tsp/5g	12	0	236	0.4	57	0	3.1
Blueberry, M&S*	1 Tsp/8g	15	0	206	0.3	51.1	0.1	1.3
Cherry, Morello, Tart, Full Flavoured, M&S*	1 Tsp/5g	13	0	256	0.4	62.6	0.3	0.8
Hedgerow, TTD, Sainsbury's*	1 Tbsp/15g	41	0	276	0.5	68.2	0.1	0.5
Morello Cherry, Waitrose*	1 Tbsp/15g	39	0	258	0.4	64.2	0	1.4
Plum, TTD, Sainsbury's*	1 Tbsp/23g	56	0.1	243	0.5	59.6	0.5	0.9
Raspberry, Average	*1 Tbsp/15g*	*37*	*0.1*	*249*	*0.6*	*61*	*0.3*	*1.3*
Raspberry, Seedless, Smooth & Sharp, M&S*	1 Tsp/5g	13	0	252	0.5	61.1	0.3	1.2
Rhubarb & Ginger, M&S*	1 Tbsp/15g	29	0	194	0.3	47.9	0.1	1
Strawberry, Average	*1 Tbsp/15g*	*37*	*0*	*250*	*0.4*	*61.6*	*0.1*	*0.5*
Strawberry, Specially Selected, Aldi*	1 Serving/15g	38	0.1	252	0.5	63	0.5	0.5
CONSOMME								
Average	*1oz/28g*	*3*	*0*	*12*	*2.9*	*0.1*	*0*	*0*
Beef, Canned, Sainsbury's*	1 Can/415g	46	0	11	2	0.7	0	0
Beef, Luxury, with Sherry, Baxters*	1 Can/415g	62	0	15	2.7	1	0	0
COOKIES								
All Butter, Almond, Italian Style, M&S*	1 Cookie/23g	120	6.4	515	6.7	59.4	27.6	3.6
All Butter, Ginger Bread, M&S*	1 Cookie/23g	102	5	445	4.3	57.5	21.8	2.4
All Butter, Italian Style Sorrento Lemon, M&S*	1 Cookie/24g	120	6.4	500	4.9	60.4	26.7	2.1
All Butter, Melting Moment, M&S*	1 Cookie/23g	110	6.4	470	4.5	51.5	27.5	3.4
All Butter, Sultana, TTD, Sainsbury's*	1 Cookie/17g	79	3.8	476	5.4	62.7	22.6	2
Almond, Ose*	1 Cookie/10g	46	1.4	456	8.4	74	14	0
Apple & Raisin, Go Ahead, McVitie's*	1 Cookie/15g	66	1.9	443	5.3	76.8	12.7	3.4
Apple Crumble, M&S*	1 Cookie/26g	90	0.5	345	4.6	76.8	2	2.9
Big Milk Chocolate Chunk, Cookie Coach*	1 Cookie/35g	174	8.8	497	6.2	61.4	25.1	0
Bounty, Mars*	1 Cookie/46g	215	9.6	468	5.7	63.4	20.9	0
Brazil Nut, Prewett's*	1 Cookie/50g	122	7.4	244	2.6	25.2	14.8	1
Butter & Sultana, Sainsbury's*	1 Cookie/13g	61	2.6	473	4.5	68.4	20.1	1.6
Cheesecake, New York, Desserts, Maryland*	2 Cookies/21g	102	4.7	485	5.9	64.9	22.2	1.6
Chia & Coconut, with Afternoon Infusion, Graze*	1 Punnet/22g	118	6.9	528	5.8	53	31	5
Choc Chip & Coconut, Maryland*	1 Cookie/10g	55	2.5	512	5.1	62.9	23.7	0
Choc Chip & Hazelnut, Maryland*	1 Cookie/11g	55	2.7	513	6.3	65.3	25	0
Choc Chip, Big, Treats, Maryland*	1 Cookie/16g	85	4.6	531	5.1	61.2	29	3.2
Choc Chip, Bronte*	1 Cookie/17g	79	3.6	474	5.8	64	21.6	0

COOKIES

	Measure INFO/WEIGHT	per Measure KCAL	FAT	Nutrition Values per 100g / 100ml KCAL	PROT	CARB	FAT	FIBRE
Choc Chip, Giant, Paterson's*	1 Cookie/60g	296	15.2	493	0.1	61.3	25.3	3.2
Choc Chip, Lyons*	1 Cookie/11g	57	2.7	499	5.2	68.3	23.4	1.7
Choc Chip, Mini, Good to Go, Waitrose*	1 Bag/25g	127	6.6	508	6	60.4	26.4	2.4
Choc Chip, Parkside*	1 Cookie/11g	56	2.7	495	5.3	64.5	23.7	0
Choc Chip, Reduced Fat, Maryland*	1 Cookie/11g	51	1.9	478	5.9	73	18	0
Choc Chunk, Finest, Tesco*	1 Cookie/80g	355	14.1	445	5.7	65.3	17.7	1.8
Chocolate & Nut, Organic, Evernat*	1 Cookie/69g	337	15.6	489	7.2	64.1	22.6	0
Chocolate & Orange, COU, M&S*	1 Cookie/26g	90	0.7	350	5.7	77.2	2.6	3.2
Chocolate Chip & Caramel, Bites, Maryland*	5 Cookies/20g	103	5.3	513	5.7	61.8	26.4	3
Chocolate Chip & Hazelnut, Extra Special, Asda*	1 Cookie/25g	130	8.1	516	6	51	32	2.5
Chocolate Chip, Asda*	1 Cookie/12g	57	2.9	497	5	63	25	2.6
Chocolate Chip, Average	***1 Cookie/10g***	***49***	***2.5***	***489***	***5.5***	***64.1***	***24.7***	***2.9***
Chocolate Chip, BGTY, Sainsbury's*	1 Cookie/17g	72	2	428	4.5	75.6	11.9	2.5
Chocolate Chip, Chips Ahoy*	1 Cookie/11g	55	2.8	500	6	65	25	3
Chocolate Chip, Co-Op*	1 Cookie/11g	55	2.6	500	5	65	24	1
Chocolate Chip, Double, Protein, Quest*	1 Cookie/59g	240	16	407	25.4	33.9	27.1	17
Chocolate Chip, Dough, Otis Spunkmeyer*	1 Cookie/38g	160	8	421	5.3	60.5	21	2.6
Chocolate Chip, Free From, Sainsbury's*	1 Cookie/19g	93	4.6	498	6.5	61.4	24.4	3.3
Chocolate Chip, Free From, Tesco*	1 Cookie/12g	59	2.6	488	5.2	65.6	22	3.4
Chocolate Chip, GF, Organic, Dove's Farm*	1 Cookie/17g	77	3.1	451	4.3	66.9	18.5	0
Chocolate Chip, GFY, Asda*	1 Cookie/10g	48	2	463	5	68	19	3.5
Chocolate Chip, Gluten & Wheat Free, Lovemore*	1 Cookie/17g	81	4.5	483	3.8	57.8	26.8	3.5
Chocolate Chip, Handbaked, Border*	1 Cookie/15g	72	3.4	480	5.9	67.4	22.6	0
Chocolate Chip, High Protein, Dr Zak's*	1 Cookie/60g	214	6.4	356	25	48	10.7	2.3
Chocolate Chip, Low Price, Sainsbury's*	1 Cookie/11g	54	2.3	500	7	70.1	21.3	2.5
Chocolate Chip, Lyons*	1 Cookie/12g	56	2.5	483	5.6	66.5	21.6	1.7
Chocolate Chip, M&S*	1 Cookie/12g	59	3	495	5.7	62.1	24.8	2.7
Chocolate Chip, Maryland*	1 Cookie/11g	53	2.5	487	5.4	63.8	22.6	3.5
Chocolate Chip, McVitie's*	1 Cookie/11g	54	2.8	496	5.8	60.2	25.8	3
Chocolate Chip, Mini, Bites, Tesco*	1 Cookie/13g	61	2.7	469	5.6	64.5	20.7	1.4
Chocolate Chip, Mini, McVitie's*	1 Bag/40g	196	9.2	491	5.5	65.1	23.1	2.8
Chocolate Chip, Morrisons*	1 Cookie/10g	52	2.5	502	5	66.2	24.1	1.3
Chocolate Chip, Organic, Sainsbury's*	1 Cookie/17g	89	4.9	530	5	61.8	29.2	0.3
Chocolate Chip, Organic, Tesco*	1 Cookie/17g	88	4.7	520	4	63.3	27.4	2.8
Chocolate Chip, Sondey Grandino*	1 Cookie/23g	113	5.8	502	7	58	26	0
Chocolate Chip, Tesco*	1 Cookie/11g	54	2.7	493	5.8	61.2	24.3	3.2
Chocolate Chip, Value, Tesco*	1 Cookie/11g	56	2.9	512	4.8	64.8	26	1.6
Chocolate Chip, Weight Watchers*	1 Cookie/11g	49	1.9	443	7.6	65.4	17.2	4.6
Chocolate Chunk & Hazelnut, Tesco*	1 Cookie/22g	118	6.7	538	6.2	60.2	30.3	1.9
Chocolate Chunk & Hazelnut, TTD, Sainsbury's*	1 Cookie/25g	132	7.7	527	6.7	54.2	30.8	3.3
Chocolate Chunk, All Butter, M&S*	1 Cookie/24g	120	6	500	5.2	62.4	25.2	2.9
Chocolate Chunk, Cadbury*	1 Cookie/22g	119	6.9	540	6.5	58	31.2	0
Chocolate Fruit & Nut, Extra Special, Asda*	1 Cookie/25g	125	7.1	509	6	56	29	2
Chocolate Orange, Half Coated, Finest, Tesco*	1 Cookie/22g	107	5.6	488	4.9	59.6	25.5	1.2
Chocolate Thin Crisp, Simply Food, M&S*	1 Pack/23g	100	2	435	4.4	78.3	8.7	4.4
Chocolate, Belgian, Extra Special, Asda*	1 Cookie/26g	138	8	535	6	58	31	2
Chocolate, Brownie, White Choc Chunk, Maryland*	1 Cookie/18g	89	4.6	493	6	58	25.6	2.8
Chocolate, Dark, & Ginger, Free From, Finest, Tesco*	1 Cookie/19g	92	4.2	485	4.6	66	22	2.1
Chocolate, Double, Sainsbury's*	1 Cookie/45g	202	8.5	450	5.8	63.1	18.9	2
Chocolate, Double, Tesco*	1 Cookie/42g	187	8.1	447	5.8	60.8	19.4	3.2
Chocolate, Milk, Free From, Tesco*	1 Cookie/20g	100	6.1	500	5.6	50.4	30.7	4.1
Chocolate, Quadruple, Finest, Tesco*	1 Cookie/25g	128	6.9	512	6.3	58.3	27.5	3
Chocolate, Soft, American Style, Budgens*	1 Cookie/50g	216	9.3	431	5.1	60.8	18.6	2.2

C

COOKIES

INFO/WEIGHT	Measure	per Measure		Nutrition Values per 100g / 100ml				
		KCAL	FAT	KCAL	PROT	CARB	FAT	FIBRE
Chocolate, Triple, Half Coated, Finest, Tesco*	1 Cookie/25g	131	7.3	525	5.7	58.7	29.3	2.3
Chocolate, Triple, Wheat, & GF, Finest, Tesco*	1 Cookie/19g	97	5	508	5.8	60.4	26.2	3.5
Chunkie Extremely Chocolatey, Fox's*	1 Cookie/26g	130	6.8	506	6.2	61	26.3	2.6
Chunkie, Chocolatey, Extremely, Fox's*	1 Cookie/25g	129	6.3	509	5.6	63	25	2.6
Cocoa, Organic, Bites, No Junk, Organix*	1 Bag/25g	105	3.2	421	7	69	13	5.5
Cocoa, Uglies, Lily O'briens*	1 Cookie/20g	100	6	500	7.5	60	30	2.5
Coconut & Raspberry, GF, Sainsbury's*	1 Cookie/20g	102	5.9	511	5.9	56	29.3	6.7
Coconut, Gluten-Free, Sainsbury's*	1 Cookie/20g	103	6.1	516	5.6	54.4	30.7	4.1
Cranberry & Orange, Finest, Tesco*	1 Cookie/26g	125	5.8	490	4.1	67.4	22.6	3.2
Crunchy Muesli, Mini, Shapers, Boots*	1 Pack/30g	134	4.5	448	6.7	71	15	1.8
Dairy Milk, with Chocolate Chunks, Dairy Milk, Cadbury*	1 Cookie/45g	210	9.3	467	6	63.6	20.6	1.4
Danish Butter, Tesco*	1 Cookie/26g	133	6.6	516	4.7	66.7	25.6	1.3
Dark Chocolate Chunk & Ginger, The Best, Morrisons*	1 Cookie/25g	126	6.4	503	4.6	63.7	25.5	2.8
Double Choc Chip, Giant, Paterson's*	1 Cookie/60g	293	15.2	489	0.3	61.3	25.3	3.7
Double Choc Chip, Mini, M&S*	1 Cookie/22g	108	5.2	490	5.3	63.6	23.7	1.8
Double Choc Chip, Tesco*	1 Cookie/11g	55	2.7	500	4.2	65.3	24.7	3
Double Choc Chip, Weight Watchers*	1 Cookie/11g	49	1.9	443	7.6	65.4	17.2	4.6
Double Choc, Maryland*	1 Cookie/10g	51	2.6	510	5.2	64.4	25.7	0
Double Choc, Minis, Maryland*	1 Mini Bag/20g	100	5	503	5.7	62.3	24.9	3.6
Double Chocolate & Nuts, Bens Cookie*	1 Cookie/85g	364	17.4	428	8.7	71.2	20.5	2.8
Double Chocolate & Walnut, Soft, Tesco*	1 Cookie/25g	116	6.4	463	5.8	52.1	25.7	4.7
Double Chocolate Chip, Co-Op*	1 Cookie/17g	87	4.6	510	5	63	27	2
Double Chocolate Chip, Organic, Waitrose*	1 Cookie/18g	96	5.6	535	5.1	58.6	31	1.9
Double Chocolate Chip, Treat Yourself, Spar*	1 Cookie/20g	94	5	470	5.5	56	25	2.5
Eton Mess, Finest, Tesco*	1 Cookie/66g	281	9.7	426	5.1	67.6	14.7	1.4
Farmbake, Arnotts*	1 Cookie/13g	61	2.4	470	5	68.4	18.7	0
Finest White Chocolate & Honeycomb, Bakery, Tesco*	1 Cookie/65g	290	11.2	446	5.3	67.1	17.2	0.9
Flapjack, Fruity, Truly Irresistible, Co-Op*	1 Cookie/25g	116	5.1	464	5.2	64	20.4	2.4
Fortune, Average	*1 Cookie/8g*	*30*	*0.2*	*378*	*4.2*	*84*	*2.7*	*1.6*
Fruit & Oat, Soft, Diet Chef Ltd*	1 Cookie45g	198	9.1	440	4.8	61.9	20.2	4.3
Fruit, Giant, Cookie Coach*	1 Cookie/60g	280	13.2	466	4.9	62	22	0
Fudge Brownie American Cream, Sainsbury's*	1 Cookie/12g	60	2.8	499	4.8	67.9	23.2	2.2
Galaxy, Galaxy, Mars*	1 Cookie/46g	207	8	451	5.6	67.3	17.4	0
Ginger & Brazil Nut, Organic, Dove's Farm*	1 Cookie/17g	79	3.5	464	5	65	20.5	4.8
Ginger & Choc Chip, BGTY, Sainsbury's*	1 Cookie/17g	69	3.2	415	5.8	55.3	19	12.1
Ginger, GF, Barkat*	1 Cookie/17g	85	4.4	501	3.2	63.8	25.9	0
Ginger, Low Fat, M&S*	1 Cookie/23g	82	1	358	5.1	74.9	4.3	2.4
Gman, Gingerbread, GF, Barkat*	2 Cookies/34g	167	9.3	490	15.8	49.5	27.3	6
Hazelnut, GF, Organic, Dove's Farm*	1 Cookie/17g	79	3.7	463	4.8	61.5	21.9	1.8
Honey, Lemon & Ginger, Nothing Naughty*	1 Cookie/60g	246	9	410	2.9	64.4	15	0
Lemon Zest, GF, Organic, Dove's Farm*	1 Cookie/17g	80	3.1	473	3.3	73.7	18.3	0
Maple Syrup, & Pecan, Finest, Tesco*	1 Cookie/25g	127	6.6	507	6.7	59.9	26.4	1.7
Milk Chocolate Chunk, Average	*1 Cookie/25g*	*129*	*6.9*	*515*	*6.6*	*60*	*27.6*	*1.6*
Milk Chocolate, Classic, Millie's Cookies*	1 Cookie/45g	190	10.2	422	5.1	49.3	22.7	1.3
Oat & Cranberry, BGTY, Sainsbury's*	1 Cookie/28g	126	5	449	6.8	65	18	5.1
Oat & Raisin, Health Matters*	1 Cookie/8g	33	0.7	414	7	76.6	8.8	3.3
Oat & Treacle, TTD, Sainsbury's*	1 Cookie/25g	121	5.9	482	5.7	61.8	23.6	3.7
Oat & Raisin, Bites, Tesco*	1 Cookie/5g	25	1	458	6.1	65.2	18.5	2.9
Oat & Raisin, GF, Prewett's*	1 Cookie18g	80	2.7	442	6.2	63	15	5.1
Oat & Sultana, Free From, Sainsbury's*	1 Cookie/19g	87	3.7	462	6.2	62.6	19.8	4.2
Oat, & Raisin, Free From, Finest, Tesco*	1 Cookie/19g	80	2.8	422	6.2	63	15	5.1
Oat, Crunchy, Grandma Wilds*	1 Cookie/15g	75	3.8	498	6.5	59.5	25.3	0
Oat, Giant Jumbo, Paterson's*	1 Cookie/60g	299	16.2	499	0.4	58.4	27	3.2

	Measure INFO/WEIGHT	per Measure KCAL	FAT	Nutrition Values per 100g / 100ml KCAL	PROT	CARB	FAT	FIBRE
COOKIES								
Oatflake & Raisin, Waitrose*	1 Cookie/17g	80	3.8	469	5.8	61.7	22.1	4.7
Oreo, Mini, Oreo*	1 Pack/25g	120	4.8	480	4.8	70	19.2	2.4
Oreo, Mint, Mondelez*	1 Cookie/11g	53	2.2	479	5.2	69	20	3
Oreo, Nabisco*	1 Cookie/11g	52	2.3	471	5.9	70.6	20.6	2.9
Pecan & Maple, Mini, Bronte*	1 Pack/100g	509	27.3	509	5.4	60.3	27.3	1.6
Pecan, & Caramel, Co-Op*	1 Cookie/25g	123	5.5	493	6	67	22	1.5
Pineapple, Coconut & White Chocolate, M&S*	1 Cookie/23g	119	5.7	518	5.1	56.7	24.9	2.9
Raisin & Cinnamon, Low Fat, M&S*	1 Cookie/22g	78	0.9	355	6.2	73	4.1	3.2
Raspberry, & Chocolate, Wonders, Maryland*	1 Cookie/18g	90	4.6	502	4.7	60.5	25.9	3.3
Red Velvet, Filled, Bakery, Tesco*	1 Cookie/42g	170	5.5	405	4.6	66.6	13.1	1.3
Stem Ginger, Aldi*	1 Cookie/13g	58	2.4	463	3.6	68.5	19.4	0
Stem Ginger, All Butter, Deluxe, Lidl*	1 Cookie/17g	80	3.6	468	5.1	62	21	5.4
Stem Ginger, Deluxe, Lidl*	1 Cookie/17g	80	3.6	468	5.1	62	21	5.4
Stem Ginger, Free From, Asda*	1 Cookie/19g	89	3.6	467	3	69	19	4.1
Stem Ginger, Free From, Sainsbury's*	1 Cookie/19g	89	3.6	476	4.1	70.8	19	2.7
Stem Ginger, Less Than 5% Fat, M&S*	1 Cookie/22g	79	0.9	360	6.2	73.9	4.3	3
Stem Ginger, Reduced Fat, Waitrose*	1 Cookie/17g	75	2.7	448	4.5	71	16.2	1.6
Stem Ginger, Tesco*	1 Cookie/20g	98	4.8	489	4.2	64	24	2
Stem Ginger, TTD, Sainsbury's*	1 Cookie/25g	124	6.2	496	4.9	62.3	24.7	2.2
Sticky Toffee, Finest, Tesco*	1 Cookie/63g	258	9.4	410	4.5	63.5	15	1.5
Sugar Free, Maryland*	2 Cookie/22g	94	4.8	433	6.1	60.6	22.3	3.6
Sultana, & Oat, Tesco*	1 Cookie/20g	91	3.9	454	5.5	61.6	19.7	4.4
Sultana, All Butter, Reduced Fat, M&S*	1 Cookie/17g	70	2.4	420	4.9	68.6	14.2	2.6
Sultana, Deluxe, Lidl*	1 Cookie/17g	77	3.2	453	5.3	64.7	18.8	2.9
Sultana, Soft & Chewy, Sainsbury's*	1 Cookie/25g	104	3.5	414	4.4	67.8	13.9	2.5
Toffee Popcorn, Butter Buds*	1 Cookie/40g	184	7.6	459	4.2	66.8	19	1.4
Treacle & Oat, All Butter, Finest, Tesco*	1 Cookie/20g	100	5	500	4.8	62.9	25	2.1
Triple Chocolate, Belgian, Bakery, Finest, Tesco*	1 Cookie/65g	310	14.9	478	6.1	60.1	23	2.9
Triple Chocolate, TTD, Sainsbury's*	1 Cookie/72g	344	16.5	478	5.8	61.2	22.9	2
Wheelies, Hutchinson's*	1 Pack/30g	146	5.4	486	6.8	73.5	17.9	0
White Chocolate & Cranberry, Devondale*	1 Cookie/65g	300	15.3	462	4.7	60.7	23.5	2.1
White Chocolate & Cranberry, Kate's Cakes Ltd*	1 Serving/100g	389	13.4	389	4.7	62.3	13.4	2
White Chocolate & Raspberry, Finest, Tesco*	1 Cookie/76g	304	9.6	400	5.2	66.3	12.6	2.4
White Chocolate, Asda*	1 Cookie/54g	256	11.9	474	5	64	22	2.1
White Chocolate, Chunk, Average	**1 Cookie/25g**	**124**	**6.2**	**498**	**5.5**	**62.8**	**24.8**	**1**
White Chocolate, Maryland*	1 Cookie/10g	51	2.5	512	5.7	64	25	0
White Chocolate, TTD, Sainsbury's*	1 Cookie/25g	126	6.4	504	5.5	62.5	25.8	1.2
COQ AU VIN								
658, Oakhouse Foods Ltd*	1 Serving/400g	728	39.6	182	14	7.9	9.9	2.8
Chicken, Parsley Box*	1 Pack/270g	221	6.8	82	14	0.9	2.5	0.4
Diet Chef Ltd*	1 Pack/300g	285	13.2	95	7.7	6.1	4.4	2.2
Donald Russell*	1 Pack/250g	230	7.2	92	10.7	3.5	2.9	0.4
Tesco*	½ Pack/229g	295	16.7	129	12.8	2.6	7.3	0.4
CORDIAL								
Apple & Mango, Hi Juice, As Prepared, Morrisons*	1 Serving/250ml	69	0	28	0	6.7	0	0.1
Apple, Crushed, & Cinnamon, Diltued, Robinson's*	1 Serving/200ml	32	0	16	0	3.8	0	0
Apple, Crushed, & Cinnamon, Undiluted, Robinson's*	1 Serving/15ml	17	0	112	0	26.6	0	0
Blackcurrant, New Zealand Honey Co*	1 Serving/30ml	109	0.3	363	1	88	1	0
Blueberry, & Passion Fruit, Sugar Free, Diluted, Mi Wadi*	1 Serving/200ml	4	0	2	0	0	0	0
Cox's Apple & Plum, Diluted, Bottle Green*	1 Serving/10ml	3	0	29	0	7.2	0	0
Elderflower, Made Up, Bottle Green*	1 Glass/200ml	46	0	23	0	5.6	0	0
Elderflower, Undiluted, Waitrose*	1 Serving/20ml	22	0	110	0	27.5	0	0
Honey, Lemon, & Ginger, Undiluted, Belvoir Fruit Farms*	1 Serving/15ml	31	0	207	0	52.2	0	0

C

C

	Measure INFO/WEIGHT	per Measure KCAL	FAT	Nutrition Values per 100g / 100ml KCAL	PROT	CARB	FAT	FIBRE
CORDIAL								
Lemon & Lime, High Juice, M&S*	1 Glass/250ml	75	0	30	0	7	0	0
Lime Juice, Concentrated	*1 Serving/20ml*	*22*	*0*	*112*	*0.1*	*29.8*	*0*	*0*
Lime Juice, Diluted	*1 Glass/250ml*	*55*	*0*	*22*	*0*	*6*	*0*	*0*
Lime Juice, Waitrose*	1 Serving/20ml	21	0	104	10	23.7	0	0
Lime with Aromatic Bitters & Ginger, Sainsbury's*	1 Serving/40ml	12	0.1	29	0	6.9	0.3	0.3
Lime, Crushed, & Mint, Diluted, Robinson's*	1 Serving/200ml	34	0	17	0	4.1	0	0
Lime, Juice, Diluted, Rose's*	1 Serving/250ml	52	0	21	0	4.9	0	0
Lime, Sainsbury's*	1 Serving/50ml	14	0	27	0	6.2	0	0
Lime, Tesco*	1 Pint/74ml	8	0	11	0.2	0.5	0	0
Lime, with Sweetener, No Added Sugar, Diluted, Co-Op*	1 Serving/200ml	4	1	2	0.5	0.5	0.5	0.5
Pear, & Elderflower, Pressed, Diluted, Robinsons*	1 Serving/200ml	36	0	18	0	4.2	0	0
Plum, Apple, & Rosehip, Superfruit, Undiluted, Fiovana*	1 Serving/36ml	18	0	49	0	9.8	0	0
Pomegranate & Elderflower, Bottle Green*	1 fl oz/30ml	9	0	30	0	7	0	0
CORIANDER								
Leaves, Dried, Average	*1oz/28g*	*78*	*1.3*	*279*	*21.8*	*41.7*	*4.8*	*0*
Leaves, Fresh, Average	*1 Bunch/20g*	*5*	*0.1*	*23*	*2.1*	*3.7*	*0.5*	*2.8*
CORN								
Baby, & Mange Tout, Eat Fresh, Tesco*	1 Serving/100g	31	0.2	31	2.9	3.3	0.2	2.1
Baby, Average	*1 Serving/80g*	*21*	*0.3*	*26*	*2.5*	*3.1*	*0.4*	*1.7*
Baby, Canned, Drained, Average	*1 Serving/80g*	*18*	*0.3*	*23*	*2.9*	*2*	*0.4*	*1.5*
Cob, Kebabs, Waitrose*	1 Cob/140g	168	3.2	120	4.2	19.6	2.3	2.2
Cobs, Boiled, Weighed with Cob, Average	*1 Ear/200g*	*78*	*1.7*	*39*	*1.5*	*6.8*	*0.8*	*0.8*
Cobs, Mini, Boiled, Morrisons*	1 Cob/80g	64	1.5	80	3.6	9.5	1.9	5.1
Cobs, Mini, Supersweet, Whole, Four Seasons, Aldi*	1 Mini Cob/80g	38	0.9	47	2.1	5.6	1.1	3
Cobs, with Butter, From Restaurant, Average	*1 Ear/146g*	*155*	*3.4*	*106*	*3.1*	*21.9*	*2.4*	*0*
Crack'd, Coconut, Pot, Made Up, Wicked Kitchen, Tesco*	1 Pot/340g	425	17.7	125	2.3	16.6	5.2	1.3
Creamed Style, Green Giant*	1 Can/418g	238	2.1	57	1.2	11.9	0.5	3
Creamed, Canned, Libby's*	¼ Can/102g	84	0.9	82	1.8	15.6	0.9	2.3
Roasted, Smokehouse BBQ, Crunch, Alesto, Lidl*	1 Serving/31g	130	3.2	419	8.9	69	10.4	7
CORN CAKES								
& Lentil, Lightly Salted, Tesco*	1 Lentil Cake/8g	31	0.2	383	19	68.5	2.7	4.4
M&S*	½ Pack/85g	238	17	280	6.4	19.8	20	3.4
Organic, Kallo*	1 Cake/7g	26	0.1	383	7.6	83.6	1.1	7.2
Slightly Salted, Mrs Crimble's*	1 Pack/28g	104	0.9	380	7.9	80	3.4	5.4
The Best, Morrisons*	1 Corn Cake/7g	29	0.2	390	7.7	80.1	3.3	4.4
with Chai Seeds, Kallo*	1 Cake/7g	27	0.2	389	8	81	2.4	0
CORNED BEEF								
Average	*1 Slice/35g*	*75*	*4.3*	*214*	*25.9*	*0.7*	*12.2*	*0*
Lean, Healthy Range, Average	*1 Slice/30g*	*57*	*2.6*	*191*	*27*	*1*	*8.7*	*0*
Reduced Salt, Canned, Princes*	1 Can/340g	741	44.2	218	24.8	0.5	13	0
Sliced, Premium, Average	*1 Slice/31g*	*69*	*3.9*	*222*	*26.6*	*0.5*	*12.6*	*0*
Slices, Iceland*	1 Slice/25g	52	2.7	210	26.6	1	10.9	1
CORNFLOUR								
Average	*1 Tsp/5g*	*18*	*0.1*	*355*	*0.6*	*86.9*	*1.2*	*0.1*
COULIS								
Mango, Passion Fruit, & Yuzu, Waitrose*	1 Tbsp/15ml	21	0.1	141	0.9	31.7	0.7	2.2
Passsion Fruit & Mango, TTD, Sainsbury's*	1 Tbs/15ml	23	0.1	155	1.2	34.7	1	0.9
Raspberry, Scottish, & Vanilla, Waitrose*	1 Tbsp/15ml	20	0	134	0.4	31.4	0.2	2.7
Raspberry, TTD, Sainsbury's*	1 Tbsp/15ml	25	0.1	165	0.4	39.1	0.6	1.4
COURGETTE								
& Mixed Vegetable, Selection, M&S*	1 Pack/100g	123	0.4	123	2	3.3	0.4	2.3
Baby, Raw, Average	*1 Courgette/29g*	*6*	*0.1*	*22*	*2*	*2*	*0.5*	*1.2*
Courgetti, Italian, Tomato, Pot, Bol*	1 Pot/380g	441	18.2	116	2.5	15	4.8	1.4

	Measure INFO/WEIGHT	per Measure KCAL	FAT	Nutrition Values per 100g / 100ml KCAL	PROT	CARB	FAT	FIBRE
COURGETTE								
Fried, Average	*1oz/28g*	*18*	*1.3*	*63*	*2.6*	*2.6*	*4.8*	*1.2*
Raw, Average	*1 Whole/224g*	*40*	*0.9*	*18*	*1.8*	*1.8*	*0.4*	*0.9*
Spaghetti, Waitrose*	½ Pack/80g	16	0.3	20	1.8	1.8	0.4	1.2
Spirals, Tomato, & Basil, Vegetable Pot, Tesco*	1 Pot/230g	94	0.8	41	2.5	5.4	0.4	3
COUS COUS								
Cauliflower, & Broccoli, Waitrose*	½ Pack/110g	43	1	39	4	2.4	0.9	2.8
Cooked, Average	*1 Tbsp/15g*	*24*	*0.3*	*158*	*4.3*	*31.4*	*1.9*	*1.3*
Cooked, From Restaurant, Average	*1 Cup/157g*	*176*	*0.3*	*112*	*3.8*	*23.2*	*0.2*	*1.4*
Coriander & Lemon, As Consumed, Sainsbury's*	½ Pack/140g	195	1	139	4.8	27.5	0.7	1.9
Dry, Average	*1 Serving/50g*	*178*	*0.7*	*356*	*13.7*	*72.8*	*1.5*	*2.6*
Fruity, Sainsbury's*	1 Portion/100g	194	4.5	194	4.4	33.2	4.5	1.7
Giant, Cooked, Sainsbury's*	1 Serving/130g	126	2.1	97	3.6	16.2	1.6	1.7
Giant, Dry, Sainsbury's*	1 Serving/38g	126	2.1	332	12.4	55.5	5.5	5.8
Giant, Tesco*	1 Pack/220g	350	14.4	160	4.1	20.7	6.6	1.2
Giant, with Butternut Squash, & Feta, Co-Op*	1 Pack/218g	246	7.6	113	4.5	13.3	3.5	5.5
Harissa, Style, Savoury, Sainsbury's*	1 Serving/260g	434	12	167	4.7	26.8	4.6	1.3
Moroccan Spiced, Fruity, Waitrose*	1 Serving/78g	146	3.7	187	4.5	29.2	4.8	4.4
Moroccan, Medley, Ainsley Harriott*	½ Sachet/130g	178	2	137	5.4	25.4	1.5	2.2
Moroccan, Style, Fruity, M&S*	1 Serving/200g	370	5.4	185	3.4	36.7	2.7	3.4
Moroccan, Style, Spiced, Meadow Fresh, Lidl*	1 Pack/280g	456	14.8	163	3	25	5.3	1.6
Moroccan, Style, TTD, Sainsbury's*	¼ Pot/100g	203	4.7	203	5.1	33.1	4.7	3.7
Mushroom, Prepared, without Oil or Butter, Tesco*	½ Pack/140g	194	1.3	139	4.3	27.7	0.9	1.4
Pearl, Cooked, Artisan Grains*	1 Serving/100g	114	0.5	114	3.8	23	0.5	0.9
Pepper, Red & Yellow, Chargrilled, Tesco*	1 Pack/200g	212	3.6	106	4.6	17.8	1.8	0.5
Spice, Sensation, Batchelors*	1 Pack/120g	163	1.1	136	4.7	26.3	0.9	1.8
Sundried Tomato, & Garlic, Sainsbury's*	½ Pack/140g	167	1.4	119	4.1	22.5	1	1.9
Tomato, & Basil, Made Up, Tesco*	1 Serving/200g	348	16.6	174	3.9	21	8.3	3.4
Tomato, & Mediterranean Herb, Made Up, Co-Op*	½ Pack/138g	189	1.5	137	5.3	26	1.1	1.6
Tomato, & Onion, Dry Weight, Waitrose*	1 Pack/110g	376	4	342	12.6	64.9	3.6	5.1
Tomato, Mediterranean, GFY, Asda*	½ Pack/141g	192	1.3	136	5	27	0.9	1.7
Tomato, Sun Dried, CBY, Asda*	1 Pack/310g	515	12.1	166	4.6	26.2	3.9	4
Tomato, Sundried, & Garlic, Newgate, Lidl*	1 Serving/135g	181	1.5	134	4.5	25.7	1.1	1.7
Vegetable, & Olive Oil, Chargrilled, Delphi*	½ Pot/75g	105	2.9	140	3.8	22.5	3.9	1.9
Vegetable, Chargrilled, Morrisons*	1 Serving/225g	227	5.4	101	3.3	16.5	2.4	1.3
Vegetable, Chargrilled, Smoky, Finest, Tesco*	½ Pack/125g	194	5.6	156	4.3	23.2	4.5	2.6
Vegetable, Roasted, Cooked, Ainsley Harriott*	1 Serving/130g	180	2	138	5.6	25.5	1.5	2.6
Vegetable, Roasted, Dry, Ainsley Harriott*	½ Sachet/50g	180	2	360	14.6	66.4	4	6.8
Vegetable, Roasted, Snack Salad Pot, HL, Tesco*	1 Pack/60g	213	2.4	355	15.1	64.6	4	4.2
Vegetable, Roasted, Waitrose*	1 Serving/200g	328	13.2	164	3.9	22	6.6	0.9
Vegetable, Spicy, GFY, Asda*	½ Pack/55g	71	0.6	129	4.7	25	1.1	2
Vegetable, Spicy, Morrisons*	1 Pack/110g	187	5.5	170	5.1	26.2	5	2.9
Vegetable, Sweet, CBY, Asda*	1 Serving/100g	120	0	120	2.9	14.8	0	0
Vegetable, Chargrilled, M&S*	1 Serving/200g	200	3	100	3.9	17.3	1.5	1.6
with Barrel Aged Feta, Toasted, Finest, Tesco*	½ Pack/90g	183	8.6	203	8.9	19.5	9.5	2.1
CRAB								
Boiled, Meat Only, Average	*1 Tbsp/40g*	*51*	*2.2*	*128*	*19.5*	*0*	*5.5*	*0*
Cornish 50/50, Seafood & Eat It*	1 Pot/100g	144	5.8	144	21.6	1.2	5.8	0.5
Cornish Potted, Seafood & Eat It*	1 Pack/100g	235	17.5	235	15	5.1	17.5	0.8
Crab, Classic, Shippam's Foods*	1 Jar/75g	74	1.4	98	15.2	4.7	1.8	0
Dressed, Average	*1 Can/43g*	*66*	*3.4*	*154*	*16.8*	*4.1*	*7.9*	*0.2*
Meat in Brine, Average	*½ Can/60g*	*41*	*0.2*	*69*	*15.6*	*0.8*	*0.4*	*0.1*
Meat, Raw, Average	*1oz/28g*	*28*	*0.2*	*100*	*20.8*	*2.8*	*0.6*	*0*

C

	Measure INFO/WEIGHT	per Measure KCAL	FAT	Nutrition Values per 100g / 100ml KCAL	PROT	CARB	FAT	FIBRE
CRAB CAKES								
Goan, M&S*	1 Pack/190g	228	7.6	120	8	12.9	4	1.8
Iceland*	1 Serving/18g	52	3.2	288	7.2	25.6	18	1.3
Shetland Isles, Dressed, TTD, Sainsbury's*	1 Cake/75g	130	8.3	174	12.4	6	11.1	0.5
Tesco*	1 Serving/130g	281	16	216	11	15.4	12.3	1.1
Thai Style, TTD, Sainsbury's*	1 Cake/141g	297	14.1	210	8.7	20.5	10	1.8
CRAB STICKS								
Average	*1 Stick/15g*	*14*	*0*	*94*	*9.1*	*13.9*	*0.3*	*0*
CRACKERBREAD								
Original, Ryvita*	1 Cracker/5g	20	0.2	390	10.5	77.5	3.7	2.5
Quinoa, Red, & Sesame, Protein, Ryvita*	1 Slice/10g	37	0.5	368	20.7	53.2	4.9	14.1
Wholegrain, Ryvita*	1 Cracker/5g	19	0.2	379	11.3	70.9	3.9	7.3
CRACKERS								
All Butter, Cheese, Oat, Nibbles, Finest, Tesco*	1 Oat Nibble/7g	39	2.6	563	13.1	43.3	36.9	2.8
Ancient Grains Crackers, Kirkland*	3 Crackers/18g	90	4	500	11.1	66.7	22.2	0
Bath Oliver, Jacob's*	1 Cracker/12g	52	1.6	432	9.6	67.6	13.7	2.6
Bean Mix, Habas Tapas, Graze*	1 Punnet/30g	131	3.8	438	11.7	68.9	12.8	1.5
Beetroot, & Seed, Finest, Tesco*	2 Crackers/15g	75	3.7	497	12.2	53.1	24.8	6.4
Black Olive, M&S*	1 Cracker/4g	20	1	485	8.3	59.4	23.5	4.3
Black Pepper for Cheese, Ryvita*	1 Cracker/7g	27	0.2	384	13.2	72.9	2.9	6.8
Black Pepper, Savoury, Gourmet, Specially Selected, Aldi*	1 Cracker/5g	24	1.1	490	8.6	62	22	3.2
Bran, Jacob's*	1 Cracker/7g	32	1.3	454	9.7	62.8	18.2	3.2
Buckwheat & Chia, Rude Health*	1 Cracker/7g	29	0.7	388	14	56	8.8	15
Butter Puff, Sainsbury's*	1 Cracker/10g	54	2.7	523	10.4	60.7	26.5	2.5
Butter Puffs, Jacob's*	1 Cracker/11g	55	2.7	502	9.3	59	24.8	3.1
Caramelised Onion, Ciabatta, Jacob's*	1 Cracker/10g	43	1	426	12.5	68.6	10.3	4.3
Carrot Crunch, Sweet & Smokey, Graze*	1 Punnet/28g	140	8.1	499	13	42	29	11
Charcoal, Wafer, Miller's Damsel*	1 Cracker/5g	21	0.7	420	13.8	59.5	13.9	0
Cheddar, Goldfish, Pepperidge Farm*	1 Pack/43g	200	7	465	11.6	65.1	16.3	2.3
Cheese & Onion, Crispy, Bites, Ritz*	1 Bag/23g	109	4.8	474	7	63	21	2.7
Cheese & onion, Triangles, Eat Well, M&S*	1 Bag/30g	128	3.3	425	9.8	69.4	11	4.7
Cheese Thins, Asda*	1 Cracker/4g	21	1.3	532	12	49	32	0
Cheese Thins, Cheddar, The Planet Snack Co*	1 Serving/30g	153	8.8	509	11.5	50.1	29.2	2.1
Cheese Thins, Co-Op*	1 Cracker/4g	21	1.3	530	12	49	32	3
Cheese Thins, Mini, Snack Rite*	1 Bag/30g	144	6.8	480	12.9	55.9	22.7	2.5
Cheese Thins, Tesco*	1 Biscuit/4g	20	1.2	543	11.3	47.5	33.7	2.5
Cheese Thins, Waitrose*	1 Cracker/4g	21	1.2	545	11.9	52.6	31.9	2.5
Cheese, Cheddar, Crispies, TTD, Sainsbury's*	1 Thin/4g	21	1.5	576	14.2	39	40.4	2.2
Cheese, Mini, Heinz*	1 Pack/25g	108	3.6	433	9.4	68.6	14.6	0.6
Cheese, Oat Bakes, Nairn's*	1 Bag/30g	130	4.7	432	15	57.4	15.8	1.3
Cheese, Protein, Weight Watchers*	1 Pack/18g	71	1.7	394	22.8	51.1	9.4	7.2
Cheese, Ritz*	1 Cracker/4g	17	0.9	486	10.1	55.9	24.7	2.2
Chips, Cheddar & Chive, Vita-Wheat, Arnotts*	1 Serving/18g	81	2.5	452	8.5	70.2	14	4.4
Chips, Honey & Soy, Arnotts*	1 Serving/18g	86	3.6	480	6.8	66	20	3.5
Chives, Jacob's*	1 Cracker/6g	28	1	457	9.5	67.5	16.5	2.7
Choice Grain, Jacob's*	1 Cracker/8g	32	1.1	427	9	65.5	14.3	5.4
Ciabatta, Sundried Tomato & Basil, Jacobs*	1 Cracker/10g	42	1	424	12.4	68.5	10.2	4.3
Corn Thins, 97% Fat Free, Real Foods*	1 Cracker/6g	23	0.2	378	10.2	81.7	3	8.6
Corn Thins, Real Foods*	1 Serving/6g	22	0.2	378	10.2	81.7	3	8.6
Cream Cheese & Onion Flavour, Bakefuls, Ritz*	1 Bag/23g	109	4.8	474	7	63	21	2.7
Cream, Aldi*	1 Cracker/8g	36	1.2	456	9.1	71.7	14.7	3
Cream, Asda*	1 Cracker/8g	35	1.2	443	10	67	15	0
Cream, Average	*1 Cracker/7g*	*31*	*1.1*	*440*	*9.5*	*68.3*	*16.3*	*2.2*
Cream, BGTY, Sainsbury's*	1 Cracker/8g	32	0.6	400	10.9	71.7	7.7	3.1

CRACKERS

INFO/WEIGHT	Measure	per Measure KCAL	per Measure FAT	Nutrition Values per 100g / 100ml KCAL	PROT	CARB	FAT	FIBRE
Cream, Choice Grain, Jacob's*	1 Cracker/7g	30	0.9	400	9	64.5	11.8	7
Cream, Jacob's*	1 Cracker/8g	35	1.1	440	10	67.7	13.5	3.8
Cream, Light, Jacob's*	1 Cracker/8g	31	0.5	388	10.6	72.2	6.3	4.1
Cream, Morrisons*	1 Cracker/8g	36	1.2	446	9.6	68.5	14.8	2.7
Cream, Sainsbury's*	1 Cracker/8g	35	1.3	422	9.5	66.7	15.2	2.8
Cream, Tesco*	1 Cracker/8g	37	1.2	454	10.1	68.2	14.8	3.6
Crispy Cheese, M&S*	1 Cracker/4g	20	1	470	9.4	58.1	22.1	3
Crispy Chickpea, M&S*	¼ Pack/25g	99	1.4	396	17.6	67.8	5.5	2.5
Crispy, Salt & Vinegar Flavour, Walkers*	1 Serving/30g	130	4.5	434	6.9	66	15	3.6
Crunchy Grain, Breaks, Ritz*	5 Crackers/33g	143	5.8	440	8.6	60	18	3.3
Cruskits, Arnotts*	2 Cruskits/12g	40	0.2	331	9	63.7	1.5	0
Extra Wheatgerm, Hovis*	1 Serving/6g	27	1.1	447	10.2	60	18.5	4.4
Flamed Baked, Traditional English, Water, Rakusen's*	1 Cracker/20g	79	1.1	394	8.6	75.8	5.5	3.3
Flatbread, Multigrain, Carr's*	1 Cracker/10g	42	0.7	411	11	73.8	6.8	5.3
Flatbread, Multigrain, Jacob's*	1 Cracker/10g	42	0.7	411	11	73.8	6.8	5.3
Flax, Pumpkin, Organic, Raw Health*	1 Cracker/12g	64	5	533	19	8	42	21
Garlic & Herb, Jacob's*	1 Cracker/10g	45	1.7	450	10	68.3	16.7	3.3
Garlic, CBY, Asda*	2 Biscuits/12g	58	2.6	483	7	63.3	21.5	4.2
Ham, & Cheese, Shapes, Arnotts*	1 Pack/25g	117	4.6	468	10.3	63.7	18.2	0
Harvest Grain, Sainsbury's*	1 Cracker/6g	27	1.1	458	8.5	64.5	18.4	4.1
Herb & Onion, 99% Fat Free, Rakusen's*	1 Cracker/5g	18	0	360	9.1	82.6	1	3.9
Herb & Onion, Trufree*	1 Cracker/6g	25	0.7	418	2.5	75	12	10
Herbs & Spice Selection, Jacob's*	1 Cracker/6g	27	0.9	451	9.5	68	15.7	2.7
Japanese Beef Teriyaki, Sensations, Walkers*	1 Serving/24g	118	6.3	490	1.4	62	26	3.5
Light & Crispy, Sainsbury's*	1 Cracker/11g	42	1.2	384	11.3	61	10.5	13
Lightly Salted, Crispy, Sainsbury's*	1 Cracker/5g	25	1.3	533	7.8	62.6	27.9	2.1
Lightly Salted, Italian, Jacob's*	1 Cracker/6g	26	0.8	429	10.3	67.6	13	2.9
Louisiana Wild Rice & Beans, Graze*	1 Pack/30g	136	5.7	454	17	49	19	8.8
Matzo, Whole Wheat, Organic, Yehuda Matzot*	1 Matzo/35g	117	0.7	334	13.4	77.2	1.9	11.3
Matzos, Egg, Aviv*	1 Matzo/34g	132	1	388	11	78	2.8	0
Matzos, Flame Baked, Rakusen's*	1 Cracker/21g	75	0.2	357	10	79	1	4.3
Matzos, Tea, Flamed Baked, Round, Rakusen's*	1 Cracker/5g	19	0	382	9.9	85.7	0.8	3.7
Mediterranean Tomato & Herb, Oat Bakes, Nairn's*	1 Bag/30g	129	4.7	431	8.1	64.2	15.8	8.3
Mediterranean, Jacob's*	1 Cracker/6g	27	1	450	9.7	66.5	16.1	2.7
Mini, Snackers, Kosher for Passover, Rakusen's*	1 Pack/85g	303	0.8	357	10	79	1	4.3
Mixed Seed, Multi Grain, Asda*	1 Cracker/6g	28	1.1	445	11	62	17	4.4
Multi Seed, Thins, Ryvita*	1 Thin/9g	39	1.3	434	16.4	56.2	14.1	8.1
Multi-grain, Aldi, Savour Bakes, Aldi*	1 Cracker/5g	20	0.8	404	8.3	55	16.8	5.1
Multigrain, Corn Thins, Real Foods*	1 Cracker/6g	23	0.2	388	10.9	71	3.7	10.3
Multigrain, Morrisons*	10 Crackers/20g	76	2.2	379	8.8	61.3	11	5.1
Multigrain, Tesco*	1 Cracker/5g	24	1	477	8.8	60.8	20.8	5.7
Naan, Multiseed, Tesco*	1 Cracker/3g	14	0.6	477	11.4	61.2	20	3.2
Naan, Tandoori, Tesco*	1 Cracker/2g	11	0.4	451	10.9	65.8	15.4	2.9
Oat & Wheat, Weight Watchers*	4 Crackers/20g	74	0.5	370	10.5	75	2.5	4
Olive Oil & Oregano, Mediterreaneo, Jacob's*	1 Cracker/6g	25	0.7	412	12.4	65.5	11.2	6
Oriental, Asda*	1 Serving/30g	115	6	383	1.7	49	20	4.3
Original, Breaks, Ritz*	1 Cracker/6g	29	1.1	460	8.4	65	18	3.5
Paprika, & Nigella Seed, The Best, Morrisons*	1 Cracker/7g	31	1.2	448	10	61.4	16.9	4.9
Pizza Flavour, Mini, Sainsbury's*	1 Serving/25g	113	4	454	7.6	68.7	15.9	2.7
Poppy & Sesame Seed, Sainsbury's*	1 Cracker/4g	20	1	482	9.5	57	23	4.2
Poppy Oat, Cracker Selection, TTD, Sainsbury's*	1 Cracker/4g	19	0.7	467	9.8	65	17.7	4.1
Ritz, Mini, Kraft*	1 Bag/25g	126	6	504	7.9	63	24	2
Ritz, Original, Jacob's*	1 Cracker/3g	17	1	509	6.9	55.6	28.8	2

	Measure	per Measure		Nutrition Values per 100g / 100ml				
	INFO/WEIGHT	KCAL	FAT	KCAL	PROT	CARB	FAT	FIBRE

CRACKERS

Rosemary, CBY, Asda*	1 Cracker/6g	29	1.2	486	6.5	68.3	20.2	2.4
Rosemary, Sainsbury's*	1 Cracker/6g	30	1.4	502	7.8	65.1	22.7	3.1
Rye Cakes, Lightly Salted, Ryvita*	1 Cake/6g	23	0.1	363	8.9	69.9	2	13.7
Rye, Organic, Dove's Farm*	1 Cracker/7g	28	1	393	7	58.4	14.6	8.7
Salada Original, Arnotts*	4 Crackers/16g	68	1.6	427	10.4	71.5	10	3.9
Salt & Black Pepper, Jacob's*	1 Cracker/6g	27	1	457	9.5	67.5	16.5	2.7
Salt & Black Pepper, Eat Well, M&S*	1 Pack/25g	106	3.7	422	9.6	62.9	14.7	5.1
Salt & Pepper, Sainsbury's*	1 Cracker/6g	29	1.3	504	8.1	65.8	22.5	3.2
Salted, Ritz, Nabisco*	1 Cracker/3g	17	0.9	493	7	57.5	26.1	2.9
Sea Salt & Vinegar Flavour, Bakefuls, Ritz*	1 Bag/23g	108	4.8	471	7	61	21	2.8
Sea Salt, Tesco*	5 Crackers/30g	149	7	496	8.1	61.8	23.5	2.8
Seeded, Gail's*	1 Cracker/10g	40	2.2	396	12	33.2	22.2	7.6
Seeds, & Sea Salt, Snacks, Finn Crisp*	1 Serving/30g	111	2.4	371	12	53	8.1	19
Selection, Finest, Tesco*	1 Serving/30g	136	4.3	452	9.6	71	14.4	0
Sesame & Poppy Thins, Tesco*	1 Cracker/4g	20	1	485	9.9	57.6	23.5	4.4
Smokehouse BBQ Crunch, Graze*	1 Box/31g	137	4.7	441	10	62	15	5.4
Sour Cream & Garlic, Crostini, Mix, Graze*	1 Punnet/25g	133	8	531	15	44	32	4
Spicy Indonesian Vegetable, Waitrose*	1 Pack/60g	295	16.3	492	1.2	60.6	27.2	2.2
Sweet Chilli, Dipping, Tesco*	1 Cracker/3g	12	0.5	470	9.3	63.2	19.6	2
Sweet Chilli, Oat Bakes, Nairn's*	1 Bag/30g	128	4	426	8.1	68.4	13.3	7.2
Sweet Chilli, Thins, Ryvita*	1 Thin/8g	31	0.1	382	12	77.5	1.5	5.2
Tarallini with Fennel Seeds, Crosta & Mollica*	1 Cracker/4g	21	0.9	529	8.2	67.5	22	4.2
Thai Spicy Vegetable, Sainsbury's*	1 Pack/50g	231	10.4	462	7.2	61.5	20.8	2.6
The British Barbecue, Graze*	1 Punnet/25g	127	8	508	17.4	36.8	32.2	7.4
Thins, Thai Sweet Chilli, Crisps, Jacob's*	1 Pack/25g	119	4.8	476	8.2	65.6	19.3	3.1
Tuc, Cheese Sandwich, Jacob's*	1 Cracker/14g	72	4.3	531	8.4	53.8	31.4	0
Tuc, Cheese, Mini, Jacobs*	¼ Pack/50g	242	11.5	485	9.2	59	23	2.4
Tuc, Jacob's*	1 Cracker/5g	25	1.4	518	6.9	54.2	29.9	2.6
Tuc, Mini with Sesame Seeds, Jacob's*	1 Biscuit/2g	10	0.5	523	9.7	63.1	25.8	3.9
Water Biscuits, High Bake, M&S*	1 Cracker/5g	22	0.4	409	9.8	75.1	6.8	3.9
Waterthins, Wafers, Philemon*	1 Crackers/2g	7	0.1	392	10.6	77.9	3.6	5
Wheat, Tesco*	6 Crackers/30g	139	5.6	464	11.2	60.2	18.8	4.6
Wheaten, M&S*	1 Cracker/4g	20	0.9	450	10.2	57	20.2	5
Wholemeal, Tesco*	1 Cracker/7g	29	1	414	9.4	60.6	14.9	10.4

CRANBERRIES

& Raisins, Dried, Sweetened, Ocean Spray*	1 Serving/50g	163	0.2	326	0.1	80.3	0.5	4.6
& White Chocolate, Shot, Asda*	1 Pack/25g	94	2	375	2.8	71	8.1	3
Dried, Reduced Sugar, Craisins, Ocean Spray*	1 Serving/30g	75	0.3	250	0	82.5	0.9	25
Dried, Sweetened, Average	*1 Serving/10g*	*34*	*0.1*	*335*	*0.3*	*81.1*	*0.8*	*4.4*
Fresh, Raw, Average	*1oz/28g*	*4*	*0*	*15*	*0.4*	*3.4*	*0.1*	*3*
Frozen, Sainsbury's*	1 Portion/80g	18	0.1	22	0.4	3.4	0.1	3

CRAYFISH

Raw	*1oz/28g*	*19*	*0.2*	*67*	*14.9*	*0*	*0.8*	*0*
Tail, Big & Juicy, Waitrose*	½ Pack/70g	52	0.5	75	17.1	0.1	0.7	0.5
Tails, Chilli & Garlic, Asda*	1 Serving/140g	133	4.3	95	16	1.1	3.1	0.8

CREAM

Aerosol, Average	*1oz/28g*	*87*	*8.7*	*309*	*1.8*	*6.2*	*30.9*	*0*
Aerosol, Reduced Fat, Average	*1 Serving/55ml*	*33*	*3*	*60*	*0.6*	*2*	*5.4*	*0*
Brandy, Extra Thick, TTD, Sainsbury's*	1 Serving/30ml	131	12.3	436	1.4	10.4	40.8	0.5
Brandy, Really Thick, Finest, Tesco*	½ Pot/125ml	579	49.5	463	1.3	19.7	39.6	0
Chantilly, TTD, Sainsbury's*	2 Tbsp/30g	136	14	455	1.4	6.9	46.8	0
Clotted, Cornish, Finest, Tesco*	1 Serving/30g	176	19	587	1.6	2.3	63.5	0
Clotted, Fresh, Average	*1 Serving/28g*	*162*	*17.5*	*579*	*1.6*	*2.3*	*62.7*	*0*

	Measure INFO/WEIGHT	per Measure KCAL	per Measure FAT	Nutrition Values per 100g / 100ml KCAL	PROT	CARB	FAT	FIBRE
CREAM								
Coconut, Soya, Cuisine, Alpro*	1 Tbsp/15g	15	1.3	100	1.2	2.3	8.8	0
Double, Average	*1 Tbsp/15ml*	*68*	*7.3*	*452*	*1.6*	*2.4*	*48.4*	*0*
Double, Brandy, Waitrose*	1 Serving/30ml	138	12.4	460	1.3	14.4	41.4	0
Double, Extra Thick, Fresh, Asda*	1 Serving/30ml	135	14.4	449	1.7	2.6	48	0
Double, Reduced Fat, Average	*1 Serving/30g*	*73*	*7*	*243*	*2.7*	*5.6*	*23.3*	*0.1*
Extra Thick, with Baileys, Baileys*	1 fl oz/30ml	129	11.6	431	1.5	13.4	38.6	0
Goat's, Double, St Helen's Farm*	1 Tbsp/15g	67	7.2	449	1.7	2.6	48	0
Oat Alternative, Dairy Free, Oatly*	1 Carton/250ml	375	32.5	150	1	6	13	0.8
Pistachio, Petit Pot, La Laitiere, Nestle*	1 Pot/100g	184	10.3	184	4.6	18.8	10.3	0
Real Dairy, Lighter, Spray, Tesco*	1 Spray/13g	29	2.4	221	2.5	11	18.6	0
Real Dairy, Spray, Tesco*	1 Portion/13g	44	4.4	338	2.2	5.9	34	0
Single, Average	*1 Tbsp/15ml*	*28*	*2.7*	*188*	*2.6*	*3.9*	*18*	*0.1*
Single, Extra Thick, Average	*1 Serving/38ml*	*72*	*6.9*	*192*	*2.7*	*4.1*	*18.4*	*0*
Single, Soya, Fresh, Plant Based, Cuisine, Alpro*	1 Tbsp/15g	18	1.5	122	2	4.5	10.2	0.4
Single, Soya, UHT, Plant Based, Cuisine, Alpro*	1 Tbsp/15g	23	2.2	151	2	1.2	15	0.3
Soured, Fresh, Average	*1 Tsp/5ml*	*10*	*0.9*	*191*	*2.7*	*3.9*	*18.4*	*0*
Soured, Reduced Fat, Average	*1 Tsp/5ml*	*6*	*0.4*	*119*	*5.2*	*6.7*	*8.6*	*0.4*
Squirty, Reduced Fat, Asda*	1 Serving/13g	29	2.4	225	2.6	11	19	0
Strawberry, Light, Real Dairy, Uht, Anchor*	1 Serving/13g	25	2.1	198	2.6	8.7	17	0
Whipping, Average	*1 Tbsp/15ml*	*52*	*5.5*	*348*	*2.1*	*3.2*	*36.4*	*0*
CREAM ALTERNATIVE								
Single, Oatly*	½ Carton/125ml	188	16.2	150	1	6	13	0.7
CREAM SODA								
American with Vanilla, Tesco*	1 Glass/313ml	75	0	24	0	5.9	0	0
Barr's*	1 Can/330ml	33	0	10	0.5	2.2	0	0
Diet, Sainsbury's*	1 Serving/250ml	2	0	1	0	0	0	0
Shapers, Boots*	1 Bottle/300ml	3	0	1	0	0	0	0
Traditional Style, Tesco*	1 Can/330ml	139	0	42	0	10.4	0	0
CREME BRULEE								
Average	*1 Serving/100g*	*313*	*26*	*313*	*3.8*	*15.7*	*26*	*0.2*
Dine in Dessert, M&S*	1 Dessert/89g	186	13.1	210	4.9	14.2	14.8	0.5
French, Pots, Tesco*	1 Pot/100g	324	26	324	4.3	18	26	0.5
Gastropub, M&S*	1 Brulee/84g	285	24.6	340	3.1	15.7	29.3	0.7
M&S*	1 Pot/100g	360	32.6	360	3.3	13	32.6	0
Reduced Fat, M&S*	1 Serving/89g	186	13.1	210	4.9	14.2	14.8	0.5
CREME CARAMEL								
Asda*	1 Pot/100g	113	2.6	113	2.4	20	2.6	0
Average	*1 Serving/128g*	*140*	*2.8*	*109*	*3*	*20.6*	*2.2*	*0*
La Laitiere*	1 Pot/100g	135	4	135	5	20	4	0
Lidl*	1 Pot/89g	79	0.7	89	2.3	18.1	0.8	0.1
Tesco*	1 Pot/100g	115	1.6	115	2.8	21.8	1.6	0
CREME EGG								
Cadbury*	1 Egg/40g	177	6	440	3.2	73	15	0.4
Minis, Cadbury*	1 Egg/12g	50	1.9	435	4.2	67	16.5	0.5
CREME FRAICHE								
Average	*1 Pot/295g*	*1067*	*112.2*	*362*	*2.2*	*2.6*	*38*	*0*
French, Smooth & Tangy, Waitrose*	1 Serving/30g	116	12.3	386	2	2.3	41	0
Half Fat, Average	*1 Tbsp/15g*	*27*	*2.4*	*181*	*3.1*	*5.5*	*16.2*	*0*
Low Fat, Average	*1 Tbsp/30ml*	*43*	*3.6*	*143*	*3.3*	*5.6*	*12.1*	*0.1*
Oat, Creamy, Oatly*	1 Tbsp/15ml	27	2.2	177	1	9.1	15	1
CREPES								
Chocolate Filled, Tesco*	1 Crepe/32g	137	5.2	429	5.9	63.5	16.2	3
Galette, Buckwheat, Average	*1 Serving/100g*	*161*	*1.7*	*161*	*5.8*	*30.2*	*1.7*	*1*

C

CREPES

	Measure INFO/WEIGHT	per Measure KCAL	FAT	Nutrition Values per 100g / 100ml KCAL	PROT	CARB	FAT	FIBRE
Mushroom, M&S*	1 Pack/186g	195	4.5	105	5.7	17.1	2.4	2.5

CRISPBAKES

Cheddar & Onion, Cooked, Free From, Tesco*	1 Bake/125g	291	15.1	232	7.1	22.8	12.1	2
Cheddar Style, & Spring Onion, Free From, Sainsbury's*	1 Crispbake/110g	259	16.2	235	3.4	21.5	14.7	1.8
Cheese & Onion, Tesco*	2 Bakes/116g	233	12.6	201	5.4	18.6	10.9	3.3
Cheese & Onion, Meat Free, Morrisons*	1 Bakes/136g	282	13.8	207	1.5	23.5	10.1	4.9
Cheese & Onion, Ovenbaked, Iceland*	1 Crispbake/77g	145	5.3	189	4.8	25.9	6.9	2.3
Cheese, Spring Onion & Chive, Sainsbury's*	1 Bake/107g	232	10.2	216	6.4	25.1	9.5	2.2
Dutch, Asda*	1 Bake/8g	31	0.3	388	14.7	74.9	3.3	4.2
Dutch, Co-Op*	1 Crispbake/10g	38	0.4	375	16	69.6	3.5	6.5
Dutch, HL, Tesco*	1 Bake/8g	30	0.2	385	14.7	74.9	2.7	4.2
Dutch, Original, Van Der Meulen*	1 Crispbake/8g	30	0.2	386	14.4	73.4	3.1	3.4
Dutch, Sainsbury's*	1 Bake/10g	38	0.5	392	14.5	72.3	5	5.8
Dutch, Tesco*	1 Crispbake/10g	40	0.5	397	13.6	71.7	5.3	4.2
Mature Cheddar, Crispy Thins, TTD, Sainsbury's*	1 Thin/4g	21	1.5	581	14.2	38.3	40.6	2.8
Minced Beef, M&S*	1 Bake/113g	226	12.3	200	10	15.6	10.9	1.5
Roast Vegetable & Basil, Cauldron Foods*	1 Bake/115g	242	11	210	3.5	26	9.6	2.9
Vegetable, M&S*	1 Bake/114g	200	10.3	175	2.5	19.2	9	2.6

CRISPBREAD

3 Grain 3 Seed, Foodie Market, Aldi*	1 Crispbread/25g	109	4.2	436	15	52	17	8.8
3 Grain, Foodie Market, Aldi*	1 Crispbread/25g	113	4.7	461	15	49	19	10
3 Grains & 3 Seeds, Organic, Dr Karg*	1 Crispbread/25g	114	4.8	455	16	50	19	9.9
3 Seed, Classic, Gourmet, Dr Karg*	1 Bread/25g	108	4.9	430	16.5	46.6	19.7	10.9
Apple & Cinnamon, Ryvita*	1 Crispbread/15g	54	0.2	356	7.2	72.5	1.6	11.8
Charcoal, & Rye, Sourdough, Peters Yard*	1 Crispbread/3g	13	0.2	381	11.3	77.1	5.5	10.9
Chia Seed, & Buckwheat, Protein, Ryvita*	1 Crispbread/10g	38	0.4	371	21.5	56.9	3.7	12
Chickpea, Mung Bean & Chive, Easy Bean*	1 Crispbread/22g	93	4.1	422	12.8	50.6	18.6	6.9
Corn, Orgran*	1 Bread/5g	18	0.1	360	7.5	83	1.8	3
Cracked Black Pepper, Thins, Ryvita*	1 Slice/10g	35	0.2	344	8.8	66.6	1.6	14.5
Dark Rye, Ryvita*	1 Bread/10g	34	0.1	342	8.5	66.5	1.2	15.2
Fibre Plus, Wholegrain with Sesame, Wasa*	1 Bread/10g	35	0.7	350	13	47	7	24
Five Seed, Bites, Knacks, Peters Yard*	1 Portion/25g	99	2.3	397	14	69.6	9.2	10.3
Fruit Crunch, Ryvita*	1 Slice/12g	45	0.7	358	8.3	61.8	5.4	14.9
GF	*1 Serving/8g*	*25*	*0.1*	*331*	*6.4*	*72.9*	*1.5*	*0*
GF, Lovemore*	1 Crispbread/6g	23	0.1	385	8	85	1	2
Knacke, Trader Joe's*	1 Crispbread/25g	118	5.1	462	16	50	20	0
Mini, Sesame & Linseed, Dr Karg*	1 Crispbread/3g	13	0.4	424	12.1	57.6	12.1	9.1
Mixed Grain, Jacobs*	1 Cracker/10g	41	1.3	436	9.1	66.7	13.9	4.2
Multigrain, Deli, Ryvita*	1 Slice/11g	41	0.8	370	11.2	56	7.2	18.3
Multigrain, Rye, Crunchy, Ryvita*	1 Crispbread/10g	37	0.5	354	12.8	55.7	5.1	17.2
Multigrain, Ryvita*	1 Slice/11g	41	0.8	370	11.2	56	7.2	18.3
Original Rye, Thin, Finn Crisp*	1 Slice/6g	22	0.2	339	10	59	2.6	20
Original Rye, Wasa*	1 Bread/11g	35	0.2	315	9	67	1.4	14
Original, Ryvita*	1 Crispbread/10g	35	0.2	350	8.5	66.9	1.7	16.5
Pink & Black Peppercorn, Sourdough, Peter's Yard*	1 Crispbread/8g	30	0.3	374	12.5	68.2	3.7	8.8
Pink Peppercorn, Sourdough, Peters Yard*	1 Crispbread/4g	13	0.1	369	11.3	77.2	3.5	8.4
Provita*	1 Bread/6g	26	0.6	416	12.5	68.4	9.9	0
Pumpkin Seeds & Oats, Rye, Deli, Ryvita*	1 Crispbread/12g	46	0.9	370	11.2	56	7.2	18.3
Pumpkin Seeds & Oats, Ryvita*	1 Slice/13g	46	0.8	366	13.5	54.7	6.6	16.8
Roasted Onion, Organic, Dr Karg*	1 Bread/25g	98	3.7	390	15.8	48.5	14.8	12.9
Rounds, Multigrain, Finn Crisp*	1 Bread/13g	41	0.8	330	13	56	6	18
Rounds, Wholegrain Wheat, Finn Crisp*	1 Bread/13g	45	0.7	360	11	66	5.9	10
Rye, Original, Tesco*	1 Crispbread/9g	32	0.3	357	11.6	62.4	2.8	18

	INFO/WEIGHT	KCAL	FAT	KCAL	PROT	CARB	FAT	FIBRE
CRISPBREAD								
Salt & Vinegar, Minis, Ryvita*	1 Pack/24g	90	1.9	376	8.2	74	7.8	11.4
Scan Bran, Slimming World*	1 Slice/10g	31	0.5	310	14.9	29	5.3	42.1
Seeded, Spelt, Organic, Dr Karg*	1 Bread/25g	108	4.5	430	17.2	44.4	18	11.2
Seeded, Thyme, & Sea Salt, Fro*	1 Crispbread/20g	100	6.8	500	17	29	34	7.3
Sesame & Rye, Tesco*	1 Biscuit/9g	34	0.8	385	12.5	55.6	8.7	17.2
Sesame, Ryvita*	1 Bread/10g	37	0.7	373	10.5	58.3	7	17.5
Sesame, Savour Bakes, Aldi*	1 Crispbread/9g	31	0.5	344	10	57.8	5.6	15.6
Sesame, Simply, Ryvita*	1 Crispbread/10g	40	0.7	383	13.4	57.5	6.9	18.5
Sour Cream & Onion, Mini, The Foodie Market, Aldi*	1/6 Pack/25g	107	3.8	427	14	54	15	7.9
Sourdough, Original, Peter's Yard*	1 Crispbread/3g	11	0.1	381	12.9	68.3	4.1	9.5
Spelt, Cheese, Sunflower Seeds, Organic, Dr Karg*	1 Bread/25g	103	4.5	411	19.2	42.8	18.1	10.4
Sport, Wasa*	1 Bread/15g	46	0.2	310	9	64	1.5	16
Sunflower Seeds & Oats, Ryvita*	1 Bread/12g	46	1.1	384	9.7	58.4	9	15.3
Super Chia, GF, Semper*	1 Crispbread/14g	50	0.4	357	5.3	72	3.2	9.4
Sweet Chilli, Minis, Ryvita*	1 Pack/24g	90	1.8	376	8.5	75.9	7.4	10.3
Sweet Onion, Ryvita*	1 Crispbread/12g	43	0.2	356	9	70.6	1.4	12.6
Sweet Onion, Wholegrain Rye, Deli, Ryvita*	1 Crispbread/10g	37	0.1	365	9	70.6	1.4	12.6
Thin Crisps, Original Taste, Finn Crisp*	1 Bread/6g	20	0.2	320	11	63	2.4	19
Toasted Corn, Orgran*	1 Crispbread/15g	55	0.2	367	6.7	75.5	1.4	1.9
Wheat, Morrisons*	1 Crispbread/8g	28	0.3	377	11.5	73.1	3.4	4.2
Whole Grain, Crispy, Thin, Kavli*	3 Breads/15g	50	0.3	333	10	70	1.7	12.7
Wholemeal Rye, Organic, Kallo*	1 Bread/10g	31	0.2	314	9.7	65	1.7	15.4
Wholemeal, Light, Allinson*	1 Bread/5g	17	0.1	349	11.7	69.7	2.6	11
Wholemeal, Rye with Milk, Grafschafter*	1 Bread/9g	29	0.1	316	11.4	64	1.6	15
CRISPS								
Apple, Air Dried, & Cinnamon, Spare Snacks*	1 Pack/22g	75	0.1	342	1.9	76.4	0.4	14.2
Apple, Dried, Snapz*	1 Pack/15g	52	0	344	2	77	0	14.7
Apple, Eat Smart, Morrisons*	1 Pack/20g	68	0.1	338	1.9	75.3	0.7	11.4
Apple, Thyme & Sage, M&S*	1 Bag/55g	253	13.4	460	5.5	55.3	24.3	6.1
Bacon, Crispies, Sainsbury's*	1 Bag/25g	117	5.7	468	19.9	45.8	22.8	4.8
Bacon, Rashers, BGTY, Sainsbury's*	1 Pack/10g	34	0.2	340	10.8	70.3	1.6	3.5
Bacon, Rashers, COU, M&S*	1 Pack/20g	72	0.6	360	9.4	77.5	2.9	3.5
Bacon, Rashers, Iceland*	1 Bag/75g	330	13.2	440	8.3	61.9	17.6	2.9
Bacon, Rashers, Snackrite, Aldi*	1 Bag/18g	89	4.3	496	5.6	63	24	1.7
Bacon, Rice Bites, Asda*	1 Bag/30g	136	4.8	452	7	70	16	0.4
Bacon, Shapers, Boots*	1 Bag/23g	99	3.4	431	8	66	15	3
Bacon, Sizzler, Ridge Cut, McCoys*	1 Bag/32g	165	9.7	516	7.1	53.6	30.3	3.9
Bacon, Sizzler, Ridged, Snackrite, Aldi*	1 Pack/30g	160	9.3	532	7.2	55	31	3.9
Bacon, Smoky, BGTY, Sainsbury's*	1 Bag/25g	118	5.9	472	6.5	58.5	23.6	5.7
Bacon, Smoky, Golden Wonder*	1 Bag/25g	131	8.4	523	5.9	49.1	33.7	2
Bacon, Smoky, Ridges, Popchips*	1 Bag/23g	99	3.4	430	6.2	64	15	3.7
Bacon, Smoky, Select, Tesco*	1 Bag/25g	134	8.7	536	6.4	49	34.9	4.3
Bacon, Smoky, Snackrite, Aldi*	1 Bag/25g	130	7.2	522	6	57	29	3.3
Bacon, Smoky, Sunseed Oil, Walkers*	1 Bag/35g	183	11.4	530	6.5	51	33	4
Bacon, Smoky, Tayto*	1 Bag/35g	184	11.9	526	7.6	47.3	34	4.5
Baked, Average	*1 Bag/25g*	*93*	*1.5*	*374*	*6.5*	*73.5*	*5.9*	*5.8*
Barbecue, Corn Chips, Popchips*	1 Bag/17g	73	2.9	430	6	65	17	1.6
Barbecue, Handcooked, Tesco*	1 Bag/40g	187	10	468	6.6	53.8	25.1	5.2
Barbecue, Pop Outs, Passions, Aldi*	1 Pack/100g	422	13	422	5.8	69	13	3
Barbecue, Potato Crisps, Popchips*	1 Pack/23g	97	3.4	420	5.7	62	15	3.9
Barbecue, Savoury Snacks, Weight Watchers*	1 Pack/22g	81	1.9	366	18.6	61	8.7	6.1
Barbecue, Sticky, Oven Baked, Walkers*	1 Pack/25g	109	3.4	435	6.8	68.4	13.5	6.3
BBQ Pulled Pork, Trending Tastes, Walkers*	1 Pack/32g	161	8.7	497	5.4	56	27	4.3

CRISPS

INFO/WEIGHT	per Measure KCAL	FAT	KCAL	PROT	CARB	FAT	FIBRE
	Measure		**Nutrition Values per 100g / 100ml**				
CRISPS							
BBQ, Bangin', Mountain Chips, Muscle Moose*	1 Pack/23g	93	2.1	406	22	55	9.1	7.9
BBQ, Southern Style, Bugles, Walkers*	1 Pack/20g	105	6	525	6.5	56	30	3.5
BBQ, Stackers, Snackrite, Aldi*	1 Serving/25g	134	8.5	538	3.1	53	34	4
Beef, & Horseradish, Hand Cooked , Deluxe, Lidl*	1 Pack/25g	121	6.8	484	7	50.5	27.1	5.1
Beef, & Horseradish, Roast, Tyrrells*	¼ Pack/38g	165	10.1	439	5.3	41.7	26.9	4.7
Beef, & Mustard, Roast, Thick Cut, Brannigans*	1 Bag/40g	203	12	507	7.6	51.7	30	3.7
Beef, & Onion Flavour, Average	**1 Bag/25g**	**131**	**8.3**	**524**	**6.5**	**50**	**33.1**	**4.3**
Beef, & Onion, Tayto*	1 Bag/35g	184	11.9	526	7.6	47.3	34	4.5
Beef, & Onion, Walkers*	1 Bag/33g	171	10.7	525	6.5	50	33	4
Beef, & Red Wine, Specially Selected, Aldi*	1 Serving/25g	130	7.3	519	5.1	59	29	2.5
Beef, Angus, & English Mustard, Furrows, Tyrrells*	1 Bag/40g	201	11.3	502	6.8	52.2	28.2	0
Beef, Barbecue, Select, Tesco*	1 Pack/25g	134	8.7	536	6.4	49.2	34.8	4.4
Beef, Chinese Sizzling, McCoys*	1 Bag/35g	177	10.6	506	6.9	51.8	30.2	4
Beef, Maize & Potato, Happy Shopper*	1/3 Pack/23g	120	6.7	520	7.3	58	29	1.6
Beef, Roast, English, & Yorkshire Pudding, Walkers*	1 Bag/35g	180	11.3	522	6.6	50.4	32.7	4
Beef, Roast, Monster Claws, Snackrite, Aldi*	1 Pack/17g	87	4.4	511	6.3	62	26	1.2
Beef, Space Raiders, KP Snacks*	1 Pack/13g	64	2.9	495	6.5	65.3	22.8	1
Beefy, Smiths, Walkers*	1 Bag/25g	133	9.2	531	4.3	45.2	37	0
Beetroot, & Parsnip, Vegetable, Nims*	1 Pack/18g	58	0.4	325	11	54	2.5	21
Beetroot, Eat Smart, Morrisons*	1 Pack/20g	63	0.1	313	15.1	52	0.4	20.5
Black Pepper, Forno, Lay's*	1 Pack/170g	731	20.9	430	5.6	74	12.3	3.6
Brussels Sprout, Walkers*	1 Bag/25g	126	6.7	504	6	57.2	26.8	4.4
Bugles, Cheese Flavour, Walkers*	1 Pack/30g	158	8.8	525	7	56.9	29.3	3
Bunny Bites, Original Flavour, Tesco*	1 Pack/19g	100	5.7	526	2.5	59.9	30.1	2.6
Carrot, Eat Smart, Morrisons*	1 Pack/200g	63	0.3	316	5.5	61.9	1.3	17.2
Cheddar, & Bacon, Temptingly, Walkers*	1 Pack/32g	169	10	520	6.2	52.3	30.9	4.2
Cheddar, & Chive, Mature, Kettle Chips*	1 Serving/50g	239	12.7	478	8.1	54.4	25.4	5
Cheddar, & Chive, Mature, Tyrrells*	1 Serving/30g	134	6.9	447	6.9	53.7	23.1	2.4
Cheddar, & Onion, Crinkles, Walkers*	1 Pack/28g	150	9.3	538	6	51.5	33.3	3.5
Cheddar, & Onion, Hand Cooked, Aldi*	1 Pack/150g	753	41.8	502	7.7	54.9	27.9	4
Cheddar, & Red Onion Chutney, Sensations, Walkers*	1 Bag/40g	198	11.2	495	6.5	54	28	4.5
Cheddar, & Red Onion, Mature, Finest, Tesco*	1 Bag/40g	208	8.3	519	5.1	58.6	20.8	2.5
Cheddar, & Jalapeno, Popchips*	1 Pack/85g	351	12.8	413	6.4	64	15	4.2
Cheddar, Mature, & Red Onion, Hand Cooked, M&S*	1 Pack/40g	206	11.7	515	7.8	52.5	29.2	5.6
Cheese & Onion, 30% Less Fat, Sainsbury's*	1 Pack/25g	115	5.4	459	7.5	58.1	21.8	5.4
Cheese & Onion, Crinkle Cut, Low Fat, Waitrose*	1 Bag/25g	122	5.8	490	7.7	62.6	23.2	4.7
Cheese & Onion, GFY, Asda*	1 Pack/26g	122	5.7	470	7	61	22	4.2
Cheese & Onion, KP Snacks*	1 Bag/25g	134	8.7	534	6.6	48.7	34.8	4.8
Cheese & Onion, M&S*	1 Bag/25g	134	8.9	535	5.5	48.8	35.5	5
Cheese & Onion, Max, Walkers*	1 Pack/50g	266	16.4	533	6.8	51	32.9	2.9
Cheese & Onion, Organic, Tesco*	1 Bag/25g	128	8.2	514	5.2	49.9	32.6	7
Cheese & Onion, Red Onion, Extra Crunchy, Walkers*	1 Serving/30g	140	6.3	468	6.8	60.6	20.9	4.9
Cheese & Onion, Rings, Crunchy, Shapers, Boots*	1 Bag/15g	56	0.4	374	5.9	81	2.9	2
Cheese & Onion, Sainsbury's*	1 Bag/25g	132	8.7	527	4.6	48.8	34.8	3.9
Cheese & Onion, Sprinters*	1 Bag/25g	137	9.2	549	5.4	49.4	36.6	0
Cheese & Onion, Squares, Walkers*	1 Bag/25g	108	4.5	430	6.5	61	18	5.5
Cheese & Onion, Value, Tesco*	1 Bag/20g	108	7.2	541	6	48.3	36	4.8
Cheese & Onion Flavour, Asda*	1 Bag/25g	130	7.8	519	5.6	53.6	31.4	3.7
Cheese & Onion, Baked, Walkers*	1 Bag/32g	164	5.1	436	6.7	68.6	13.6	6.2
Cheese & Onion, Crinkle, Seabrook*	1 Pack/32g	170	10.5	536	5.9	51.1	33.1	5.2
Cheese & Onion, Discos, KP Snacks*	1 Pack/28g	146	8.2	520	5.1	59.1	29.3	2.5
Cheese & Onion, Golden Wonder*	1 Bag/25g	132	8	530	6.1	53	31.9	3
Cheese & Onion, Hand Cooked, Ten Acre*	1 Bag/40g	201	11.5	503	6.6	51.8	28.7	6.2

CRISPS

	Measure INFO/WEIGHT	per Measure KCAL	FAT	KCAL	PROT	CARB	FAT	FIBRE
Cheese & Onion, Handcooked, Fairfields Farm*	1 Pack/40g	207	12.4	518	8.2	53.5	31.1	5
Cheese & Onion, Lights, Walkers*	1 Bag/24g	113	5	470	7.5	62	21	5
Cheese & Onion, Oven Baked, Asda*	1 Bag/25g	95	2	380	5.1	72	8	3.3
Cheese & Onion, Oven Baked, Tesco*	1 Bag/25g	102	1.6	410	5.3	74.7	6.6	7.7
Cheese & Onion, Pom Bear, Intersnack Ltd*	1 Bag/19g	95	5.3	498	3.8	58.1	27.8	3.2
Cheese & Onion, Snackrite, Aldi*	1 Pack/25g	137	8.2	548	7.2	55	33	1.5
Cheese & Onion, Sunseed Oil, Walkers*	1 Bag/33g	171	10.7	525	7	50	33	4
Cheese & Onion, Tesco*	1 Pack/25g	135	8	535	5.4	54.8	31.8	3.2
Cheese Curls, Asda*	1 Pack/17g	87	4.9	511	3.8	59.7	28.6	1.7
Cheese Curls, Asda*	1 Bag/16g	87	5.3	541	3.6	57	33	1.7
Cheese Curls, Bobby's*	1 Bag/40g	225	14.8	563	7.6	50.1	36.9	0
Cheese Curls, Morrisons*	1 Bag/17g	95	6.1	557	3.1	54.8	35.6	2.6
Cheese Curls, Shapers, Boots*	1 Pack/14g	68	3.8	489	4.5	57	27	2.7
Cheese Curls, Tesco*	1 Bag/14g	75	4.5	520	4.5	54.4	31.1	1.9
Cheese Curls, Tesco*	1 Pack/17g	90	5.4	530	3.5	56	32	1.9
Cheese Curls, Weight Watchers*	1 Pack/20g	78	1.7	392	5	73.8	8.6	3.4
Cheese Puffs, Co-Op*	1 Bag/60g	321	20.4	535	3	54	34	2
Cheese Tasters, M&S*	1 Pack/30g	156	8.7	521	8.2	56.2	29	1
Cheese, & Chives, Mature, Potato Chips, Tyrrells*	1 Bag/50g	261	14	522	6.1	56.5	27.9	0
Cheese, & Chives, Walkers*	1 Bag/33g	172	10.7	530	6.5	50	33	4.1
Cheese, Moments, Smiths*	1 Pack/28g	148	9.2	530	8	50	33	2
Cheese, Space Raiders, KP Snacks*	1 Bag/16g	76	3.5	473	7.1	61.6	22	3.1
Chicken & Thyme, Oven Baked, Walkers*	1 Pack/25g	109	3.4	436	7.1	68	13.6	6.1
Chicken Katsu Curry, Ridge Cut, M&S*	1 Pack/40g	202	11.6	506	7.5	51	28.9	5.7
Chicken Wings, Hot, Strong, Max, Walkers*	1 Bag/30g	160	9.9	532	6.3	51	33	3
Chicken, & Thyme, Oven Roasted, Tesco*	1 Pack/150g	728	40.5	485	6.5	54	27	4.5
Chicken, Chargrilled, Ridge Cut, McCoys*	1 Pack/32g	167	10	521	7	52.9	31.3	4
Chicken, Chargrilled, Ridged, Snackrite, Aldi*	1 Pack/30g	157	9	524	6.5	54	30	4
Chicken, Coronation, Walkers*	1 Bag/25g	131	8.2	525	6.5	50	33	4
Chicken, Firecracker, McCoys*	1 Bag/35g	177	10.3	506	6.2	54	29.5	4
Chicken, Roast, Select, Tesco*	1 Bag/25g	134	8.8	536	6.6	48.6	35	4.4
Chicken, Roast, Snack Rite*	1 Bag/25g	132	8.3	526	5.3	51.3	33.3	0
Chilli & Garlic, Hot & Spicy, Kolak Snack Foods*	1 Pack/25g	134	8.3	536	6.4	51	33.1	4.4
Chilli, & Lemon, Houmous Chips, Eat Real*	1 Serving/28g	126	4.8	449	6.5	68.4	17	4.5
Chilli, & Lemon, Lentil Chips, Eat Real*	1 Serrving/28g	130	5.4	466	9.3	66	19.5	3.2
Chilli, & Lime, Quinoa Chips, Eat Real*	1 Pack/30g	165	8.7	549	7	66.2	28.9	2.5
Chilli, & Lime, Strong, Max, Walkers*	1 Pack/30g	160	9.9	532	6.6	50.9	32.9	3.1
Chilli, & Lime, Thai, Oven Baked, Fusions, Walkers*	1 Bag/25g	108	3.4	434	6.7	68.3	13.5	6.3
Chilli, Cheese, Hummus Chips, Eat Real*	1 Pack/45g	213	10.4	474	6.5	57.2	23	5.8
Chilli, Haze, Chickpea Puffs, Organic, Hippeas*	1 Serving/22g	90	3.9	408	13.5	49.6	17.5	7.9
Chilli, Spiced, McCoys*	1 Bag/35g	175	10.1	500	6.1	54.2	28.8	4.2
Chipotle BBQ Pulled Pork, Ridged, The Best, Morrisons*	1 Serving/25g	122	6.7	488	6	53.2	26.8	6
Coconut, & Rice, Cheese Flavour, Puffs, Ape*	1 Bag/25g	115	4.2	462	7.9	68.5	16.7	2.8
Coconut, & Rice, Lightly Salted, Puffs, Ape*	1 Serving/20g	92	3.3	462	7.9	68.5	16.7	2.8
Coconut, & Rice, Thai Chilli, Puffs, Ape*	1 Sm Bag/25g	115	4.2	462	7.9	67.1	16.7	3
Corn Chips, Fritos*	1 Pack/43g	240	15	565	4.7	56.5	35.3	0
Corn Snacks, Crispy, Bugles*	1 Bag/20g	102	5.6	508	4.8	60.7	28	1.4
Cream Cheese, & Chive, Waffles, Spar*	1 Pack/27g	132	6.8	488	4.2	60.7	25.3	1.3
Cream Cheese, & Onion, Crisp & Thin, Ritz*	1 Serving/30g	135	4.8	450	5.7	68	16	5.1
Creamy Dill, Houmous Chips, Eat Real*	1 Serving/28g	126	4.8	449	6.5	68.4	17	4.5
Creamy Dill, Lentil Chips, Eat Real*	1 Serving/28g	130	5.4	466	9.3	66	19.5	3.2
Crinkle Cut, Lower Fat, No Added Salt, Waitrose*	1 Bag/40g	193	10	483	6.5	58	25	3.9
Crinklys, Baked, Cheese & Onion, Jacob's*	1 Pack/25g	122	5.4	489	8.5	63.4	21.6	2.9

CRISPS

INFO/WEIGHT	Measure	per Measure KCAL	per Measure FAT	Nutrition per 100g KCAL	PROT	CARB	FAT	FIBRE
Crinklys, Baked, Chilli Beef, Jacob's*	1 Pack/25g	123	5.6	492	8.3	63.2	22.2	2.6
Crinklys, Baked, Salt & Vinegar, Jacob's*	1 Pack/25g	122	5.4	488	8.1	63.5	21.5	2.6
Crunchers, BBQ, Smokehouse, Ufit*	1 Bag/27g	107	2.6	395	36	36	9.5	11
Crunchy Sticks, Ready Salted, M&S*	1 Pack/75g	398	24.8	530	5.6	52.2	33	3.8
Crunchy Sticks, Ready Salted, Tesco*	1 Serving/25g	119	5.9	475	5.6	60.3	23.5	3
Crunchy Sticks, Salt & Vinegar, Sainsbury's*	1 Bag/25g	118	6.1	474	5.9	58	24.3	2.4
Crunchy Sticks, Salt & Vinegar, Value, Tesco*	1 Bag/22g	112	5.7	509	5	64	25.8	0.8
Duck & Hoisin, Crispy, Walkers*	1 Bag/25g	131	8.2	523	5.8	51.5	32.6	4
Extreme Fitness & Sport, May & Raeburn*	1 Pack/15g	55	0.8	367	78	0.5	5.6	2.1
Fajita, Far Out, Chickpea Puffs, Organic, Hippeas*	1 Bag/22g	90	3.8	410	13.7	49.9	17.4	7.9
Fig, Banana, Crunchy, Emily Crisps Ltd*	1 Pack/18g	81	2.3	448	4	78.8	13	2
Four Cheese & Red Onion, Sensations, Walkers*	1 Bag/40g	194	10.8	485	6.5	54	27	4.5
French Fries, Crispy, Ready Salted, Asda*	1 Bag/18g	82	3.8	458	4.4	62	21	3.9
Fromage, 3-D Bugles, Benenuts*	1 Serving/30g	160	9.6	535	5.5	56	32	2.1
Fromage, O Smaku, Walkers*	1 Pack/40g	208	12.4	521	6.2	52	31	4.3
Garlic & Herbs Creme Fraiche, Kettle Chips*	1 Bag/50g	248	14.2	497	6	54.7	28.3	4.2
Green Onion, Lay's*	1 Pack/40g	210	12.4	526	6.4	53	31	4.4
Guinness, Burts*	1 Bag/40g	206	11.5	514	5.1	58.6	28.8	2.5
Ham, & English Mustard Flavour, Real*	1 Bag/35g	176	9.9	502	6.2	53.9	28.2	4.2
Ham, & Mustard, Salty Dog*	1 Pack/40g	192	10.8	480	7.5	54.5	27.1	4.2
Ham, & Pickle, Smoked, Thick Cut, Brannigans*	1 Bag/40g	203	11.9	507	7	52.8	29.8	3.8
Ham, Canadian, Seabrook*	1 Pack/30g	159	9.8	531	5.7	50.9	32.7	5.1
Ham, Honey Roast, Hand Cooked, Finest, Tesco*	1 Serving/25g	130	7.3	515	5.1	58.6	28.8	2.5
Ham, Sabor a Jamon, Ruffles*	1 Pack/45g	236	14.6	524	6.4	49.6	32.4	4.2
Hint of Salt, Natural Sea Salt, Walkers*	1 Pack/25g	126	7	506	6	54.3	28.3	4.7
Hoops, Ready Salted, Snackrite, Aldi*	1 Bag/25g	124	6	494	3.3	65	24	2.6
Hot & Spicy Salami, Tesco*	1 Bag/50g	216	18	431	26.2	0.7	35.9	0
Hummus Bites, The Foodie Market, Aldi*	1 Bag/20g	94	4.2	468	7.9	59	21	6.1
Jalapeno, & Cheese, Strong, Max, Walkers*	1 Pack/30g	159	9.9	531	6.5	51	33	3.1
Lamb & Mint, Slow Roasted, Sensations, Walkers*	1 Bag/35g	170	9.4	485	6.5	54	27	4.5
Lant Chips, Ikea*	1 Serving/25g	126	6.9	505	8.3	55.9	27.6	4.5
Lentil Chips, Sour Cream, & Chive, Proper Chips*	1 Pack/20g	93	3.9	466	9.8	63	19.3	1
Lentil Curls, Sour Cream & Chive, Sainsbury's*	1 Pack/20g	95	4.1	476	10.5	61.3	20.3	3.1
Lentil Curls, Sour Cream, & Chive, Tesco*	1 Pack/20g	90	3.1	448	11.3	64.1	15.6	3.3
Marmite, Sunseed, Walkers*	1 Bag/33g	168	9.9	517	7.3	51.1	30.5	4.3
Matar Paneer, Crispeas, Piper's*	1 Pacl/21g	91	3.5	433	19	45.7	16.7	11.4
Multigrain Bites, Lightly Sea Salted, Snaktastic, Lidl*	1 Pack/25g	114	4.4	454	6.3	65	17.7	4.6
Multigrain Waves, Smokey Bacon, Golden Wonder*	1 Pack/19g	80	2.2	422	7.5	69.7	11.8	3.6
Multigrain Waves, Sour Cream & Black Pepper, Tesco*	1 Bag/20g	97	4.6	483	6.4	60.4	23.1	3.9
Multigrain Waves, Sweet Chilli, Tesco *	1 Pack/20g	96	4.6	480	6.5	59.5	23	4
Munchos, Cheese & Onion, Eta*	1 Pack/14g	65	2.4	461	7.6	68.5	17.1	0
Naked, Tyrrells*	1 Pack/150g	680	36.8	453	5.6	50.8	24.5	0
Nature, Sibell*	1 Serving/25g	139	8.9	555	5.2	51.1	35.6	4.6
Oat, Snackers, Smoked Paprika, GF, Nairn's*	1 Bag/23g	101	4	440	9.7	56.6	17.4	9.3
Olive Oil, Mozzarella & Oregano, Walkers*	1 Serving/30g	152	8.7	505	6.5	54	29	4
Onion Rings, Corn Snacks, Average	**1 Bag/25g**	**122**	**6.1**	**486**	**5.8**	**60.9**	**24.2**	**2.7**
Onion Rings, Johnnys, Golden Cross*	1 Pack/16g	84	4.7	525	5.3	60.4	29.4	1.2
Onion Rings, M&S*	1 Pack/40g	186	8.6	465	5.2	62.1	21.5	4.3
Onion Rings, Tayto*	1 Pack/17g	82	4.1	484	3	63.4	24	2.4
Onion Rings, Tesco*	1 Serving/25g	129	6.8	515	6	61	27.1	1.7
Onion, Pickled, Golden Wonder*	1 Bag/25g	131	8.5	524	5.6	49	34	2
Onion, Pickled, Space Raiders, KP Snacks*	1 Bag/13g	64	2.9	495	6.5	65.3	22.8	1
Onion, Pickled, Sunseed, Walkers*	1 Bag/33g	171	10.7	525	6.5	50	33	4

CRISPS

	Measure INFO/WEIGHT	per Measure KCAL	FAT	Nutrition Values per 100g / 100ml KCAL	PROT	CARB	FAT	FIBRE
Paprika, Corn Snacks, Shapers, Boots*	1 Pack/13g	64	3.5	494	8.7	54	27	2.2
Paprika, Hand Cooked, M&S*	1 Pack/40g	210	12.5	524	5.9	52.3	31.3	4.5
Paprika, Max, Walkers*	1 Bag/50g	265	16.3	530	6.5	51.2	32.6	3.1
Pastrami & Cheese, Crinkle, M&S*	1 Bag/25g	120	5.9	485	6.5	61	24	3.5
Pea Snacks, Snackrite, Aldi*	1 Pack/21g	87	2.7	415	20	49	13	13
Peanut Puffs, Roasted, Ellert*	1 Serving/25g	125	6	500	13	56	24	4.1
Peanut, Supersize Flips, McEnnedy American Way, Lidl*	1 Portion/30g	147	7.2	491	14	11	24	0
Pear, Fruit, Nims*	1 Pack/22g	78	0.2	353	4	76	1	12
Pigs in Portionets, Walkers*	1 Bag/25g	126	6.7	504	6	56.8	26.8	4.4
Pineapple, & Beetroot, Nims*	1 Pack/22g	73	0.2	333	9	67	1	14
Plain, Quinoa Chips, Eat Real*	1 Serving/30g	159	8.6	531	7.1	62.3	28.7	2.4
Pom Bear, Original, Intersnack Ltd*	1 Bag/19g	100	5.3	528	3.2	64	28	2.4
Pop Corn, Sweet & Salty, Corners*	1 Pack/85g	389	12.3	458	4.8	76.4	14.5	1.1
Pop Oats, Sour Cream, & Chive, Nairn's*	1 Pack/20g	83	1.8	416	7.7	73.7	8.9	5.3
Pop Outs, Brown Rice, & Kale, Snackrite, Aldi*	1 Pack/23g	93	1.8	404	8.7	73.9	7.8	5.6
Popchips, Sea Salt & Vinegar	1 Serving/23g	95	3.2	411	5.1	63	14	4
Popped, Cheese & Onion, Weight Watchers*	1 Pack/20g	82	1.9	409	20	57.4	9.3	8
Popped, Crazy Hot, Ridges, Popchips*	1 Sm Pack/28g	118	4.2	420	6.7	60	15	4.1
Potato	*1oz/28g*	*148*	*9.6*	*530*	*5.7*	*53.3*	*34.2*	*5.3*
Potato Squares, Ready Salted, Sainsbury's*	1 Bag/50g	192	8	384	6.5	53.8	15.9	7.8
Potato Twirls, Sainsbury's*	1 Serving/50g	218	7.3	435	3	72.8	14.6	3.1
Potato Zoo, Crispy Potato Animals, Kids, Tesco*	1 Bag/30g	57	1.9	190	2.5	24.5	6.3	2.1
Potato, Baked, COU, M&S*	1 Bag/25g	88	0.6	350	8.5	76.4	2.3	5.7
Potato, Low Fat	*1oz/28g*	*128*	*6*	*458*	*6.6*	*63.5*	*21.5*	*5.9*
Potato, Tyrrells*	1 Pack/261g	1362	72.8	522	6.1	56.5	27.9	0
Prawn Cocktail, Crusti Croc, Lidl*	1 Pack/25g	136	8.2	546	5.3	55.1	33	3.9
Prawn Cocktail, Flavour, Seabrook*	1 Bag/30g	163	10.1	544	5.7	49.2	33.7	4.5
Prawn Cocktail, Golden Wonder*	1 Bag/25g	131	7.7	521	5.3	53.9	30.8	3.5
Prawn Cocktail, Hand Cooked, M&S*	1 Pack/40g	205	11.5	512	7.1	54.4	28.7	3.8
Prawn Cocktail, Lites, Shapers, Boots*	1 Bag/21g	92	3.8	438	5.1	64	18	4.1
Prawn Cocktail, Snaktastic, Lidl*	1 Pack/25g	134	8	535	5.9	54	32	3.5
Prawn Cocktail, Spirals, Shapers, Boots*	1 Bag/15g	73	3.8	489	3.3	61	25	3
Prawn Cocktail, Sunseed Oil, Walkers*	1 Bag/33g	171	10.7	525	6.5	50	33	4
Prawn Cocktail, Tayto*	1 Bag/35g	185	12.3	526	7.5	46.6	35	4.5
Prawn Crackers, Tesco*	1 Pack/40g	220	13.3	550	2.2	60.4	33.2	0.6
Prawn Marie Rose, Finest, Tesco*	1 Serving/25g	129	7.7	517	7.4	50.3	30.7	4.7
Prawn, Melts, Snackrite, Aldi*	1 Pack/16g	78	4.5	504	0.6	59	29	0.6
Prawn, Spirals, Shapers, Boots*	1 Pack/100g	468	22	468	3.1	64	22	2.8
Pretzel, Salted, Original, Pretzel Crisps*	1 Serving/28g	100	0	357	7.1	85.7	0	3.6
Puffs, Black Eyed Peas, Cheese, Bepps*	1 Pack/22g	91	3.7	414	15	54.5	16.6	4.4
Quinoa, & Poppy Seed, Chorizo & Goats Cheese, Tesco*	1 Bag/25g	115	4	461	10.7	66.6	16.1	3.4
Ready Salted, Crinkle Cut, Reduced Fat, Tesco*	1 Pack/25g	118	5.4	474	5.6	61.3	21.8	4.9
Ready Salted, Ruffles, Ruffles*	1 Serving/30g	160	10.1	533	6.5	48.8	33.7	4.5
Reggae Reggae, Grove Cut, Levi Roots*	1 Pack/40g	200	11.5	500	5.1	58.6	28.8	2.5
Rice Chips, Sour Cream & Black Pepper, Co-Op*	1 Pack/27g	109	1.8	404	9.8	74	6.6	4.6
Rice Chips, Sweet Chilli, Co-Op*	1 Pack/27g	109	1.8	404	9.4	75	6.5	4.2
Rice, & Corn, Snacks, Snaktastic, Lidl*	1 Pack/26g	109	2.4	419	7.4	76.2	9.1	1.2
Ridge Cut, BBQ Rib, Asda*	1 Pack/27g	139	7.8	514	7.9	54	29	4.5
Roast Chicken & Thyme, Oven Baked, Fusions, Walkers*	1 Pack/25g	109	3.4	436	7.1	68	13.6	6.1
Rough Cuts, Chargrilled Steak, Golden Wonder*	1 Pack/25g	124	6.6	497	7.1	55.7	26.6	2.8
Rough Cuts, Cheese & Onion, Golden Wonder*	1 Pack/25g	124	6.8	495	6.9	54.6	27	2.6
Salt & Vinegar, Sea Salt, Handcooked, Real *	1 Bag/35g	179	10.2	512	5.6	54.6	29.2	4.2
Salt & Pepper, Black, Cracked, Hand Cooked, M&S*	1 Bag/40g	206	11.8	516	7.5	52.2	29.5	6

CRISPS

INFO/WEIGHT	Measure	per Measure KCAL	FAT	Nutrition Values per 100g / 100ml KCAL	PROT	CARB	FAT	FIBRE
Salt & Pepper, Black, Handcooked, M&S*	1 Bag/40g	180	9.2	450	5.7	55	22.9	5.2
Salt & Pepper, Indian Black, Pipers Crisps*	1 Pack/40g	195	11.6	487	6.6	49.9	29	0
Salt & Peppercorn, Black, Delux, Lidl*	1 Pack/25g	123	6.1	492	6.4	57.2	24.4	4.8
Salt & Vinegar, Asda*	1 Bag/25g	130	8.5	522	6	48	34	4.2
Salt & Vinegar, Balsamic, Cracker, Jacob's*	1 Serving/25g	118	4.8	470	5.2	67	19.3	2.4
Salt & Vinegar, Balsamic, Delux, Lidl*	1 Pack/25g	121	6.3	484	6	56.8	25.2	4.4
Salt & Vinegar, Balsamic, Handcooked, M&S*	1 Bag/40g	208	12.1	521	6.7	52.8	30.4	4.6
Salt & Vinegar, Balsamic, Kettle Chips*	1 Bag/40g	204	11.2	509	5.7	55.8	28.1	4.9
Salt & Vinegar, Chiplets, M&S*	1 Pack/50g	220	9.4	440	5.7	61.3	18.9	4.7
Salt & Vinegar, Cider Vinegar & Sea Salt, Tyrrells*	1 Pack/40g	192	9.8	481	7.2	60.1	24.6	2.4
Salt & Vinegar, Cider Vinegar, Crinkle Cut, Finest, Tesco*	¼ Pack/38g	186	10	495	6.7	54.6	26.7	4.5
Salt & Vinegar, Crinkle, M&S*	1 Pack/25g	120	5.9	485	6.5	61	24	3.5
Salt & Vinegar, Fries, COU, M&S*	1 Bag/25g	85	0.4	340	5	80	1.6	4
Salt & Vinegar, Golden Wonder*	1 Bag/25g	130	8.5	522	5.4	48.5	34	2
Salt & Vinegar, Lights, Walkers*	1 Bag/28g	133	6.2	475	7	62	22	4.5
Salt & Vinegar, M&S*	1 Bag/25g	131	8.6	525	5.4	48.8	34.5	4.6
Salt & Vinegar, Malt, Hunky Dorys*	1 Serving/25g	132	7.9	527	5.1	54.7	31.4	0
Salt & Vinegar, Malt, Ridge Cut, McCoys*	1 Bag/32g	169	9.9	529	6.5	54	31	3.9
Salt & Vinegar, Morrisons*	1 Bag/25g	129	7.8	515	4.9	53.9	31.1	3.6
Salt & Vinegar, Sainsbury's*	1 Bag/25g	130	8.8	522	4.1	46.9	35.3	3.9
Salt & Vinegar, Sea Salt, Cider Vinegar, TTD, Sainsbury's*	1/3 Pack/50g	245	14.3	489	5.5	52.7	28.5	6.1
Salt & Vinegar, Sea Salt, Crisp & Thin, Ritz*	1 Serving/30g	134	4.8	445	5.6	67	16	5.3
Salt & Vinegar, Snack Rite*	1 Bag/25g	127	8.2	508	4.7	48.1	33	0
Salt & Vinegar, Snaktastic, Lidl*	1 Pack/25g	130	7.8	520	5.6	52	31.2	3.6
Salt & Vinegar, Tayto*	1 Bag/35g	184	11.9	526	7.6	47.3	34	4.5
Salt & Shake, Walkers*	1 Pack/24g	128	7.8	533	6.2	52.2	32.3	4.4
Salt & Vinegar, Average	**1 Bag/25g**	**130**	**8.2**	**519**	**5.5**	**50.3**	**32.9**	**3.4**
Salt & Vinegar, Baked, Walkers*	1 Pack/38g	150	3	400	6	73.5	8.1	4.6
Salt & Vinegar, Crinkle Cut, Reduced Fat, Lidl*	1 Pack/25g	116	5.2	464	6.7	60.6	20.8	3.6
Salt & Vinegar, Crinkle Cut, Seabrook*	1 Pack/25g	126	7.2	502	5.9	52.9	28.7	3.9
Salt & Vinegar, Discos, KP Snacks*	1 Bag/28g	145	8.3	517	4.7	58.3	29.5	2.3
Salt & Vinegar, Distinctively, Walkers*	1 Pack/33g	169	10	519	5.9	52.6	30.8	4.2
Salt & Vinegar, Oven Baked, Asda*	1 Bag/25g	95	2	380	5.1	72	8	2.9
Salt & Vinegar, Reduced Fat, Crinkle, M&S*	1 Pack/40g	183	7.7	457	6.8	61.9	19.2	4.5
Salt & Vinegar, Spirals, Shapers, Boots*	1 Pack/15g	73	3.8	486	3	61	25	3.4
Salt & Vinegar, Squares, Walkers*	1 Bag/28g	122	5	443	6.5	61	18	5.5
Salt & Vinegar, Sunseed Oil, Walkers*	1 Bag/33g	171	10.7	525	6.5	50	33	4
Salt & Vinegar, Thick Ridged, Snackrite, Aldi*	1 Bag/30g	159	9.3	529	5.8	55	31	3.4
Salt & Vinegar, Vibes, Chickpea Puffs, Organic, Hippeas*	1 Pack/22g	90	3.8	408	12.7	50.4	17.2	7.1
Salt Your Own, Excluding Salt, Aldi*	1 Pack/24g	130	8.1	536	6	52.6	33.5	4.5
Salt Your Own, Sainsbury's*	1 Pack/24g	127	7.9	520	5	52.2	32.3	3.7
Salt Your Own, Snackrite, Aldi*	1 Pack/24g	130	8.1	536	6	52.6	33.5	4.5
Salt, & Black Pepper, Popchips*	1 Bag/23g	94	3.2	410	5.6	62	14	4.2
Salt, & Vinegar, Sea, Ridges, Popchips*	1 Pack/23g	98	3.4	426	5.4	68	15	3.7
Salted, 30% Less Fat, Sainsbury's*	1 Serving/25g	122	5.6	486	7.3	63.7	22.4	8.2
Salted, Average	**1 Bag/25g**	**127**	**7.4**	**508**	**6.1**	**53.4**	**29.7**	**4**
Salted, Baked, Walkers*	1 Pack/25g	104	2.1	417	6.2	76.2	8.3	4.8
Salted, Co-Op*	1 Bag/25g	131	8.5	525	6	51	34	3
Salted, Crinkle Cut, Lights, Snackrite, Aldi*	1 Bag/25g	122	5.8	486	7	61	23	3.7
Salted, Crushed Natural Sea Salt, Darling Spuds*	1 Bag/40g	195	12	488	5.6	53.4	30	4.5
Salted, Deep Ridge, Walkers*	1 Pack/28g	148	9	529	6.4	51.1	32.1	4.6
Salted, Everyday Value, Tesco*	1 Pack/18g	100	6.1	535	5	52.8	32.7	3.8
Salted, Golden Wonder*	1 Bag/25g	135	8.8	539	5.5	49.9	35.3	2

CRISPS

	Measure INFO/WEIGHT	per Measure KCAL	per Measure FAT	Nutrition Values per 100g / 100ml KCAL	PROT	CARB	FAT	FIBRE
Salted, Lightly, Deluxe, Lidl*	1 Pack/25g	123	6.4	492	6.3	56	25.8	5.1
Salted, Lightly, Handcooked, Finest, Tesco*	1 Bag/40g	206	11.5	515	5.1	58.6	28.8	2.5
Salted, Lightly, Kettle Chips*	1 Serving/50g	256	15	513	5.8	51.5	30.1	6.5
Salted, Lightly, Potato Thins, LC, Tesco*	1 Pack/20g	72	0.4	360	5.1	79.5	2	4.2
Salted, Lights, Simply, Walkers*	1 Bag/24g	113	5.3	470	7	61	22	5
Salted, M&S*	1 Bag/25g	136	9.2	545	5.6	47.8	36.6	4.9
Salted, Morrisons*	1 Bag/25g	134	8.7	536	4.9	50.9	34.8	4.3
Salted, Oven Baked, Tesco*	1 Bag/25g	95	1.9	380	4.4	73.1	7.7	8.4
Salted, Potato Chips, Tesco*	1 Bag/25g	136	8.3	544	6.4	52.4	33.2	4.4
Salted, Potato Rings, Sainsbury's*	1 Serving/50g	257	14.2	514	3.2	61.5	28.4	1.8
Salted, Reduced Fat, Crinkle, M&S*	1 Pack/40g	188	8.2	471	6.3	62.8	20.6	4.6
Salted, Reduced Fat, Tesco*	1 Pack/25g	114	6.2	456	6.3	52	24.7	5.9
Salted, Ridge Cut, McCoys*	1 Bag/49g	257	15.6	524	6.6	52.6	31.9	4.1
Salted, Sainsbury's*	1 Bag/25g	132	8.1	530	5	52.5	32.5	3.7
Salted, Sea, Anglesey Sea Salt, Red Sky*	1 Serving/40g	185	8.7	463	6.8	59.8	21.8	5
Salted, Sea, Crinkle Cut, Seabrook *	1 Bag/32g	165	10	517	5.7	53.7	31.1	0
Salted, Sea, Furrows, Tyrells *	1 Serving/30g	143	7.2	476	6.2	59.9	23.9	0
Salted, Sea, Hand Cooked, Specially Selected, Aldi*	¼ Lge Bag/38g	182	9	486	6.2	59	24	4.5
Salted, Sea, Houmous Chips, Eat Real*	1 Serving/28g	126	4.8	449	6.5	68.4	17	4.5
Salted, Sea, Lentil Chips, Eat Real*	1 Serving/28g	133	5.9	478	8	62.1	21	4.5
Salted, Sea, Lightly, Hand Cooked, English, Tyrrells*	1 Pack/25g	125	6.4	501	5.9	49	25.4	5.3
Salted, Sea, Lightly, Potato Chips, Hand Fried, Burts*	¼ Bag/50g	252	13.8	504	6.4	57.4	27.7	0
Salted, Sea, Lightly, Potato Chips, Tyrrells*	1 Pack/150g	740	38.1	493	7.7	58.9	25.4	2.6
Salted, Sea, Popchips*	1 Bag/23g	94	3.2	410	5.5	62	14	4.3
Salted, Sea, Potato, Mackies*	1 Pack/40g	200	10.8	499	7.4	55	27	4.5
Salted, Squares, Walkers*	1 Pack/25g	109	4.8	435	6.5	60	19	6
Salted, Sunseed Oil, Walkers*	1 Bag/33g	175	11.1	537	5.9	49.7	34.1	4.2
Salted, Tesco*	1 Bag/25g	140	8.5	545	5	55.4	33.2	1.8
Scampi, Smiths, Walkers*	1 Bag/27g	134	7	496	13	52.5	26	0
Sea Salt & Malt Vinegar, Baked, M&S*	1 Serving/30g	149	7.9	497	5.4	57.1	26.5	4.2
Sea Salt & Malt Vinegar, Handcooked, Real*	1 Pack/35g	173	8.9	494	6.8	57.9	25.3	3.5
Shells, Prawn Cocktail, Asda*	1 Bag/18g	90	5.3	501	4.6	54.9	29.2	6.2
Smoked Chipotle Chilli, Kent Crisps*	1 Pack/40g	208	11.5	519	5.1	58.6	28.8	2.5
Smoky Bacon Flavour, Average	*1 Bag/25g*	*132*	*8.4*	*527*	*6.2*	*49.7*	*33.7*	*3.2*
Smoky Chilli Chicken, Muchos, McCoys*	1 Serving/30g	152	7.8	507	6.1	60	26	2.9
Snax, Original, Asda*	1 Serving/25g	126	6.5	504	4.5	61	26	4.2
Sour Cream & Chive, Popped, Snaktastic, Lidl*	1 Pack/25g	110	3.8	438	6.1	67	15	5.3
Sour Cream & Onion, Potato Chips, Popchips*	1 Pack/23g	95	3.5	413	28.3	69.6	15.2	4.3
Sour Cream, & Chilli Lentil Curls, M&S*	1 Pack/60g	243	5.2	405	13.6	65.3	8.7	4.3
Sour Cream, & Chive Flavour, Average	*1 Bag/25g*	*127*	*7.7*	*508*	*6.8*	*50.7*	*30.9*	*4.6*
Sour Cream, & Chive, Baked, Walkers*	1 Pack/38g	148	3.2	395	7	73	8.5	5
Sour Cream, & Chive, Crinkle, Reduced Fat, M&S*	1 Bag/40g	187	8.1	468	6.7	62.2	20.3	4.6
Sour Cream, & Chives, Quinoa Chips, Eat Real*	1 Pack/30g	165	8.6	550	8	66.4	28.8	2.5
Sour Cream, & Onion, Corn Chips, Popchips*	1 Pack/17g	72	2.9	422	6.5	65	17	1.9
Sour Cream, & Chive, Hummus Chips, Eat Real*	1 Pack/45g	213	10.4	474	6.7	58	23	5.8
Sour Cream, & Mexican Lime, Deluxe, Lidl*	1 Serving/25g	124	5.8	496	6	63.2	23.3	4.5
Sour Cream, & Onion, Stackers, Snackrite, Aldi*	1 Serving/25g	139	9.2	557	3.1	52	37	2.8
Spicy Sriracha, Trending Tastes, Walkers*	1 Pack/33g	160	8.7	491	5.6	55	26.7	4.3
Spicy, Mix Ups, Walkers*	¼ Pack/30g	148	7.2	492	6.4	60	24	3.6
Spring Onion, Tayto*	1 Bag/35g	184	11.9	526	7.6	47.3	34	4.5
Steak, Chargrilled, Max, Walkers*	1 Bag/55g	289	18.2	525	6.5	50	33	4
Steak, Flame Grilled, Argentinean, Walkers*	1 Bag/35g	182	11.3	520	6.5	50.7	32.4	4.2
Steak, Flame Grilled, Ridge Cut, McCoys*	1 Bag/47g	250	14.7	526	6.9	53	31	3.9

C

CRISPS	Measure INFO/WEIGHT	per Measure KCAL	FAT	Nutrition Values per 100g / 100ml KCAL	PROT	CARB	FAT	FIBRE
Steak, Flamed Grilled, Max, Walkers*	1 Pack/50g	266	16.4	533	6.5	51.6	32.8	2.8
Steak, T Bone, Bubble Chips, Roysters*	1 Pack/28g	151	8.9	540	5.5	55	32	2.6
Sticks, Salt & Vinegar, Asda*	1 Serving/25g	126	6.2	504	5.2	63	25	2
Sunbites, Cheddar & Caramelised Onion, Walkers*	1 Bag/25g	120	5.4	480	7.6	60.8	21.6	6.4
Sundried Tomato, & Garlic, Quinoa Chips, Eat Real*	1 Bag/30g	145	6.3	482	7.3	62.4	21	5.1
Sweet & Salty, Katy's Kettle Corn, Popchips*	1 Serving/28g	128	4	455	6.9	65.9	14.1	5.4
Sweet & Smokin', Hippeas*	1 Pack/22g	90	3.8	411	13.2	51.1	17.4	7.3
Sweet Chilli, & Red Pepper, Potato Chips, Tyrrells*	¼ Pack/37g	180	9.2	481	7.9	59.7	24.5	2.4
Sweet Chilli, & Irish Red Pepper, Keoghs*	1 Bag/50g	263	13.2	526	7.2	49	26.5	5
Sweet Chilli, Average	*1 Bag/25g*	*115*	*5.6*	*461*	*5.1*	*59.9*	*22.6*	*4.6*
Sweet Chilli, Crinkle Cut, Finest, Tesco*	1 Serving/25g	124	6.6	497	7.5	54.5	26.6	4.9
Sweet Chilli, Hand Cooked, M&S*	1 Pack/40g	207	12.1	517	6.1	52.8	30.2	4.6
Sweet Chilli, Lentil, Curls, Bites, Kettle Chips*	1 Pack/22g	94	2.6	428	13.2	65	11.9	4
Sweet Chilli, Mountain Chips, Muscle Moose*	1 Pack/23g	93	2.1	405	22	55	9.1	8.4
Sweet Chilli, Multigrain, Waves, Sainsbury's*	1 Pack/20g	104	5.6	520	6.3	58.6	28	4
Sweet Chilli, Thai, Lentil Waves, Burts*	1 Pack/20g	91	3.3	453	11.7	62.6	16.3	4.9
Sweet Chilli, Thai, Sensations, Walkers*	1 Bag/40g	198	9.9	494	6.9	59	24.7	3.7
Sweet Chilli, Thai, Velvet Crunch, King*	1 Pack/20g	81	1.9	404	1.6	77.5	9.7	2
Sweet Potato, Chipotle & Creme Fraiche, Kettle Chips*	1 Serving/30g	158	9.7	527	6.9	49.8	32.4	3.9
Sweet Potato, Lightly Salted, Baked, Kettle Chips*	1 Serving/20g	82	2.7	409	6.3	60	13.4	11.6
Tangy Toms, Red Mill*	1 Bag/15g	76	4.1	507	6	60	27.3	0.7
Thai Bites, Mild, Jacob's*	1 Bag/25g	93	0.8	373	6.9	79	3.3	1
Thai Curry, & Coriander, Tyrrells*	1 Pack/50g	261	14	522	6.1	56.5	27.9	5.4
Thai Sweet Chilli, Finlays, Aldi*	1 Serving/25g	126	6.8	503	8.3	54	27	5.3
Thick Cut, Guiness, Burts*	1 Bag/40g	208	11.5	519	5.1	58.6	28.8	2.5
Tomato & Basil, Houmous Chips, Eat Real*	1 Serving/28g	126	4.8	449	6.5	68.4	17	4.5
Tomato & Basil, Lentil Chips, Eat Real*	1 Serving/28g	130	5.4	466	9.3	66	19.5	3.2
Tomato & Herbs, Baked Fusions, Snacks, Walkers*	1 Pack/25g	109	3.4	434	6.7	68.3	13.5	6.4
Tomato Ketchup, Golden Wonder*	1 Bag/25g	135	8	521	5.1	54	30.8	3.6
Treble Crunch, Farmhouse Cheddar & Spring Onion, Tayto*	1 Pack/20g	99	5	494	5.6	60.2	25	0
Turkey, & Stuffing, Walkers*	1 Bag/25g	126	6.8	504	6.4	56.4	27.2	4.4
Twirls, Salt & Vinegar, Happy Shopper*	1/3 Pack/20g	96	3.9	480	3	70	19.5	2.5
Twirls, Salt & Vinegar, Sainsbury's*	½ Bag/40g	167	5.6	418	3	70.1	14	3
Twirls, Salt & Vinegar, Tesco*	1 Bag/80g	349	14	436	3.9	65.8	17.5	2.4
Unsalted, Seabrook*	1 Bag/30g	163	10.7	544	5.7	47.9	35.8	4.1
Vegetable, Average	*1 Bag/25g*	*118*	*7.4*	*470*	*4.1*	*46.5*	*29.6*	*12.1*
Vegetable, Crunchy, Asda*	½ Bag/50g	251	12	502	1.4	70	24	6
Vegetable, Finest, Tesco*	1 Serving/50g	203	12.8	406	5	39	25.5	14.6
Vegetable, Waitrose*	1 Pack/100g	490	35.2	490	4.7	38.5	35.2	13
Veggie & Kale, Straws, Eat Real*	1 Bag/22g	109	5.6	497	3.1	65.1	25.5	2.8
Veggie Puffs, Roast Beef, The Foodie Market, Aldi*	1 Pack/21g	87	2.8	414	21.9	45.7	13.3	11.9
Wasabi, Strong, Max, Walkers*	1 Pack/30g	160	9.9	534	6.3	51.7	32.9	2.9
Wheat Crunchies, Golden Wonder*	1 Pack/35g	172	8.7	491	11.1	55.9	24.8	0
Worcester Sauce, Sunseed Oil, Walkers*	1 Bag/33g	168	9.9	516	6.2	52	30.5	4.3
CRISPY PANCAKE								
Beef Bolognese, Findus*	1 Pancake/65g	104	2.6	160	6.5	25	4	1
Chicken, Bacon & Sweetcorn, Findus*	1 Pancake/63g	101	2.5	160	5.5	26	4	1.1
Minced Beef, As Consumed, Findus*	1 Pancake/115g	178	2.9	155	6.2	26	2.5	1.9
Three Cheeses, As Consumed, Findus*	2 Pancakes/107g	183	3.6	171	6.5	28	3.4	1.4
CROISSANT								
All Butter, Bakers Selection, Asda*	1 Croissant/40g	164	8.4	412	6.9	48	21	1.9
All Butter, Finest, Tesco*	1 Croissant/62g	258	14.3	415	7.9	42.9	23.1	1.9
All Butter, M&S*	1 Croissant/40g	179	10.8	447	10.1	40.1	27	1.6

CROISSANT	Measure INFO/WEIGHT	per Measure KCAL	FAT	Nutrition Values per 100g / 100ml KCAL	PROT	CARB	FAT	FIBRE
All Butter, Mini, Sainsbury's*	1 Croissant/30g	126	7	420	8.1	42.9	23.4	2.6
All Butter, Reduced Fat, Tesco*	1 Croissant/52g	164	5.5	315	7.5	47.4	10.6	1.8
All Butter, Sainsbury's*	1 Croissant/44g	166	7.5	377	9	46.2	17	1.3
All Butter, Tesco*	1 Croissant/44g	168	7.5	383	9	47.2	17	2.6
Almond, Bakery, Tesco*	1 Crossant/84g	342	17.7	407	9.3	43.8	21	2.4
Asda*	1 Croissant/47g	190	9.9	405	9	45	21	0
Average	*1 Croissant/50g*	*180*	*10.2*	*360*	*8.3*	*38.3*	*20.3*	*1.6*
Butter, Bakery, Tesco*	1 Croissant/72g	285	13.7	396	9.3	46.1	19	1.6
Butter, Charentes, Waitrose*	1 Croissant/41g	176	9.7	430	8.7	44.2	23.8	2.4
Butter, Morrisons*	1 Croissant/44g	196	12.5	446	9.3	38.2	28.4	2
Cheese & Ham, Delice de France*	1 Serving/91g	225	12.3	247	7	24.4	13.5	2.5
Cheese & Ham, Mini, Waitrose*	1 Croissant/17g	64	4.1	383	13.2	28.1	24.6	3
Chocolate Filled, All Butter, Finest, Tesco*	1 Croissant/75g	267	11.3	355	7.4	45.9	15.1	2.8
Flaky Pastry with a Plain Chocolate Filling, Tesco*	1 Croissant/83g	369	20.8	445	8.6	45	25.1	2.6
French Butter, You Count, Love Life, Waitrose*	1 Croissant/44g	168	7.4	382	9.8	46.4	16.8	3.1
Ham, & Cheese, Gail's*	100g	302	19.7	302	14	17.8	19.7	0
Hazelnut Creme Filling, Maitre Jean Pierre, Lidl*	1 Croissant/48g	235	14.4	490	6	47.3	30	2.9
Hazlenut, Waitrose*	1 Croissant/95g	466	29.9	490	8.3	41.6	31.5	3.6
Low Fat, M&S*	1 Croissant/49g	195	7.8	398	9.8	52.9	15.9	1.8
Mini, Lidl*	1 Croissant/30g	112	5	373	7.8	48	16.6	0
Plain, H.W. Nevill's, Tesco*	1 Croissant/40g	150	6.4	375	7.2	48.9	16.1	2.9
Reduced Fat, Asda*	1 Croissant/44g	159	6.5	361	9.7	47.2	14.8	2
Sainsbury's*	1 Croissant/40g	172	9.5	429	6.7	46.4	23.7	1.8
TTD, Sainsbury's*	1 Croissant/60g	264	15.7	440	9.7	40.6	26.1	0
Wholesome, Sainsbury's*	1 Croissant/44g	192	12.1	436	8.8	38.3	27.5	4
with Cocoa Filling, Max, 7 Days*	1 Croissant/28g	128	7.8	456	6	44	28	0
CROQUETTES								
Cauliflower Cheese, Spicy, Veggie, Morrisons*	½ Pack/112g	159	6.3	142	3.8	17.6	5.6	3
Cheese, Cheddar, Inspired Cuisine, Aldi*	1 Croquette/42g	129	7.1	306	7.2	24	17	2.5
Cod, & Chorizo, Chunky, Captain Birds Eye, Birds Eye*	2 Croquettes/95g	179	6.3	188	10	21	6.6	2.1
Potato, Asda*	3 Croquettes/81g	144	5.7	177	2	26.5	7	2.2
Potato, Birds Eye*	1 Croquette/29g	44	1.7	152	2.6	22.6	5.7	1.2
Potato, Chunky, Aunt Bessie's*	3 Croquettes/119g	192	9.5	162	2.3	19	8	2.8
Potato, Cooked, Sainsbury's*	2 Croquettes73g	157	7.6	214	2.9	26	10.3	2.6
Potato, Fried in Blended Oil, Average	*1 Croquette/80g*	*171*	*10.5*	*214*	*3.7*	*21.6*	*13.1*	*1.3*
Potato, Frozen, HFC, Tesco*	1 Serving/128g	266	11.7	208	3.3	26.5	9.1	3.2
Potato, Tesco*	1 Croquette/40g	83	3.6	208	3.9	26.6	9.1	2
Potato, Waitrose*	1 Croquette/30g	47	2.4	157	3	17.9	8.1	1.5
Serrano Ham & Manchego, World Cafe, Waitrose*	½ Pack/78g	238	14	305	8.4	26.1	18	2.6
with Meat, U Jedrusia*	1 Croquette/80g	205	9.6	256	10	25	12	1.9
CROSTINI								
Tomato, & Olive, Piccolo*	1 Pack/100g	427	12	427	11	67	12	3.8
with Goats Cheese & Red Onion Chutney, Waitrose*	1 Crostini/17g	47	1.3	274	9.1	33.5	7.8	3.1
with Oregano, Crosta & Mollica*	1 Pack/150g	726	21.2	484	11.7	74.2	14.1	6.4
CROUTONS								
Black Pepper, & Sea Salt, Crunchy & Spicy, 1, Waitrose*	1 Serving/25g	114	4.2	454	11.6	61.5	17	4.5
Fresh, M&S*	1 Serving/10g	53	3.3	530	11.4	50	32.8	3.2
Garlic, Waitrose*	1 Serving/40g	209	12	522	10.8	52.1	30	2.7
Herb, Sainsbury's*	1 Serving/15g	64	1.7	429	13.4	68.2	11.4	2.8
Lightly Sea Salted, Asda*	1 Serving/20g	83	1.9	414	12.9	69.7	9.3	4.3
Prepacked, Average	*1 Serving/15g*	*74*	*3.6*	*495*	*10.8*	*58.7*	*24*	*2.6*
Sea Salt, & Black Pepper, Belbake, Lidl*	1 Serving/20g	92	3.2	461	11	66	16	4.4
Sun Dried Tomato, Sainsbury's*	¼ Pack/15g	75	3.8	497	11.7	55.2	25.5	2.5

C

	Measure INFO/WEIGHT	per Measure KCAL	FAT	Nutrition Values per 100g / 100ml KCAL	PROT	CARB	FAT	FIBRE
CRUDITES								
Selection, Prepared, M&S*	1 Serving/250g	75	1	30	1.4	5.8	0.4	2
Vegetable Sticks, Average	*1 Serving/100g*	*24*	*0.2*	*24*	*0.7*	*4.5*	*0.2*	*1.9*
with Cheese & Chive Dip, Tesco*	1 Pack/115g	132	10.5	115	1.6	5.9	9.1	1.5
with Soured Cream & Chive, Reduced Fat, Dip, Tesco*	1 Pack/53g	30	1.6	56	1.8	5	3	1.9
CRUMBLE								
Almond, & Apricot, Devondale*	1 Cake/80g	314	13.2	392	3.6	57	16.5	9.8
Apple, & Blackberry, Bramley, BGTY, Sainsbury's*	1 Crumble/120g	217	3.2	181	1.7	35.8	2.7	2.2
Apple, & Blackberry, M&S*	1 Serving/135g	398	15.1	295	3.5	44.9	11.2	1.6
Apple, & Blackberry, Sainsbury's*	1 Serving/110g	232	6.2	211	3	37.1	5.6	2.1
Apple, & Blackberry, Tesco*	1/6 Pie/90g	286	11.7	318	3	45.8	13	2.8
Apple, & Custard, Asda*	1 Serving/125g	250	8.8	200	2.3	32	7	0
Apple, & Blackberry, Waitrose*	¼ Crumble/125g	296	9.8	236	2.9	37.6	7.8	2.1
Apple, 633, Oakhouse Foods Ltd*	1 Pack/150g	259	11.8	173	2.3	24.6	7.9	1.8
Apple, Average	*1 Serving/240g*	*497*	*12*	*207*	*0.9*	*40.5*	*5*	*1.1*
Apple, Basics, Sainsbury's*	¼ Crumble/125g	235	4.9	188	1.7	36.5	3.9	1.2
Apple, Blackberry & Plum, Bramley, Finest, Tesco*	½ Pack/175g	396	14.9	226	2.6	33.5	8.5	2.6
Apple, Bramley, 2 Pots, Sainsbury's*	1 Pot/116g	303	9.5	261	2.6	43.2	8.2	2.1
Apple, Bramley, CBY, Asda*	1 Serving/100g	257	8.4	257	2.5	41.8	8.4	2.3
Apple, Bramley, Favourites, M&S*	1 Serving/140g	390	13.8	279	4.6	43.2	9.9	1.2
Apple, Bramley, M&S*	1 Serving/149g	387	13.7	260	4.3	40.3	9.2	1.1
Apple, Bramley, Tesco*	1/3 Pack/155g	378	14.9	244	2.8	36.7	9.6	1.8
Apple, Fresh, Chilled, Tesco*	¼ Pack/135g	342	11.2	253	3	40.6	8.3	1.8
Apple, Sainsbury's*	1 Crumble/565g	1034	32.8	183	2.3	30.5	5.8	2.9
Apple, Slices, Frozen, Tesco*	1 Slice/54g	173	8	321	4.9	40.6	14.9	2.8
Apple, Waitrose*	1 Serving/125g	310	2.9	248	2.2	54.5	2.3	1.2
Apple, with Custard, Green's*	1 Serving/79g	171	5.3	216	1.9	37	6.7	1.2
Apple, with Custard, Individual, Sainsbury's*	1 Pudding/120g	286	13.9	238	2	31.4	11.6	2.4
Apple, with Sultanas, Weight Watchers*	1 Dessert/110g	196	4.3	178	1.4	34.2	3.9	1.3
Blackcurrant, & Apple, Devondale*	1 Cake/80g	314	13.2	393	3.6	57	16.5	9.8
Fruit	*1 Portion/170g*	*337*	*11.7*	*198*	*2*	*34*	*6.9*	*1.7*
Fruit, Wholemeal	*1oz/28g*	*54*	*2*	*193*	*2.6*	*31.7*	*7.1*	*2.7*
Fruit, with Custard	*1 Serving/270g*	*463*	*17.6*	*171*	*2.4*	*27*	*6.5*	*1.3*
Gooseberry, M&S*	1 Serving/133g	379	14.2	285	3.5	43.3	10.7	1.7
Plum, & Cherry, 775, Wiltshire Farm Foods*	1 Serving/120g	248	7.4	194	2.3	34	5.8	0
Rhubarb, Average	*1 Portion/150g*	*330*	*11.1*	*220*	*2.7*	*35.5*	*7.4*	*1.9*
Rhubarb, M&S*	1 Serving/133g	366	13.2	275	3.4	42.6	9.9	1.4
Rhubarb, Sainsbury's*	1 Serving/50g	112	2.8	224	3.1	40.4	5.6	1.8
Rhubarb, Tesco*	1 Serving/136g	318	10.6	234	3.6	36.1	7.8	2.5
CRUMBLE MIX								
Luxury, Tesco*	¼ Pack/55g	243	9	441	5.7	67.9	16.3	3.2
Topping, Sainsbury's*	1 Serving/47g	188	9.2	401	5.9	50.3	19.6	5.3
CRUMPETS								
Asda*	1 Crumpet/45g	85	0.4	188	6	39	0.9	2.1
Bakers Selection, Asda*	1 Crumpet/50g	106	0.6	211	6.7	42	1.2	2.7
Buttermilk, TTD, Sainsbury's*	1 Crumpet/52g	102	0.6	195	6.5	38.5	1.1	2.6
Co-Op*	1 Crumpet/40g	70	0.3	175	7	35	0.7	2
Essential, Waitrose*	1 Crumpet/52g	94	0.6	182	6.5	35.1	1.1	2.6
Golden Sun, Lidl*	1 Crumpet/43g	83	0.7	193	7.8	37.1	1.6	1.6
Morrisons*	1 Crumpet/40g	90	0.2	225	7.8	47.2	0.5	3.2
Premium, Sainsbury's*	1 Crumpet/50g	96	0.7	191	6.1	38.6	1.4	1.7
Rowan Hill Bakery, Lidl*	1 Crumpet/44g	78	0.5	178	5.5	34.5	1.2	0
Sourdough, TTD, Sainsbury's*	1 Crumpet/55g	93	0.3	169	5.6	34.1	0.6	2.4
Sourdough, Waitrose*	1 Crumpet/55g	95	0.4	172	5.6	34.9	0.7	2

	Measure INFO/WEIGHT	per Measure KCAL	FAT	Nutrition Values per 100g / 100ml KCAL	PROT	CARB	FAT	FIBRE
CRUMPETS								
Square, Tesco*	1 Crumpet/60g	101	0.5	168	6.3	33.8	0.8	2.7
Thins , Kingsmill*	1 Thin/27g	54	0.3	199	6.9	39.3	1.1	2.3
Toasted, Average	**1 Crumpet/40g**	**80**	**0.4**	**199**	**6.7**	**43.4**	**1**	**2**
Toasted, Tesco*	1 Crumpet/55g	106	0.6	193	5.8	39.1	1	2.2
Waitrose*	1 Crumpet/62g	116	0.7	188	6.3	37.9	1.2	2.1
Warburton's*	1 Crumpet/55g	97	0.4	176	6	35.3	0.8	1.9
Wholemeal, Bakers Selection, Asda*	1 Crumpet/50g	94	0.4	189	7.3	36	0.8	3.7
CRUNCHIE								
Blast, Cadbury*	1 Serving/42g	199	8.3	480	4.7	69.6	20.1	0.7
Cadbury*	1 Bar/40g	185	7.5	465	4	69.5	18.9	0.5
Nuggets, Cadbury*	1 Bag/125g	569	20.5	455	3.8	73.1	16.4	0
Treat Size, Cadbury*	1 Bar/17g	80	3.1	470	4	71.5	18.4	0
CUCUMBER								
Average	**1 Serving/80g**	**8**	**0.1**	**10**	**0.7**	**1.5**	**0.1**	**0.6**
Baby, Pickled, Always Fresh*	1 Serving/30g	14	0.1	47	2	8	0.3	0
Baby, Raw, Tesco*	2 Cucumbers/80g	12	0.5	16	1	1.2	0.6	0.7
Crunchies with a Yoghurt & Mint Dip, Shapers, Boots*	1 Serving/110g	35	1	32	2.1	3.7	0.9	0.8
Mini, Love Me Tender*	1 Cucumber/33g	6	0.2	19	0.7	3.5	0.5	0.5
CUMIN								
Seeds, Whole, Average	**1 Tsp/2g**	**8**	**0.5**	**375**	**17.8**	**44.2**	**22.7**	**10.5**
CUPCAKES								
Assorted, Sainsbury's*	1 Cupcake/38g	130	2.3	341	2.2	69.3	6.1	0.4
Carrot, Average	**1 Cupcake/40g**	**157**	**8.6**	**392**	**3.6**	**45.4**	**21.6**	**0.6**
Celebration, Tesco*	1 Cupcake/61g	310	17.8	510	2.6	58.5	29.3	1
Chocolate Filled, Free From, Tesco*	1 Cupcake/52g	238	13.1	459	3.4	53.6	25.3	1.6
Chocolate Fudge, Party Pack, Tesco*	1 Cupcake/63g	300	17.5	476	4.2	50.7	27.8	3
Chocolate Iced, Chocolate Buttons, Party Selection, Tesco*	1 Cupcake/32g	144	7.6	450	4.4	54.1	23.6	1.5
Chocolate, Average	**1 Cupcake/40g**	**159**	**6.4**	**398**	**3.5**	**59.9**	**16**	**1.2**
Chocolate, COU, M&S*	1 Cupcake/45g	130	1.3	290	4.6	62.2	2.8	4.3
Chocolate, Fabulous Bakin' Boys*	1 Cupcake/34g	152	8.1	448	4	54	24	1
Chocolate, Lyons*	1 Cupcake/39g	125	1.8	321	2.4	67.5	4.6	0.8
Chocolate, Mini, GF, Free From, Morrisons*	1 Cupcake/18g	79	3.7	438	4.9	57.3	20.5	2.3
Chocolate, Mini, Weight Watchers*	1 Cupcake/20g	87	4.3	426	6.1	52	21.1	1.8
Chocolate, Party Platter, Holly Lane, Aldi*	1 Cupcake/55g	268	16	487	3.1	53	29	1.4
Chocolate, Party Selection, Tesco*	1 Cupcake/47g	230	13.3	486	3.3	54.1	28	2.5
Cookies & Cream, Secret Chocolate Centre, Tesco*	1 Cupcake/69g	335	20	485	2.7	52.2	29	1
Funcakes, Mini, Peppa Pig*	1 Cupcake/26g	104	5	400	3.2	53.5	19.1	0
Iced Cupcake, Gluten & Wheat Free, Lovemore*	1 Cupcake/33g	138	6.3	418	2.1	54.5	19	0.4
Lemon, Average	**1 Cupcake/40g**	**184**	**10.1**	**461**	**3**	**55.5**	**25.3**	**1.1**
Lemon, COU, M&S*	1 Cupcake/43g	130	0.9	305	3.3	68.1	2.1	2
Lemon, Healthy Option, Average	**1 Cupcake/40g**	**131**	**1.5**	**328**	**2.7**	**68.9**	**3.7**	**5.2**
Milkshake Flavour, Mini, Co-Op*	1 Cupcake/22g	23	1.3	106	0	9.5	5.8	0
Red Velvet, Party Pack, Tesco*	1 Cupcake/62g	308	17.5	497	2.5	58	28.3	2.6
Red Velvet, Tesco*	1 Cupcake/63g	308	16.6	490	3.1	59.3	26.4	1.2
Sponge Top, Individual, Tesco*	1 Cupcake/50g	220	10.5	443	3	59.5	21.1	1.3
Strawberry & Cream, Party Pack, Tesco*	1 Cupcake/65g	316	17.8	486	2.5	56.8	27.3	1.8
Strawberry, Party Selection, Tesco*	1 Cupcake/46g	229	13.3	496	2	55.8	28.8	2.8
Toffee, Thorntons*	1 Cupcake/80g	330	16	412	2.4	56	20	0
Unicorn, Tesco*	1 Cupcake/63g	316	17.6	502	3.2	58.6	28	1.1
Vanilla, & Chocolate, Mini, Waitrose*	1 Cupcake/21g	93	4.8	441	4.1	53.7	22.9	2.2
Vanilla, Mini, GF, Free From, Morrisons*	1 Cupcake/18g	29	4.1	162	3.5	60.3	22.8	0.8
Vanilla, Party Platter, Holly Lane, Aldi*	1 Cupcake/57g	282	16	494	2.6	56	28	2.1
Vanilla, Party Selection, Tesco*	1 Cupcake/46g	230	13.1	495	2.6	57.2	28.1	1.5

C

	Measure INFO/WEIGHT	per Measure KCAL	per Measure FAT	Nutrition Values per 100g / 100ml KCAL	PROT	CARB	FAT	FIBRE
CUPCAKES								
White Chocolate, & Vanilla, Tesco*	1 Cupcake/76g	390	22.5	513	1.7	59.7	29.6	0.8
White Iced, with Sugar Strands, Party Selection, Tesco*	1 Cupcake/33g	142	6.7	430	4.2	57.1	20.2	1.4
CURACAO								
Average	***1 Pub Shot/35ml***	***109***	***0***	***311***	***0***	***28.3***	***0***	***0***
CURLY WURLY								
Cadbury*	1 Bar/26g	118	4.7	453	3.1	70	18	0.7
Squirlies, Cadbury*	1 Squirl/3g	13	0.5	442	3.5	69.2	17.3	0.8
CURRANTS								
Average	***1oz/28g***	***75***	***0.1***	***267***	***2.3***	***67.8***	***0.4***	***1.9***
CURRY								
& Chips, Curry Sauce, Chipped Potatoes, Kershaws*	1 Serving/330g	391	8.2	118	10	14	2.5	2
Aubergine	***1oz/28g***	***33***	***2.8***	***118***	***1.4***	***6.2***	***10.1***	***1.5***
Aubergine, Masala, TTD, Sainsbury's*	½ Pack/115g	135	11.4	117	2.9	4.1	9.9	5.8
Beef, Sainsbury's*	1 Serving/400g	552	32.8	138	10.7	5.4	8.2	0.9
Beef, Thai, Finest, Tesco*	1 Serving/500g	770	29	154	9	16.5	5.8	1.2
Beef, with Rice, Iceland*,	1 Pack/500g	580	14.5	116	5	16.7	2.9	1.5
Blackeye Bean, Gujerati	***1oz/28g***	***36***	***1.2***	***127***	***7.2***	***16.1***	***4.4***	***2.8***
Cabbage	***1oz/28g***	***23***	***1.4***	***82***	***1.9***	***8.1***	***5***	***2.1***
Cauliflower & Potato	***1oz/28g***	***17***	***0.7***	***59***	***3.4***	***6.6***	***2.4***	***1.8***
Cauliflower, & Chickpea, Lovely Vegetables, M&S*	1 Serving/390g	351	13.6	90	2.9	11.2	3.5	3.7
Cauliflower, & Paneer, Charlie Bigham's*	1 Serving/403g	480	28.2	119	5.6	10	7	0
Cauliflower, Chickpea, & Potato, Vegan, Waitrose*	½ Pack/205g	166	7.4	81	3.2	6.4	3.6	5.2
Chana Saag, Slimming World*	1 Pack/350g	256	4.9	73	4.4	7.3	1.4	6.8
Chennai Dhal, Chickpea, Mumbai Street Food, Iceland*	1 Meal/181g	174	8	96	4.3	8	4.4	4
Chick Pea, Whole, Average	***1oz/28g***	***50***	***2.1***	***179***	***9.6***	***21.3***	***7.5***	***4.5***
Chick Pea, Whole, Basic, Average	***1oz/28g***	***30***	***1***	***108***	***6***	***14.2***	***3.6***	***3.3***
Chicken, & Rice, Calorie Controlled, Tesco*	1 Pack/325g	299	4.6	92	5.1	14.3	1.4	1.1
Chicken, & Rice, Calorie Counted, Asda*	1 Pack/350g	283	3.6	81	4.6	13.1	1	0.9
Chicken, & Rice, Dinner, Tesco*	1 Pack/500g	520	12	104	8.2	11.7	2.4	1.3
Chicken, & Rice, HFC, Tesco*	1 Pack/402g	476	12.3	118	5.2	16.8	3	1.3
Chicken, & Rice, Microwaved, Asda*	1 Pack/400g	588	22.2	148	5.5	18	5.6	1.8
Chicken, & Vegetable, Green Thai, with Rice, Tesco*	1 Serving/346g	339	3.5	98	6.1	15.8	1	0.9
Chicken, Butter Masala, Asda*	½ Pack/189g	261	14.4	138	13	4.3	7.6	0.7
Chicken, Butter, & Rice, Taste of India, Tesco*	1 Pack/427g	624	29.9	146	6.4	12.8	7	3.1
Chicken, Butter, Takeaway, Tesco*	½ Pack/175g	224	13.3	128	7.9	6.4	7.6	1.2
Chicken, Chinese Style, Musclefood*	1 Serving/293g	264	5.3	90	14.9	3.4	1.8	0.5
Chicken, Chinese with Rice, Ready Meal, Average	***1 Serving/450g***	***490***	***11.5***	***109***	***7.2***	***14.1***	***2.6***	***1.3***
Chicken, Chinese, Morrisons*	1 Pack/340g	347	15.6	102	10.3	5	4.6	0.8
Chicken, Chinese, Takeaway, Tesco*	½ Pack/182g	191	8.6	105	9.7	5.7	4.7	0.5
Chicken, Coconut, with Jasmine Rice, Tesco*	1 Pack/420g	482	8.8	115	7.1	16.7	2.1	0.4
Chicken, Dhansak, Kit, Musclefood*	1 Serving/506g	349	0.5	69	11.7	4.5	0.1	2.3
Chicken, Fruity, Meal for One, M&S*	1 Pack/400g	508	15.6	127	6.7	15.6	3.9	1.1
Chicken, Fruity, Mini Meal, M&S*	1 Pack/200g	262	7.4	131	8.2	15.7	3.7	1.1
Chicken, Garlic, Cook*	1 Pack/320g	358	13.7	112	10.7	7.5	4.3	0.5
Chicken, Green Thai Style & Sticky Rice, Asda*	1 Pack/450g	585	10.8	130	7	20	2.4	0.1
Chicken, Green Thai, BFY, M&S*	1 Pack/395g	383	5.9	97	7.8	12.7	1.5	1
Chicken, Green Thai, Charlie Bigham's*	½ Pack/300g	342	21	114	8.7	4.8	7	0
Chicken, Green, Thai, Jasmine Rice, Sainsbury's*	½ Pack/188g	184	4.7	98	7.9	10.5	2.5	1.3
Chicken, Hot, Can, Tesco*	1 Can/418g	514	26.3	123	9.7	6.9	6.3	0.9
Chicken, Jamaican, with Rice, Well & Good, Co-Op*	1 Pack/350g	287	2.8	82	6.8	11	0.8	1.6
Chicken, Kashmiri, Waitrose*	1 Serving/400g	640	36.4	160	14.5	5	9.1	0.6
Chicken, Katsu, with Sticky Rice, Taste of Japan, Tesco*	1 Pack/341g	460	9.2	135	6.1	21.3	2.7	0.4
Chicken, Makhani, with Pilaf Rice, Oh So Lean*	1 Pack/400g	400	10.4	100	9.6	10	2.6	0

CURRENT

	Measure INFO/WEIGHT	per Measure KCAL	FAT	Nutrition Values per 100g / 100ml KCAL	PROT	CARB	FAT	FIBRE
CURRY								
Chicken, Malaysian, Finest, Tesco*	1 Pack/375g	375	8.3	100	7.4	12.2	2.2	0.8
Chicken, Mild, Canned, Bilash, Aldi*	½ Can/200g	180	7.6	90	9.5	4.5	3.8	0.7
Chicken, Mild, with Fluffy Rice, M&S*	1 Pack/225g	238	5.8	106	6.9	13.3	2.6	0.9
Chicken, Panang, Taste Thailand, Banquet Box, M&S*	½ Pack/115g	170	11.2	148	10.9	5.2	9.7	1.2
Chicken, Piri Piri, & Cajun Rice, Asda*	1 Pack/380g	410	8.7	108	6.7	14	2.3	2.6
Chicken, Red Thai, with Jasmine Rice, Finest, Tesco*	1 Pack/413g	719	28.5	174	8.4	19.1	6.9	0.9
Chicken, Red Thai, with Rice, G&B, Asda*	1 Pack/361g	350	9	97	5.8	12	2.5	1.1
Chicken, Sweet & Sour, Chinese, Tesco*	1 Pack/507g	684	21.8	135	6.6	16.7	4.3	1.6
Chicken, Thai Green, Calorie Counted, Asda*	1 Pack/363g	370	6.5	102	7.1	14	1.8	0.8
Chicken, Thai Green, Charlie Bigham's*	1 Serving/303 g	373	23	123	9.2	5.3	7.6	0
Chicken, Thai Green, Frozen, Tesco*	1 Serving/334g	387	6.7	116	7	16.4	2	2
Chicken, Thai Green, Just Cook, Tesco*	1 Pack/304g	392	10.6	129	8.1	15.7	3.5	1.3
Chicken, Thai Green, Rice, Pot, Musclefood*	1 Serving/309g	272	2.2	88	10.8	8.8	0.7	1.8
Chicken, Thai Green, Taste of Thailand, Tesco*	½ Pack/223g	258	14.9	116	8.1	5.2	6.7	1.1
Chicken, Thai Red, & Fragrant Rice, Charlie Bigham's*	1 Serving/417 g	604	30.4	145	6.7	13.6	7.3	0
Chicken, Thai Red, & Jasmine Rice, BFY, M&S*	1 Pack/380g	441	10.3	116	8.1	14.3	2.7	0.8
Chicken, Thai Red, Curry Meal Box, Tesco*	½ Pack/167g	195	10.3	117	10.1	4.8	6.2	1
Chicken, Thai Red, Takeaway, Tesco*	½ Pack/193g	233	13.1	121	8.9	5.7	6.8	0.5
Chicken, Thai, Green, & Jasmine Rice, Ready Meal	*1 Serving/450g*	*520*	*17.2*	*116*	*7.7*	*12.6*	*3.8*	*1.1*
Chicken, Thai, Green, No Rice, Average	*1 Serving/200g*	*174*	*7*	*87*	*8.2*	*5*	*3.5*	*1.4*
Chicken, Thai, Green, Taste Thailand, Banquet Box, M&S*	½ Pack/115g	155	11	135	8.9	2.7	9.6	1.1
Chicken, Thai, Red, & Jasmine Rice, Ready Meal	*1 Serving/450g*	*500*	*15.3*	*111*	*7.5*	*12.6*	*3.4*	*1*
Chicken, Thai, Red, & Rice, Ready Meal, Healthy	*1 Serving/400g*	*400*	*7.8*	*100*	*6.4*	*14*	*2*	*1*
Chicken, Thai, Red, & Sticky Rice, Ready Meal	*1 Serving/450g*	*527*	*15.7*	*117*	*6.7*	*14.2*	*3.5*	*1.7*
Chicken, Thai, Red, HE, Tesco*	1 Pack/380g	373	5	105	6.4	15.4	1.4	2.5
Chicken, Thai, Red, No Rice, Average	*1 Serving/200g*	*194*	*6.9*	*97*	*7.2*	*9*	*3.4*	*1.4*
Chicken, Tikka, Biryani, Tesco*	1 Pack/365g	599	13.9	164	10.2	20.7	3.8	3.5
Chicken, with Rice, & Veg, Balanced 2 Go, Oh So Lean*	1 Pack/400g	374	4.1	94	10.2	11.5	1	0
Chicken, with Rice, Average	*1 Serving/400g*	*465*	*11*	*116*	*5.1*	*17.8*	*2.8*	*0.8*
Chicken, with Rice, Basics, Sainsbury's*	1 Pack/343g	477	9.3	139	6	21.7	2.7	1.7
Chicken, Yellow Thai Style, HL, Tesco*	1 Pack/450g	504	12.2	112	9.3	12.6	2.7	0.5
Coconut Chicken, & Brown Rice, As Consumed, Morrisons*	1 Pack/300g	390	11.7	130	8	14.9	3.9	1.6
Cod, Squid, & King Prawn, Keralan, Waitrose*	½ Pack/185g	211	9.6	114	13.5	3	5.2	0.6
Courgette, & Potato	*1oz/28g*	*24*	*1.5*	*86*	*1.9*	*8.7*	*5.2*	*1.2*
Fish, & Vegetable, Bangladeshi, Average	*1oz/28g*	*33*	*2.4*	*117*	*9.1*	*1.4*	*8.4*	*0.5*
Fish, Bangladeshi, Average	*1oz/28g*	*35*	*2.2*	*124*	*12.2*	*1.5*	*7.9*	*0.3*
Fish, Coconut, Creamy, My Goodness, Sainsbury's*	1 Pack/373g	362	7.1	97	5.3	14.2	1.9	1.1
Fish, Goan, with Basmati Rice, Hello Fresh*	1 Serving/719g	561	26.9	78	4.7	6	3.7	0
Fish, Red Thai, Waitrose*	1 Pack/500g	275	11	55	5.2	3.7	2.2	1
Fish, Thai Red, & Snap Peas, Musclefood*	1 Pack/350g	315	6.3	90	7.1	11.1	1.8	0.8
Fish, Yellow Thai, Asian Fusion, Waitrose*	½ Pack/175g	222	15.8	127	6.8	3.9	9	1.4
Goan, Fish, Charlie Bigham's*	1 Serving/400 g	484	19.2	121	6.2	13.5	4.8	0
Gobi, Sri Lankan, Vegan, Hi Five*	1 Pack/500g	270	15	54	2	6	3	2
Green, Thai, Coconut, Bol*	1 Pack/345g	307	8.3	89	1.9	14.1	2.4	1.7
Haddock, & Tomato, Mild, Gousto*	1 Portion/448g	538	16.1	120	6.5	16	3.6	0.7
Indonesian, with Coconut, & Cauliflower, One Pot, Aldi*	1 Pot/367g	367	14	100	0.5	3.5	3.8	0.4
Jackfruit, Thai Green, with Rice, Soulful Food Co*	1 Pot/380g	319	17.1	84	1.5	10.6	4.5	2.3
Katsu, Chicken, & Rice, G&B, Asda*	1 Pack/370g	388	8.1	105	9.4	11	2.2	1.4
Katsu, Sweet Potato, Plant Kitchen, M&S*	1 Pack/400g	536	16.8	134	3.2	19.8	4.2	2
Korma, Red, Hyderabad, Meal Kit, The Spice Tailor*	½ Pack/150g	218	12.2	145	3.1	9.6	8.1	2.1
Lamb, & Potato, 385, Wiltshire Farm Foods*	1 Serving/210g	334	23	159	8.9	6.2	11	1.7
Lamb, Aromatic, BFY, M&S*	1 Pack/380g	388	9.1	102	9	9.2	2.4	3.7
Lamb, Hot, M&S*	½ Can/213g	320	19.6	150	14.9	6	9.2	2.3

CURRY

INFO/WEIGHT	Measure	per Measure KCAL	FAT	Nutrition Values per 100g / 100ml KCAL	PROT	CARB	FAT	FIBRE
Lentil, Canned, Creationz, Heinz*	1 Can/390g	277	3.9	71	4	10.4	1	2.3
Lentil, Tomato, Creamy, Punjabi, Tasty Bite*	½ Pack/142g	136	6.1	96	4.2	8.2	4.3	3.6
Mango Masala, with Pilaf Rice, Oh So Lean*	1 Pack/380g	441	3.4	116	2.3	25.3	0.9	0
Mushroom, & Pea, Masala, Indian, Sainsbury's*	1 Pack/300g	264	14.7	88	3.3	5.2	4.9	5.1
Mutton, wiith Rice, Island Delight*	1 Pack/400g	548	18.4	137	9	15.6	4.6	0
Paneer, & Sweet Potato, Kofte Biryani, Everdine*	1 Serving/450g	562	22.1	125	3.8	13.1	4.9	6.7
Paneer, Spiced Chilli, Bowl, Vegetarian, Indian, Waitrose*	1 Pack/300g	387	13.5	129	6.2	14.9	4.5	2.1
Pav Bhaji, Kohinoor*	1 Pack/300g	282	16.2	94	2.3	10.4	5.4	2.8
Peanut, Chickpea, Red Rice, West African*	1 Pot/380g	346	11	91	3.5	15	2.9	4
Potato & Pea	*1oz/28g*	*26*	*1.1*	*92*	*2.9*	*13*	*3.8*	*2.4*
Prawn, & Mushroom	*1oz/28g*	*47*	*4*	*168*	*7.3*	*2.5*	*14.4*	*1*
Prawn, Coconut & Lime, King, Sainsbury's*	½ Pack/351g	207	8.8	59	3.7	5.4	2.5	1
Prawn, Goan, King, M&S*	1 Pack/400g	680	44.4	170	5.1	11.6	11.1	1.5
Prawn, King, Taste Sri Lanka, M&S*	1 Pack/350g	413	23.4	118	6.3	7.3	6.7	1.6
Prawn, Malay, King, Waitrose*	1 Pack/350g	364	19.2	104	6.6	7.1	5.5	0.9
Prawn, Red Thai, King, City Kitchen, Tesco*	1 Pack/385g	460	14.4	119	4.5	16.7	3.7	1
Prawn, Red Thai, Sainsbury's*	1 Pack/300g	546	39.6	182	6.3	9.4	13.2	1.7
Prawn, Sri Lankan, Giraffe*	1 Pack/368g	497	24.3	135	4	13.8	6.6	2.1
Prawn, Takeaway, Average	*1 Serving/350g*	*410*	*29.8*	*117*	*8.2*	*2.2*	*8.5*	*2*
Prawn, Yellow Thai, Cook*	1 Serving/295g	215	8	73	6.4	5.7	2.7	0.4
Red Kidney Bean, Punjabi	*1oz/28g*	*30*	*1.6*	*106*	*4.7*	*10.1*	*5.6*	*3.8*
Red Thai, Vegetarian, Tesco*	1 Pack/429ml	588	21.9	137	5.4	17.3	5.1	1.6
Roasted Veg, & Chickpea, Mild, 602, Oakhouse Foods Ltd*	1 Serving/400g	408	10.8	102	3.1	15.6	2.7	1.6
Root, Ruby 7, Microwaved, Mumbai Street Food, Iceland*	1 Meal/224g	222	14.8	99	1.7	7.1	6.6	1.8
Salmon, Green, Waitrose*	1 Pack/401g	581	40.5	145	9.1	4.5	10.1	2.7
Sambhar Mix, Lentil & Vegetable, Fudco*	1 Box/100g	354	13.2	354	13.6	45.3	13.2	9.6
Sri Lankan Sambar, Pot, Bol*	1 Pot/345g	310	8.6	90	5.3	9.4	2.5	4.4
Sri Lankan Veg, Weight Watchers*	1 Pack/380g	171	6.1	45	1.5	5.2	1.6	2
Sweet Potato, & Cashew, Plant Kitchen, M&S*	1 Pack/340g	411	10.9	121	4.4	16.7	3.2	3.8
Sweet Potato, Slimfree, Aldi*	1 Pack/500g	250	3	50	2.3	6.5	0.6	4.8
Sweet Potato, What's Cooking, Lidl*	1 Serving/550g	335	7.3	61	2.6	7.9	1.3	3.3
Thai Green, Rice, & Quinoa, Made Up, Prep Co*	1 Pot/251g	274	5.8	109	2.4	19	2.3	1.7
Thai Green, Veggie, Organic, Pot, Clive's*	1 Pot/400g	268	14	67	2.1	5.6	3.5	0
Thai, Chickpea, & Sweet Potato, Veggie Bowl, Birds Eye*	1 Pack/370g	459	10.7	124	3.8	19	2.9	3.1
Thai, Coconut, Veg Pot, Vegan, Bol*	1 Pot/345g	307	8.3	89	1.9	14.1	2.4	1.7
Thai, Green, & Jasmine Rice, Plant Kitchen, M&S*	1 Pack/400g	596	24.8	149	3.6	18.8	6.2	1.7
Thai, Red, Coconut, Bol*	1 Serving/345g	297	7.6	86	3	12.4	2.2	2.2
Tofu, Red Thai, 1, Waitrose*	½ Pack/175g	345	25.9	197	8.7	6.7	14.8	1.1
Tomato, Lentil, & Chickpea, Cauliflower, Soulful Food Co*	1 Pot/380g	224	4.6	59	2.6	11	1.2	2.5
Vegetable, & Chickpea, Cook*	1 Serving/330g	224	6.3	68	3.2	7.9	1.9	3.3
Vegetable, Canned, Sainsbury's*	½ Can/200g	200	12.2	100	1.4	9.8	6.1	1.8
Vegetable, Canned, Tesco*	1 Can/400g	308	11.2	77	2	9.7	2.8	2.4
Vegetable, Frozen, Mixed Vegetables, Average	*1oz/28g*	*25*	*1.7*	*88*	*2.5*	*6.9*	*6.1*	*0*
Vegetable, in Sweet Sauce, Average	*1 Serving/330g*	*162*	*6.9*	*49*	*1.4*	*6.7*	*2.1*	*1.3*
Vegetable, Indian Meal for One, Tesco*	1 Serving/200g	218	14.4	109	2	9	7.2	1.2
Vegetable, Indian, Sainsbury's*	½ Pack/200g	206	14.6	103	2.5	6.8	7.3	4.6
Vegetable, Indian, Tesco*	1 Serving/225g	257	17.8	114	2.1	8.6	7.9	1.6
Vegetable, Malay, Giraffe*	1 Pack/380g	471	36.1	124	2.2	6.2	9.5	2.4
Vegetable, Medium, Tesco*	1 Pack/350g	326	21.7	93	2.3	7.1	6.2	1.9
Vegetable, Pakistani, Average	*1oz/28g*	*17*	*0.7*	*60*	*2.2*	*8.7*	*2.6*	*2.2*
Vegetable, Red Thai, with Brown Rice, Aldi*	1 Pack/380g	293	14.4	77	1.9	7.9	3.8	2
Vegetable, Red Thai, with Rice, Tesco*	1 Pack/385g	381	11.5	99	4.4	12.6	3	2.1
Vegetable, Sabzi Tarkari, Patak's*	1 Pack/400g	500	31.2	125	2.5	11.1	7.8	2.2

	Measure INFO/WEIGHT	per Measure KCAL	FAT	Nutrition Values per 100g / 100ml KCAL	PROT	CARB	FAT	FIBRE
CURRY								
Vegetable, South Indian, Weight Watchers*	1 Pack/400g	256	7.6	64	2.7	7.9	1.9	2.4
Vegetable, South Indian, Weight Watchers, Heinz*	1 Pack/400g	256	7.6	64	2.7	7.9	1.9	2.4
Vegetable, Takeaway, Average	*1 Serving/330g*	*346*	*24.4*	*105*	*2.5*	*7.6*	*7.4*	*0*
Vegetable, Takeaway, Tesco*	1 Pack/385g	262	13.1	68	2.3	5.8	3.4	2.7
Vegetable, Thai Red, with Brown Rice, Soulful Food Co*	1 Pot/380g	262	13.7	69	2.1	6.1	3.6	1.8
Vegetable, with Rice, Healthy Range, Average	*1 Serving/400g*	*351*	*4.6*	*88*	*2.3*	*16.8*	*1.1*	*1.9*
Vegetable, with Rice, Ready Meal, Average	*1 Serving/400g*	*408*	*12*	*102*	*3.3*	*16.4*	*3*	*0*
Vegetable, with Yoghurt, Average	*1oz/28g*	*17*	*1.1*	*62*	*2.6*	*4.6*	*4.1*	*1.4*
Vegetable, Yellow Thai, Sainsbury's*	1 Pack/400g	624	48.8	156	2.2	9.4	12.2	1.1
Vegetable, Yellow, Cook*	1 Serving/270g	367	25.1	136	2.4	10	9.3	1.6
Yellow, Thai, Deliciously Ella*	½ Pack/200g	232	19	116	2.1	4.7	9.5	1.9
CURRY LEAVES								
Fresh	*1oz/28g*	*23*	*0.3*	*81*	*6.6*	*11*	*1.1*	*0*
CURRY PASTE								
Balti, Sainsbury's*	¼ Jar/50g	73	4.9	147	3.4	7.6	9.9	6.7
Curry, Katsu, Mild, M&S*	¼ Jar/48g	88	4.2	186	4.8	19.6	8.8	4.7
Green Thai, Average	*1 Tsp/5g*	*6*	*0.4*	*128*	*2.1*	*11.7*	*7.9*	*3.1*
Gulyaskrem Cispos, Le Gusto*	1 Serving/15g	18	1	118	2	9	7	0
Jalfrezi, Patak's*	1 Serving/30g	96	8.1	320	3.7	14.2	26.9	5.6
Korma, Asda*	1 Tube/100g	338	23.5	338	5.1	26.6	23.5	1.2
Madras, Cumin & Chilli, Hot, Patak's*	¼ Jar/70g	202	18.1	289	4.7	7.6	25.9	10.8
Madras, Pot, Patak's*	½ Pot/35g	98	8.1	279	4.4	7	23.1	0
Massaman, Thai, Pot, Blue Dragon*	½ Pot/25g	89	6.8	357	4.9	24	27	0
Mild, Coriander & Cumin, Original, Patak's*	1 Serving/35g	99	8.6	283	4.8	9.1	24.6	10.7
Red, Thai, Average	*1 Tsp/5g*	*7*	*0.5*	*132*	*2.3*	*9.5*	*9.1*	*3*
Rogan Josh, Tomato & Paprika, Patak's*	1 Serving/30g	119	11	397	4.1	12.7	36.7	5.9
Thai Yellow, Mae Ploy*	1 Serving/30g	30	0	100	10	20	0	10
Tikka Masala, Coriander & Lemon, Medium, Patak's*	1 Serving/30g	111	9.5	369	3.8	16.9	31.8	2.9
Tikka Masala, Spice, Patak's*	1 Tbsp/15g	40	3.4	270	3	7.8	22.9	6.8
Tikka, M&S*	¼ Jar/50g	110	7.8	219	2.8	13.8	15.5	6.4
Tom Yum, Thai Taste*	1 Tsp/13g	35	2	269	5.4	30.8	15.4	7.7
Yellow Thai, Tesco*	1 Tbsp/15g	15	0.6	100	1.9	13.6	4.1	4.9
Yellow, Thai, Barts*	1 Serving/30g	84	3.8	281	2.7	30.4	12.8	8.3
CURRY POWDER								
Average	*1 Tsp/2g*	*6*	*0.3*	*325*	*12.7*	*41.8*	*13.8*	*0*
CUSTARD								
Banana Flavour, Ambrosia*	1 Sm Pot/135g	139	3.9	103	2.9	16.1	2.9	0
Canned, Essential, Waitrose*	¼ Can/100g	101	3.2	101	2.7	15.3	3.2	0
Canned, Ready to Serve, Stockwell & Co., Tesco*	½ Can/193g	131	1.7	68	2.6	12.4	0.9	0
Chocolate Flavour, Ambrosia*	1 Pot/150g	177	4.4	118	3	20	2.9	0.7
Chocolate Flavour, Pot, Average	*1 Pot/125g*	*138*	*3.4*	*111*	*3.1*	*18.2*	*2.7*	*0.6*
Instant, Just Add Water, Made Up, Weight Watchers*	1 Serving/145g	93	0.6	64	1.2	13.9	0.4	0.9
Instant, Low Fat, Made Up, Morrisons*	1/3 Pack/142g	85	2.6	60	0.9	10	1.8	0.1
Instant, Mix, As Sold, Smart Price, Asda*	1 Pack/70g	204	2.7	291	2.6	61.3	3.9	0
Low Fat, Average	*1/3 Pot/141g*	*116*	*1.6*	*82*	*2.9*	*15*	*1.2*	*0*
Low Fat, Salco, Lidl*	1 Pot/150g	135	2.4	90	2.7	15.9	1.6	0.5
Powder	*1 Tsp/5g*	*18*	*0*	*354*	*0.6*	*92*	*0.7*	*0.1*
Ready to Eat. Low Fat, Pot, Tesco*	1 Pot/150g	132	2	88	3.2	15.9	1.3	0
Ready To Serve, Aldi*	¼ Pot/125g	152	7.2	122	2.7	15	5.8	0
Ready to Serve, Average	*1 Serving/50g*	*59*	*2.3*	*118*	*3.3*	*16.1*	*4.6*	*0.2*
Ready to Serve, Canned, Everyday Value, Tesco*	½ Can/192g	133	1.3	69	2.8	12.9	0.7	0
Salted Caramel Flavour, Morrisons*	½ Pot/150g	167	4.8	111	2.9	17.4	3.2	0.5
Soya, Vanilla, Dairy Free, Deliciously, Alpro*	1 Tbsp/15g	12	0.3	81	3	13.3	1.8	0.5

C

	Measure INFO/WEIGHT	per Measure KCAL	FAT	Nutrition Values per 100g / 100ml KCAL	PROT	CARB	FAT	FIBRE
CUSTARD								
Toffee Flavour, Ambrosia*	1 Pot/150g	156	4.2	104	2.8	17	2.8	0
Vanilla Flavour, Pot, Average	*1 Pot/125g*	*128*	*3.5*	*102*	*2.8*	*16.4*	*2.8*	*0*
Vanilla, Low Fat, Fresh, Waitrose*	1/5 Pot/100g	104	2.4	104	3.5	17.1	2.4	0
Vanilla, Oat, Oatly*	¼ Pack/63g	97	6.2	155	1	15	10	0
Vanilla, TTD, Sainsbury's*	1 Pot/150g	312	23.2	208	2.5	14.7	15.5	0.1
CUSTARD APPLE								
Cherimoya, Weighed without Skin & Seeds, Average	*1 Serving/312g*	*234*	*2.1*	*75*	*1.6*	*17.7*	*0.7*	*3*
CUTLETS								
Nut, Goodlife*	1 Cutlet/88g	283	19.4	322	9.1	21.8	22	3.4
Nut, Meat Free, Tesco*	1 Cutlet/82g	198	12.2	241	6.8	15.7	14.9	8.7
Nut, Retail, Fried in Vegetable Oil, Average	*1 Cutlet/90g*	*260*	*20.1*	*289*	*4.8*	*18.7*	*22.3*	*1.7*
Nut, Retail, Grilled, Average	*1 Cutlet/90g*	*191*	*11.7*	*212*	*5.1*	*19.9*	*13*	*1.8*
Nut, Vegetarian, Oven Baked, Asda*	1 Cutlet/83g	213	14.9	258	7.2	13	18	8
Nut, Vegetarian, Sainsbury's*	1 Cutlet/87g	234	15.6	269	3.9	20.2	17.9	5.6

C

	Measure INFO/WEIGHT	per Measure KCAL	FAT	Nutrition Values per 100g / 100ml KCAL	PROT	CARB	FAT	FIBRE
DAB								
Raw	*1oz/28g*	*21*	*0.3*	*74*	*15.7*	*0*	*1.2*	*0*
DAHL								
Black, Ultimate, Jamie Oliver*	1 Serving/125g	162	6.1	130	6.8	13	4.9	3.9
Cauliflower, & Lentil, Deliciously Ella*	½ Pack/222g	200	11.8	90	3.4	6.2	5.3	2.3
Cauliflower, Roasted, & Butternut Squash, Sainsbury's*	1 Pack/350g	245	6.6	70	3.4	8.2	1.9	3.5
Channa, Jane Plan*	1 Pack/220g	326	18.5	148	3.9	12	8.4	4.4
Coconut, with Roasted Tofu, Plant Kitchen, M&S*	1 Pack/350g	406	20.3	116	6.9	7.7	5.8	2.8
Lentil, & Spinach, Tideford*	½ Pot/300g	117	6.3	39	1.4	3.1	2.1	0.9
Lentil, with Chunky Vegetables, Indian Style, Aldi*	1 Pot/380g	304	11.4	80	4.1	6.9	3	4.6
Tarka, Indian, Waitrose*	1 Pack/300g	432	21.9	144	6.5	7.2	7.3	11.6
Vegetable, & Red Lentil, North Indian, Soulful Food Co*	1 Pot/380g	376	16	99	10.9	10.9	4.2	1.5
DAIM								
Mondelez*	1 Bar/28g	148	8.7	530	2.9	59	31	1.2
DAIRYLEA DUNKERS								
with Jumbo Tubes, Kraft*	1 Pack/43g	108	5.1	255	9.1	27	12	0.9
with Ritz Crackers, Dairylea, Kraft*	1 Tub/46g	118	5.5	258	9.6	26	12	2.2
DAMSONS								
Raw, Weighed with Stones, Average	*1oz/28g*	*9*	*0*	*31*	*0.4*	*7.7*	*0*	*1.4*
Raw, Weighed without Stones, Average	*1oz/28g*	*11*	*0*	*38*	*0.5*	*9.6*	*0*	*1.8*
DANDELION & BURDOCK								
Barr*	1 Bottle/250ml	40	0	16	0	4	0	0
Fentiman's*	1 Serving/200ml	94	0	47	0	10.6	0	0
Fermented, Botanical, Fentiman's*	1 Bottle/275ml	130	0	47	0	11.6	0	0
Original, Ben Shaws*	1 Can/440ml	128	0	29	0	7	0	0
Sparkling, Diet, Morrisons*	1 Glass/200ml	2	0	1	0	0.3	0	0
DANISH PASTRY								
Apple & Cinnamon, Danish Twist, Entenmann's*	1 Serving/52g	150	1	288	5.6	62	1.9	1.5
Apple & Sultana, Tesco*	1 Pastry/72g	293	16.4	407	5.4	45	22.8	1.4
Apple Danish, Bakery, Waitrose*	1 Pastry/123g	400	22.2	325	5.1	35.7	18	2.4
Apple, Fresh Cream, Sainsbury's*	1 Pastry/67g	248	14.6	368	3.1	40.2	21.6	0.4
Average	*1 Pastry/110g*	*411*	*19.4*	*374*	*5.8*	*51.3*	*17.6*	*1.6*
Cherry & Custard, Bar, Tesco*	1 Bar/350g	910	49	260	3.5	29.9	14	7.7
Custard, Bar, Sara Lee*	¼ Bar/100g	228	6.4	228	6.6	36.1	6.4	0.8
Fruit Bears Claw , Waitrose*	1 Pastry/97g	339	15.8	349	4.6	45	16.3	2
Fruit Filled, Average	*1 Pastry/94g*	*335*	*15.9*	*356*	*5.1*	*47.9*	*17*	*0*
Maple, & Pecan, Plait, Frozen, Tesco*	1 Pastry/78g	348	22.8	447	5.6	39	29.3	2.7
Toasted Pecan, Danish Twist, Entenmann's*	1 Slice/48g	171	7.6	351	7	47.2	15.6	1.4
DATES								
Dried, Average	*1 Date/5g*	*13*	*0*	*266*	*2.8*	*64.1*	*0.4*	*4.1*
Dried, Medjool, Average	*1 Date/20g*	*56*	*0.1*	*279*	*2.2*	*69.3*	*0.3*	*4.3*
Fresh, Raw, Yellow, Average	*1 Date/20g*	*21*	*0*	*107*	*1.3*	*27.1*	*0.1*	*1.5*
Medjool, Stuffed with Walnuts, Tesco*	2 Dates/40g	98	2.3	245	4.4	44	5.7	3.4
Milk Chocolate Coated, Julian Graves*	1 Pack/200g	768	22.6	384	4.5	66	11.3	2.6
Milk Chocolate Covered, Holland & Barrett*	1 Date/17g	65	1.9	384	4.5	66	11.3	2.6
DELI FILLER								
Cheese & Onion, Essential, Waitrose*	1 Pot/170g	692	64.8	407	10.8	4.5	38.1	1.5
Chicken & Bacon, Co-Op*	1 Pack/200g	420	29.6	210	17.6	1	14.8	2.6
King Prawn & Avocado, M&S*	1 Pack/170g	425	38.8	250	9.5	1.4	22.8	0.5
Prawn & Mayonnaise, M&S*	1 Serving/60g	150	13.8	250	11.3	1	23	0.5
Prawn Cocktail, Eat Well, M&S*	½ Pot/85g	119	7.3	140	9.1	6.4	8.6	0.6
DESSERT								
After Eight, Dark Chocolate & Mint, Nestle*	1 Pot/70g	125	4.9	178	4.2	25.3	7	0
Apple Crumble, Sainsbury's*	1 Pot/136g	291	10.5	214	3.2	33	7.7	2.7

DESSERT

INFO/WEIGHT	Measure	per Measure		Nutrition Values per 100g / 100ml				
		KCAL	FAT	KCAL	PROT	CARB	FAT	FIBRE
Banana Split	**1 Serving/175g**	**368**	**25.5**	**210**	**2.2**	**18**	**14.6**	**0.2**
Banoffee, Layered, Sainsbury's*	1 Pot/115g	270	14.7	235	2.2	27.8	12.8	1
Banoffee, Sainsbury's*	1 Pot/140g	360	19.1	257	2.7	30.9	13.6	1.3
Banoffee, Weight Watchers*	1 Dessert/81g	170	3.6	210	4.9	37.7	4.4	1.4
Blueberry, Muffin, Tesco*	1 Pot/91g	265	18.7	291	2	24.5	20.6	3
Cappuccino, Italian, Co-Op*	1 Pack/90g	256	10.8	285	5	39	12	0.1
Caramel, Crunch, Weight Watchers*	1 Serving/89g	174	2.6	196	4.6	37.9	2.9	1.7
Caramel, Pots Of Joy, Dairy Milk, Cadbury*	1 Pot/70g	150	7.3	215	2.5	27.1	10.5	0.1
Caramel, Soya, Creamy, Sweet, Alpro*	1 Pot/125g	106	2.2	85	3.2	13.7	1.8	0.5
Caramel, Soya, Dairy Free, Organic, Provamel*	1 Pot/125g	125	2.2	100	3	17.8	1.8	0.5
Choc Delight, Brooklea, Aldi*	1 Pot/80g	74	1.2	92	4.5	15	1.5	0.6
Chocolate & Caramel, Fix, Mullerlight, Muller*	1 Pot/80g	70	1.5	88	3	14.2	1.9	0
Chocolate Fix, Belgian, with Mint, Mullerlight, Muller*	1 Pot/100g	97	2.9	97	3.5	14.7	2.9	0
Chocolate, & Caramel, Semifreddo, Waitrose*	1 Slice/64g	217	12.3	342	3.4	37.4	19.4	2.1
Chocolate, & Summer Fruits, Specially Selected, Aldi*	1 Dessert/95g	277	16.2	292	1.8	32	17	2.7
Chocolate, Banoffee, Gu*	1 Pot/85g	325	21.5	382	3.9	35	25.3	1
Chocolate, Belgian, Sweetheart, Specially Selected, Aldi*	1 Dessert/70g	258	16.1	369	5.5	33	23	3
Chocolate, Brownie, Double, Weight Watchers*	1 Pot/86g	167	3.3	194	5.1	33.7	3.8	2.4
Chocolate, Buttons, Cadbury*	1 Pack/100g	275	14.5	275	5	30.5	14.5	0
Chocolate, Buttons, Milk, Cadbury*	1 Pot/100g	280	14.9	280	6.2	30.8	14.9	0
Chocolate, Buttons, Twin Pot, Cadbury*	1 Pot/90g	220	11.7	245	4.4	27.5	13	0.6
Chocolate, Creme, King Frais, Lidl*	1 Pot/125g	131	3.6	105	2.6	17	2.9	0
Chocolate, Dark, & Mint, Aldi*	1 Pot/190g	256	11.4	135	3.2	17	6	0.9
Chocolate, Dark, Soya, Alpro*	1 Pot/125g	118	2.9	94	3	14.7	2.3	1.4
Chocolate, Delights, Shape, Danone*	1 Pot/110g	109	2.4	99	3.3	16.3	2.2	0.6
Chocolate, Everyday Value, Tesco*	1 Pot/100g	121	4	121	2.7	18.4	4	0.4
Chocolate, Fix, Mullerlight, Muller*	1 Pot/100g	94	1.9	94	3.2	15.2	1.9	0
Chocolate, Frappe, Skinny, COU, M&S*	1 Pot/100g	116	2.6	116	6.2	16.9	2.6	0.5
Chocolate, Little Choc Pots, The Coconut Collaborative*	1 Pot/45g	103	5.8	228	2.5	24.8	13	1.5
Chocolate, Mousse Cake, Weight Watchers*	1 Dessert/75g	148	2.2	198	5.9	37.1	2.9	1
Chocolate, Muffin, LC, Tesco*	1 Pot/108g	140	2.4	130	4.3	22.6	2.2	1.3
Chocolate, Muffin, Skinny, Low Fat, COU, M&S*	1 Pot/110g	154	3.1	140	5.2	23.5	2.8	0.5
Chocolate, Muffin, Tesco*	1 Serving/104g	354	21.2	340	3.5	35.5	20.4	2.1
Chocolate, Muffin, Waitrose*	1 Serving/110g	138	3	126	5.2	20	2.7	0.4
Chocolate, Orange, Pots of Joy, Terry's*	1 Pot/70g	150	7.3	215	3.7	26	10.5	0.1
Chocolate, Pots Of Joy , Dairy Milk, Cadbury*	1 Pot /70g	158	8.2	225	4.2	25.6	11.7	0.1
Chocolate, Salted Caramel, Pot, M&S*	1 Pot/85g	341	25	401	5.2	30.3	29.4	0
Chocolate, Soya, Dairy Free, Organic, Provamel*	1 Pot/125g	111	3	89	3	13.6	2.4	1
Chocolate, Soya, Silky Smooth, Alpro*	1 Pot/125g	104	2.4	83	3	13	1.9	1.1
Chocolate, Toffee, Weight Watchers*	1 Dessert/89g	177	4	197	4.3	34.9	4.5	2.2
Chocolate, Twin Hearts, M&S*	1 Heart/85g	313	21.9	368	4.3	29.1	25.8	1.3
Chocolate, White Buttons, Pots of Joy, Cadbury*	1 Pot /70g	158	6.6	225	4.8	30.4	9.4	0
Chocolate, Fudge, Pot, Fabulous, Thorntons*	1 Pot /65g	168	10.4	258	5.5	22.7	16	0
Cocoa, Postre, Organic, Vrai*	1 Dessert/125g	155	3.5	124	5.4	18.8	2.8	0.9
Coffee Creme, Bonne Maman*	1 Serving/90g	180	12.7	200	2.2	16	14.1	0.3
Cookie Dough, Ed's Diner*	1 Dessert/100g	307	17	307	5	32.5	17	1.6
Cookies & Cream, Chaos Pot, Tesco*	½ Pot/96g	324	22.5	338	4.6	26.9	23.4	0.9
Creme Caramel, Sainsbury's*	1 Pot/100g	116	1.6	116	2.6	22.9	1.6	0
Fudge, Cadbury*	1 Pot/90g	216	11.2	240	4.1	28.5	12.4	0
Gulabjam Indian, Waitrose*	1 Pot/180g	479	15.5	266	4.8	42.9	8.6	0.6
Jaffa Cake, COU, M&S*	1 Serving/120g	138	3.1	115	2.4	20.1	2.6	1
Jaffa, COU, M&S*	1 Pot/107g	155	4.9	145	3.4	22.4	4.6	0.5
Jaffa, Skinny, M&S*	1 Pot/107g	167	4	156	2.7	27	3.7	1.7

	Measure INFO/WEIGHT	per Measure KCAL	FAT	Nutrition Values per 100g / 100ml KCAL	PROT	CARB	FAT	FIBRE
DESSERT								
Key Lime Pie	**1 Serving/125g**	**431**	**25**	**344**	**4.1**	**37.9**	**20**	**1.4**
Lemon, & Raspberry Semifreddo, Waitrose*	1 Slice/63g	193	12.3	305	1.9	30.4	19.4	0.5
Lemon, Mousse Cake, Weight Watchers*	1 Serving/90g	130	2.4	144	3.2	26.7	2.7	0.5
Lemon, Posset, Creamy, Pot, Love Something*	1 Pot/90g	290	22.5	322	1.4	23	25	0.1
Lemon, Sicilian, & Raspberry, Buche, Finest, Tesco*	1 Slice/72g	155	10.3	215	3.8	17.1	14.3	1.3
Liegeois, DÃƒÆ'Ã‚Â©lisse*	1 Pot/100g	134	5.5	134	3	18	5.5	0.5
Mandarin, COU, M&S*	1 Serving/150g	195	5.7	130	1	22	3.8	0.1
Millionaire's Shortbread, M&S*	1 Dessert/120g	440	27.8	365	3.2	35.5	23.1	1
Mississippi Mud Pie	**1 Serving/125g**	**480**	**32**	**384**	**5.3**	**33.1**	**25.6**	**1.8**
Mochi, Mixed, Royal Family*	1 Mochi/30g	109	3.3	363	5.5	64	10.9	0
Raspberry, Royale, Essential, Waitrose*	1 Pot/150g	216	10.6	144	1.1	18.9	7.1	0.5
Rolo, Nestle*	1 Pot/70g	170	8.3	243	3.3	30.8	11.9	0.5
Salted Caramel, Pot, The Coconut Collaborative*	1 Pot/45g	130	6.3	288	2	37	14	3.1
Strawberry, & Raspberry, Charlotte, COU, M&S*	1 Pot/110g	153	1.2	139	2.1	29.7	1.1	1.1
Tiramisu	**1 Serving/150g**	**420**	**20.8**	**280**	**4.4**	**34**	**13.9**	**0.8**
Toffee, Cheesecake, Individual, Dessert Menu, Aldi*	1 Dessert/100g	266	12	266	2.5	36	12	0.5
Toffee, Fudge , Pot, Fabulous, Thorntons*	1 Pot/65g	178	10.5	274	4.8	27.3	16.1	0
Toffee, with Biscuit Pieces, Iced, Weight Watchers*	1 Pot/57g	93	2.7	163	2.7	26.2	4.8	0.2
Trifle, Chocolate, Cadbury*	1 Pot /90g	234	13.8	260	4.8	22.5	15.3	0
Vanilla, & Caramel, Little Desserts, Petits Filous, Yoplait*	1 Pot/50g	75	2.6	150	4.7	21	5.3	0.2
Vanilla, Choc Fudge, Non Dairy Soya, Frozen, Tofutti*	1 Tub/500ml	825	45	165	1.6	20	9	0.4
Vanilla, Soya, Heavenly Velvet, Alpro*	1 Pot/125g	94	2.8	75	3.7	9.5	2.2	1
DHAL								
Black Gram, Average	**1oz/28g**	**21**	**1**	**74**	**4.2**	**7**	**3.4**	**1.7**
Chick Pea	**1oz/28g**	**42**	**1.7**	**149**	**7.4**	**17.7**	**6.1**	**3.8**
Lentil, Red Masoor & Tomato with Butter, Average	**1oz/28g**	**26**	**1.4**	**94**	**4**	**9.7**	**4.9**	**0.9**
Lentil, Red Masoor & Vegetable, Average	**1oz/28g**	**31**	**1.1**	**110**	**5.8**	**14.7**	**3.8**	**1.8**
Lentil, Red Masoor with Vegetable Oil, Average	**1oz/28g**	**48**	**2.2**	**172**	**7.6**	**19.2**	**7.9**	**1.8**
Lentil, Red Masoor, Punjabi, Average	**1oz/28g**	**39**	**1.3**	**139**	**7.2**	**19.2**	**4.6**	**2**
Lentil, Red Masoorl & Mung Bean, Average	**1oz/28g**	**32**	**1.9**	**114**	**4.8**	**9.9**	**6.7**	**1.6**
Lentil, Tesco*	1 Serving/200g	248	13.2	124	5.1	10.6	6.6	2.5
Mung Bean, Bengali	**1oz/28g**	**20**	**0.9**	**73**	**4.2**	**7.4**	**3.3**	**1.7**
Mung Beans, Dried, Boiled in Unsalted Water	**1oz/28g**	**26**	**0.1**	**92**	**7.8**	**15.3**	**0.4**	**0**
Split Peas, Yellow, Chana, Asda*	1 Serving/275g	300	19.2	109	2.6	9	7	1.8
Tarka, Asda*	½ Pack/150g	216	12	144	6	12	8	6
Tarka, M&S*	1 Serving/250g	235	8.8	94	4.3	9.4	3.5	3.7
Vegetable, Microwaved, Slimming World*	1 Pack/350g	259	2.1	74	5.4	8.3	0.6	7
DHANSAK								
Butternut, Slim Cook, Tesco*	1 Pack/485g	364	3.9	75	3.8	10.5	0.8	5.1
Chicken with Bagara Rice, Waitrose*	1 Pack/450g	549	8.1	122	8.2	18.2	1.8	1.2
Vegetable, Curry, Microwaved, Slimzone, Asda*	1 Portion/459g	225	2.3	49	2.5	7.7	0.5	2.6
Vegetable, Sainsbury's*	1 Serving/200g	148	5.6	74	3.1	8.9	2.8	2.8
DILL								
Dried, Average	**1 Tsp/1g**	**3**	**0**	**253**	**19.9**	**42.2**	**4.4**	**13.6**
Fresh, Average	**1 Tbsp/3g**	**1**	**0**	**25**	**3.7**	**0.9**	**0.8**	**2.5**
DIP								
Allioli, Garlic, Creamy, Chovi*	1 Serving/10g	75	8.2	746	1.1	1.3	81.9	0.1
Aubergine, Fresh, Waitrose*	1 Serving/85g	159	12.8	187	2.5	10.5	15	1.7
Aubergine, Greek Style, Yarden*	1 Serving/30g	58	4.9	192	2	9.2	16.3	0
Baba Ganoush, Sabra*	1 Serving/75g	188	17.6	251	3.9	4.4	23.5	0
Bean, Mexican, Doritos, Walkers*	1 Tbsp/20g	18	0.7	89	2.7	12.1	3.3	2.4
Beetroot, & Mint, Meadow Fresh, Lidl*	¼ Pack/50g	58	3	116	3.1	10.6	6	3.6
Beetroot, & Mint, The Deli, Aldi*	¼ Pot/50g	66	3.8	131	3.5	10	7.6	4.2

DIP

INFO/WEIGHT	Measure	per Measure KCAL	per Measure FAT	Nutrition Values per 100g / 100ml KCAL	PROT	CARB	FAT	FIBRE
Blue Cheese, Fresh, Sainsbury's*	1/5 Pot/34g	115	11.7	337	3.6	3.1	34.5	0.1
Butternut Squash, & Cumin, Sainsbury's*	¼ Pot/45g	33	1.8	74	3.5	4.2	3.9	4
Caramel, Salted, for Mini Doughnuts, Tesco*	1 Dip/3g	11	0.3	386	2.9	68.7	11.1	0
Cheese & Chive, 50% Less Fat, Asda*	1 Pot/125g	261	21.5	209	4.5	9	17.2	0
Cheese & Chive, 50% Less Fat, Morrisons*	1 Serving/50g	86	6.4	172	8.8	5.2	12.7	0.2
Cheese & Chive, Mature Cheddar, Fresh, Waitrose*	½ Pot/85g	393	40.5	462	5.8	2.4	47.7	1.7
Cheese & Chive, Asda*	1 Serving/43g	190	19.6	447	4.9	3.4	46	0
Cheese & Chive, Tesco*	¼ Pack/50g	148	13.9	296	3.8	7.5	27.8	0.2
Chilli Cheese, Asda*	1 Serving/50g	131	11	262	8	8	22	1.1
Chilli, M&S*	1 Pot/35g	103	0.1	295	0.4	73.2	0.2	0.4
Cracked Corn, Hella Hot, Wicked Kitchen, Tesco*	1 Serving/30g	27	1.3	90	2	10.2	4.3	1.2
Edamame, & Ginger, Meadow Fresh, Lidl*	¼ Pot/50g	59	3	118	3.3	10.6	5.9	4.6
Edamame, Thai Spiced, TTD, Sainsbury's*	¼ Pot/43g	140	12.7	329	7.3	6	29.8	4
Endamame & Pea, Waitrose*	¼ Pot/51g	85	5.9	166	6.3	8	11.6	2
Feta Cheese, Fresh, Tesco*	1oz/28g	81	7.1	288	6.8	7.9	25.5	0.7
Frijolemole, Cannellini Bean & Chick Pea, Waitrose*	¼ Pot/50g	104	7.6	208	4.3	12.2	15.2	2.6
Garlic & Herb, Big Dipper, Morrisons*	¼ Pot/75g	278	28.1	370	1.3	6.9	37.5	0.4
Garlic & Herb, Reduced Fat, M&S*	1 Serving/10g	10	0.4	95	6	8.1	4	0.5
Garlic & Herb, Tesco*	¼ Pack/43g	257	27.8	604	0.9	3.2	65.4	0.3
Garlic & Herb	*1 Serving/100g*	*584*	*62.4*	*584*	*1.4*	*4.1*	*62.4*	*0.2*
Garlic, & Onion, 30% Less Fat, Asda*	1 Serving/30g	50	3.9	166	3.9	8.2	13	0.5
Garlic, Takeaway Pizza, Goodfella's*	1 Pot/18g	57	5.4	319	0.3	12	30	0
Guacamole, Tex-Mex Multipack Selection, Tesco*	½ Pot/53g	76	6.8	142	1.1	4	12.8	3
Jalapeno, Chilli Cheese, Tex-Mex Selection, Tesco*	½ Pot/53g	147	13.6	276	4.7	6.6	25.6	0.3
Jalapeno, Greek Yoghurt, Skotidakis*	1 Tbsp/15g	25	1.8	167	6.7	13.3	11.7	0
Nacho Cheese, Average	*1 Serving/50g*	*175*	*17.2*	*350*	*6.3*	*3.4*	*34.4*	*0.9*
Nacho Cheese, Doritos, Walkers*	1 Serving/40g	92	8.1	231	3.4	8.5	20.2	0.6
Nacho Cheese, Sainsbury's*	1 Serving/50g	244	25.1	487	4.8	3.9	50.2	0
Nacho Cheese, Tex-Mex Multipack Selection, Tesco*	1 Tub/125g	619	62	495	5.9	5.8	49.6	0
Onion & Garlic, Average	*1 Tbsp/15g*	*62*	*6.4*	*410*	*1.7*	*4.8*	*42.7*	*0.4*
Onion & Garlic, HL, Tesco*	1 Serving/43g	80	7.2	188	2.5	6.3	17	0.1
Onion, & Garlic, The Deli, Aldi*	¼ Pot/50g	159	15.5	318	1.7	7.5	31	0.5
Onion, Three, Toasted, Wicked Kitchen, Tesco*	½ Pot/85g	269	26.3	317	2.2	7.6	30.9	0.3
Pea & Spinach, Tesco*	¼ Pot/46g	34	1	75	4	7.7	2.1	4.4
Pea, & Mint, The Deli, Aldi*	¼ Pack/50g	52	3	103	3.3	6.4	6.1	4.4
Pea, & Spinach, Tesco*	¼ Pot/46g	61	4	132	3.1	8.6	8.6	3.9
Pea, Yogurt & Mint, Sainsbury's*	¼ Pack/50g	119	10.8	238	3.4	7.5	21.6	2.1
Peanut, Satay Selection, Occasions, Sainsbury's*	1 Serving/2g	4	0.2	186	7.1	13.8	11.4	1.1
Pecorino, Basil & Pine Nut, Fresh, Waitrose*	½ Pot/85g	338	33.7	398	5.1	5.1	39.7	0
Red Pepper, Meadow Fresh, Lidl*	¼ Pot/50g	59	3	118	3.3	10.6	5.9	4.6
Red Pepper, Sainsbury's*	1 Pot/100g	103	4	103	2.3	14.6	4	0
Red Pepper, Smoky, Gazpacho, Graze*	1 Punnet/23g	54	1.3	242	5.7	40.1	5.9	3.7
Red Pepper, The Deli, Aldi*	¼ Pot/50g	60	3	119	3.6	11	6	4
Salsa, Chunky Tomato, Tesco*	1 Pot/170g	68	2.2	40	1.1	5.9	1.3	1.1
Salsa, Chunky, Fresh, Sainsbury's*	1 Serving/100g	51	1.7	51	1.1	7.8	1.7	1.2
Salsa, Hot, Doritos, Walkers*	1 Jar/300g	99	0.3	33	1.1	6.4	0.1	0.9
Salsa, Hot, Snaktastic, Lidl*	1 Serving/50g	17	0.1	34	1.3	6.1	0.2	1.5
Salsa, Mango, Ginger & Chilli, Spiced, Weight Watchers*	1 Serving/56g	48	0.1	85	1	19.9	0.2	2.6
Salsa, Mild, Asda*	1 Portion/100g	47	0.3	47	1.4	8.7	0.3	1.8
Salsa, Mild, Doritos, Walkers*	1 Tbsp/30g	9	0.1	30	0.8	6	0.3	1.5
Sour Cream & Chive, BGTY, Sainsbury's*	¼ Pot/57g	101	8.4	176	2.2	7.3	14.6	0.5
Sour Cream & Chive, Classic, Tesco*	¼ Pot/50g	124	11.9	249	2	6.6	23.8	0.2
Sour Cream & Chive, Doritos, Walkers*	1 Tbsp/20g	52	4.9	258	1.9	6.9	24.7	1.9

	Measure INFO/WEIGHT	per Measure KCAL	FAT	Nutrition Values per 100g / 100ml KCAL	PROT	CARB	FAT	FIBRE
DIP								
Sour Cream & Chive, Fresh, Tesco*	½ Pot/75g	305	31.8	407	2.1	4.1	42.4	0
Sour Cream & Chive, Half Fat, Waitrose*	½ Pot/85g	133	9.9	157	5.5	7.6	11.6	0.1
Sour Cream & Chive, Mexican Style, Morrisons*	¼ Pack/25g	68	7	274	2.2	3.4	27.9	0.4
Sour Cream & Chive, Morrisons*	1 Serving/100g	317	32.6	317	2.6	3.3	32.6	0
Sour Cream & Chive, Reduced Fat, Tesco*	¼ Pot/50g	80	6.1	159	4.2	7.9	12.2	0.2
Sour Cream & Chive, Sainsbury's*	1 Serving/50g	141	13.8	282	3.1	5.4	27.5	0.1
Sour Cream & Chive, Average	**1 Tbsp/15g**	**48**	**4.8**	**317**	**3.2**	**4**	**32**	**0.3**
Sour Cream & Chive, M&S*	½ Pack/57g	218	22.5	383	2.2	4.9	39.4	0.1
Sour Cream, Tesco*	1 Serving/38g	111	11.2	297	3.4	3.9	29.8	0.2
Soy, Gyoza Selection, Tesco*	1 Pot/30g	30	0.2	100	1.7	21.4	0.7	0.7
Sweetcorn, & Chilli, Tesco*	¼ Pot/46g	53	1.6	115	2.9	17.3	3.4	1.7
Taramasalata, Sainsbury's*	¼ Pot/57g	267	26.6	465	3.3	8.6	46.3	0.5
Thousand Island, HL, Tesco*	1 Serving/31g	57	4.6	183	2.5	9.6	14.9	0.3
Thousand Island, M&S*	1oz/28g	69	6.2	245	2.1	9.4	22.2	0.7
Tortilla Chips, Cool Flavour, Big, Morrisons*	½ Pack/100g	453	22	453	6.4	57.4	22	8.1
Yoghurt & Cucumber, & Mint, Tesco*	1oz/28g	34	2	121	7	7.2	7.1	0.6
DOLMADES								
Stffed Vine Leaves, Delphi*	1 Dolmade/30g	36	0.8	119	2.2	21.9	2.5	1.1
Stuffed with Rice, M&S*	1 Leaf/38g	40	1.6	105	2.6	14.2	4.1	1.2
DOPIAZA								
Chicken, Indian, Waitrose*	½ Pack/175g	243	14.5	139	10.2	5	8.3	1.6
Chicken, M&S*	1 Pack/350g	402	21.4	115	11.5	3.7	6.1	2.5
Chicken, Slimming World*	1 Pack/500g	335	6	67	9.1	4.2	1.2	1.6
Mushroom, Retail	**1oz/28g**	**19**	**1.6**	**69**	**1.3**	**3.7**	**5.7**	**1.1**
DORITOS								
Chilli Heatwave, Walkers*	1 Bag/30g	148	7.6	495	6.3	57.3	25.3	6.7
Cool Spice 3ds, Walkers*	1 Bag/24g	108	4.3	450	8	64	18	4.4
Cool, Original, Walkers*	1 Bag/40g	197	10	492	5.7	58	25	5.9
Dippas, Hint of Lime, Walkers*	1 Bag/35g	173	8.8	495	7	60	25	3.5
Dippas, Lightly Salted, Dipping Chips, Walkers*	1 Serving/25g	128	6.8	510	6.5	60	27	3
Lighly Salted, Corn Chips, Doritos*	1 Bag/30g	149	7.1	497	6.9	62.9	23.6	3.3
Tangy Cheese, Walkers*	1 Bag/40g	200	10.8	500	7	57	27	3
DOUBLE DECKER								
Cadbury*	1 Bar/54.5g	253	9.3	464	3.7	73	17	1.6
Dinky Deckers, Cadbury*	1 Piece/5g	22	0.8	456	4.2	71	17	1.5
Snack Size, Cadbury*	1 Bar/36g	165	7.4	465	4.8	64.5	20.9	0
DOUGH BALLS								
with Garlic & Herb Butter, Aldi*	1 Ball/12g	45	2.2	365	7.7	46.7	18.2	1.8
with Garlic Butter Dip, Supermarket, Pizza Express*	4 Balls/44g	137	1.3	311	10.8	59	3	2.5
DOUGHNUTS								
Beignets, De Crevette, Carrefour*	½ Pack/70g	158	4.6	225	8	33	6.6	1.2
Chocolate, Bakery, Tesco*	1 Doughnut/66g	250	12.8	379	6.6	43.5	19.4	2.2
Chocolate, Iced, Ring, Bakery, Sainsbury's*	1 Doughnut/55g	212	10.3	386	6.3	47.4	18.8	1
Custard Filled, Average	**1 Doughnut/75g**	**268**	**14.2**	**358**	**6.2**	**43.3**	**19**	**0**
Custard, Sainsbury's*	1 Doughnut/70g	172	7.5	246	5.1	32.3	10.7	2.3
Custard, Tesco*	1 Doughnut/70g	199	7.4	284	6.8	39.5	10.6	1.8
Glazed, Bakery, Tesco*	1 Doughnut/52g	202	10.1	389	6.5	45.9	19.5	2
Glazed, Ring, Bakery, Sainsbury's*	1 Doughnut/62g	229	12	369	5.5	42.8	19.3	1.1
Jam, & Cream, Asda*	1 Doughnut/41g	139	7.4	336	4.9	39	18	0.6
Jam, & Cream, Cream Cake Selection, Tesco*	1 Doughnut/71g	225	10.2	317	6	40.4	14.4	1
Jam, Bakery, Tesco*	1 Doughnut/70g	225	7.6	321	5.6	49.2	10.9	2
Jam, Filled, Average	**1 Doughnut/75g**	**252**	**10.9**	**336**	**5.7**	**48.8**	**14.5**	**0**
Jam, M&S*	1 Doughnut/49g	141	2	287	5	57.6	4	1.3

D

	Measure INFO/WEIGHT	per Measure KCAL	FAT	Nutrition Values per 100g / 100ml KCAL	PROT	CARB	FAT	FIBRE
DOUGHNUTS								
Mini, Ring, Bites, Sugar Coated, Simply Doughnuts*	1 Ring/12g	57	3.5	474	6.9	43	29	0
Mini, Sainsbury's*	1 Doughnut/14g	53	2.7	379	5.2	47.9	18.9	2.1
Oreo, CSM, UK LTD*	1 Doughnut/72g	326	19.5	453	5	46.8	27	1.1
Plain, Ring, Average	*1 Doughnut/60g*	*238*	*13*	*397*	*6.1*	*47.2*	*21.7*	*0*
Raspberry Jam, Sainsbury's*	1 Doughnut/58g	203	8.9	350	5.5	46.4	15.3	2.3
Ring, Iced, Average	*1 Doughnut/70g*	*268*	*12.2*	*383*	*4.8*	*55.1*	*17.5*	*0*
Ring, Mini, Bakers Selection, Asda*	1 Doughnut/13g	55	2.8	409	5.2	49	21	1.4
Ring, Sugar, Tesco*	1 Doughnut/56g	234	15.9	419	6.2	33.6	28.4	2.1
Selection, Bakers Selection, Asda*	1 Doughnut/75g	273	17.9	365	4.5	32	24	1.4
Strawberry, Iced, Ring, Bakery, Tesco*	1 Doughnut/58g	248	14.3	428	5.4	45.3	24.7	1.4
Strawberry, Iced, Ring, Mini, Bakery, Tesco*	1 Doughnut/15g	62	3.1	415	4.9	51.5	20.8	1.3
Sugar, Ring, Bakery, Sainsbury's*	1 Doughnut/51g	222	14	435	5.7	40.7	27.4	2.1
Vanilla, Bakery, Sainsbury's*	1 Doughnut/66g	248	12.9	376	6.1	42.7	19.6	2
White Iced, Ring, Bakery, Sainsbury's*	1 Doughnut/55g	211	10.2	383	7	46.4	18.6	1
Yum Yums, Glazed, Sweet, Waitrose*	1 Doughnut/45g	172	10	382	4	41.6	22.2	2
Yum Yums, M&S*	1 Doughnut/37g	155	8.9	420	4.9	45.7	23.9	1.6
DOVER SOLE								
Fillet, Raw, Average	*1oz/28g*	*25*	*0.5*	*89*	*18.1*	*0*	*1.8*	*0*
DR PEPPER*								
Coca-Cola*	1 Bottle/500ml	145	0	29	0	7.2	0	0
Zero, Coca-Cola*	1 Can/330ml	2	0	0	0	0	0	0
DRAGON FRUIT								
Raw, Edible Portion, Average	*1 Serving/100g*	*41*	*0.5*	*41*	*0.7*	*9.6*	*0.5*	*3.6*
DRAMBUIE								
39% Volume	*1 Pub Shot/35ml*	*125*	*0*	*358*	*0*	*23*	*0*	*0*
DRESSING								
French, Style, BGTY, Sainsbury's*	1 Tbsp/15ml	11	0.4	76	0.7	12.6	2.5	0.5
Avocado, & Garlic, Eta*	1 Serving/25ml	85	8.2	337	0.8	10.3	32.6	0
Balsamic, & Olive Oil, Sainsbury's*	1 Serving/25ml	104	10.4	415	0.9	9.4	41.8	0.2
Balsamic, & Olive Oil, Tesco*	1 Tbsp/15ml	45	4.2	297	1.1	10.6	27.8	0
Balsamic, Fig Glaze, Tesco*	1 Tbsp/15ml	31	0	208	1.4	47.9	0	0
Balsamic, Glaze, Odysea *	1 Tsp/5ml	9	0	171	0.5	40	0	0
Balsamic, Italian, Loyd Grossman*	1 Serving/10g	36	3.4	357	0.9	13.1	33.5	0.1
Balsamic, Sweet, BGTY, Sainsbury's*	1 Tsp/5g	3	0	61	0.5	13.6	0.5	0.5
Balsamic, Vinaigrette, Newman's Own*	1 Tbsp/15ml	56	5.7	372	0.1	7.2	38.2	0.5
Balsamic, Vinegar, Asda*	1 Tsp/5ml	7	0.2	146	0.5	27	4	0
Balsamic, Vinegar, Morrisons*	1 Serving/15ml	17	0.2	111	0.1	22.9	1.6	0.1
Blue Cheese, Counted, Eat Smart, Morrisons*	1 Tbsp/15ml	14	0.5	93	2.8	12.2	3.1	0.5
Blue Cheese, Hellmann's*	1 Tbsp/15g	69	7.1	459	0.7	6.3	47.2	1.1
Blue Cheese, Salad, Waitrose*	1 Serving/50g	265	25.2	530	2.1	17.3	50.3	4.1
Caesar, 95% Fat Free, Tesco*	1 Tsp/6g	5	0.2	88	4.1	8.9	3.7	0.3
Caesar, Asiago, Briannas*	1 Tbsp/15ml	70	7.5	467	3.3	3.3	50	0
Caesar, Chilled, Reduced Fat, Tesco*	1 Tsp/5ml	13	1.2	252	6.5	3.1	23.7	0.1
Caesar, Classic, Sainsbury's*	1 Tsp/5ml	22	2.3	442	2.7	4.6	45.9	0.5
Caesar, Creamy, M&S*	1 Tbsp/15ml	66	6.5	437	2.6	9.1	43.1	1
Caesar, Fat Free, Average	*1 Tsp/5g*	*4*	*0.2*	*84*	*4.6*	*11*	*4.1*	*0.2*
Caesar, Finest, Tesco*	1 Tbsp/15ml	72	7.6	477	1.9	2.8	50.9	0.2
Caesar, Hellmann's*	1 Tsp/6g	30	3.1	499	2.5	4.5	51.7	0.3
Caesar, LC, Tesco*	1 Serving/15g	9	0.2	60	1.5	9.5	1.5	0.5
Caesar, Less Than 3% Fat, BGTY, Sainsbury's*	1 Serving/20g	10	0.4	48	0.8	7	1.9	0.3
Caesar, Low Fat, Average	*1 Tsp/5g*	*4*	*0.1*	*77*	*2.3*	*11.1*	*2.6*	*0.2*
Caesar, Original, Cardini's*	1 Serving/10g	56	6	555	2.3	1.5	60	0.2
Caesar, Skinny Sauce, The Skinny Food Co.*	1 Tbsp/15ml	0	0	0	0	0	0	0

D

DRESSING	Measure INFO/WEIGHT	per Measure KCAL	FAT	Nutrition Values per 100g / 100ml KCAL	PROT	CARB	FAT	FIBRE
Caesar, Tesco*	1 Tbsp/15ml	65	6.8	435	0.9	5.4	45.1	0.3
Caesar, The Best, Morrisons*	1 Tbsp/15ml	48	4.7	322	3.2	7.1	31.1	0.6
Caesar, Waitrose*	1 Serving/15ml	72	7.6	479	4.5	0.9	50.8	0.2
Caesar, with Smoked Garlic, Hellmann's*	1 Tbsp/15ml	35	3.3	231	2	6.4	22	0
Chilli, & Balsamic, Glaze, Jamie Oliver*	1 Tbsp/15ml	32	0	212	0.2	50	0	0
Chilli, & Herb, Morrisons*	1 Tbsp/15ml	21	1.1	140	1.1	17	7.3	0.9
Cucumber, & Mint, M&S*	1 Tbsp/15ml	46	3.9	305	0.7	16.7	26.1	0.1
French, Chilled, Tesco*	1 Tbsp/15ml	63	5.9	421	1.1	15.1	39.6	0
French, Classic, Fresh, M&S*	1 Serving/10ml	52	5.3	515	0.6	8.2	53.1	0.2
French, Classics, M&S*	1 Tbsp/15ml	77	8	516	0.6	8.2	53.1	0.2
French, Fresh, Organic, Sainsbury's*	1 Tbsp/15ml	45	4.6	301	0.4	5.5	31	0.4
French, Fresh, Sainsbury's*	1 Tbsp/15ml	64	6.7	429	0.6	6.6	44.6	0.6
French, LC, Tesco*	1 Tbsp/16g	8	0.3	50	0.8	7.6	1.6	1.1
French, Reduced Fat, M&S*	1 Tbsp/15g	10	0.4	70	0.7	11.5	2.8	0.7
French, Reduced Fat, Tesco*	1 Tbsp/15ml	10	0.2	65	0.5	13	1.3	0
French, Tesco*	1 Serving/25ml	110	11.2	441	0.7	7.2	44.9	0.2
French, Virtually Fat Free, Aldi*	1 Serving/10g	3	0	33	0.9	6.7	0.3	1.1
Garlic & Herb, Eat Smart, Morrisons*	1 Tbsp/15ml	10	0.5	66	1.2	7.5	3.1	0.5
Garlic & Herb, Tesco*	1 Tbsp/15g	32	3	210	0.9	5.8	20.2	0.8
Honey & Mustard, Dijon, Wholegrain, Loyd Grossman*	1oz/28g	93	8.9	331	1.2	9.9	31.8	1.3
Honey & Mustard, BGTY, Sainsbury's*	1 Tbsp/15g	12	0.2	78	0.5	16.1	1.3	0.5
Honey & Mustard, Counted, Morrisons*	1 Tbsp/15ml	12	0.5	79	1.4	10	3.1	1.8
Honey & Mustard, Finest, Tesco*	1 Serving/25ml	72	5.6	288	1.7	19.6	22.5	0.7
Honey & Mustard, Hellmann's*	1 Serving/15ml	27	0.2	182	0.7	13.7	1.6	0.3
Honey & Mustard, M&S*	1 Tbsp/15ml	47	3.8	313	2.7	16.8	25.5	2.8
Honey & Mustard, Tesco*	1 Tbsp/15ml	33	2.3	220	0.8	18.8	15.2	2.5
Honey, Orange & Mustard, BGTY, Sainsbury's*	1 Tbsp/15ml	16	0.4	105	1.8	18.6	2.5	1.8
House, Classic, Salad, Hellmann's*	1 Tbsp/15ml	38	3.9	254	0.5	5.7	26	0
House, Light, Supermarket, Pizza Express*	1 Tbsp/15ml	45	4.5	300	0.7	4.3	30	0.3
House, Supermarket, Pizza Express*	1 Tbsp/15ml	62	6.6	415	0.7	3.3	44	0.3
Italian, Newman's Own*	1 Tbsp/15g	55	5.7	367	0.3	5.5	38.3	1
Lemon & Cracked Black Pepper, GFY, Asda*	1 Tbsp/15g	9	0	57	0.2	14	0	0.3
Lemon, & Black Pepper, Fat Free, Tesco*	1 Tbsp/15ml	11	0	74	0.1	17.8	0.1	0.9
Mary Berry*	1 Serving/15g	77	6.6	513	0.8	28.5	44	0.1
Oil & Lemon	*1 Tbsp/15g*	*97*	*10.6*	*647*	*0.3*	*2.8*	*70.6*	*0*
Salad, Lemon, & Thyme, Specially Selected, Aldi*	1 Tbsp/15ml	23	1.2	157	0.5	21	7.9	1.2
Super Nutty, Soy, Wholefood, M&S*	1 Pack/230g	301	11.7	131	5.3	12.8	5.1	6.1
Sweet Chilli, & Coriander, Sainsbury's*	1 Tbsp/15g	38	2.4	255	1.1	26.5	16	0.5
Thousand Island	*1 Tsp/6g*	*19*	*1.8*	*323*	*1.1*	*12.5*	*30.2*	*0.4*
Thousand Island, Hellmann's*	1 Tbsp/15ml	36	3	238	1	14	20	0
Thousand Island, Reduced Calorie	*1 Tsp/6g*	*12*	*0.9*	*195*	*0.7*	*14.7*	*15.2*	*0*
Thousand Island, Walden Farms*	2 Tbsps/30ml	3	0	9	0	4.3	0	1
Yoghurt & Mint, PB, Waitrose*	1 Serving/100ml	130	2.6	130	4.6	22.1	2.6	0.7
Yoghurt & Mint, Crucials*	1 Tbsp/15g	58	5.9	387	1.4	6.2	39.5	0.4
DRIED FRUIT								
Apricots, Soft, Alesto, Lidl*	1 Serving/30g	81	0.1	269	2	61.3	0.3	6.4
Fruity Biscuit Shot, Whitworths*	1 Pack/25g	93	2.1	372	2.8	69.2	8.4	4.5
Pineapple, Sweetened, Whitworths*	1 Bag/35g	122	0.1	350	0.4	86.3	0.2	0.5
Raisin & Chocolate, Shot, Whitworths*	1 Pack/25g	91	2.3	364	4	63.2	9.2	5.6
Trail Mix, Kick Start, Wholefoods, Asda*	1 Serving/50g	194	10.2	387	10.9	40	20.4	10.7
Tropical Mix, Alesto, Lidl*	1 Serving/25g	104	4.8	416	3.4	55.9	19	4
DRIED FRUIT MIX								
5 Fruits, Ready to Eat, Sundora*	½ Pack/100g	233	0.4	233	1.6	58.4	0.4	6.8

	Measure INFO/WEIGHT	per Measure KCAL	FAT	Nutrition Values per 100g / 100ml KCAL	PROT	CARB	FAT	FIBRE
DRIED FRUIT MIX								
Average	*1 Tbsp/25g*	*67*	*0.1*	*268*	*2.3*	*68.1*	*0.4*	*2.2*
Berry, Love Life, Waitrose*	1 Serving/30g	89	0.3	296	1.9	70	0.9	3
Garden of England, Graze*	1 Punnet/25g	70	0.2	280	1	71.2	0.7	5.6
Luxury, Co-Op*	1 Serving/40g	114	0.2	285	2	68	0.6	4
Scandinavian Forest, Graze*	1 Punnet/28g	79	0.2	282	2	71	0.6	8
Sultanas Raisins & Cranberries, Dunnes*	1 Handful/15g	47	0.1	315	2	80.2	0.9	4.7
Sultanas, Currants, Raisins & Citrus Peel, Asda*	1 Serving/100g	283	0.5	283	2.6	67	0.5	1.7
Tesco*	1 Tbsp/25g	71	0.1	284	2.3	67.9	0.4	2.2
Tropical Sundae, Graze*	1 Punnet/29g	86	0.3	299	2.7	72.7	1	8.5
DRIFTER								
Nestle*	1 Finger/20g	99	4.3	484	4.1	68.9	20.9	1.2
DRINK								
Aloe Vera, Mango, Say Aloe*	1 Bottle/500ml	160	0	32	0	7.9	0	0
Aperitif, Bitter, Non Alcoholic, AEcorn *	1 Measure/60ml	28	0	47	0.4	8.6	0	0
Apple, & Cucumber, Mojo*	1 Bottle/250ml	72	0	29	0.4	6.6	0	0
Arancia Rossa, Soda, Vive, Aldi*	¼ Bottle/250ml	10	1.2	4	0.5	0.7	0.5	0.5
Bubblegum, Sparkling, Barr's*	1 Can/330ml	7	0	2	0	0	0	0
Bubbly, Wild Elderflower, Luscombe*	1 Bottle/270ml	86	0.8	32	0.2	7.2	0.3	0
Citrus, & Ginger, Hot Shot, M&S*	1 Shot/100ml	32	0.1	32	0.7	6.9	0.1	0.4
Dark Muscovado, Spirit Mixer, Schweppes*	1 Can/150ml	50	0	33	0	7.9	0	0
Elderflower, Gently Sparkling, Fentiman's*	1 Bottle/275ml	77	0	28	0	6.9	0	0
Fizzio Zero, Tesco*	1 Serving/250ml	1	0	0	0	0.1	0	0
G&T, Reduced Calorie, Low Alcohol, Tesco*	1 Can/250ml	12	0	5	0	0	0	0
Limone e Menta, Sparkling, Vive, Aldi*	1 Serving/250ml	5	1.2	2	0.5	0.5	0.5	0.5
Malted, Instant, As Sold, Morrisons*	1 Serving/30g	130	2.7	433	8.3	79	9	1.3
Pineapple, Soda, Old Jamaica*	1 Can/330ml	66	0.3	20	0.1	4.9	0.1	0
Raspberry, Isotonic, Sports, Tesco*	1 Bottle/500ml	115	0	23	0	5.3	0	0
Shake, Vanilla Chai, Plant Protein, For Goodness Shakes*	1 Bottle/330ml	99	0.3	30	6	0.9	0.1	1.2
Turmeric, & Cayenne, Shot, Eat Well, M&S*	1 Bottle/100ml	42	0.1	42	0.3	10	0.1	0.6
DRINK MIX								
Spritz, Pink Grapefruit, & Vodka, Kalosa Natural Spritz*	1 Bottle/275ml	99	0	36	0	0	0	0
DRINKING CHOCOLATE								
Made Up with Semi-Skimmed Milk, Average	*1 Mug/227ml*	*129*	*4.3*	*57*	*3.5*	*7*	*1.9*	*0.2*
Made Up with Skimmed Milk, Average	*1 Mug/227ml*	*100*	*1.1*	*44*	*3.5*	*7*	*0.5*	*0*
Made Up with Whole Milk, Average	*1 Mug/227ml*	*173*	*9.5*	*76*	*3.4*	*6.8*	*4.2*	*0.2*
DRIPPING								
Beef	*1oz/28g*	*249*	*27.7*	*891*	*0*	*0*	*99*	*0*
DUCK								
Breast, Meat Only, Cooked, Average	*1oz/28g*	*48*	*2*	*172*	*25.3*	*1.8*	*7*	*0*
Breast, Meat Only, Raw, Average	*1 Serving/160g*	*206*	*6.8*	*128*	*22.6*	*0*	*4.2*	*0.2*
Breast, Roast, & Blueberries, Everdine*	1 Serving/450g	436	18.4	97	6	7.7	4.1	2.9
Confit, Roasted, with Juniper, Cook*	1 Serving/250g	368	18.8	147	13.8	6.1	7.5	0.5
Duck, Sainsbury's*	1 Serving/15g	135	15	900	0.5	0.5	100	0.5
Leg, Meat & Skin, Average	*1oz/28g*	*80*	*5.6*	*286*	*17.2*	*0.5*	*20*	*0.4*
Raw, Meat, Fat & Skin	*1oz/28g*	*109*	*10.4*	*388*	*13.1*	*0*	*37.3*	*0*
Roasted, Meat Only, Weighed with Fat, Skin & Bone	*1 Serving/100g*	*41*	*2.2*	*41*	*5.3*	*0*	*2.2*	*0*
Roasted, Meat, Fat & Skin	*1oz/28g*	*118*	*10.7*	*423*	*20*	*0*	*38.1*	*0*
Vegetarian, Shredded Hoisin, Cooked, Linda McCartney*	½ Pack/167g	317	12.9	190	22.1	5.9	7.7	3.9
Vegetarian, Shredded, Hoisin, Frozen, Linda McCartney*	1 Serving/75g	159	6.5	212	24.7	6.7	8.7	4.4
DUCK AROMATIC								
Crispy, ¼, Hoisin Sauce & 6 Pancakes, Tesco*	1/6 Pack/40g	92	3.3	231	13.3	25.3	8.3	1
Crispy, ¼, Hoisin Sauce, Pancakes, M&S*	½ Pack/155g	290	12.1	187	10.5	18.1	7.8	1
Crispy, ½, Duck & Pancakes, M&S*	½ Pack/311g	590	26.7	190	13.9	14	8.6	2.1

D

	Measure INFO/WEIGHT	per Measure KCAL	per Measure FAT	Nutrition Values per 100g / 100ml KCAL	PROT	CARB	FAT	FIBRE
DUCK AROMATIC								
Crispy, ½, Hoisin Sauce, & 12 Pancakes, Tesco*	3 Pancakes/106g	263	9.5	248	17.9	23.4	8.9	1
DUCK CANTONESE								
Style, Roast, Tesco*	1 Pack/300g	375	6.9	125	8.2	17.9	2.3	0.5
DUCK IN								
Chinese Barbecue, Wings, Sainsbury's*	1 Serving/175g	430	25	246	19.4	9.7	14.3	0
Orange Sauce, Breast, Simply, Gressingham Foods*	½ Pack/175g	254	11.9	145	15.9	5.1	6.8	0.4
Orange Sauce, Roast, a L'Orange, M&S*	½ Pack/259g	482	26.9	186	16.2	6.5	10.4	0.8
Plum Sauce, with Egg Fried Rice, Serves 1, Sainsbury's*	1 Pack/450g	738	18.9	164	6.2	24	4.2	2.8
DUCK PEKING								
Crispy, Aromatic, Sainsbury's*	½ Pack/300g	1236	110.7	412	19.5	0.6	36.9	0.1
DUCK WITH								
Port & Orange Sauce, Legs, Slow Cooked, M&S*	½ Pack/158g	265	16.9	168	14.8	3	10.7	0.5
Pancakes & Hoisin Sauce, M&S*	1 Pack/80g	136	3.2	170	13	19.9	4	0.9
DUMPLINGS								
Average	**1oz/28g**	**58**	**3.3**	**208**	**2.8**	**24.5**	**11.7**	**0.9**
Dim Sum, Assorted Stuffing, Steamed, Restaurant	**1 Serving/100g**	**230**	**8.2**	**230**	**7.9**	**32**	**8.2**	**3**
Dim Sum, Chicken, Asian Fusion, Waitrose*	1 Dumpling/20g	30	0.4	152	9.5	22.8	2.2	1.4
Dim Sum, Chicken, Steamed, Restaurant	**1 Serving/100g**	**230**	**5.9**	**230**	**7.5**	**37**	**5.9**	**2.1**
Dim Sum, Chinese, Deep Fried, Restaurant	**1 Serving/100g**	**430**	**23**	**430**	**4.9**	**50**	**23**	**1.8**
Dim Sum, From Restaurant, Average	**1 Piece/12g**	**50**	**2.4**	**433**	**28.9**	**31.3**	**20.4**	**0**
Dim Sum, Meat Dumpling, Deep Fried, Restaurant	**1 Serving/100g**	**340**	**16**	**340**	**4.9**	**43**	**16**	**1**
Dim Sum, Pork, Restaurant, Average	**1 Serving/100g**	**270**	**7.3**	**270**	**7.3**	**43**	**7.3**	**1.6**
Dim Sum, Prawn, Steamed, Eat Well, M&S*	1 Dim Sum/20g	28	0.2	138	6.7	25.1	1.1	0.6
Dim Sum, Steamed, Prawn, M&S*	6 Dim Sum/120g	222	3.2	185	1.1	39	2.7	1.5
Dim Sum, Vegetable & Meat, Steamed, Restaurant	**1 Serving/100g**	**240**	**7.9**	**240**	**5.9**	**37**	**7.9**	**2.5**
Dim Sum, Wonton, Deep Fried, Restaurant	**1 Serving/100g**	**430**	**29**	**430**	**9.7**	**32**	**29**	**1.2**
Gyoza, Vegetable, in Broth, The City Kitchen*	1 Pack/355g	270	8.5	76	2.1	10.7	2.4	1.6
Gyozas, Chicken, Microwaved, Iceland*	1 Gyozas/18g	31	0.5	176	8.3	28	2.7	3.3
Homestyle, Baked Weight, Frozen, Aunt Bessie's*	1 Dumpling/53g	177	7.9	337	5.4	47	15	3.5
Mix, Cooked as Directed, Aunt Bessie's*	2 Dumpling/53g	126	4.9	238	4.5	33	9.2	2.4
Pierogi, Meat Filled, U Jedrusia*	6 Dumplings/118g	252	10	214	10	23	8.5	2.4
Pierogi, Ruskie, Jawo*	1/3 Pack/150g	266	4.5	177	8	29	3	0
Pork & Garlic Chive, Waitrose*	1 Pack/115g	215	8.1	187	9.4	20.4	7	1.1
Prawn Sui Mai, Selection, M&S*	6 Sui Mai/120g	143	0.8	119	9.4	13.3	0.7	1.5
Prawn, Siu Mai, Chinese, M&S*	1 Dumpling/20g	22	0.3	108	9.4	13.3	1.6	1.5
Vegetable, Steamed, Bibigo*	1 Dumpling/28g	29	1.9	103	6.9	18.5	6.7	1.4

D

	Measure INFO/WEIGHT	per Measure KCAL	FAT	Nutrition Values per 100g / 100ml KCAL	PROT	CARB	FAT	FIBRE
EASTER EGG								
Aero, Medium, Egg Shell Only, Aero, Nestle*	1 Egg/131g	702	38.9	534	6.2	59.9	29.6	1.6
After Eight Giant Chocolate Egg, Nestle*	¼ Egg /50g	274	16.8	547	5.5	51.8	33.7	7.1
Artisanal, Belgian, Egg Shell Only, Guylian*	1 Easter Egg/70g	386	23.8	552	7.2	53	34	0
Butterscotch, Medium, Egg Shell Only, Green & Black's*	1 Egg/165g	914	57.8	554	8.8	50	35	2.5
Buttons, Chocolate Egg Shell Only, Cadbury*	1 Sm Egg/100g	537	31	537	7.3	56	31	2.1
Caramel, Chocolate Egg Shell Only, Cadbury*	1 Lge Egg/343g	1801	102.9	525	7.5	56.8	30	0.7
Chick, Dairy Milk, Chocolate Egg Shell Only, Cadbury*	1 Egg/167g	877	50.1	525	7.5	56.8	30	0.7
Chocolate Egg Shell Only, Dairy Milk, Cadbury*	1 Lg Egg/343g	1818	104.6	530	7.6	56.5	30.5	0.7
Chocolate Egg Shell Only, Small, Dairy Milk, Cadbury*	1 Egg/72g	386	22.3	537	7.3	56	31	2.1
Chocolate Orange, Terry's*	1 Egg/196g	1015	52.9	518	8.1	59	27	2.3
Chocolate, Free From, Sainsbury's*	1 Egg/100g	581	35.8	581	3	59.5	35.8	4.5
Chocolate, Milk, Organic, Egg Shell Only, Green & Black's*	¼ Egg/41g	230	14.8	561	9.8	48	36	2.8
Creme Egg, Chocolate Egg Shell Only, Cadbury*	1 Egg/178g	956	55.2	537	7.3	56	31	2.1
Crunchie, Cadbury*	1 Lge Egg/200g	1072	61.9	537	7.3	56	31	2.1
Dairy Milk, Caramel, Egg Shell Only, Cadbury*	1 Egg/176g	945	54.6	537	7.3	56	31	2.1
Dark Chocolate, 70%, Green & Black's*	1 Med Egg/160g	952	69	580	9.1	36	42	10
Disney, Nestle*	1 Egg/65g	342	18.9	526	6.3	59.7	29.1	0.6
Ferrero Rocher, Egg Shell Only, Ferrero*	1 Egg/175g	1064	80.2	608	7.3	39.8	45.8	0
Flake, Chocolate Egg Shell Only, Cadbury*	1 Lge Egg/200g	1074	62	537	7.3	56	31	2.1
Freddo Faces, Chocolate Egg Shell Only, Cadbury*	1 Egg/72g	382	22	530	7.6	56.5	30.5	0.7
Galaxy Ripple Indulgence, with Chocolate Egg, Mars*	1 Egg/198g	1045	57.4	528	7.1	58.9	29	1.6
Kinder Surprise, Ferrero*	1 Egg/100g	579	36.2	579	8.8	53.9	36.2	0
Kit Kat, Chunky, Nestle*	1 Med Egg/107g	572	31.5	534	6.1	60.4	29.4	1.5
Lindor, Milk Chocolate, Egg Shell Only, Lindt*	1 Egg/230g	1240	71.3	539	7.1	57	31	0
Malteser, Malteaster, Egg Shell Only, Mars*	1 Egg/149g	785	43.2	527	7	59	29	0
Maltesers, Bunny, Egg Shell Only, Mars*	1 Egg/175g	922	50.8	527	7	59	29	0
Maltesers, Truffles, Egg Shell Only, Mars*	1 Egg/175g	922	50.8	527	6.7	59	29	0
Milk Chocolate, Classic Collection, Thorntons*	1 Egg/205g	1078	61.5	526	6.1	57	30	0
Milk Chocolate, Nestle*	½ Egg/42g	205	9.7	489	5	65.2	23.1	0.5
Milk Chocolate, Swiss, Hollow, M&S*	1 Egg/18g	100	6.3	555	6.7	53.2	34.8	2.5
Milk, & Ruby, Fruit & Nut, Half, The Best, Morrisons*	1 Egg/310g	1674	102.6	540	7.4	51.6	33.1	2.9
Milky Bar, Nestle*	¼ Egg/18g	97	5.7	543	10.6	53.1	31.7	0
Mini Eggs, Chocolate Egg Shell Only, Cadbury*	¼ Egg/25g	134	7.7	537	7.3	56	31	2.1
Mini, Oodles of Eggs, Hotel Chocolat*	1 Egg/18g	99	6.2	558	6.8	53	35	2.3
Minstrels, Egg Shell Only, Galaxy, Mars*	1 Egg/200g	1056	58	528	7.1	58.9	29	0
Mint Collection, Dark, Thorntons*	¼ Egg/41g	215	13.4	531	6.3	47	33	0
Mint, Lindor, Egg Shell Only, Lindt*	1 Egg/200g	1078	62	539	7.1	57	31	0
Munchies, Egg Shell Only, Nestle*	1 Egg/184g	981	54	534	6.1	60.4	29.4	1.5
Oreo, Cadbury*	1 Egg/31g	175	11.2	563	5	55	36	1.4
Quality Street, Egg Shell Only, Quality Street, Nestle*	1 Egg/204g	1090	60	534	6.1	60.4	29.4	1.5
Reeses, Egg Shell Only, Hershey*	1 Egg/172g	855	50.2	497	7.1	61.1	29.2	0
Roses, Chocolate Egg Shell Only, Cadbury*	1 Egg/200g	1060	61	530	7.6	56.5	30.5	0.7
Smarties, Nestle*	¼ Egg/31g	160	8.4	524	6	62	27.7	1.4
Smarties, Orange, Egg Shell Only, Smarties, Nestle*	1 Egg/184g	981	54	534	6.1	60.4	29.4	1.5
Snickers, Egg Shell Only, Mars*	1 Egg/178g	940	51.6	528	7.1	58.9	29	0
Twirl, Chocolate Egg Shell Only, Cadbury*	1 Lge Egg/325g	1745	100.8	537	7.3	56	31	2.1
White Chocolate, Thorntons*	1 Egg/360g	1958	109.1	544	5.5	62.2	30.3	2.1
Wispa, Chocolate Egg Shell Only, Cadbury*	1 Egg/200g	1074	62	537	7.3	56	31	2.1
ECLAIR								
Caramel, Asda*	1 Eclair/58g	215	15.1	371	5.6	29	26	0.7
Chocolate, 25% Less Fat, Sainsbury's*	1 Eclair/58g	171	9.3	295	6.8	31.1	16	1.2
Chocolate, Asda*	1 Eclair/33g	144	11	436	6.7	27.3	33.3	4.8
Chocolate, Belgian, & Cream, Essential, Waitrose*	1 Eclair/39g	148	9.5	379	6.2	33	24.4	1.6

	Measure INFO/WEIGHT	per Measure KCAL	FAT	Nutrition Values per 100g / 100ml KCAL	PROT	CARB	FAT	FIBRE
ECLAIR								
Chocolate, Belgian, Fresh Cream, Tesco*	1 Eclair/61g	233	15.4	382	7.3	30.6	25.3	1
Chocolate, Fresh Cream, M&S*	1 Eclair/44g	170	12.2	390	6.3	28.4	27.9	2
Chocolate, Fresh Cream, Sainsbury's*	1 Eclair/35g	130	8.3	372	6.5	32.2	23.8	1.5
Chocolate, Frozen, Free From, Tesco*	1 Eclair/25g	81	4.2	327	4.1	38.9	17	0.8
Chocolate, Frozen, Morrisons*	1 Eclair/31g	116	9.6	374	5	18.8	31	1.3
Chocolate, Mini, Iceland*	1 Eclair/12g	49	3.6	418	5.3	29.3	30.8	1
EEL								
Cooked or Smoked, Dry Heat, Average	*1 Serving/100g*	*236*	*15*	*236*	*23.6*	*0*	*15*	*0*
Jellied, Average	*1oz/28g*	*26*	*1.9*	*93*	*8*	*0*	*6.7*	*0*
Raw, Average	*1oz/28g*	*32*	*2.1*	*113*	*11.1*	*0*	*7.6*	*0*
EGG SUBSTITUTE								
Easy Egg, Vegan, Dry , Orgran*	1 Serving/50g	175	1.6	350	14.9	46.8	3.2	16
Vegan Egg, Follow Your Heart*	1 Serving/10g	40	1.7	401	5	0	17	40
EGGS								
Araucana, Bluebell, Free Range, Finest, Tesco*	1 Egg/50g	66	4.5	131	12.6	0.1	9	0
Blue, Old Cotswold Legbar, Clarence Court*	1 Egg/60g	79	5.4	131	12.4	0	9	0
Duck, Boiled & Salted, Weight with Shell	*1 Egg/75g*	*148*	*11.6*	*198*	*14.6*	*0*	*15.5*	*0*
Duck, Whole, Raw, Weight with Shell	*1 Egg/75g*	*122*	*8.8*	*163*	*14.3*	*0*	*11.8*	*0*
Free Range, Large, Weight with Shell	*1 Egg/68g*	*97*	*6.8*	*143*	*12.6*	*0.8*	*9.9*	*0*
Fried in Veg Oil, Average	*1 Med/60g*	*107*	*8.3*	*179*	*13.6*	*0.7*	*13.9*	*0*
Fried, without Fat, Average	*1 Med/60g*	*104*	*7.6*	*174*	*15*	*0.7*	*12.7*	*0*
Goose, Whole, Fresh, Raw, Weight with Shell	*1 Egg/144g*	*232*	*16.6*	*161*	*12.1*	*1.2*	*11.5*	*0*
Large, Weight with Shell	*1 Egg/68g*	*97*	*6.8*	*143*	*12.6*	*0.8*	*9.9*	*0*
Medium, Boiled, Weight with Shell	*1 Egg/60g*	*86*	*6*	*143*	*12.6*	*0.8*	*9.9*	*0*
Medium, Weight with Shell	*1 Egg/56g*	*80*	*5.6*	*143*	*12.6*	*0.8*	*9.9*	*0*
Poached, Weight with Shell	*1 Med/58g*	*83*	*5.8*	*143*	*12.6*	*0.8*	*9.9*	*0*
Quail, Ready To Eat, Clarence Court *	4 Eggs/33g	51	3.7	154	13.1	0.5	11.1	0
Quail, Whole, Raw, Weight with Shell	*1 Egg/13g*	*20*	*1.4*	*151*	*12.9*	*0.4*	*11.1*	*0*
Ready Scrambled, Easy Egg Co*	1 Pack/125g	144	9.9	115	7.9	2.9	7.9	0.5
Savoury, Bites, Mini, Sainsbury's*	1 Bite/12g	34	2.1	285	9.4	21.1	17.9	1.2
Savoury, Mini, Tesco*	1 Egg/20g	55	3.5	274	9.2	20.2	17.4	2.3
Savoury, Vegetarian, Mini, Quorn*	1 Egg/20g	51	2.3	257	15	21	11.5	4.6
Scotch, Asda*	1 Egg/114g	286	19.2	251	11.2	13.7	16.8	1.4
Scotch, Cumberland, Waitrose*	1 Egg/114g	243	14.3	214	13	12.1	12.6	1.6
Scotch, Finest, Tesco*	1 Egg/114g	280	20.1	247	11.6	10.4	17.7	1.1
Scotch, Free Range, Sainsbury's*	1 Egg/113g	284	19	252	12.4	12.5	16.9	2.5
Scotch, Lincolnshire, M&S*	1 Egg/114g	306	21.1	268	12	12.8	18.5	1.2
Scotch, Morrisons*	1 Egg/114g	286	19.1	251	11.2	13.7	16.8	1.4
Scotch, Retail	*1 Egg/120g*	*301*	*20.5*	*251*	*12*	*13.1*	*17.1*	*0*
Scrambled, 1 Minute, Musclefood*	1 Serving/125g	144	9.9	115	7.9	2.9	7.9	0.5
Scrambled, Average	*1 Lge Egg/68g*	*97*	*6.8*	*143*	*12.6*	*0.8*	*9.9*	*0*
Very Large, Average, Weight with Shell	*1 Egg/78g*	*112*	*7.8*	*143*	*12.6*	*0.8*	*9.9*	*0*
White, Free Range, Liquid, Two Chicks*	3 Tbsp/45g	23	0	50	10.5	1	0	0
Whites Only, Raw, Average	*1 Lg Egg/33g*	*17*	*0.1*	*52*	*10.9*	*0.7*	*0.2*	*0*
Yolks, Raw	*1 Yolk/17g*	*55*	*4.5*	*322*	*15.9*	*3.6*	*26.5*	*0*
ELK								
Raw, Meat only	*1 Serving/100g*	*111*	*1.4*	*111*	*23*	*0*	*1.4*	*0*
Roasted, Meat only	*1 Serving/100g*	*146*	*1.9*	*146*	*30.2*	*0*	*1.9*	*0*
ENCHILADAS								
3 Bean, Ready Meal, Average	*1 Pack/400g*	*505*	*16.6*	*126*	*4.4*	*16.9*	*4.2*	*3.2*
Beans, & Rice, Big Bros, Wicked Kitchen, Tesco*	1 Pack/404g	565	15.3	140	4.2	20.5	3.8	3.4
Chicken, Average	*1 Serving/295g*	*483*	*18.8*	*164*	*11.6*	*16*	*6.4*	*1.7*
Chicken, Diner Specials, M&S*	½ Pack/227g	340	12	150	9.9	15.4	5.3	2

E

	Measure INFO/WEIGHT	per Measure KCAL	FAT	Nutrition Values per 100g / 100ml KCAL	PROT	CARB	FAT	FIBRE
ENCHILADAS								
Chicken, in a Spicy Salsa & Bean Sauce, Asda*	½ Pack/212g	373	17	176	10	16	8	0
Chicken, Lidl*	½ Pack/228g	483	15.5	212	17.1	19.7	6.8	2
Spicy, Three Bean, Cooked, CBY, Asda*	1 Pack/400g	466	15.9	117	4.4	13.7	4	4.1
with Cheese & Beef, From Restaurant	**1 Serving/295g**	**496**	**27.1**	**168**	**6.2**	**15.9**	**9.2**	**0**
with Cheese, From Restaurant	**1 Serving/163g**	**319**	**18.8**	**196**	**5.9**	**17.5**	**11.6**	**0**
ENDIVE								
Raw	**1oz/28g**	**2**	**0**	**8**	**1.1**	**0.6**	**0.1**	**1.3**
ENERGY DRINK								
1899, Original, Morrisons*	1 Can/250ml	58	0	23	0	5	0	0
Average	**1 Can/250ml**	**118**	**0**	**47**	**0**	**11.4**	**0**	**0**
Cherry, Lucozade*	1 Bottle/500ml	345	0	69	0	17.1	0	0
Citrus Blast, Soft Drink, Mountain Dew, Britvic*	1 Bottle/500ml	240	0	48	0	13	0	0
Gym Drink, Citrus Blend, iPro Sport*	½ Bottle/250ml	62	0	25	0	6	0	0
KX, Sugar Free, Diet, Tesco*	1 Can/250ml	5	0	2	0	0	0	0
Light, Energetica, Mercadona*	1 Can/250ml	7	0	3	0	0	0	0
Monster*	1 Can/500ml	240	0	48	0	12	0	0
Origin, Relentless*	1 Can/500ml	110	0	22	0	6.1	0	0
Protein, Fresubin*	1 Bottle/200g	300	13.4	150	10	12	6.7	0
Red Devil, Britvic*	1 Can/250ml	160	0	64	0.4	15.1	0	0
Red Thunder, Diet, Low Calorie, Aldi*	1 Can/250ml	5	0	2	0.1	0	0	0
Relentless, Original, Relentless*	1 Can/500ml	230	0	46	0	10.4	0	0
Sparkling Orange, Dual Energy, Powerade*	1 Bottle/500ml	225	0	45	0	10.5	0	0
Sugar Free, Boost Drinks Ltd*	1 Can/250ml	5	0	2	0	0	0	0
Sugar Free, Diet, Mountain Dew, Britvic*	1 Can/440ml	3	0	1	0	0	0	0
Ultra Red, Zero Sugar Plus Calorie, Monster*	1 Can/500ml	15	0	3	0	0.9	0	0
Ultra Violet, Monster*	1 Can/500ml	15	0	3	0	1.4	0	0
Ultra, Zero Calorie, Monster*	1 Can/500ml	10	0	2	0	0.9	0	0
ENERGY GEL								
Isotonic, Apple, Go, Science in Sport*	1 Serving/60ml	90	0.1	144	0	36	0.1	0.1
Isotonic, Blackcurrant, Go, Science in Sport*	1 Pack/60ml	86	0.1	144	0	36	0.1	0.1
Isotonic, Cherry, Go, Science in Sport*	1 Serving/60ml	86	0	144	0	36	0	0.1
Isotonic, Lemon & Lime, Go, Science in Sport*	1 Serving/60ml	90	0.1	144	0	36	0.1	0.1
Isotonic, Orange, Go, Science in Sport*	1 Serving/60ml	90	0	144	0	36	0	0.1
Isotonic, Pink Grapefruit, Go, Science in Sport*	1 Pack/60ml	87	0.1	144	0	36	0.1	0
Isotonic, Tropical, Go, Science in Sport*	1 Serving/60ml	90	0.1	144	0	36	0.1	0.1
Isotonic, Vanilla, Go, Science in Sport*	1 Serving/60ml	87	0	144	0	36	0	0.1
ESCALOPE								
Escalope, Average	**1 Escalope/138g**	**341**	**19.3**	**247**	**13.5**	**16.7**	**14**	**0.6**
Escalope, Lemon & Pepper, Average	**1 Escalope/143g**	**371**	**22.6**	**260**	**12.6**	**16.7**	**15.8**	**0.4**
Vegetarian, Garlic & Herb, Quorn*	1 Escalope/140g	293	16.5	209	8.9	16.9	11.8	3.8
Vegetarian, Garlic & Mushroom, Creamy, Quorn*	1 Escalope/120g	259	12.3	216	10.4	18.8	10.3	3.7
Vegetarian, Gruyere Cheese, Quorn*	1 Escalope/110g	267	15.4	243	10	18	14	2.6
Vegetarian, Lemon & Black Pepper, Quorn*	1 Escalope/110g	256	12.9	233	9.6	20.5	11.7	2.1
Vegetarian, Mozzarella & Pesto, Quorn*	1 Escalope/120g	271	15.6	226	10	15	13	4.5
Vegetarian, Turkey Style, Sage & Onion, Quorn*	1 Escalope/100g	188	9.8	188	10	15	9.8	4.5

E

	Measure INFO/WEIGHT	per Measure KCAL	FAT	Nutrition Values per 100g / 100ml KCAL	PROT	CARB	FAT	FIBRE
FAGGOTS								
Pork, West Country Sauce, Six Pack, Cooked, Mr Brains*	2 Faggots/218g	190	4.8	87	6	10	2.2	0
FAJITA								
Chicken, Average	*1 Serving/240g*	*357*	*12.8*	*149*	*10.2*	*15*	*5.4*	*2.3*
Chicken, Crispy, Old El Paso*	1 Fajita/70g	183	5.4	263	7.6	41	7.8	1.8
Chicken, M&S*	1 Pack/230g	345	12.2	150	8.6	17.7	5.3	1
Meal Kit, Mexican StyleMade Up, CBY, Asda*	¼ Pack/120g	280	6.6	234	6	39	5.5	2.3
Meal Kit, Mild, Tesco*	1 Wrap/59g	144	3.4	247	6.9	40.5	5.8	2.5
Meal Kit, Roasted Tomato, & Pepper, Old El Paso*	1 Fajita/63g	143	2.5	227	6.6	40.1	3.9	2.7
Meal Kit, Sizzling, Smoky BBQ, As Sold, Old El Paso*	1 Fajita/63g	141	2.3	224	6.8	40	3.7	1.8
Vegetable	*1 Serving/275g*	*472*	*14.9*	*172*	*4.9*	*25.6*	*5.4*	*1.9*
FALAFEL								
& Houmous, Snack Pot, Tesco*	1 Pack/106g	354	26.2	324	8.4	14.5	24	8.4
& Tabbouleh, Co-Op*	1 Pack/250g	308	13.8	123	5.5	9.7	5.5	6.5
12 pack, Sainsbury's*	1 Falafel/17g	48	2.6	281	6.8	25.2	15.5	6.4
Balls, Meat Free, Meat Free, Tesco*	3 Balls/67g	135	5.3	205	7.1	21.7	8.1	6.3
Beetroot, & Feta, World Deli, Waitrose*	1 Falafel/21g	59	3.3	279	7.5	25.1	15.5	4.6
Beetroot, Quinoa, & Kale, Love Your Veg!, Sainsbury's*	1 Falafel/26g	61	2.2	231	9.2	27	8.4	5.5
Beetroot, with Red Pepper, & Chilli, Gosh*	4 Falafel/88g	150	6	170	5.4	25.1	6.8	6.4
Butternut Squash, with Spiced Couscous, G&B, Asda*	1 Pack/367g	341	7.7	93	3.2	14	2.1	3.6
Chickpea, Cumin, & Coriander, Goodlife*	1 Falafel/19g	39	2	207	7.9	14.1	10.4	12.6
Fresh Herb, M&S*	1 Falafel/18g	45	2.2	248	8.3	22.6	12	8.1
Fried in Vegetable Oil, Average	*1 Falafel/25g*	*45*	*2.8*	*179*	*6.4*	*15.6*	*11.2*	*3.4*
Mediterranean, Aldi*	1 Pack/200g	470	24	235	6.4	21	12	7.6
Mediterranean, with Chickpea, & Parsley, Gosh!*	1 Falafel/22g	53	2.5	241	7	30.9	11.5	7.1
Mini, M&S*	1 Falafel/14g	43	2.5	310	7.9	28.1	18.4	2.6
Mix, Organic, Quick & Easy, Hale & Hearty*	1 Pack/200g	646	11	323	19.2	43.8	5.5	10.7
Moroccan, Gluten & Milk Free, Free From, Morrisons*	1 Falafel/24g	63	2.4	263	5.8	34	10.1	6.4
Shawarma, Everdine*	1 Serving/450g	590	18.4	131	4.5	16.7	4.1	5
Sweet Potato, Meat Free, Vegan, Tesco*	3 Falafels/62g	123	6.2	199	4.2	18.1	10	9.6
FANTA								
Fruit Twist, Coca-Cola*	1 Serving/250ml	65	0	26	0	6.4	0	0
Grap, Zero	1 Can/325ml	13	0	4	0	0.7	0	0
Icy Lemon, Coca-Cola*	1 Can/330ml	112	0	34	0	8.3	0	0
Icy Lemon, Zero, Coca-Cola*	1 Can/330ml	7	0	2	0	0.2	0	0
Lemon, Coca-Cola*	1 Can/330ml	165	0	50	0	12	0	0
Orange, Coca-Cola*	1 Can/330ml	63	0	19	0	4.6	0	0
Orange, Zero, Coca-Cola*	1 Can/330ml	11	0	3	0	0.5	0	0
Pink Grapefruit, Zero Sugar, Coca-Cola*	1 Can/330ml	10	0	3	0	0.3	0	0
Red Fruits, Coca-Cola*	1 Serving/100ml	37	0	37	0	9	0	0
FARFALLE								
Bows, Dry, Average	*1 Serving/75g*	*265*	*1.4*	*353*	*11.4*	*72.6*	*1.9*	*1.9*
FENNEL								
Florence, Boiled in Salted Water	*1oz/28g*	*3*	*0.1*	*11*	*0.9*	*1.5*	*0.2*	*2.3*
Florence, Raw, Unprepared, Average	*1 Bulb/250g*	*24*	*0.4*	*10*	*0.7*	*1.4*	*0.2*	*1.9*
Florence, Steamed	*1 Serving/80g*	*9*	*0.2*	*11*	*9*	*1.5*	*0.2*	*2.3*
FENUGREEK								
Leaves, Raw, Fresh, Average	*10g*	*4*	*0*	*35*	*4.6*	*4.8*	*0.2*	*1.1*
FETTUCCINE								
Edamame & Mung Bean, Explore Asian*	¼ Pack/50g	168	2.1	335	47.2	16.8	4.2	20.6
Slim Pasta, Eat Water*	½ Pack/100g	9	0	9	0.2	0	0	4
with Tomato & Mushroom, Easy Cook, Napolina*	1 Pack/120g	461	8.6	384	11.8	67.9	7.2	0
FIG ROLLS								
Asda*	1 Biscuit/19g	71	1.7	372	4.8	68	9	0

F

	Measure INFO/WEIGHT	per Measure KCAL	per Measure FAT	Nutrition Values per 100g / 100ml KCAL	PROT	CARB	FAT	FIBRE
FIG ROLLS								
Jacob's*	1 Biscuit/17g	66	1.5	386	3.4	72.2	8.6	3
Sainsbury's*	1 Biscuit/19g	67	1.6	360	4.3	64.5	8.7	3.4
FIGS								
Dried, Average	**1 Fig/14g**	**32**	**0.1**	**232**	**3.6**	**53.2**	**1.1**	**8.6**
Dried, Partially Rehydrated, Soft, Asda*	1 Serving/30g	71	0.4	237	3.3	49	1.5	6.9
Dried, with Honey, Intermarche *	4 Figs/30g	80	0.4	268	3.2	57.1	1.2	8.4
Raw, Fresh, Average	**1 Fig/35g**	**16**	**0.1**	**45**	**1.3**	**9.8**	**0.2**	**1.5**
FISH								
Char, Arctic, Whole, Raw	**1 Serving/100g**	**137**	**6**	**137**	**20.8**	**0**	**6**	**0**
Chargrills, Sun Ripened Tomato, Basil, Birds Eye*	1 Chargrill/163g	127	2.5	75	14	1.4	1.5	0.5
Fillet, Battered Or Breaded, & Fried, From Restaurant	**1 Portion/256g**	**594**	**31.5**	**232**	**14.7**	**17**	**12.3**	**0.5**
Fillets, Crispy, Sweet Chilli, Oven Baked, Gastro, Youngs*	1 Fillet/144g	311	13.4	216	12.3	20.3	9.3	0.9
Fillets, Fishless, Battered, Totally Vegan, Quorn*	1 Fillet/97g	202	8.3	209	4.5	27	8.6	2.9
Fillets, Fishless, Breaded, Totally Vegan, Quorn*	1 Fillet/91g	165	2.6	181	4.5	32	2.8	5.2
Fillets, Lemon & Pepper, Youngs*	1 Fillet/130g	283	16.7	218	10.3	15.3	12.9	4.3
Goujons, Vegetarian, Vivera*	1 Goujon/35g	87	3.5	248	13	25	10	2.7
Grouper	**1 Serving/100g**	**92**	**1**	**92**	**19.4**	**0**	**1**	**0**
Pie Mix, Ocado*	1 Pack/320g	410	18.2	128	19	0	5.7	0
Pie Mix, Seasonal, Sainsbury's*	1 Pack/320g	480	28.2	150	17.7	0	8.8	0
White, Fillets, Frozen, Bay Fishmongers, Tesco*	1 Fillet/104g	77	0.6	74	17.2	0	0.6	0
White, Smoked, Average	**1 Serving/100g**	**108**	**0.9**	**108**	**23.4**	**0**	**0.9**	**0**
FISH & CHIPS								
Haddock, Chunky Chips, & Mushy Peas, Gastropub, M&S*	1 Pack/425g	654	25.1	154	7.2	17	5.9	2.2
Mini Meal, 093, Wiltshire Farm Foods*	1 Serving/185g	255	8.3	138	6.9	17.7	4.5	2.8
Takeaway or Fast Food, Average	**1 Serving/469g**	**998**	**115.6**	**213**	**17.7**	**45.7**	**24.6**	**2.6**
with Mushy Peas, Kershaws*	1 Pack/315g	450	18.3	143	6.4	16.4	5.8	1.6
FISH CAKES								
Breaded, Oven Baked, Youngs*	2 Cakes/96g	184	8.7	192	8	18.9	9.1	1.2
Cod, Melting Middle, Oven Baked, Gastro, Youngs*	1 Cake/132g	246	12.7	186	8.6	15.9	9.6	1
Cod, & Parsley, Waitrose*	1 Cake/85g	147	6.5	173	9.2	16.9	7.6	1.1
Cod, & Chorizo, Aldi*	1 Cake/137g	266	11.5	194	11	18	8.4	1.3
Cod, & Chorizo, Chunky, The Best, Morrisons*	1 Cake/139g	270	12.8	194	10.4	17	9.2	1.1
Cod, & Chorizo, Finest, Tesco*	1 Cake/131g	222	9.4	170	11.6	13.8	7.2	1.6
Cod, & Parsley Sauce, The Best, Morrisons*	1 Cake/150g	278	13	185	10.2	16.1	8.7	0.7
Cod, Baked, (2 Pack), Tesco*	1 Cake/135g	255	9.9	189	9.1	21.1	7.3	3.2
Cod, Breaded, Lighthouse Bay, Lidl*	1 Cake/132g	224	8.4	170	9.7	17.5	6.4	1.6
Cod, Chunky, Breaded, Chilled, Youngs*	1 Cake/90g	192	11.5	213	9.5	14.9	12.8	1.2
Cod, Fillet, GF, Made Without Wheat, M&S*	1 Cake/85g	145	6.7	171	8.3	16	7.9	1.4
Cod, HFC, Tesco*	2 Cakes/96g	173	6.7	181	8.6	20.2	7	1.4
Cod, Homemade, Average	**1 Cake/50g**	**120**	**8.3**	**241**	**9.3**	**14.4**	**16.6**	**0.7**
Cod, M&S*	1 Cake/85g	153	7.8	180	8.9	15.4	9.2	1.3
Cod, Melt in the Middle, Specially Selected, Aldi*	1 Cake/141g	261	13.7	185	8.1	16	9.7	0.6
Cod, Mornay, Easy to Cook, Waitrose*	1 Cake/149g	248	9.4	166	10.6	16.2	6.3	1.4
Cod, Sweet Potato, & Chilli, Finest, Tesco*	1 Cake/136g	203	6.4	149	8.4	17.1	4.7	2.3
Cod, with Parsley Sauce, Melt in the Middle, Deluxe, Lidl*	1 Cake/138g	255	10.6	185	8	20.3	7.7	1.2
Fried in Blended Oil	**1 Cake/50g**	**109**	**6.7**	**218**	**8.6**	**16.8**	**13.4**	**0**
Frozen, Average	**1 Cake/85g**	**112**	**3.3**	**132**	**8.6**	**16.7**	**3.9**	**0**
Haddock, & Vintage Cheddar, Smoked, Saucy Fish Co*	1 Cake/135g	220	7.6	163	9.7	18	5.6	0.9
Haddock, & Cheddar, Smoked, Melting Middle, Co-Op*	1 Cake/135g	259	11.9	192	9.1	19	8.8	1
Haddock, Fillet, Smoked, Morrison's*	1 Cake/130g	238	9.1	183	11.7	17.7	7	1.6
Haddock, GF, Free From, Sainsbury's*	1 Cake/129g	233	10.4	180	10.6	15.8	8	1
Haddock, Melting, Cheddar & Leek, TTD, Sainsbury's*	1 Cake/138g	276	13.5	200	9.7	17.8	9.8	0.9
Haddock, Sainsbury's*	1 Cake/135g	253	10	188	10.8	18.7	7.4	1.5

	Measure INFO/WEIGHT	per Measure KCAL	FAT	Nutrition Values per 100g / 100ml KCAL	PROT	CARB	FAT	FIBRE
FISH CAKES								
Haddock, Smoked, Breaded, Asda*	1 Cake/90g	202	11.7	225	9	18	13	1.6
Haddock, Smoked, Cheddar, & Leek, TTD, Sainsbury's*	1 Cake/138g	276	13.5	200	9.7	17.8	9.8	0.9
Haddock, Smoked, Extra Special, Asda*	1 Cake/115g	218	10.9	190	12.8	13.2	9.5	1.3
Haddock, Smoked, M&S*	1 Cake/85g	153	8	180	10.6	13.4	9.4	2.6
Prawn, & Sweet Potato, Cajun, Waitrose*	1 Cake/138g	187	4.7	136	8.1	17.2	3.4	2.3
Prawn, Cod, Sweet Potato, & Sweet Chilli, Co-Op*	1 Cake/135g	255	8.8	189	6.1	26	6.5	1.6
Prawn, Thai Style, Finest, Tesco*	1 Cake/135g	196	6.8	145	9.5	14.6	5	1.8
Salmon, & Dill, Waitrose*	1 Cake/85g	206	11.9	242	11.5	17.5	14	1.8
Salmon, & Broccoli, Morrisons*	1 Cake/110g	211	10.3	191	9	16.7	9.3	2.2
Salmon, Asda*	1 Cake/132g	266	11.9	202	11	18	9	1.5
Salmon, Cod, Haddock, & Cheddar, The Best, Morrisons*	1 Cake/137g	228	9.3	167	13.2	12.6	6.8	1.4
Salmon, Homemade, Average	*1 Cake/50g*	*136*	*9.8*	*273*	*10.4*	*14.4*	*19.7*	*0.7*
Salmon, Morrisons*	1 Cake/90g	241	11.8	268	10.1	27.6	13.1	1.5
Salmon, Scottish, Sainsbury's*	1 Cake/130g	276	13.8	212	11.7	17	10.6	1
Salmon, Spinach & Sicilian Lemon, Finest, Tesco*	1 Cake/145g	290	16.2	200	9.9	14.3	11.2	1.4
Salmon, Thai Style, with Sweet Chilli Sauce, Waitrose*	½ Pack/135g	238	9.3	176	10.7	17.1	6.9	1.7
Thai Style, Slimming World*	1 Cake/140g	119	2	85	12	5.2	1.4	1.9
FISH FINGERS								
Chunky, Cooked, Tesco*	2 Fingers/98g	230	10	235	13.2	21.6	10.2	1.3
Chunky, Extra Large, Captain Birds Eye, Birds Eye*	2 Fingers/120g	247	9.6	206	13	20	8	0.8
Cod, 100% Cod Fillet, Tesco*	1 Finger/30g	53	2.2	177	12.4	14.9	7.5	1.4
Cod, Breaded, Chunky, Waitrose*	1 Finger/64g	136	5.3	213	13.4	21	8.3	0.5
Cod, Fillet, Chunky, Finest, Tesco*	2 Fingers/115g	225	8.7	196	12.2	19.1	7.6	1
Cod, Fillets, Asda*	1 Finger/31g	66	3.1	214	13	18	10	0
Cod, Fried in Blended Oil, Average	*1 Finger/28g*	*67*	*3.9*	*238*	*13.2*	*15.5*	*14.1*	*0.6*
Cod, Frozen, Average	*1 Finger/28g*	*48*	*2.2*	*170*	*11.6*	*14.2*	*7.8*	*0.6*
Cod, Grilled, Average	*1 Finger/28g*	*56*	*2.5*	*200*	*14.3*	*16.6*	*8.9*	*0.7*
Cod, HFC, Tesco*	3 Fingers/70g	162	7.6	231	14.5	18.1	10.9	1.4
Cod, Sainsbury's*	1 Finger/28g	53	2.1	190	12.5	17.7	7.7	1
Cod, Youngs*	1 Finger/24g	50	2	209	13.3	19.8	8.3	0.8
Fishless, Squeaky Bean*	1 Finger/27g	68	3	250	13	24	11	3
Free From, Sainsbury's*	1 Finger/30g	56	2.3	188	11.4	18	7.8	0.7
Haddock, Chunky, Panko Breaded, Gastro, Youngs*	2 Fingers/78g	154	7	198	13.1	15.7	9	0.9
Haddock, Fillet, Chunky, TTD, Sainsbury's*	2 Fingers/113g	244	10.3	216	13.8	19.3	9.1	0.6
Haddock, Fillets, Asda*	1 Finger/30g	62	2.7	205	14	17	9	0
Haddock, in Crispy Batter, Birds Eye*	1 Finger/30g	56	2.3	188	14.3	15.1	7.8	0.7
Iceland*	1 Finger/23g	44	2	192	11.5	17.3	8.5	1.3
Pollock, Sainsbury's*	3 Fingers/85g	160	6.7	188	13	15.9	7.9	0.8
Vegetarian, Fishless, Vegan, Quorn*	1 Finger/20g	37	1.4	187	4.4	24.1	7.1	4.7
FISH IN								
Butter Sauce, Steaks, Ross*	1 Serving/140g	111	4	84	10.6	3.6	3	0.3
Butter Sauce, Steaks, Youngs*	1 Serving/140g	102	2.9	73	9.6	3.7	2.1	0.5
Parsley Sauce, Steaks, Ross*	1 Serving/150g	123	5.6	82	9.1	3.1	3.7	0.1
FIVE SPICE								
Powder, Sharwood's*	1 Tsp/2g	3	0.2	172	12.2	11.6	8.6	23.4
FLAKE								
Dipped, Cadbury*	1 Bar/41g	215	12.5	530	7.6	56.1	30.8	0.8
Luxury, Cadbury*	1 Bar/45g	240	13.6	533	7.3	57.8	30.2	0
Praline, Cadbury*	1 Bar/38g	201	12.9	535	7.7	49.5	34.3	0
FLAN								
Pastry with Fruit	*1oz/28g*	*33*	*1.2*	*118*	*1.4*	*19.3*	*4.4*	*0.7*
Sponge with Fruit	*1oz/28g*	*31*	*0.4*	*112*	*2.8*	*23.3*	*1.5*	*0.6*

F

	Measure INFO/WEIGHT	per Measure KCAL	FAT	Nutrition Values per 100g / 100ml KCAL	PROT	CARB	FAT	FIBRE
FLAN CASE								
Sponge, Average	**1oz/28g**	**90**	**1.5**	**320**	**7**	**62.5**	**5.4**	**0.7**
FLAPJACK								
Lemon Curd, Graze*	1 Punnet/53g	248	12.7	468	6	60	24	6
All Butter, Sainsbury's*	1 Flapjack/35g	156	8	446	5.7	54.5	22.8	2.7
All Butter, Squares, M&S*	1 Flapjack/34g	150	7.2	441	6.2	56.2	21.2	4.4
All Butter, Topped with Caramel, Spar*	1 Bar/65g	292	12.9	449	5	60.5	19.9	3.8
Apple & Raspberry, Fox's*	1 Flapjack/26g	105	5	403	4.8	52.5	19.4	3.7
Apple & Cinnamon, Graze*	1 Punnet/52g	236	12	453	5	54	23	5
Apricot & Raisin, Waitrose*	1 Flapjack/38g	143	4.2	376	4.7	64.3	11.1	5.8
Average	*1 Sm/50g*	*242*	*13.3*	*484*	*4.5*	*60.4*	*26.6*	*2.7*
Berry, Protein, Bar, Graze*	1 Punnet/53g	246	12.7	465	15	45	24	5.4
Bites, Sainsbury's*	1 Bite/17g	74	3.4	435	5.3	56	20	4.8
Caramel Bake, The Handmade Flapjack Company*	1 Flapjack/90g	375	13	417	6	65.6	14.5	0
Caramel Fudge, Wholebake*	1 Flapjack/80g	369	18.4	461	6.2	56.2	23	4
Cherry Bakewell, Iced, Devondale*	1 Flapjack/95g	432	21.9	455	3.7	54	23.1	2.6
Chocolate Chip, Boots*	1 Flapjack/75g	313	11.2	417	5.6	65	15	3.5
Chocolate Chip, Devondale*	1 Flapjack/95g	434	24.7	457	4.3	49	26	3.6
Chocolate Dipped, M&S*	1 Flapjack/96g	442	21.5	460	6.1	61.3	22.4	3
Chocolate, Belgian, M&S*	1 Bar/80g	372	19.8	465	5.5	52.9	24.7	4.6
Chunky Chocolate, M&S*	1 FlapJack/80g	348	15.1	435	5.8	59.9	18.9	2.2
Cranberry, & Orange, Free From, Tesco*	1 Flapjack/30g	131	5.5	440	5.9	60.4	18.5	4.3
Cranberry, Apple & Raisin, LC, Tesco*	1 Flapjack/30g	98	1.7	325	5.7	63.1	5.6	5.7
Dark Chocolate, Delectable , Thomas J Fudge*	1 Flapjack/36g	171	7.4	476	5.5	64.9	20.6	0
Fruity, M&S*	1 Flapjack/68g	287	11.7	422	5.5	59.3	17.2	4.1
Golden Oaty Fingers, Tesco*	1 Flapjack/34g	142	5.7	420	5.7	59.7	16.8	3.7
Golden Oaty, Fingers, Fabulous Bakin' Boys*	1 Finger/28g	130	6.8	464	4.5	60.2	24.3	3.1
Granola, Traybake, Tesco*	1 Serving/46g	202	9.5	440	7.1	54	20.6	5
Hobnobs, Milk Chocolate, McVitie's*	1 Flapjack/35g	155	6	443	5.8	64.2	17.2	4.2
Honey, Norfolk Cake Co*	1 Serving/100g	425	20	425	6.5	50.8	20	0
Jaffa Cake, Graze*	1 Punnet/53g	242	12.7	457	6	53	24	5
Lemon Drizzle, Graze*	1 Punnet/53g	248	12.7	468	5.9	54	24	5.8
Lemon, Lively, Retail, Graze*	1 Slice/17g	80	4.1	468	5.9	54	24	5.8
M&S*	1 Flapjack/53g	228	10.1	430	6	59.1	19	3.5
Milk Chocolate, Bites, Bakery, Sainsbury's*	1 Bite/16g	74	3.4	452	6.4	58.3	20.7	3.7
Mince Pie, Graze*	1 Punnet/52g	234	10.9	450	4.9	63	21	6.3
Mini, Sainsbury's*	1 Slice/15g	65	2.9	431	5.6	59.3	19	2.7
Morning Berry, Protein, Trek*	1 Bar/40g	172	7.7	431	20.4	42.2	19.3	4.7
Oat, GF, Hale & Hearty*	1 Cake/36g	165	9.1	457	6.8	55.1	25.2	8.9
Oat, Morrisons*	1 Flapjack/50g	228	11	455	5.8	56.3	22.1	3.9
Protein, Cocoa, Vanilla, Retail, Graze*	1 Flapjack/53g	248	13.3	467	17	47	25	5.4
Raspberry Preserve, The Handmade Flapjack Company*	1 Flapjack/90g	310	2.1	345	6.4	74.4	2.4	0
Slices, Free From, Tesco*	1 Flapjack/30g	132	5.8	442	6.2	59	19.3	4
Sultana, & Cherry, Bar, Holland & Barrett*	1 Bar/60g	247	10.2	412	6.3	54	17	8.3
Summer Berry, Graze*	1 Punnet/52g	230	10.9	442	5	56	21	5
Toffee, Finest, Tesco*	1 Flapjack/35g	156	6.7	446	4.9	63.6	19.1	1.3
FLATBREAD								
Cheddar, & Tomato, Cooked, Sainsbury's*	¼ Pack/56g	153	3.8	284	11.6	42.4	7	2.2
Cheddar, Mature, & Garlic, Finest, Tesco*	¼ Flatbread/66g	188	6.3	285	7.2	41.8	9.6	2.6
Cheese, & Tomato, Tesco*	¼ Flatbread/54g	158	3.5	291	11.6	45.7	6.4	1.9
Chicken, Chargrilled, COU, M&S*	1 Pack/163g	245	3.1	150	10.8	23	1.9	5.2
Chicken, Harissa, & Roasted Vegetable, M&S*	1 Pack/186g	342	4.8	184	10.7	19.7	2.6	0
Chicken, Mexican, Stonebaked, Finest, Tesco*	1 Pack/155g	280	5.1	180	11.7	25.1	3.3	1.6
Chicken, Moroccan, Shapers, Boots*	1 Pack/164g	289	2.1	176	9.8	30	1.3	2.2

F

FLATBREAD	Measure INFO/WEIGHT	per Measure KCAL	FAT	Nutrition Values per 100g / 100ml KCAL	PROT	CARB	FAT	FIBRE
Chicken, Tikka, BGTY, Sainsbury's*	1 Flatbread/186g	292	4.5	157	11.6	20.5	2.4	3.5
Chicken, Tikka, Shapers, Boots*	1 Flatbread/175g	270	4.9	154	11	21	2.8	1.7
Chicken, with Mango Salsa, Jerk Style, Chargrilled, M&S*	1 Flatbread/200g	300	7.6	150	12.5	15.4	3.8	2.6
Crispy, Marmite*	2 Flatbreads/18g	79	2.7	441	20.1	57.4	15.1	0
Feta, COU, M&S*	1 Pack/180g	225	4	125	6.3	20.6	2.2	1.9
Garlic, & Cheese, Co-Op*	1 Serving/66g	194	4.4	294	9.5	39	6.7	1.9
Garlic, Deep Filled, Tesco*	¼ Flatbread/61g	170	4	278	9	44.1	6.5	3.6
Goats Cheese, Butternut Squash, & Beetroot, Tesco*	1 Pack/164g	378	13.6	231	5.9	31.8	8.3	2.6
Ham, & Emmental, Smoked, Fold, Delicious, Boots*	1 Fold/165g	394	16.5	239	12	24	10	3.6
Pizza, Meat, Spicy, Asda*	1 Pizza/234g	589	19.9	252	12	31	8.5	2.3
Plain, Thins, Deli Kitchen*	1 Flatbread/35g	103	1.9	295	8.5	51.4	5.3	4.1
Pork, Bramley Apple, & Stuffing, Tesco Finest*	1 Pack/201g	385	4.8	192	8.1	33.8	2.4	1.9
Prawn, Tikka, King, Waitrose*	1 Pack/165g	257	3.3	156	9.4	25.1	2	1.5
Rosemary, & Sea Salt, GF, Nairn's*	1 Flatbread/13g	54	1.8	430	9	63	14.2	7.2
Rosemary, & Sea Salt, Thins, Ryvita*	1 Slice/7g	28	0.4	401	14.8	70.8	5.4	5.2
Salami, Calabrese, Carlos, Aldi*	½ Pizza/181g	490	21.7	271	10	30	12	1.7
Village Lavash, Ulta Thin, Yeast Free, Dina Foods Ltd*	1 Flatbread/110g	289	1.1	263	11.2	52.3	1	4.6
FLAXSEED								
Golden, Ground, P H Foods*	1 Serving/10g	51	4.2	514	18.3	1.6	42.2	27.3
Milled, Holland & Barrett*	1 Tbsp/15g	84	5.6	560	20	4.7	37.3	30.6
Milled, Organic, Linwoods*	1 Tsp/5g	25	2	508	22.1	3	40	23.7
FLOUR								
Arrowroot, Average	*1oz/28g*	*100*	*0*	*357*	*0.3*	*88.2*	*0.1*	*3.4*
Bread, White, Strong, Average	*1oz/28g*	*94*	*0.4*	*336*	*11.8*	*68.4*	*1.5*	*3.4*
Brown, Chapati, Average	*1 Tbsp/20g*	*67*	*0.2*	*333*	*11.5*	*73.7*	*1.2*	*0*
Brown, Wheat	*1oz/28g*	*90*	*0.5*	*323*	*12.6*	*68.5*	*1.8*	*6.4*
Chakki Wheat Atta, Whole Wheat, Pillsbury*	1 Portion/30g	98	0.5	327	12	65	1.7	0
Chick Pea	*1oz/28g*	*88*	*1.5*	*313*	*19.7*	*49.6*	*5.4*	*10.7*
Coconut, Average	*1 Serving/100g*	*344*	*13.6*	*344*	*18.2*	*15.4*	*13.6*	*43.8*
Plain, Average	*1oz/28g*	*98*	*0.4*	*349*	*10.3*	*73.8*	*1.5*	*2.2*
Rice	*1 Tsp/5g*	*18*	*0*	*366*	*6.4*	*80.1*	*0.8*	*2*
Soya, Low Fat, Average	*1oz/28g*	*99*	*2*	*352*	*45.3*	*28.2*	*7.2*	*13.5*
Speciality GF, Dove's Farm*	1 Serving/100g	353	1.8	353	4.7	85.2	1.8	2.7
Spelt, Average	*1 Serving/57g*	*216*	*1.7*	*381*	*14.3*	*74.5*	*3*	*6.4*
White, Average	*1oz/28g*	*89*	*0.3*	*319*	*9.8*	*66.8*	*1*	*2.9*
White, Chapati, Average	*1 Tbsp/20g*	*67*	*0.1*	*335*	*9.8*	*77.6*	*0.5*	*0*
White, Self Raising, Average	*1oz/28g*	*94*	*0.4*	*336*	*9.9*	*71.8*	*1.3*	*2.9*
White, Self Raising, Gluten & Wheat Free, Dove's Farm*	1 Serving/100g	344	1	344	5.5	78.1	1	1.4
Wholemeal, Average	*1oz/28g*	*87*	*0.6*	*312*	*12.6*	*61.9*	*2.2*	*9*
FOOL								
Apricot, Fruit, Tesco*	1 Pot/113g	200	12.7	177	2.6	16.4	11.2	0.3
Apricot, Spanish, The Best, Morrisons*	1 Pot/114g	198	11.6	174	2.7	17.5	10.2	0.5
Fruit, Average	*1 Pot/120g*	*196*	*11.2*	*163*	*1*	*20.2*	*9.3*	*1.2*
Gooseberry, Fabulously Fruity, Sainsbury's*	1 Pot/113g	197	11.6	173	2.7	17.1	10.2	1.2
Gooseberry, Fruit, Co-Op*	1 Pot/114g	211	11.4	185	3	22	10	1
Gooseberry, Tesco*	1 Pot/112g	225	14.1	200	3	17.8	12.5	0.7
Lemon, Fruit, BGTY, Sainsbury's*	1 Pot/113g	94	3.8	83	3.4	9.7	3.4	0.3
Lemon, Signature, Morrisons*	1 Pot/114g	213	11.8	187	3	20	10.4	0.5
Raspberry, Fruit, Tesco*	1 Pot/113g	234	12.8	207	2.6	23.6	11.3	0.3
Rhubarb, Fruit, Waitrose*	1 Pot/114g	182	12.9	160	2.7	11.9	11.3	0.3
Rhubarb, Timberly, Fabulously Fruity, Sainsbury's*	1 Pot/113g	167	11.7	147	2.4	10.9	10.3	0.5
Strawberry, Fruit, BGTY, Sainsbury's*	1 Pot/120g	100	3.1	83	3.7	11.1	2.6	0.8
Strawberry, Fruit, Co-Op*	1 Pot/114g	188	10.3	165	2	18	9	0.8

	Measure INFO/WEIGHT	per Measure KCAL	per Measure FAT	Nutrition Values per 100g / 100ml KCAL	PROT	CARB	FAT	FIBRE
FRANKFURTERS								
Average	*1 Sausage/42g*	*123*	*11.2*	*292*	*12*	*1.3*	*26.6*	*0*
Chicken, Halal, Tahira*	1 Sausage/34g	64	4.7	187	11.5	4.5	13.7	0
Vegetarian, Quorn*	1 Sausage/45g	92	6.3	205	13.5	4.5	14	3.5
Vegetarian, Tivall*	1 Sausage/30g	73	4.8	244	18	7	16	3
FRAZZLES								
Bacon, Smith's, Walkers*	1 Bag/23g	113	5.3	488	7.5	62	23	1.3
FRENCH FRIES								
Cheese & Onion, Walkers*	1 Pack/22g	95	3.5	430	5	66	16	5
Ready Salted, Walkers*	1 Bag/21g	91	3.4	434	5	65	16	5
Salt & Vinegar, Walkers*	1 Bag/22g	95	3.5	430	5	66	16	5
Worcester Sauce, Walkers*	1 Bag/22g	96	3.5	435	5	65	16	5
FRENCH TOAST								
Asda*	1 Toast/8g	30	0.4	381	10	74	5	4
Bacon, & Maple, Gail's*	100g	310	21.6	310	11.8	16.7	21.6	0.8
Blueberry & Blackcurrant Compote, Gail's*	100g	275	19.4	275	8	16.6	19.4	0.6
Sainsbury's*	1 Toast/8g	31	0.5	382	10	72	6.6	5
FRIES								
As Sold, Aunt Bessie's*	1 Serving/100g	150	3.7	150	2.4	26	3.7	1.9
Butternut, Crinkle Cut, Oven Cooked, Morrisons*	½ Pack/83g	58	0.7	70	2.2	11.7	0.9	3.1
Chips, From Restaurant, Average	*1 Serving/105g*	*294*	*16.3*	*280*	*3.3*	*34*	*15.5*	*2.1*
Criss Cross, Oven Baked, Iceland*	1 Serving/125g	324	14.1	259	3.5	33.7	11.3	4.4
Curly, Cajun, Weighed Frozen, McCain*	1 Portion/100g	156	8.7	156	1.6	17.7	8.7	1.8
Curly, Lightly Seasoned, McCain*	1 Serving/125g	239	10.8	191	2.3	25.1	8.6	2.4
Curly, Southern Style, Tesco*	1 Serving/50g	95	2.8	189	2.6	29.6	5.6	4.9
Dirty, Cheesy, M&S*	½ Pack/250g	518	30	207	7	16.7	12	2
Extra Chunky, Oven Baked, Homefries, McCain*	1 Serving/200g	306	6.2	153	3.2	28	3.1	2.3
Pizza, Cheesy, Loaded, Cheese & Tomato Sauce, M&S*	½ Pack/240g	372	16.3	155	5.2	17.2	6.8	2
Seasoned, Frozen, Ovenbaked, Asda*	1/6 Pack/125g	286	10.9	229	3.1	33	8.7	3
Skin On, Bacon Flavour, Oven Baked, Asda*	¼ Pack/77g	144	5.7	186	2.1	26	7.4	2.8
Skin On, Crispy, McCain*	1 Serving/125g	222	7.8	178	2.4	27	6.2	2.6
Skin on, Ovenbaked, Iceland*	1/10 Bag/100g	204	6.9	204	3.3	30.6	6.9	3.2
Steak, Golden, Ore-ida*	1 Serving/84g	80	3	95	1.2	15.5	3.6	2.4
Sweet Potato, Crispy, McCain*	1 Serving/125g	170	5.7	136	1.6	20.4	4.6	3.5
Sweet Potato, Crispy, Tesco*	½ Pack/150g	320	18.2	213	2.6	21.6	12.1	3.8
Sweet Potato, Oven Baked, CBY, Asda*	1 Serving/125g	188	6.5	150	5.6	19	5.2	2.4
Sweet Potato, Prefried & Frozen, Cooked, Sainsbury's*	1 Serving/125g	297	14.7	237	2.4	28.3	11.7	4.6
Sweet Potato, Ready to Roast, Cooked, Sainsbury's*	½ Pack/116g	201	8.3	174	2.1	23.7	7.2	3.2
Sweet Potato, Slims Kitchen *	1 Bowl/340g	578	25.5	170	1.5	22	7.5	0
FRISPS								
Tangy Salt & Vinegar, KP Snacks*	1 Bag/30g	160	10	532	5	52.6	33.5	2.9
Tasty Cheese & Onion, KP Snacks*	1 Bag/28g	150	9.4	537	5.5	53.2	33.6	3.2
FRITTATA								
Goats Cheese, & Butternut Squash, Chef Select, Lidl*	1 Pack/130g	189	10.1	145	8.9	9.1	7.8	1.4
Spinach & Courgette, Meat Free, Tesco*	1 Frittata/120g	199	12.8	166	5.8	10.2	10.7	2.9
Vegetable, CBY, Asda*	1 Frittata/150g	183	7.8	122	6.2	12.1	5.2	1
Veggie, Ella's Kitchen*	1 Frittata/25g	24	1.3	95	6.5	6.2	5.1	0.9
FRITTERS								
Courgette, Pea, & Mint, Waitrose*	½ Pack/70g	155	9.7	221	4.9	17.7	13.9	3.4
Fritters, Hormel Foods*	1 Fritter/80g	221	14.5	276	10.2	18.1	18.1	2.2
Sweetcorn, & Courgetti, Tesco*	1 Fritter/63g	89	3.4	142	2.5	18.5	5.5	4.1
Sweetcorn, Tesco*	1 Fritter/25g	53	2.9	212	5.2	19.9	11.5	4.1
FROMAGE FRAIS								
0% Fat, Vitalinea, Danone*	1 Tbsp/28g	14	0	50	7.4	4.7	0.1	0

FROMAGE FRAIS	Measure INFO/WEIGHT	per Measure KCAL	FAT	Nutrition Values per 100g / 100ml KCAL	PROT	CARB	FAT	FIBRE
Apricot, Creamfields*	1 Pot/50g	41	0.4	83	6.9	11.7	0.9	0.1
Apricot, Summer Fruit, Layered, Weight Watchers*	1 Pot/90g	44	0.1	49	5.6	6	0.1	0.2
Blackberry, Berry Fruits, Layered, Weight Watchers*	1 Pot/100g	49	0.2	49	5.5	5.7	0.2	0.4
Fabby, Loved By Kids, M&S*	1 Pot/43g	45	1.6	105	6.2	12.3	3.7	0
Fat Free, Average	*1 Pot/60g*	*35*	*0.1*	*58*	*7.7*	*6.8*	*0.2*	*0*
High Protein,, Tesco*	1 Serving/30g	16	0	54	8.8	4.6	0	0
Kids, Yeo Valley*	1 Serving/90g	111	4.8	123	6.6	12.6	5.3	0
Milbona, Lidl*	1 Pot/50g	44	1	88	5.6	11.5	2.1	0.5
Munch Bunch, Nestle*	1 Pot/42g	44	1.3	105	6.7	12.6	3	0
Peach, Summer Fruit, Layered, Weight Watchers*	1 Pot/90g	44	0.1	49	5.6	6	0.1	0.3
Plain, Average	*1oz/28g*	*32*	*2*	*113*	*6.8*	*5.7*	*7.1*	*0*
Raspberry, Berry Fruits, Layered, Weight Watchers*	1 Pot/90g	44	0.1	49	5.6	5.9	0.1	0.4
Raspberry, Creamfields*	1 Pot/50g	40	0.4	80	6.9	11.2	0.8	0.2
Raspberry, Value, Tesco*	1 Serving/60g	56	0.8	93	7.2	13.5	1.3	0
Strawberry Cheesecake, Dessert Selection, Sainsbury's*	1 Pot/90g	95	2.2	106	5.8	15.3	2.5	0.1
Strawberry, 99.9% Fat Free, Onken*	1 Serving/50g	46	0	91	6.9	15.3	0.1	0
Strawberry, Apricot & Raspberry, Everyday Essentials, Aldi*	1 Pot/55g	46	0.8	83	6.8	10	1.5	0.5
Strawberry, Organic, Yeo Valley*	1 Pot/90g	116	5.4	129	6.3	12.5	6	0.2
Strawberry, Petits Filous, Yoplait*	1 Pot/50g	52	1.4	104	6.7	12.6	2.9	0.2
Strawberry, Pouches, Fruit King, Milbona, Lidl*	1 Pouch/80g	90	2.4	112	6.4	14.9	3	0.5
Strawberry, Thomas the Tank Engine, Yoplait*	1 Pot/50g	50	0.6	101	6.8	15.4	1.3	0
Strawberry, Value, Tesco*	1 Pot/60g	55	0.8	92	7.2	13	1.3	0
Wildlife, Strawberry, Raspberry Or Peach, Yoplait*	1 Pot/50g	46	0.6	93	7.1	13.2	1.3	0.2
with Fruit, Average	*1 Avg Pot/90g*	*74*	*2.2*	*83*	*6.1*	*9*	*2.5*	*0.8*
with Fruit, Healthy Range, Average	*1 Avg Pot/90g*	*40*	*0.1*	*45*	*5.8*	*5.1*	*0.2*	*0.3*
FROZEN YOGHURT								
Black Cherry, M&S*	1 Pot/125g	164	1.4	131	3.1	27.1	1.1	0.5
Cherry Garcia, Low Fat, Ben & Jerry's*	1 Serving/100g	143	2.4	143	3	26	2.4	1
Chocmoo, Yoomoo*	1 Serving/100g	142	1.7	142	3.5	26	1.7	4.1
Chocolate, Average	*1 Portion/100g*	*120*	*1.9*	*120*	*4.3*	*22*	*1.9*	*2.1*
Chocolate, Belgian, Calorie Controlled, Love Life, Waitrose*	1/6 Pot/54g	74	1.4	137	6.6	21.6	2.6	0.4
Chocolate, Pinkberry*	1 Sm Pot/140g	168	2.1	120	5	23	1.5	2
Chocolate, Snog*	1 Serving/100g	109	1.6	109	4.5	19.9	1.6	1.7
Coconut, Pinkberry*	1 Sm Pot/140g	196	0	140	4	30	0	0
Frae*	1 Sm/83ml	56	0	67	2.4	12	0	0
Green Tea, Pinkberry*	1 Sm Pot/100g	110	0	110	4	25	0	0
Little Coconutters, Mini, Sticks, The Coconut Collaborative*	1 Stick/45ml	81	3.4	180	1.8	20.5	7.5	1.2
Mango, Pinkberry*	1 Sm Cup/140g	140	0	100	3	23	0	0
Nakedmoo, Yoomoo*	1 Serving/125g	168	2	134	3.3	24.5	1.6	4.1
Natural, Average	*1 Portion/100g*	*101*	*0.8*	*101*	*3.8*	*19.9*	*0.8*	*0.9*
Original, Pinkberry*	1 Sm Pot/140g	140	0	100	3	21	0	0
Phish Food, Lower Fat, Ben & Jerry's*	½ Pot/211g	464	10.6	220	4	40	5	1.5
Raspberry Snowconut, The Coconut Collaborative*	1 Serving/200ml	378	15	189	1.8	21.2	7.5	1.2
Raspberry, Handmade Farmhouse, Sainsbury's*	1 Serving/100g	132	3.8	132	2.7	21.8	3.8	2.2
Strawberry Cheesecake, Low Fat, Ben & Jerry's*	1 Serving/100g	170	3	170	4	31	3	1
Strawberry, Average	*1 Portion/100g*	*114*	*2.2*	*114*	*2.6*	*21.2*	*2.2*	*0.5*
Strawberry, Lolly, Yoomoo *	1 Lolly/57g	73	0.8	128	2.8	25.5	1.4	0.5
Strawberry, Tesco*	1 Pot/60g	82	1.3	136	2.6	26.5	2.2	0.8
Tropical, Lolly, Yoomoo *	1 Lolly/57g	74	0.8	130	2.9	26.1	1.4	0.6
Vanilla, Less Than 5% Fat, Tesco*	1 Pot/120g	179	2.9	149	8.1	23.8	2.4	0.7
FRUIT								
Apple, Apricot, & Strawberry, Pots, Aldi*	1 Pot/100g	55	0.9	55	0.5	10	0.9	1.9
Apple, Pineapple & Grape, Ready to Eat, Sainsbury's*	1 Pack/180g	94	0.2	52	0.5	8.3	0.1	1.3

F

	Measure INFO/WEIGHT	per Measure KCAL	FAT	Nutrition Values per 100g / 100ml KCAL	PROT	CARB	FAT	FIBRE
FRUIT								
Apples & Grape, Snack Pack, Goodness for Kids, Tesco*	1 Pack/80g	44	0.1	55	0.3	12.3	0.1	2.6
Bananas & Berries, Eat Well, M&S*	1 Pack/160g	96	0.3	60	0.9	13.1	0.2	1
Berry Medley, Freshly Prepared, M&S*	1 Pack/180g	90	0.4	50	0.7	10.9	0.2	2.9
Fabulous Fruity Fingers, Melon & Mango, M&S*	1 Pack/240g	96	0.5	40	0.6	8.2	0.2	1
Fingers, Melon & Pineapple, Sainsbury's*	1 Pack/240g	74	0.2	31	0.5	6.5	0.1	0.8
Mango, Pineapple, & Orange Melon, Fingers, M&S*	½ Pack/120g	54	0.2	45	0.6	9.1	0.2	2.3
Melon & Grape Pot, Co-Op*	1 Pot/130g	39	0.1	30	0.6	6.9	0.1	0.7
Mixed, Fresh, Tesco*	1 Pack/200g	70	0.4	35	0.8	7.4	0.2	1.4
Mixed, Pieces, in Orange Jelly, Fruitini, Del Monte*	1 Can/140g	94	0.1	67	0.3	15.8	0.1	0
Orchard, Frozen, British, Delicious & Colourful, Waitrose*	½ Pack/150g	60	0.2	40	0.6	7.7	0.1	2.7
Paws, Raspberry, & Blueberry, Arctic, Bear*	1 Bag/20g	54	0	275	1.9	62.2	0.2	8
Peach Pieces in Fruit Juice, Tesco*	1 Pot/125g	60	0	48	0.4	11.7	0	1
Peach, & Nectarine, Slices, Frozen, Sainsbury's*	1 Serving/80g	34	0.4	42	1.2	8.1	0.5	1.8
Peach, Slices, Frozen, Sainsbury's*	1 Serving/80g	30	0	37	1	7.6	0	1.5
Pear, Plum, Figs, & Blackberries, Waitrose*	1 Serving/80g	34	0.2	43	0	9.4	0.2	2.1
Peel, Candied, Average	**1 Serving/30g**	**86**	**0**	**286**	**0.3**	**80.8**	**0**	**5**
Pineapple Fingers, Snack Pack, Goodness for Kids, Tesco*	1 Pack/70g	31	0.1	44	0.4	10.1	0.2	2
Pink Lady Apple & Grape, Snack Pack, On The Go, Tesco*	1 Pack/80g	44	0.1	55	0.3	12.3	0.1	2.6
Red, Mixed, Mercadona*	1 Serving/80g	31	0	39	0.9	5.5	0	0
Summer Berries, M&S*	1 Pack/160g	80	0.3	50	0.7	10	0.2	3
Tropical in Juice, Dole*	1 Pot/113g	59	0	52	0.3	14.2	0	1.8
FRUIT & NUT MIX								
Alesto, Lidl*	1 Serving/30g	150	9.5	500	10.7	39.7	31.7	6.7
Almonds, Cashews, & Berry Mix, Waitrose*	1 Serving/30g	153	9.8	510	14.5	35.8	32.8	7.2
Apple, & Carrot, with Chia, Defence, Graze*	1 Punnet/40g	169	8	422	9.6	56	20	11
Billionaires Shortbread, Graze*	1 Serving/43g	197	10.7	459	8.6	56	25	6.5
Chocolate, & Hazelnut, Shots, Whitworths*	1 Pack/25g	99	3.5	397	5.7	59.9	14	4.2
Seeds, Nuts, & Sultanas, Sprinkle, Good Health, Waitrose*	1 Serving/30g	183	15.4	609	18.6	15	51.2	6.8
Bounty Hunter, Graze*	1 Punnet/31g	147	8.3	474	4	54.4	26.8	5.6
Chocolate, On the Go, Sainsbury's*	1 Serving/30g	109	3.1	363	5.1	60.1	10.2	5.1
Daily Vigour Mix, Waitrose*	1 Pack/50g	265	18.8	530	14.6	30	37.6	6.4
Honeycomb Crunch, Graze*	1 Punnet/40g	181	9.7	446	9	50	24	4
Marvellous Macaroon, Graze*	1 Punnet/28g	157	10.9	562	11	41	39	6
Nuts & Raisins, Mixed, Natural, Love Life, Waitrose*	1 Serving/50g	258	16.4	515	16.5	38.4	32.8	7.2
Salted Caramel, Nibbles, Nak'd*	1 Bag/40g	138	4.7	345	6.6	56.1	11.8	3.3
Strawberry Milkshake, Graze*	1 Pack/39g	148	3.9	380	2	72	10	2
Trail Mix, Average	**1oz/28g**	**121**	**8**	**432**	**9.1**	**37.2**	**28.5**	**4.3**
Unsalted, Tesco*	1 Serving/25g	112	4.6	449	12.6	58.1	18.5	12.2
FRUIT & SEED MIX								
Cranberry, Goji, & Seeds, The Good Snack Company*	1 Pack/50g	226	11.5	451	13.6	46.2	23	5.7
FRUIT COCKTAIL								
Cocktail de Fruits Rouges, U*	1 Serving/300g	126	0	42	1	6.4	0	3
Fresh & Ready, Sainsbury's*	1 Pack/300g	117	0.3	39	0.6	9	0.1	1.2
in Apple Juice, Asda*	1/3 Can/80g	40	0.1	50	0.3	12	0.1	1.6
in Fruit Juice, Sainsbury's*	1 Serving/198g	97	0.2	49	0.3	11.9	0.1	1.3
in Juice, Del Monte*	1 Can/415g	203	0.4	49	0.4	11.2	0.1	0
in Light Syrup, Princes*	1 Serving/206g	64	0	31	0.4	7.3	0	1
in Syrup, Morrisons*	½ Can/205g	129	0.2	63	0.3	14.9	0.1	0
in Syrup, Smart Price, Asda*	1 Can/411g	173	0.4	42	0.3	10	0.1	1.6
Tropical, Canned, Asda*	½ Can/200g	120	0	60	0	15	0	1.6
FRUIT COMPOTE								
Apple, & Pear, No Added Sugar, Andros*	1 Tbsp/15g	7	0	46	0.2	9.6	0.3	2.1
Apple, Strawberry & Blackberry, Organic, Yeo Valley*	½ Pot/112g	73	0.1	65	0.5	15.5	0.1	1.9

F

	Measure INFO/WEIGHT	per Measure KCAL	FAT	Nutrition Values per 100g / 100ml KCAL	PROT	CARB	FAT	FIBRE
FRUIT COMPOTE								
Apricot & Prune, Yeo Valley*	1 Pot/225g	207	0.2	92	0.6	22.3	0.1	1.6
Blackcurrant, & Cassis, British, TTD, Sainsbury's*	1 Tbsp/35g	52	0.4	147	1.8	31	1.2	2.7
Rhubarb, Bonne Maman*	1 Thin Spread/7g	7	0	103	0.5	24	0.1	2
Strawberry & Raspberry, M&S*	1 Serving/80g	72	0.1	90	0.7	23.5	0.1	2.3
FRUIT FLAKES								
Blackcurrant with Yoghurt Coating, Fruit Bowl*	1 Bag/21g	95	4	453	1.3	69	19	3.9
Raspberry with Yoghurt Coating, Fruit Bowl*	1 Serving/21g	95	4	453	1.3	69	19	3.9
Strawberry with Yoghurt Coating, Fruit Bowl*	1 Serving/21g	95	4	453	1.3	69	19	3.9
FRUIT GUMS								
Rowntree's*	1 Tube/49g	170	0.1	344	4.8	81.3	0.2	0
FRUIT MIX								
Apple, & Strawberry, Pot, Market Street , Morrisons*	1 Serving/125g	61	0.6	49	0.6	9.8	0.5	1.2
Date, & Banana, Dried, Asda*	1 Serving/30g	117	4.2	389	2.9	61	14	5.5
Exotic, Frozen, Tesco*	1 Serving/80g	33	0	41	0.6	8.7	0	1.9
Melon, & Grape, Snack Pot, Boots*	½ Pack/45g	15	0	34	0.4	7.5	0.1	0.7
Melon, & Mango, Morrisons*	1 Pot/150g	52	0.2	35	0.6	7.3	0.1	1.2
Nectarines, Grapes, & Raspberries, with Jelly, M&S*	1 Pack/330g	198	1	60	0.8	12.3	0.3	1.1
Pineapple, Melon, Mango, Tesco*	1 Pack/440g	242	0.9	55	1.1	11.4	0.2	1.3
Plum, & Berries, Eat Well, M&S*	1 Serving/100g	41	0.2	41	0.8	7.8	0.2	2.3
Plum, Pomegranate, & Blueberry, Market Street, Morrisons*	1 Serving/80g	38	0.1	47	0.6	10	0.1	1.8
Red, Frozen, Crops*	3 Tbsp/80g	28	0.1	35	1	5.2	0.1	4.6
Sour Mango Tangtastic, Graze*	1 Pack/34g	110	0.2	323	1.3	79.8	0.6	2
Summer Fruits, British, Frozen, Waitrose*	1 Pack/380g	99	0.8	26	1	5.2	0.2	5.5
Summer Fruits, Frozen, Asda*	1 Serving/100g	28	0	28	0.9	6	0	2.5
Summer Fruits, Frozen, Sainsbury's*	1 Serving/80g	43	0.1	54	0.9	6.9	0.1	2
Watermelon, & Mango, Fingers, Tesco*	½ Pack/136g	64	0.4	47	0.5	9.8	0.3	1.6
FRUIT PUREE								
Apple & Blueberry, Organic, Clearspring*	1 Tub/100g	76	0.3	76	0.4	17.8	0.3	0
Apple & Peach, Organix*	1 Pot/100g	49	0.3	49	0.6	11	0.3	2.1
Banana, Apple & Apricot, Organix*	1 Pot/100g	68	0.4	68	0.8	15.4	0.4	2
FRUIT SALAD								
Apple, Melon, & Berries, Nutritious, Boots*	1 Pack/257g	118	0.8	46	0.6	9.4	0.3	1.8
Apple, Orange, Pineapple & Grape, Morrisons*	1 Serving/64g	40	0.1	62	0.8	13.1	0.1	2.6
Apple, Pineapple & Grape, Sweet & Tangy, Sainsbury's*	1 Pack/180g	70	0.2	39	0.5	8.3	0.1	1.3
Autumn, Fresh, M&S*	½ Pack/160g	64	0.2	40	0.7	9.4	0.1	2.9
Berry, Seasonal, Asda*	1 Pack/300g	93	0.3	31	0.6	7	0.1	2.1
Chunky in Fruit Juice, Canned, John West*	1 Can/411g	193	0.8	47	0.4	11	0.2	0.8
Citrus, Fresh, M&S*	½ Pack/225g	79	0.2	35	0.9	7.7	0.1	1.5
Classic, Fresh, Prepared, Sainsbury's*	1 Pack/320g	157	0.3	49	0.6	10.3	0.1	2
Classic, Waitrose*	1 Pack/330g	162	0.7	49	0.8	10.4	0.2	1.2
Dried, M&S*	½ Pack/125g	269	0.5	215	1.8	51.4	0.4	5.9
Exotic with Melon, Mango, Kiwi Fruit & Grapes, Asda*	1 Pot/300g	141	0.9	47	0.6	10.5	0.3	1.4
Exotic, Fresh, Tesco*	1 Serving/225g	86	0.4	38	0.7	8.4	0.2	1.5
Exotic, Fully Prepared, Sainsbury's*	1 Serving/200g	74	0.4	37	0.6	8.3	0.2	1.3
Exotic, Waitrose*	1 Pack/300g	126	0.6	42	0.6	9.5	0.2	1.1
Fresh for You, Tesco*	1 Pack/160g	59	0.3	37	0.6	8.2	0.2	1.1
Fresh, Morrisons*	1 Tub/350g	150	0.4	43	0.7	9.9	0.1	0
Fresh, Tesco*	1 Pack/200g	84	0.4	42	0.7	9.3	0.2	1.5
Freshly Prepared, M&S*	1 Pack/350g	140	0.7	40	0.5	9.3	0.2	1
Frozen, Tesco*	1 Serving/80g	26	0.4	32	0.5	6.1	0.5	1.7
Fruity Cocktail, M&S*	1 Serving/80g	33	0.1	41	0.6	8.5	0.1	1.7
Grapefruit & Orange, Fresh, M&S*	1 Serving/250g	88	0.2	35	0.9	7.4	0.1	1.6
Homemade, Unsweetened, Average	*1 Serving/140g*	*77*	*0.1*	*55*	*0.7*	*13.8*	*0.1*	*1.5*

FRUIT SALAD	Measure INFO/WEIGHT	per Measure KCAL	per Measure FAT	KCAL	PROT	CARB	FAT	FIBRE
FRUIT SALAD								
Juicy Melon, Pineapple & Grapes, Asda*	1 Pot/300g	111	0.3	37	0.5	8.4	0.1	0.9
Kiwi, Pineapple & Grape, Fresh Tastes, Asda*	1 Pack/200g	106	0.6	53	0.6	11	0.3	1.8
Layered, Tropical Rainbow, Freshly Prepared, M&S*	1 Pack/375g	206	1.1	55	0.7	12.6	0.3	1.7
Mango, Kiwi, Blueberry & Pomegranate, Fresh, M&S*	1 Pack/350g	210	1	60	0.9	13.4	0.3	2.4
Melon & Red Grape, Freshly Prepared, M&S*	1 Pack/450g	158	0.4	35	0.5	8.4	0.1	0.7
Melon & Mango, Shapers, Boots*	1 Pack/80g	29	0.1	36	0.6	7.8	0.1	1.2
Melon, & Grape, Sainsbury's*	1 Pack/159g	59	0.8	37	0.6	7.8	0.5	1.2
Melon, Grape, Kiwi, Strawberry, & Pomegranate, Tesco*	1 Serving/95g	42	0	44	0.8	9.6	0	1.2
Melon, Kiwi, Grapes & Pomegranate Seeds, Morrisons*	1 Pack/400g	152	1.2	38	0.7	8.2	0.3	1.2
Melon, Pineapple & Grapes, Fresh, Tesco*	1 Pack/300g	120	0.3	40	0.5	9.2	0.1	1
Mixed, Average	**1 Bowl/100g**	**42**	**0.2**	**42**	**0.6**	**9.4**	**0.2**	**1.5**
Mixed, Food to Go, M&S*	1 Pack/400g	400	1.2	100	0.9	23.3	0.3	2.8
Mixed, Fresh, Sainsbury's*	1 Pack/200g	84	0.4	42	0.7	9.4	0.2	1.9
Mixed, Tesco*	1 Pack/225g	86	0.4	38	0.7	8.3	0.2	1.3
Nectarine, Melon, Strawberry, & Blueberry, Morrisons*	1 Pot/230g	78	0.5	34	0.9	6.7	0.2	1.1
Oranges, Apple, Pineapple & Grapes, Fresh, Asda*	1 Pack/260g	120	0.3	46	0.6	10.5	0.1	2.1
Pineapple, Apple & Strawberries, Tesco*	1 Pack/190g	80	0.2	42	0.4	9.8	0.1	1.4
Pineapple, Mango & Passion Fruit, Prepared, M&S*	1 Pack/400g	200	0.8	50	0.7	10.8	0.2	1.8
Pineapple, Melon & Grape, Eat Well, M&S*	1 Pot/120g	52	0.1	43	0.5	9.3	0.1	1.4
Pineapple, Melon, & Mango, Nutritious, Boots*	1 Pack/250g	111	0.5	44	0.6	9.2	0.2	1.6
Pineapple, Melon, Kiwi & Blueberry, Shapers, Boots*	1 Pack/179g	75	0.4	42	0.6	8.7	0.2	1.4
Pineapple, Melon, Mango, Apple, Kiwi, & Blueberries, M&S*	1 Pack/185g	87	0.6	47	0.6	9.7	0.3	1.7
Pineapple, Strawberry, Grape & Carrot, M&S*	1 Pack/240g	101	1	42	0.6	8.3	0.4	1.4
Plum, Blackberries, & Fig, Tesco*	1 Pot/260g	109	0.5	42	0.8	8.2	0.2	2.5
Plum, Blackberry, Seasonal Opal Apple, Tesco*	1 Pack/105g	51	0.3	49	0.6	9.8	0.3	2.1
Rainbow Layers, Tesco*	1 Pack/270g	122	0.5	45	0.5	9.8	0.2	1.1
Rainbow, Fresh, Tesco*	1 Tub/270g	105	0.5	39	0.5	8.8	0.2	0.9
Seasonal Melon & Grapes, Asda*	½ Pack/200g	66	1	33	0.5	7.5	0.5	0.4
Seasonal, Fresh, Asda*	1 Pack/125g	55	0.1	44	0.5	10.4	0.1	1.2
Selection, M&S*	½ Pack/275g	140	0.8	51	0.6	10.3	0.3	2.1
Summer, Red, Fresh, M&S*	1 Pack/400g	160	0.8	40	0	10	0.2	1.2
Sunshine, Fresh, M&S*	1 Serving/200g	70	0.2	35	0	8.3	0.1	1.3
Tropical in Light Syrup, Passion Fruit Juice, Tesco*	½ Can/216g	130	0.2	60	0.3	14.1	0.1	1.1
Tropical Mix, Tesco*	½ Pack/140g	71	0.3	51	0.5	11	0.2	1.5
Tropical, Fresh, Asda*	1 Pack/400g	164	0.8	41	0.7	9	0.2	1.8
Tropical, Fruit Snacks, Frozen, Sainsbury's*	1 Serving/175g	79	0.2	45	0.7	10.4	0.1	1.6
Tropical, Tropical Harvest*	1 Serving/100g	52	0	52	0.3	12.8	0	1.4
Virgin Trains*	1 Serving/140g	56	0.1	40	0.4	10	0.1	0.8
FRUIT SHOOT								
Apple & Blackcurrant, Robinson's*	1 Bottle/200ml	10	0	5	0.1	0.8	0	0
FRUIT SPREAD								
Cherries & Berries, Organic, Meridian Foods*	1 Tbsp/15g	16	0	109	0.5	26	0.3	1.1
Cherry & Berry, Meridian Foods*	1 Serving/10g	14	0.1	138	0.7	33.7	0.6	3.2
Seville Orange, Weight Watchers*	1 Tsp/15g	17	0	111	0.2	27.5	0	0.3
FRUIT WINDERS								
Strawberry, Kellogg's*	1 Roll/17g	67	1.4	393	0.2	79	8	2
FU YUNG								
Chicken, Chinese Takeaway, Tesco*	1 Pack/350g	315	3.5	90	5.6	14.5	1	0.8
Egg, Average	**1oz/28g**	**67**	**5.8**	**239**	**9.9**	**2.2**	**20.6**	**1.3**
FUDGE								
All Butter, Finest, Tesco*	1 Sweet/10g	43	1.4	429	1.3	73.4	14.5	0
Butter Tablet, Thorntons*	1oz/28g	116	3.1	414	0.9	77.6	11.1	0
Butter, Milk, Thorntons*	1 Sweet/13g	60	2.5	462	3.7	68.5	19.2	0

F

	Measure INFO/WEIGHT	per Measure KCAL	FAT	Nutrition Values per 100g / 100ml KCAL	PROT	CARB	FAT	FIBRE
FUDGE								
Cadbury*	1 Bar/25g	118	4	445	2.5	74.5	15	0.5
Chocolate, Average	*1 Sweet/30g*	*132*	*4.1*	*441*	*3.3*	*81.1*	*13.7*	*0*
Chocolate, Thorntons*	1 Bag/100g	459	19.1	459	3.1	69	19.1	0.6
Chunks for Baking	*1 Serving/100g*	*428*	*12.2*	*428*	*1.7*	*77.2*	*12.2*	*0.6*
Clotted Cream, Sainsbury's*	1 Sweet/8g	35	0.9	430	1.9	81.5	10.7	0.7
Dairy, Co-Op*	1 Sweet/9g	39	1.2	430	2	76	13	0
Dairy, Morrisons*	3 Sweets/24g	107	3.6	447	1.8	76.1	14.9	0.5
Minis, Cadbury*	1 Piece/5g	23	0.9	455	2.6	73	17	0.7
Salted Caramel, Fudgelicious, Ryedale Farm*	1 Piece/9g	43	1.8	473	2.1	72	20	0
Vanilla, Bar, M&S*	1 Bar/43g	205	10	476	3.7	63	23.3	0.4
Vanilla, Julian Graves*	1 Serving/10g	41	1	407	1	78.9	9.7	0
Vanilla, Thorntons*	1 Bag/100g	465	21.9	465	1.8	65.9	21.9	0
FUSILLI								
Chickpea, GF, Cooked, Ugo*	½ Pack/255g	428	7.9	168	9.8	22.4	3.1	5.7
Cooked, Average	*1 Serving/210g*	*248*	*1.4*	*118*	*4.2*	*23.8*	*0.6*	*1.2*
Dry, Average	*1 Serving/90g*	*316*	*1.4*	*352*	*12.3*	*72*	*1.6*	*2.2*
Fresh, Cooked, Average	*1 Serving/200g*	*329*	*3.6*	*164*	*6.4*	*30.6*	*1.8*	*1.8*
Fresh, Dry, Average	*1 Serving/75g*	*208*	*2*	*277*	*10.9*	*53.4*	*2.7*	*2.1*
GF, Cooked, Free From, Sainsbury's*	1 Serving/200g	340	2.4	170	3.3	36	1.2	0.9
GF, Dry, Free From, Morrisons*	1 Serving/75g	258	0.8	344	5.6	77.1	1.1	1.9
Green Pea, Organic, Uncooked, Napolina*	1 Serving/75g	99	0.1	132	9.2	20.4	0.1	6.9
Red Lentil, Dry, Cook Italian*	1 Serving/80g	283	1.6	354	23	58	2	6
Tricolore, Dry, Average	*1 Serving/75g*	*264*	*1.3*	*351*	*12.2*	*71.8*	*1.7*	*2.7*
Whole Wheat, Dry Weight, Average	*1 Serving/90g*	*290*	*2.1*	*322*	*13.1*	*62.3*	*2.3*	*9*
Wholegrain Spelt, Cooked, Sainsbury's*	1 Serving/75g	120	0.8	160	6.2	30.3	1	2.6
FYBOGEL								
Lemon, Reckitt Benckiser*	1 Serving/4g	4	0	95	2.4	11.3	1.1	64.8
Orange, Reckitt Benckiser*	1 Serving/4g	5	0	106	2.4	12.7	1.1	64.4

F

	Measure INFO/WEIGHT	per Measure KCAL	per Measure FAT	Nutrition Values per 100g / 100ml KCAL	PROT	CARB	FAT	FIBRE
GALANGAL								
Raw, Root, Average	*100g*	*71*	*0.6*	*71*	*1.2*	*15.3*	*0.6*	*2.4*
GALAXY								
Caramel Crunch, Promises, Mars*	1 Bar/100g	540	31.8	540	6.1	57.5	31.8	0
Caramel, Mars*	1 Bar/49g	254	13	518	5.8	64.2	26.4	0
Cookie Crumble, Mars*	1 Bar/114g	627	37.6	550	6.2	56	33	1.9
Hazelnut, Mars*	1 Piece/6g	37	2.5	582	7.8	49.4	39.2	0
Roasted Hazelnut, Darker Collection, Galaxy, Mars*	1 Serving/21g	117	7.4	555	6.7	51	35	0
GAMMON								
Breaded, Average	*1oz/28g*	*34*	*0.9*	*120*	*22.5*	*1*	*3*	*0*
Honey & Mustard, Average	*½ Pack/190g*	*294*	*13.5*	*155*	*19.1*	*3.6*	*7.1*	*0.1*
Joint, Boiled, Average	*1 Serving/60g*	*122*	*7.4*	*204*	*23.3*	*0*	*12.3*	*0*
Joint, Honey Glaze, Just Cook, Sainsbury's*	1/3 Pack/123g	242	12.8	197	23.4	2.1	10.4	0
Joint, Raw, Average	*1 Serving/100g*	*138*	*7.5*	*138*	*17.5*	*0*	*7.5*	*0*
Joint, with Honey Glaze, Tesco*	¼ Pack/124g	186	2.6	150	27.4	4.9	2.1	0.6
Shank, with Maple, & Balsamic, Finest, Tesco*	1 Pack/347g	587	15.3	169	25.5	6.6	4.4	0.5
Steak, Hawaiian Style, with Cheese, & Pineapple, Aldi*	1½ Pack/170g	238	8.5	140	20	3.3	5	0.5
Steaks, Honey Roast, Average	*1 Steak/100g*	*142*	*5.3*	*142*	*21.5*	*2.3*	*5.3*	*0*
Steaks, Smoked, Average	*1 Steak/110g*	*150*	*5.5*	*137*	*22.7*	*0.1*	*5*	*0.1*
Steaks, with Pineapple & Mango Salsa, Easy, Waitrose*	1 Steak/163g	239	11.6	146	14.1	6.5	7.1	0.5
Vegetarian, Roast, Quorn*	¼ Roast/100g	141	4.4	141	17.6	3.8	4.4	7.6
GARAM MASALA								
Dry, Ground, Average	*1 Tbsp/15g*	*57*	*2.3*	*379*	*15.6*	*45.2*	*15.1*	*0*
GARLIC								
Black	*1 Clove/5g*	*13*	*0*	*264*	*13.3*	*53.3*	*0*	*20*
Powder, Average	*1 Tsp/3g*	*7*	*0*	*246*	*18.7*	*42.7*	*1.2*	*9.9*
Raw, Average	*1 Clove/3g*	*3*	*0*	*98*	*7.9*	*16.3*	*0.6*	*2.1*
Very Lazy, The English Provender Co.*	1 Tsp/3g	3	0	111	6	20.9	0.4	3
Wild	*1 Leaf/1g*	*0*	*0*	*23*	*2.8*	*1.7*	*0.6*	*1.9*
GARLIC PUREE								
Average	*1 Tbsp/18g*	*68*	*6*	*380*	*3.5*	*16.9*	*33.6*	*0*
in Vegetable Oil, GIA*	1 Tsp/5g	12	0.9	248	3.6	18.8	17.7	0
with Tomato, GIA*	10g	7	0.1	70	5.1	0.5	1.2	0
GATEAU								
Black Forest, 500g Size, Tesco*	1 Cake/500g	1125	55	225	4	27.1	11	1.8
Black Forest, 702, Oakhouse Foods Ltd*	1 Portion/125g	400	27.2	320	3.4	27.5	21.8	1.3
Black Forest, Dome, Tesco*	1 Dome/600g	1626	68.4	271	4	37.4	11.4	1.6
Black Forest, M&S*	1/8 Cake/77g	207	10.9	269	3.1	31.6	14.1	1.5
Black Forest, Mini, Tesco*	1 Serving/55g	136	5.1	247	5.7	35.3	9.2	1
Black Forest, Sara Lee*	1 Serving/80g	221	9.8	276	3.6	37.9	12.3	1.2
Caramel, Salted, Dome, Frozen, Tesco*	1 Serving/78g	233	9.9	298	4.2	41.2	12.7	0.9
Caramel, Salted, Profiterole, Tesco*	1 Slice/88g	248	13.6	282	4.3	31	15.5	0.9
Chocolate Layer, M&S*	1 Serving/86g	278	15.7	323	4.2	35.9	18.3	0.9
Chocolate, & Vanilla, Ice Cream, Iceland*	1 Serving/130g	252	12.2	194	3.3	24.1	9.4	0.6
Chocolate, Double, Frozen, Tesco*	1/5 Gateau/70g	115	4.4	255	5.5	34.2	9.8	3.5
Chocolate, Rich, Tesco*	1 Slice/84g	210	8.6	251	5.1	32.9	10.2	3.4
Chocolate, Swirl, Tesco*	1 Serving/83g	230	13.3	277	3.8	29.3	16	0.2
Strawberry, Co-Op*	1 Serving/77g	222	12.9	288	5.1	29.2	16.7	1
Strawberry, Double, Sara Lee*	1/8 Cake/199g	533	24.3	268	3.2	36.2	12.2	0.6
Strawberry, Frozen, Tesco*	1 Serving/75g	144	6.2	192	2.6	26.3	8.3	0.7
Swiss, Cadbury*	1/6 Gateau/60g	228	10.1	380	5.2	52	16.8	0.9
GHEE								
Butter	*1oz/28g*	*251*	*27.9*	*898*	*0*	*0*	*99.8*	*0*
Vegetable	*1oz/28g*	*251*	*27.8*	*895*	*0*	*0*	*99.4*	*0*

	Measure INFO/WEIGHT	per Measure		Nutrition Values per 100g / 100ml				
		KCAL	FAT	KCAL	PROT	CARB	FAT	FIBRE
GHERKINS								
Pickled, Average	*1 Gherkin/36g*	*4*	*0*	*12*	*0.8*	*2.1*	*0.1*	*1*
Pickled, with Chilli, Bramwells, Aldi*	1 Gherkin/20g	3	0.1	16	0.9	2.6	0.4	1
GIN								
& Diet Tonic, Can, Greenalls*	1 Can/250ml	95	0	38	0	0	0	0
& Tonic, Canned, Ready to Drink, M&S*	1 Can/250ml	175	0.8	70	0.2	5.6	0.3	0.1
& Tonic, Premixed, Flor De Sevilla, Tanqueray*	1 Bottle/275ml	190	0	69	0	6.6	0	0
37.5% Volume	*1 Pub Shot/35ml*	*72*	*0*	*207*	*0*	*0*	*0*	*0*
40% Volume	*1 Pub Shot/35ml*	*78*	*0*	*224*	*0*	*0*	*0*	*0*
41% Volume	*1 Pub Shot/35ml*	*83*	*0*	*237*	*0*	*0*	*0*	*0*
Average, 43%	*1 Serving/25ml*	*60*	*0*	*241*	*0*	*0*	*0*	*0*
Citrus, Grove 42, Non Alcoholic, Seedlip Ltd*	1 Shot/30ml	0	0	0	0	0	0	0
Gordons & Schweppes Slimline Tonic, Canned, Diageo*	1 Can/250ml	75	0	30	0	0	0	0
Gordons & Schweppes Tonic, Canned, Diageo*	1 Can/250ml	152	0	61	0	6.2	0	0
Pink, & Tonic, Mixed, Can, Gordons*	1 Can/250ml	168	0	67	0	8.7	0	0
Rose, Premium, Bosford*	1 Single/25ml	66	0	262	0	0	0	0
GINGER								
Chunks, Crystallised, Julian Graves*	1 Serving/10g	28	0	283	0.2	70.1	0.2	1.5
Ground, Average	*1 Tsp/2g*	*5*	*0.1*	*258*	*7.4*	*60*	*3.3*	*0*
Minced, Lee Kum Kee*	1 Tsp/10g	1	0	14	0.5	2.9	0.5	0
Root, Raw, Pared, Average	*1 Tsp/2g*	*2*	*0*	*81*	*1.8*	*18*	*0.8*	*2*
Root, Raw, Unprepared, Average	*1 Tsp/2g*	*1*	*0*	*74*	*1.7*	*16.3*	*0.7*	*1.8*
Stem in Sugar Syrup, Sainsbury's*	1 Ball/10g	29	0	292	0.5	71.3	0.5	1.6
Very Lazy, The English Provender Co.*	1 Tsp/5g	3	0	52	0.7	10.9	0.8	0.8
GINGER ALE								
American, Tesco*	1 Glass/250ml	58	0	23	0	5.5	0	0
Dry	*1 Glass/250ml*	*38*	*0*	*15*	*0*	*3.9*	*0*	*0*
Dry, Sainsbury's*	1 Glass/250ml	95	0.2	38	0.1	9.1	0.1	0.1
Orange, Light Spiced, Fever-Tree*	1 Serving/200ml	36	0	18	0	4.3	0	0
Refreshingly Light, Fever-Tree*	1 Bottle/200ml	36	0	18	0	4.6	0	0
GINGER BEER								
Alcoholic, Crabbies*	1 Bottle/500ml	254	0	51	0	7.1	0	0
Classic, Schweppes*	1 Can/330ml	115	0	35	0	8.4	0	0
D & G Old Jamaican*	1 Can/330ml	211	0	64	0	16	0	0
Diet, Crabbies*	1 Bottle/700ml	7	0	1	0	0	0	0
Light, Belvoir Fruit Farms*	1 Serving/200ml	42	0	21	0	4.4	0	0
Light, Waitrose*	1 Glass/250ml	2	0.2	1	0	0	0.1	0.1
No Added Sugar, Canned, Tesco*	1 Can/330ml	3	0.3	1	0	0.1	0.1	0.1
Rhubarb, Sparkling, No Added Sugar, M&S*	1 Can/250ml	2	0.2	1	0.1	0.1	0.1	0.1
Scottish Raspberry, John Crabbie & Co*	1 Serving/200ml	64	0	32	0	7.9	0	0
Traditional, Fentiman's*	1 Bottle/275ml	130	0	47	0	11.3	0	0
GINGER WINE								
Green Ginger Wine & Scots Whisky, Crabbies*	1 Glass/125ml	192	0	153	14.3	14.3	0	0
Green, Crabbies*	1 Serving/125ml	202	0	162	0	21.8	0	0
GINGERBREAD								
Average	*1oz/28g*	*106*	*3.5*	*379*	*5.7*	*64.7*	*12.6*	*1.2*
Bunny, Mini, Co-Op*	1 Biscuit/11g	48	1.2	435	5.7	78	11	1.8
Iced, Alan Avocado, Waitrose*	1 Biscuit/75g	320	8.2	427	3.1	78.2	10.9	0
Iced, Anna the Llama, Waitrose*	1 Biscuit/40g	172	4.4	429	2.8	78.8	10.9	0
Iced, Cheeky Monkey, Waitrose*	1 Biscuit/50g	214	5.4	428	3	78.5	10.9	0
Iced, Sarah The Dinosaur, Waitrose*	1 Biscuit/30g	127	3.3	422	4.5	75.1	11.1	0
Man, Free From, Co-Op*	1 Biscuit/25g	115	3.7	461	4.2	77	15	1.3
GIRASOLE								
Ricotta, & Spinach, Creamy, Specially Selected, Aldi*	½ Pack/155g	312	15.5	201	7.1	19	10	2.2

G

	Measure INFO/WEIGHT	per Measure KCAL	FAT	Nutrition Values per 100g / 100ml KCAL	PROT	CARB	FAT	FIBRE
GIRASOLE								
Spinach, Buffalo Ricotta, & Pine Nuts, Finest, Tesco*	½ Pack/150g	276	13	184	7.4	16.4	8.7	5.7
GNOCCHI								
Asparagus, & Pesto, Cook*	1 Pack/270g	332	7.6	123	4.4	2.2	2.8	3.1
Bacon, Mascarpone, Green Beans, & Tomato, Hello Fresh*	1 Serving/495g	861	43.1	174	5.7	18	8.7	0
Chorizo, Spinach, & Courgette, Hello Fresh*	1 Portion/514g	714	28	139	5	17.3	5.4	0
Di Patate, Italfresco*	½ Pack/200g	296	0.4	148	3.3	33.2	0.2	0
Fresh, Cooked, Essential, Waitrose*	¼ Pack/134g	242	0.5	181	4.7	39	0.4	1
Fresh, Italian, Chilled, Sainsbury's*	½ Pack/250g	355	1.2	142	2.5	29.9	0.5	4
Pesto, Creamy, with Courgette, & Tomatoes, Hello Fresh*	1 Serving/436g	580	31.1	133	4.4	14.5	7.1	0
Potato, & Quinoa, GF, Sottolestelle*	½ Pack/250g	385	0.5	154	1.6	36	0.2	1
Potato, Cooked, Average	*1 Serving/150g*	*200*	*0*	*133*	*0*	*33.2*	*0*	*0*
Tomato, & Mozzarella, Italiamo, Lidl*	1 Serving/250g	365	4.8	146	3.5	28	1.9	2.3
GOAT								
Meat, Uncooked	*1 Serving/100g*	*109*	*2.3*	*109*	*20.6*	*0*	*2.3*	*0*
GOJI BERRIES								
Average	*1 Serving/100g*	*287*	*0.7*	*287*	*6.6*	*65.1*	*0.7*	*6.8*
Dried, Tesco*	½ Pack/50g	181	0.9	362	14	70	1.8	5
Organic, Unsweetened, KoRo*	1 Serving/30g	103	0.4	343	13	64.1	1.2	2
GOOSE								
Meat & Skin, Roasted	*½ Goose/774g*	*2361*	*169.5*	*305*	*25.2*	*0*	*21.9*	*0*
Meat, Raw	*1 Portion/185g*	*298*	*13*	*161*	*23*	*0*	*7*	*0*
Meat, Roasted	*1 Portion/143g*	*340*	*18.1*	*238*	*29*	*0*	*12.7*	*0*
GOOSEBERRIES								
Dessert, Raw, Tops & Tails Removed	*1oz/28g*	*11*	*0.1*	*40*	*0.7*	*9.2*	*0.3*	*2.4*
Stewed with Sugar	*25g*	*14*	*0.1*	*54*	*0.7*	*12.9*	*0.3*	*4.2*
Stewed without Sugar	*25g*	*4*	*0.1*	*16*	*0.9*	*2.5*	*0.3*	*4.4*
GOULASH								
Beef with Tagliatelle, COU, M&S*	1 Pack/360g	414	8.3	115	8.5	14.5	2.3	1
Beef, Average	*1 Serving/300g*	*310*	*9.5*	*103*	*8.1*	*10.4*	*3.2*	*0.9*
Beef, Finest, Tesco*	½ Pack/300g	297	9.3	99	11.6	6.2	3.1	0.6
Meatball, Beef, with Rice, Hello Fresh*	1 Serving/796g	621	20	78	5.5	8.8	2.5	0
GRAINS								
Italian Infused, Pesto-ey, Merchant Gourmet*	1 Pack/250g	452	12.7	181	6.1	25.8	5.1	3.4
Moroccan Style, M&S*	1 Pack/290g	447	6.4	154	4.7	26.3	2.2	5.1
Quinoa & Lentils, Persian Style, Merchant Gourmet*	½ Pack/125g	220	3.5	176	6.7	28.6	2.8	4.9
Super, Garlic, & Ginger, Tilda*	½ Pack/110g	183	6.6	166	4.6	22.6	6	1.6
Tomato, & Herb, with Buckwheat, Spelt, & Bulgur, Twistd*	½ Pack/125g	181	3.4	145	4.8	23	2.7	5.2
Wheatberries, & Kale, Sainsbury's*	½ Pack/150g	195	6.8	130	6.6	12	4.5	7.6
Wonder, Mediterranean, Stir & Eat, Quorn*	1 Pot/200g	212	4	106	5.5	14	2	4.9
GRAPEFRUIT								
in Juice, Canned, Average	*1/3 Can/179g*	*82*	*0.1*	*46*	*0.5*	*10.6*	*0*	*0.4*
in Syrup, Average	*1oz/28g*	*19*	*0*	*69*	*0.5*	*16.8*	*0.1*	*0.5*
Raw, Flesh Only, Average	*½ Fruit/160g*	*48*	*0.2*	*30*	*0.8*	*6.8*	*0.1*	*1.3*
Raw, Weighed with Skin & Seeds, Average	*1 Lge/340g*	*54*	*0.2*	*16*	*0.3*	*4*	*0*	*0.6*
Ruby Red in Juice, Average	*1 Serving/135g*	*54*	*0.1*	*40*	*0.6*	*9.4*	*0*	*0.5*
GRAPES								
Black, Seedless, Sable, TTD, Sainsbury's*	1 Serving/80g	56	0.4	70	0.5	15.4	0.5	0.7
Candy Floss, Seedless, Raw, Tesco*	1 Serving/80g	58	0.1	73	0.6	17	0.1	0.6
Cotton Candy, 1, Waitrose*	1 Serving/80g	53	0.1	66	0.4	15.4	0.1	0.9
Cotton Candy, Black, Seedless, Finest, Tesco*	1 Portion/80g	53	0.1	66	0.4	15.4	0.1	0.7
Green, Average	*1 Grape/5g*	*3*	*0*	*62*	*0.4*	*15.2*	*0.1*	*0.7*
Red & Green Selection, Average	*1 Grape/5g*	*3*	*0*	*62*	*0.4*	*15.2*	*0.1*	*0.8*
Red, Average	*1 Grape/5g*	*3*	*0*	*65*	*0.4*	*15.8*	*0.1*	*0.6*

G

	Measure INFO/WEIGHT	per Measure KCAL	FAT	Nutrition Values per 100g / 100ml KCAL	PROT	CARB	FAT	FIBRE
GRAPES								
Sable, 1, Waitrose*	1 Pack/400g	264	0.4	66	0.4	15.4	0.1	0.9
Sable, Finest, Tesco*	1 Serving/80g	53	0.1	66	0.4	15.4	0.1	0.7
Seedless, Red, Average	*1 Grape*	*4*	*0*	*74*	*0.6*	*17*	*0.3*	*0.6*
GRAPPA								
Average	*1 Serving/30ml*	*85*	*0*	*283*	*0*	*6.7*	*0*	*0*
GRATIN								
Broccoli, & Cauliflower, Creamy, Iceland*	1 Gratin/112g	204	17.1	182	3.1	7	15.3	1.9
Butternut Squash, Creamy Pecorino Sauce, Finest, Tesco*	½ Pack/164g	202	13.1	123	3.9	7.1	8	3.4
Chicken, & Leek, Cooked, Fresh Ideas, Morrisons*	½ Pack/178g	288	11.7	162	21.3	4.1	6.6	0.7
Crab, & Lobster Mac & Cheese, Iceland*	1 Pot/100g	148	7.1	155	7.4	14	7.4	1.5
Fish, Smoked, Champ, & Greens, Gousto*	1 Serving/370g	400	11.1	108	8.4	12.8	3	0.9
Haddock, Smoked, & Bacon, 419, Oakhouse Foods Ltd*	1 Serving/400g	496	19.2	124	8.9	9.9	4.8	1.2
Haddock, Smoked, Frozen, Tesco*	1 Pot/90g	145	9.2	162	12.4	4.5	10.3	1.1
Ham, Wiltshire Cured, Specially Selected, Aldi*	1 Pack/400g	616	28	154	7.6	14	7	1.6
Leek, & Carrot, Findus*	1 Pack/400g	440	26	110	3.5	9.5	6.5	0
Leek, & Potato, Goats Cheese, & Spinach, Hello Fresh*	1 Serving/627g	740	44.1	118	4.5	11	7	0
Potato, & Onion, Frozen, Picard*	1 Pack/220g	341	22	155	4.9	10.4	10	1.6
Potato, & Spinach, M&S*	1 Serving/225g	259	16	115	2.9	9.1	7.1	1.3
Potato, Cheesy, Ovenbaked, Asda*	½ Pack/200g	179	8	90	1.7	11	4	1.4
Potato, Creamy, M&S*	½ Pack/225g	360	25	160	2.2	11.9	11.1	0.9
Potato, Dauphinoise, Finest, Tesco*	1 Gratin/107g	210	14.1	196	3.3	15	13.1	2
Potato, Tasty, Aldi*	½ Pack/180g	187	7	104	2.4	14	3.9	2.2
Spinach & Cheese, Gratin, Oven Baked, Gastro, Youngs*	1 Pack/337g	442	21.9	131	8.3	9.3	6.5	0.9
Vegetable, Root, Finest, Tesco*	½ Pack/214g	365	23.9	171	2.4	14	11.2	2
GRAVY								
Beef, Aunt Bessie's*	1 Serving/100g	73	5.3	73	1	5.3	5.3	0.5
Beef, Favourite, Granules, Made Up, Bisto*	1 Serving/50ml	13	0.5	26	0	4.2	1	0
Beef, Free From, Sainsbury's*	½ Pack/151g	47	1.5	31	1.5	4.1	1	0.2
Beef, Fresh, Sainsbury's*	1 Serving/83ml	47	2.7	56	2.4	4.5	3.2	0.6
Beef, Granules, Dry, Tesco*	1 Serving/6g	29	2.1	480	5.5	36.4	34.7	1.5
Beef, Granules, Made Up, Tesco*	1 Serving/140ml	48	3.6	35	0.3	2.6	2.5	0.1
Beef, Roast, Best in Glass Jar, Made Up, Bisto*	1 Serving/70ml	21	0.3	30	0.3	6.1	0.4	0
Beef, Roast, Traditional, Finest, Tesco*	¼ Pot/125g	68	3	54	2.4	5.5	2.4	0.3
Beef, with Winter Berry & Shallot, Made Up, Oxo*	1 Serving/105ml	24	0.3	23	0.6	4.3	0.3	0.1
Chicken, & Hint of Sage & Onion, Granules, Oxo*	1 Serving/30g	95	1.8	316	11.1	54.2	6.1	0.7
Chicken, & Turkey, Christmas, TTD, Sainsbury's*	¼ Pot/112g	66	1.7	59	6.9	4.2	1.5	0.5
Chicken, Finest, Tesco*	¼ Pouch/88ml	38	1.1	43	2.3	5.6	1.3	0
Chicken, Granules For, Dry Weight, Bisto*	1 Serving/20g	80	3.2	400	1.9	62.5	15.8	0.2
Chicken, Granules, Dry, Average	*1 Tsp/4g*	*17*	*0.9*	*428*	*4.5*	*49.4*	*23.6*	*1.2*
Chicken, Granules, Made Up, Average	*1 Serving/50ml*	*15*	*0.8*	*30*	*0.4*	*3.6*	*1.5*	*0.1*
Chicken, Granules, Made Up, Smart Price, Asda*	1 Serving/100ml	34	2.3	34	0.2	3	2.3	0.1
Chicken, Organic, Kallo*	1 Serving/75ml	259	1.7	345	1.6	79.1	2.3	0.4
Granules, Beef, Original, Made Up, Goldenfry Foods Ltd*	1 Serving/50ml	17	1.2	34	1	3.2	2.4	1
Granules, Beef, Reduced Salt, Made Up, Tesco*	1 Serving/75ml	25	1.6	33	0.1	3.4	2.1	0.1
Granules, Dry, Bisto*	1 Serving/10g	38	1.6	384	3.1	56.4	16.2	1.5
Granules, Instant, Made Up	*1oz/28g*	*10*	*0.7*	*34*	*0.3*	*3*	*2.4*	*0*
Granules, Low Salt, Organic, Made Up	1 Serving/70ml	22	0.8	32	0.3	5.1	1.2	0
Granules, Made Up, Oxo*	1 Serving/150ml	28	0.4	19	0.6	3.4	0.3	0
Granules, Meat, Made Up, Newgate, Lidl*	1 Serving/50ml	14	0.9	27	0.2	2.5	1.9	0.8
Granules, Onion, Dry	1 Tbsp/15g	17	1.1	116	1.9	10.9	7.5	1.9
Granules, Stockwell & Co., Tesco*	1 Tbsp/15g	5	0.3	34	0.2	3.4	2.2	0.1
Lamb, Granules, As Prepared, Best, Bisto*	1 Serving/50ml	13	0.5	26	1	5.4	1	1
Lamb, Granules, Dry, Average	*1 Tsp/4g*	*14*	*0.3*	*344*	*10.8*	*56.2*	*8.4*	*2.8*

G

	Measure INFO/WEIGHT	per Measure KCAL	FAT	Nutrition Values per 100g / 100ml KCAL	PROT	CARB	FAT	FIBRE
GRAVY								
Lamb, Roast, Bisto*	1 Serving/20g	60	0.9	302	3.4	62.3	4.3	0
Meat, Granules, As Consumed, Quixo, Aldi*	1 Serving/70ml	24	1.6	34	0.5	3.1	2.3	0.5
Meat, Granules, Made Up, Asda*	1 Serving/100ml	38	2.4	38	0.6	4	2.4	0.1
Meat, Granules, Made Up, Sainsbury's*	1 Serving/100ml	37	2.4	37	0.4	3.5	2.4	0.1
Onion, Caramelised, Made Up, Bisto*	1 Serving/50ml	14	0.2	29	0.1	6.1	0.4	0.1
Onion, Fresh, Asda*	1/6 Pot/77g	30	1.6	39	1.7	3.3	2.1	0.4
Onion, Granules, Dry Weight, Bisto*	4 Tsp/20g	78	2.9	391	2.4	62.3	14.7	2.3
Onion, Granules, Made Up, Bisto*	1 Serving/50ml	14	0.3	28	0.2	5.6	0.6	0
Onion, Rich, M&S*	½ Pack/150g	60	1.8	40	2	5.9	1.2	0.3
Pork, & Sage, Roast, Classic, Dry, Schwartz*	1 Pack/25g	88	1.4	354	11.8	63.8	5.8	0
Pork, Best, Made Up, Bisto*	1 Serving/50ml	13	0.5	26	1	5.8	1	1
Pork, Roast, Best, in Glass Jar, Dry Weight, Bisto*	4 Tsp/20g	67	0.9	333	5.7	66.6	4.7	0.8
Powder, GF, Dry, Allergycare*	1 Tbsp/10g	26	0	260	0.3	63.8	0.4	0
Powder, Made Up, Sainsbury's*	1 Serving/100ml	15	0.1	15	0.4	3.2	0.1	0.1
Reduced Salt, Granules, Chicken, As Prepared, Bisto*	1 Tsp/5g	1	0	28	1	4.4	1	1
Reduced Salt, Granules, Chicken, Dry Weight, Bisto*	1 Tsp/5g	21	0.8	415	2.3	65.5	15.6	1.7
Turkey, Finest, Tesco*	¼ Pouch/88ml	49	1.4	56	3.9	6.4	1.6	0
Turkey, Rich, Ready to Heat, Schwartz*	1 Pack/200g	62	2.4	31	1.9	3.1	1.2	0.5
Vegetable, Granules, Dry Weight, Bisto*	1 Tsp/4g	15	0.5	380	2.1	63	13.3	4.5
Vegetable, Granules, Made Up, Bisto*	1 Serving/50ml	14	0.2	28	0.2	5.6	0.4	0.2
Vegetarian, Granules, Dry Weight, Bisto*	1 Serving/28g	100	3.7	356	2.7	56	13.3	4.5
Vegetarian, Granules, Made Up, Sainsbury's*	1 Serving/50ml	16	1.1	32	0.2	2.8	2.2	0.8
GROUSE								
Meat Only, Roasted	*1oz/28g*	*36*	*0.6*	*128*	*27.6*	*0*	*2*	*0*
GUACAMOLE								
Average	*1 Tbsp/17g*	*33*	*3.3*	*194*	*1.6*	*3.4*	*19.2*	*2.4*
Dip, Tesco*	¼ Pot/41g	58	5.2	142	1.1	4	12.8	3
Reduced Fat, Dip, BGTY, Sainsbury's*	¼ Pot/43g	62	5.7	146	1.3	2.9	13.5	4
Squeezy, Old El Paso*	1 Tbsp/15g	14	0.9	96	1.3	7.4	6.3	2.4
Style, Topping, Dip, Discovery*	1 Seving/37g	29	2.1	79	1.2	6	5.6	1.2
GUAVA								
Canned in Syrup	*1oz/28g*	*17*	*0*	*60*	*0.4*	*15.7*	*0*	*3*
Raw, Flesh Only, Average	*1 Fruit/55g*	*37*	*0.6*	*68*	*3*	*14*	*1*	*5*
GUINEA FOWL								
Boned & Stuffed, Fresh, Fayrefield Foods*	1 Serving/325g	650	39.3	200	19.1	3.3	12.1	0.5
Fresh, Free Range, without Giblets, No.1, Waitrose*	1 Portion/193g	368	16.9	191	27.6	0.5	8.8	0.6
GUMS								
American Hard, Sainsbury's*	1 Sweet/6g	22	0	360	0.1	90	0.1	0
American Hard, Tesco*	1 Serving/200g	646	0	323	0	80.8	0	0
Milk Bottles, Bassett's*	1 Pack/25g	88	0.4	353	6.2	78.3	1.6	0
Milk Bottles, Milk Flavour, Asda*	1 Pack/100g	369	2.3	369	7	80	2.3	0.4

G

	Measure INFO/WEIGHT	per Measure KCAL	FAT	Nutrition Values per 100g / 100ml KCAL	PROT	CARB	FAT	FIBRE
HADDOCK								
Battered, Essential, Waitrose*	1 Fillet/121g	221	11.1	182	13.6	11.1	9.1	0.8
Beer Battered, Bubbly, Scottish , Waitrose*	1 Portion/177g	389	20.5	220	14.7	13.5	11.6	1.2
Fillet, Battered, Goujons, Tesco*	1 Pack/184g	552	30	300	12.3	25.3	16.3	1.4
Fillets, Battered, Average	*1oz/28g*	*64*	*3.4*	*228*	*13.4*	*16.3*	*12.2*	*1.1*
Fillets, Battered, Crisp & Golden, Waitrose*	1 Fillet/139g	264	11.5	190	13.5	14.7	8.3	0.9
Fillets, Breaded, Ocean Trader, Lidl*	1 Fillet/119g	236	9	198	14	17	7.6	3
Fillets, in Breadcrumbs, Average	*1 Fillet/125g*	*253*	*12.4*	*203*	*13.5*	*14.9*	*9.9*	*1.2*
Fillets, Lightly Dusted, Tesco*	1 Fillet/115g	182	6.7	158	15.3	10.9	5.8	0.6
Fillets, Raw, Average	*1 Fillet/140g*	*111*	*1.2*	*79*	*17.7*	*0.2*	*0.8*	*0*
Fillets, Smoked, Cooked, Average	*1 Pack/300g*	*337*	*7.7*	*112*	*21.9*	*0.4*	*2.6*	*0.1*
Fillets, Smoked, Raw, Average	*1 Pack/227g*	*190*	*1*	*84*	*19.9*	*0.1*	*0.4*	*0.2*
Florentine, with Garlic & Herb Potato, Gastropub, M&S*	1 Pack/370g	492	29.2	133	7.7	7.4	7.9	0.7
Flour, Fried in Blended Oil	*1oz/28g*	*39*	*1.1*	*138*	*21.1*	*4.5*	*4.1*	*0.2*
Goujons, Batter, Crispy, M&S*	1 Serving/100g	250	14.1	250	11.7	18.5	14.1	0.8
HAGGIS								
Premium, Canned, Grants*	½ Can/392g	823	41.9	210	10.4	16.9	10.7	2.3
Slices, Uncooked, Malcolm Allan*	1 Slice/56g	178	11.8	318	10.4	21.6	21.1	0
Traditional, Average	*1 Serving/454g*	*1119*	*66.5*	*246*	*12.4*	*17.2*	*14.6*	*1*
Vegetarian, Macsween*	1/3 Pack/151g	412	24.6	273	6	22.9	16.3	0
HAKE								
Fillets, in Breadcrumbs, Average	*1oz/28g*	*66*	*3.7*	*234*	*12.9*	*16*	*13.4*	*1*
Goujons, Average	*1 Serving/150g*	*345*	*17.8*	*230*	*12.4*	*18.6*	*11.9*	*1.3*
Raw, Average	*1oz/28g*	*28*	*0.6*	*100*	*20.1*	*0*	*2.2*	*0*
HALIBUT								
Cooked, Dry Heat, Average	*1oz/28g*	*38*	*1.1*	*135*	*24.6*	*0.4*	*4*	*0*
Raw	*1oz/28g*	*28*	*0.5*	*101*	*21.1*	*0*	*1.9*	*0*
HALVA								
Average	*1oz/28g*	*107*	*3.7*	*381*	*1.8*	*68*	*13.2*	*0*
HAM								
Applewood Smoked, Average	*1 Slice/28g*	*31*	*0.8*	*112*	*21.2*	*0.6*	*2.8*	*0.2*
Baked, Average	*1 Slice/74g*	*98*	*3.7*	*133*	*21*	*1*	*5*	*0*
Black Forest, Slices, Dulano, Lidl*	1 Slice/11g	26	1.6	240	25	1	15	0.5
Boiled, Average	*1 Pack/113g*	*154*	*6.5*	*136*	*20.6*	*0.6*	*5.8*	*0*
Breaded, Average	*1 Slice/37g*	*57*	*2.3*	*155*	*23.1*	*1.8*	*6.3*	*1.6*
Breaded, Dry Cured, Average	*1 Slice/33g*	*47*	*1.8*	*142*	*22.2*	*1.4*	*5.4*	*0*
Brunswick, Average	*1 Slice/20g*	*32*	*1.8*	*160*	*19.5*	*0.6*	*8.8*	*0*
Cooked, Sliced, Average	*1 Slice/17g*	*18*	*0.5*	*109*	*19*	*1*	*3.2*	*0.1*
Crumbed, Sliced, Average	*1 Slice/28g*	*33*	*0.9*	*117*	*21.5*	*0.9*	*3.1*	*0*
Danish, Average	*1 Slice/11g*	*14*	*0.6*	*125*	*18.4*	*1*	*5.4*	*0*
Dry Cured, Average	*1 Slice/18g*	*26*	*1*	*144*	*22.4*	*1*	*5.6*	*0.2*
Extra Lean, Average	*1 Slice/11g*	*10*	*0.2*	*90*	*18*	*1.4*	*1.4*	*0*
Gammon, Breaded, Average	*1 Serving/25g*	*31*	*0.8*	*122*	*22*	*1.5*	*3.1*	*0*
Gammon, Dry Cured, Sliced, Average	*1 Slice/33g*	*43*	*1.4*	*131*	*22.9*	*0.4*	*4.2*	*0*
Gammon, Honey Roast, Average	*1 Serving/60g*	*81*	*2.8*	*134*	*22.4*	*0.4*	*4.8*	*0*
Gammon, Smoked, Average	*1 Slice/43g*	*59*	*2.1*	*137*	*22.3*	*0.7*	*4.9*	*0.2*
German Black Forest, Average	*½ Pack/35g*	*93*	*6*	*267*	*27.2*	*1.3*	*17*	*0.5*
Hock, Cooked, Shredded, Sainsbury's*	½ Pack55g	100	4.1	182	27.6	0.5	7.5	1
Hock, in Parsley Sauce, Classic, Waitrose*	1 Pack/368g	320	13.6	87	6.6	6.3	3.7	1.2
Hock, Mustard Sauce, with Mash, & Peas, Tesco*	1 Pack/450g	387	13	86	7.5	6.8	2.9	1.4
Hock, Pulled, M&S*	1 Pack/100g	165	6.5	165	26.5	0.1	6.5	0.1
Honey & Mustard, Average	*1oz/28g*	*39*	*1.2*	*140*	*20.8*	*4.6*	*4.3*	*0*
Honey Roast, Average	*1 Slice/20g*	*25*	*0.8*	*123*	*20.3*	*1.6*	*3.8*	*0.1*
Honey Roast, Dry Cured, Average	*1 Slice/33g*	*46*	*1.5*	*140*	*22.7*	*2.3*	*4.4*	*0.2*

H

	Measure INFO/WEIGHT	per Measure KCAL	per Measure FAT	Nutrition Values per 100g / 100ml KCAL	PROT	CARB	FAT	FIBRE
HAM								
Honey Roast, Lean, Average	*1 Serving/25g*	*28*	*0.8*	*111*	*18.2*	*2.7*	*3.1*	*0*
Honey Roast, Wafer Thin, Average	*1 Slice/10g*	*11*	*0.3*	*113*	*17.4*	*3.7*	*3.2*	*0.3*
Jamon, Iberico de Bellota, Hand Carved, 1, Waitrose*	¼ Pack/16g	56	3.9	344	31.5	0.7	23.7	0.9
Joint, Cured, Roasted, Average	*1 Serving/100g*	*138*	*5.2*	*138*	*21.7*	*1*	*5.2*	*0.1*
Joint, Roast, Christmas, Tesco*	1/6 Joint/167g	225	10.8	135	17.9	1.1	6.5	0
Lean, Average	*1 Slice/18g*	*19*	*0.4*	*104*	*19.5*	*1.1*	*2.4*	*0.3*
Oak Smoked, Average	*1 Slice/20g*	*26*	*0.9*	*130*	*21*	*1*	*4.7*	*0.3*
Parma, Average	*1 Slice/10g*	*21*	*1.1*	*213*	*29.3*	*0*	*10.6*	*0*
Parma, Premium, Average	*1 Slice/14g*	*36*	*2.3*	*258*	*27.9*	*0.3*	*16.1*	*0*
Peppered, Average	*1 Slice/12g*	*13*	*0.3*	*110*	*18.5*	*2*	*2.7*	*0*
Prosciutto, Average	*1 Slice/12g*	*27*	*1.5*	*226*	*28.7*	*0*	*12.4*	*0.4*
Pulled, in Mustard Sauce, BFY, M&S*	1 Pack/400g	304	10	76	6	6.9	2.5	0.9
Pulled, in Mustard Sauce, Mash, Beans, & Carrots, Tesco*	1 Pack/368g	309	9.9	84	6.5	7.6	2.7	1.4
Serrano, Average	*1 Slice/20g*	*46*	*2.4*	*230*	*30.5*	*0.4*	*11.8*	*0*
Smoked, Average	*1 Slice/18g*	*21*	*0.7*	*117*	*19.7*	*0.9*	*3.7*	*0*
Smoked, Black Treacle, & Stout, Specially Selected, Aldi*	1 Serving/30g	44	1.8	146	21	1.9	6	0.5
Smoked, Dry Cured, Average	*1 Slice/28g*	*38*	*1.2*	*137*	*23*	*1.4*	*4.4*	*0.2*
Smoked, Wafer Thin, Average	*1 Serving/40g*	*41*	*1.2*	*102*	*17.7*	*1.2*	*2.9*	*0.2*
Thick Cut, Average	*1 Slice/74g*	*94*	*2.9*	*127*	*22.4*	*0.6*	*3.9*	*0.1*
Tinned, Average	*½ Can/100g*	*136*	*8.8*	*136*	*12.2*	*2*	*8.8*	*0*
Torchon, Aldi*	1 Slice/50g	58	1.4	116	22	1	2.8	0.5
Vegetarian, Slices, Deli, Wafer Thin, Deli, Quorn*	1/3 Pack/60g	66	1.3	110	16	6.5	2.2	5.8
Vegetarian, Slices, Quorn*	¼ Pack/25g	30	0.5	122	16	6.5	2.2	5.8
Wafer Thin, Average	*1 Slice/10g*	*10*	*0.3*	*101*	*17.9*	*1.4*	*2.6*	*0.1*
Wiltshire Cured, Plckle Glazed, Sliced, Waitrose*	1 Slice/32g	45	1.7	139	21.1	1.1	5.4	0.6
Wiltshire, Average	*1oz/28g*	*41*	*1.7*	*148*	*23.1*	*0*	*6*	*0*
Wiltshire, Breaded, Average	*1oz/28g*	*41*	*1.4*	*145*	*23.9*	*1*	*5*	*0*
Yorkshire, Cured, Slices, Delicatessen, Tesco*	1 Slice/95g	132	1.8	139	19.4	0.2	1.9	22
Yorkshire, Slices, Deli, Morrisons*	1 Slice/40g	59	1.7	148	26.3	0.9	4.2	0.5
HARIBO*								
American Hard Gums, Haribo*	1 Pack/175g	630	3.3	360	0.3	85.5	1.9	0.2
Cola Bottles, Fizzy, Haribo*	1 Pack/175g	595	0.4	340	6.3	78.3	0.2	0.3
Cola Bottles, Haribo*	1 Pack/16g	56	0	348	7.7	78.9	0.2	0.3
Dolly Mixtures, Haribo*	1 Pack/175g	719	8.4	411	1.8	90.2	4.8	0.2
Fantasy Mix, Haribo*	1 Pack/100g	344	0.2	344	6.6	79	0.2	0.3
Fruitilicious, 30% Less Sugar, Haribo*	¼ Bag/30g	85	0.2	282	6.4	54	0.5	0
Gold Bears, Haribo*	1 Pack/100g	343	0.5	343	6.9	77	0.5	0
Happy Cherries, Haribo*	1 Serving/40g	139	0.1	348	7.7	78.9	0.2	0.3
Horror Mix, Haribo*	1 Pack/100g	344	0.2	344	6.6	79	0.2	0.3
Jelly Babies, Haribo*	1oz/28g	97	0.1	348	4.5	82.1	0.2	0.5
Jelly Beans, Haribo*	1 Pack/100g	379	0.2	379	0.6	93.8	0.2	0.1
Kiddies Super Mix, Haribo*	1 Pack/100g	344	0.2	344	6.6	79	0.2	0.3
Liquorice Favourites, Haribo*	1 Serving/40g	143	1.2	357	2.8	78.8	3	2.3
Liquorice with Stevia, Stevi-Lakritz, Haribo*	¼ Bag/25g	46	0	185	8.1	16	0.1	48.6
Magic Mix, Haribo*	1oz/28g	102	0.5	366	5.4	82	1.9	0.3
Maoam Stripes, Haribo*	1 Chew/7g	27	0.4	384	1.2	81.7	6.1	0.3
Mega Roulette, Haribo*	1oz/28g	97	0.1	348	7.7	78.9	0.2	0.3
Milky Mix, Haribo*	1 Pack/175g	607	0.4	347	7.1	79.6	0.2	0.4
Pontefract Cakes, Haribo*	1 Serving/40g	118	0.1	296	5.3	68.2	0.2	0.5
Snakes, Haribo*	1 Snake/8g	28	0	348	7.7	78.9	0.2	0.3
Starmix, Haribo*	1 Pack/100g	344	0.2	344	6.6	79	0.2	0.3
Tangfastics, Haribo*	1 Pack/100g	359	2.3	359	6.3	78.3	2.3	0.5
Tropifruit, Haribo*	1oz/28g	97	0.1	348	4.5	82.1	0.2	0.5

H

	Measure INFO/WEIGHT	per Measure KCAL	FAT	Nutrition Values per 100g / 100ml KCAL	PROT	CARB	FAT	FIBRE
HARISSA PASTE								
Average	*1 Tsp/5g*	*6*	*0.3*	*123*	*2.9*	*12.9*	*6.7*	*2.8*
HASH								
Beef, Corned, 303, Oakhouse Foods Ltd*	1 Serving/400g	428	17.2	107	6.7	9.3	4.3	2
Beef, in Gravy, & Buttery Potato & Onion, Gastropub, M&S*	1 Pack/400g	432	16	108	9	8.1	4	1.7
Chicken, & Stuffing, Dinner, M&S*	1 Pack/400g	480	18.4	120	8	10.9	4.6	1.3
Corned Beef, Homestyle, Hormel*	1 Can/400g	644	40.7	161	7.2	9.8	10.2	0.8
Steak, Hash, Extra Special, Asda*	1 Pack/354g	450	11	127	7.5	16	3.1	2.4
Steak, in London Porter Gravy, British, TTD, Sainsbury's*	1 Pack/400g	408	13.6	102	8.5	8.5	3.4	1.4
HASH BROWNS								
Cauliflower, Strong Roots*	1 Piece/40g	74	4.3	185	1.7	19.4	10.7	1.8
Fries, Oven Baked, Iceland*	1 Serving/150g	375	15	250	3.4	34.7	10	3.5
Homestyle, Aunt Bessie's*	2 Pieces/98g	182	9.2	186	1.6	23	9.4	1.9
Oven Baked, Weighed Cooked, McCain*	1 Piece/37g	64	2.4	170	1.8	24.9	6.4	2.7
Oven Baked, Weighed Frozen, McCain*	1 Piece/40g	60	2.4	150	1.6	21.3	6	2.1
Potatoes, From Restaurant, Average	*1 Portion/150g*	*489*	*32.5*	*326*	*2.6*	*32.1*	*21.6*	*2.7*
Uncooked, Average	*1 Piece/45g*	*78*	*3.7*	*173*	*2*	*22.5*	*8.3*	*1.9*
HAZELNUTS								
Blanched, Average	*1 Serving/25g*	*164*	*15.9*	*656*	*15.4*	*5.8*	*63.5*	*6.5*
Chopped, Average	*1 Serving/10g*	*67*	*6.4*	*666*	*16.8*	*5.6*	*64*	*6.6*
Whole, Average	*10 Whole/10g*	*66*	*6.4*	*655*	*15.4*	*5.8*	*63.5*	*6.5*
HEART								
Lambs, Average	*1 Heart/75g*	*92*	*4.5*	*122*	*16*	*1*	*6*	*0*
Ox, Raw	*1oz/28g*	*23*	*0.8*	*82*	*14.4*	*0*	*2.8*	*0*
Ox, Stewed	*1oz/28g*	*44*	*1.4*	*157*	*27.8*	*0*	*5.1*	*0*
HERRING								
Bismarck, in Tangy Marinade, Ocean Sea, Lidl*	1/3 Pack/80g	112	7.3	140	14.1	0.1	9.1	0
Canned in Tomato Sauce, Average	*1oz/28g*	*57*	*4.3*	*204*	*11.9*	*4.1*	*15.5*	*0.1*
Fillets, Marinated, in Cream Sauce, Lisner*	1 Serving/70g	201	18.8	287	5.4	5.9	26.8	0
Fillets, Raw, Average	*1 Herring/100g*	*139*	*9.4*	*139*	*13.8*	*0*	*9.4*	*0*
Fillets, Smoked, & Peppered, Sainsbury's*	½ Pack/80g	163	8.7	204	22.8	3.5	10.9	0
Grilled, Average	*1oz/28g*	*51*	*3.1*	*181*	*20.1*	*0*	*11.2*	*0*
in Dill Marinade, Drained, Elsinore*	1 Jar/140g	336	15.4	240	9.8	27	11	0
Pickled in Mustard Sauce, Abba*	1 Serving/58g	150	10.9	260	7	16	19	0
Pickled, Average	*1oz/28g*	*42*	*2.9*	*149*	*8.1*	*5.5*	*10.3*	*0*
HONEY								
Acacia Blossom, Sainsbury's*	1 Serving/24g	81	0	339	0.1	84.7	0.1	0.3
Clear, with a Hint of Cinnamon, Rowse*	1 Tbsp/15g	49	0.1	329	0.5	81.5	0.5	0.5
Greek, Waitrose*	1 Tsp/6g	18	0	307	0.4	76.4	0	0
Manuka, New Zealand, M&S*	1 Tsp/5g	17	0	348	0.1	86.9	0.1	0.3
Pure, Clear, Average	*1 Tbsp/20g*	*63*	*0*	*315*	*0.5*	*78.5*	*0*	*0*
Pure, Set, Average	*1 Tbsp/20g*	*62*	*0*	*312*	*0.4*	*77.6*	*0*	*0*
Raw, British Wildflower, Hilltop*	1 Tsp/5g	17	0	333	0.2	83.1	0.2	0
Scottish Heather, Waitrose*	1 Serving/20g	61	0	307	0.4	76.4	0	0
Soft Set, British, Hilltop Honey*	1 Tbsp/15g	50	0	333	0.2	83.1	0.2	0.5
Spanish Orange Blossom, Sainsbury's*	1 Tbsp/15g	51	0	339	0.1	84.7	0	0.3
HONEYCOMB								
Natural, Epicure*	1 Serving/100g	290	4.6	290	0.4	74.4	4.6	0
HOOCH*								
Vodka, Calculated Estimate, Hooch*	1 Bottle/330ml	145	0	44	0.3	5.1	0	0
HORLICKS								
Malted Drink, Chocolate, Extra Light, Dry Weight, Horlicks*	1 Serving/32g	95	2.5	296	9.2	47	7.8	17.3
Malted Drink, Light, Dry Weight, Horlicks*	1 Serving/32g	116	1.2	364	14.8	72.2	3.8	1.9
Malted Drink, Light, Made Up, Horlicks*	1 Mug/200ml	116	1.2	58	2.4	11.6	0.6	0.3

H

	Measure INFO/WEIGHT	per Measure KCAL	FAT	Nutrition Values per 100g / 100ml KCAL	PROT	CARB	FAT	FIBRE
HORLICKS								
Powder, Made Up with Semi-Skimmed Milk	*1 Mug/227ml*	*184*	*4.3*	*81*	*4.3*	*12.9*	*1.9*	*0*
Powder, Made Up with Whole Milk	*1 Mug/227ml*	*225*	*8.9*	*99*	*4.2*	*12.7*	*3.9*	*0*
HORSERADISH								
Cream, Strong, Tracklement's*	1 Tsp/5g	15	1.3	299	4.3	7.5	26.5	4.9
Creamed, Sainsbury's*	1 Tsp/10ml	25	1.4	253	2.8	26.9	14.3	2.3
Prepared, Average	*1 Tsp/5g*	*1*	*0*	*28*	*2*	*5*	*0.1*	*2.8*
HOT CHOCOLATE								
Belgian Choc & Butterscotch, Made Up, Options*	1 Sachet/11g	39	0.9	353	2.7	52	8.1	8.5
Belgian Choc, Options*	1 Sachet/11g	40	0.8	365	8.9	59	7.3	0
Cadbury*	1 Serving/12g	44	0.7	370	6.3	73.3	5.9	0
Caramel, Whittards of Chelsea*	1 Serving/20g	71	1.5	355	7.5	64.5	7.5	13
Choc Mint, Highlights, Made Up, Cadbury*	1 Serving/200ml	40	1.4	20	1	2.5	0.7	0.3
Choca Mocha Drink, Options, Ovaltine*	1 Sachet/11g	39	1.3	359	14.1	50.1	11.4	7
Chocolate Au Lait, Options, Ovaltine*	1 Sachet/10g	36	1	355	11.8	54.5	10	7.3
Cocoa, Lidl*	1 Serving/20g	77	1.2	386	6.1	74.1	6.2	0
Dairy Fudge, Highlights, Dry Weight, Cadbury*	1 Serving/11g	38	1.2	347	16	41	11	9.7
Dairy Fudge, Highlights, Made Up, Cadbury*	1 Serving/200ml	40	1	20	1	2.7	0.5	0.2
Dark, Bournville, Highlights, Made Up, Cadbury*	1 Serving/200ml	35	0.9	18	1.2	2	0.4	0
Dreamy Caramel, Options, Ovaltine*	1 Sachet/11g	39	0.9	354	12.3	48.5	7.8	0
Drink, Organic, Green & Black's*	1 Tsp/5g	20	0.4	396	8.6	67	7.5	12
Fairtrade, Whittards of Chelsea*	4 Tsp/20g	68	0.8	342	7.8	69	3.9	10.9
From Coffee Shop, Waitrose*	1 Serving/298ml	217	5.9	73	3.6	10.9	2	0
Galaxy, Mars*	1 Sachet/25g	97	1.9	386	4.8	71.9	7.7	4.7
Highlights, Instant, Made Up, Cadbury*	1 Cup/200ml	40	1.4	20	1	2.5	0.7	0.3
Instant Break, Cadbury*	1 Sachet/28g	119	3.9	425	10.9	64.2	14	0
Instant, Highlights, Cadbury*	1 Sachet/22g	80	2.8	364	17.3	44.6	12.7	0
Instant, Powder, As Prepared with Hot Water, Morrisons*	1 Serving/230ml	108	1.1	47	1	9.5	0.5	0.5
Instant, Tesco*	1 Serving/30g	120	2.5	401	7.1	71.6	8.4	5.4
Low Calorie, Dry Weight, As Sold, Average	*1 Sachet/11g*	*41*	*1.2*	*374*	*14.6*	*50*	*10.7*	*11.1*
Luxury, Skinny, Whittards of Chelsea*	1 Serving/28g	92	0.8	328	12.9	67.1	2.8	13.5
Made Up, Tassimo, Suchard*	1 Serving/280ml	88	2.4	31	0.3	5.5	0.9	0.2
Maltesers, Malt Drink, Instant, Made Up, Mars*	1 Serving/220ml	104	3	47	0.9	7.7	1.4	0
Mint Madness, Belgian, Options, Ovaltine*	1 Sachet/11g	38	0.8	348	12.3	49.2	6.9	20
Mint, Highlights, Cadbury*	1 Serving/200ml	40	1.4	20	1	2.5	0.7	0
Outrageous Orange, Options, Ovaltine*	1 Serving/11g	38	0.8	348	12.3	49.3	6.9	20
Powder, Tresor, Monbana*	1 Scoop/28g	107	2	382	6.5	68	7	0
San Cristobal, Cafe Direct*	1 Serving/40g	158	3.4	396	8.9	65	8.4	0
Spanish, El Canario*	1 Serving/50g	170	1.4	340	5.5	72.1	2.9	3.1
Tempting Toffee, Options, Ovaltine*	1 Sachet/11g	43	1	391	13.6	66.4	9.1	0
Velvet, Cadbury*	1 Serving/28g	136	6.9	487	8.6	57.8	24.6	2
Wicked White, Options, Ovaltine*	1 Sachet/11g	44	1.1	398	10.5	64.6	10	3.7
Wispa, Hot Frothy, Cadbury*	1 Sachet/27g	107	1.4	395	11	74	5.3	2.9
HOT DOG								
Jumbo, in Brine, Ye Olde Oak*	1 Hot Dog/50g	74	4.8	149	11	4.5	9.5	0
Plain, From Restaurant, Average	*1 Hot Dog/98g*	*242*	*14.5*	*247*	*10.6*	*18.4*	*14.8*	*0*
Sausage, American Style, Average	*1 Hot Dog/75g*	*180*	*14.3*	*241*	*11.6*	*6.2*	*19*	*0*
Sausage, Average	*1 Hot Dog/23g*	*40*	*3*	*175*	*10.8*	*4.3*	*12.8*	*0.3*
Vegetarian, Meat Free, Sainsbury's*	1 Sausage/30g	72	5.1	240	17.4	3.8	16.8	2
Vegetarian, Tesco*	1 Sausage/30g	66	4.7	222	17.1	1.6	15.8	2.2
HOT POT								
Beef, Classic, 800g, Asda*	1 Serving/400g	400	20.8	100	5.7	7.1	5.2	1.2
Beef, Minced, Bisto*	1 Pack/375g	363	13.5	97	4.1	11.3	3.6	1.4
Beef, Minced, Classic, Asda*	1 Pack/400g	424	18.4	106	6.8	8.7	4.6	1.1

H

INFO/WEIGHT	Measure	per Measure KCAL	FAT	Nutrition Values per 100g / 100ml KCAL	PROT	CARB	FAT	FIBRE

HOT POT

	Measure INFO/WEIGHT	KCAL	FAT	KCAL	PROT	CARB	FAT	FIBRE
Beef, Minced, Frozen, Tesco*	1 Pack/360g	377	10.1	105	5.2	11.7	2.8	1.6
Beef, Minced, HFC, Tesco*	1 Pack/362g	347	10	96	5.2	11.7	2.8	1.6
Beef, Minced, Iceland*	1 Pack/500g	500	20	100	2.8	12.1	4	1.8
Beef, Minced, Sainsbury's*	1 Pack/450g	464	22.1	103	5.3	9.5	4.9	2.2
Beef, Weight Watchers*	1 Pack/320g	231	7.7	72	3.6	8.4	2.4	1.6
Chicken, & Mushroom, HL, Tesco*	1 Serving/450g	369	6.8	82	6.3	11.8	1.5	0.5
Chicken, Chunky, Weight Watchers*	1 Pack/320g	275	9	86	4.7	10.4	2.8	0.6
Chicken, Co-Op*	1 Pack/340g	289	10.2	85	6	9	3	0.7
Chicken, Calorie Controlled, Eat Smart, Morrisons*	1 Pack/350g	217	1.8	62	7.3	6.6	0.5	0.9
Chicken, Honey & Mustard, 417, Oakhouse Foods Ltd*	1 Serving/440g	629	36.9	143	6	9.8	8.4	1.3
Chicken, Sainsbury's*	1 Pack/400g	340	11	85	5.2	9.8	2.8	1.3
Chicken, Weight Watchers*	1 Pack/320g	296	6.7	93	6.3	11.8	2.1	1.1
Lamb, Diet Chef Ltd*	1 Pack/300g	276	5.4	92	8.9	10.1	1.8	3
Lamb, Keema, Microwaved, Mumbai Street Food, Iceland*	1 Meal/231g	296	15.5	128	5.6	9.6	6.7	3
Lamb, Lancashire, with Wilted Greens, Gousto*	1 Portion/474g	474	19	100	6.5	9.9	4	0.9
Lamb, Minced, & Vegetable, COU, M&S*	1 Pack/400g	340	10.8	85	5.7	12.5	2.7	1.8
Lamb, Minced, Classic Kitchen, Tesco*	1 Pack/434g	389	10.8	90	5.2	11	2.5	1.3
Lamb, Minced, Morrison*	1 Pack/400g	376	11.6	94	4.1	11.7	2.9	2.2
Lamb, Shank, Extra Special, Asda*	1 Pack/450g	508	20.2	113	10.2	7.8	4.5	1.3
Lamb, with Parsley & Thyme Crumb, Tesco*	1 Pack/342g	551	30.1	161	4.9	14.5	8.8	1.9
Lancashire, 305, Oakhouse Foods Ltd*	1 Serving/400g	344	14	86	5.6	7.4	3.5	1.1
Lancashire, M&S*	1 Pack/450g	441	13.5	98	8.4	8.8	3	1.3
Lancashire, Tesco*	½ Pack/225g	205	7	91	6	9.7	3.1	0.5
Lancashire, with Sliced Potatoes, Cooked, Aldi*	1 Pot/450g	460	17	108	7.3	9.3	4	2.7
Potato, Slim & Save*	1 Pack/40g	147	2.2	368	36	26.6	5.5	11.3
Quorn, Vegetarian, Wiltshire Farm Foods*	1 Serving/341g	307	5.5	90	3.3	14	1.6	0
Sausage, & Vegetable, Vegetarian, Linda McCartney*	1 Pot/400g	516	20.4	129	6.4	15.7	5.1	2.3
Vegetable, 468, Oakhouse Foods Ltd*	1 Meal/400g	284	8.4	71	1.6	10.9	2.1	1.3
Vegetarian, Quorn*	1 Pack/400g	252	8	63	3.3	8	2	1.9

HOUMOUS

	Measure INFO/WEIGHT	KCAL	FAT	KCAL	PROT	CARB	FAT	FIBRE
Beetroot, Asda*	1 Serving/30g	57	3.9	191	5.3	11	13	5.6
Beetroot, Roasted, & Mint, Sainsbury's*	¼ Pot/50g	130	10.2	261	5.8	11.5	20.3	4.9
Caramelised Onion, Co-Op*	¼ Pack/43g	106	8.1	249	6.3	11	19	6.3
Classic, Sainsburys*	¼ Pot/58g	161	12.8	278	6.7	10.6	22	5.3
Classic, Snappable, Pots, Sainsbury's*	1 Pot/40g	111	8.8	278	6.7	10.6	22	5.3
Extra Virgin Olive Oil, TTD, Sainsbury's*	¼ Pot/43g	133	11.3	310	6.3	10.2	26.2	3.8
Jalapeno, Mexican, Morrisons*	¼ Pot/50g	162	13.6	325	7.5	9.8	27.3	5.1
Jalapeno, Pepper, Hot & Spicy, Tesco*	¼ Pot/46g	104	6.8	227	8.1	12.8	14.9	4.8
Kalamata Olive, Organic, Daylesford*	¼ Pack/50g	71	4.6	142	4.3	11.7	9.1	5
Lemon & Coriander, Sainsbury's*	¼ Tub/50g	146	12.6	291	7	9.1	25.1	6
Lemon & Coriander, M&S*	½ Pack/100g	296	24.5	296	6.5	9.1	24.5	6.3
Lemon & Coriander, Tesco*	¼ Pot/46g	116	8.9	253	6.8	9.9	19.4	5.8
Lentil, Original, Pulse*	1 Serving/30g	70	4.1	232	8.5	15.3	13.8	6.5
Moroccan, Inspired, Finest, Tesco*	¼ Pot/43g	130	10.7	305	5.3	12	25.1	4.7
Moroccan, Sainsbury's*	¼ Pot/50g	114	8.3	229	6	11.1	16.6	5.5
Onion, Caramelised, Tesco*	¼ Pack/46g	118	8.9	256	5.2	12.4	19.4	5.8
Onion, Caramelised, The Deli, Aldi*	½ Pack/42g	94	5.9	224	7.4	15	14	4.1
Organic, Clive's*	1 Serving/30g	68	5.2	228	7.6	9.3	17.2	0
Organic, M&S*	1 Serving/25g	83	7.4	332	7.2	5.9	29.4	7.3
Red Pepper, & Chilli, Chargrilled, 30% Less Fat, Asda*	1 Serving/50g	116	8.2	233	7.5	11.5	16.4	4.9
Red Pepper, Meadow Fresh, Lidl*	1 Serving/50g	158	12.9	307	7.1	11	25	5
Red Pepper, Reduced Fat, Tesco*	1 Serving/20g	44	2.9	220	7.7	11.9	14.4	5.7
Red Pepper, Roasted, Reduced Fat, M&S*	¼ Pack/50g	91	5.5	182	5.8	12.7	11	4.5

H

	Measure INFO/WEIGHT	per Measure KCAL	FAT	Nutrition Values per 100g / 100ml KCAL	PROT	CARB	FAT	FIBRE
HOUMOUS								
Red Pepper, Roasted, Sainsbury's*	½ Pot/100g	317	27.2	317	6.2	9	27.2	5.7
Reduced Fat, Average	**1 Tbsp/30g**	**72**	**5**	**241**	**9.2**	**13.3**	**16.8**	**3.6**
Reduced Fat, Mini Pot, Tesco*	1 Sm Pot/70g	118	6.4	168	6.2	12.7	9.2	4.7
Reduced Fat, with Crunchy Carrot Sticks, M&S*	1 Pack/130g	157	9.9	121	3.3	7.8	7.6	3.9
Smoked, Moorish*	1 Pack/150g	448	36.3	299	7.1	11.5	24.2	3.4
Sweet Chilli, Morrisons*	1 Serving/20g	58	4.1	290	7.1	17.5	20.3	4.3
Sweet Chilli, Sainsbury's*	¼ Pot/50g	151	11.8	302	5.8	14.1	23.6	4.8
Sweet Chilli, Tesco*	¼ Pot/46g	106	6.8	231	7.1	15	14.7	5.2
Sweet Chilli, The Deli, Aldi*	¼ Pot/50g	125	8	250	7.7	16	16	5.3
Turmeric, Organic, Daylesford*	¼ Pot/50g	90	5.8	181	6.4	8	11.6	9.7
Turmeric, Pickled Red Cabbage, & Pomegranate, Waitrose*	½ Pack/75g	205	15.8	273	5.7	13.3	21	4
HULA HOOPS								
BBQ Beef, KP Snacks*	1 Bag/24g	120	5.8	500	3.8	65	24	2.2
Beef Puft, Hula Hoops*	1 Pack/15g	72	3	478	9	64	20	4
Beef, 55% Less Saturated Fat, KP Snacks*	1 Pack/34g	172	9	505	3.7	61.8	26.4	2.2
Beef, Big Hoops, Hula Hoops*	1 Pack/50g	250	12	499	3.8	65	24	2.8
Cheese & Onion 55% Less Saturated Fat, KP Snacks*	1 Bag/34g	175	9.7	515	3.6	61	28.5	1.9
Cheese & Onion, KP Snacks*	1 Pack/24g	120	5.8	502	3.8	66	24	2.5
Original, 55% Less Saturated Fat, KP Snacks*	1 Bag/34g	172	8.8	507	3.3	63	26	2.2
Ready Salted, Puft, KP Snacks*	1 Pack/15g	72	3.2	482	8.3	64	21	4
Salt & Vinegar, 50% Less Saturated Fat, KP Snacks*	1 Pack/25g	128	7	510	3.1	60.9	28.2	1.8
Salt & Vinegar, KP Snacks*	1 Pack/24g	122	5.8	507	3.4	66	24	2.2
Salt & Vinegar, Puft, KP Snacks*	1 Pack/15g	72	3	478	8.1	63	20	3.9
Spicy, Big, KP Snacks*	1 Serving/30g	162	10.8	541	4.9	44	36	8.2
Sweet Chilli, Puft, KP Snacks*	1 Pack/15g	71	3	474	8.1	64	20	4
Tangy Cheese, Flavarings, KP Snacks*	1 Serving/30g	161	10.8	538	5	44	36	8.1

H

ICE CREAM

	Measure INFO/WEIGHT	per Measure KCAL	FAT	Nutrition Values per 100g / 100ml KCAL	PROT	CARB	FAT	FIBRE
Praline, Carte d'Or*	1 Serving/100g	225	11	225	4	27	11	0
Baked Alaska, Ben & Jerry's*	1 Serving/100g	260	15	260	4	29	15	0.1
Banana, Pot, Yeo Valley*	1 Pot/100g	171	5.6	171	3.6	26.1	5.6	0.2
Bananas Foster, Haagen-Dazs*	1 Serving/125ml	260	15	208	3.2	22.4	12	0
Banoffee Fudge, Sainsbury's*	1/8 Pot/67g	119	4	178	2.8	28.7	5.9	0.2
Banoffee, Haagen-Dazs*	1 Serving/120ml	274	15.6	228	4	23	13	0
Bar, Belgian Chocolate & Vanilla, Giant, M&S*	1 Bar/120g	384	26.3	320	3.5	27.7	21.9	0.1
Belgian Chocolate, Haagen-Dazs*	1 Sm Tub/78g	249	16.2	318	4.6	28.4	20.7	0
Belgian Milk Chocolate, Tesco*	1 Lolly/75g	241	15.4	321	3	31.2	20.5	0
Berry Neighbourly, Ben & Jerry's*	1 Scoop/44g	123	7	279	3.5	29	16	0
Birthday Cake, Asda*	1 Scoop/50ml	42	0.8	83	4.1	12	1.7	4.5
Birthday Cake, High Protein, Halo Top*	1 Scoop/50g	30	1	59	4	12	2	2.5
Black Treacle, Northern Bloc*	1 Sm Tub/120ml	149	5.2	124	2.9	19.6	4.3	0
Blondie Brownie, Ben & Jerry's*	1 Scoop/43g	109	6	253	4.2	29	14	0
Blueberries & Cream, Minicup, Haagen-Dazs*	1 Minicup/87g	212	14	244	4.1	20.3	16.1	0.5
Blueberry, Gelateria, Carte d'Or*	2 Scoops/56g	110	4.1	190	28	31	7	0
Bob Marleys One Love, Ben & Jerry's*	1 Scoop/45g	123	6.3	273	3.2	33	14	0
Bounty, Mini Bar, Mars*	1 Bar/25ml	72	4.8	288	4.5	24.8	19	1
Caffe Latte, The Best, Morrisons*	1/5 Tub/100ml	144	6.6	144	2.9	18	6.6	0.4
Candy Bar, Halo Top*	¼ Tub/118g	90	3.7	76	4.3	14	3.1	2.3
Cappuccino, Tesco*	1 Scoop/54g	121	4.5	224	2.3	34.8	8.3	0.2
Cappuccino, Thorntons*	1oz/28g	61	3.6	218	4.4	20.7	12.9	0
Caramel Biscuit & Cream, Minicup, Haagen-Dazs*	1 Minicup/87g	249	16.1	286	4.6	25.5	18.4	0.1
Caramel Chew Chew, Classic Mix, Minicup, Ben & Jerry's*	1 Minicup/100g	271	15	271	3.6	30	15	0
Caramel Craze, Organic, Tesco*	1 Serving/100g	253	15.3	253	3.3	25.5	15.3	0
Caramel Sensation, Baileys*	1 Ice Cream/73g	262	16.8	359	3.2	34	23	0
Caramel Swirl, Gelato, Haagen-Dazs*	1 Mini Tub/72g	139	5.3	193	5.1	23.2	7.4	6.4
Caramel, Chew Chew, Ben & Jerry's*	1 Scoop/45g	122	6.8	270	3.5	28	15	0
Caramel, Cookie Fix, Moophoria, Ben & Jerry's*	2 Scoops/61g	128	4.3	210	3.5	33	7	0
Caramel, Pecan, Jude's*	1 Scoop/50g	90	5.2	180	3	18.6	10.3	0
Caramel, with Caramel Pieces, Carte d'Or*	1 Serving/100g	230	7.4	230	2.9	38	7.4	0
Caramella, Sundae, Tesco*	1 Sundae/80g	165	5.5	205	2.2	32.9	6.8	1.9
Caramella, Tesco*	1 Serving/51g	120	5.5	235	2.6	32	10.7	1.1
Cheesecake Brownie, Ben & Jerry's*	1 Serving 100g	260	16	260	4	26	16	0
Cheesecake, Strawberry, Haagen-Dazs*	2 Scoops/86g	226	12.3	262	3.8	29.4	14.3	0.4
Choc Choc Chip, Minicup, Haagen-Dazs*	1 Minicup/87g	245	15.9	281	4.5	24.3	18.2	0.9
Chocolate & Orange, Organic, Green & Black's*	1 Serving/100g	248	14.1	248	5	25.3	14.1	0.1
Chocolate Brownie, Salted Caramel, Kelly's Of Cornwall*	1 Serving/125ml	161	7.3	129	2.1	16.6	5.8	0.8
Chocolate Chip Cookie Dough, Halo Top*	1 Serving/118g	90	3.1	76	3.9	14	2.6	2.5
Chocolate Chip, Baskin Robbins*	1 Serving/75g	170	10	227	4	24	13.3	0
Chocolate Drizzle, Gelato, Mini Cup, Haagen-Dazs*	1 Mini Tub/72g	137	4.9	190	5.9	22.4	6.8	7.5
Chocolate Flavour, Average	*1 Serving/70g*	*149*	*7.9*	*212*	*4.1*	*23.7*	*11.3*	*0.6*
Chocolate Flavour, Soft Scoop, Sainsbury's*	1 Serving/70g	122	5.2	174	3.1	23.6	7.5	0.3
Chocolate Honeycomb, Co-Op*	¼ Pot/81g	186	10.5	230	4	26	13	0.3
Chocolate Salted Caramel, Minicup, Haagen-Dazs*	1 Minicup/87g	250	15.2	287	4.3	27.5	17.5	1.4
Chocolate, & Toasted Almond, Nobo*	1 Serving/100ml	191	14	191	2.9	13.4	14	0
Chocolate, Caramel, Cookie Dough, Topped, Ben & Jerry's	1 Scoop/45g	137	7.6	305	3.9	33	17	0
Chocolate, Creamy, Breyer's Delights*	1 Serving/100ml	62	1.7	62	3.9	9.3	1.7	0
Chocolate, Dairy Free, Halo Top*	¼ Tub/119g	70	3.1	59	2.3	11	2.6	2.2
Chocolate, Double, Belgian, Pot, Yeo Valley*	1 Pot/100g	212	9.5	212	4.6	26.2	9.5	1.6
Chocolate, Finest, Tesco*	1 Scoop/70g	254	17.7	363	4.4	28.9	25.3	1.1
Chocolate, Fudge, Brownie, Ben & Jerry's*	1 Scoop/42g	102	5.4	245	4.2	29	13	0
Chocolate, Fudge, Brownie, Non-Dairy, Ben & Jerry's*	1 Scoop/40g	88	4.3	222	2.9	26	11	0

I

ICE CREAM

	Measure INFO/WEIGHT	per Measure KCAL	FAT	Nutrition Values per 100g / 100ml KCAL	PROT	CARB	FAT	FIBRE
Chocolate, Gelatelli, Lidl*	1 Portion/50g	126	6.8	251	3.8	27.3	13.6	2.1
Chocolate, Haagen-Dazs*	1 Serving/120ml	269	18	224	4	19	15	0
Chocolate, Heavenly, Non Dairy, Swedish Glace, Wall's*	1 Serving/100g	206	11	206	3.3	23	11	0
Chocolate, High Protein, Halo Top*	1 Scoop/50g	34	1.2	68	4.2	11	2.3	1.5
Chocolate, Inspiration, Gelateria, Carte d'Or*	1 Serving/100g	210	9	210	3.5	28	9	0
Chocolate, Organic, Green & Black's*	1 Serving/125g	310	17.6	248	5	25.3	14.1	1.1
Chocolate, Santo Domingo, 1, Waitrose*	1 Serving/66g	220	16.4	333	4.5	22.8	24.8	0.5
Chunky Monkey, Non-Dairy, Ben & Jerry's*	1 Scoop/42g	109	5.8	262	2.4	30	14	0
Cinnamon Oat Cluster, High Protein, Breyer's Delights*	1 Scoop/50ml	34	0.8	68	4.1	10	1.7	0
Cinnamon Roll, Tub, Halo Top*	1 Serving/118g	90	3	76	4	15	2.5	2.5
Cioccolato, UAU!, Sammontana*	1 Serving/63g	84	1.6	134	8	17	2.6	4.1
Clotted Cream, Cornish, Kelly's Of Cornwall*	1 Serving/125g	282	18.6	226	2.9	20.1	14.9	0.1
Coconut, Alpro*	1 Serving/100g	167	8.2	167	0.2	16.1	8.2	12.5
Coconut, Carte d'Or*	1 Serving/100ml	125	7.1	125	1.8	14	7.1	0.5
Coconut, Toasted, Dairy Free, Halo Top*	1 Scoop/50g	34	1.8	68	2.2	14	3.5	4.2
Coffee Coffee Chip, Baskin Robbins*	1 Scoop/112g	264	15	236	3.8	25	13.4	0
Coffee Cupcake, High Protein, Breyer's Delights*	1 Scoop/50ml	33	0.6	66	4	10	1.3	0
Coffee, Finest, Tesco*	¼ Pot/93g	236	14.9	254	4.9	22.5	16	0
Coffee, Haagen-Dazs*	1 Serving/120ml	271	18.4	226	4.1	17.9	15.3	0
Coffee, Waitrose*	¼ Tub/125ml	292	16.4	234	3.6	25.4	13.1	0
Cookie Dough, Asda*	1 Scoop/50ml	42	1.4	84	3.8	11	2.8	3.4
Cookie Dough, Ben & Jerry's*	1 Scoop/43g	115	6.4	270	4	30	15	0
Cookie Dough, Choc Chip, High Protein, Giannis, Aldi*	1 Tub/273g	352	11.5	129	6.6	16	4.2	0.6
Cookie Dough, S'wich Up, Ben & Jerry's*	1 Scoop/41g	117	6.5	290	4.2	31	16	0
Cookie Dough, Tesco*	1 Serving/125g	301	14.2	241	3.3	31	11.4	0.6
Cookies & Cream, Breyer's Delights*	1 Scoop/50ml	35	1	70	3.9	11	1.9	0
Cookies & Cream, Haagen-Dazs*	1 Sm Tub/100ml	226	14.7	226	4	19.5	14.7	0
Crunchie, Blast, Cadbury*	1 Lolly/100ml	230	13.9	230	2.8	23.1	13.9	0.1
Dairy Cornish, Tesco*	1 Serving/49g	112	6	228	3.2	24.7	12.3	0.1
Dairy, Flavoured	*1oz/28g*	*50*	*2.2*	*179*	*3.5*	*24.7*	*8*	*0*
Dark Chocolate, & Almonds, Minicup, Haagen-Dazs*	1 Minicup/87g	252	16.6	289	5	23.1	19	2.6
Dark Chocolate, Lolly, Minis, Multipack, Aldi*	1 Lolly/35g	131	8.8	373	3.8	31	25	2.3
Double Chocolate, Nestle*	1 Serving/78g	248	14.3	320	4.8	33.7	18.4	0
Dulce De Leche, Minicup, Haagen-Dazs*	1 Minicup/87g	231	13.6	265	4.4	26.7	15.6	0.1
Eton Mess, Gelateria, Carte d'Or*	1 Serving/100g	181	5.8	181	2.2	30	5.8	0
Eton Mess, Kelly's Of Cornwall*	1 Serving/125ml	261	10.1	209	3.1	30.7	8.1	0.4
Exotic, Solero, Wall's*	1 Lolly/68g	98	2.1	144	1.7	27	3.1	0
Fig & Orange Blossom Honey, Waitrose*	1 Serving/100g	219	11.8	219	3.9	24.3	11.8	0.4
Fruit & Fresh Tropical, Carte d'Or*	1 Serving/83g	154	7.1	185	2.5	24.5	8.5	0
Galaxy, Mars*	1 Bar/60ml	203	13.4	339	4.7	29.7	22.4	0
Gelato, Vanilla	**1 Serving/100g**	**162**	**7.2**	**162**	**2.4**	**22.6**	**7.2**	**0.3**
Gingerbread, Specially Selected, Aldi*	1 Scoop/64g	169	8.3	264	4	33	13	0.6
Gingerbread, with Toffee Sauce, Sticky, Kelly's Of Cornwall*	1 Scoop/50g	62	3	123	1.8	15.3	6	0.1
Greek Yoghurt & Honey, Carte d'Or*	1 Serving/55g	114	4.8	207	2.7	29	8.8	0
Half Baked, Ben & Jerry's*	1 Scoop/41g	107	5.3	262	4.1	32	13	0
Hazelnut Chocolate, Alpro*	1 Serving/100g	177	9.4	177	0.8	17.2	9.4	8.6
Home Sweet Honeycomb, Ben & Jerry's*	1 Scoop/43g	114	6.4	266	3.8	30	15	0
Honeycomb & Caramel, Dairy, Sainsbury's*	2 Scoops/76g	180	8	236	3.2	32	10.5	0.6
Honeycomb Harvest, Mackies*	1 Serving/100g	209	10	209	4	25	10	0
Hunky Punky Chocolate, Dairy Free, Booja-Booja*	1 Tub/500ml	685	35	137	3.3	17	7	0
Karamel Sutra, Ben & Jerry's*	1 Scoop/43g	112	6	260	4	27	14	0
Kulfi Ice, Almond & Pistachio, Tubzee*	1 Stick/62g	102	4.3	165	3.6	21.8	6.9	0.5
Kulfi Ice, Original, Tubzee*	1 Scoop/50g	82	3.4	165	3.6	21.8	6.9	0.5

ICE CREAM

INFO/WEIGHT	Measure	per Measure		Nutrition Values per 100g / 100ml				
		KCAL	FAT	KCAL	PROT	CARB	FAT	FIBRE
Lavazza, Carte d'Or*	1 Serving/55g	120	5.4	218	3.5	29	9.9	0
Lemon Curd Swirl, Duchy Originals*	¼ Pot/101g	247	14.2	245	3.7	25.8	14.1	0
Lemon Meringue Bar, Heston from Waitrose, Waitrose*	1 Serving/60g	108	2.8	181	1.8	32	4.7	1.5
Lemon Meringue Pie, Aunt Bessie's*	1 Serving/50g	101	4.6	202	3.6	26	9.1	0.1
Lemon Tart, Dessert, Carte d'Or*	1 Dessert/130g	212	9.6	163	1.6	22	7.4	0
Lemon, Haagen-Dazs*	1 Serving/120ml	144	0.2	120	0.3	29.3	0.2	0
Light Chocolate Ices, Co-Op*	1 Ice/62g	121	8.1	195	2	18	13	0.5
Luscious Mint Choc Chip, Morrisons*	1 Serving/50g	99	5.2	198	2.9	23.1	10.5	0.7
Lychee Cream & Ginger, Haagen-Dazs*	1 Serving/120ml	258	12.7	215	3.6	26.1	10.6	0
Madagascan Vanilla, Pot, Yeo Valley*	1 Pot/100g	112	6.3	112	2.4	11.4	6.3	0
Magnum, Chocolate, & Hazelnut Praline, Tub, Wall's*	2 Scoops/100g	233	16	233	3	19	16	0
Magnum, Classic, Tub, Wall's*	1 Scoop/50g	108	7	217	2.4	21	14	0
Magnum, White, Tub, Wall's*	1 Scoop/50g	109	6.5	218	2.5	23	13	0
Maltesers, Mars*	1 Scoop/50g	64	3	128	1.4	17	6	0
Mango & Raspberry, Minicup, Haagen-Dazs*	1 Minicup/87g	211	11.5	243	3.3	27.2	13.3	0.6
Mango, 98% Fat Free, Bulla*	1 Serving/70g	94	1.1	134	4.2	25.4	1.6	0
Mango, Swirl, Passionate, Alpro*	1 Scoop/50g	76	3	153	2.1	16.9	6	10.5
Maple & Walnut, American, Sainsbury's*	1/8 Pot/68g	121	4.9	179	3.1	25.6	7.2	0.2
Milk Chocolate, & Chopped Almonds, Minis, Lolly, Aldi*	1 Lolly/38g	144	9.5	380	4.5	34	25	1.1
Milk Chocolate, Minis, Lolly, Multipack, G, Aldi*	1 Lolly/34g	120	7.5	353	3.4	35	22	0.5
Mince Pie, Farmhouse Dairy, TTD, Sainsbury's*	¼ Pot/100g	272	14.9	272	4.5	29.3	14.9	1.3
Mince Pie, Finest, Tesco*	¼ Pack/188g	476	22.1	254	3.9	33	11.8	1.1
Mini Mix, Chocolate Coated, Gelatelli, Lidl*	1 Lolly/36g	123	7.8	342	3.9	32	21.8	1.2
Mini Mix, Sorbet Coated, Gelatelli, Lidl*	1 Lolly/40g	64	2.4	160	1.7	24.7	5.9	0.6
Mint & Chocolate Flavour, Average	*1 Serving/70g*	*129*	*6.3*	*184*	*3*	*22.6*	*9*	*1.2*
Mint & Chocolate, Sainsbury's*	1 Serving/71g	137	6.7	192	3.4	23.5	9.4	0.4
Mint Chip, Breyer*	1 Serving/100ml	68	2.1	68	4	10	2.1	0
Mint Choc Chip Soft Scoop, Asda*	1 Serving/46g	86	4.1	189	2.9	24	9	0.3
Mint Chocolate Chip, Baskin Robbins*	1 Scoop/113g	270	16	239	4.4	24.8	14.2	0.9
Mint Chocolate, with Dark Chocolate Pieces, Carte D'or*	2 Scoops/50g	109	5.5	218	2.8	28	11	0
Mint, Majestic Luxury, Iceland*	1 Serving/80g	269	14.6	337	3.8	39.3	18.3	1.3
Mint, Viennetta, Wall's*	1 Scoop/50g	125	8	250	2.5	25	16	0
Minter Wonderland, Ben & Jerry's*	1 Scoop/44g	117	7.5	266	4	24	17	0
Mocha Coffee Indulgence, Sainsbury's*	¼ Pot/82g	178	10.6	217	3.2	22.1	12.9	0.1
My Carte D'or, Chocolate, Carte d'Or*	1 Tub/200ml	220	11	110	1.8	12.5	5.5	0.4
Neapolitan, Average	*1 Serving/70g*	*111*	*4.6*	*158*	*3.1*	*21.9*	*6.5*	*0.6*
Neapolitan, Brick, Tesco*	1 Serving/50g	82	3.4	163	3.3	21.9	6.9	0.4
Neapolitan, Soft Scoop, Sainsbury's*	1 Serving/75g	124	5.2	165	2.8	22.8	6.9	0.2
Neopolitian, Soft Scoop, Tesco*	1 Serving/43g	70	3	163	3.3	21.9	6.9	0.4
Non-Dairy, Reduced Calorie	*1oz/28g*	*33*	*1.7*	*119*	*3.4*	*13.7*	*6*	*0*
Oatmeal, High Protein, Halo Top*	1 Scoop/50ml	30	1	59	4	13	1.9	2.5
Organic, Madagascan Vanilla, Yeo Valley*	1 Serving/40ml	45	2.5	112	2.4	11.4	6.3	0.1
Panna Cotta, & Raspberry Swirl, Haagen-Dazs*	1 Serving/120ml	250	14.9	208	3.2	21	12.4	0
Peanut Butter Crunch, Haagen-Dazs*	2 Scoops/100g	343	24.4	343	8.4	21.7	24.4	1.7
Peanut Butter Cup, Ben & Jerry's*	1 Scoop/43g	138	9	320	7	25	21	0
Peanut Butter Cup, Dairy Free, Halo Top*	1 Scoop/50g	34	1.6	68	2.5	13	3.3	3.9
Peanut Butter, & Cookies, Non-Dairy, Ben & Jerry's*	1 Scoop/41g	113	6.5	280	4.3	29	16	0
Peanut Butter, Asda*	1 Scoop/50ml	38	1.1	75	3.7	9.3	2.2	4.6
Peanut Butter, High Protein, Morrisons*	1 Scoop/50ml	36	1.4	71	4.2	11.4	2.7	0.4
Peanut Chip, Vegan, Northern Bloc*	1 Sm Tub/120ml	163	5.6	136	3	20.2	4.7	0
Phish Food, Ben & Jerry's*	1 Scoop/43g	116	5.2	270	3.5	36	12	0
Pistachio, Haagen-Dazs*	1 Serving/120ml	276	18.8	230	4.4	17.7	15.7	0
Pistachio, Joe Deluccis Gelato*	1 Scoop/70g	148	6.6	211	2.4	28	9.4	0

ICE CREAM

INFO/WEIGHT	Measure KCAL	FAT	Nutrition Values per 100g / 100ml KCAL	PROT	CARB	FAT	FIBRE
Praline, Green & Black's*	1 Sm Pot/100g	191	10.8	191	3.5	20	10.8	0.9
Pralines & Cream, Haagen-Dazs*	1 Sm Tub/78g	213	12.9	272	3.9	27.2	16.5	0
Protein, Chocolate, WheyHey*	1 Scoop/50ml	42	1.8	84	6.9	7.8	3.7	1.1
Protein, Salted Caramel, WheyHey*	1 Scoop/50ml	38	1.7	76	7.1	7.2	3.4	0.1
Protein, Vanilla, WheyHey*	1 Pot/150ml	149	4.4	99	13.4	7.8	2.9	0
Raspberries, Clotted Cream, Waitrose*	1 Tub/500ml	790	39.5	158	2.9	18.9	7.9	0.1
Raspberry Ripple Brick, Tesco*	1 Serving/48g	71	2.9	148	2.6	20.8	6	0.2
Raspberry Ripple, Average	***1 Serving/70g***	***93***	***3.3***	***134***	***1.9***	***20.8***	***4.7***	***0.1***
Raspberry Ripple, Soft Scoop, Asda*	1 Scoop/46g	78	3.2	170	2.5	24	7	0.3
Raspberry Ripple, Soft Scoop, Tesco*	1 Scoop/25g	39	1.5	157	2.5	23	6.1	0.2
Raspberry, Delightful, Non Dairy, Swedish Glace, Wall's*	1 Serving/100g	211	9.4	211	2.6	29	9.4	0
Really Creamy Chocolate, Asda*	1 Serving/100g	227	11	227	4.1	28	11	0.4
Really Creamy Toffee, Asda*	1 Serving/120ml	146	6	122	1.8	17.5	5	0.1
Red Berries, Solero, Wall's*	1 Lolly/75g	111	2	148	1.4	29	2.7	0
Red Velvet, Halo Top*	1 Scoop/50g	38	1.2	76	4.2	14	2.5	2.5
Rhubarb Crumble, Aunt Bessie's*	1 Serving/50g	96	4.4	192	3.8	25	8.7	0.2
Rocky Road, Sainsbury's*	1/8 Pot/67g	137	4.9	205	3.8	30.9	7.3	1
Rum & Raisin, Haagen-Dazs*	1 Serving/120ml	264	17.6	220	3.4	18.6	14.7	0
Rum & Raisin, TTD, Sainsbury's*	¼ Pot/100g	220	10.4	220	3.8	27.7	10.4	1
Run & Raisin, with West Indies Rum, Carte d'Or*	1 Serving/100g	201	7.5	201	2.6	25	7.5	0
Salted Caramel Cake, High Protein, Breyers Delights*	1 Scoop/50ml	34	0.7	68	4	10.6	1.3	0
Salted Caramel, Almond, Alpro*	1 Scoop/50g	90	4.4	181	0.8	18.5	8.8	12.3
Salted Caramel, Brownie, Topped, Ben & Jerry's*	1 Scoop/45g	134	8	301	4.2	30	18	0
Salted Caramel, High Protein, Giannis, Aldi*	1 Scoop/50g	56	1.5	113	6.7	14	3	0.6
Salted Caramel, Irish, Nobo*	1 Serving/100ml	190	11.5	190	1.4	18.9	11.5	0
Salted Caramel, Minicup, Haagen-Dazs*	1 Minicup/87g	246	15	282	4.1	27.8	17.2	0
Salted Caramel, Tesco*	1 Lolly/68g	224	12.4	330	3.6	37.1	18.3	1.2
Salted Caramel, The Best, Morrisons*	1 Serving/100ml	188	11.5	188	2.8	17.9	11.5	0.5
Sea Salt Caramel, Dairy Free, Halo Top*	1 Scoop/50g	34	1.2	68	2.2	14	2.5	4
Sea Salt Caramel, Halo Top*	1 Scoop/50ml	58	1.8	116	7.2	23.2	3.6	4.4
Sea-Salted Caramel, Pot, Yeo Valley*	1 Pot/100g	189	7.1	189	3.3	27.6	7.1	0.1
Smarties Ice Cream Pot, Nestle*	1 Pot/69g	151	5.7	218	4.4	33.6	8.2	0
Smarties, Nestle*	1 Serving/50g	125	6	250	3.6	32.3	11.9	0.2
Sofa So Good , Ben & Jerry's*	1 Scoop/43g	110	5.5	259	4	31	13	0
Speculoos? Specu-Love, Ben & Jerry's*	1 Scoop/42g	129	8.3	310	3.8	28	20	0
Spice & All Things N'ice, Ben & Jerry's*	1 Scoop/50g	116	9	233	3.9	27	18	0
Stem Ginger with Belgian Chocolate, Waitrose*	1 Lolly/110g	255	14.4	232	2.9	25.5	13.1	1.7
Sticky Toffee Pudding, Co-Op*	1 Scoop/50g	110	5	220	1.9	30	10	0.6
Sticky Toffee, Cream O' Galloway*	1 Serving/30g	80	4.4	266	4.7	28.7	14.7	0
Strawberries & Cream, Minicup, Haagen-Dazs*	1 Minicup/87g	211	13.5	243	3.9	21.8	15.5	0.3
Strawberries & Cream, Haagen-Dazs*	1 Scoop/50g	122	7.8	244	3.9	22.2	15.5	0.3
Strawberry & Cream, Mivvi, Nestle*	1 Serving/60g	118	4.6	196	2.6	29.4	7.6	0.2
Strawberry Cheesecake, Ben & Jerry's*	1 Serving 100g	240	14	240	3	27	14	0
Strawberry Cheesecake, Co-Op*	1/6 Pot/86g	163	6	190	3	29	7	0.2
Strawberry, & Yuzu, Vegan, Northern Bloc*	1 Sm Tub/120ml	103	0	86	0	21.5	0	0
Strawberry, Carte d'Or*	1 Scoop/50g	46	1.4	91	1.4	15	2.9	0
Strawberry, Iced Dessert, Free From, Sainsbury's*	1 Serving/67g	106	6.3	159	1.7	16.4	9.5	0.5
Strawberry, Les Classiques, From Multipack, Carte d'Or*	1 Portion/50g	84	3	167	2.8	25	5.9	0
Strawberry, Pot, Yeo Valley*	1 Pot/100g	91	1.9	91	3.1	15.2	1.9	0
Strawberry, Soft Scoop, Tesco*	1 Serving/46g	78	3.4	170	2.8	23.1	7.4	0.1
Summer Berries & Cream, Minicup, Haagen-Dazs*	1 Minicup/88g	225	14.1	255	3	24.4	16	0.8
Taste of Carrot Cake, Iced Dessert, Perfect World*	1 Tub/120ml	170	12	142	3.1	14	10	2.6
Tiramisu, Haagen-Dazs*	1 Serving/120ml	303	19.6	253	3.8	22.7	16.3	0

ICE CREAM	Measure INFO/WEIGHT	per Measure KCAL	FAT	Nutrition Values per 100g / 100ml KCAL	PROT	CARB	FAT	FIBRE
Toffee & Honeycomb Sundaes, Weight Watchers*	1 Pot/98g	119	1.8	122	1.7	18.1	1.8	5.9
Toffee & Vanilla, Sainsbury's*	1 Serving/71g	146	6.8	205	3.1	26.7	9.5	0.1
Toffee Fudge, Soft Scoop, Asda*	1 Serving/50g	92	3.5	185	2.6	28	7	0
Toffee Vanilla, HE, Tesco*	1 Serving/73g	106	1.8	145	2.5	28.1	2.5	0.5
Triple Chocolate, Carte d'Or*	1 Serving/58g	122	5.7	210	3.7	27	9.8	0
Triple Chocolate, Dairy, Morrisons*	1 Serving/100g	233	10.8	233	3.8	30	10.8	0.4
Vanilla & Cinnamon, Finest, Tesco*	1 Serving/50g	114	7.4	229	3.9	20.2	14.7	0.4
Vanilla & Caramel, Tesco*	1 Scoop/53g	117	4.4	222	2.4	34.5	8.3	0.1
Vanilla Bean, Light, Deluxe, Lidl*	1 Serving/64g	110	2.5	172	4.7	26.6	3.9	0
Vanilla Bean, Purbeck*	1 Serving/100g	198	11.5	198	4.8	18.7	11.5	0
Vanilla Caramel Brownie, Haagen-Dazs*	1 Serving/150g	410	24.8	273	4.5	26.8	16.5	0
Vanilla Caramel Brownie, Minicup, Haagen-Dazs*	1 Minicup/83g	228	13.7	275	4.4	26.9	16.5	0.4
Vanilla Flavour, Soft Scoop, Sainsbury's*	1 Serving/71g	96	3.9	136	2.9	18.8	5.5	0.2
Vanilla Florentine, Specially Selected, Aldi*	1 Scoop/62g	148	7.4	238	4.4	28	12	0.7
Vanilla with Strawberry Swirl, Mini Tub, Weight Watchers*	1 Mini Tub/57g	81	2.2	142	2.5	23.4	3.9	0.2
Vanilla, & Chocolate Sauce, Organic, Green & Black's*	1 Serving/71g	170	9.8	240	4.3	24.6	13.9	0.6
Vanilla, & Chocolate, Viennetta, Wall's*	1 Serving/100ml	125	7	250	2.5	27	14	0
Vanilla, & Coconut, Nobo*	1 Serving/100ml	176	12.2	176	1.4	13.4	12.2	0
Vanilla, Alpro*	1 Serving/100g	166	8	166	2.3	16.4	8	9.8
Vanilla, Bean, Halo Top*	1 Serving/118ml	70	2	59	3.9	12	1.7	2.5
Vanilla, Ben & Jerry's*	1 Mini Tub/112g	258	16.8	230	4	20	15	0.1
Vanilla, Clotted Cream, 817, Oakhouse Foods Ltd*	1 Serving/76g	145	8	191	4.3	21.4	10.6	0.1
Vanilla, Dairy Milk, Cadbury*	1 Serving/120g	259	13.9	216	3.5	26	11.6	0.1
Vanilla, Dairy, Average	*1 Scoop/40g*	*80*	*4.4*	*201*	*3.5*	*23.6*	*11*	*0.7*
Vanilla, Dairy, Finest, Tesco*	1 Serving/92g	227	16	247	4.5	18	17.4	0.3
Vanilla, Dairy, Organic, Yeo Valley*	1 Serving/100g	206	11.2	206	4.9	21.3	11.2	0
Vanilla, Haagen-Dazs*	1oz/28g	70	4.8	250	4.5	19.7	17.1	0
Vanilla, High Protein, Asda*	1 Scoop/50g	35	0.9	70	3.9	9.9	1.8	2.7
Vanilla, Homemade, The Original, Blue Bell*	1 Serving/88g	180	9	205	4.6	22.7	10.2	0
Vanilla, Les Classiques, From Multipack, Carte d'Or*	1 Portion/50g	86	3.3	172	2.1	26	6.6	0
Vanilla, Light, Soft Scoop, Wall's*	1 Serving/100g	139	5.9	139	3	17	5.9	0
Vanilla, Low Fat, Average	*1 Scoop/50g*	*59*	*1.7*	*118*	*2.3*	*19.4*	*3.4*	*0.6*
Vanilla, Low Fat, Weight Watchers*	1 Scoop/125ml	75	2.1	60	1.1	9.7	1.7	0.1
Vanilla, Mackies*	1 Serving/100g	193	11	193	4	18	11	0
Vanilla, Madagascan, Light, 4.5% Fat, Carte d'Or*	1 Serving/100g	140	4.5	140	2.1	21	4.5	4
Vanilla, Madagascan, Low Sugar, Oppo*	1 Scoop/50g	36	1.8	72	3.5	9	3.7	0
Vanilla, Made with Madagascan Vanilla, Sainsbury's*	1 Serving/56g	101	4	181	3	25.6	7.2	0.6
Vanilla, Ms Mollys*	1 Scoop/40g	58	1.9	146	2.5	23.1	4.7	0.6
Vanilla, Non-Dairy, Average	*1 Serving/60g*	*107*	*5.2*	*178*	*3.2*	*23.1*	*8.7*	*0*
Vanilla, Really Creamy, Asda*	1 Serving/50g	98	5	196	3.5	23	10	0.1
Vanilla, Smart Price, Asda*	1 Scoop/40g	55	2.4	137	2.8	19	6	0.2
Vanilla, Smooth, Soy, Non Dairy, Swedish Glace, Wall's*	1 Scoop/50g	46	1.6	91	0.5	15	3.1	0
Vanilla, Soft Scoop, Tesco*	1 Serving/45g	69	2.3	153	2.5	23.6	5.2	0.7
Vanilla, Soft Scoop, Wall's*	1 Serving/100g	187	9.1	187	3	23	9.1	0
Vanilla, Toffee Crunch, Ben & Jerry's*	1 Tub/407g	1099	65.1	270	4	29	16	0.5
Vanilla, Vanilla Collection, Minicup, Haagen-Dazs*	1 Minicup/87g	217	14.7	249	4.3	19.9	16.9	0
Vanilla, Very, Soft Scoop, Iceland*	1 Scoop/42g	70	2.8	167	2.4	23.8	6.7	0.6
Vanilla, Waitrose*	1 Serving/100ml	156	10.8	156	2.6	12	10.8	0
Venezuelan Chocolate, Truly Irresistible, Co-Op*	1 Serving/100g	329	21	329	4.5	30	21	0.5
White Chocolate, Minis, Lolly, Multipack, G, Aldi*	1 Lolly/35g	128	8.4	366	3.2	34	24	0.5
with Cherry Sauce, Tesco*	1 Scoop/56g	114	4.1	204	2.1	32.4	7.3	0.2
ICE CREAM BAR								
Bounty, 100 Ml Bar, Mars*	1 Bar/100ml	278	18.5	278	3.4	24.7	18.5	0.7

ICE CREAM BAR

INFO/WEIGHT	Measure	per Measure		Nutrition Values per 100g / 100ml				
		KCAL	FAT	KCAL	PROT	CARB	FAT	FIBRE
Chocolate Covered	*1 Bar/40g*	*128*	*9.3*	*320*	*5*	*24*	*23.3*	*0*
Crunchie, Cadbury*	1 Bar/60ml	165	9.7	275	3	29.5	16.2	0.5
Dairy Milk, Caramel, Cadbury*	1 Bar/60ml	175	10.3	290	3.6	30.2	17.1	0
Dairy Milk, Lolly, Cadbury*	1 Lolly/100g	235	15	235	3	25.1	15	0
Maltesers, Mars*	1 Bar/45ml	113	7	252	2.9	25	15.6	0.7
Snickers, Mars*	1 Bar/53ml	179	10.4	337	6.5	33.2	19.6	0
Twix, Mars*	1 Serving/43ml	128	7.3	301	4	32	17.1	1.2

ICE CREAM CONE

INFO/WEIGHT	Measure	per Measure		Nutrition Values per 100g / 100ml				
		KCAL	FAT	KCAL	PROT	CARB	FAT	FIBRE
Average	*1 Cone/75g*	*140*	*6.4*	*186*	*3.5*	*25.5*	*8.5*	*0*
Choc Chip with Hazelnut, Flirt, Cornetto, Wall's*	1 Cone/70g	223	11.2	320	4	40	16	0
Chocolate & Nut, Co-Op*	1 Cone/110g	307	17	279	3.9	31	15.5	0.6
Chocolate & Vanilla, Good Choice, Iceland*	1 Cone/110ml	161	7.2	146	2.7	22.9	6.5	0.8
Chocolate Fudge, Gooey, Extreme, Nestle*	1 Cone/73g	218	10.4	299	3.8	37.4	14.3	2.5
Chocolate, & Caramel, Crunch, Cornetto, Wall's*	1 Cornetto/75g	247	15	329	3.6	34	20	0
Chocolate, Mini, Cornetto, Wall's*	1 Cone/36g	110	5.9	300	3.5	34	16	2
Chocolate, Vanilla & Hazelnut, Sainsbury's*	1 Cone/62g	190	10.5	306	4.5	33.9	16.9	0.6
Cookies & Cream, Tesco*	1 Cone/71g	197	7.9	277	3.9	39.8	11.1	1.4
Cornet, Wafer Cone, Askeys*	1 Cone/4g	13	0.1	376	10.7	77.6	2.5	0
Cornetto, GFY, Asda*	1 Cone/67g	162	6	241	3	37	9	0.1
Cornetto, Wall's*	1 Cone/75g	195	9.7	260	3.7	34.5	12.9	0
Cup Cornet, Wafer Cone, Askeys*	1 Cone/4g	13	0.1	376	10.7	77.6	2.5	0
Dairy Milk Buttons, Cadbury*	1 Cone/100ml	204	10.4	204	0	24.6	10.4	0.6
Extreme Raspberry, Cornetto, Nestle*	1 Cone/76g	177	6.2	233	2.4	36.4	8.2	1.5
Flake 99, Cadbury*	1 Cone/125ml	238	12	190	2.6	23.1	9.6	0.5
Mint Choc Chip, Iceland*	1 Cone/72g	210	9.4	292	3.3	40.4	13	1
Mint, Cornetto, Wall's*	1 Cornetto/60g	169	8.4	282	3.4	37	14	0
Peanut Butter, Love, Cornetto, Wall's*	1 Cornetto/75g	245	15	326	3.3	33	20	0
Salted Butter Caramel, Gelatelli*	1 Cone/76g	216	8.1	284	3.6	43.4	10.6	0
Salted Caramel, & White Chocolate, Extreme, Nestle*	1 Cone/73g	209	9.3	286	3.3	39.3	12.7	0.8
Strawberry & Vanilla, Iceland*	1 Serving/70g	182	7.6	260	3.3	37.5	10.8	0.7
Strawberry & Vanilla, Tesco*	1 Cone/69g	181	7	262	3.3	39	10.1	0.8
Strawberry, Cornetto, Wall's*	1 Cornetto/75g	198	8.2	264	2.1	40	11	0
Strawberry, Swirl Top, Co-Op*	1 Cone/75g	200	8.2	267	3	40	11	0.6
Toffee & Vanilla, Giannis, Aldi*	1 Cone/71g	195	7.1	275	4.5	42	10	0.6
Toffee, & Vanilla, Free From, Tesco*	1 Cone/65g	185	8.9	285	2.1	38	13.7	0.6
Toffee, & Vanilla, Sainsbury's*	1 Cone/72g	176	6.8	244	2.8	37.1	9.4	0.5
Vanilla, & Strawberry Sauce, Dairy Free, Swedish Glace*	1 Cone/105g	207	8.2	197	1.3	30	7.8	0
Vanilla, & Chocolate, Classico, Cornetto, Wall's*	1 Cornetto/60g	178	9.6	296	3.1	33	16	0

ICE CREAM ROLL

INFO/WEIGHT	Measure	per Measure		Nutrition Values per 100g / 100ml				
		KCAL	FAT	KCAL	PROT	CARB	FAT	FIBRE
Arctic, Average	*1 Serving/70g*	*140*	*4.6*	*200*	*4.1*	*33.3*	*6.6*	*0*

ICE CREAM SANDWICH

INFO/WEIGHT	Measure	per Measure		Nutrition Values per 100g / 100ml				
		KCAL	FAT	KCAL	PROT	CARB	FAT	FIBRE
'Wich, Ben & Jerry's*	1 Pack/117g	398	19.9	340	4	44	17	1
Cookie, Chocolate Chip, Dark, Gelatelli, Lidl*	1 Sandwich/65g	233	11	359	4.9	45.7	16.9	0
Neapolitan, Gelatelli, Lidl*	1 Sandwich/106g	233	9.5	220	4.9	29	9	1.9

ICE CREAM STICK

INFO/WEIGHT	Measure	per Measure		Nutrition Values per 100g / 100ml				
		KCAL	FAT	KCAL	PROT	CARB	FAT	FIBRE
Belgian Milk Chocolate Ices , Waitrose*	1 Bar/62g	208	12.7	338	4	33.5	20.6	1.6
Black Forest, Majestic, Iceland*	1 Ice Cream/63g	210	13.2	333	3.4	30.8	20.9	3.6
Chocolate, & Almond, Tesco*	1 Stick/77g	268	18	348	4.5	29.2	23.4	1.2
Chocolate, Feast, Wall's*	1 Lolly/70g	245	16.1	350	3.6	31	23	0
Chocolate, Milk, & Almond, Mini Belgian, Morrisons*	1 Stick/35g	126	8.2	360	4.1	32.8	23.3	1.1
Chocolate, Milk, Mini Belgian Selection, Morrisons*	1 Stick/35g	117	7.3	334	3	33.5	20.8	0.5
Chocolate, Milk, Mini, Tesco*	1 Lolly/35g	119	7.7	341	3.1	31.9	22.2	0.9
Chocolate, Milk, Rich, Mini Belgian Selection, Morrisons*	1 Stick/35g	117	7.4	334	3.4	32.3	21	1.2

I

	Measure INFO/WEIGHT	per Measure KCAL	per Measure FAT	Nutrition Values per 100g / 100ml KCAL	PROT	CARB	FAT	FIBRE
ICE CREAM STICK								
Chocolate, Mini Milk, Wall's*	1 Lolly/23g	32	0.7	138	4.4	22	3.2	0
Chocolate, White, Mini Belgian Selection, Morrisons*	1 Stick/35g	119	7.5	340	3	33.7	21.5	0.2
Chocolate, White, Tesco*	1 Lolly/75g	255	17.5	341	3.3	29.4	23.4	0
Coconut, & Vanilla, The Coconut Collaborative*	1 Lolly/81g	230	14.3	284	1.3	25.9	17.7	8.3
Dark Chocolate, & Nordic Berry, Nuii*	1 Ice Cream/66g	241	15.2	365	3.8	33	23	3.3
Peanut Butter, Haagen-Dazs*	1 Ice Cream/70g	290	22.1	414	8.4	23.1	31.5	2.3
Peanut Butter, Swirl, Halo Top*	1 Bar/58g	100	5	172	9.1	16	8.6	6.9
Raspberry, & Chocolate, Triple Dipped, Majestic, Iceland*	1 Ice Cream/69g	267	17.3	386	3.3	36.2	25	1.8
Salted Caramel, & Australian Macadamia, Nuii*	1 Ice Cream/68g	246	14.3	361	3.8	38	21	0.8
Speculoos, Caramel Biscuti, & Cream, Haagen-Dazs*	1 Bar/70g	258	18.4	369	4.9	28.1	26.3	0.1
Stem Ginger, 1, Waitrose*	1 Ice Cream/79g	287	17.2	364	4.1	37.5	21.8	0.6
Strawberry, Refreshing, Non Dairy, Swedish Glace, Wall's*	1 Lolly/37g	117	7.8	317	2.3	29	21	0
Vanilla, Chocolate Covered, Swedish Glace, Wall's*	1 Ice Cream/37g	105	6.6	285	1	30	18	0
Vanilla, Mini Milk, Wall's*	1 Lolly/23g	30	0.7	130	3.9	22	3.1	0
ICE LOLLY								
Assorted, Iceland*	1 Lolly/51g	33	0	65	0	16.2	0	0
Baby, Tesco*	1 Lolly/32g	26	0	80	0.1	20	0	0.1
Blackcurrant Split, Iceland*	1 Lolly/75g	61	2.4	81	1.1	12	3.2	0.1
Blackcurrant, Dairy Split, Sainsbury's*	1 Lolly/73ml	88	2.6	121	1.8	20.4	3.6	0.1
Blackcurrant, Ribena*	1 Lolly/35ml	25	0	68	0	16.4	0	0
Blue Raspberry, & Tangy Cherry, Shockwave, Ice King*	1 Lolly/50g	38	0	76	0	18.8	0	0.2
Bubblegum, Calippo, Wall's*	1 Calippo/106g	90	0.5	85	0.5	21	0.5	0
Bubblegum, Tesco*	1 Lolly/59g	60	1.1	102	1.8	19.2	1.9	0.6
Cherry Tango, Liquid Ice, Britvic*	1 Lolly/65g	84	0.1	129	0.1	31	0.1	0.2
Chocolate Wonderpops, Sainsbury's*	1 Lolly/43g	118	8.3	276	2.6	21.8	19.4	0.7
Chocolate, Plain, Mini, Tesco*	1 Lolly/31g	94	6.6	304	3.1	24.8	21.4	1.2
Chocolate, with Chocolate Coating, & Core, Tesco*	1 Lolly/47g	157	10.6	335	3.1	29.2	22.6	1.5
Cider Refresher, Treats*	1 Lolly/70ml	54	0	77	0	19.2	0	0
Coconut, Creamy, Finest, Tesco*	1 Lolly/77g	77	1.6	100	0.4	19.6	2.1	0.6
Exotic Fruit, Ice Cream, Gelatelli, Lidl*	1 Lolly/110g	148	2.8	135	1.8	25.6	2.5	0
Exotic Fruit, Mini, HL, Tesco*	1 Lolly/31g	41	0.6	131	1	26.4	2	1
Fab, Nestle*	1 Lolly/58g	82	2.9	142	0.6	23.1	5.1	0.3
Fab, Strawberry, Mini, Nestle*	1 Lolly/35ml	47	1.6	133	0.5	22.5	4.6	0.3
Frozen Yoghurt, Mango, Greek Style, Claudi & Fin*	1 Mini Lolly/26g	29	1.3	112	2.7	12.9	5.2	0.5
Fruit Blaster, Rowntree's*	1 Lolly/80ml	54	0	67	0.1	15.8	0	0.3
Fruit Flavour, Assorted, Basics, Sainsbury's*	1 Lolly/50g	33	0	66	0	16.5	0	0
Fruit Fusion, Mini, Farmfoods*	1 Lolly/45ml	36	0	79	0.2	19.2	0.1	0.2
Fruit Ices, Made with Orange Juice, Del Monte*	1 Lolly/75ml	69	0.1	92	1.2	21.5	0.1	0.2
Fruit Luxury, Mini, Co-Op*	1 Lolly/45g	58	2.7	130	2	18	6	0.2
Fruit Pastilles, Rowntree's*	1 Lolly/65ml	61	0	94	0.2	23.2	0	0
Fruit Split, Waitrose*	1 Lolly/73g	91	2.6	124	2.5	21.7	3.6	0.4
Fruits of the Forest, Ice Cream, Gelatelli, Lidl*	1 Lolly/110g	145	2.8	132	1.9	24.5	2.5	0
Fruity, Helter Skelter, Tesco*	1 Lolly/70g	51	0.1	74	0.2	18.1	0.1	0
Ice Burst, Aldi*	1 Lolly/60g	67	1.1	112	0.5	24	1.8	0.5
Icicles, All Flavours, Freezepops, Calypso*	1 Lolly/50ml	1	0	1	0	0.3	0	0
Lemon & Blackcurrant, Twister, Wall's*	1 Lolly/71g	68	0.4	96	0.7	21	0.6	0
Lemon & Lime, Mini, Calippo, Wall's*	1 Mini/78g	70	0.4	90	0.5	21	0.5	0
Lemon & Lime, Mini, Lemon Core, Twister, Wall's*	1 Mini/39g	42	0.5	107	0.6	22	1.2	0
Lemon & Lime, Mini, Strawberry Core, Twister, Wall's*	1 Mini/39g	41	0.5	105	0.6	22	1.2	0
Lemon & Lime, Twister, Wall's*	1 Lolly/71g	76	0.9	107	0.5	22	1.2	0
Lemon Sorbet, Mercadona*	1 Lolly/63g	38	0.2	61	0.5	32.4	0.3	8
Lemonade & Cola, Morrisons*	1 Lolly/55ml	36	0	65	0	16.2	0	0
Lemonade Flavour, R White*	1 Lolly/75ml	56	1.1	75	0.5	15.1	1.5	0.1

ICE LOLLY

	Measure INFO/WEIGHT	per Measure KCAL	FAT	Nutrition Values per 100g / 100ml KCAL	PROT	CARB	FAT	FIBRE
Mango & Passion Fruit Smoothie, Waitrose*	1 Lolly/73g	60	0.3	82	0.7	18.9	0.4	0.7
Milk, Blue Parrot Cafe, Sainsbury's*	1 Lolly/30ml	34	1	113	2.7	18	3.3	0.3
Mint Chocolate, Tesco*	1 Lolly/47g	160	10.9	342	2.7	30	23.2	1.1
Mixed Berry, Helter Skelter, Tesco*	1 Lolly/75g	77	0.1	104	0.1	25.5	0.1	0.1
Mixed Fruit, Vimto*	1 Lolly/45ml	39	0.2	87	0.5	20.9	0.5	0.2
Morrisons*	1 Lolly/100g	30	0	30	0	7.4	0	0
No Added Sugar, Tesco*	1 Lolly/32g	26	0	80	0.1	20	0	0.1
Nobbly Bobbly, Nestle*	1 Lolly/70ml	219	11.6	312	2.9	38.1	16.5	0.6
Orange Juice, Co-Op*	1 Lolly/73g	51	0.1	70	0.4	17	0.1	0.1
Orange Juice, Freshly Squeezed, Finest, Tesco*	1 Lolly/80ml	89	0	111	0.7	27	0	0
Orange Juice, Freshly Squeezed, Waitrose*	1 Lolly/73g	88	0.1	120	0.6	29.7	0.1	0
Orange, Average	*1 Lolly/72g*	*66*	*0*	*92*	*0.4*	*22.4*	*0*	*0.1*
Orange, Calippo, Wall's*	1 Calippo/105g	100	0.5	95	0.5	23	0.5	0
Orange, Lidl*	1 Lolly/50g	50	0	100	0.5	24.4	0	0
Orange, Mini, Calippo, Wall's*	1 Mini/79g	75	0.4	95	0.5	23	0.5	0
Pineapple & Coconut Colada, Waitrose*	1 Lolly/73ml	79	1.5	108	1	21	2.1	0.6
Pineapple, Dairy Split, Sainsbury's*	1 Lolly/72ml	84	2.6	116	1.8	19	3.6	0.1
Pineapple, Real Fruit Juice, Sainsbury's*	1 Lolly/73ml	55	0.1	76	0.1	19	0.1	0.1
Pop Up, CBY, Asda*	1 Lolly/80ml	65	0	81	0	20.1	0	0.3
Push Up, Various, Swizzels*	1 Ice Lolly/56ml	19	0	34	0	8	0	0
Raspberry, Real Fruit Juice, Sainsbury's*	1 Lolly/72g	62	0.1	86	0.3	21	0.1	0.1
Raspberry, Smoothie, Iced, Del Monte*	1 Lolly/90ml	84	0	94	0.3	22.8	0	0.8
Real Fruit, Dairy Split, Sainsbury's*	1 Lolly/73ml	100	3.1	137	2.1	22.8	4.2	0.1
Refresher, Fruit Flavour, Bassett's*	1 Lolly/45g	56	0.7	125	1.6	26	1.6	0.3
Rocket, Asda*	1 Lolly/60g	44	0.3	73	0.5	17	0.5	0.6
Rocket, Co-Op*	1 Lolly/60g	42	0	70	0	17	0	0
Rocket, Essential, Waitrose*	1 Lolly/58ml	42	0.1	72	0.4	16.8	0.2	0.7
Rocket, Sainsbury's*	1 Lolly/60g	50	0.3	83	0.5	19.9	0.5	0.5
Rocket, Tesco*	1 Lolly/60g	39	0.1	66	0.4	15.2	0.2	0.6
Scooby Doo, Freezepops, Calypso*	1 Lolly/45ml	13	0	28	0	7	0	0
Scottish Raspberry, The Best, Morrisons*	1 Lolly/73ml	63	0.1	86	0.5	20.3	0.2	0.6
Seriously Fruity, Mango Sorbet, Waitrose*	1 Lolly/100ml	79	0.3	79	0.8	18.4	0.3	0.5
Solero, Peach Organic, Solero, Wall's*	1 Solero/52g	60	0.3	115	0.5	27	0.5	0
Strawberries & Cream, Cadbury*	1 Lolly/100ml	225	11.7	225	2.9	27	11.7	0
Strawberry Split, Average	*1 Lolly/72g*	*78*	*2.3*	*108*	*1.5*	*18.5*	*3.2*	*0.2*
Strawberry Split, Co-Op*	1 Lolly/71ml	75	2.1	105	1	17	3	0.1
Strawberry, & Chocolate, with Sugar Balls, Tesco*	1 Lolly/47g	137	6.9	293	2.2	37.9	14.7	0.5
Strawberry, Blackcurrant & Vanilla, Mini, Twister, Wall's*	1 Lolly/50ml	38	0.3	77	0.7	16	0.7	0
Strawberry, Fruit Split, Iceland*	1 Lolly/73g	77	2.4	105	0.9	17.8	3.3	0.5
Strawberry, Orange & Pineapple, Rocket, Iceland*	1 Lolly/47g	38	0	81	0	20.2	0	0.1
Traffic Light, Co-Op*	1 Lolly/52g	55	0.4	105	0.4	25	0.8	0
Tropical, Giannis, Aldi*	1 Lolly/75g	112	3.2	150	1.8	26	4.3	0.6
Tropical, Mmmm, Tesco*	1 Lolly/73g	109	3.1	150	1.2	26.6	4.3	0.4
Vimto, Ice Pop, Vimto*	1 Pop/50ml	4	0	7	0	1.7	0	0
Watermelon, Rowntree's*	1 Lolly/73ml	61	0.3	83	0.1	19	0.4	0.3
Whirlz, Giannis, Aldi*	1 Lolly/50g	49	0.9	98	0	17.4	1.8	0
Zoom, Nestle*	1 Lolly/58ml	54	0.4	93	0.9	20.6	0.7	0

IRN BRU

	Measure INFO/WEIGHT	per Measure KCAL	FAT	Nutrition Values per 100g / 100ml KCAL	PROT	CARB	FAT	FIBRE
Diet, Sugar Free, Barr's*	1 Can/330ml	2	0	1	0.5	0	0	0
Original, Barr's*	1 Bottle/500ml	100	0	20	0.5	4.8	0	0

	Measure INFO/WEIGHT	per Measure KCAL	FAT	Nutrition Values per 100g / 100ml KCAL	PROT	CARB	FAT	FIBRE
JACKFRUIT								
Canned, in Water, Drained, Summer Pride*	1 Can/250g	55	0.8	22	0.8	2.3	0.3	3.2
Canned, in Water, Tesco*	½ Can/205g	78	0.2	38	0.9	5.9	0.1	5
in Chilli Sauce, Vegan, Waitrose*	1 Pot/350g	259	13	74	2.8	4.7	3.7	5.1
Pulled, BBQ, Sweet & Smoky, Sainsbury's*	½ Pack/175g	126	0.9	72	1.6	13.2	0.5	4.9
Raw, Average, Flesh Only	*1 Portion/165g*	*155*	*0.5*	*94*	*1.5*	*24.4*	*0.3*	*1.6*
Shredded, in Mexican Sauce, Vegan, Tesco*	1 Pouch/150g	117	4.6	78	2.3	8.9	3.1	2.4
Shredded, in Thai Green Sauce, Vegan, Tesco*	1 Pack/150g	120	8.8	80	1.4	4.6	5.9	1.6
JALFREZI								
Chicken, & Rice, Serves 1, Tesco*	1 Pack/509g	636	25.9	125	5.3	11.4	5.1	5.9
Chicken, & Coriander Rice, TTD, Sainsbury's*	1 Pack/473g	501	15.1	106	6.2	13.2	3.2	3.1
Chicken, & Pilau Rice, Sainsbury's*	1 Pack/417g	596	17.5	143	7	17.9	4.2	2.9
Chicken, 138, Oakhouse Foods Ltd*	1 Serving/400g	388	11.6	97	5.9	11.1	2.9	1
Chicken, Asda*	1 Pack/340g	415	20.4	122	10	7	6	1.6
Chicken, Canned, Tesco*	½ Can/200g	190	6.8	95	10.8	4.1	3.4	1.4
Chicken, Diet Chef Ltd*	1 Pack/300g	285	5.7	95	10.5	9	1.9	2.2
Chicken, Finest, Tesco*	1 Pack/350g	402	16.4	115	10.4	6.9	4.7	1.2
Chicken, Hot & Spicy, Sainsbury's*	½ Pack/200g	228	11.4	114	12.8	2.9	5.7	1
Chicken, Indian Takeaway, Tesco*	½ Pack/194g	162	7.8	84	7.1	3.9	4	1.8
Chicken, with Lemon Pilau Rice, Finest, Tesco*	1 Pack/493g	665	21.7	135	6.9	16.4	4.4	1.8
Chicken, with Pilau Rice, Charlie Bigham's*	½ Pack/422g	586	27.4	139	6.5	14.3	6.5	0
Chicken, with Pilau Rice, Indian Cuisine, Aldi*	1 Pack/450g	673	21.3	158	8.7	18	5	3.3
Chicken, with Pilau Rice, Taste of India, Tesco*	1 Pack/421g	445	10.1	106	7.3	12.2	2.4	3
Chicken, with Pilau Rice, Tesco*	1 Pack/460g	506	17.5	110	5.3	13.6	3.8	0.9
Chicken, with Rice, Ready Meal	*1 Serving/450g*	*557*	*18.9*	*124*	*6.9*	*14.5*	*4.2*	*1.5*
Chicken, with Rice, Ready Meal, Healthy Range	*1 Serving/400g*	*363*	*5.7*	*91*	*7.1*	*12.3*	*1.4*	*1.4*
Vegetable, Waitrose*	1 Pack/400g	256	16	64	2.2	4.7	4	3.7
JAM								
Apricot, Average	*1 Tbsp/15g*	*37*	*0*	*248*	*0.2*	*61.6*	*0*	*1.5*
Black Cherry, Average	*1 Tsp/5g*	*12*	*0*	*247*	*0.4*	*61.2*	*0.3*	*0.4*
Blackberry, Extra Special, Asda*	1 Tbsp/15g	29	0.1	190	0.9	45	0.7	0
Blackcurrant, Average	*1 Tbsp/15g*	*38*	*0*	*250*	*0.2*	*62.3*	*0*	*1*
Blackcurrant, Reduced Sugar, Average	*1 Tsp/6g*	*10*	*0*	*178*	*0.4*	*44.4*	*0.2*	*1*
Blueberry, Best, Hartley's*	1 Tsp/20g	49	0	244	0.3	60.6	0.1	0
Damson, Extra Fruit, Best, Hartley's*	1 Tsp/5g	12	0	244	0.2	60.8	0	0
Fig	*1 Tsp/15g*	*36*	*0*	*242*	*0.5*	*60*	*0*	*0*
Golden Peach, Rhapsodie De Fruit, St Dalfour*	1 Tsp/10g	23	0	227	0.5	56	0.1	1.3
Kiwi & Gooseberry, 66% Fruit, Asda*	1 Serving/30g	56	0.2	187	0.5	45	0.5	0
Mixed Fruit, Average	*1 Tbsp/15g*	*38*	*0*	*252*	*0.3*	*63.5*	*0*	*0.5*
Peach, & Ginger, Eswatini*	1 Tbsp/15g	38	0	252	0.5	66	0.1	0
Peach, Pure, Summerland Sweets*	1 Tsp/5g	25	0	500	0	130	0	0
Plum, & Damson, Soft Set, British, M&S*	1 Tsp/5g	13	0	264	0.4	63.7	0.5	1.3
Plum, Tesco*	1 Serving/50g	130	0	261	0.2	64.4	0	0.6
Raspberry, Average	*1 Tbsp/15g*	*36*	*0*	*239*	*0.6*	*58.6*	*0.1*	*0.9*
Raspberry, Reduced Sugar, Average	*1 Tsp/6g*	*10*	*0*	*160*	*0.5*	*39.3*	*0.2*	*0.6*
Raspberry, Seedless, Average	*1 Tsp/10g*	*26*	*0*	*257*	*0.4*	*63.6*	*0*	*0.3*
Rhubarb & Ginger, Baxters*	1 Tsp/15g	40	0	264	0.4	65	0.1	0.8
Strawberry & Redcurrant, Reduced Sugar, Streamline*	1 Tbsp/15g	29	0	192	0.4	46.8	0.3	0
Strawberry, Average	*1 Tsp/10g*	*24*	*0*	*243*	*0.3*	*60.2*	*0.1*	*0.7*
Strawberry, Reduced Sugar, Average	*1 Tbsp/15g*	*28*	*0*	*187*	*0.4*	*45.8*	*0.3*	*0.2*
Wild Blackberry Jelly, Baxters*	1 Tsp/15g	32	0	210	0	53	0	1.2
JAMBALAYA								
Cajun Chicken, Cooked, BGTY, Sainsbury's*	1 Pack/400g	381	7.2	100	6.2	12.7	1.9	3.3
Chicken & Prawn, World Cafe, Waitrose*	1 Pack/350g	413	12.2	118	5.3	15.3	3.5	2.3

J

	Measure INFO/WEIGHT	per Measure KCAL	per Measure FAT	Nutrition Values per 100g / 100ml KCAL	PROT	CARB	FAT	FIBRE
JAMBALAYA								
Chicken, Calorie Controlled, Counted, Morrisons*	1 Pack/370g	389	4.1	105	6.8	15.7	1.1	2.2
Chicken, HL, Tesco*	1 Pack/385g	319	5.2	83	7.7	9	1.3	2.1
Chicken, Ready Meal, Inspired Cuisine, Aldi*	1 Pack/400g	440	5.6	110	6.9	16	1.4	2
Ready Meal, Average	***1 Pack/450g***	***569***	***18.2***	***126***	***6.4***	***15.7***	***4***	***1.3***
JELLY								
Apple & Watermelon, Low Calorie, Hartley's*	1 Serving/175g	5	0	3	0	0.3	0	0.3
Apple, & Watermelon, 10 Cal, Hartley's*	1 Pot/175g	7	0.2	4	0.1	0.2	0.1	0
Apple, No Added Sugar, Hartley's*	1 Pot/115g	7	0.3	6	0	1.1	0.3	0
Black Forest Gateau, 10 Cal, Hartley's*	1 Pot/175g	9	0.2	5	0.1	0.2	0.1	0
Blackcurrant & Tahitian Vanilla, M&S*	¼ Pack/143g	77	0.4	54	0.3	12.1	0.3	0.6
Blackcurrant, Low Cal, Pot, Asda*	1 Pot/175g	4	0	2	0	0.5	0	0
Blackcurrant, Made Up, Rowntree's*	¼ Jelly/140ml	100	0.1	71	1.4	16.4	0.1	0
Blackcurrant, Made Up, Sainsbury's*	¼ Jelly/150g	98	0	65	1.2	15.1	0	0
Blackcurrant, Ready to Eat, Pot, Hartleys*	1 Pot/124g	51	0.1	41	0.1	9.5	0.1	0
Blackcurrant, Sugar Free, Unprepared, Rowntree's*	1 Pack/24g	73	0	305	50	25	0	25
Blueberry & Blackcurrant, 10 Cal, Hartley's*	1 Pot/175g	4	0.2	2	0.1	0.2	0.1	0.1
Bramble, Tesco*	1 Serving/100g	257	0.1	257	0.3	63.7	0.1	1.3
Cherry Flavoured, Waitrose*	1 Pot/175g	87	0.5	50	0.3	11.3	0.3	0.2
Cloudy Lemonade, Pot, Hartley's*	1 Pot/183g	11	0.9	6	0.5	0.9	0.5	0
Crystals, Strawberry, Made Up, Tesco*	1 Serving/145g	9	0	6	1.3	0.3	0	0
Exotic Fruit, M&S*	1 Pot/175g	140	0.4	80	0.1	18.9	0.2	0.9
Fresh Fruit, M&S*	1 Pot/175g	131	0.2	75	0.2	18.4	0.1	0.3
Lemon Cheesecake, 10 Cal, Hartley's*	1Pot/175g	7	0.2	4	0.1	0.1	0.1	0
Lime Flavour, Cubes, Hartley's*	1 Cube/12g	36	0	296	5.1	68.9	0	0
Lime, Made Up, Rowntree's*	¼ Jelly/140ml	100	0.1	71	1.4	16.4	0.1	0
Made Up with Water, Average	***1oz/28g***	***17***	***0***	***61***	***1.2***	***15.1***	***0***	***0***
Mandarin & Pineapple, Sainsbury's*	1 Pot/125g	95	0.1	76	0.2	18.9	0.1	1.2
Orange, 10 Cal, Hartley's*	1 Pot/175g	4	0.2	2	0.1	0.3	0.1	0
Orange, Sugar Free, Crystals, Dry Weight, Hartley's*	1 Pack/26g	66	0	254	57.4	6.1	0	0
Orange, Sugar Free, Made Up, Hartley's*	1 Serving/145g	9	0.8	6	1.3	0.5	0.5	0
Orange, Sugar Free, Rowntree's*	1 Serving/140ml	8	0	6	1.4	0.1	0	0
Orange, Unprepared, Rowntree's*	1 Square/11g	33	0	296	4.4	69.6	0	0
Orange, with Mandarin Pieces, Tesco*	1 Pot/120g	92	0.1	77	0.1	18.7	0.1	0.5
Raspberry & Elderflower, Seriously Fruity, Waitrose*	1/6 Pack/103g	71	0.3	69	2.3	13.9	0.3	0.5
Raspberry Flavour, Sugar Free, Made Up, Rowntree's*	1 Serving/140ml	9	0	6	1.4	0.1	0	0
Raspberry Flavour, Tesco*	1 Serving/34g	22	0	64	1	15	0	0.1
Raspberry Glitter, Made Up, Hartley's*	1 Serving/150g	94	0	63	0	15.4	0	0
Raspberry, Crystals, Vegetarian, Just Wholefoods*	1 Pack/85g	293	0	345	0.5	85.7	0	0
Raspberry, Individual Pot, Waitrose*	1 Pot/175g	92	1.2	53	0.3	10.7	0.7	1.1
Redcurrant, Average	***1oz/28g***	***70***	***0***	***250***	***0.2***	***64.4***	***0***	***0***
Strawberry & Raspberry, Sainsbury's*	½ Pot/280g	230	0	82	0.2	20.2	0	1.2
Strawberry Flavour, Sugar Free, Made Up, Rowntree's*	1 Serving/140ml	10	0	7	1.5	0.1	0	0
Strawberry, Glitter, Made Up, Hartley's*	1 Serving/150g	94	0	63	0	15.4	0	0
Strawberry, Sugar Free, Crystals, Dry Weight, Hartley's*	1 Sachet/26g	73	0	280	56.8	13.1	0	0
Strawberry, Unprepared, Co-Op*	1 Pack/135g	402	0.1	298	5.5	69.1	0	0
Sugar Free, Dry, Tesco*	1 Pack/13g	36	0	285	55.4	15.6	0	0.2
JELLY BABIES								
Bassett's*	1 Sweet/6g	20	0	335	3.5	79.7	0	0
M&S*	1 Pack/125g	418	0	334	5.2	78	0	0
Mini, Rowntree's*	1 Sm Bag/35g	128	0	366	4.6	86.9	0	0
JELLY BEANS								
Average	***1 Serving/100g***	***365***	***0.1***	***365***	***0.1***	***91.2***	***0.1***	***0.1***
Jelly Belly*	35 Beans/40g	140	0	350	0	90	0	0

	INFO/WEIGHT	KCAL	FAT	KCAL	PROT	CARB	FAT	FIBRE
JERKY								
Beef, BBQ Flavour, Kings*	1 Bag/40g	116	1.9	291	36.3	26.3	4.9	1.3
Beef, Honey & Chipotle, Tesco*	1 Pack/40g	123	2.2	307	29.1	34.7	5.4	1.8
Beef, Honey BBQ, Wild West*	1 Pack/70g	216	2.2	308	29.6	39.6	3.2	1.1
Salmon, Hot & Spicy, Ready To Eat, Sainsbury's*	1 Pack/55g	263	17.5	479	27.8	20.1	31.9	0.5
Vegetable, Original Flavour, Prostrips, Kings*	1 Pack/25g	97	3.1	389	19.5	41.2	12.3	0
JUICE								
12 Fruits, Multivitamins, Tropicana*	1 Glass/150ml	70	0	47	0.5	11	0	0.6
Apple & Cranberry, Average	**1 Glass/250ml**	**114**	**0**	**46**	**0.1**	**10.2**	**0**	**0**
Apple & Elderflower, Copella*	1 Glass/250ml	108	0.2	43	0.4	10.2	0.1	0
Apple & Mango, Average	**1 Glass/200ml**	**108**	**0.1**	**54**	**0.3**	**12.6**	**0**	**0.1**
Apple & Orange, Fresh Up*	1 Serving/250ml	105	0	42	0	10.3	0	0
Apple & Raspberry, Average	**1 Serving/200ml**	**89**	**0.1**	**44**	**0.4**	**10.2**	**0**	**0.2**
Apple & Cherry, Sainsbury's*	1 Serving/200ml	96	0	48	0.3	10.8	0	0.8
Apple & Mango, 100% Pressed, Tesco*	1 Glass/150ml	72	0	48	0.4	10.7	0	0.9
Apple & Mango, Pressed, Waitrose*	1 Glass/100ml	54	0	54	0.3	12.6	0	0.9
Apple & Raspberry, Tropicana*	1 Glass/150ml	72	0	48	0.2	10.5	0	0.9
Apple & Rhubarb, Caxton Vale*	1 Glass/250ml	115	1	46	0.2	9.7	0.4	0
Apple & Rhubarb, Pressed, Cawston Press*	1 Serving/200ml	92	0.8	46	0.2	9.7	0.4	0
Apple, Cloudy, Not From Concentrate, Rio D'Oro, Aldi*	1 Glass/150ml	70	0.8	47	0.5	11	0.5	0.5
Apple, Cloudy, Pressed, Copella*	1 Glass/100ml	46	0	46	0.2	10.7	0	0.7
Apple, Pink Lady, Pressed, Eat Well, M&S*	1 Bottle/300ml	153	0.6	51	0.4	11.7	0.2	0.3
Apple, Pressed, 100%, Never From Concentrate, Tesco*	1 Glass/180ml	88	0	49	0.3	11.2	0	0.5
Apple, Pure, Average	**1 Glass/250ml**	**116**	**0.1**	**47**	**0.1**	**11.2**	**0**	**0**
Apple, Pure, Value, Tesco*	1 Glass/200ml	94	0.2	47	0.1	11.1	0.1	0.1
Apple, Raspberry, & Rhubarb, Waitrose*	1 Serving/150ml	63	0	42	0.2	10.2	0	0.4
Beetroot, Apple, & Rhubarb, Morrisons*	1 Glass/150ml	68	0.2	45	0.7	9.9	0.1	0.7
Beetroot, Natural, So Organic, Sainsbury's*	1 Pack/250g	105	1.2	42	0.9	8.2	0.5	1.9
Black Cherry, & Cinnamon, The Best, Morrisons*	1 Bottle/750ml	38	0	5	0	1.2	0	0
Blueberry, Blackcurrant & Cranberry, Innocent*	1 Serving/150ml	69	0	46	0	11.3	0	0
Breakfast, Ruby, Tropicana*	1 Glass/200ml	90	0	45	0.8	9.7	0	0.7
Carrot, Average	**1 Glass/200ml**	**48**	**0.2**	**24**	**0.5**	**5.7**	**0.1**	**0**
Carrot, Orange, & Apple, Cold Pressed, B Fresh *	1 Bottle/250ml	65	0	26	0	6.2	0	0
Chia Watermelon & Pomegranate, WOW, Planet Organic*	1 Bottle/250ml	122	3.8	49	2.3	5.6	1.5	2.2
Clementine, 100% Pure Squeezed, Tesco*	1 Serving/150ml	71	0	48	0.4	10.7	0	0.2
Clementine, Morrisons*	1 Serving/100ml	48	0.1	48	0.5	10.9	0.1	0.1
Cranberry, Average	**1 Bottle/250ml**	**139**	**0.2**	**56**	**0.1**	**13.4**	**0.1**	**0.3**
Cranberry, No Added Sugar, Average	**1 Glass/200ml**	**11**	**0.1**	**6**	**0.1**	**0.8**	**0**	**0**
Exotic, No Added Sugar, Morrisons*	1 Glass/150ml	24	0	16	0	3.6	0	0
Fruit, Tropical in Sparkling Spring Water, Light, Rio*	1 Can/330ml	17	0	5	0.1	1.1	0	0
Fruit, Tropical, Pure Premium, Tropicana*	1 Glass/200ml	98	0	49	0.5	11	0	0.8
Ginger, Boost, Shot, On the Go, Sainsbury's*	1 Shot/100ml	41	0.5	41	0.5	9.9	0.5	0.5
Grape, Purple, Welch's*	1 Serving/200ml	136	0	68	0.1	16.5	0	0
Grape, Red, Average	**1 Serving/100ml**	**62**	**0**	**62**	**0.2**	**15.2**	**0**	**0**
Grape, White, Average	**1 Can/160ml**	**95**	**0.1**	**60**	**0.2**	**14.3**	**0.1**	**0.1**
Grape, White, Sparkling, Non-Alcoholic, M&S*	1 Glass/125ml	90	0.1	72	0.2	17.9	0.1	0
Grapefruit, Pink, Average	**1 Glass/200ml**	**81**	**0.1**	**40**	**0.6**	**9**	**0**	**0.2**
Grapefruit, Pure, Average	**1 Glass/200ml**	**77**	**0.2**	**38**	**0.5**	**8.5**	**0.1**	**0.1**
Lemon, Fresh, Average	**1 Lemon/36ml**	**2**	**0**	**7**	**0.3**	**1.6**	**0**	**0.1**
Lemon, from Concentrate, Asda*	1 Tsp/5ml	1	0	22	0.5	1	0.5	0.5
Lemon, The Pantry, Aldi*	1 Tbsp/15ml	3	0.1	20	0.5	1.2	0.5	0.5
Lime, Fresh, Average	**1 Tsp/5ml**	**0**	**0**	**9**	**0.4**	**1.6**	**0.1**	**0.1**
Mandarin Orange, Tropicana*	1 Serving/200ml	94	0	47	0.6	10	0	0.8
Mango, Peach, Papaya, Pure, Premium, Tropicana*	1 Glass/200ml	88	0	44	0.5	9.8	0	0.1

J

JUICE

INFO/WEIGHT	Measure	per Measure KCAL	per Measure FAT	Nutrition Values per 100g / 100ml KCAL	PROT	CARB	FAT	FIBRE
Multivitamin, Fruit, Vitafit, Lidl*	1 Carton/250ml	135	0.2	54	0.3	12.5	0.1	0.5
Orange & Pineapple, Average	*1 Glass/120ml*	*56*	*0.6*	*46*	*0.4*	*10.5*	*0.5*	*0.5*
Orange & Grapefruit, Average	*1 Glass/200ml*	*84*	*0.2*	*42*	*0.8*	*9.2*	*0.1*	*0.4*
Orange & Lime, Tropicana*	1 Serving/250ml	115	0	46	1.1	9.4	0	0.6
Orange & Mango, Average	*1 Bottle/375ml*	*176*	*0.4*	*47*	*0.5*	*10.7*	*0.1*	*0.2*
Orange & Passionfruit, Tropicana*	1 Serving/200ml	94	0	47	0.8	10	0	0.7
Orange & Raspberry, Tropicana*	1 Bottle/330ml	139	0	42	0.4	9	0	0.8
Orange 100% from Concentrate, Farmfoods*	1 Serving/200ml	84	0.2	42	0.6	9.1	0.1	0.1
Orange with Bits, Freshly Squeezed, TTD, Sainsbury's*	1 Serving/249g	132	0	53	0.7	11.4	0	0.2
Orange with Bits, Innocent*	1 Glass/250ml	120	0	48	0.8	10.9	0	0.3
Orange with Bits, Not From Concentrate, Tesco*	1 Glass/250ml	110	0	44	0.4	10.6	0	0
Orange, Apple & Mango, Calypso*	1 Carton/200ml	92	0.4	46	0	11	0.2	0.1
Orange, Freshly Squeezed, Average	*1 Serving/200ml*	*66*	*0*	*33*	*0.6*	*8.1*	*0*	*1*
Orange, Freshly Squeezed, with Bits, 1, Waitrose*	¼ Bottle/250ml	108	0.2	43	0.7	9.5	0.1	0.5
Orange, From Concentrate, Lidl*	1 Serving/200ml	86	0.2	43	0.7	8.9	0.1	0.5
Orange, Mango & Passionfruit, Pure Squeezed, Waitrose*	1 Serving/250ml	130	0.8	52	0.6	10.9	0.3	0.3
Orange, Organic, Cold Pressed, Pip organic*	1 Serving/150ml	70	0.2	47	0.6	10.8	0.1	0
Orange, Pure from Concentrate, Carton, Value, Tesco*	1 Serving/250ml	115	0	46	0.5	10.4	0	0
Orange, Pure Premium, Smooth, No Bits, Tropicana*	1 Glass/200ml	96	0	48	0.8	10	0	0.4
Orange, Pure with Bits, Average	*1 Glass/200ml*	*90*	*0.1*	*45*	*0.6*	*10.2*	*0.1*	*0.1*
Orange, Pure, Smooth, Average	*1 Glass/200ml*	*88*	*0.1*	*44*	*0.7*	*9.8*	*0*	*0.2*
Orange, Pure, Smooth, From Concentrate, Sainsbury's*	1 Serving/200ml	84	0.2	42	0.5	9.1	0.1	0.1
Orange, Smooth, Freshly Squeezed, TTD, Sainsbury's*	1 Serving/249g	132	0	53	0.7	11.4	0	0.2
Orange, Smooth, Innocent*	1 Serving/200ml	76	0	38	0.7	8.2	0	0
Orange, Smooth, Pure, From Concentrate, Iceland*	1 Serving/200ml	94	0.2	47	0.5	10.4	0.1	0
Orange, Sparkling, 55, Britvic*	1 Bottle/275ml	135	0.3	49	0.3	11.3	0.1	0.1
Orange, Squeezed, Pure, M&S*	1 Serving/100ml	42	0.1	42	0.5	9.2	0.1	0.1
Orange, with Bits, 100%, Morrisons*	1 Serving/200ml	80	0.2	40	0.6	9	0.1	0.3
Pineapple, Average	*1 Glass/200ml*	*100*	*0.1*	*50*	*0.3*	*11.7*	*0.1*	*0.2*
Pomegranate, Pomegreat*	1 Glass/200ml	88	0	44	0.1	11.1	0	0
Prune, Average	*1 Serving/200ml*	*123*	*0.1*	*61*	*0.6*	*15.3*	*0.1*	*1.8*
Sweet Carrot & Orange, Shapers, Boots*	1 Serving/250ml	100	0.4	40	0.9	8.8	0.2	0.4
Tomato from Concentrate, Sainsbury's*	1 Glass/250ml	40	0.2	16	0.7	2.7	0.1	0.7
Tomato, Average	*1 Glass/200ml*	*40*	*0.1*	*20*	*0.8*	*4*	*0*	*0.4*
Tomato, Pressed, M&S*	1 Serving/200ml	36	0.2	18	0.5	3.2	0.1	1
Tomato, Rich & Savoury, Waitrose*	1 Serving/150ml	28	0.2	19	0.7	3.4	0.1	0.9
Tomato, Vitafit, Lidl*	1 Serving/250ml	47	0.5	19	0.8	2.9	0.2	0.7
Tropical made from Concentrate, Sainsbury's*	1 Glass/250ml	120	0.2	48	0.5	10.7	0.1	0.1
Tropical, Pure, Sainsbury's*	1 Glass/200ml	104	0.2	52	0.5	12	0.1	0.1
Turmeric Booster, Cold Pressed, Moju*	1 Shot/60ml	22	0.1	36	0.9	7.5	0.1	0
Vegetable, Original, V8*	1 Glass/150ml	26	0	17	0.9	2.8	0.1	0.9
Water with Pineapple, Vita Coco*	1 Carton /330ml	82	0	25	0	6	0	0
Water, M&S*	1 Bottle/263ml	50	0.3	19	0.1	4.7	0.1	0.1
Watermelon, Mello Drinks*	1 Bottle/250ml	100	0.2	40	1	8.5	0.1	0.7

JUICE DRINK

INFO/WEIGHT	Measure	per Measure KCAL	per Measure FAT	Nutrition Values per 100g / 100ml KCAL	PROT	CARB	FAT	FIBRE
Aloe Vera, OKF*	1 Bottle/500ml	175	0	35	0	9	0	0
Apple & Blueberry, The Feel Good Drinks Co*	1 Serving/375ml	163	0.4	44	0.1	10.6	0.1	0
Apple & Raspberry, Sainsbury's*	1 Serving/200ml	112	0.2	56	0.1	13.8	0.1	0.1
Apple & Strawberry, Sainsbury's*	1 Serving/250ml	13	0.1	5	0	1	0	0
Apple & Pomegranate, Sparkling Water, Sainsbury's*	1 Serving/200ml	4	0	2	0	0.3	0	0
Apple & Raspberry, Tesco*	1 Serving/300ml	138	0	46	0.1	11.2	0	0
Apple Lemonade, Cawston Press*	1 Glass/200g	106	0.2	53	0.2	11.9	0.1	0
Apple, & Rhubarb, Sparkling, Pressed, Shloer*	1 Can/330ml	63	0	19	0.1	4.4	0	0

JUICE DRINK

	Measure INFO/WEIGHT	per Measure KCAL	FAT	Nutrition Values per 100g / 100ml KCAL	PROT	CARB	FAT	FIBRE
Apple, Plum & Pear, Pure Pressed, CBY, Asda*	1 Glass/200ml	92	0	46	0.4	10.5	0	0.2
Blackcurrant & Apple, Oasis*	1 Serving/500ml	90	0	18	0	4.1	0	0
Blackcurrant, 45% High, No Added Sugar, Asda*	1 Serving/250ml	50	1.2	20	0.5	4.5	0.5	0
Blackcurrant, Extra Light, Ribena*	1 Serving/200ml	8	0	4	0	0.5	0	0
Blackcurrant, Hi Juice, No Added Sugar, Sun Quench, Aldi*	1 Serving/200ml	52	1	26	0.5	4.9	0.5	0.5
Blood Orange, Sparkling, Aranciata Rossa, San Pellegrino*	1 Can/330ml	73	0	22	0.1	4.9	0	0
Cherry, No Added Sugar, Sainsbury's*	1 Carton/250ml	25	0.1	10	0.2	1.9	0	0
Cranberry & Raspberry, BGTY, Sainsbury's*	1 Glass/250ml	10	0.2	4	0.1	0.7	0.1	0.1
Cranberry & Raspberry, Sainsbury's*	1 Serving/250ml	105	0	42	0.1	9.9	0	0
Cranberry & Raspberry, No Add Sugar, LC, Tesco*	1 Serving/250ml	12	0	5	0	0.8	0	0
Cranberry & Raspberry, with Spring Water, Zeo*	1 Serving/275ml	33	0	12	0	2.6	0	0
Cranberry Blend, Ocean Spray*	1 Glass/250ml	148	0	59	0.1	13.9	0	0
Cranberry, & Raspberry, Tesco*	1 Serving/150ml	28	0	19	0	4.4	0	0
Cranberry, Asda*	1 Serving/200ml	40	0	20	0	4.5	0	0
Cranberry, Classic, Ocean Spray*	1 Bottle/500ml	115	0	23	0	5.8	0	0
Cranberry, Light, Classic, Ocean Spray*	1 Glass/200ml	16	0	8	0	1.4	0	0
Cranberry, No Added Sugar, BGTY, Sainsbury's*	1 Glass/200ml	4	0	2	0	0.3	0	0
Cranberry, No Added Sugar, HL, Tesco*	1 Glass/200ml	8	0	4	0	1.1	0	0
Cranberry, Original, Concentrated, Ocean Spray*	1 Serving/15ml	27	0	183	0.2	44.1	0	0
Cranberry, Tesco*	1 Serving/250ml	50	0	20	0	4.4	0	0.1
Cranberry, Waitrose*	1 Serving/250ml	145	0	58	0.1	13.9	0	0.1
Forest Fruits, Asda*	1 Serving/200ml	88	0	44	0.3	10.9	0	0.3
Fruit Shoot, My-5, Apple & Pear, Robinson's*	1 Bottle/200ml	78	0.2	39	0.2	8.9	0.1	0
Grape & Elderflower, White, Sparkling, Shloer*	1 Glass/200ml	74	0	37	0	9.2	0	0
Grape, Apple & Raspberry, Co-Op*	1 Serving/150ml	75	0	50	0.4	12	0	0.1
Grape, Apple & Raspberry, Asda*	1 Glass/200ml	82	1	41	0.5	9.8	0.5	0.5
Grape, Red, Sparkling, Shloer*	1 Glass/200ml	84	0	42	0	10.4	0	0
Grape, Rose, Sparkling, Shloer*	1 Serving/200ml	42	0	21	0.1	4.8	0	0
Grape, White, Sparkling, Light, Shloer*	1 Glass/125ml	28	0	22	0.7	5.3	0	0
Grape, White, Sparkling, Shloer*	1 Serving/120ml	59	0	49	0	11.6	0	0
Guava Exotic, Rubicon*	1 Carton/288ml	150	0.3	52	0.2	12.9	0.1	0
J20, Apple & Mango, Britvic*	1 Bottle/275ml	83	0	30	0.1	6.8	0	0.2
J20, Apple & Raspberry, Britvic*	1 Bottle/275ml	88	0	32	0.1	7.3	0	0.3
J20, Apple, & Watermelon, Spritz, Britvic*	1 Bottle/275ml	55	0	20	0	4.8	0	0
J20, Orange & Passion Fruit, Britvic*	1 Bottle/275ml	63	0	23	0	4.8	0	0
J2O, Apple & Watermelon, Sparkling, Spritz, Britvic*	1 Serving/250ml	58	0	23	0	5.4	0	0
J2O, Glitterberry, Britvic*	1 Bottle/275ml	77	0	28	0	6.4	0	0
Lemon & Lime, Light, Oasis*	1 Bottle/250ml	6	0	3	0	0.2	0	0
Lemon, & Ginger, Refresher, Innocent*	1 Bottle/400ml	56	0	14	0	3.6	0	0
Lemon, Cloudy, Lightly Carbonated, Zeo*	1 Serving/275ml	28	0	10	0.1	2.3	0	0
Lemon, Lime, & Apple, Sparkling, Bubbles, Innocent*	1 Can/333ml	90	0	27	0	6.8	0	0
Lemonade, Asda*	1 Glass/200ml	88	0	44	0.1	11	0	0
Lime, Mexican, & Elderflower, Fruit Crush, Freeway*	1 Serving/250ml	8	0.1	3	0	0.4	0	0
Lychee, Sparkling, Rubicon*	1 Can/330g	182	0	55	0	13.6	0	0
Mandarin, Detox, Vit Hit*	1 Serving/200ml	14	0.2	7	0.1	1.2	0.1	0.1
Mango, & Earl Grey Tea, Rio Doro, Aldi*	1 Bottle/ 330ml	3	0.3	1	0.1	0.3	0.1	0.1
Mango, & Passion Fruit, Still, Get More Vits*	1 Bottle/500ml	5	0	1	0	0	0	0
Mango, No Added Sugar, Morrisons*	1 Serving/150ml	21	0	14	0.1	2.8	0	0.5
Mango, Rubicon*	1 Serving/100ml	54	0.1	54	0.1	13.1	0.1	0
Mango, Sparkling, Rubicon*	1 Can/330ml	172	0	52	0	12.8	0	0
Mixed Berry Crush, Sparkling, CBY, Asda*	1 Glass/250ml	8	0	3	0	0.5	0	0
Mulled Lemonade, Sainsbury's*	1 Serving/150ml	67	0.8	44	0.5	10.8	0.5	0.5
Orange & Lime, Refresh'd, Robinson's*	1 Bottle/500ml	55	0	11	0	2.2	0	0

JUICE DRINK

	Measure INFO/WEIGHT	per Measure KCAL	per Measure FAT	Nutrition Values per 100g / 100ml KCAL	PROT	CARB	FAT	FIBRE
Orange & Lime, Sparkling, Innocent*	1 Can/330ml	93	0	28	0.6	6.5	0	0
Orange & Mango, Spring Water, Sparkling, Rubicon*	1 Bottle/500ml	15	0	3	0	0.5	0	0
Orange, Caprisun*	1 Pouch/200ml	89	0	45	0	10.8	0	0
Orange, HE, Tesco*	1 Glass/200ml	56	0.2	28	0.3	6.1	0.1	0
Orange, Juice Burst, Purity Soft Drinks Co*	1 Bottle/500ml	220	0	44	1	10.2	0	0
Orange, Mango, & Passionfruit, Morrisons*	1 Serving/200ml	6	0	3	0	0.2	0	0
Orange, Value, Tesco*	1 Glass/250ml	32	0	13	0	3.3	0	0
Orange, Zero, Vive, Aldi*	1 Serving/200g	2	1	1	0.5	0.5	0.5	0.5
Oranges & Lemons, Juicy Water*	1 Bottle/420ml	134	0	32	0	8.1	0	0
Passion Fruit, Exotic, Rubicon*	1 Serving/200ml	110	0	55	0.1	13.6	0	0
Peach & Passionfruit Fruit, Sunmagic*	1 Serving/330ml	172	0	52	0.3	13	0	0.1
Peach & Apricot, Sparkling, J2O Spritz, Britvic*	1 Serving/250ml	52	0	21	0	4.9	0	0
Peach Hibiscus, with Black Tea Extracts, Fuzetea*	1 Bottle/400ml	76	0	19	0	4.3	0	0
Peach, & Cherry, Sparkling, Perrier & Juice*	1 Serving/250ml	45	0	18	0	3.9	0	0
Pear & Raspberry, Sparkling, J2O Spritz, Britvic*	1 Serving/250ml	55	0	22	0	5.2	0	0
Pear, Partially Made with Concentrate, Tesco*	1 Glass/200ml	110	0	55	0	12.4	0	0.2
Pink Cranberry Lemonade, Diet, Sparkling, M&S*	1 Bottle/500ml	15	0.5	3	0.1	0.5	0.1	0.1
Pomegranate, Rubicon*	1 Can/330ml	108	0	54	0	13.5	0	0
Sicilian Lemon & Garden Mint, Presse, Finest, Tesco*	1 Serving/250ml	50	0	20	0	5	0	0
Strawberry, & Kiwi, Sparkling, Perrier & Juice*	1 Serving/250ml	36	0	18	0	3.8	0	0
Strawberry, & Raspberry, Sparkling, Franklin & Sons Ltd*	1 Serving/200ml	44	0	22	0	5.2	0	0
Summer Fruits, Fresh, Tesco*	1 Glass/250ml	112	0.2	45	0.1	10.8	0.1	0.3
Summer Fruits, Oasis*	1 Bottle/500ml	90	0	18	0	4.2	0	0
Tropical Fruit, No Added Sugar, Naturis*	1 Serving/100ml	24	0.1	24	0.2	5.3	0.1	0
Tropical Fruit, Tesco*	1 Glass/250ml	118	0	47	0	11.4	0	0
Tropical, Be Light, Aldi*	1 Glass/250ml	62	0.2	25	0.2	5.4	0.1	0.2
Tropical, Naturis*	1 Carton/250ml	60	0.2	24	0.2	5.3	0.1	0.5
Tropical, No Added Sugar, Tesco*	1 Carton/250ml	12	0	5	0	1.1	0	0
White Grape, Raspberry & Cranberry, Sparkling, Shloer*	1 Serving/250ml	117	0	47	0	11	0	0

J

	Measure INFO/WEIGHT	per Measure KCAL	FAT	Nutrition Values per 100g / 100ml KCAL	PROT	CARB	FAT	FIBRE
KALE								
Black, Cavolo Nero, Aldi*	1 Serving/80g	23	0.9	29	2.4	1	1.1	2.8
Curly, Boiled in Salted Water, Average	*1 Serving/60g*	*14*	*0.7*	*24*	*2.4*	*1*	*1.1*	*2.8*
Curly, Raw, Average	*1 Serving/90g*	*25*	*1.2*	*28*	*2.9*	*1.2*	*1.4*	*2.6*
KARELA								
Frozen, Shana*	1 Serving/80g	14	0.1	18	1.4	1.3	0.1	0
KATSU								
Chicken, Pot, Tesco*	1 Pack/132g	187	4.1	141	7.1	20.4	3.1	1.7
Chicken, Red Pepper, Edamame, Jasmine Rice, BFY, M&S	1 Pack/380g	372	8.7	98	8.9	9.8	2.3	1.1
Chicken, with Edamame, Rice, & Quinoa, Charlie Bigham's	1 Serving/385g	624	22.7	162	9.3	19	5.9	0
Chicken, with Jasmine Rice, & Quinoa, Charlie Bigham's*	½ Pack/386g	695	32	180	8.1	19	8.3	0
Coconut, Everdine*	1 Serving/450g	585	28.4	130	9.1	7.2	6.3	4.4
Curry, City Kitchen, Tesco*	1 Pack/350g	375	5.6	107	7	15.8	1.6	0.6
Sweet Potato, with Rice, Love Your Veg!, Sainsbury's*	1 Pack/393g	688	22	175	2.9	27.2	5.6	2.3
Yakisoba, Wasabi Co Ltd*	1 Pack/450g	891	32.8	198	8	24.6	7.3	0
KEBAB								
Beef ,& Pepper, Kofta, Waitrose*	1 Kebab/138g	223	13.9	162	14.8	2.9	10.1	0.6
Beef, BBQ, 5% Fat, Ashfield Farm, Aldi*	1 Kebab/80g	120	2.9	150	21	7.4	3.6	1.2
Beef, Kofta, Spicy, Oakhurst, Aldi*	1 Kebab/45g	112	6.8	248	20	6.5	15	2.8
Beef, Kofta, Uncooked, Tesco*	1 Kebab/73g	163	12.5	225	14	3.2	17.3	1.2
Chicken, Indian Spiced, Morrisons*	½ Pack/112g	159	2.7	142	26.7	3.1	2.4	0.5
Chicken, Shawarma, Ashfield Farm, Aldi*	½ Pack/95g	149	3.9	157	17	12	4.1	1.1
Chicken, Shish in Pitta Bread with Salad	*1 Kebab/250g*	*388*	*10.2*	*155*	*13.5*	*17.2*	*4.1*	*1*
Chicken, Shish, Meat Only, Average	*1 Kebab/250g*	*312*	*5.2*	*125*	*25.7*	*0.9*	*2.1*	*0.1*
Chicken, Spanish Style, Good to Go, Waitrose*	1 Pack/80g	148	4.6	185	18.3	13.8	5.7	2.6
Chicken, Thigh, Sticky Barbecue, M&S*	1 Pack/100g	189	6.8	189	26.3	5.7	6.8	0.1
Courgette, & Feta, Kofta, Vegetarian, Waitrose*	½ Pack/75g	166	7.8	222	5.8	24.2	10.4	4.1
Doner, Heat 'Em Up, Tesco*	1 Kebab/159g	346	10.6	218	8.4	30	6.7	2
Doner, in Pitta, with Salad, Average	*1 Serving/400g*	*1020*	*64.8*	*255*	*14.2*	*14*	*16.2*	*0.8*
Handmade, Seekh, Mumtaz*	½ Pack/94g	201	14.6	214	15.8	2.9	15.5	0
Kofta, Middle Eastern, Slimming World, Iceland*	½ Pack/150g	184	5	123	19.4	3.8	3.3	0.6
Lamb, & Chicken, Kofta, Tesco*	2 Koftas/38g	97	5.3	255	14.6	16.8	13.9	2
Lamb, Kofta, Citrus Tikka, Sainsbury's*	1 Kebab/84g	199	11.6	235	18.1	9.8	13.7	2.6
Lamb, Minted, Ashfield Farm, Aldi*	1 Kebab/54g	137	9.2	254	18.5	5.7	17	0
Lamb, Minted, Shish, As prepared, Waitrose*	1 Kebab/57g	123	7.3	217	17.2	7.9	12.9	0.1
Lamb, Shami with a Mint Raita Dip, M&S*	½ Pack/90g	189	12.1	210	12.8	9.7	13.4	3.5
Lamb, with Mint, Tesco*	1 Serving/80g	192	13.4	240	16	5.5	16.7	0.4
Pork, BBQ, Sainsbury's*	1 Serving/90g	65	2.2	72	11	1.4	2.4	0.9
Salmon, Chilli & Lime, Tesco*	2 Kebabs/78g	187	10.4	240	21.9	8.2	13.3	0
Shish, with Onions & Peppers	*1oz/28g*	*59*	*4.5*	*212*	*12.9*	*3.9*	*16.2*	*1.2*
KEDGEREE								
Average	*1oz/28g*	*48*	*2.4*	*171*	*15.9*	*7.8*	*8.7*	*0.1*
COU, M&S*	1 Pack/370g	388	8.1	105	7.6	13.7	2.2	2.1
Haddock, Smoked, Big Dish, M&S*	1 Pack/450g	585	22.5	130	8.5	13	5	1.9
KETCHUP								
Barbeque, Asda*	1 Tbsp/15g	20	0	136	0.9	33	0	0
BBQ, Heinz*	1 Serving/10g	14	0	137	1.3	31.3	0.3	0.3
Chilli, Smoked, Gran Luchito*	1 Tsp/5g	18	0	358	1.8	18.4	0.9	0
Curry, Scharf, Hela*	1 Tbsp/15g	21	0	137	0.8	30.8	0.3	0
Tomato, Average	*1 Tsp/5g*	*6*	*0*	*120*	*1.5*	*28.1*	*0.2*	*0.8*
Tomato, Reduced Sugar, Average	*1 Tbsp/10g*	*9*	*0.1*	*87*	*2*	*16.9*	*1.2*	*0.9*
KIDNEY								
Lamb, Fried, Average	*1oz/28g*	*53*	*2.9*	*188*	*23.7*	*0*	*10.3*	*0*
Lamb, Raw, Average	*1oz/28g*	*25*	*0.7*	*91*	*17*	*0*	*2.6*	*0*

K

	Measure INFO/WEIGHT	per Measure KCAL	FAT	Nutrition Values per 100g / 100ml KCAL	PROT	CARB	FAT	FIBRE
KIDNEY								
Ox, Raw	*1oz/28g*	*22*	*0.5*	*77*	*15.1*	*0*	*1.8*	*0*
Pig, Fried	*1oz/28g*	*57*	*2.7*	*202*	*29.2*	*0*	*9.5*	*0*
Pig, Raw	*1oz/28g*	*22*	*0.7*	*77*	*14*	*0*	*2.4*	*0*
Pig, Stewed	*1oz/28g*	*43*	*1.7*	*153*	*24.4*	*0*	*6.1*	*0*
Veal, Raw, Average	*1 Serving/100g*	*99*	*3.1*	*99*	*15.8*	*0.8*	*3.1*	*0*
KIEV								
Chicken, Cheese & Ham, Morrisons*	1 Kiev/128g	282	16	221	14.3	12	12.5	1.8
Chicken, COU, M&S*	1 Kiev/150g	188	2.7	125	15.8	10.8	1.8	0.5
Chicken, Creamy Peppercorn, Tesco*	1 Kiev/132g	290	17.3	220	13.1	12.1	13.1	0.6
Chicken, Garlic & Parsley Butter, Breaded, Waitrose*	1 Kiev/156g	375	21.3	241	17.5	11.1	13.7	1.4
Chicken, Garlic & Herb Sauce, Inspirations, Birds Eye*	1 Kiev/125g	305	16.5	244	12.2	18.8	13.2	0.7
Chicken, Garlic & Herb, Frozen, Birds Eye*	1 Kiev/91g	240	11.9	264	15.3	20.6	13.1	1
Chicken, Garlic & Herb, Sainsbury's*	1 Kiev/121g	350	26.2	289	13.8	9.6	21.6	0.7
Chicken, Garlic & Parsley, BGTY, Sainsbury's*	1 Kiev/125g	267	15.5	213	14.7	10.6	12.4	0.5
Chicken, Garlic Butter, HL, Tesco*	1 Kiev/106g	318	22.3	300	13.6	14	21	0.7
Chicken, Garlic, Wild, & Cornish Butter, Gastropub, M&S*	1 Kiev/225g	493	32.2	219	17.3	5	14.3	0.6
Chicken, Ham, & Cheese, Tesco*	1 Kiev/143g	307	18.6	215	14.4	9.3	13	1.3
Mushroom & Spinach, Good Life*	1 Kiev/125g	290	14	232	6.4	24.5	11.2	3.7
Vegetable, Veggie, M&S*	1 Kiev/155g	267	15.5	172	3.4	15.9	10	2.6
Vegetarian, Mini, Quorn*	1 Kiev/20g	41	2.2	207	14	13	11	6.5
with Garlic Butter, & Parsley, Kiev, Barber Foods*	1 Kiev/140g	243	15.7	243	14.3	10	15.7	0.7
KIMCHI								
Spicy, Biona Organic*	1 Serving/50g	12	0.1	24	1.1	3.7	0.2	1.8
Unpasteurised , Kim Kong*	1 Serving/15g	6	0.1	37	2.3	4.4	0.7	2.1
KIPPER								
Baked, Average	*1oz/28g*	*57*	*3.2*	*205*	*25.5*	*0*	*11.4*	*0*
Fillets in Sunflower Oil, John West*	1 Can/140g	321	23.8	229	19	0	17	0
Fillets, Raw, Average	*1 Serving/200g*	*384*	*29.1*	*192*	*14.5*	*0*	*14.6*	*0*
Fillets, Scottish, with Butter, Youngs*	1 Pack/170g	350	25.9	226	18.9	0.1	16.7	0
Fillets, Smoked with Butter, Scottish, Boil in Bag, Tesco*	1 Serving/100g	225	17.2	225	17	0	17.2	0
Grilled, Average	*1oz/28g*	*71*	*5.4*	*255*	*20.1*	*0*	*19.4*	*0*
Smoked, Average	*1 Serving/150g*	*322*	*23*	*214*	*18.9*	*0*	*15.4*	*0*
Whole, with Bone, Grilled, Average	*1 Serving/100g*	*161*	*12.2*	*161*	*12.7*	*0*	*12.2*	*0*
KIT KAT								
2 Finger, Dark, Nestle*	2 Fingers/21g	107	5.4	510	5.4	62.2	25.5	5.4
2 Finger, Nestle*	2 Fingers/21g	104	5.1	502	6.7	62.7	24.4	2.1
4 Finger, Nestle*	4 Fingers/42g	208	10.2	502	6.7	62.7	24.5	2.1
Chunky, Caramel, Nestle*	1 Bar/48g	259	15.3	539	5.2	58.6	31.8	0
Chunky, Double Caramel, Nestle*	½ Bar/21g	109	5.8	520	6.5	61	27.6	1
Chunky, Nestle*	1 Bar/40g	206	10.2	516	5.4	65.1	25.6	1.7
Chunky, Orange, Nestle*	1 Bar/48g	247	12.5	515	5.8	62	26.1	0
Chunky, Peanut, Nestle*	1 Bar/42g	226	13.2	537	8.4	54.9	31.5	0
Chunky, Snack Size, Nestle*	1 Bar/26g	133	7.1	513	6.6	60.4	27.2	1.1
Cookies & Cream, 2 Finger, Nestle*	1 Bar/21g	106	5.3	507	7.6	60.9	25.4	1.4
Dark, Mint, 2 Finger, Nestle*	1 Bar/21g	105	5.3	502	5.4	60.6	25.3	5.3
Kubes, Nestle*	1 Pack/50g	258	13.8	515	5.9	60.9	27.5	1
Lemon Drizzle, Nestle*	1 Bar/21g	105	5.1	505	6.8	63.2	24.5	2.1
Mini, Nestle*	1 Bar/15g	75	3.9	502	7.5	59.4	26	0
Orange, 2 Finger, Nestle*	2 Fingers/21g	107	5.6	507	5.5	61.7	26.5	0
Peanut Butter, Bites, Nestle*	4 Pieces/23g	121	6.5	525	10.8	55.3	28.3	2.1
Ruby, 4 Finger, Kit Kat*	1 Pack/42g	225	13	541	6.5	56.8	31.4	1.4
Senses, Nestle*	1 Bar/31g	165	9.5	531	7.5	56.3	30.7	0
White, Chunky, Nestle*	1 Bar/40g	206	10.6	516	8.1	60.8	26.4	0.5

K

	Measure INFO/WEIGHT	per Measure KCAL	FAT	Nutrition Values per 100g / 100ml KCAL	PROT	CARB	FAT	FIBRE
KIWI BERRY								
Tesco*	1 Serving/80g	70	0.5	87	1.2	17.6	0.6	3.2
KIWI FRUIT								
Fresh, Raw, Flesh & Seeds, Average	*1 Kiwi/60g*	*29*	*0.3*	*49*	*1.1*	*10.6*	*0.5*	*1.9*
Weighed with Skin, Average	*1 Kiwi/60g*	*25*	*0.3*	*42*	*0.9*	*9.1*	*0.4*	*1.6*
KOHLRABI								
Boiled in Salted Water	*1oz/28g*	*5*	*0.1*	*18*	*1.2*	*3.1*	*0.2*	*1.9*
Raw	*1oz/28g*	*5*	*0*	*16*	*1.1*	*2.6*	*0.1*	*1.5*
KOMBUCHA								
Cherry Plum, Remedy*	1 Can/250ml	25	1.2	10	0.5	2.2	0.5	0.5
Classic, Kinoko*	1 Can/330ml	86	0.3	26	0.5	4.6	0.1	0.1
Ginger & Lemon, Organic, Lo Bros Living Drinks*	1 Bottle/330ml	18	1.5	6	0.1	1.1	0.5	0.1
Raspberry, & Lemon, Lo Bros Living Drinks*	1 Bottle/330ml	30	0	9	0	1.8	0	0
KORMA								
Chicken, & Basmati Rice, Tesco*	1 Pot/350g	588	32.6	168	4.3	16.9	9.3	2.3
Chicken, & Pilau Rice, Charlie Bigham's*	1 Serving/405g	688	38.4	170	7.3	14.7	9.5	0
Chicken, & White Rice, BGTY, Frozen, Sainsbury's*	1 Pack/375g	341	3.8	91	5.6	14.9	1	0.5
Chicken, & Pilau Rice, Charlie Bigham's*	½ Pack/405g	688	38.4	170	7.3	14.7	9.5	0
Chicken, & Rice, Free From, Tesco*	1 Pack/369g	565	18.8	153	8.3	17.8	5.1	1.5
Chicken, & Rice, Indian Meal for Two, Sainsbury's*	1 Pack/500g	785	40.5	157	6.8	14.3	8.1	3.1
Chicken, Asda*	1 Pack/380g	630	41.7	166	13	3.6	11	1.8
Chicken, Indian Meal for 2, Finest, Tesco*	½ Pack/200g	348	24	174	10.3	6.2	12	2.5
Chicken, Indian Takeaway for One, Sainsbury's*	1 Serving/300g	498	30.9	166	13	5.3	10.3	1.6
Chicken, Indian Takeaway, Iceland*	1 Pack/400g	656	44	164	11.8	4.5	11	1.4
Chicken, Indian, Takeaway, Morrisons*	1 Pack/350g	532	32.2	152	11.9	4.2	9.2	2.2
Chicken, Indian, Takeaway, Tesco*	½ Pack/179g	280	18.8	156	9.7	5.2	10.5	1.1
Chicken, Indian, Waitrose*	½ Pack/175g	280	17.5	160	12.4	4.7	10	1.2
Chicken, Korma, Meal For Two, Tesco*	½ Pack/154g	245	15.4	159	12	3.5	10	3.6
Chicken, M&S*	½ Pack/200g	316	19.2	158	13.1	4.4	9.6	1
Chicken, with Peshwari Coriander Rice, Finest, Tesco*	1 Pack/550g	908	48.4	165	7.5	13.9	8.8	0.9
Chicken, with Pilau Rice, Co-Op*	1 Pack/450g	783	44.6	174	7.4	13	9.9	1.8
Chicken, with Pilau Rice, PB, Waitrose*	1 Pack/400g	452	6.8	113	8.9	15.4	1.7	1.3
Chicken, with Pilau Rice, Taste of India, Tesco*	1 Pack/426g	609	28.1	143	8.1	11.5	6.6	2.8
Chicken, with Rice, Ready Meal	*1 Pack/400g*	*740*	*34.7*	*185*	*8.4*	*18.1*	*8.7*	*1.7*
Vegetable, Indian, Amy's Kitchen*	1 Pack/270g	307	12.1	114	3.3	15	4.5	2.6
Vegetable, Ready to Cook, Fresh, Sainsbury's*	½ Pack/255g	263	17.3	103	2.8	7.7	6.8	2.1
Vegetable, Takeaway or Restaurant	*1 Serving/300g*	*336*	*13.5*	*112*	*3.4*	*15.4*	*4.5*	*2.6*
KRISPROLLS								
Cracked Wheat, Original, Pagen*	1 Krisproll/13g	48	0.9	380	12	67	7	9
Golden, Swedish Toasts, Pagen*	1 Krisproll/12g	48	1	400	11	69	8.5	5
Organic, Bio, Pagen*	1 Krisproll/12g	46	0.8	380	12	67	7	8
Swedish Toasts, Wholegrain, Pagen*	1 Toast/13g	51	0.8	390	11	67	6.5	8.5
KULFI								
Average	*1oz/28g*	*119*	*11.2*	*424*	*5.4*	*11.8*	*39.9*	*0.6*
KUMQUATS								
Raw	*1 Kumquat/20g*	*9*	*0.1*	*43*	*0.9*	*9.3*	*0.5*	*3.8*
KUNG PO								
Chicken, Sainsbury's*	½ Pack/175g	131	4.4	75	9.2	4	2.5	1
Chicken, Waitrose*	1 Pack/350g	318	3.9	91	8.2	12.1	1.1	1.2

K

	Measure INFO/WEIGHT	per Measure KCAL	FAT	Nutrition Values per 100g / 100ml KCAL	PROT	CARB	FAT	FIBRE
LAGER								
Alcohol Free, Becks*	1 Serving/275ml	55	0	20	0.7	5	0	0
Alcohol Free, Heineken*	1 Can/330ml	69	0	21	0	4.8	0	0
Amstel, Heineken*	1 Pint/568ml	227	0	40	0.5	3	0	0
Average	*½ Pint/284ml*	*117*	*0*	*41*	*0.3*	*3.1*	*0*	*0*
Basics, Sainsbury's*	1 Can/440g	71	0	16	0	1	0	0
Becks*	1 Can/275ml	113	0	41	0	3	0	0
Blanc, Kronenbourg*	½ pt/284ml	119	0	42	0	3.3	0	0
Boston, Samuel Adams*	1 Bottle/355ml	160	0	45	0	0	0	0
Bottled, Brahma*	1 Bottle/330ml	125	0	38	0	0	0	0
Budweiser, 66, Anheuser-Busch*	1 Bottle/330ml	102	0	31	0	0	0	0
Budweiser, Light, Anheuser-Busch*	1 Can/440ml	118	0	27	0.3	1.5	0	0
Can, Carlsberg*	1 Can/440ml	141	0	32	0	2	0	0
Cinque, Shepherd Neame*	1 Bottle/330ml	129	0.3	39	0.4	2.9	0.1	0
Czech, Low Alcohol, M&S*	1 Bottle/500ml	20	0	4	0	0.4	0	0
Draught, Carling*	1 Pint/568ml	189	0	33	0	1.4	0	0
Export, Carlsberg*	1 Can/440ml	185	0	42	0.4	2.8	0	0.4
Export, Foster's*	1 Pint/568ml	210	0	37	0	2.2	0	0
Foster's*	1 Pint/568ml	193	0	34	0	3.1	0	0
German, Low Alcohol, Sainsbury's*	1 Bottle/330ml	92	0.3	28	0.4	5.9	0.1	0.1
Grolsch*	1 Sm Can/330ml	145	0	44	0	2.2	0	0
Heineken v 5, Heineken*	1 Pint/568ml	256	0	45	0.5	3	0	0
Heineken*, 5%, Heineken*	1 Bottle/250ml	110	0	44	0.4	3.4	0	0
Innis & Gunn*	1 Bottle/330ml	132	0	40	0.3	3.5	0	0
Irish, 4%, Rockshore*	1 Can/500ml	160	0	32	0.4	1.9	0	0
Light, Coors*	1 Pint/568ml	170	0	30	0.3	1.5	0	0
Light, Corona*	1 Bottle/330ml	105	0	32	1.5	0	0	0
Low Alcohol	*1 Can/440ml*	*44*	*0*	*10*	*0.2*	*1.5*	*0*	*0*
Pils, Holsten*	1 Can/440ml	167	0	38	0.3	2.4	0	0
Pilsner, Efes*	1 Can/500ml	226	0	45	0	7.6	0	0
Pilsner, Premium, Bavaria*	1 Bottle/330ml	142	0	43	0.4	3.5	0	0
Pilsner, Rheinbacher, Aldi*	1 Can/500ml	135	0	27	0	0	0	0
Polish, Tyskie*	1 Can/549ml	236	0	43	0	0	0	0
Premier, Kronenbourg*	½ Pint/284ml	136	0	48	0	0	0	0
Premium	*1 Can/440ml*	*260*	*0*	*59*	*0.3*	*2.4*	*0*	*0*
Premium, French, Biere Speciale, Tesco*	1 Serving/250ml	105	0	42	0.3	3.3	0	0
Premium, Light, Amstel*	1 Can/355ml	95	0	27	0	1.4	0	0
Premium, San Miguel*	1 Bottle/330ml	148	0	45	0.3	3.7	0	0
Shandy, Traditional Style, Asda*	1 Serving/200ml	44	0	22	0	4.6	0	0
Skinny Brands*	1 Bottle/330ml	89	0.3	27	0	0.9	0.1	0
Stella Artois*	1 Can/550ml	220	0	40	0.4	3.1	0	0
Tuborg Green, Carlsberg*	1 Serving/200ml	78	0	39	0.5	2.5	0	0
Vier, Becks*	1 Bottle/275ml	110	0	40	0	3	0	0
LAKSA								
Chicken & Coconut Noodle, Cooked, Tesco*	1 Pack/351g	321	10.6	91	7.1	8.4	3	1.2
Chicken, & King Prawn, Chargrilled, Taste Singapore, M&S*	1 Pack/400g	436	21.2	109	6.2	8.7	5.3	0.9
Prawn, King, & Coconut, G&B, Asda*	1 Pack/367g	268	4.8	73	3.1	11	1.3	1.2
Thai Noodle, with Chicken, M&S*	1 Pack/400g	460	21.6	115	7	9.8	5.4	1.1
LAMB								
& Mash, Colcannon, Asda*	1 Pack/450g	392	17	92	4.4	9.3	4	0.7
Breast, Lean, Roasted, Average	*1 Serving/100g*	*273*	*18.5*	*273*	*26.7*	*0*	*18.5*	*0*
Chops, Average	*1 Chop/82g*	*190*	*13.4*	*231*	*20.6*	*0.4*	*16.4*	*0*
Chops, Minted, Average	*1 Chop/100g*	*260*	*15.1*	*260*	*25.9*	*5.1*	*15.1*	*0.3*
Chops, Rosemary, & Garlic, Barnsley, Donald Russell*	½ Pack/120g	403	31.6	336	24.7	0.2	26.3	0.1

L

	Measure INFO/WEIGHT	per Measure KCAL	per Measure FAT	Nutrition Values per 100g / 100ml KCAL	PROT	CARB	FAT	FIBRE
LAMB								
Cutlets, Neck, Raw, Lean & Fat, Weighed with Bone	1 Pack 210g	359	31.7	171	8.8	0	15.1	0
Diced, From Supermarket, Healthy Range, Average	½ Pack/200g	277	8.9	138	24.6	0.1	4.5	0
Grill Steak, Average	1oz/28g	70	4.7	250	20.2	4.4	16.9	0.4
Leg, Joint, Raw, Average	1 Joint/510g	858	45.5	168	20.9	1.4	8.9	0.2
Leg, Roasted, Lean & Fat, Average	1oz/28g	66	3.8	237	28.6	0	13.6	0
Leg, Roasted, Lean, Average	1oz/28g	58	2.7	206	29.9	0	9.6	0
Loin, Chop, Grilled, Lean & Fat, Weighed with Bone	1 Serving/100g	193	14	193	16.8	0	14	0
Loin, Chops, Raw, Lean & Fat, Weighed with Bone	1 Serving/100g	216	17.9	216	13.7	0	17.9	0
Mince, Average	1oz/28g	58	4.2	207	17.6	0.5	14.8	0
Mince, Extra Lean, Sainsbury's*	1 Serving/225g	324	11.9	144	24.1	0	5.3	0.1
Neck Fillet, Lean, Raw	1 Serving/100g	232	17.6	232	18.4	0	17.6	0
Rack, Raw, Lean & Fat	1oz/28g	79	6.7	283	17.3	0	23.8	0
Rack, Raw, Lean Only, Weighed with Bone	1oz/28g	21	1.1	73	8.6	0	4	0
Rack, Roasted, Lean	1oz/28g	63	3.6	225	27.1	0	13	0
Rack, Roasted, Lean & Fat	1oz/28g	102	8.4	363	23	0	30.1	0
Shank, in Minted Gravy, Asda*	1 Shank/267g	465	24.6	174	18	4.1	9.2	0.5
Shank, Just Cook, Sainsbury's*	1 Shank/225g	394	18.7	175	22.9	1.8	8.3	0
Shank, Minted, Cooked, Morrisons*	½ Pack/231g	466	16.6	202	29.1	5	7.2	0.2
Shank, Slow Cook, Wine & Rosemary Gravy, Sainsbury's*	½ Pack/265g	374	15.1	141	19.8	2.6	5.7	0.5
Shank, with Mint Gravy, Oakhurst, Aldi*	1 Shank/266g	357	11.7	134	22	1.1	4.4	0.5
Shoulder, Cooked, Lean & Fat	1oz/28g	84	6.3	301	24.4	0	22.5	0
Shoulder, Fillet, Average	1oz/28g	66	5.1	235	17.6	0	18.3	0
Shoulder, Raw, Average	1oz/28g	70	5.7	248	16.8	0	20.2	0
Shoulder, Roasted, Whole, Lean	1oz/28g	61	3.4	218	27.2	0	12.1	0
Steak, Leg, Raw, Average	1 Steak/150g	169	5.5	112	20	0	3.6	0
Steak, Minted, Average	1 Steak/125g	212	9	170	22.7	3.4	7.2	0.9
Steak, Raw, Average	1 Steak/140g	190	7.6	136	21.7	0.2	5.4	0
Stewing, Raw, Lean & Fat	1oz/28g	57	3.5	203	22.5	0	12.6	0
Stewing, Stewed, Lean & Fat	1oz/28g	78	5.6	279	24.4	0	20.1	0
LAMB DINNER								
Irish, Dunnes Stores*	1 Meal/500g	515	13	103	5.6	13	2.6	3.2
LAMB IN								
Garlic & Rosemary Gravy, Shank, Asda*	1 Shank/280g	451	23.2	161	19.8	1.7	8.3	0.5
Rich Minted Gravy, Shank, Morrisons*	1 Pack/400g	612	26.4	153	18.8	5.2	6.6	0
LAMB MOROCCAN								
with Cous Cous, PB, Waitrose*	1 Pack/400g	390	5.2	98	7.7	13.6	1.3	2.2
LAMB WITH								
Mint Butter, Leg Steaks, Waitrose*	1 Serving/155g	270	16.3	174	19.6	0.4	10.5	0
Mint Gravy, Leg Chops, Tesco*	1 Serving/175g	214	9.8	122	15	3.2	5.6	1.7
LANGOUSTINE								
Fishmongers, Frozen, Tesco*	½ Pack/229g	262	5.3	114	23	0.1	2.3	0.5
LARD								
Average	1oz/28g	249	27.7	891	0	0	99	0
LASAGNE								
Al Forno, Heated, Finest, Tesco*	1 Pack/400g	608	29.2	158	9.8	11.8	7.6	1.5
Al Forno, TTD, Sainsbury's*	1 Pack/400g	550	24.4	142	8.9	11.7	6.3	1.5
Asda*	1 Pack/398g	502	23.9	126	7.3	10.6	6	1.1
Beef, & Chunky Vegetable, HL, Tesco*	1 Pack/360g	356	8.9	99	6.5	12	2.5	1.2
Beef, & Italian Veg, Musclefood*	1 Serving/380g	471	16	124	10.5	9.4	4.2	3
Beef, BGTY, Sainsbury's*	1 Pack/390g	380	11.1	103	6.8	10.8	3	2.8
Beef, Calorie Controlled, As Prepared, Love Life, Waitrose*	1 Pack/400g	341	7.1	91	6.7	10.6	1.9	2.4
Beef, Cooked, Italian, Sainsbury's*	1 Serving/375g	555	32.2	148	7.8	6.8	8.6	6.7
Beef, COU, M&S*	1 Pack/365g	394	9.1	108	6.6	13.9	2.5	1.7

L

LASAGNE

	Measure INFO/WEIGHT	per Measure KCAL	FAT	Nutrition Values per 100g / 100ml KCAL	PROT	CARB	FAT	FIBRE
Beef, Counted, Morrisons*	1 Pack/328g	266	5.6	81	6.7	9.4	1.7	1.1
Beef, Frozen, Eat Smart, Morrisons*	1 Pack/315g	343	10.4	109	5.9	13.1	3.3	1.4
Beef, HFC, Tesco*	1 Pack/400g	420	13.2	105	7.6	10.6	3.3	1.3
Beef, Italian Inspired, Meal for 1, Asda*	1 Pack/450g	612	31	136	8.4	9.3	6.9	1.6
Beef, Italian, Classic, Tesco*	1 Pack/600g	948	51	158	7.5	12.7	8.5	0.5
Beef, Italian, Inspired Cuisine, Aldi*	1 Pack/450g	536	18.9	119	8.4	11	4.2	1.8
Beef, Lidl*	½ Pack/200g	256	11.8	128	6.1	12.2	5.9	1
Beef, Low Fat, Well & Good, Co-Op*	1 Pack/360g	310	6.5	86	7.1	10	1.8	0.8
Beef, Meal to Share, 800g, M&S*	½ Pack/400g	644	33.2	161	8	12.7	8.3	1.6
Beef, Oven Baked, Calorie Counted, Asda*	1 Pack/372g	357	7.8	96	6.2	13	2.1	0.5
Beef, Ready Meal, Average	*1 Serving/400g*	*553*	*24*	*138*	*8.2*	*12.7*	*6*	*1.4*
Beef, Serves 2, TTD, Sainsbury's*	½ Pack/400g	626	31.9	159	8.4	12.1	8.1	1.7
Beef, Specially Selected, Aldi*	1 Pack/800g	1192	40	149	10	15	5	2
Bolognese, Lidl*	1 Serving/200g	336	18	168	8	13.7	9	0
Butternut Squash, & Lentil, Love Your Veg!, Sainsbury's*	1 Pack/369g	310	10.3	84	3.2	10.3	2.8	2.8
Family, Big Value Pack, Iceland*	¼ Pack/237g	322	14	136	5	15.9	5.9	1.4
for Two, Charlie Bigham's*	1 Serving/369 g	601	33.9	163	6.8	10.5	9.2	0
Mushroom, & Spinach, Waitrose*	1 Pack/400g	373	14	93	3.1	12.3	3.5	1.3
Sheets, Dry, Average	*1 Sheet/20g*	*70*	*0.3*	*349*	*11.9*	*72.1*	*1.5*	*2.9*
Sheets, Wholewheat, Sainsbury's*	1 Serving/63g	216	1.4	346	12.7	64.8	2.3	7.8
Spinach, & Ricotta, Finest, Tesco*	1 Pack/350g	584	37.1	167	6.1	11.7	10.6	1.2
Topped with Cheese Alternative, Plant Kitchen, M&S*	1 Pack/400g	372	7.6	93	5.3	12.3	1.9	2.9
Vegetable, Healthy Range, Average	*1 Serving/400g*	*318*	*8.2*	*80*	*3.5*	*11.8*	*2.1*	*1.5*
Vegetable, Mediterranean, COU, M&S*	1 Pack/360g	306	9.7	85	3.4	11.5	2.7	1.4
Vegetable, Ready Meal, Average	*1 Serving/400g*	*408*	*17.6*	*102*	*4.1*	*12.4*	*4.4*	*1*
Vegetable, Roasted, M&S*	1 Pack/400g	408	14.4	102	3.6	13.2	3.6	1.4
Vegetarian, Butternut Squash, Ovenbaked, Asda*	1 Pack/400g	376	13.1	92	2.4	13	3.2	0.6
Vegetarian, Meat Free, Quorn*	½ Pack/250g	251	8.8	109	4.5	13.1	3.8	2.5
Vegetarian, Vegetable, Meat Free, Tesco*	1 Pack/349g	305	5.9	87	3.6	13.4	1.7	2

LAVERBREAD

Average	*1oz/28g*	*15*	*1*	*52*	*3.2*	*1.6*	*3.7*	*0*

LEEKS

Boiled, Average	*1oz/28g*	*6*	*0.2*	*21*	*1.2*	*2.6*	*0.7*	*1.7*
Creamed, Frozen, Waitrose*	1 Serving/225g	115	5.4	51	1.8	5.5	2.4	0
Raw, Unprepared, Average	*1 Leek/166g*	*37*	*0.8*	*22*	*1.6*	*2.9*	*0.5*	*2.2*

LEMON

Fresh, Raw, Average	*1 Slice/5g*	*1*	*0*	*18*	*0.9*	*2.9*	*0.3*	*2.1*
Peel, Raw, Average	*1 Tbsp/6g*	*3*	*0*	*47*	*1.5*	*16*	*0.3*	*10.6*
Zest, Average	*1 Tsp/2g*	*2*	*0*	*100*	*0*	*25*	*0*	*0*

LEMON CURD

Average	*1 Tbsp/15g*	*44*	*0.7*	*294*	*0.7*	*62.9*	*4.7*	*0.1*
Luxury, Average	*1 Tsp/7g*	*23*	*0.6*	*326*	*2.8*	*59.7*	*8.4*	*0.1*

LEMON GRASS

Easy, Asda*	1 Tsp/10g	5	0.1	52	0.4	7.4	1.2	5.2

LEMON SOLE

Fillets, Raw, Average	*1 Serving/220g*	*177*	*2.8*	*81*	*17*	*0.2*	*1.3*	*0.3*
Goujons, Average	*1 Serving/150g*	*359*	*18.3*	*239*	*13.9*	*18.5*	*12.2*	*1*
Grilled, Average	*1oz/28g*	*27*	*0.5*	*97*	*20.2*	*0*	*1.7*	*0*
in Breadcrumbs, Average	*1 Fillet/142g*	*322*	*17.4*	*228*	*13.7*	*15.7*	*12.3*	*1*

LEMONADE

7 Up, Free, Britvic*	1 Bottle/500ml	10	0	2	0	0	0	0
7 Up, Zero, Britvic*	1 Can/330ml	6	0	2	0.1	0.1	0	0
7-Up, Light, Britvic*	1 Can/330ml	4	0	1	0.1	0.2	0	0

L

	Measure INFO/WEIGHT	per Measure KCAL	FAT	Nutrition Values per 100g / 100ml KCAL	PROT	CARB	FAT	FIBRE
LEMONADE								
Average	*1 Glass/250ml*	*52*	*0.2*	*21*	*0.1*	*5*	*0.1*	*0.1*
Cloudy, Diet, Sparkling, M&S*	1 Serving/250ml	8	0.2	3	0.1	0.1	0.1	0.1
Diet, Average	*1 Glass/250ml*	*4*	*0.1*	*2*	*0.1*	*0.2*	*0*	*0*
Diet, Premium, Tesco*	1 Glass/250ml	8	0	3	0.1	0.4	0	0
Diet, Toppers, Aldi*	1 Glass/100ml	1	0	1	0	0	0	0
Diet, Traditional Style, Tesco*	1 Glass/200ml	6	0	3	0	0.8	0	0
Low Calorie, Smart Price, Asda*	1 Glass/250ml	1	0	0	0	0.1	0	0
Pink, No Added Sugar, Tesco*	1 Glass/250ml	8	0.2	3	0.1	0.3	0.1	0.1
Pink, Still, Pure Premium, Tropicana*	1 Serving/200ml	90	0	45	0.2	10	0	0.7
Pink, Zero Calories, Lucozade*	1 Bottle/380ml	8	0	2	0.1	0.1	0	0
R White*	1 Glass/250ml	65	0	26	0.1	6.2	0	0
Raspberry, R White*	1 Can/330ml	56	0	17	0	3.9	0	0
Schweppes*	1 Glass/250ml	45	0	18	0	4.2	0	0
Schweppes*	1 Can/150ml	27	0	18	0	4.2	0	0
Slimline, Schweppes*	1 Glass/300ml	6	0	2	0	0	0	0
Still, Freshly Squeezed, M&S*	½ Bottle/250ml	100	0.5	40	0.1	9	0.2	0.5
Sugar Free, Everyday Value, Tesco*	1 Glass/250ml	1	0	0	0	0	0	0
TTD, Sainsbury's*	1 Serving/248g	159	0	64	0.1	14.8	0	0.2
Victorian, Fentiman's*	1 Bottle/275ml	130	0	47	0	11.3	0	0
LEMSIP								
Beechams*	1 Sachet/3g	11	0	387	0	100	0	0
LENTILS								
Beluga, No Added Sugar or Salt, Drained, Biona Organic*	½ Can/240g	226	0	94	6	14	0	7
Black Beluga, Ready to Eat, Merchant Gourmet*	1 Serving/63g	92	0.8	147	10.9	20.5	1.2	5.2
Good Grains, Aldi*	1 Pack/250g	242	5.2	97	6.6	10	2.1	5
Green & Brown, Dried, Boiled in Salted Water, Average	*1 Tbsp/30g*	*32*	*0.2*	*105*	*8.8*	*16.9*	*0.7*	*3.8*
Green or Brown in Water, Tinned, Average	*½ Can/132g*	*131*	*0.8*	*99*	*8.1*	*15.4*	*0.6*	*3.8*
Green or Brown, Dried, Average	*1 Serving/50g*	*150*	*0.8*	*301*	*22.8*	*49.8*	*1.5*	*9.6*
Green, Dried, Cooked, Sainsbury's*	1 Serving/80g	83	1.8	104	7.4	10.5	2.2	6.2
Green, Organic, Canned, Eat Wholesome*	¼ Can/100g	54	0.3	54	4	6.8	0.3	4
Puy, Green, Dry, Average	*1 Serving/100g*	*306*	*1.4*	*306*	*24.7*	*49.5*	*1.4*	*10.3*
Red, Boiled in Unsalted Water, Average	*1oz/28g*	*28*	*0.1*	*102*	*7.6*	*17.5*	*0.4*	*2.6*
Red, Split, Wholefoods, Tesco*	1 Serving/80g	81	0.3	102	7.6	16	0.4	1.9
LETTUCE								
Average, Raw	*½ Cup/28g*	*4*	*0.1*	*13*	*1*	*1.7*	*0.3*	*1.1*
Curly Leaf, Sainsbury's*	1 Serving/80g	11	0.4	14	0.8	1.7	0.5	0
Iceberg, Chopped, Nature's Pick, Aldi*	1 Serving/80g	10	0.4	13	0.8	2.4	0.5	0.5
Lamb's, Average	*1 Serving/80g*	*12*	*0.2*	*14*	*1.4*	*1.6*	*0.2*	*1*
Little Gem, Average	*1 Lettuce/90g*	*14*	*0.4*	*15*	*0.8*	*1.8*	*0.5*	*0.7*
Radicchio, Red, Raw, Average	*1 Head/220g*	*29*	*0.2*	*13*	*1.4*	*1.6*	*0.1*	*3*
Red Gem, Tesco*	½ Lettuce/45g	7	0.2	15	0.8	1.7	0.5	0.9
Romaine, Average	*1 Serving/80g*	*12*	*0.4*	*15*	*0.9*	*1.7*	*0.5*	*0.7*
Romaine, Hearts, Average	*1 Serving/80g*	*12*	*0.4*	*16*	*0.9*	*1.7*	*0.6*	*1*
Romaine, Sweet, Average	*1 Serving/80g*	*12*	*0.4*	*16*	*0.9*	*1.6*	*0.6*	*0.8*
Round, Average	*1 Serving/80g*	*10*	*0.2*	*13*	*1.4*	*2.2*	*0.2*	*1.1*
Sweet Gem, TTD, Sainsbury's*	1 Serving/100g	15	0.5	15	0.8	1.7	0.5	0.9
LILT								
Fruit Crush, Coca-Cola*	1 Can/330ml	66	0	20	0	4.6	0	0
Fruit Crush, Zero, Coca-Cola*	1 Can/330ml	12	0	4	0	0.3	0	0
Zero, Coca-Cola*	1 Can/330ml	10	0	3	0	0.3	0	0
LIME								
Peel, Raw	*1 Tbsp/6g*	*3*	*0*	*47*	*1.5*	*16*	*0.3*	*10.6*
Raw, Flesh Only, Average	*1 Lime/71g*	*18*	*0.1*	*25*	*0.6*	*8.8*	*0.2*	*2.4*

L

	Measure INFO/WEIGHT	per Measure KCAL	per Measure FAT	Nutrition Values per 100g / 100ml KCAL	PROT	CARB	FAT	FIBRE
LIME								
Zest, Average	*1 Tsp/2g*	*2*	*0*	*100*	*0*	*25*	*0*	*0*
LINGUINE								
Cooked	*1 Serving/100g*	*133*	*0.7*	*133*	*5.1*	*26.3*	*0.7*	*1.1*
Crab, Rocket & Chilli, Italian, Heated, Finest, Tesco*	1 Serving/352g	410	12.7	117	5.7	14.8	3.6	1
Dry, Average	*1 Serving/100g*	*352*	*2.2*	*352*	*13.1*	*70*	*2.2*	*2.8*
Fresh, Dry, Average	*1 Pack/250g*	*681*	*6.5*	*272*	*12.3*	*51.7*	*2.6*	*4*
Prawn, Creamy, Calorie Counted, Asda*	1 Pack/338g	318	7.1	94	4.7	13	2.1	1.2
Prawn, in a White Wine Sauce, Microwaved, HL, Tesco*	1 Pack/340g	326	7.5	96	4.5	14.2	2.2	0.8
Prawn, King, COU, M&S*	1 Meal/360g	400	9	111	5.9	16.4	2.5	0.8
Prawn, King, White Wine, & Chilli Sauce, No.1, Waitrose*	1 Pack/375g	413	12.4	110	5.5	13.6	3.3	2
Salmon, Smoked, Sainsbury's*	1 Serving/400g	586	28.8	146	6.2	14.2	7.2	1.2
Spinach, & Prawn, G&B, Asda*	1 Pack/371g	338	6.7	91	4	14	1.8	1.7
with Scallops, Pancetta & Peas, Spirit of Summer, M&S*	1 Pack/380g	521	14.8	137	7	17.6	3.9	1.8
LINSEEDS								
Average	*1 Tsp/5g*	*23*	*1.7*	*464*	*21.7*	*18.5*	*33.5*	*26.3*
Golden, Asda*	1 Serving/25g	122	8.5	490	28	0.9	34	34
LION BAR								
Mini, Nestle*	1 Bar/16g	80	3.6	486	4.6	67.7	21.7	0
Nestle*	1 Bar/52g	248	11.2	478	6.5	64.6	21.6	0
Peanut, Nestle*	1 Bar/40g	195	10	488	8.1	57.1	25	2.3
LIQUEURS								
Amaretto, Average	*1 Pub Shot/25ml*	*97*	*0*	*388*	*0*	*60*	*0*	*0*
Aperol, Cocktail Mixer, Aperol*	1 Serving/150ml	142	0	95	0	6.7	0	0
Chambord*	1 Serving/35ml	79	0	225	0	29.3	0	0
Cointreau, Specialite De France	*1 Serving/37ml*	*80*	*0*	*215*	*0*	*8.5*	*0*	*0*
Cream, Average	*1 Shot/25ml*	*81*	*4*	*325*	*0*	*22.8*	*16.1*	*0*
Grand Marnier*	1 Pub Shot/35ml	94	0	268	0	22.9	0	0
High Strength, Average	*1 Shot/25ml*	*78*	*0*	*314*	*0*	*24.4*	*0*	*0*
Kirsch, Average	*1 Shot/25ml*	*67*	*0*	*267*	*0*	*20*	*0*	*0*
LIQUORICE								
Allsorts, Average	*1 Sm Bag/56g*	*195*	*2.9*	*349*	*3.7*	*76.7*	*5.2*	*2*
Allsorts, Bassett's*	1 Pack/225g	855	11	380	5.6	77.8	4.9	1.6
Catherine Wheels, Barratt*	1 Wheel/22g	65	0.1	290	3.8	67.2	0.3	0.7
Catherine Wheels, Sainsbury's*	1 Wheel/17g	49	0.1	286	3.8	67.2	0.3	0.7
Original, Soft Eating, Sugar Free, Darrell Lea*	3 Pieces/25g	70	1	280	4	72	4	0
Panda*	1 Bar/32g	109	0.2	340	3.8	78	0.5	0
Raspberry, All Natural, Panda*	1 Bar/32g	98	0.1	307	3.6	72	0.4	0.9
Shapes, Average	*1oz/28g*	*78*	*0.4*	*278*	*5.5*	*65*	*1.4*	*1.9*
Strawberry, Sticks of Ace, Epic Snacks*	1 Serving/25g	101	0.8	403	2.8	89	3.2	1
Sweet, Sugar Free, Dominion, Aldi*	1/3 Pack/25g	56	0.1	224	0.5	77	0.5	6.3
Torpedos, Panda*	1 Serving/25g	92	0	366	1.9	88	0.2	1.4
LIVER								
Calves, Fried	*1oz/28g*	*49*	*2.7*	*176*	*22.3*	*0*	*9.6*	*0*
Calves, Raw	*1oz/28g*	*29*	*1*	*104*	*18.3*	*0*	*3.4*	*0*
Chicken, Cooked, Simmered, Average	*1 Serving/100g*	*167*	*6.5*	*167*	*24.5*	*0.9*	*6.5*	*0*
Chicken, Fried, Average	*1oz/28g*	*47*	*2.5*	*169*	*22.1*	*0*	*8.9*	*0*
Chicken, Raw, Average	*1oz/28g*	*26*	*0.6*	*92*	*17.7*	*0*	*2.3*	*0*
Lamb's, Braised, Average	*1 Serving/100g*	*220*	*8.8*	*220*	*30.6*	*2.5*	*8.8*	*0*
Lamb's, Fried, Average	*1oz/28g*	*66*	*3.6*	*237*	*30.1*	*0*	*12.9*	*0*
Lamb's, Raw, Average	*1 Serving/125g*	*171*	*7.8*	*137*	*20.3*	*0*	*6.2*	*0*
Ox, Raw	*1oz/28g*	*43*	*2.2*	*155*	*21.1*	*0*	*7.8*	*0*
Pig's, Raw	*1oz/28g*	*32*	*0.9*	*113*	*21.3*	*0*	*3.1*	*0*
Pig's, Stewed	*1 Serving/70g*	*132*	*5.7*	*189*	*25.6*	*3.6*	*8.1*	*0*

L

INFO/WEIGHT	Measure	per Measure		Nutrition Values per 100g / 100ml				
		KCAL	FAT	KCAL	PROT	CARB	FAT	FIBRE
LIVER								
Veal, Deluxe, Lidl*	1 Slice/150g	188	5.2	125	19.6	3.8	3.5	0
LIVER & BACON								
with Colcannon Mash, 659, Oakhouse Foods Ltd*	1 Meal/400g	416	12.4	104	10	8.4	3.1	1.2
& Onions, Cook*	1 Portion/280g	372	21.3	133	11.8	4.3	7.6	0.5
Meal for One, M&S*	1 Pack/452g	430	16.7	95	7	8	3.7	1.2
Mini, Frozen, Waitrose*	1 Pack/250g	277	12	111	5.6	10.6	4.8	1.3
with Fresh Mashed Potato, Waitrose*	1 Pack/400g	416	17.2	104	7.3	9	4.3	1.3
with Mash, Mini Meals, Tesco*	1 Pack/234g	262	9.1	112	5.8	12.9	3.9	1.1
with Mash, Serves 1, Classic, Sainsbury's*	1 Pack/450g	448	18.7	103	6.4	8.6	4.3	2.5
LIVER SAUSAGE								
Average	*1 Slice/10g*	*22*	*1.5*	*216*	*15.3*	*4.4*	*15.2*	*0.2*
LLAMA								
Steak, Average	*1 Steak/150g*	*158*	*2*	*105*	*23*	*0.2*	*1.3*	*0*
LOBSTER								
Boiled, Average	*1oz/28g*	*29*	*0.4*	*103*	*22.1*	*0*	*1.6*	*0*
Dressed, Canned, John West*	1 Can/43g	45	2.1	105	13	2	5	0
Raw, Average	*1 Serving/100g*	*92*	*1.4*	*92*	*18.7*	*0.3*	*1.4*	*0*
Thermidor, M&S*	1 Serving/140g	287	19.2	205	10.7	9.7	13.7	0
LOGANBERRIES								
Raw	*1oz/28g*	*5*	*0*	*17*	*1.1*	*3.4*	*0*	*2.5*
LOLLIPOPS								
Assorted, Co-Op*	1 Lolly/10g	40	0	400	0	97	0	0
Chupa Chups*	1 Lolly/12g	47	0	388	0	95	0.3	0
Cremosa, Sugar Free, Chupa Chups*	1 Lolly/10g	28	0.5	275	0.2	92.5	5.4	0
Double, Swizzels*	1 lolly/50g	20	0	41	0	7	0	0
Drumsticks, Swizzels*	1 Lolly/12g	50	0.7	413	0.4	87.9	6.1	0
Refreshers, Bassett's*	1 Lolly/6g	25	0	417	0	108.3	0	0
LOQUATS								
Raw	*1oz/28g*	*5*	*0*	*18*	*0.4*	*4*	*0.1*	*0*
LOZENGES								
Blackcurrant Flavour, Fishermans Friend, Lofthouses*	1 Lozenge/1g	3	0	251	0.1	97.2	1.3	0
Original Extra Strong, Fishermans Friend, Lofthouses*	1 Lozenge/1g	4	0	382	0.3	94.9	0	0.5
Original, Victory V*	1 Lozenge/3g	9	0	350	0	91	0	0
LUCOZADE								
Apple Blast, Lucozade*	1 Serving/200ml	70	0	35	0	8.4	0	0
Energy, Original, GlaxoSmithKline UK Limited*	1 Bottle/380ml	266	0	70	0	17.2	0	0
Orange Energy Drink, GlaxoSmithKline UK Limited*	1 Bottle/500ml	350	0	70	0	17.2	0	0
Orange, Sport Lite, GlaxoSmithKline UK Limited*	1 Serving/500g	50	0	10	0	2	0	0
Raspberry Sport Body Fuel, GlaxoSmithKline UK Limited*	1 Bottle/500ml	140	0	28	0	6.4	0	0
Zero Calories, Lucozade*	1 Serving/250ml	10	0	4	0.1	0.5	0	0
LUNCHEON MEAT								
Pork, Average	*1oz/28g*	*81*	*6.8*	*288*	*13.3*	*4*	*24.3*	*0*
LYCHEES								
Fresh, Raw, Flesh Only	*1oz/28g*	*16*	*0*	*58*	*0.9*	*14.3*	*0.1*	*0.7*
in Juice, Amoy*	1oz/28g	13	0	46	0.4	10.9	0	0
in Syrup, Average	*1oz/28g*	*19*	*0*	*69*	*0.4*	*17.7*	*0*	*0.4*
Raw, Weighed with Skin & Stone	*1oz/28g*	*6*	*0*	*22*	*0.3*	*5.5*	*0.1*	*0.2*

L

M

M&M'S

INFO/WEIGHT	Measure	per Measure		Nutrition Values per 100g / 100ml				
		KCAL	FAT	KCAL	PROT	CARB	FAT	FIBRE
Bar, Milk, Crispy, M&M's, Mars*	½ Bar/75g	407	23.2	543	6.3	58	31	0
Bar, Milk, Hazelnut, M&M's, Mars*	½ Bar/83g	460	28.9	558	6.5	54	35	0
Bar, Milk, M&M's, Mars*	1 Serving/21g	113	6.6	548	6.2	58	32	0
Bar, Milk, Peanut, M&M's, Mars*	½ Bar/83g	460	28.9	558	7.6	53	35	0
Caramel, Crunchy, Limited Edition, M&M's, Mars*	1 Pack/36g	172	6.6	478	3.7	73.5	18.4	0
Crispy, Mars*	1 Serving/36g	179	8.8	498	4.1	63.9	24.4	2.7
Mars*	1 Pack/45g	218	9.7	485	5	68	21.5	0
Mini, Mars*	1 Sm Pack/36g	176	8.4	489	6.3	63.6	23.2	0
Peanut Butter, Mars*	1 Pack/46g	240	14	520	8.7	56.3	30.3	2.2
Peanut, M&M's, Mars*	1 Bag/45g	230	11.7	512	9.8	59	26	0
Salted Caramel, M&M's, Mars*	1 Serving/36g	172	6.5	474	4.4	71	18	0

MACADAMIA NUTS

INFO/WEIGHT	Measure	KCAL	FAT	KCAL	PROT	CARB	FAT	FIBRE
Plain, Average	*1 Pack/100g*	*750*	*77.6*	*750*	*7.9*	*4.8*	*77.6*	*5.3*
Roasted, Salted, Average	*6 Nuts/10g*	*75*	*7.8*	*748*	*7.9*	*4.8*	*77.6*	*5.3*

MACARONI

INFO/WEIGHT	Measure	KCAL	FAT	KCAL	PROT	CARB	FAT	FIBRE
Dry, Average	*1oz/28g*	*99*	*0.5*	*354*	*11.9*	*73.5*	*1.7*	*2.6*
GF, Dry, Free From, Morrisons*	1 Serving/75g	258	0.8	344	5.6	77.1	1.1	1.9

MACARONI CHEESE

INFO/WEIGHT	Measure	KCAL	FAT	KCAL	PROT	CARB	FAT	FIBRE
& Mushroom, Vegan, Waitrose*	1 Pack/260g	320	13.5	123	4	14.1	5.2	2.1
Bites, Mac N Cheese, Crispy, M&S*	½ Pack/100g	255	13.8	255	7.9	23.9	13.8	1.6
Canned	*1oz/28g*	*39*	*1.8*	*138*	*4.5*	*16.4*	*6.5*	*0.4*
Canned, Sainsbury's*	½ Can/200g	181	7.8	91	2.4	11.1	3.9	0.9
Cheddar, Vintage, Rich & Creamy, TTD, Sainsbury's*	1 Pack/375g	703	33.5	197	8.2	18.8	9.4	2.1
Chilled, HFC, Tesco*	1 Pack/400g	540	16.4	135	5.6	18	4.1	1.9
Creamy & Cheese, Made Up, Tesco*	½ Pack/195g	258	3.7	132	4.9	23	1.9	1.4
Creamy, Weight Watchers*	1 Pack/360g	344	9.7	96	4.4	12.9	2.7	1
Iceland*	1 Pack/500g	650	20.5	130	4.8	18	4.1	0.9
Italian, Tesco*	1 Pack/450g	764	25.8	169	7.3	21.6	5.7	1.1
Meal for One, M&S*	1 Pack/400g	684	30.8	171	7.7	17.3	7.7	0.6
Mini, Frozen, Waitrose*	1 Pack/235g	428	19.5	182	8	18.3	8.3	1
Ready Meal, Average	*1 Serving/400g*	*580*	*25.5*	*145*	*6*	*15.8*	*6.4*	*1*
Rice, GF, Amy's Kitchen*	1 Pack/257g	416	18.2	162	6.3	18	7.1	0.4
Triple, Finest, Tesco*	1 Pack/400g	645	22.2	174	7.3	22	6	1.4
Waitrose*	1 Pack/350g	466	32.9	133	6.8	5.2	9.4	0
with Cauliflower, & Squash, Italian, Waitrose*	1 Pack/400g	752	38	188	4.8	20.3	9.5	0.8
with Ham, & Cauliflower, Cook*	1 Pack/300g	306	9.6	102	6.5	12.7	3.2	1.7
with Pancetta, Crispy, for One, Charlie Bigham's*	1 Serving/361g	740	44.8	205	9.3	13.7	12.4	0

MACARONS

INFO/WEIGHT	Measure	KCAL	FAT	KCAL	PROT	CARB	FAT	FIBRE
Brioche Pasquier*	1 Macaron/10g	46	2.4	456	9.8	50.3	23.5	0

MACAROONS

INFO/WEIGHT	Measure	KCAL	FAT	KCAL	PROT	CARB	FAT	FIBRE
Coconut, Gail's*	100g	471	26.1	471	6.1	49.3	26.1	7.2
Coconut, Mini, Sainsbury's*	1 Macaroon/22g	100	5.3	445	3.9	51.6	23.4	6.3
Coconut, Tesco*	1 Macaroon/33g	143	6.3	432	4.5	58	19	5.5
French, Average	*1 Serving/60g*	*225*	*11*	*375*	*6.7*	*46.7*	*18.3*	*3.3*

MACKEREL

INFO/WEIGHT	Measure	KCAL	FAT	KCAL	PROT	CARB	FAT	FIBRE
Atlantic, Raw, Average	*1 Fillet/75g*	*154*	*10.4*	*205*	*18.6*	*0*	*13.9*	*0*
Fillets, Canned, in BBQ Sauce, Smokehouse, John West*	1 Can/115g	239	13.8	208	13	12	12	0
Fillets, in a Hot Chilli Dressing, Princes*	1 Pack/125g	370	33.8	296	13.3	0	27	0
Fillets, in Brine, Average	*1 Can/88g*	*206*	*15.3*	*234*	*19.4*	*0*	*17.4*	*0*
Fillets, in Mustard Sauce, Average	*1 Can/125g*	*274*	*19.4*	*219*	*14.1*	*5.4*	*15.5*	*0*
Fillets, in Olive Oil, Average	*1 Serving/50g*	*149*	*12.2*	*298*	*18.5*	*1*	*24.4*	*0*
Fillets, in Spicy Tomato Sauce, Average	*1oz/28g*	*56*	*3.9*	*199*	*14.3*	*3.8*	*14*	*0*
Fillets, in Sunflower Oil, Average	*1 Can/94g*	*262*	*20.6*	*279*	*20.2*	*0.2*	*21.9*	*0.2*

	Measure INFO/WEIGHT	per Measure		Nutrition Values per 100g / 100ml				
		KCAL	FAT	KCAL	PROT	CARB	FAT	FIBRE
MACKEREL								
Fillets, in Teriyaki Sauce, Boneless & Skinless, Tesco*	1 Can/125g	320	20.3	255	12.6	13.4	16.2	2
Fillets, in Tomato Sauce, Average	*1 Can/125g*	*251*	*18.3*	*200*	*14.3*	*2.7*	*14.7*	*0*
Fillets, Smoked, Average	*1 Fillet/75g*	*251*	*21.1*	*334*	*19.7*	*0.5*	*28.2*	*0.3*
Fillets, Smoked, Skinless, Average	*1 Fillet/65g*	*215*	*17*	*330*	*20.9*	*2.8*	*26.1*	*0.4*
Fried in Blended Oil	*1oz/28g*	*76*	*5.5*	*272*	*24*	*0*	*19.5*	*0*
Grilled	*1oz/28g*	*67*	*4.8*	*239*	*20.8*	*0*	*17.3*	*0*
King, Raw	*1 Fillet/198g*	*208*	*4*	*105*	*20.3*	*0*	*2*	*0*
Raw with Skin, Weighed with Bone, Average	*1oz/28g*	*64*	*4.7*	*227*	*18.9*	*0*	*16.8*	*0*
Smoked, Peppered, Average	*1oz/28g*	*87*	*7*	*310*	*20.4*	*0.3*	*25.2*	*0.2*
Whole, Raw, Average	*1 Serving/100g*	*156*	*11.4*	*156*	*13.3*	*0*	*11.4*	*0*
MADRAS								
Beef, Indian, Takeaway, CBY, Asda*	½ Pack/200g	246	14.2	123	8.9	4.7	7.1	2.5
Beef, Tesco*	1 Pack/460g	616	37.7	134	10.6	4.5	8.2	1.2
Beef, with Pilau Rice, Finest, Tesco*	1 Pack/418g	643	19.7	154	8.3	18.5	4.7	2.1
Chicken, M&S*	1 Pack/400g	492	25.2	123	12.7	2.7	6.3	2.2
Chicken, M&S*	1 Pack/400g	472	23.2	118	12.9	2.5	5.8	1.9
Chicken, Sainsbury's*	1 Pack/400g	532	29.6	133	11	4.5	7.4	1.9
Chicken, Taste of India, Tesco*	½ Pack/215g	275	14.2	128	10.2	5.7	6.6	2.7
Chicken, Waitrose*	1 Pack/400g	672	42	168	14.6	3.7	10.5	1.8
MAGNUM								
Almond, Mini, Wall's*	1 Mini/55g	155	9.4	281	3.9	27	17	0
Almond, Vegan, Wall's*	1 Magnum/90g	248	16.2	276	2.2	26	18	0
Almond, Wall's*	1 Magnum/73g	243	14.6	332	4.8	32	20	0
Bites, After Dinner Classic, Wall's*	1 Bite/29g	102	6.9	353	4	30	24	0
Caramel, Double, Mini, Wall's*	1 Mini/50g	174	10	348	3.2	37	20	0
Caramel, Double, Wall's*	1 Magnum/73g	246	14.6	338	3.2	36	20	0
Chocolate, Double, Mini, Wall's*	1 Mini/50g	182	11.5	365	4	33	23	0
Chocolate, Double, Wall's*	1 Magnum/69g	248	15.9	359	4.1	33	23	0
Classic, Mini, Wall's*	1 Mini/50g	168	11	336	3.7	31	22	0
Classic, Vegan, Wall's*	1 Magnum/90g	234	14.3	261	1.3	27	16	0
Classic, Wall's*	1 Magnum/79g	244	15	309	3.6	29	19	1.2
Dark, Mini, Wall's*	1 Mini/50g	165	11	329	3.8	29	22	0
Double Coconut, Wall's*	1 Magnum/88g	239	14.1	272	3.2	27	16	0
Espresso, Black, Mini, Wall's*	1 Mini/50g	159	10.5	317	3.7	29	21	0
Espresso, Black, Wall's*	1 Magnum/82g	237	15.6	289	3.4	27	19	0
Honeycomb, Wall's*	1 Magnum/78g	240	13.2	308	3.6	35	17	0
Mint, Mini, Wall's*	1 Mini/50g	165	10.5	330	4.2	30	21	0
Mint, Wall's*	1 Magnum/78g	244	14	313	3.1	33	18	0
Peanut Butter, Double, Mini, Wall's*	1 Mini/50g	173	11	346	4.3	32	22	0
Peanut Butter, Double, Wall's*	1 Magnum/73g	245	15.3	336	4.2	32	21	0
Pistachio, Wall's*	1 Magnum/75g	250	15.8	333	4.2	30	21	0
Raspberry, Pink, Mini, Wall's*	1 Mini/50g	166	11.5	332	2.9	31	23	0
Raspberry, Pink, Wall's*	1 Magnum/73g	239	15.3	328	2.9	30	21	0
Strawberry, & White, Wall's*	1 Magnum/88g	250	13.2	284	3	34	15	0
White, Mini, Wall's*	1 Mini/55g	137	8.3	248	2.8	26	15	0
White, Wall's*	1 Magnum/79g	239	14.2	303	3.5	33	18	0
MAKHANI								
Chicken, Morrisons*	½ Pack/175g	301	18.6	172	9.8	8.4	10.6	2
Chicken, Sainsbury's*	½ Pack/199g	313	21.3	157	12.2	2.9	10.7	2.5
Chicken, Tikka, & Pilau Rice, BGTY, Sainsbury's*	1 Pack/400g	448	4	112	8.3	17.5	1	1.9
Chicken, Tikka, Waitrose*	1 Pack/400g	560	30.4	140	14	3.8	7.6	2.1
Prawn, King, Curry, M&S*	1 Pack/400g	732	51.6	183	8	8.1	12.9	1

M

M

	Measure INFO/WEIGHT	per Measure KCAL	per Measure FAT	Nutrition Values per 100g / 100ml KCAL	PROT	CARB	FAT	FIBRE
MALTESERS								
MaltEaster, Chocolate Bunny, Mars*	1 Bunny/29g	157	9	541	7.1	57	31	0
Mini Bunnies, Mars*	1 Bunny/12g	64	3.6	534	8	53.5	30.2	0
MANDARIN ORANGES								
in Juice, Average	*1oz/28g*	*11*	*0*	*39*	*0.7*	*9*	*0*	*0.5*
in Light Syrup, Average	*1 Can/298g*	*201*	*0.1*	*68*	*0.6*	*16*	*0*	*0.1*
Weighed with Peel, Average	*1 Sm/50g*	*14*	*0*	*27*	*0.7*	*6.2*	*0.1*	*0.9*
MANGE TOUT								
& Sugar Snap Peas, Tesco*	1 Pack/150g	102	0.6	68	7	9.2	0.4	3.8
Boiled in Salted Water	*1oz/28g*	*7*	*0*	*26*	*3.2*	*3.3*	*0.1*	*2.2*
Raw, Average	*1 Serving/80g*	*25*	*0.2*	*31*	*3.5*	*4*	*0.2*	*1.1*
Stir-Fried in Blended Oil	*1oz/28g*	*20*	*1.3*	*71*	*3.8*	*3.5*	*4.8*	*2.4*
MANGO								
Dried, Average	*1 Serving/50g*	*174*	*0.5*	*347*	*1.4*	*83.1*	*1*	*4.9*
in Syrup, Average	*1oz/28g*	*22*	*0*	*80*	*0.3*	*20.5*	*0*	*0.9*
Ripe, Raw, Weighed with Skin & Stone, Average	*1 Mango/225g*	*60*	*0.2*	*27*	*0.3*	*6.5*	*0.1*	*1.2*
Ripe, Raw, without Peel & Stone, Flesh Only, Average	*1 Mango/207g*	*118*	*0.4*	*57*	*0.7*	*14.1*	*0.2*	*2.6*
MANGOSTEEN								
Raw, Fresh, Average	1 Serving/80g	50	0.5	63	0.6	15.6	0.6	5.1
MARINADE								
Barbeque, Sticky, Sainsbury's*	¼ Jar/77g	112	2.8	145	0.8	26.7	3.6	1
Cajun Spice, The English Provender Co.*	1 Serving/50g	94	6.7	187	1.3	15.3	13.4	1.6
Sticky Barbecue, Tesco*	¼ Jar/70g	80	0.1	115	0.7	26.7	0.2	0.6
Tandoori, Oven Bake, Pataks*	½ Pack/60g	65	4.1	109	3	7.9	6.8	0
Tandoori, Spice, Patak's*	1 Tbsp/15g	15	0.4	99	3.5	10.1	2.7	5.9
Texan, Hickory Style, BBQ, Quick, Batts, Lidl*	1 Serving/16g	29	0.1	181	1.2	42.5	0.6	3.1
MARJORAM								
Dried	*1 Tsp/1g*	*2*	*0*	*271*	*12.7*	*42.5*	*7*	*0*
MARMALADE								
3 Fruit, Thick Cut, Waitrose*	1 Tsp/15g	39	0	262	0.4	64.8	0.1	0.7
Blood Orange, TTD, Sainsbury's*	1 Tbsp/15g	40	0	264	0.3	65.7	0	0.8
Lemon & Lime, Average	*1 Tbsp/20g*	*53*	*0*	*267*	*0.2*	*66.4*	*0.1*	*0.4*
Lemon with Shred, Average	*1 Serving/20g*	*50*	*0*	*248*	*0.2*	*61.6*	*0*	*0.6*
Lime with Shred, Average	*1 Tbsp/15g*	*39*	*0*	*261*	*0.2*	*65*	*0.1*	*0.4*
Onion, Organic, Duchy Originals*	1 Serving/40g	103	1	257	1	57.8	2.4	2.6
Onion, Red, Stokes*	1 Tbsp/15g	37	0	244	1.2	57.2	0.1	1.3
Orange & Ginger, Average	*1 Tbsp/15g*	*40*	*0*	*264*	*0.2*	*65.7*	*0.1*	*0.3*
Orange & Tangerine, Tiptree, Wilkin & Sons*	1 Tsp/15g	40	0	268	0	67	0	0
Orange with Shred, Average	*1 Tsp/5g*	*13*	*0*	*263*	*0.2*	*65.2*	*0*	*0.3*
Orange, Reduced Sugar, Average	*1 Tbsp/15g*	*26*	*0*	*170*	*0.4*	*42*	*0.1*	*0.6*
Orange, Shredless, Average	*1 Tsp/10g*	*26*	*0*	*261*	*0.2*	*65*	*0*	*0.1*
Thick Cut, Maribel*	1 Tsp/5g	12	0	240	0.2	58.3	0.1	1.5
MARMITE*								
Yeast Extract, Marmite*	1 Tsp/9g	23	0	260	34	30	0.5	3.5
MARROW								
Boiled, Average	*1oz/28g*	*3*	*0.1*	*9*	*0.4*	*1.6*	*0.2*	*0.6*
Raw	*1oz/28g*	*2*	*0*	*6*	*0.3*	*1.2*	*0.1*	*0.3*
MARS								
Bar, 5 Little Ones, Mars*	1 Piece/8g	38	1.5	477	4.5	73.6	18.3	0
Bar, Duo, Mars*	1 Pack/78.8g	355	13.3	450	4.3	69.3	16.9	0
Bar, from Multipack (39.4g bar), Mars*	1 Bar/39.4g	177	6.6	448	4.4	69.3	16.7	0
Bar, Funsize, Mars*	1 Bar/18g	80	2.8	443	3.9	70.7	15.7	0
Bar, Protein, Mars*	1 Bar/57g	200	4.6	351	33	39	8.1	0
Bar, Snacksize (33.8g bar), Mars*	1 Bar/33.8g	151	5.7	448	4.3	69	17	0

	Measure INFO/WEIGHT	per Measure KCAL	FAT	Nutrition Values per 100g / 100ml KCAL	PROT	CARB	FAT	FIBRE
MARS								
Bar, Standard, Single, Mars*	1 Bar/51g	228	8.5	448	4.4	69.3	16.7	0
Choc Brownie, Bar, Mars*	1 Bar/51g	231	9.4	452	4.6	66	18.3	0
MARSHMALLOWS								
Average	*1 Mallow/5g*	*16*	*0*	*327*	*3.9*	*83.1*	*0*	*0*
Chocolate Covered, Ptasie Mleczko, E Wedel*	1 Mallow/11g	47	2.3	441	2.8	57	22	2.6
Chocolate Mallows, Cadbury*	1 Mallow/13g	56	2.2	435	4.7	64.7	17.4	0.8
Dark Chocolate Covered, Mister Choc, Lidl*	1 Mallow/25g	95	2.5	380	4	68	10	0
Fat Free, Tesco*	1 Mallow/7g	24	0	339	3.4	80.8	0.2	0.5
Gourmet, Belinda Clark*	1 Square/6g	17	0	280	2.1	68	0	0
Haribo*	1 Mallow/5g	16	0	330	3	80	0	0
No Added Sugar, Sainsbury's*	1 Mallow/2g	5	0	206	3.3	77	0.1	0
Pink & White, Co-Op*	1 Mallow/7g	24	0	340	3	82	0	0
Pink & White, Waitrose*	1 Mallow/8g	26	0	327	3.8	77.4	0.1	0.5
Princess*	1 Mallow/5g	16	0	314	3.4	80	0	0
Raspberry & Cream, Sainsbury's*	1 Mallow/7g	23	0	330	4.1	78.5	0	0.5
Sainsbury's*	1 Mallow/7g	23	0	330	4.1	78.5	0	0.5
Snowballs, Lees*	1 Snowball/18g	79	3	432	3.4	65.2	16.6	3.9
Soft Mallow Pieces, Mr Mallo*	1 Pack/80g	273	0	341	4.2	81	0	0
MARZIPAN								
Bar, Chocolate, Plain, Thorntons*	1 Bar/46g	206	8	448	5.2	69.1	17.4	2
Dark Chocolate, Thorntons*	1 Serving/46g	207	8	451	5.2	69.4	17.4	2.1
Eggs, in Dark Chocolate, Favorina, Lidl*	1 Egg/20g	91	4	454	6.1	62.2	19.9	4.9
Plain, Average	*1oz/28g*	*115*	*4*	*412*	*5.8*	*67.5*	*14.2*	*1.7*
MASALA								
Chickpea, & Potato, with Cauliflower Rice, Sainsbury's*	1 Pack/518g	671	21.5	130	3.3	17.9	4.2	3.7
Keema, Vegetable, Love Your Veg!, Sainsbury's*	1 Pack/382g	401	19.5	105	2.8	10.1	5.1	3.6
Prawn Mango, Waitrose*	½ Pack/175g	175	11.2	100	5.8	4.3	6.4	1.3
Vegetable, Indian, Sainsburys*	1 Pack/300g	273	17.7	91	2.2	5.5	5.9	3.7
MAYONNAISE								
Average	*1 Tsp/5g*	*35*	*3.8*	*690*	*0.9*	*1.6*	*75.5*	*0*
Branston, with a Twist of Pesto, Crosse & Blackwell*	1 Tbsp/30ml	124	11.6	412	1.2	14.1	38.6	0.2
Extra Light, Average	*1 Tbsp/33g*	*34*	*2*	*102*	*0.7*	*10.5*	*6.2*	*0.8*
French, Light, Sainsbury's*	1 Serving/15ml	46	4.7	307	0.4	6.1	31.1	0.2
Garlic, Retail, Average	*1 Tsp/11g*	*44*	*4.4*	*403*	*1.2*	*8.6*	*40.3*	*0*
Garlic, Roasted, Tiptree, Wilkin & Sons*	1 Tbsp/15g	114	12.6	762	1.6	0	84	0
Reduced Calorie, Average	*1 Tsp/6g*	*18*	*1.7*	*301*	*0.7*	*8.9*	*29*	*0.1*
Truffle, M&S*	1 Tsp/5g	34	3.7	687	1.3	4.4	73.6	1
Vegan, Hellmann's*	1 Serving/15g	98	10.8	654	0.5	3.9	72	0
Vegenaise, Organic, Follow Your Heart*	1 Tbsp/15g	93	10	622	0.8	3.6	67	0
with a Spark of Chilli, Hellmann's*	1 Tbsp/15ml	41	4	276	0.8	7.5	27	0.3
with Dijon Mustard, Hellmann's*	1 Tbsp/15ml	32	3	210	2.9	5.1	19.7	0
MEAL REPLACEMENT								
Banana Flavour Shake, Celebrity Slim*	1 Sachet/55g	214	2.4	389	34.5	51.5	4.4	0.6
Bars, Crispy Caramel Flavour, Slim & Save*	1 Bar/45g	169	5.3	377	26.7	37.5	11.8	6.9
Bars, Lemon, White Chocolate Coated, Slim & Save*	1 Bar/45g	167	4.8	372	24.3	41.8	10.7	5.6
Breakfast Shake, Chocolate, Be Fast*	1 Bottle/250ml	200	3.8	80	3.3	12	1.5	2.5
Brownie, Chocolate, Meal, Diet Now*	1 Pack/55g	200	5.4	364	30.4	35.1	9.9	6.2
Cake, Salted Caramel, Meal, Diet Now*	1 Pack/57g	205	5.4	362	29.6	36.4	9.5	6.1
Caramel Flavour Shake, Celebrity Slim*	1 Pack/55g	212	2.4	385	34.2	50.9	4.4	0.6
Chocolate Flavour Shake, Celebrity Slim*	1 Sachet/55g	211	2.5	383	34	49.1	4.6	2.2
Chocolate, Slender Shake, Boots*	1 Serving/30g	116	2.1	385	15	60	7	11
Chocolate, Weight Loss Shake, As Consumed, Yokobe*	1 Serving/300ml	302	7.2	101	9.6	9.4	2.4	1.4
Drink, Berry, Ready To Drink, Huel*	1 Bottle/500ml	400	18.5	80	4	6.8	3.7	1

MEAL REPLACEMENT

	Measure INFO/WEIGHT	per Measure KCAL	FAT	Nutrition Values per 100g / 100ml KCAL	PROT	CARB	FAT	FIBRE
Pasta, Carbonara, Diet Now*	1 Pack/56g	201	5.2	361	30.1	36	9.3	6.5
Pie, Cottage, Diet Now*	1 Pack/39g	140	3.2	359	33.3	33.3	8.2	10.3
Porridge, Apple & Cinnamon, Diet Now*	1 Serving/40g	143	3.7	354	30.9	32.7	9.2	8.4
Powder, Pro Recover, Chocolate, CNP Professional*	2 Scoops/80g	302	2.6	378	29	57	3.2	2
Powder, PROMR, High Protein, CNP Professional*	1 Pack/72g	255	1.9	354	58	25	2.7	3.6
Shake, Caramel, Diet Now*	1 Pack/34g	131	2.9	385	36.8	37.7	8.6	4.6
Shake, Chocolate Orange, Diet Now*	1 Pack/38g	150	4.6	395	32.9	33.7	12.1	8.7
Shake, Chocolate Orange, New You Plan *	1 Pack/38g	150	4.6	400	33.3	34.1	12.2	8.8
Shake, Chocolate, Advantage, Atkins*	1 Serving/34g	121	4.2	361	49	8.1	12.5	15.5
Shake, Chocolate, Original, Mediterranean Style, Fast 800*	1 Serving/50g	198	9.8	397	46.1	9.8	19.6	14.7
Shake, Chocolate, Ready to Drink, Advantage, Atkins*	1 Carton/330ml	172	9.2	52	6	0.6	2.8	1.2
Shake, Chocolate, Rich, Great Shape, Asda*	1 Bottle/330ml	198	6.3	60	5.2	4.8	1.9	1.5
Shake, Cookies & Cream, Slim Fast*	1 Bottle/325ml	205	5.2	63	4.6	6.6	1.6	1.5
Shake, Herbalife*	1 Serving/250ml	245	6.4	98	10	8.8	2.6	1
Shake, Latte, Smooth, Great Shape, Asda*	1 Bottle/330ml	208	6.9	63	5.5	4.8	2.1	1.6
Shake, Lemon Cheesecake, Exante*	1 Serving/51g	201	6.6	394	33.5	34.7	13	8.2
Shake, Original Flavour, Huel*	1 Serving/125g	500	16.5	400	29.6	36.7	13.2	7.9
Shake, Strawberry, Delight, Great Shape, Asda*	1 Serving/330ml	198	6.3	60	5.1	5.1	1.9	1.2
Shake, Strawberry, Diet Now*	1 Serving/35g	132	3	377	35.7	35.7	8.5	7.4
Shake, Vanilla, Diet Now*	1 Sachet/35g	134	3.4	389	32.7	38.9	9.8	7.2
Shake, Vanilla, Fast800*	1 Serving/50g	196	9.5	392	44	12.6	19	13.1
Shake, Vanilla, Herbalife*	2 Scoops/25g	90	1	360	36	52	4	12
Shake, Vanilla, Ready to Drink, Advantage, Atkins*	1 Carton/330ml	175	8.9	53	6.2	0.6	2.7	0.9
Shake, Vanillla, Smooth, Great Shape, Asda*	1 Bottle/330ml	198	6.3	60	5.1	5.1	1.9	1.2
Shake, Weight Loss, Strawberry, As Sold, XLS-Nutrition*	1 Serving/40g	151	2.7	377	53.3	21.1	6.7	7.6
Soup, Chicken, Noodle, Curry, Diet Now*	1 Pack/55g	201	5.1	366	30.7	36.4	9.3	6.9
Strawberry Flavour Shake, Celebrity Slim*	1 Sachet/55g	214	2.4	389	34.4	51.6	4.4	0.6
Ultra Slim, Ready to Drink, Strawberry, Tesco*	1 Carton/330ml	231	3	70	4.2	10.5	0.9	1.5
Ultra Slim, Ready to Drink, Vanilla, Tesco*	1 Carton/330ml	224	3	68	4.2	10.5	0.9	1.5
Ultra-Slim, Ready to Drink, Chocolate, Tesco*	1 Carton/330ml	214	3.6	65	4	9.8	1.1	1.3
Vanilla Flavour Shake, Celebrity Slim*	1 Sachet/55g	215	2.4	391	34.2	52	4.4	0.6

MEAT LOAF

	Measure INFO/WEIGHT	per Measure KCAL	FAT	Nutrition Values per 100g / 100ml KCAL	PROT	CARB	FAT	FIBRE
Beef & Pork, Co-Op*	¼ Loaf/114g	314	25.1	275	13	7	22	1
Iceland*	1 Serving/150g	332	23.6	221	10.8	9.3	15.7	0.9
Turkey & Bacon, Tesco*	1 Serving/225g	400	22.3	178	14.7	7.4	9.9	1.1

MEATBALLS

	Measure INFO/WEIGHT	per Measure KCAL	FAT	Nutrition Values per 100g / 100ml KCAL	PROT	CARB	FAT	FIBRE
Al Forno, Charlie Bigham's*	½ Pack/324g	532	32.4	164	7	11.5	10	1.1
Beef, Aberdeen Angus, 12 Pack, Waitrose*	1 Meatball/36g	93	7.1	259	18	2.3	19.8	0.1
Beef, As Sold, Tesco*	1 Meatball/28g	78	6.2	277	16.6	2.3	22.3	0.9
Beef, Ashfield Farm, Aldi*	1 Meatball/20g	45	2.7	232	23	3.9	14	0.5
Beef, in Onion & Ale Gravy, Classic Kitchen, Tesco*	½ Pack/224g	331	17.6	148	10.5	8.5	7.9	0.5
Beef, in Tomato Sauce, with Parmigiano, Sainsbury's*	½ Pack/217g	467	33	215	13.8	5.5	15.2	0.5
Beef, Italian Style, As Consumed, Morrisons*	3 Meatballs/104g	235	14.7	226	19.7	4.5	14.1	0.9
Beef, Mini, Oven Cooked, Finest, Tesco*	5 Meatballs/72g	149	8.2	207	21.8	4	11.4	0.8
Beef, Sainsbury's*	1 Meatball/24g	59	4	251	19.6	4.8	16.9	0.5
Beef, Skinny, Mini, 24, M&S*	½ Pack/120g	132	2.9	110	17.9	4.3	2.4	0.5
Beef, with Italian Herbs, Finest, Tesco*	4 Meatballs/83g	184	11.2	222	23.6	1.6	13.5	0.1
Chicken, in Tomato Sauce, Average	**1 Can/392g**	**580**	**32.9**	**148**	**7.7**	**10.4**	**8.4**	**0**
Pork, & Beef, Swedish Style, Tesco*	1 Meatball/14g	34	2.5	245	14.3	6.5	17.7	2
Pork, & Beef, Swedish, Smorgasbord *	¼ Pack/100g	265	20	265	13	9.4	20	0
Pork, Duchy Originals, Waitrose*	5 Meatballs/68g	184	12.6	270	21.7	4	18.6	0
Pork, Italian, Al Forno, Sainsbury's*	1 Pack/450g	644	23.8	143	6.1	17.6	5.3	1.4
Swedish Style, Meat Free, Green Cuisine, Birds Eye*	½ Pack/140g	325	19.6	232	16	8	14	4.8

	Measure INFO/WEIGHT	per Measure KCAL	per Measure FAT	Nutrition Values per 100g / 100ml KCAL	PROT	CARB	FAT	FIBRE
MEATBALLS								
Swedish, Average	*¼ Pack/88g*	*198*	*13.8*	*224*	*14*	*7.4*	*15.7*	*1.3*
Tomato, Spicy, Vegetarian, The Deli, Aldi*	3 Balls/63g	126	5.7	200	5.5	20	9.1	7.5
Turkey, Marinara, Frozen, Microwaved, Slimzone, Asda*	1 Pack/500g	448	4.1	99	7.1	14	0.9	2.6
Vegetarian, Super Greens Balls, as Sold, Heck*	1 Ball/28g	43	0.5	153	6.5	30.3	1.8	5.4
Vegetarian, Swedish Style, Quorn*	½ Bag/150g	195	6.9	130	13.2	7.4	4.6	3
Vegetarian, Swedish, Frozen, Quorn*	¼ Pack/75g	98	3.5	130	13.2	7.4	4.6	3
with Veggies, & Tomato Sauce, Ella's Kitchen*	1 Meatball/26g	21	0.5	82	7.2	8.5	2.1	1.5
MELBA TOAST								
Asda*	1 Slice/3g	13	0.2	395	12	76	4.8	4.6
Average	*1 Serving/3g*	*13*	*0.2*	*396*	*12*	*76*	*4.9*	*4.6*
NUME, Morrisons*	6 Slices/20g	77	0.5	384	11.8	76.9	2.4	3.9
Original, Thins, Van Der Meulen*	1 Thin/3g	13	0.1	384	11.8	76.9	2.4	3.9
Thinly Sliced Toasted Wheat Bread, Sainsbury's*	1 Slice/3g	12	0.1	374	13.1	75.1	2.4	4.6
MELON								
Cantaloupe, Flesh Only, Average	*½ Melon/255g*	*87*	*0.5*	*34*	*0.8*	*8.2*	*0.2*	*0.9*
Cantaloupe, Weighed with Rind, Average	*1 Wedge/100g*	*18*	*0.2*	*18*	*0.4*	*4.2*	*0.2*	*0.4*
Galia	*1 Serving/240g*	*60*	*0.1*	*25*	*0.8*	*5.8*	*0*	*0.2*
Honeydew, & Cantaloupe, Morrisons*	1 Pot/320g	64	0.3	20	0.4	3.9	0.1	1
Honeydew, Raw, Flesh Only, Average	*1oz/28g*	*8*	*0*	*30*	*0.7*	*7*	*0.1*	*0.5*
Medley, Pre Packed, Average	*1 Pack/240g*	*66*	*0.3*	*27*	*0.6*	*6*	*0.1*	*0.5*
MELON & GRAPES								
Fresh, Tesco*	1 Pack/300g	105	0.3	35	0.6	7.2	0.1	1.2
Meadow Fresh, Lidl*	1 Pack/200g	84	0.4	42	0.8	8.9	0.2	0.5
MERINGUE								
Average	*1 Meringue/8g*	*30*	*0*	*379*	*5.3*	*95.4*	*0*	*0*
Bombe, Raspberry & Vanilla, M&S*	1 Bombe/100g	155	1.8	155	3.4	33.3	1.8	2.6
Coffee Fresh Cream, Asda*	1 Meringue/28g	109	4.7	396	3.8	57	17	0.3
Cream, Fresh, Sainsbury's*	1 Meringue/35g	142	5.1	407	3.5	65.4	14.6	0.5
Cream, M&S*	1 Meringue/34g	145	7.6	425	4.1	52.6	22.2	1.4
Mini, M&S*	1 Meringue/4g	15	0	395	6.1	91.6	0	0.2
Nests, Average	*1 Nest/16g*	*63*	*0*	*397*	*4.8*	*93.3*	*0.1*	*0.1*
Nests, Bakery, Sainsbury's*	1 Nest/12g	47	0.1	395	4.6	93.9	0.5	0.5
Nests, M&S*	1 Nest/12g	47	0	390	6.1	91.6	0	0
Nests, Mini, Tesco*	1 Nest/5g	19	0	386	4.8	91.2	0.2	0
Nests, Waitrose*	1 Nest/16g	62	0	386	4.8	91.2	0.2	0
Shells, Mini, Asda*	1 Shell/4g	16	0	395	4.3	94	0	0.6
Shells, Mini, Waitrose*	1 Shell/5g	19	0	386	4.8	91.2	0.2	0
Strawberry, Mini, The Best, Morrisons*	1 Meringue/5g	21	0	394	5.1	92.6	0.3	0
Toffee Cream, Tesco*	1 Meringue/30g	114	5	380	4.2	52.9	16.5	0
MIDGET GEMS								
M&S*	1 Bag/113g	367	0.1	325	6.3	75.1	0.1	0
Smart Price, Asda*	1 Pack/178g	586	0.2	329	6	76	0.1	0
MILK								
Almond, & Rice, Almond Dream*	1 Glass/95ml	36	1.2	38	0.6	5.2	1.3	0.4
Almond, Dark Chocolate, Alpro*	1 Serving/200ml	94	2.6	47	0.8	7.6	1.3	0.8
Almond, Original, Actileaf, Aldi*	1 Serving/200ml	56	2.8	28	0.6	3.2	1.4	0
Almond, Original, Alpro*	1 Serving/200ml	48	2.2	24	0.5	3	1.1	0.2
Almond, Original, Fresh, Alpro*	1 Serving/200ml	48	22	24	0.5	3	11	0.2
Almond, Original, Roasted, Alpro*	1 Serving/100ml	22	1.1	22	0.4	2.4	1.1	0.4
Almond, Unsweetened, Breeze, Blue Diamond*	1 Serving/250ml	32	2.8	13	0.5	0.2	1.1	0.3
Almond, Unsweetened, Innocent*	1 Serving/200ml	74	6.8	37	1.4	0.3	3.4	0
Almond, Unsweetened, Roasted, Alpro*	1 Serving/200ml	26	2.2	13	0.4	0	1.1	0.4
Almond, Unsweetened, Roasted, Fresh, Alpro*	1 Serving/200ml	26	2.2	13	0.4	0	1.1	0.4

MILK

	Measure INFO/WEIGHT	per Measure KCAL	per Measure FAT	KCAL	PROT	CARB	FAT	FIBRE
Almond, Unsweetened, Sainsbury's*	1 Serving/200ml	36	2.6	18	0.5	1.1	1.3	0
Almond, Unsweetened, UHT, Tesco*	1 Serving/125ml	20	1.2	16	0.6	1.1	1	0
Almond, Unsweetened, Unroasted, Alpro*	1 Serving/200ml	26	2.6	13	0.5	0	1.3	0.2
Alternative, Original, Good Hemp*	1 Glass/250ml	90	6	36	1.3	2.2	2.4	0.2
Chocolate, M&S*	½ Bottle/500ml	360	9	72	3.3	10.2	1.8	0.9
Coconut, & Almond, Fresh, Alpro*	1 Serving/200ml	48	2.6	24	0.3	2.6	1.3	0
Coconut, Asia Specialities, Aldi*	1 Serving/100ml	176	18	176	1.5	2.2	18	0.5
Coconut, Average	*1 Can/400ml*	*698*	*69.7*	*174*	*1.4*	*2.9*	*17.4*	*2.9*
Coconut, Canned, Pride*	½ Can/200ml	284	30	142	1	1.6	15	0
Coconut, Canned, Sainsbury's*	1 Can/400ml	764	72.8	191	0.9	5.7	18.2	0.5
Coconut, Canned, Tesco*	¼ Can/100ml	151	15	151	0.9	3.2	15	0
Coconut, Chocolate, Alpro*	1 Serving/200ml	82	2.2	41	0.4	7	1.1	0
Coconut, Ga-Ti, Thai Taste*	1 Can/400ml	696	72	174	0	2.9	18	0
Coconut, Half Fat, Waitrose*	½ Can/135ml	92	8.1	68	0.7	2.7	6	0
Coconut, KTC*	1 Can/400ml	516	73.2	129	1.3	1.8	18.3	0
Coconut, Light, Tesco*	1 Can/400ml	244	24	61	0.4	1.3	6	0
Coconut, Lighter, Sainsbury's*	¼ Can/100ml	75	6.5	75	0.9	2.9	6.5	0.5
Coconut, Milk Free, Free From, Asda*	1 Serving/250ml	50	2.8	20	0.5	2	1.1	0.5
Coconut, Organic, Tesco*	1/8 Can/49g	85	8.3	175	1.8	2.7	17	1.3
Coconut, Original, Fresh, Alpro*	1 Serving/200ml	40	1.8	20	0.1	2.7	0.9	0
Coconut, Pure, Kefir Cultures, Drink, Rhythm Health*	1 Bottle/126g	43	2.5	34	0.8	2.8	2	1.7
Coconut, Reduced Fat, Amoy*	1 Tin/400ml	440	44	110	1	2	11	1
Coconut, Reduced Fat, Average	*1 Serving/100g*	*104*	*10*	*104*	*1*	*2.4*	*10*	*0.4*
Coconut, Reduced Fat, Canned, Essential, Waitrose*	1 Can/400ml	244	24	61	0	1.8	6	0
Coconut, Sweetened, Sainsbury's*	1 Serving/250ml	45	2.5	18	0.5	2.2	1	0.5
Coconut, Unsweetened, UHT, Alpro*	1 Serving/200ml	28	2.4	14	0.1	0.4	1.2	0
Condensed, Caramel, Carnation, Nestle*	1 Serving/50g	148	3	296	5.5	55.1	6	0
Condensed, Semi Skimmed, Sweetened	*1oz/28g*	*75*	*0.1*	*267*	*10*	*60*	*0.2*	*0*
Condensed, Skimmed, Unsweetened, Average	*1oz/28g*	*30*	*1.1*	*108*	*7.5*	*10.5*	*4*	*0*
Condensed, Squeezy, Carnation, Nestle*	1 Serving/50g	162	4	325	7.3	56	8	0
Condensed, Whole, Sweetened, Average	*1oz/28g*	*93*	*2.8*	*333*	*8.5*	*55.5*	*10.1*	*0*
Dried, Skimmed, Average	*1oz/28g*	*99*	*0.3*	*355*	*35.4*	*52.3*	*0.9*	*0*
Dried, Whole, Average	*1oz/28g*	*137*	*7.4*	*490*	*26.3*	*39.4*	*26.3*	*0*
Evaporated, Average	*1 Serving/85g*	*136*	*7.6*	*160*	*8.2*	*11.6*	*9*	*0*
Evaporated, Reduced Fat, Average	*1oz/28g*	*33*	*1.5*	*118*	*7.4*	*10.5*	*5.2*	*0*
Goat's, Semi Skimmed, St Helen's Farm*	1 Serving/200ml	88	3.2	44	3	4.3	1.6	0
Goat's, Skimmed, St Helen's Farm*	1 Serving/200ml	60	0.2	30	3	4.3	0.1	0
Goat's, Whole, St Helen's Farm*	1 Serving/200ml	122	7.2	61	2.8	4.3	3.6	0
Goats, Pasteurised	*1 fl oz/30ml*	*18*	*1*	*60*	*3.1*	*4.4*	*3.5*	*0*
Gold Top, Original, Graham's*	1 Tbsp/15ml	12	0.8	80	3.7	4.7	5	0
Kefir, Bibi's Homemade*	1 Glass/210g	128	7.4	61	3.3	4.3	3.5	0
Kefir, Starter Culture, Nourish*	1 Sachet/5g	18	0	360	40	40	0	0
Oat, Original, Alpro*	1 Serving/200ml	88	3	44	0.3	6.8	1.5	1.4
Powder, Instant, Skimmed, Basics, Sainsbury's*	1 Serving/60g	209	0.4	349	35.6	50.4	0.6	0
Rice, Organic, Provamel*	1 Serving/250ml	122	3.8	49	0.1	9.5	1.5	0
Rice, Original, Alpro*	1 Glass/200ml	94	2	47	0.1	9.5	1	0
Rice, Original, Rice Dream*	1 Serving/150ml	70	1.5	47	0.1	9.4	1	0.1
Semi Skimmed, Average	*1fl oz/30ml*	*15*	*0.5*	*49*	*3.4*	*5*	*1.7*	*0*
Semi Skimmed, Long Life, Average	*1fl oz/30ml*	*15*	*0.5*	*49*	*3.4*	*5*	*1.7*	*0*
Semi Skimmed, Low Lactose, Lactofree, Arla*	1 Glass/125ml	50	1.9	40	3.6	3	1.5	0
Semi Skimmed, UHT, Viva*	1 Serving/200ml	94	3	47	3.6	4.8	1.5	0
Skimmed, Average	*1 Pint/568ml*	*194*	*0.5*	*34*	*3.3*	*5*	*0.1*	*0*
Skimmed, Lactofree, Arla*	1 Serving/200ml	62	1	31	3.7	2.8	0.5	0

MILK

INFO/WEIGHT	Measure	per Measure KCAL	FAT	Nutrition Values per 100g / 100ml KCAL	PROT	CARB	FAT	FIBRE
Skimmed, Long Life, Mootrition*	1 Serving/200ml	66	0.2	33	3.5	4.5	0.1	0
Skimmed, Proactiv, Actively Lowers Cholesterol, Flora*	1 Serving/100ml	35	0.3	35	3.2	4.8	0.3	0
Skimmed, Uht, Average	*1fl oz/30ml*	*10*	*0*	*34*	*3.4*	*5*	*0.1*	*0*
Soy, Reg, Good Hope*	1 Serving/100ml	38	1.7	38	3	3	1.7	0
Soya, Banana Flavour, Provamel*	1 Serving/250ml	195	5.5	78	3.8	10.4	2.2	0.6
Soya, Chocolate, Alpro*	1 Serving/200ml	122	3.6	61	3.1	7.8	1.8	0.9
Soya, Chocolate, UHT, Alpro*	1 Serving/200ml	122	3.6	61	3.1	7.8	1.8	0.9
Soya, Fat Free, Original, So Good Beverages*	1 Serving/250ml	100	0.2	40	3.6	6.4	0.1	0
Soya, Flavoured, Average	*1 Glass/250ml*	*100*	*4.2*	*40*	*2.8*	*3.6*	*1.7*	*0*
Soya, Growing Up Drink, Low in Sugars, Alpro*	1 Serving/200ml	128	4.4	64	2.5	8.3	2.2	0.4
Soya, Light, Alpro*	1 Serving/200ml	54	2.4	27	2.1	1.6	1.2	0.9
Soya, Light, Fresh, Alpro*	1 Serving/200ml	44	2.4	22	2	0.1	1.2	1.2
Soya, No Added Sugar, Unsweetened, Average	*1 Serving/250ml*	*85*	*4.8*	*34*	*3.3*	*0.9*	*1.9*	*0.4*
Soya, Original, Alpro*	1 Serving/200ml	88	3.8	44	3.3	3	1.9	0.6
Soya, Original, Fresh, Alpro*	1 Serving/200ml	78	3.6	39	3	2.5	1.8	0.5
Soya, Original, Fresh, Organic, Alpro*	1 Serving/200ml	76	3.4	38	3	2.4	1.7	0.5
Soya, Strawberry, Alpro*	1 Serving/200ml	124	3.6	62	3.3	7.6	1.8	0.5
Soya, Sweetened, Actileaf, Aldi*	1 Serving/200ml	98	5.2	49	3.5	2.6	2.6	0.5
Soya, Sweetened, Average	*1 Glass/200ml*	*94*	*4.2*	*47*	*3.4*	*3.7*	*2.1*	*0.4*
Soya, Sweetened, Calcium Enriched, Average	*1 Glass/200ml*	*91*	*3.9*	*46*	*3.4*	*3.7*	*2*	*0.3*
Soya, Sweetened, UHT, Tesco*	1 Serving/200ml	84	3.8	42	3.4	2.6	1.9	0.6
Soya, Unsweetened, Actileaf, Aldi*	1 Serving/200ml	68	4.2	34	3.4	0.5	2.1	0.5
Soya, Unsweetened, Dairy Free, Just Free, Lidl*	1 Serving/200ml	66	3.8	33	3.4	0.2	1.9	0.6
Soya, Unsweetened, Organic, Waitrose*	1 Serving/60ml	19	1.1	31	3.3	0.2	1.9	0
Soya, Unsweetened, Smart Price, Asda*	1 Serving/250ml	80	4.8	32	3.3	0.5	1.9	0.5
Soya, Unsweetened, Uht, Everyday Value, Tesco*	1 Serving/250ml	72	4	29	2.9	0.4	1.6	0.5
Soya, Unsweetened, Uht, Organic, Tesco*	1 Serving/150ml	50	2.8	33	3.4	0.4	1.9	0.6
Soya, Vanilla, Alpro*	1 Serving/200ml	108	3.4	54	3	6.5	1.7	0.5
Soya, Vitasoy*	1 Serving/250ml	130	3.8	52	3	5.5	1.5	2
Soya, Wholebean, Unsweetened, Alpro*	1 Serving/200ml	66	3.6	33	3.3	0	1.8	0.6
Soya, Wholebean, Unsweetened, Fresh, Alpro*	1 Serving/200ml	66	3.6	33	3.3	0	1.8	0.6
Soya, Wholebean, Unsweetened, Organic, Alpro*	1 Serving/200ml	66	3.6	33	3.3	0	1.8	0.6
Strawberry Flavoured, Essential, Waitrose*	1 Glass/200ml	136	3.4	68	3.3	9.5	1.7	0.5
Strawberry, Flavoured, M&S*	1 Serving/200ml	142	3.6	71	3.2	10.6	1.8	0.5
Whole, Average	*1 Serving/200ml*	*134*	*7.8*	*67*	*3.3*	*4.7*	*3.9*	*0*
Whole, Lactose Free, Lactofree, Arla*	1 Serving/200ml	114	7	57	3.4	2.8	3.5	0

MILK DRINK

INFO/WEIGHT	Measure	per Measure KCAL	FAT	Nutrition Values per 100g / 100ml KCAL	PROT	CARB	FAT	FIBRE
Banana, Breakfast, Fuel 10K*	1 Carton/330g	218	4.6	66	6.1	6.7	1.4	1
Breakfast, Chocolate, Protein, Fuel 10K*	1 Carton/330ml	208	3.3	63	6.1	6.9	1	1
Chocolate Coconut, Free From, Tesco*	1 Serving/250ml	125	5.4	49	0.4	6.8	2.1	0.7
Chocolate Sterilised Skimmed, Happy Shopper*	1 Bottle/500ml	295	1.5	59	3.6	10.4	0.3	0
Chocolate, Break Time, Arla*	1 Bottle/500ml	290	1.5	58	3.6	10.2	0.3	0
Chocolate, Brekkie, Up & Go, Life Health Foods*	1 Carton/330ml	218	3.3	66	3.8	9.1	1	2.4
Chocolate, Spar*	1 Serving/500ml	290	1.5	58	3.6	10.2	0.3	0
Chocolatte, Cafe Met*	1 Bottle/290ml	174	4.1	60	3.7	9.1	1.4	0.3
Kefir, Baked, Bio-tiful Dairy*	1 Bottle/500g	305	15.5	61	3.3	5	3.1	0
Kefir, Honey, & Ginger, Bio-tiful*	1 Serving/250ml	161	6.8	64	2.9	7.1	2.7	0
Kefir, Milko*	1 Serving/100ml	46	1.5	46	3.6	4.6	1.5	0
Kefir, Organic, Bio-tiful Dairy*	1 Serving/250g	145	7.5	58	3.2	4.6	3	0
Oat, Oat Dream*	1 Serving/200ml	56	1.4	28	0.4	4.8	0.7	0
Original, Mars*	1 Serving/330g	284	6.9	86	3.1	13.7	2.1	0
Shake, Strawberry, Ready to Drink, Atkins*	1 Bottle/330ml	163	9	49	4.6	0.9	2.7	1.5
Strawberry Flavoured, Goodness for Kids, Tesco*	1 Bottle/330ml	248	5.6	75	4	9.9	1.7	0.4

M

MILK DRINK

	Measure INFO/WEIGHT	per Measure KCAL	FAT	Nutrition Values per 100g / 100ml KCAL	PROT	CARB	FAT	FIBRE
Strawberry, Flavoured, Asda*	1 Bottle/330ml	211	3.6	64	3.6	10	1.1	0.5
Vanilla, Breakfast, Protein, Fuel 10K*	1 Carton/330ml	218	4.6	66	6.1	6.7	1.4	1

MILK SHAKE

Banana Flavour, Frijj*	1 Bottle/500ml	325	4.5	65	3.7	10.5	0.9	0
Banana Flavour, Spar*	1 Bottle/500ml	250	0.5	50	3.3	9.1	0.1	0
Banana, Yazoo, Campina*	1 Bottle/200ml	120	2.4	60	3.1	9.6	1.2	0
Chocolate Flavour, BGTY, Sainsbury's*	1 Bottle/500ml	290	2.5	58	5.3	8	0.5	0.9
Chocolate Flavour, Diet Chef Ltd*	1 Drink/330ml	210	2.3	64	4.1	8.5	0.7	1.9
Chocolate Flavoured, Fresh, Thick, Frijj*	1 Bottle/500ml	350	5	70	3.5	11.7	1	0
Chocolate, Asda*	1 Serving/250ml	198	9.2	79	4.4	7	3.7	0.4
Chocolate, Belgian, M&S*	1 Bottle/300ml	360	14.4	120	4.2	14.6	4.8	0.7
Chocolate, Dry, Cadbury*	1 Serving/14g	54	0.9	387	7.7	64	6.3	21
Chocolate, Fudge, Cowbelle, Aldi*	1 Serving/100ml	74	1.3	74	4.5	11	1.3	0.5
Chocolate, High Protein, Musclefood*	1 Bottle/250ml	143	1	57	8.5	4.9	0.4	0
Chocolate, Mint, Yazoo*	1 Bottle/400ml	260	6	65	3.3	9.1	1.5	0
Chocolate, Protein, Ufit*	1 Bottle/310ml	170	3.1	55	7.1	3.6	1	1.2
Chocolate, Soy, Good Hope*	1 Serving/250ml	180	6	72	3	10	2.4	0
Powder, Made Up with Semi-Skimmed Milk	**1 Serving/250ml**	**172**	**4**	**69**	**3.2**	**11.3**	**1.6**	**0**
Powder, Made Up with Whole Milk	**1 Serving/250ml**	**218**	**9.2**	**87**	**3.1**	**11.1**	**3.7**	**0**
Protein, Supplement, USN*	1 Bottle/310ml	145	0.3	47	8.1	3.4	0.1	0
Raspberry & Strawberry, Protein 20g, Arla*	1 Serving/225ml	171	3.6	76	9	6.5	1.6	0
Strawberry & Raspberry, Syrup, Robinson's*	1 Serving/50ml	20	0.7	39	2.9	4	1.4	0
Strawberry Flavour, Thick, Low Fat, Frijj*	1 Bottle/250ml	155	2	62	3.4	10.1	0.8	0
Strawberry, British, M&S*	1 Bottle/300ml	270	10.2	90	4	10.8	3.4	0.1
Strawberry, Diet Chef Ltd*	1 Drink/330g	225	3	68	4.2	10.5	0.9	1.5
Strawberry, High Protein, Breakfast, Ufit*	1 Bottle/310ml	189	4.6	61	4.9	5.7	1.5	2.7
Strawberry, High Protein, For Goodness Shakes*	1 Bottle/475ml	206	0.5	43	5.3	5.3	0.1	0.1
Strawberry, Protein, Euro Shopper*	1 Bottle/330ml	148	1.6	45	6.2	5.1	0.5	0.5
Strawberry, Yazoo, Campina*	1 Bottle/475ml	300	6	60	3.1	9.5	1.2	0
Thick, Milky Way, Mars*	1 Bottle/440ml	282	4.8	64	3.4	10	1.1	0.7
Vanilla, Diet Chef Ltd*	1 Pack/330ml	225	3	68	4.2	10.5	0.9	1.5
White Chocolate, & Vanilla, M&S*	1 Bottle/300ml	315	12.9	105	3.8	12.4	4.3	0.6

MILKY BAR

Buttons, Nestle*	1 Pack/14g	78	4.6	543	10.6	53.1	31.7	0
Chunky, Nestle*	¼ Bar/38g	207	12	547	7.3	58.4	31.7	0
Crunchies, Nestle*	1 Pack/30g	168	10.4	560	7	54.9	34.7	0
Egg, White Chocolate, Nestle*	1 Egg/65g	353	20.6	543	10.6	53.1	31.7	0
Funsize (17g), Mars*	1 Bar/17g	75	2.7	449	3.8	71.8	16.3	0.6
Mini Eggs, Nestle*	1 Pack/90g	443	18.5	492	7	69.4	20.6	0
Munchies, Nestle*	1 Serving/70g	392	24.3	560	7	54.9	34.7	0.1
Nestle*	1 Sm Bar/13g	68	4	547	7.3	58.4	31.7	0

MILKY WAY

Fun Size, Mars*	1 Bar/17g	75	2.7	447	3.8	71.6	16.2	0
Funsize (15.5g), Mars*	1 Bar/16g	69	2.5	446	3.9	71.6	16.3	0.6
Mars*	1 Bar/22g	96	3.3	446	3.9	72.4	15.5	0.6

MINCEMEAT

Average	**1oz/28g**	**77**	**1.2**	**274**	**0.6**	**62.1**	**4.3**	**1.3**
Sainsbury's*	1 Tbsp/20g	58	0.6	291	1.2	62.3	3.1	1.4
Traditional, Robertson*	1 Tbsp/24g	68	0.6	285	0.8	63.5	2.7	2.5

MINSTRELS

Galaxy, Mars*	1 Serving/39g	196	8.6	498	5.2	69.1	21.9	0

MINT

Dried, Average	**1 Tsp/5g**	**14**	**0.2**	**279**	**24.8**	**34.6**	**4.6**	**0**

	Measure INFO/WEIGHT	per Measure KCAL	FAT	Nutrition Values per 100g / 100ml KCAL	PROT	CARB	FAT	FIBRE
MINT								
Fresh, Average	*2 Tbsp/3.2g*	*1*	*0*	*43*	*3.8*	*5.3*	*0.7*	*0*
MINTS								
After Dinner, Dark, Elizabeth Shaw*	1 Sweet/9g	42	2.1	469	2.8	62.5	23.1	0
Butter Mintoes, M&S*	1 Sweet/9g	35	0.6	391	0	84	6.8	0
Butter Mintoes, Tesco*	1 Sweet/7g	24	0.5	349	0	71.3	7.1	0
Clear, Co-Op*	1 Sweet/6g	24	0	395	0	98	0	0
Cream, Luxury, Thorntons*	1 Sweet/13g	62	3.1	477	4.2	62.3	23.8	2.3
Creams, Bassett's*	1 Sweet/11g	40	0	365	0	91.8	0	0
Curiously Strong, M&S*	1 Sweet/1g	4	0	390	0.4	97.5	0	0
Everton, Co-Op*	1 Sweet/6g	25	0.2	410	0.6	92	4	0
Extra Strong, Peppermint, Trebor*	1 Mint/2g	10	0	395	0.3	98.5	0	0
Extra Strong, Spearmint, Trebor*	1 Pack/44g	174	0	395	0.4	98.7	0	0
Extra Strong, Trebor*	1 Pack/13g	30	0	235	0.4	97	0.2	0
Glacier, Fox's*	1 Sweet/5g	19	0	386	0	96.4	0	0
Humbugs, Co-Op*	1 Sweet/8g	34	0.6	425	0.6	89.9	7	0
Humbugs, Grumpy Old Gits, Spencer & Fleetwood Ltd*	1 Sweet/25g	92	0.4	366	0.2	87.5	1.5	0
Humbugs, M&S*	1 Sweet/9g	37	0.4	407	0.6	91.1	4.4	0
Humbugs, Thorntons*	1 Sweet/9g	31	0.4	340	1	87.8	4.4	0
Imperials, Co-Op*	1 Sweet/3g	12	0	395	0.3	98	0.2	0
Imperials, M&S*	1 Sweet/3g	12	0	391	0	97.8	0	0
Imperials, Sainsbury's*	1 Sweet/3g	10	0	374	0	92.1	0	0
Imperials, Tesco*	1 Sweet/3g	12	0	397	0.6	98.7	0	0
Mento, Sugar Free, Mentos*	1 Sweet/2g	5	0.1	260	1	87	5.5	0
Mighties, Sugar Free, Trebor*	1 Sweet/1g	1	0	235	0.4	97	0.2	0
Mint Assortment, M&S*	1 Sweet/7g	26	0.5	375	0.4	78.2	6.9	0
Peppermints, Strong, Altoids*	1 Sweet/1g	3	0	385	0.5	96	0	0
Soft, Trebor*	1 Pack/48g	182	0	380	0	94.9	0	0
Softmints, Peppermint, Trebor*	1 Pack/48g	170	0	355	0	88.9	0	0
Softmints, Spearmint, Trebor*	1 Pack/45g	170	0	375	0	94.3	0	0
Thins, Chocolate, Waitrose*	1 Thin/5g	27	1.3	509	4.2	69.6	23.8	0.2
MIRIN								
Mikawa, Organic, Clearspring*	1 Tbsp/15ml	24	0.1	163	0.5	39	0.4	0
Rice Wine, Sweetened, Average	*1 Tbsp/15ml*	*35*	*0*	*231*	*0.2*	*41.6*	*0*	*0*
MISO								
Average	*1oz/28g*	*57*	*1.7*	*203*	*13.3*	*23.5*	*6.2*	*0*
Paste, Red, AKA, Unpasteurised, Organic, Miso Tasty*	1 Tbsp/15g	31	0.8	208	10	25.3	5.6	4.1
Paste, Sainsbury's*	¼ Jar/25g	22	0.6	89	4.6	9.7	2.5	4.4
White, Sweet, Organic, Clearspring*	1 Tbsp/15g	26	0.6	171	7.7	26	4	0.6
MIXED HERBS								
Average	*1 Tsp/5g*	*13*	*0.4*	*260*	*13*	*37.5*	*8.5*	*6.7*
MOLASSES								
Average	*1 Tsp/5g*	*13*	*0*	*266*	*0*	*68.8*	*0.1*	*0*
MONKEY NUTS								
without Shell, Average	*1oz/28g*	*158*	*13.4*	*565*	*25.6*	*8.2*	*48*	*6.3*
MONKFISH								
Grilled	*1oz/28g*	*27*	*0.2*	*96*	*22.7*	*0*	*0.6*	*0*
Raw	*1oz/28g*	*18*	*0.1*	*66*	*15.7*	*0*	*0.4*	*0*
MONSTER MUNCH								
Pickled Onion, Walkers*	1 Std Bag/22g	108	5.5	490	6	60	25	1.7
Roast Beef, Walkers*	1 Std Bag/22g	108	5.5	490	7	59	25	1.7
Spicy, Walkers*	1 Std Bag/25g	125	7.2	500	5	55	29	1.3
MOUSSAKA								
182, Oakhouse Foods Ltd*	1 Meal/400g	588	39.6	147	7.3	7.6	9.9	0.7

M

M

MOUSSAKA

	Measure INFO/WEIGHT	per Measure KCAL	FAT	Nutrition Values per 100g / 100ml KCAL	PROT	CARB	FAT	FIBRE
Beef, & Lamb, Waitrose*	1 Pack/323g	387	19.4	120	6.2	9.5	6	1.5
Beef, BGTY, Sainsbury's*	1 Pack/400g	300	10.4	75	6.1	6.8	2.6	1.2
Charlie Bigham's*	½ Pack/328g	425	27.8	130	6.1	6.9	8.5	0
for One, Charlie Bigham's*	1 Serving/340 g	442	29.2	130	6	6.9	8.6	0
for Two, Charlie Bigham's*	1 Serving/327 g	425	27.8	130	6.1	6.9	8.5	0
Lamb, BGTY, Sainsbury's*	1 Pack/400g	296	10.4	74	5	6.1	2.6	3
Lamb, Finest, Tesco*	½ Pack/334g	513	36.5	154	6.4	6.6	10.9	1.5
Lamb, Gastropub, M&S*	1 Pack/409g	528	31.5	129	6.2	7.5	7.7	2.2
Lamb, Serves 2, TTD, Sainsbury's*	½ Pack/400g	546	33.7	141	7.2	8	8.7	1.2
Vegetable, COU, M&S*	1 Pack/400g	280	10.8	70	2.7	9.1	2.7	2.4
Vegetarian, Quorn*	1 Pack/400g	364	16.4	91	3.6	9.8	4.1	1.2

MOUSSE

	Measure INFO/WEIGHT	per Measure KCAL	FAT	Nutrition Values per 100g / 100ml KCAL	PROT	CARB	FAT	FIBRE
Aero Chocolate, Nestle*	1 Pot/58g	101	3	174	4.8	27.3	5.1	1.1
Apricot, Lite, Onken*	1 Pot/150g	156	2.2	104	4.6	18	1.5	0.3
Banoffee, COU, M&S*	1 Pot/70g	102	1.5	145	2.9	28.8	2.1	1.5
Blackcurrant, Onken*	1 Pot/150g	210	10.2	140	5.2	14.6	6.8	0
Cappuccino, Essential, Waitrose*	1 Pot/100g	279	16.7	279	4.2	27.7	16.7	0.5
Caramel, Meringue, Cadbury*	1 Pot/65g	181	6.7	277	4.6	42.4	10.3	1
Cherry, & Kirsch, Finest, Tesco*	1 Pot/100g	195	11.6	195	2.7	19.6	11.6	0.5
Chocolate	***1 Pot/60g***	***83***	***3.2***	***139***	***4***	***19.9***	***5.4***	***0***
Chocolate, & Hazelnut, Creamy, Dr Oetker*	1 Pot/115g	158	6.9	137	3.3	17.6	6	0.6
Chocolate, & Hazelnut, Onken*	1 Pot/125g	171	7.5	137	3.3	17.8	6	0
Chocolate, & Mint, COU, M&S*	1 Pot/70g	84	1.8	120	6.2	18.7	2.5	1
Chocolate, & Orange, COU, M&S*	1 Pot/70g	77	1.8	110	5.9	16	2.6	0.9
Chocolate, & Vanilla, Belgian, Weight Watchers*	1 Pot/80g	106	2.2	132	4.4	22.2	2.8	0.9
Chocolate, Asda*	1 Pot/61g	134	6.1	219	3.7	26	10	1
Chocolate, Belgian, Finest, Tesco*	1 Pot/100g	285	18.2	285	6.2	23.9	18.2	0.4
Chocolate, Belgian, Fix, Mullerlight, Muller*	1 Pot/100g	95	2.7	95	3.4	15	2.7	0
Chocolate, Belgian, Pud, Muller*	½ Pot/100g	177	6.3	177	5.3	24.8	6.3	0
Chocolate, BGTY, Sainsbury's*	1 Pot/63g	83	1.8	133	4.9	21.8	2.9	0.5
Chocolate, Bonne Maman*	1 Pot/70g	206	15.9	295	3.6	18.8	22.7	0.8
Chocolate, Cadbury*	1 Pot/55g	107	4.5	195	6.1	24.6	8.2	0
Chocolate, Finest, Tesco*	1 Pot/82g	321	26.4	391	3.7	21.7	32.2	0
Chocolate, GFY, Asda*	1 Pot/60g	70	1.7	117	4.8	17.9	2.9	3.5
Chocolate, Iceland*	1 Pot/62g	113	4.3	183	4	26.3	6.9	0
Chocolate, Light, Asda*	1 Mousse/60g	65	1.4	109	4.9	16	2.3	1.4
Chocolate, Low Fat, Danette, Danone*	1 Pot/60g	73	1.1	121	5.1	20.8	1.9	1.5
Chocolate, Milk, M&S*	1 Pot/90g	180	7.8	200	5.3	24.8	8.7	1.5
Chocolate, Minty, Bubbly, Dessert, Aero, Nestle*	1 Pot/58g	108	5.9	186	4.6	18.9	10.2	0.3
Chocolate, Plain, Low Fat, Nestle*	1 Pot/120g	71	0.9	59	2.4	10.4	0.8	1
Chocolate, Sainsbury's*	1 Pot/63g	119	5.3	190	4.7	23.8	8.5	1
Chocolate, Tesco*	1 Pot/60g	120	5	200	3.6	27.6	8.4	0.9
Chocolate, Value, Tesco*	1 Pot/63g	101	3.3	161	4.9	23.3	5.2	1.3
Chocolate, White, Bubbly, Dessert, Aero, Nestle*	1 Pot/58g	99	4.4	170	4.3	21	7.5	0.2
Chocolate, with Mini Chunks of, Dairy Milk, Cadbury*	1 Pot/100g	215	9.9	215	6.1	25.7	9.9	0
Chocolate, with Vanilla Layer, Cadbury*	1 Pot/100g	162	6.1	162	4.8	21.9	6.1	0
Cocoa, Vegan, Sugar Free, As Prepared, Eco Free From*	1 Serving/80g	74	1.8	92	2.7	13.4	2.3	3.5
Lemon, COU, M&S*	1 Pot/70g	91	1.8	130	3.1	23.7	2.5	0.6
Lemon, Dessert, Sainsbury's*	1 Pot/63g	114	5.9	182	3.6	20.7	9.4	0.6
Lemon, Low Fat, Morrisons*	1 Pot/63g	99	5.8	158	3.7	15.4	9.3	0.3
Lemon, Sicillian, Deluxe, Lidl*	1 Pot/100g	210	12.4	210	2.6	22	12.4	0.5
Lemon, Ski, Nestle*	1 Tub/60g	76	2.8	127	3.7	17.6	4.7	0
Lemon, with Meringue Style Sauce, Ski, Nestle*	1 Pot/60g	81	2.8	137	3.1	19.8	4.8	0

	Measure INFO/WEIGHT	per Measure KCAL	FAT	Nutrition Values per 100g / 100ml KCAL	PROT	CARB	FAT	FIBRE
MOUSSE								
Raspberry, Ripple, Ms Mollys*	1 Tub/50g	80	3.4	161	3.3	21.5	6.7	0.7
Raspberry, Ripple, Value, Tesco*	1 Pot/47g	70	2.9	149	2.1	21.3	6.1	0.1
Raspberry, Ripple, Value, Tesco*	1 Mousse/47g	77	3.1	163	2.9	23	6.6	0.3
Rolo, Nestle*	1 Pot/50g	80	3	158	4.7	21.6	5.9	0
Strawberry, Asda*	1 Pot/64g	107	5.8	167	3.5	18	9	0.2
Strawberry, Layered, Co-Op*	1 Pot/100g	120	3	120	3	19	3	0.2
Strawberry, Light, Muller*	1 Pot/150g	147	0.6	98	4.3	19.4	0.4	0
Strawberry, Ski, Nestle*	1 Tub/60g	77	3.1	128	3.8	16.6	5.2	0
Strawberry, Tesco*	1 Pot/60g	97	4.6	162	2.7	20.2	7.7	0.5
Strawberry, with Strawberry Sauce, Ski, Nestle*	1 Pot/60g	79	3.1	131	3.1	18.1	5.2	0
Summer Fruits, Light, Muller*	1 Pot/149g	143	0.6	96	4.3	18.7	0.4	0
Toffee, M&S*	1 Pot/90g	180	7.2	200	4.5	27.6	8	0.6
Vanilla, Finesse, Aero, Rowntree's*	1 Pot/57g	127	8.3	223	3.7	18.8	14.6	0
White Chocolate & Raspberry, Gu*	1 Pot/83g	225	14.6	271	1.9	28.4	17.6	4.1
White Chocolate, Finest, Tesco*	1 Pot/92g	436	34.5	474	3.9	30.2	37.5	0
MUFFIN								
All Butter, M&S*	1 Muffin/65g	175	4.7	270	10.3	40.8	7.3	2.1
Ancient Grain, Rankin Selection*	1 Muffin/70g	212	3.6	303	10.7	49.4	5.2	7.8
Banana Pecan, Organic, Honeyrose Bakery*	1 Muffin/110g	300	12.6	273	4.1	38.3	11.5	4.3
Blueberry, American Style, Aldi*	1 Muffin/85g	344	17.3	405	4.3	51.2	20.3	0
Blueberry, American Style, Sainsbury's*	1 Muffin/72g	256	13.1	355	5.1	42.7	18.2	1.9
Blueberry, Asda*	1 Muffin/77g	273	13.1	353	5	45	17	1.3
Blueberry, Bakery, Tesco*	1 Muffin/82g	307	13.1	374	4.3	52.2	16	1.9
Blueberry, Big, Asda*	1 Muffin/105g	342	11.2	326	7.5	49.8	10.7	2.3
Blueberry, Breakfast, Weetabix*	1 Muffin/92g	249	7.3	270	6	42.1	7.9	3.4
Blueberry, GF, Genius*	1 Muffin/95g	352	16.2	370	3.6	51	17.1	1.6
Blueberry, M&S*	1 Muffin/75g	255	12.6	340	4.9	41.9	16.8	1.3
Blueberry, McVitie's*	1 Muffin/80g	328	18.6	405	4.7	47.9	23	1.3
Blueberry, Mini, Tesco*	1 Muffin/28g	104	5.4	370	5.6	43.5	19.3	1.2
Blueberry, PB, Waitrose*	1 Muffin/100g	225	2.2	225	4.6	46.5	2.2	1.8
Blueberry, Waitrose*	1 Muffin/65g	239	9.2	367	4.7	55.2	14.2	1.7
Brown, Bottom, Rowan Hill Bakery, Lidl*	1 Muffin/65g	160	1.6	246	9.6	44.1	2.4	5
Buttermilk, Rankin Selection*	1 Muffin/70g	210	3.7	300	8.6	55.4	5.3	2.4
Caramel, Cadbury*	1 Muffin/116g	535	30.3	461	5.9	50.8	26.1	0
Caramel, Salted, Filled, Tesco*	1 Muffin/82g	320	15.5	390	4.7	49.5	18.9	1.6
Caramel, Salted, TTD, Sainsbury's*	1 Muffin/113g	447	22	396	4.8	49.6	19.5	1.5
Cheese, & Courgette, Ella's Kitchen*	1 Muffin/25g	59	3	237	8.3	25.4	12	1.2
Chocolate Chip, BGTY, Sainsbury's*	1 Muffin/75g	282	12.3	376	5.2	51.8	16.4	1.6
Chocolate Chip, Double, Co-Op*	1 Muffin/60g	246	12.6	410	6	49	21	3
Chocolate Chip, Double, Mini, Asda*	1 Muffin/19g	76	3.7	400	7.4	48.5	19.6	2.7
Chocolate Chip, Double, Tesco*	1 Muffin/100g	360	17.9	360	6.1	44.9	17.9	5.4
Chocolate Chip, Mini, Asda*	1 Muffin/22g	77	2.9	349	7	51	13	2.1
Chocolate Chip, Mini, BGTY, Sainsbury's*	1 Muffin/30g	130	6.7	434	5.5	52.1	22.5	0.8
Chocolate Chip, Mini, Essential, Waitrose*	1 Muffin/27g	108	5.1	399	5.9	49.8	19	2.5
Chocolate Chip, Mini, Tesco*	1 Muffin/25g	108	5.6	436	5	52.5	22.5	1.6
Chocolate Chip, Plain, Tesco*	1 Muffin/72g	270	12.7	375	5	48.1	17.6	1.4
Chocolate, Double, Mini, M&S*	1 Muffin/32g	133	6.9	416	5.4	49.8	21.7	1.1
Cinnamon, & Sultana, Morrisons*	1 Muffin/74g	199	1.1	269	7.6	54.7	1.5	3.1
English	1 Muffin/57g	120	1	211	7	43.9	1.8	1.8
English, Egg, Cheese, & Sausage, From Restaurant	**1 Muffin/165g**	**487**	**30.9**	**295**	**13.1**	**18.8**	**18.7**	**0**
English, Gluten, Wheat & Milk Free, Free From, Livwell*	1 Muffin/50g	160	4.9	320	4.6	52.8	9.8	3.2
English, Kingsmill*	1 Muffin/75g	167	1.4	222	9.7	40.4	1.8	2.6
English, Mild Red Cheddar Cheese, Extra Special, Asda*	1 Muffin/70g	201	4.7	288	11	45	6.7	2.7

M

MUFFIN

INFO/WEIGHT	Measure	per Measure KCAL	per Measure FAT	Nutrition KCAL	Values PROT	per 100g CARB	/ 100ml FAT	FIBRE
English, Tesco*	1 Muffin/72g	158	1.1	219	8.4	41.7	1.5	2.7
English, White, Butter, Waitrose*	1 Muffin/62g	165	2.2	266	10	47.7	3.5	1.9
Halloween, Asda*	1 Muffin/84g	346	16.8	412	4.8	53	20	1.3
Lemon & Poppy Seed, Entenmann's*	1 Muffin/105g	417	20.3	397	5.6	52.8	19.3	2.5
Lemon & Poppy Seed, Waitrose*	1 Muffin/121g	460	23.1	380	4.3	46.8	19.1	1.8
Lemon Curd, Patisserie, TTD, Sainsbury's*	1 Muffin/108g	418	20.9	386	5.4	47.1	19.3	1.4
Mini, Tesco*	1 Muffin/28g	120	6.3	428	6.4	50	22.6	1.2
Muesli, Breakfast, Love Life, Waitrose*	1 Muffin/68g	216	6.2	318	9.1	50	9.1	3.4
Orange, Apricot & Almond, Organic, Honeyrose Bakery*	1 Muffin/110g	312	11.4	284	3.5	44.2	10.4	1.9
Oven Bottom, Aldi*	1 Muffin/68g	173	1	255	10	50.4	1.5	2.2
Oven Bottom, Asda*	1 Muffin/65g	175	1.8	269	9	51	2.7	2.1
Oven Bottom, Warburton's*	1 Muffin/63g	173	2.7	274	10.4	49.4	4.3	2.3
Plain, Co-Op*	1 Muffin/60g	135	1.1	225	11.2	41.3	1.9	2.4
Plain, Prepared From Recipe, Average	*1 Muffin/57g*	*169*	*6.5*	*296*	*6.9*	*41.4*	*11.4*	*2.7*
Raspberry, Cream, Sainsbury's*	1 Muffin/90g	314	19.8	349	3.9	33.8	22	1.3
Raspberry, PB, Waitrose*	1 Muffin/101g	220	2.1	219	4.7	45.4	2.1	3.7
Sausage, Breakfast, All Day, Rustlers*	1 Pack/155g	386	13.8	249	11.8	29	8.9	0
Sourdough, Toasting, Specially Selected, Aldi*	1 Muffin/68g	158	1.3	232	9.5	43	1.9	3.2
Strawberry, & White Chocolate, Bakers Selection, Asda*	1 Muffin/82g	353	17.2	430	4.2	56	21	2.3
Toasting, Warburton's*	1 Muffin/64g	138	1	216	8.9	41.4	1.6	2.9
Vanilla, & Choc Chip, GFY, Asda*	1 Muffin/59g	152	1.3	260	7	53	2.2	1.6
White Chocolate, & Strawberry Filled, Tesco*	1 Muffin/103g	415	20.3	405	5.2	51.3	19.8	1.3
White Chocolate, Chunk Lemon, Mini, M&S*	1 Muffin/26g	106	5	409	5.7	52.4	19.3	1.2
White, M&S*	1 Muffin/60g	135	1.1	225	11.2	43.7	1.9	2.9
White, Soft, Hovis*	1 Muffin/60g	145	1.7	241	8.9	44	2.8	2.4
White, Tesco*	1 Muffin/72g	173	2.3	240	11.3	41.6	3.2	2.8
Wholemeal, Tesco*	1 Muffin/65g	130	1.3	200	12.6	32.9	2	5.7

MULBERRIES

INFO/WEIGHT	Measure	per Measure KCAL	per Measure FAT	KCAL	PROT	CARB	FAT	FIBRE
Raw	*1oz/28g*	*10*	*0*	*36*	*1.3*	*8.1*	*0*	*0*

MULLET

INFO/WEIGHT	Measure	per Measure KCAL	per Measure FAT	KCAL	PROT	CARB	FAT	FIBRE
Grey, Grilled	*1oz/28g*	*42*	*1.5*	*150*	*25.7*	*0*	*5.2*	*0*
Red, Grilled	*1oz/28g*	*34*	*1.2*	*121*	*20.4*	*0*	*4.4*	*0*

MUNCHIES

INFO/WEIGHT	Measure	per Measure KCAL	per Measure FAT	KCAL	PROT	CARB	FAT	FIBRE
Original, Tube, Nestle*	1 Pack/55g	266	12.3	487	5.4	64.6	22.5	1.4

MUSHROOMS

INFO/WEIGHT	Measure	per Measure KCAL	per Measure FAT	KCAL	PROT	CARB	FAT	FIBRE
Breaded, Average	*3 Mushroom/51g*	*77*	*2.9*	*152*	*4.3*	*20.8*	*5.7*	*0.6*
Breaded, Crispy, in Panko Crumb, M&S*	½ Pack/100g	214	11.7	214	4.9	21.1	11.7	2.3
Breaded, Garlic, Average	*3 Mushroom/50g*	*92*	*4.9*	*183*	*5.2*	*18.7*	*9.7*	*1.7*
Button, Raw, Average	*1 Serving/50g*	*7*	*0.2*	*15*	*2.3*	*0.5*	*0.4*	*1.2*
Chestnut, Average	*1 Med/5g*	*1*	*0*	*13*	*1.8*	*0.4*	*0.5*	*0.6*
Chinese, Dried, Raw	*1oz/28g*	*80*	*0.5*	*284*	*10*	*59.9*	*1.8*	*0*
Closed Cup, Average	*1 Handful/30g*	*4*	*0.2*	*14*	*1.8*	*0.4*	*0.5*	*1.1*
Common, Boiled in Salted Water, Average	*1oz/28g*	*3*	*0.1*	*11*	*1.8*	*0.4*	*0.3*	*1.1*
Common, Fried, Average	*1oz/28g*	*44*	*4.5*	*157*	*2.4*	*0.3*	*16.2*	*1.5*
Common, Raw, Average	*1 Serving/80g*	*18*	*0.3*	*22*	*3.1*	*3.3*	*0.3*	*1*
Creamed, Average	*1oz/28g*	*23*	*1.5*	*82*	*1.3*	*6.8*	*5.5*	*0.5*
Dried	*1oz/28g*	*45*	*1.7*	*159*	*21.8*	*4.8*	*6*	*13.3*
Enoki, Average	*1 Serving/80g*	*34*	*0*	*42*	*3*	*7*	*0*	*3*
Flat, Large, Average	*1 Mushroom/52g*	*10*	*0.3*	*20*	*3.3*	*0.5*	*0.5*	*0.7*
Garlic, Average	*½ Pack/150g*	*159*	*14*	*106*	*2.1*	*3.7*	*9.3*	*1.7*
Garlic, Breaded, Frozen, Tesco*	1 Serving/54g	96	3	179	5.3	25.5	5.6	3
Garlic, Creamy, Extra Special, Asda*	½ Pack/146g	121	7.9	83	4.2	2	5.4	5
Oyster, Average	*1 Serving/80g*	*10*	*0.2*	*13*	*1.4*	*1.4*	*0.2*	*1.1*

MUSHROOMS	Measure INFO/WEIGHT	per Measure KCAL	FAT	Nutrition Values per 100g / 100ml KCAL	PROT	CARB	FAT	FIBRE
Porcini, Wild, Dried, Merchant Gourmet*	1 Pack/50g	154	1.1	307	29.6	34.1	2.2	16.5
Portobello, Raw, Average	*1 Mushroom/50g*	*7*	*0.2*	*14*	*1.8*	*0.4*	*0.5*	*1.1*
Portobello, with Chorizo, & Cheddar, The Best, Morrisons*	½ Pack/79g	100	5.8	126	8.7	5.1	7.4	2.1
Shiitake, Cooked	*1oz/28g*	*15*	*0.1*	*55*	*1.6*	*12.3*	*0.2*	*0*
Shiitake, Dried, Raw	*1oz/28g*	*83*	*0.3*	*296*	*9.6*	*63.9*	*1*	*0*
Shreds, BBQ, & Greens, Chinese, Wicked Kitchen, Tesco*	1 Serving/356g	467	11.1	131	4.4	19.8	3.1	3
Sliced, Average	*1oz/28g*	*3*	*0.1*	*12*	*1.8*	*0.4*	*0.3*	*1.1*
Straw, Canned, Drained	*1oz/28g*	*4*	*0.1*	*15*	*2.1*	*1.2*	*0.2*	*0*
Stuffed, Cheese, & Garlic, Mini, Nature's Pick, Aldi*	1 Pack/210g	275	14.7	131	5.5	10	7	2.3
Stuffed, Cheese, & Garlic, with Breadcrumbs, Sainsbury's*	1 Mushroom/110g	173	5.7	157	9.4	16	5.2	0
Stuffed, Cream Cheese, & Garlic, Tesco *	1 Mushroom/100g	138	10.1	138	4.1	7	10.1	1.2
Stuffed, Garlic, Cream Cheese, Herb, Breadcrumbs, Aldi*	½ Pack/125g	184	10.1	147	6.4	11	8.1	2.2
Stuffed, SunDried Tomato, Red Pepper, Lattice, Morrisons*	1 Mushroom/92g	116	6.5	126	4.4	10.5	7.1	1.1
Stuffed, with Chorizo, & Spinach, Asda*	½ Pack/80g	90	5	112	8	4.7	6.3	2.3
Stuffed, with Leek & Wensleydale, Loved by Us, Co-Op*	1 Mushroom/100g	85	3.6	85	4.3	7.8	3.6	2.1
MUSSELS								
Boiled, Flesh Only, Average	*1 Mussel/2g*	*2*	*0.1*	*104*	*16.7*	*3.5*	*2.7*	*0*
Boiled, Weighed in Shell, Average	*1 Mussel/7g*	*2*	*0.1*	*28*	*4.5*	*0.9*	*0.7*	*0*
Pickled, Drained, Average	*1oz/28g*	*32*	*0.6*	*112*	*20*	*1.5*	*2.2*	*0*
Raw, Weighed in Shell, Average	*1oz/28g*	*7*	*0.2*	*23*	*3.4*	*1*	*0.7*	*0*
MUSSELS IN								
Garlic Butter Sauce, Average	*½ Pack/225g*	*179*	*11.5*	*80*	*6.4*	*2*	*5.1*	*0.2*
Green Curry Sauce, Scottish, Fishmonger, Aldi*	½ Pack/140g	116	5.6	83	7.9	3.9	4	0.5
Oil, Smoked, Canned, Drained, John West*	1 Can/60g	117	7.3	196	19.9	1.6	12.2	0
Scottish, in Garlic Butter, Waitrose*	½ Pack/120g	108	7.4	90	6.7	1.6	6.2	0.6
Scottish, in White Wine & Cream, Waitrose*	½ Pack/129g	110	4.3	85	6.6	6.8	3.3	0.6
Seasoned White Wine Sauce, Bantry Bay*	1 Serving/450g	270	9	60	6.3	4.1	2	0.1
White Wine & Garlic Sauce , Scottish, Tesco*	1 Pouch/155g	130	6.2	84	9.8	1.9	4	0.6
White Wine Sauce, Sainsbury's*	½ Pack/250g	215	10.2	86	6.4	5.6	4.1	0.7
MUSTARD								
American, Average	*1 Tsp/5g*	*5*	*0.2*	*102*	*4.4*	*10.5*	*5*	*2.5*
Coarse Grain, Average	*1 Tsp/5g*	*7*	*0.4*	*141*	*7.7*	*8.4*	*8.3*	*5.9*
Dijon, Average	*1 Tsp/5g*	*8*	*0.6*	*163*	*7.4*	*7.7*	*11.3*	*1.1*
English, Average	*1 Tsp/5g*	*9*	*0.4*	*173*	*6.8*	*19.2*	*7.6*	*1.2*
French, Average	*1 Tsp/5g*	*5*	*0.3*	*106*	*5.4*	*8.1*	*5.6*	*1.8*
German Style, Sainsbury's*	1 Serving/10g	9	0.6	92	5.5	2.8	6.5	0
Honey, Colman's*	1 Tsp/6g	12	0.5	208	7.4	24	8.2	0
Powder, Average	*1 Tsp/3g*	*15*	*0.9*	*452*	*28.9*	*20.7*	*28.7*	*0*
Smooth, Average	*1 Tsp/8g*	*11*	*0.7*	*139*	*7.1*	*9.7*	*8.2*	*0*
Whole Grain, Average	*1 Tsp/8g*	*11*	*0.8*	*140*	*8.2*	*4.2*	*10.2*	*4.9*
MUSTARD CRESS								
Raw	*1oz/28g*	*4*	*0.2*	*13*	*1.6*	*0.4*	*0.6*	*1.1*

M

	Measure INFO/WEIGHT	per Measure KCAL	per Measure FAT	Nutrition Values per 100g / 100ml KCAL	PROT	CARB	FAT	FIBRE
NACHOS								
Beef, Chilli, Asda*	1 Serving/200g	208	10	104	10	4.7	5	0.8
Cheesy, with Salsa, & Soured Cream, Sainsbury's*	½ Pack/170g	449	26.9	264	8.8	21.5	15.8	1.4
Chilli, Sainsbury's*	½ Pack/250g	695	32.2	278	10.9	29.5	12.9	1.3
Kit, Old El Paso*	½ Pack/260g	598	26	230	4	31	10	0
with Cheese, From Restaurant, Average	*1 Nacho/16g*	*49*	*2.7*	*306*	*8*	*32.2*	*16.8*	*0*
NASI GORENG								
Indonesian, Asda*	1 Pack/360g	778	22.7	216	7.4	32.3	6.3	1.3
Slimming World*	1 Pack/550g	495	3.3	90	6.8	13.5	0.6	1.6
Vitasia, Lidl*	1 Bowl/250g	438	11	175	7.3	25.8	4.4	1.1
NECTARINES								
Fresh, Raw, Weighed with Stone, Average	*1 Med/140g*	*50*	*0.1*	*36*	*1.2*	*8*	*0.1*	*1.1*
NESQUIK								
Chocolate Flavour, Powder, Dry Weight, Nesquik, Nestle*	1 Serving/15g	56	0.5	372	3	82.9	3.1	6.5
Strawberry Flavour, Powder, Dry Weight, Nesquik, Nestle*	1 Serving/15g	59	0	393	0	98.1	0	0
NETTLES								
Raw, Average	1 Serving/80g	34	0.1	42	2.7	7	0.1	6.9
NIK NAKS								
Cream 'n' Cheesy, KP Snacks*	1 Bag/34g	196	13	575	5.2	52.7	38.1	0.2
Nice 'n' Spicy, KP Snacks*	1 Bag/30g	171	11.5	571	4.6	51.6	38.4	1.6
Rib 'n' Saucy, Golden Wonder*	1 Sm Bag/25g	143	9.4	571	4.5	53.7	37.6	0.5
Scampi 'n' Lemon, KP Snacks*	1 Bag/25g	143	9.4	573	4.9	53.1	37.5	0.1
NOODLES								
Bacon, Dry Supernoodles, Weight, Batchelors*	1 Pack/100g	526	23.6	526	9.4	69.2	23.6	1.6
Beef, BBQ, Instant, Cooked, Aldi*	1 Serving/324g	515	19.4	159	3.7	21.9	6	1.1
Beef, BBQ, Made Up, Supernoodles, Batchelors*	½ Pack/150g	250	11.1	167	3.2	21.3	7.4	1
Beef, Chilli, Ramen, M&S*	1 Pack/484g	532	17.4	110	8.1	11.9	3.6	0.8
Beef, Korean Style, Slimming World*	1 Pack/550g	468	3.3	85	7.5	11.8	0.6	1.4
Beef, Oriental, GFY, Asda*	1 Pack/400g	372	6.8	93	7.4	12.1	1.7	1.7
Beef, Teriyaki, 606, Oakhouse Foods Ltd*	1 Meal/325g	292	4.9	90	6.1	12.4	1.5	0.6
Beef, Teriyaki, Taste of Japan, Tesco*	½ Pack/221g	253	9.1	114	6.9	12	4.1	0.9
Chicken, & Coconut & Lime, Fuller Longer, M&S*	1 Pack/390g	448	17.6	115	8.7	10	4.5	1.6
Chicken, & Ham, Dry Weight, Supernoodles, Batchelors*	1 Pack/100g	472	20.2	472	9.4	63.2	20.2	1.5
Chicken, & Herb, Made Up, Supernoodles, Batchelors*	1 Pack/170g	322	1.6	189	6.1	39.2	0.9	1.2
Chicken, & Noodle, Sweet Chilli, Tesco*	1 Pot/240g	323	4.3	134	6.4	22.5	1.8	1.3
Chicken, & Red Thai, Easy Steam, Tesco*	1 Serving/400g	556	28.4	139	10.3	8.6	7.1	1.1
Chicken, & Sweetcorn, Snack Pot, Morrisons*	1 Pot/247g	249	1.5	101	4.1	19.8	0.6	1.6
Chicken, & Mushroom, Snack, Made Up, Aldi*	1 Serving/299g	341	7.8	114	18.7	0.5	2.6	2
Chicken, & Prawn, Chinese, Tesco*	½ Pack/298g	307	7.2	103	2.3	16.2	2.4	3.5
Chicken, Chinese, Asda*	1 Pot/302g	305	4.2	101	6	16	1.4	0.8
Chicken, Chinese, Fresh Ideas, Morrisons*	1 Pack/400g	94	1.8	94	7.2	11.3	1.8	1.7
Chicken, Curry Flavour, Instant, Sainsbury's*	1 Pack/85g	167	6.2	196	4.6	27.9	7.3	0.8
Chicken, Feel Good, Bang Bang, Ko-Lee*	1 Pot/65g	281	9.8	433	9	64	15	4
Chicken, Firecracker, Made Up, Naked Noodle, Symingtons	1 Pot/338g	301	2	89	2.7	17.5	0.6	1.3
Chicken, Flavour, 3 Minute, Dry, Blue Dragon*	1 Pack/85g	403	18.2	475	9.3	61.2	21.4	0
Chicken, Flavour, Dry, Princes*	1 Pack/85g	395	16	465	10	63.8	18.8	0
Chicken, Flavour, Instant, Cooked, Smart Price, Asda*	1 Serving/246g	293	11.1	111	2.8	14.9	4.2	1
Chicken, Flavour, Instant, Made Up, Tesco*	½ Pack/168g	285	10.6	170	4.1	23.7	6.3	1.5
Chicken, Flavour, Instant, Sainsbury's*	1 Pack/335g	549	21.4	164	4.4	22.3	6.4	1.3
Chicken, Hot, Instant, Rollton*	1 Pack/60g	270	11.8	450	8.7	58	19.7	3
Chicken, Instant, Cooked, Aldi*	½ Pack/150g	248	10.6	165	3.3	21	7.1	1.3
Chicken, Instant, Made Up, Everyday Value, Tesco*	1 Pack/265g	437	15.6	165	3.8	19.4	5.9	3.2
Chicken, Instant, Made Up, HFC, Tesco*	1 Pack/176g	220	7.7	125	3.4	16.4	4.4	3.2
Chicken, Instant, Mama*	1 Pack/350g	238	10.2	68	1.2	9.2	2.9	0

NOODLES

	Measure INFO/WEIGHT	per Measure KCAL	FAT	Nutrition Values per 100g / 100ml KCAL	PROT	CARB	FAT	FIBRE
Chicken, Kimchi, As Prepared, Mr Noodles*	1 Bowl/484g	353	18.4	73	2.2	5.1	3.8	4.7
Chicken, Made Up, Supernoodles, Batchelors*	1 Serving/150g	264	11.8	176	3.1	23	7.9	0.4
Chicken, Oriental Style, Instant, Cooked, Koka*	1 Pack/485g	393	16.5	81	1.9	10.4	3.4	0.5
Chicken, Pad Thai, Cook*	1 Serving/240g	396	8.9	165	7.2	26.5	3.7	1.6
Chicken, Peri Peri, Super Noodles, Batchelors*	1 Pack/290g	440	18.8	152	3.1	19.5	6.5	1.3
Chicken, Pot, Made Up, Super Noodles, Batchelors*	1 Pot/265g	353	14.9	133	2.5	17.7	5.6	0.9
Chicken, Satay, Fresh Ideas, Morrisons*	1 Pack/400g	468	11.2	117	8.9	13	2.8	2.2
Chicken, Snack Stop, Made Up, Mug Shot, Symingtons*	1 Pack/233g	175	1.2	75	2.3	14	0.5	1.2
Chicken, Spicy, & King Prawn, Bowl, Tesco*	1 Pack/355g	353	2.2	100	7.1	15.2	0.6	2.3
Chicken, Spicy, with Veg, Balanced 2 Go, Oh So Lean*	1 Pack/400g	640	4.8	160	14.9	20	1.2	0
Chicken, Sweet Chilli, Cooked, My Goodness, Sainsbury's*	1 Pack/380g	321	5.5	87	5.9	11.6	1.5	2
Chicken, Teriyaki, Cook*	1 Pack/300g	330	6	110	7.8	16.8	2	2.9
Chicken, Teriyaki, Pot, Tesco*	1 Pot/300g	315	4.8	105	5.8	15.9	1.6	1.8
Chicken, Teriyaki, The City Kitchen*	1 Pack/347g	399	6.6	115	8.2	16	1.9	0.9
Chicken, Thai Green, Cook*	1 Pack/329g	306	9.5	93	7.2	10.6	2.9	2.3
Chicken, Tikka Masala, Made Up, Mug Shot, Symingtons*	1 Pot/256g	200	2.8	78	2.2	14.5	1.1	0.7
Chinese, & Veggies, Cashew Cream Sauce, Amy's Kitchen*	1 Pack/271g	490	21.9	181	6	21	8.1	2
Chow Mein, Classic, As Prepared, Fusian, Maggi*	½ Pack/190g	273	11.8	144	3.3	18	6.2	1.7
Chow Mein, Made Up, Supernoodles, Batchelors*	½ Pack/150g	262	11.8	175	3	23	7.9	0.4
Chow Mein, Sainsbury's*	1 Pack/125g	136	2.2	109	3.9	19.2	1.8	0.8
Chow Mein, Snack in a Pot, LC, Tesco*	1 Pot/235g	235	1.2	100	3.7	19.4	0.5	1.8
Crispy, Dry, Blue Dragon*	1 Box/125g	438	0.6	350	2.4	84	0.5	0
Curry, Instant, Sainsbury's*	1 Pack/335g	412	15.4	123	2.6	17.8	4.6	0.1
Curry, Instant, Vitasia, Lidl*	1 Pack/108g	124	5.3	115	2.5	15.3	4.9	0
Curry, Mild, Dry Weight, Supernoodles, Batchelors*	½ Pack/50g	260	11.7	520	9.4	67.8	23.4	1.4
Curry, Mild, Made Up, Supernoodles, Batchelors*	1 Serving/100g	157	6.7	157	3.2	20.9	6.7	1
Curry, Singapore, Made Up, Naked Noodle Snack Pot*	1 Pot/329g	270	2	82	2.9	15.7	0.6	0.9
Curry, Spicy, Pot, Made Up, HFC, Tesco*	1 Pot/277g	283	8	102	2.3	16.3	2.9	0.7
Duck, Hoisin, Shredded, Tesco*	1 Pack/388g	384	10.1	99	5.6	12.3	2.6	2
Duck, Shredded, Hoisin, G&B, Asda*	1 Pack/367g	396	6.2	108	5.8	17	1.7	1.8
Egg, & Bean Sprouts, Cooked, Tesco*	1 Pack/250g	238	5.2	95	4.4	14.6	2.1	1.5
Egg, Asda*	¼ Pack/176g	319	1.1	181	5.4	38	0.6	0.8
Egg, Boiled	*1oz/28g*	*17*	*0.1*	*62*	*2.2*	*13*	*0.5*	*0.6*
Egg, Chilli & Ginger, Asian Fusion, Waitrose*	½ Pack/137g	188	3.3	137	4.4	24	2.4	0.8
Egg, Coconut, & Lemongrass, Waitrose*	½ Pack/121g	176	6.2	145	3.6	19.9	5.1	2.7
Egg, Dry, Average	*1 Block/63g*	*218*	*1.2*	*348*	*12.1*	*70.1*	*1.9*	*2.6*
Egg, Fine Thread, Dry, M&S*	1 Serving/63g	220	0.6	350	14.3	71.6	0.9	5.1
Egg, Fine, Blue Dragon*	1 Serving/100g	356	1.7	356	13.8	70	1.7	3.4
Egg, Fine, Dry Weight, Sharwood's*	1 Block/63g	216	1.3	346	12	70	2.1	2.5
Egg, Fine, Fresh, M&S*	1 Pack/275g	330	6.1	120	4.4	20.7	2.2	1.5
Egg, Fine, Morrisons*	¼ Pack/184g	232	0.9	126	4.6	24.8	0.5	1.9
Egg, Fine, Waitrose*	¼ Pack/63g	221	1.6	353	15	67.3	2.6	3.8
Egg, Free Range, Asda*	1 Serving/125g	209	4.9	167	5.1	27	3.9	1.8
Egg, Free Range, Fresh, Sainsbury's*	½ Pack/205g	340	7	166	5	28	3.4	1.8
Egg, Free Range, Morrisons*	1 Pack/300g	372	8.7	124	4.9	19.7	2.9	1.3
Egg, Fresh, Tesco*	½ Pack/205g	287	3.9	140	4.9	25.3	1.9	2
Egg, M&S*	½ Pack/110g	165	1.9	150	4.9	38	1.7	2.8
Egg, Medium, Asda*	1 Serving/83g	125	0.7	150	4.8	31	0.8	1.3
Egg, Medium, Co-Op*	¼ Pack/144g	168	0.9	117	4.5	23	0.6	1.4
Egg, Medium, Dry Nests, Cooks' Ingredients, Waitrose*	1 Nest/54g	189	0.9	350	13.2	70.4	1.7	2.4
Egg, Medium, Dry, Blue Dragon*	1 Serving/50g	158	1.2	317	10.1	62.3	2.4	3.1
Egg, Medium, Dry, Sharwood's*	1 Serving/63g	229	1.4	367	13.2	71.2	2.3	4.1
Egg, Medium, Sainsbury's*	1 Serving/63g	236	1.2	375	12.5	76.4	1.9	1.3

NOODLES

	Measure INFO/WEIGHT	per Measure KCAL	FAT	Nutrition Values per 100g / 100ml KCAL	PROT	CARB	FAT	FIBRE
Egg, Raw, Medium, Waitrose*	¼ Pack/63g	221	1.6	353	15	67.3	2.6	3.8
Egg, Singapore Curry, Made Up, Aldi*	1 Pot/338g	341	1.9	88	2.7	18	0.5	1
Egg, Thick, Dry Weight, Sharwood's*	1 Serving/63g	214	1.1	342	10.8	71	1.7	2.5
Egg, Tossed in Sesame Oil, Asda*	½ Pack/150g	174	10.5	116	2.3	11	7	0.6
Fried, Average	*1oz/28g*	*43*	*3.2*	*153*	*1.9*	*11.3*	*11.5*	*0.5*
Glass, Dry Weight	*1 Serving/100g*	*351*	*0.1*	*351*	*0.1*	*86.1*	*0.1*	*0.5*
Konjac, Raw, Asian Cuisine, Clean Foods*	1 Serving/100g	6	0	6	1	0	0	3.6
Madras, Mighty Spicy, Made Up, Mug Shot, Symingtons*	1 Pot/320g	278	1	87	2.5	18.1	0.3	0.8
Medium, Soft, Ready to Wok, Asia Specialities, Aldi*	1 Serving/150g	232	0.9	155	6.6	30	0.6	1.6
Nest, Medium, Cooked, Waitrose*	1 Nest/63g	88	0.3	139	5	28.6	0.5	0.6
Pad Thai, GF, Amy's Kitchen*	1 Pack/268g	407	8.8	152	4.1	26	3.3	1.1
Pad Thai, Ribbon, Ready to Wok, Sharwood's*	1 Serving/150g	206	1.7	137	5	26.3	1.1	1
Pad Thai, Rice, M&S*	½ Pack/137g	246	4	179	3.7	33.4	2.9	2.3
Pad Thai, with Mixed Vegetables, Fit Kitchen*	1 Pack/380g	327	6.8	86	8.3	10	1.8	2
Plain, Boiled	*1oz/28g*	*17*	*0.1*	*62*	*2.4*	*13*	*0.4*	*0.7*
Plain, Dry	*1oz/28g*	*109*	*1.7*	*388*	*11.7*	*76.1*	*6.2*	*2.9*
Pork, Spicy BBQ, Snack Pot, Tesco*	1 Pack/280g	351	7.3	125	4.8	19.7	2.6	2
Prawn, Chilli, King, Finest, Tesco*	1 Pack/400g	340	8	85	4	11.9	2	0.9
Prawn, Hot & Sour, King, Bowl, My Goodness, Sainsbury's*	1 Pack/360g	324	3.2	90	4.7	15.1	0.9	1.1
Prawn, King, Laksa, Slimming World*	1 Pack/550g	346	3.8	63	4.5	8.8	0.7	1.5
Prawn, King, Singapore, Free From, Tesco*	1 Pack/338g	352	11.8	104	3.8	13.8	3.5	1.2
Prawn, Tiger, Stir Fry, Tesco*	1 Pack/400g	596	14.8	149	6	23	3.7	2.7
Ramen, Morrisons*	1/3 Pack/83g	289	0.7	348	11.1	72.7	0.8	2.8
Ribbon, Ready to Wok, Shangri-la*	1 Serving/150g	234	2.2	156	6.2	31	1.5	2.2
Ribbon, Soft, Sharwood's*	1 Portion/150g	225	1.8	150	5.7	25.7	1.2	6.6
Rice, Cooked	*1 Cup/176g*	*192*	*0.4*	*109*	*0.9*	*24.9*	*0.2*	*1*
Rice, Dry, Amoy*	1oz/28g	101	0.3	361	6.5	86.6	1	0
Rice, Dry, Blue Dragon*	1 Serving/30g	113	0	376	7	84	0	0
Rice, Fresh, Sainsbury's*	½ Pack/150g	202	3.3	135	2.2	25.9	2.2	1.4
Rice, in Curry Sauce, Instant, Made Up, Free From, Tesco*	1 Pot/374g	292	0.7	78	1.6	17	0.2	1
Rice, Oriental, Thai, Stir Fry, Dry Weight, Sharwood's*	1 Serving/63g	226	0.6	361	6.5	86.8	1	2.4
Rice, Singapore, Market St, Morrisons*	¼ Pack/90g	192	6.2	214	3.5	33.4	6.9	1.9
Rice, Stir Fry, Tesco*	½ Pack/190g	304	10.8	160	2	24.8	5.7	1
Rice, Vermicelli, Mama*	1 Serving/45g	166	0.4	370	7	81	1	0
Rice, with Spring Onions, Fresh Tastes, Asda*	½ Pack/188g	248	4.1	132	2.2	25.9	2.2	1.4
Rogan Josh, Spicetastic, Made Up, Mug Shot, Symingtons*	1 Serving/249g	207	0.7	83	2.3	17.4	0.3	0.8
Singapore, BGTY, Sainsbury's*	1 Pack/369g	317	10	86	7.2	8.2	2.7	2.1
Singapore, Sainsbury's*	1 Pack/450g	540	18	120	6.4	13.3	4	2.7
Singapore, Style, Asda*	1 Pack/400g	688	32	172	7	18	8	1
Singapore, Style, Sainsbury's*	½ Pack/150g	320	10.8	214	3.2	33.2	7.2	1.3
Singapore, Vegetable, Love Your Veg!, Sainsbury's*	1 Pack/350g	357	17.5	102	3.1	10.4	5	1.6
Singapore, with Chicken, G&B, Asda*	1 Pack/365g	383	5.5	105	5.4	17	1.5	1
Singapore, with Chicken, Pork, Egg, & Prawns, M&S*	1 Pack/400g	560	25.6	140	5.7	14.1	6.4	1.4
Soba, with Yakisoba Sauce, Instant, Made Up, Nissin*	1 Pot/180g	394	17.6	219	5.3	26.1	9.8	0
Straight to Wok, Medium, Amoy*	1 Pack/150g	240	2.2	160	5.8	31.7	1.5	0
Straight to Wok, Rice, Amoy*	1 Pack/150g	174	0.2	116	1.6	27.4	0.1	0
Straight to Wok, Singapore, Amoy*	1 Serving/150g	206	3.3	137	6.4	21.6	2.2	2.8
Straight to Wok, Thread, Fine, Amoy*	1 Pack/150g	237	3.9	158	5	28.7	2.6	0
Straight to Wok, Udon, Amoy*	1 Pack/150g	212	2	141	4.4	28.8	1.3	0
Sweet & Sour, Asian, Veggie Bowl, Birds Eye*	1 Meal/380g	323	6.8	85	3.5	12.8	1.8	1.7
Sweet Chilli, Thai, Dry Weight, Supernoodles, Batchelors*	1 Pack/85g	292	1	343	10.6	72.5	1.2	3
Sweet Chilli, Thai, Made Up, Aldi*	1 Pot/338g	301	1.7	89	2.9	18	0.5	1
Teriyaki, Japanese, Made Up, Naked Noodle, Symingtons*	1 Pot/327g	268	2	82	2.9	15.8	0.6	0.7

	Measure INFO/WEIGHT	per Measure KCAL	FAT	Nutrition Values per 100g / 100ml KCAL	PROT	CARB	FAT	FIBRE
NOODLES								
Thai, Style, Sainsbury's*	1 Pack/340g	381	7.8	112	3.3	19.4	2.3	0.7
Thai, Style, Snack, Cupshotz, Aldi*	1 Pack/55g	215	2.8	391	11.4	71.4	5.1	6.9
Tom Yum, Vegetable, Made Up, Kabuto Noodles*	1 Pot/405g	263	0.8	65	1.3	14.6	0.2	0.5
Udon, Japanese, & Dashi Soup Stock, Yutaka*	1 Pack/230g	290	1.2	126	3	26.8	0.5	0
Udon, Japanese, Sainsbury's*	1 Serving/150g	210	2.7	140	3.9	27.1	1.8	1.2
Udon, Style, Thick, Ready to Wok, Sharwood's*	1 Pack/150g	233	0.6	155	5.4	32.5	0.4	2.1
Udon, Wheat, Organic, Explore Asian*	1 Serving/56g	202	1.2	361	14.3	71.4	2.1	1.8
Udon, Wholesome, Good Health, Waitrose*	½ Pack/126g	201	2.1	160	4.7	31	1.7	1
Udon, Yasai Yaki, Allplants*	½ Pack/380g	494	24.3	130	4.4	12	6.4	2.1
Wheat, High Protein, Tesco*	1 Pack/300g	459	3.3	153	9.4	25.4	1.1	1.8
Wholewheat, Cooked Weight, Sharwoods*	1 Portion/161g	215	1.5	134	5	24.8	0.9	2.7
Wholewheat, Dry, Sharwoods*	1 Portion/63g	224	1.4	356	13	66.2	2.3	9.2
Wholewheat, Dry, Tesco*	¼ Pack/66g	227	0.9	342	14.2	64.2	1.4	7.7
Wholewheat, Straight to Wok, Asda*	½ Pack/152g	225	1.2	148	4.9	29	0.8	2.8
NOUGAT								
Average	*1 Sm Bar/28g*	*108*	*2.4*	*384*	*4.4*	*77.3*	*8.5*	*0.9*
Raspberry & Orange Hazelnut, Thorntons*	1 Sweet/9g	39	1.8	433	4.8	60	20	2.2
Soft, Bar, Bassett's*	1 Bar/25g	94	1	375	4	82	4	0
NUT ROAST								
Average	*1 Serving/200g*	*704*	*51.4*	*352*	*13.3*	*18.3*	*25.7*	*4.2*
Kale, & Broccoli, Vegetarian, Tesco*	½ Pack/122g	226	12.1	185	5.9	13.7	9.9	8.8
Lentil, Average	*1oz/28g*	*62*	*3.4*	*222*	*10.6*	*18.8*	*12.1*	*3.8*
Sweet Potato, & Maple Carrot, Loaf, Sainsbury's*	¼ Loaf/100g	202	12.4	202	9.3	9.6	12.4	7.5
Vegan, GF, Clive's*	1 Serving/140g	216	13.7	154	5.1	20.8	9.8	0
Vegan, Good Health, Waitrose*	½ Pack/143g	315	19.7	220	11.3	7.6	13.8	9.9
NUTMEG								
Ground, Average	*1 Tsp/3g*	*16*	*1.1*	*525*	*5.8*	*45.3*	*36.3*	*0*
NUTS								
Cashews & Peanuts, Honey Roasted, Average	*1 Serving/50g*	*290*	*21.4*	*579*	*21.6*	*26.6*	*42.9*	*4.2*
Chilli, & Lime, Protein, The Foodie Market, Aldi*	1 Pack/25g	154	12.5	614	25	12	50	7.4
Collection, Spiced, Tesco*	1 Serving/25g	148	11.6	592	15.8	23.2	46.6	8.1
Mixed	*1 Pack/40g*	*243*	*21.6*	*607*	*22.9*	*7.9*	*54.1*	*6*
Mixed, Almonds, Brazil, Hazel & Walnuts, M&S*	1 Serving/25g	168	16	670	16	4.8	64	5.4
Mixed, Natural, Asda*	1 Snack/30g	197	18.8	656	18	4.3	62.7	7.4
Mixed, Natural, Luxury, Tesco*	1oz/28g	179	16.2	639	22.6	6.9	57.9	5.6
Mixed, Roasted, & Salted, On the Go, Sainsbury's*	1 Serving/30g	186	15.6	620	23.1	10.5	52	8.9
Mixed, Roasted, Salted, Waitrose*	1 Pack/200g	1252	116.8	626	13.7	11.3	58.4	4.4
Selection, Roasted, Finest, Tesco*	1 Serving/30g	200	17.9	665	18.7	9.8	59.6	7.4
Selection, Roasted, with Cornish Sea Salt, Finest, Tesco*	1 Serving/30g	194	17.4	648	16	11	58	8.9
NUTS & RAISINS								
Mixed, Average	*1 Serving/30g*	*144*	*10.2*	*481*	*14.1*	*31.5*	*34.1*	*4.5*
Mixed, Grazin', Holland & Barrett*	1 Pack/200g	888	62	444	8.8	34	31	3.4
Mixed, Natural Selection, Aldi*	1 Serving/30g	146	9.3	488	14	35	31	5.2
Peanuts, Mixed, Average	*1 Pack/40g*	*174*	*10.4*	*435*	*15.3*	*37.5*	*26*	*4.4*
Peanuts, Posh, & Ritzy Raisins, Holland & Barrett*	1 Pack/40g	152	6.2	379	8	54.5	15.4	3
Yoghurt Coated, Waitrose*	1 Serving/50g	264	18.4	527	10.9	38.2	36.7	3
NUTS & SEEDS								
Paprkia, Smoky, Crunch, Tesco*	1 Pack/35g	152	4.8	434	18	54.5	13.7	10.2
Trail Mix, Natural Days*	1 Serving/30g	133	7.2	442	12	42	24	6

N

	Measure INFO/WEIGHT	per Measure KCAL	FAT	Nutrition Values per 100g / 100ml KCAL	PROT	CARB	FAT	FIBRE
OAT CAKES								
Ancient Grain, Nairn's*	1 Oatcake/8g	37	1.4	444	13.5	55.3	16.8	8.8
Cheese, GF, Nairn's*	1 Oatcake/9g	45	2.3	498	14.8	44.4	25.7	7.3
Cheese, Nairn's*	1 Oatcake/8g	39	2.3	471	13.2	43.3	27.2	6.8
Fine Milled, Nairn's*	1 Oatcake/8g	35	1.7	449	10.5	52.6	21.8	8.6
Fruit, & Seed, On the Go, Nairn's*	1 Oatcake/13g	57	2	437	9.6	60.2	15.5	9.2
Herb & Pumpkin Seed, Nairn's*	1 Oatcake/10g	43	2.1	426	12.2	46.8	21.1	13
Highland, Walkers*	1 Oatcake/12g	54	2.5	451	10.3	56	20.6	6.7
Northstaffs Oatcake Bakers Ltd*	1 Oatcake/67g	125	2.3	187	5.8	31.2	3.5	3.9
Oatmeal, Rough, Nairn's*	1 Oatcake/11g	45	1.8	431	10.2	58.6	17.3	8
Oatmeal, Rough, Organic, Nairn's*	1 Oatcake/10g	43	1.7	418	10.2	57.7	16.3	7.5
Original, Scottish, Macleans*	1 Oatcake/8g	37	1.6	489	13.2	54.9	21.4	12
Orkney, Thick, Stockan's*	1 Oatcake/25g	122	4.6	489	9.8	68	18.2	6.8
Orkney, Thin, Stockan's*	1 Oatcake/13g	65	2.9	501	10.4	62.4	22	6
Retail, Average	*1 Oatcake/13g*	*57*	*2.4*	*441*	*10*	*63*	*18.3*	*2*
Rough Scottish, Sainsbury's*	1 Oatcake/11g	51	2.1	462	12.3	59.9	19.3	6.5
Rough with Olive Oil, Paterson's*	1 Oatcake/13g	55	2.1	440	11.7	54.7	17	0
Rough, Sainsbury's*	1 Oatcake/10g	47	2	454	9.8	55.4	19.2	10
Rough, Scottish, Morrisons*	2 Oatcakes/21g	95	4.2	456	9.9	54.7	20	9
Rough, Scottish, Tesco*	1 Oatcake/10g	45	1.9	435	11.4	55.3	18.4	8
Scottish, Asda*	1 Oatcake/13g	58	2.3	461	11	59	18	9.8
Scottish, Rough, Waitrose*	1 Oatcake/13g	55	2.3	438	10.4	57.4	18.5	8
Scottish, Tower Gate, Lidl*	1 Oatcake/13g	60	2.5	465	10	60	19	6.8
Seeded, Aldi*	1 Oatcake/10g	46	2	443	11	52	19	10
Seeded, Scottish, Rivercote, Lidl*	1 Oatcake/11g	48	2.1	461	11	54.9	19.9	9.1
Traditional, M&S*	1 Oatcake/11g	49	2	445	11	59.3	18.3	6.6
OAT DRINK								
Barista Edition, Oatly*	100ml	59	3	59	1	6.6	3	0.8
Healthy, Enriched, Oatly*	1 Serving/250ml	112	3.8	45	1	6.5	1.5	0.8
Oat Milk, Organic, Healthy, Oatly*	1 Serving/250ml	100	1.2	40	1	6.7	0.5	0.8
OCTOPUS								
Chunks in Olive Oil, Palacio De Oriente*	1 Tin/111g	148	4	133	21.6	4.5	3.6	0
Raw	*1oz/28g*	*18*	*0.3*	*66*	*14.1*	*0*	*1*	*0*
OIL								
Avocado, Olivado*	1 Tsp/5ml	40	4.4	802	0	0	88	0
Black Truffle, Grapeseed, Cuisine Perel*	1 Tsp/5ml	43	5	857	0	7.1	100	0
Chilli, Average	*1 Tsp/5ml*	*41*	*4.6*	*824*	*0*	*0*	*91.5*	*0*
Coconut, Average	*1 Tsp/5ml*	*45*	*5*	*899*	*0*	*0*	*99.9*	*0*
Coconut, Cold Pressed, Virgin, Waitrose*	1 Tbsp/15g	135	15	900	0	0	100	0
Cod Liver, Average	*1 Capsule/1g*	*9*	*1*	*900*	*0*	*0*	*100*	*0*
Corn, Average	*1 Tsp/5ml*	*43*	*4.8*	*864*	*0*	*0*	*96*	*0*
Evening Primrose, Average	*1 Serving/1g*	*9*	*1*	*900*	*0*	*0*	*100*	*0*
Fish, Average	*1 Serving/1g*	*9*	*1*	*900*	*0*	*0*	*100*	*0*
Flax Seed, Average	*1 Tbsp/15ml*	*124*	*13.9*	*829*	*0*	*0*	*92.6*	*0*
Garlic, Infuse, Fry Light*	1 Spray/0.2ml	1	0.1	507	0	0.4	52.9	0
Grapeseed, Average	*1 Tsp/5ml*	*43*	*4.8*	*866*	*0*	*0*	*96.2*	*0*
Groundnut, Average	*1 Tsp/5ml*	*41*	*4.6*	*824*	*0*	*0*	*91.8*	*0*
Hazelnut, Average	*1 Tsp/5ml*	*45*	*5*	*899*	*0*	*0*	*99.9*	*0*
Mustard, Average	*1 Serving/100g*	*884*	*100*	*884*	*0*	*0*	*100*	*0*
Olive, Average	*1 Tsp/5ml*	*43*	*4.7*	*855*	*0*	*0*	*94.9*	*0*
Olive, Basil Infused, Tesco*	1 Serving/20ml	180	20	900	0	0	100	0
Olive, Extra Virgin, Average	*1 Tsp/5ml*	*42*	*4.7*	*848*	*0*	*0*	*94.5*	*0*
Olive, Garlic, Average	*1 Tbsp/15ml*	*127*	*14.1*	*848*	*0*	*0*	*94.3*	*0*
Olive, Mild, Average	*1 Tbsp/15ml*	*129*	*14.4*	*862*	*0*	*0*	*95.7*	*0*

	Measure INFO/WEIGHT	per Measure KCAL	FAT	Nutrition Values per 100g / 100ml KCAL	PROT	CARB	FAT	FIBRE
OIL								
Olive, Spray, Average	**10 Sprays/2ml**	**10**	**1.1**	**508**	**0**	**0**	**54.6**	**0**
Palm, Average	**1 Tsp/5ml**	**45**	**5**	**899**	**0**	**0**	**99.9**	**0**
Peanut, Average	**1 Tsp/5ml**	**45**	**5**	**899**	**0**	**0**	**99.9**	**0**
Rapeseed, Average	**1 Tbsp/15ml**	**130**	**14.4**	**864**	**0**	**0**	**96**	**0**
Rapeseed, Spray, Everyday, Borderfields*	1 Spray/0g	2	0.2	824	0	0	92	0
Rice Bran, Average	**1 Tbsp/14g**	**120**	**13.6**	**884**	**0**	**0**	**100**	**0**
Sesame, Average	**1 Tsp/5ml**	**45**	**5**	**892**	**0.1**	**0**	**99.9**	**0**
Sunflower, Average	**1 Tsp/5ml**	**43**	**4.8**	**869**	**0**	**0**	**96.6**	**0**
Sunflower, Spray, Fry Light*	1 Spray/0.2ml	1	0.1	519	0	0.2	53.9	0
Ultimate Blend, Udo's Choice*	1 Capsule/1ml	9	1	900	1.3	0	96.8	0
Vegetable, Average	**1 Tbsp/15ml**	**129**	**14.3**	**858**	**0**	**0**	**95.3**	**0**
Walnut, Average	**1 Tsp/5ml**	**45**	**5**	**899**	**0**	**0**	**99.9**	**0**
OKRA								
Boiled in Unsalted Water, Average	**1 Serving/80g**	**22**	**0.7**	**28**	**2.5**	**2.7**	**0.9**	**3.6**
Raw, Average	**1 Serving/80g**	**18**	**0.6**	**23**	**2.1**	**2.2**	**0.7**	**3**
Stir-Fried in Corn Oil, Average	**1 Serving/80g**	**215**	**20.9**	**269**	**4.3**	**4.4**	**26.1**	**6.3**
OLIVES								
Black & Green, with Greek Feta Cheese, Tesco*	1 Pot/100g	200	20.1	200	3.4	0.3	20.1	4.6
Black, Pitted, Average	**½ Jar/82g**	**135**	**13.3**	**164**	**1**	**3.5**	**16.2**	**3.1**
Green, Filled, Red Pepper, In Brine, Drained, Lyttos, Aldi*	1 Serving/30g	50	5	166	0.5	2.7	16.7	1.6
Green, Garlic Stuffed, Asda*	1 Olive/3g	6	0.6	174	1.8	3.5	17	0
Green, Manzanilla, Stuffed with Jalapeno, Fragata *	½ Can/100g	169	18	169	0.8	0	18	0
Green, Pimento Stuffed, With Gouda & Cumin, Unearthed*	1 Serving/30g	65	6	217	6.6	1	20	2.6
Green, Pitted, Average	**1 Olive/3g**	**4**	**0.4**	**130**	**1.1**	**0.9**	**13.3**	**2.5**
Green, Pitted, with Mixed Herbs, Sainsbury's*	1 Serving/15g	27	2.7	178	1.2	0.6	18.1	4
Green, Stuffed with Almonds, Pitted, Waitrose*	1 Serving/50g	90	8.4	180	3.8	3.2	16.9	2.5
Halkidiki, Stuffed with Garlic, Tesco*	¼ Pack/40g	66	6.7	164	1.3	0.3	16.8	3
Kalamata, in Brine, Drained, Finest, Tesco*	1 Serving/30g	79	8.3	264	1.5	1.2	27.7	1.9
Kalamata, Pitted, Greek, Drained, Sainsbury's*	1 Serving/15g	31	3.2	205	1.6	0.5	21.4	3.2
Manzanilla, Pitted, with Garlic & Herbs, Sainsbury's*	1 Serving/60g	111	11.3	184	1.3	1.6	18.7	2.2
Marinated, Mixed, M&S*	1 Serving/20g	33	3	165	1.6	6.5	14.9	3
Marinated, Selection, M&S*	4 Olives/20g	44	4.4	225	1.4	3.9	22.6	2.1
Mixed, Chilli & Garlic, Asda*	1 Serving/30g	43	4.7	144	0.9	0	15.6	6.1
Mixed, Mediterranean, Morrisons*	1 Serving/30g	74	7.7	248	1	1.6	25.8	2.9
Mixed, with Rosemary, & Black Pepper, Unearthed*	1 Serving/30g	64	6.6	213	1.4	2.1	22	2.9
Selection, Co-Op*	1 Serving/30g	68	6.9	225	1	2	23	2
OMELETTE								
Cheese & Mushroom, Apetito*	1 Serving/320g	486	25	152	6.2	14.4	7.8	1.9
Cheese, 2 Egg, Average	**1 Omelette/180g**	**479**	**40.7**	**266**	**15.9**	**0**	**22.6**	**0**
Cheese, Asda*	1 Omelette/87g	244	19.1	281	15	3.8	22	1.4
Cheese, HFC, Tesco*	1 Omelette/95g	214	16.4	226	13.2	4.1	17.3	0.6
Ham & Mushroom, Farmfoods*	1 Omelette/120g	200	16.7	167	8.7	1.8	13.9	0.1
Mushroom & Cheese, Tesco*	1 Omelette/120g	248	21.5	207	9.8	1.6	17.9	0.2
Plain, 2 Egg	**1 Omelette/120g**	**229**	**19.7**	**191**	**10.9**	**0**	**16.4**	**0**
Potato, Spanish, Waitrose*	1 Pack/500g	710	40	142	6.9	9.5	8	0.5
Spanish	**1oz/28g**	**34**	**2.3**	**120**	**5.7**	**6.2**	**8.3**	**1.4**
Spanish, Potato, Rapido, Unearthed*	1 Pack/250g	410	27.2	164	5.2	10.5	10.9	2.2
Spanish, Red Pepper, Unearthed*	1 Omelette/250g	415	23.5	166	5	14	9.4	2.2
ONION POWDER								
Average	**1 Tsp/2g**	**7**	**0**	**341**	**10.4**	**79.1**	**1**	**15.2**
ONION RINGS								
Battered, Free From, Tesco*	3 Rings/63g	190	9.5	303	3.1	37.3	15.2	2.1
Battered, Mini, Frozen, Tesco*	4 Rings/34g	87	3.9	259	4.2	32.8	11.6	3.3

	Measure INFO/WEIGHT	per Measure KCAL	FAT	Nutrition Values per 100g / 100ml KCAL	PROT	CARB	FAT	FIBRE
ONION RINGS								
Battered, Oven Baked, Tesco*	1 Serving/50g	110	5	219	3.9	28.4	10	3.5
Battered, Sainsbury's*	1 Ring/12g	32	1.4	265	3.8	34.4	11.6	4.1
Beer Battered, Frozen, Tesco*	3 Rings/75g	213	10	284	4.6	36	13.3	0.8
Beer Battered, Mash Direct*	½ Pack/100g	283	10.3	283	2.6	23.9	10.3	2.7
Breaded & Fried, From Restaurant	***1 Ring/12g***	***40***	***2.2***	***332***	***4.5***	***37.7***	***18.7***	***0***
Breaded, Asda*	1 Serving/67g	180	7.4	267	4.3	36	11	3.3
Breaded, Iceland*	1 Ring/11g	33	1.7	293	4.4	34.2	15.4	2.7
Oven Crisp Batter, Tesco*	1 Ring/17g	44	1.9	259	4.1	34.4	11.2	2.1
Whole, Battered, Frozen, Aunt Bessies*	5 Rings/90g	195	10.8	217	2.5	24	12	1.8
ONIONS								
Baked	***1oz/28g***	***29***	***0.2***	***103***	***3.5***	***22.3***	***0.6***	***3.9***
Boiled in Unsalted Water	***1oz/28g***	***5***	***0***	***17***	***0.6***	***3.7***	***0.1***	***0.7***
Dried, Raw, Average	***1oz/28g***	***88***	***0.5***	***313***	***10.2***	***68.6***	***1.7***	***12.1***
Flakes, Dried, Average	***1 Tbsp/15g***	***52***	***0.1***	***349***	***9***	***83.3***	***0.5***	***9.2***
Fried, Average	***1oz/28g***	***46***	***3.1***	***164***	***2.3***	***14.1***	***11.2***	***3.1***
Pickled, Average	***1 Onion/15g***	***3***	***0***	***19***	***0.7***	***4.1***	***0.1***	***0.6***
Raw, Average	***1 Med/180g***	***69***	***0.4***	***38***	***1.2***	***7.9***	***0.2***	***1.3***
Red, Raw, Average	***1 Med/180g***	***66***	***0.4***	***37***	***1.2***	***7.9***	***0.2***	***1.5***
Spring, Raw, Average	***1 Med/15g***	***4***	***0.1***	***24***	***1.9***	***2.9***	***0.5***	***1.4***
ORANGE CURD								
Jaffa, Luxury, Waitrose*	1 Tbsp/15g	54	1.5	357	3	63.5	10.1	0.1
ORANGES								
Blood, Average	***1 Orange/140g***	***82***	***0***	***58***	***0.8***	***13.3***	***0***	***2.5***
Fresh, Weighed with Peel, Average	***1 Med/220g***	***97***	***0.5***	***44***	***0.9***	***10.8***	***0.2***	***3.2***
Fresh, without Peel, Average	***1 Med/154g***	***97***	***0.5***	***63***	***1.3***	***15.5***	***0.3***	***4.5***
Peel Only, Raw, Average	***1 Tbsp/6g***	***6***	***0***	***97***	***1.5***	***25***	***0.2***	***10.6***
Ruby Red, Tesco*	1 Med/130g	51	0.1	39	1.1	8.5	0.1	1.7
Segments, Canned, in Fruit Juice, Trout Hall*	1 Serving/138g	47	0.7	34	0.7	7.7	0.5	0.3
Segments, in Juice, Canned, Morrisons*	1 Portion/80g	36	0.1	45	0.4	10.3	0.1	0.5
OREGANO								
Dried	***1 Tsp/1g***	***3***	***0.1***	***306***	***11***	***49.5***	***10.3***	***0***
Fresh	***1 Tsp/1.3g***	***1***	***0***	***66***	***2.2***	***9.7***	***2***	***0***
OSTRICH								
Steak, Fillet, Klein Karoo*	1 Fillet/125g	141	2.6	113	23.1	1	2.1	1
Steaks, in Marrakesh Marinade, South African, Deluxe*	1 Steak/150g	158	1.4	105	20	4.1	0.9	0
OVALTINE*								
Chocolate, Light, Ovaltine*	1 Serving/20g	76	1.2	380	8.5	70.5	6	4.5
Chocolate, Light, Sachet, Ovaltine*	1 Sachet/25g	96	1.5	384	7.4	73	5.9	4.7
Hi Malt, Light, Instant Drink, Ovaltine*	1 Sachet/20g	72	1.2	358	9.1	67.1	5.9	2.8
Powder, Made Up with Semi-Skimmed Milk, Ovaltine*	1 Mug/227ml	179	3.9	79	3.9	13	1.7	0
Powder, Made Up with Whole Milk, Ovaltine*	1 Mug/227ml	220	8.6	97	3.8	12.9	3.8	0
OXTAIL								
Raw	***1oz/28g***	***18***	***1.1***	***65***	***7.6***	***0***	***3.8***	***0***
Stewed, Bone Removed	***1oz/28g***	***68***	***3.8***	***243***	***30.5***	***0***	***13.4***	***0***
OYSTERS								
Raw, Shelled, Shucked	***1 Oyster/14g***	***9***	***0.2***	***65***	***10.8***	***2.7***	***1.3***	***0***

O

	Measure INFO/WEIGHT	per Measure		Nutrition Values per 100g / 100ml				
		KCAL	FAT	KCAL	PROT	CARB	FAT	FIBRE
PAELLA								
Chicken, & Chorizo, & Prawn, City Kitchen, Tesco*	1 Pack/400g	540	20	135	4.7	17	5	1.4
Chicken, & Prawn, King, BFY, M&S*	1 Pack/390g	425	8.6	109	8.3	13.4	2.2	1.2
Chicken, & Prawn, Spanish, Inspirations, Birds Eye*	1 Serving/345g	410	12.1	119	6.1	15	3.5	1.4
Chicken, & Chorizo, Rice Pot, Tesco*	1 Pack/330g	469	10.6	142	5.5	22	3.2	1.4
Chicken, & Chorizo, SlimWell, Aldi*	1 Pack/500g	430	3.5	86	5.7	13	0.7	2.4
Chicken, & Prawn, King, Mix, Simply Bistro, Aldi*	½ Bag/309g	303	4	98	5.3	16	1.3	1.6
Chicken, & Prawn, Slim Choice, Sainsbury's*	1 Pack/500g	425	3	85	6.2	13.1	0.6	1.3
Chicken, & Prawn, Slim Cook, Tesco*	1 Pack/500g	380	3	76	6.2	10.5	0.6	2.3
Chicken, Chorizo & King Prawn, Finest, Tesco*	1 Pack/450g	590	14	131	6.2	18.9	3.1	1.1
Chicken, King Prawn, & Chorizo, Truly Irresistible, Co-Op*	1 Pack/400g	512	12	128	6.8	17.5	3	1.2
PAIN AU CHOCOLAT								
All Butter, Tesco*	1 Pain/58g	235	11.6	406	8.3	46.8	20	3
Average	***1 Pastry/60g***	***253***	***13.7***	***422***	***8***	***45.8***	***22.8***	***3.1***
M&S*	1 Pastry/60g	210	11.5	350	5.9	38	19.2	1.6
Mini, Asda*	1 Pastry/23g	96	5.5	420	8	43	24	3.3
Sainsbury's*	1 Pastry/58g	241	13.8	415	7.9	42.5	23.7	3.3
Waitrose*	1 Pastry/52g	226	12.7	435	8.3	44.2	24.4	2.9
PAIN AU RAISIN								
Bakery, Sainsbury's*	1 Pastry/100g	335	14.5	335	6	44.6	14.5	1.4
Bakery, Tesco*	1 Pastry/107g	351	14.7	328	6.9	43.3	13.7	1.8
Takeaway, Average	***1 Pastry/100g***	***313***	***13.2***	***313***	***5.2***	***43***	***13.2***	***1.3***
Twist, Extra Special, Asda*	1 Pastry/110g	421	20.9	383	7	46	19	2.5
PAK CHOI								
Raw, Average	***1 Leaf/14g***	***2***	***0***	***11***	***1.3***	***1.9***	***0.2***	***0.9***
PAKORA								
Bhaji, Onion, Fried in Vegetable Oil	***1oz/28g***	***76***	***4.1***	***271***	***9.8***	***26.2***	***14.7***	***5.5***
Bhajia, Potato Carrot & Pea, Fried in Vegetable Oil	***1oz/28g***	***100***	***6.3***	***357***	***10.9***	***28.8***	***22.6***	***6.1***
Bhajia, Vegetable, Retail	***1oz/28g***	***66***	***4.1***	***235***	***6.4***	***21.4***	***14.7***	***3.6***
Chicken, Indian, Sainsbury's*	½ Pack/45g	95	3.3	211	27.7	7.8	7.4	1
Chicken, Taste of India, Tesco*	1 Pack/150g	345	10.8	230	26.6	13.8	7.2	1.8
Vegetable, Indian Starter Selection, M&S*	1 Pakora/20g	43	0.6	214	1.2	4.1	3.2	0.9
PANCAKE								
Asda*	1 Pancake/23g	59	1.6	254	4.8	43	7	4
Blueberry, Tesco*	1 Pancake/75g	195	3.1	260	4.8	49.5	4.1	2
Buttermilk, Giant , Village Bakery, Aldi*	1 Pancake/65g	146	1.8	225	6.7	42	2.8	1.7
Buttermilk, Large, Tesco*	1 Pancake/65g	176	3.9	270	6.7	46.8	6	1.2
Cheese, Mushroom, & Spinach, Vegetarian, Waitrose*	1 Pack/260g	530	31.2	204	8.2	14.6	12	2.6
Maple & Raisin, M&S*	1 Pancake/35g	102	2.4	290	5.6	50.4	6.9	2.2
Mini, Scotch, Tesco*	1 Pancake/16g	44	0.9	277	6.7	50	5.6	1.4
Plain, Prepared From Recipe, Average	***1 Pancake/38g***	***86***	***3.7***	***227***	***6.4***	***28.3***	***9.7***	***0***
Raisin & Lemon, Asda*	1 Serving/30g	92	2.4	304	6	52	8	1.4
Raisin & Lemon, Sainsbury's*	1 Pancake/35g	95	1.5	272	6.3	51.8	4.4	2.2
Ready Made, Average	***1 Sm/30g***	***77***	***1.9***	***258***	***6.1***	***44.2***	***6.4***	***1.7***
Savoury, Made with Skimmed Milk, Average	***6"Pancake/77g***	***192***	***11.3***	***249***	***6.4***	***24.1***	***14.7***	***0.8***
Scotch	***1 Pancake/50g***	***146***	***5.8***	***292***	***5.8***	***43.6***	***11.7***	***1.4***
Scotch, Hovis*	1 Pancake/30g	88	2.5	295	5.5	48.1	8.4	2.3
Scotch, M&S*	1 Pancake/34g	95	1.4	280	6.5	54.5	4	1.6
Scotch, Morrisons*	1 Pancake/28g	82	1.8	294	6.3	51.9	6.4	1.6
Scotch, Sainsbury's*	1 Pancake/30g	78	1.3	260	5.9	48.8	4.4	1
Scotch, Tesco*	1 Pancake/30g	81	2	271	5.5	46.7	6.5	1.8
Sweet, Dessert Menu*	1 Pancake/63g	167	7.5	267	5.1	35	12	0.6
Syrup, Tesco*	1 Pancake/30g	80	2.5	265	4.7	42.1	8.2	1.5
Vegetable Roll	***1 Roll/85g***	***185***	***10.6***	***218***	***6.6***	***21***	***12.5***	***0***

	Measure INFO/WEIGHT	per Measure KCAL	FAT	Nutrition Values per 100g / 100ml KCAL	PROT	CARB	FAT	FIBRE
PANCAKE								
with Syrup, American Style, Large, Tesco*	1 Pancake/38g	102	1.3	268	5.1	54.2	3.4	0.9
PANCAKE MIX								
Slender, Dry, Protein World*	1 Serving/50g	172	1.5	343	21.4	57.3	3	2.9
PANCETTA								
Average	*½ Pack/65g*	*212*	*18.7*	*326*	*17*	*0.1*	*28.7*	*0*
PANINI								
Cheese, Tesco*	1 Panini/100g	249	9.1	249	10.5	31.3	9.1	3.1
Chicken, & Pesto, Rustlers*	1 Panini/143g	415	19.6	290	13.3	27.8	13.7	0
Chicken, Arrabiata, Ginsters*	1 Panini/200g	489	16.8	245	12.8	29.4	8.4	2.4
Chicken, Chargrilled, Mozzarella, & Pesto, Udo's Choice*	1 Panini/170g	389	14.6	229	16.4	21.6	8.6	2
Ham, & Cheese, Ginsters*	1 Panini/200g	567	25.6	283	13.3	28.7	12.8	1.6
Mozzarella, & Tomato, M&S*	1 Serving/176g	484	28.5	275	11.3	21.3	16.2	2.1
Tuna, & Sweetcorn, Tesco*	1 Serving/250g	559	16.4	224	12	29.3	6.6	1.4
PANNA COTTA								
BGTY, Sainsbury's*	1 Pot/150g	150	2.8	100	2.4	18.2	1.9	1.4
Caramel, Sainsbury's*	1 Serving/120g	319	15.1	266	4	31.8	12.6	0.7
Raspberry, COU, M&S*	1 Pot/140g	146	3.5	104	2.6	17.5	2.5	0.6
Raspberry, Hotel Chocolat*	1 Serving/30g	162	11.2	541	6	45.6	37.4	0
Raspberry, Pot, The Coconut Collaborative*	1 Pot/65g	132	9.1	203	1.6	18	14	1.2
Sainsbury's*	1 Pot/100g	304	15.7	304	3	41.5	15.7	4
Strawberry, COU, M&S*	1 Pot/145g	145	3.8	100	2.6	15.7	2.6	0.8
PAPAYA								
Dried, Pieces, Nature's Harvest*	1 Serving/50g	178	0	355	0.2	85.4	0	2.6
Raw, Flesh Only, Average	*1 Serving/140g*	*37*	*0.1*	*26*	*0.4*	*6.6*	*0.1*	*1.2*
PAPPARDELLE								
Egg, Dry, Average	*1 Serving/100g*	*364*	*3.7*	*364*	*14.1*	*68.5*	*3.7*	*2.1*
PAPRIKA								
Average	*1 Tsp/2g*	*6*	*0.3*	*289*	*14.8*	*34.9*	*13*	*0*
PARATHA								
Average	*1 Paratha/80g*	*258*	*11.4*	*322*	*8*	*43.2*	*14.3*	*4*
Roti, Plain, Crown Farms*	1 Slice/80g	250	10	312	5	46.2	12.5	1.2
PARCELS								
Chicken, & Bacon, Sainsbury's*	½ Pack/170g	406	28.6	239	21.9	0.1	16.8	0
Chicken, & Bacon, Specially Selected, Aldi*	1 Parcel/190g	572	34.2	301	12	22	18	0.5
Feta, & Spinach, Filo, Sainsbury's*	1 Parcel/27g	83	5.6	307	5.8	23.8	20.7	1.8
Goats Cheese, & Caramelised Onion, Asda*	1 Parcel/22g	71	4.2	325	6.6	30	19	2.3
Salmon, Puff Pastry, Cream Cheese Sauce & Dill, Tesco*	1 Parcel/124g	334	19.4	269	10.7	20.5	15.6	1.8
PARSLEY								
Dried	*1 Tsp/1g*	*2*	*0.1*	*181*	*15.8*	*14.5*	*7*	*26.9*
Fresh, Average	*1 Tbsp/3.8g*	*1*	*0*	*27*	*2.4*	*2.2*	*1*	*4*
Root, Raw, Average	*1 Avg Root/33g*	*18*	*0.2*	*55*	*2.3*	*12.3*	*0.6*	*4.3*
PARSNIP								
Boiled, Average	*1 Serving/80g*	*53*	*1*	*66*	*1.6*	*12.9*	*1.2*	*4.7*
Honey Glazed, Roast, Baked, Aunt Bessie's*	1 Serving/100g	158	12	158	1.1	8.6	12	5.1
Honey Roasted, Tesco*	½ Pack/142g	159	5	112	1.2	16.8	3.5	4.2
Raw, Unprepared, Average	*1 Serving/100g*	*62*	*1*	*62*	*1.7*	*11.6*	*1*	*4.3*
PARTRIDGE								
Meat Only, Roasted	*1 Partridge/260g*	*551*	*18.7*	*212*	*36.7*	*0*	*7.2*	*0*
PASSATA								
Italian, Rustica, TTD, Sainsbury's*	1 Bottle/430g	155	6.9	36	1.1	3.7	1.6	1
Italian, with Onion & Garlic, Classic, Sainsbury's*	¼ Carton/125g	29	0.6	23	1.3	3.6	0.5	1.2
Italian, with Onion, & Garlic, Sainsbury's*	1 Pack/390g	117	2	30	1.9	4.3	0.5	1.5
Mutti Di Pomodoro , Mutti*	1/5 Jar/140g	50	0.4	36	1.6	5.1	0.3	0

P

	Measure INFO/WEIGHT	per Measure KCAL	FAT	Nutrition Values per 100g / 100ml KCAL	PROT	CARB	FAT	FIBRE
PASSATA								
Napolina*	1 Bottle/690g	172	0.7	25	1.4	4.5	0.1	0
Smart Price, Asda*	1 Serving/100g	30	0.1	30	1.1	5.6	0.1	0.9
Soffritto, Napolina*	1/3 Jar/143g	57	1.7	40	2.4	3.9	1.2	2
Tomato, Freshona, Lidl*	1 Carton/500g	170	2.5	34	1.5	4.6	0.5	1.3
PASSION FRUIT								
Raw, Fresh, Average	*1 Fruit/18g*	*7*	*0.1*	*36*	*2.6*	*5.8*	*0.4*	*3.3*
Weighed with Skin, Average	*1 Fruit/30g*	*7*	*0.1*	*22*	*1.6*	*3.5*	*0.2*	*2*
PASTA								
Alphabet Shapes, Dry, Sainsbury's*	1 Serving/70g	223	1	319	10.2	65	1.4	2.8
Cappelletti, Prosciutto, Italian, Sainsbury's*	½ Pack/200g	362	9.4	181	9.6	23.9	4.7	2.2
Cheese, & Tomato, Taste Buds, Tiny Taste Buds, M&S*	1 Pack/225g	250	7.4	111	5.3	14.5	3.3	1.2
Cheese, Leek, & Ham, Pasta n Sauce, Batchelors*	½ Pack/184g	235	3.9	128	5	21.9	2.1	0.7
Cheese, Macaroni, Dry, Pasta n Sauce, Batchelors*	1 Pack/108g	402	5.1	372	17.2	65.2	4.7	2.7
Chicken, & Chorizo, Average	*1 Pack/400g*	*174*	*5.7*	*174*	*10.1*	*20.3*	*5.7*	*1.5*
Chicken, & Chorizo, Quadrotti, TTD, Sainsbury's*	1 Pack/320g	616	25.3	192	9.6	19.5	7.9	2.4
Chicken, & Bacon, Italian, Iceland*	1 Pack/400g	492	11.6	123	6.8	16.9	2.9	1
Chicken, & Mushroom, Free From, Tesco*	1 Pack/373g	393	5.6	105	4.4	18.1	1.5	0.9
Chicken, Chilli, Spicy, Tesco*	1 Pack/275g	387	4.4	141	6.2	24.4	1.6	2.1
Chicken, Ham, & Vegetable, Slimming World*	1 Pack/550g	500	4.4	91	8.3	11.5	0.8	2.1
Chicken, Peri Peri, No Mayonnaise, Tesco*	1 Pack/300g	363	5.1	121	4.3	21.4	1.7	1.4
Chicken, Pesto, & Tomato, Fresh Ideas, Morrisons*	1 Pack/388g	1808	39.6	466	7.1	15.7	10.2	3.9
Chicken, Piri Piri, On the Go, Sainsbury's*	1 Pack/350g	514	10.8	147	7.7	21.2	3.1	1.9
Chicken, Roast, As Consumed, Mug Shot, Symingtons*	1 Serving/258g	201	2.6	78	2.8	14.2	1	0.5
Chicken, Tomato, & Basil, Tesco*	1 Pack/300g	471	11.1	157	6.7	23.3	3.7	1.6
Chorizo, with Chickpea Crumb, Musclefood*	1 Serving/297g	345	11	116	5.8	14	3.7	2.4
Gemelli, Egg, Fresh, Sainsbury's*	1 Serving/100g	193	1.8	193	7.5	36	1.8	1.3
Green Pea, GF, As Prepared, Love Life, Waitrose*	1 Serving/175g	276	1.6	158	10.5	24.1	0.9	5.5
Green Pea, GF, Dry, Free From, Morrisons*	1 Serving/75g	262	1.1	349	18.5	61.1	1.5	9.1
Margherite, Basil, & Pinenut, TTD, Sainsbury's*	½ Pack/125g	259	10.9	207	7.8	23.5	8.7	1.5
Meat Feast, Microwaved, Slimming World*	1 Pack/550g	478	7.2	87	7.3	10.9	1.3	1.3
Orzo, Dry, Average	*1 Serving/100g*	*348*	*1.5*	*348*	*12.4*	*71.9*	*1.5*	*3*
Pennette Rigate, Di Lenticchie, & Riso, Rosse, Dry, Rummo	1 Serving/60g	217	1.8	361	6	67.4	3	4.4
Pesto, with Semi Dried Tomatoes, Tesco*	1 Pack/225g	432	18.2	192	5.6	23.4	8.1	1.7
Porcini Mushroom, & Truffle, Filled, Fresh, Bertagni*	1 Pack/250g	762	37.5	305	9.5	32	15	3
Pumpkin, & Pine Nut, Stuffed, Fiorelli, Fresh, Waitrose*	½ Pack/125g	225	7.5	180	8	22.3	6	2.3
Tomato 'n' Herb, Mug Shot, Symingtons*	1 Serving/253g	223	2	88	3	16.6	0.8	1
Tuna, & Sweetcorn, Tesco*	½ Pot/150g	253	11.6	169	6.5	17.9	7.7	0.9
Vegetable, Mediterranean, Cooked, BGTY, Sainsbury's*	1 Pack/400g	347	5.5	89	2.8	15.2	1.4	1.9
Wholewheat, Cooked, Tesco*	1 Serving/200g	284	1.8	142	5.7	27.9	0.9	4.5
PASTA BAKE								
Bacon & Leek, Average	*1 Serving/400g*	*633*	*32.3*	*158*	*6.7*	*14.8*	*8.1*	*1.3*
Beef, Bolognese, Meal to Share, M&S*	½ Pack/400g	700	30.8	175	9.3	16.6	7.7	1.2
Cheese, & Tomato, Italiano, Tesco*	1 Bake/300g	354	12.6	118	3.9	16.1	4.2	1
Chicken, & Bacon, Asda*	¼ Pack/374g	610	26.2	163	9	16	7	4.1
Chicken, & Bacon, Average	*1 Serving/400g*	*627*	*28.7*	*157*	*9*	*13.7*	*7.2*	*1.6*
Chicken, & Bacon, Taste of Italy, Tesco*	1 Pack/429g	627	19.3	146	11	15	4.5	0.9
Chicken, & Penne, Italian, Mulkerns*	1 Serving/430g	305	3.9	71	6.7	9.1	0.9	0
Chicken, Bacon & Mushroom, Average	*1 Serving/400g*	*632*	*29.2*	*158*	*7.8*	*15.1*	*7.3*	*2.3*
Chicken, Pesto, & Mozzarella, Meal to Share, M&S*	½ Pack/400g	632	24.4	158	8.3	16.7	6.1	1.3
Mac 'n' Greens, Slimming World*	½ Pack/275g	190	1.1	69	3.9	11.5	0.4	1.7
Meat Feast, Average	*1 Serving/400g*	*601*	*21.4*	*150*	*5.8*	*19.2*	*5.4*	*1.4*
Pepperoni, Taste of Italy, Tesco*	1 Pack/450g	651	23.3	145	5.9	18	5.2	1.1
Sausage, Average	*1 Serving/400g*	*591*	*24*	*148*	*5.5*	*17.7*	*6*	*1.9*

P

	Measure INFO/WEIGHT	per Measure KCAL	FAT	Nutrition Values per 100g / 100ml KCAL	PROT	CARB	FAT	FIBRE
PASTA BAKE								
Tomato, & Bacon, Creamy, Italian, Asda*	1 Serving/125g	131	11.2	105	2	3.9	9	0.6
Tomato, & Mozzarella, Average	**1 Serving/400g**	**500**	**12.4**	**125**	**5.3**	**17.3**	**3.1**	**1.5**
Tomato, & Pepperoni, Spicy, Asda*	1 Pack/440g	431	26.4	98	1.1	10	6	1.2
Tomato, & Mozzarella, Taste of Italy, Tesco*	1 Pack/450g	535	13.7	119	5	17	3	1.8
Tomato, Creamy, Dolmio*	1 Serving/125g	141	9	113	2.3	8.4	7.2	0
Tuna, & Sweetcorn, Average	**1 Pack/400g**	**423**	**22.4**	**106**	**5**	**8.6**	**5.6**	**1.9**
Tuna, Aldi*	1 Pack/400g	568	16	142	7.9	18	4	1.1
Vegetable, M&S*	1 Pack/350g	396	13.3	113	4.4	14.5	3.8	1.4
PASTA QUILLS								
Dry, Average	**1 Serving/75g**	**256**	**0.9**	**342**	**12**	**72.3**	**1.2**	**2**
GF, Salute*	1 Serving/75g	269	1.4	359	7.5	78	1.9	0
PASTA SALAD								
Cheese, Average	**1 Serving/370g**	**782**	**56.8**	**211**	**5.5**	**12.8**	**15.4**	**1.2**
Chicken, & Bacon, Caesar, Asda*	1 Pack/300g	552	30	184	6.9	16	10	1.2
Chicken, & Bacon, Caesar, Tesco*	1 Pack/265g	418	18.3	158	11.5	12.1	6.9	0.7
Chicken, & Bacon, Tesco*	½ Pack/233g	487	28.6	209	6.6	17.6	12.3	0.9
Chicken, Bacon, & Sweetcorn, M&S*	1 Pack/380g	680	33.1	179	8.2	16.1	8.7	1.7
Chicken, Honey & Mustard, Sainsbury's*	1 Pack/350g	649	34	185	7	16.6	9.7	1.8
Chicken, Spicy, On the Go, Sainsbury's*	1 Pot/300g	455	10.8	152	6.4	22.7	3.6	1.5
Chicken, Sweet Chilli, Asda*	1 Pack/225g	259	5.4	115	5.2	17	2.4	2.5
Chicken, Tomato, & Basil, 205g Pot, M&S*	1 Pack/205g	340	14.6	166	8	16.7	7.1	1.4
Chicken, Tomato, & Basil, 380g Pot, M&S*	1 Pot/380g	559	21.7	147	7.9	15.3	5.7	1.6
Chicken, Tomato, & Basil, Tesco*	1 Pack/260g	235	3.9	90	7.7	10.8	1.5	1.1
Feta, & Slow Roasted Tomato, M&S*	1 Pack/190g	344	13.3	181	6.5	22.3	7	2.5
Goats Cheese, & Mixed Pepper, Sainsbury's*	1 Pack/200g	366	18.8	183	6.4	18.2	9.4	1.5
Ham, & Cheese, Asda*	½ Pack/160g	213	10.7	133	4.9	12	6.7	1.8
Mozzarella, Basil, & Tomato, On the Go, Sainsbury's*	1 Pack/260g	437	16.1	168	6.6	20.4	6.2	1.9
Pesto, Creamy, Pot, Diet Chef*	1 Pot/248g	236	3.7	95	3.6	16.2	1.5	1
Pesto, Spicy Chilli, Sainsbury's*	¼ Pot/63g	170	12.3	272	3.8	20.1	19.6	1.6
Prawn Cocktail, Layered, Shapers, Boots*	1 Pot/210g	181	5.2	86	3.6	13	2.5	1.3
Prawn, Growers Selection, Asda*	1 Pack/380g	365	9.1	96	5.1	13	2.4	1.2
Prawn, Layered , On the Go, Sainsbury's*	1 Pack/380g	464	16.3	122	5.2	14.8	4.3	1.8
Prawn, Morrison's*	1 Pack/250g	528	35.5	211	3.7	16.5	14.2	1.1
Spinach, & Pine Nut, Sainsbury's*	½ Pot/100g	226	11.6	226	6.4	23	11.6	2.2
Tomato, & Basil, Sainsbury's*	1 Serving/83g	121	3.4	145	3.7	22.7	4.1	1.6
Tomato, & Pepper, Roast, Orzo, TTD, Sainsbury's*	½ Pot/150g	234	8.4	156	3.6	22.1	5.6	1.7
Tuna, & Sweetcorn, HE, Tesco*	1 Pot/200g	230	5.4	115	5.7	17	2.7	1.3
Tuna, & Sweetcorn, Meadow Fresh, Lidl*	½ Pack/190g	272	19	143	17.5	31.2	10	3
Tuna, & Sweetcorn, On the Go, Sainsbury's*	1 Pack/300g	492	17.1	164	5.9	21.6	5.7	1.4
Vegetable, Chargrilled, & Tomato, Shapers, Boots*	1 Pack/175g	187	5.4	107	2.8	17	3.1	1.5
Vegetable, Chargrilled, Sainsbury's*	1 Serving/178g	192	4.8	108	2.7	15.9	2.7	4.7
PASTA SAUCE								
Amatriciana, Italiano, Tesco*	½ Pot/175g	124	6.6	71	4.1	5.3	3.8	0.9
Amatriciana, M&S*	1 Jar/340g	425	32.3	125	3.4	6.3	9.5	2.9
Arrabbiata, Finest, Tesco*	½ Pot/175g	214	10.5	122	3.7	13	6	1.1
Arrabbiata, Fresh, Tesco*	½ Pot/175g	84	3.2	48	0.8	6.7	1.8	0.9
Arrabiata, Barilla*	1 Serving/100g	47	3	47	1.5	3.5	3	0
Arrabiata, Fresh, Co-Op*	½ Pot/150g	82	4.5	55	1	5	3	1
Arrabiata, GFY, Asda*	1 Serving/350g	133	3.9	38	1.1	6	1.1	0
Aubergine, & Mascarpone, Roasted, Stir Through, M&S*	½ Jar/95g	111	8.9	117	1	6.3	9.4	1.7
Bacon, Smoked, & Tomato, Stir-In, Dolmio*	1 Pot/150g	142	8.2	95	5	5.7	5.5	1.2
Bacon, Smoky, Loyd Grossman*	½ Jar/175g	142	8.4	81	3	6.1	4.8	0.8
Bolognese, Extra Onion & Garlic, Dolmio*	1 Serving/125g	51	0.8	41	1.4	6.6	0.6	1

PASTA SAUCE

	Measure INFO/WEIGHT	per Measure KCAL	FAT	Nutrition Values per 100g / 100ml KCAL	PROT	CARB	FAT	FIBRE
Bolognese, Free From, Tesco*	¼ Jar/125g	63	0.9	51	1.9	8.4	0.7	1.5
Bolognese, Garlic & Onion, Intense, Dolmio*	1 Jar/500g	210	1	42	1.7	7.4	0.2	1.8
Bolognese, Mushroom, Chunky, Dolmio*	½ Jar/375g	165	0.8	44	1.7	7.9	0.2	2
Bolognese, Organic, Seeds of Change*	1 Jar/500g	290	6	58	1.3	10.4	1.2	0.8
Bolognese, Original, Light, Low Fat, Dolmio*	1 Serving/125g	41	0.1	33	1.2	6	0.1	1.3
Bolognese, Original, Sainsbury's*	¼ Jar/136g	90	2.9	66	1.9	9.9	2.1	1.3
Bolognese, Smooth, Hidden Vegetables, Dolmio*	1 Portion/125g	60	1	48	1.4	7.7	0.8	1.9
Bolognese, Tesco*	1 Serving/100g	41	0.7	41	1.4	6.6	0.7	1.3
Bolognese, Tomato, Beef & Red Wine, Fresh, Waitrose*	1 Pot/350g	290	15.8	83	5.7	4.2	4.5	1.3
Bolognese, with Beef, Tesco*	½ Pack/175g	170	10	97	5.6	4.7	5.7	2.1
Cacciatore, Fresh, Sainsbury's*	½ Pot/150g	152	8.8	101	5.4	8.1	5.9	1.5
Carbonara, Asda*	½ Pot/175g	359	29.8	205	7	6	17	0.1
Carbonara, Co-Op*	½ Pot/150g	270	25.5	180	3	4	17	0.1
Carbonara, Creamy, Dolmio Express, Dolmio*	1 Pack/150g	166	13.2	111	3.3	4.7	8.8	0.1
Carbonara, Creamy, Stir in Sauce, Dolmio*	1 Serving/75g	98	8	130	3.3	5.2	10.6	0.2
Carbonara, Italian, Fresh, Sainsbury's*	½ Pot/176g	209	16.3	119	5.4	3.4	9.3	0.9
Cheese, Four, Sainsbury's*	1 Serving/150g	296	25.5	197	6.6	4.5	17	0.8
Cheese, Fresh, PB, Waitrose*	½ Pot/175g	144	5.1	82	6.1	7.9	2.9	0.5
Cheese, Three, Co-Op*	1 Pack/300g	405	27	135	6	6	9	0.1
Lasagne, Tomato, Red, Ragu, Knorr*	1 Jar/500g	215	0	43	1.1	9.7	0	1.1
Lasagne, White, Morrisons*	½ Jar/215g	245	20.2	114	2	5.2	9.4	0.5
Lasagne, White, Ragu, Knorr*	1 Jar/475g	755	72.2	159	0.5	5.1	15.2	0.3
Mac & Cheese, Pasta Bake, Sainsbury's*	¼ Jar/118g	176	14.9	149	1.8	6.9	12.6	0.5
Mediterranean, Fresh, Waitrose*	1 Pot/350g	214	13.6	61	1.4	5	3.9	2.4
Mushroom, & Cream, M&S*	1oz/28g	45	4	160	1.5	6.6	14.3	0.6
Mushroom, Creamy, Dolmio*	1 Pack/150g	166	15	111	1.3	3.7	10	0
Mushroom, Creamy, Express, Dolmio*	1 Serving/150g	160	14.4	107	1.4	3.8	9.6	0
Mushroom, Italian, Sainsbury's*	1 Serving/85g	56	1.8	66	2	9.8	2.1	1.7
Mushroom, Sainsbury's*	1 Serving/100g	66	2.1	66	2	9.8	2.1	1.7
Mushroom, Tesco*	1/6 Jar/120g	48	0.6	40	1.2	6.9	0.5	1.5
Napoletana, Fresh, Sainsbury's*	1oz/28g	25	1.6	91	1.9	7.9	5.8	1.1
Napoletana, M&S*	½ Jar/170g	126	7.8	74	1.9	4.5	4.6	3.7
Napoletana, Sainsbury's*	½ Pot/150g	126	8.4	84	1.9	6.6	5.6	0.9
Olive, & Tomato, Sacla*	½ Jar/95g	182	17.8	192	1.5	2.9	18.7	2.8
Pepperonata, Waitrose*	½ Pot/175g	128	7.9	73	1.5	6.2	4.5	0.8
Pomodoro, & Chianti, The Best, Morrisons*	½ Pack/175g	119	5.8	68	1.7	6.8	3.3	1.9
Pomodoro, Cirio*	1 Serving/200g	116	4.6	58	1.4	8.4	2.3	0
Provencale, Carrefour*	¼ Jar/105g	49	1	47	1.5	6.9	1	2.2
Puttanesca, Loyd Grossman*	½ Jar/175g	117	6	67	1.4	5.5	3.4	0.7
Red Pepper, & Tomato, Roasted, Finest, Tesco*	1 Serving/145g	117	7.8	81	1.2	6.8	5.4	2.2
Red Pepper, Sweet, Loyd Grossman*	1 Jar/350g	304	19.6	87	1.7	7.3	5.6	1.2
Sweet Pepper, Tesco*	½ Pot/77g	47	1.8	61	1.3	8.2	2.4	0.7
Tomato, & Basil, Dolmio*	1 Serving/170g	95	3.6	56	1.4	7.9	2.1	0
Tomato, & Basil, Loyd Grossman*	½ Jar/175g	107	6	61	1.5	5.8	3.4	0.8
Tomato, & Basil, Morrisons*	½ Jar/140g	76	0.7	54	1.7	10.1	0.5	1.3
Tomato, & Basil, Sun Dried, Organic, Seeds of Change*	½ Jar/100g	155	13.1	155	1.6	7.7	13.1	0
Tomato, & Basil, Sun Ripened, Dolmio*	1 Serving/150g	117	6.9	78	1.3	7.9	4.6	0
Tomato, & Basil, Sun Ripened, Express, Dolmio*	1 Pouch/170g	88	2.7	52	1.5	7.9	1.6	0
Tomato, & Chilli, Pour Over, M&S*	1 Jar/330g	231	12.5	70	1.3	7.6	3.8	1.8
Tomato, & Chilli, Whole Cherry Tomatoes, Classic, Sacla*	½ Jar/175g	238	19.2	136	2	7.2	11	3.1
Tomato, & Garlic, CBY, Asda*	½ Jar/160g	74	0.8	46	1.6	7.9	0.5	1.7
Tomato, & Garlic, Roasted, CBY, Asda*	1 Pot/350g	122	2.1	35	1.5	5	0.6	1.7
Tomato, & Garlic, Roasted, Loyd Grossman*	½ Jar/175g	133	5.6	76	2	9	3.2	1.4

	Measure INFO/WEIGHT	per Measure		Nutrition Values per 100g / 100ml				
		KCAL	FAT	KCAL	PROT	CARB	FAT	FIBRE
PASTA SAUCE								
Tomato, & Herb, Sainsbury's*	¼ Jar/125g	70	1.8	56	2	7.9	1.4	2
Tomato, & Mascarpone, Finest, Tesco*	1 Serving/175g	135	8.8	77	2.7	5.4	5	0.8
Tomato, & Mascarpone, Fresh, Sainsbury's*	1 Serving/150g	177	15.4	118	2.2	4.2	10.3	1.1
Tomato, & Mascarpone, Italiano, Tesco*	½ Pot/175g	168	12.2	96	2.8	5.5	7	0.7
Tomato, & Mascarpone, Sainsbury's*	½ Pot/150g	137	9.9	91	2.1	5.9	6.6	1.2
Tomato, & Mascarpone, Tesco*	¼ Jar/125g	101	5.2	81	1.4	8.8	4.2	1
Tomato, & Mascarpone, Waitrose*	½ Pot/175g	184	14.7	105	1.9	5.5	8.4	1.1
Tomato, & Mushroom, Wild, Loyd Grossman*	½ Jar/175g	107	6	61	1.4	5.8	3.4	0.6
Tomato, & Onions, Original, Morrisons*	1 Serving/125g	51	1.4	41	1.4	6.3	1.1	1.2
Tomato, & Parmesan, Cherry, Seeds of Change*	1 Serving/175g	103	5.1	59	1.5	5.9	2.9	1.3
Tomato, & Parmesan, Seeds of Change*	1 Serving/150g	100	4.4	67	2.5	7.8	2.9	1.1
Tomato, & Ricotta, Italian, Sainsbury's*	1 Pack/390g	238	11.7	61	2.5	6.1	3	1.2
Tomato, & Tuna, Loyd Grossman*	½ Jar/175g	154	7.7	88	4.4	7.5	4.4	0.8
Tomato, & Basil, Fresh, Co-Op*	1 Pot/300g	135	4.8	45	1.6	4.5	1.6	3.3
Tomato, & Herb, HFC, Tesco*	¼ Jar/110g	36	0.8	33	0.8	5.5	0.7	0.8
Tomato, & Herb, Pasta Bake, Free From, Asda*	¼ Jar/125g	159	12.5	127	1.4	7.7	10	0.5
Tomato, & Mascarpone, Chef Select, Lidl*	½ Pot/175g	150	10.7	86	1.4	5.8	6.1	1.2
Tomato, & Mascarpone, Co-Op*	½ Pot/150g	130	8.4	87	2.4	5.5	5.6	2.3
Tomato, Bacon, & Mushroom, Asda*	½ Pot/50g	33	1.8	66	2.5	6	3.6	0
Tomato, Courgette, & Basil, Veggie Goodness, Dolmio*	½ Pack/170g	70	1.2	41	1.7	6.2	0.7	1.4
Tomato, Mushroom, & Smoked Garlic, Zest*	½ Jar/170g	153	12.2	90	1	4.9	7.2	0
Tomato, Onion, & Garlic, Baresa, Lidl*	1 Jar/500g	240	2.5	48	2.1	7.8	0.5	1.8
Tomato, Sun Dried, Stir In, Light, Dolmio*	1 Serving/75g	62	3.5	83	1.7	9.8	4.7	0
Tomato, with Basil Pesto, Rich, Express, Dolmio*	1 Pack/170g	146	10	86	2	6.2	5.9	0
Vegetable, Chargrilled, Stir-In, Sainsbury's*	½ Pot/75g	67	3.5	89	1.7	8.5	4.7	2.8
Vegetable, Chunky, Tesco*	1 Jar/500g	235	5	47	1.8	6.8	1	1.8
Vegetable, Mediterranean, Organic, Seeds of Change*	1 Jar/350g	210	10.2	60	1.2	6.6	2.9	1.4
Vegetable, Mediterranean, Tesco*	1 Serving/166g	95	2.8	57	1.4	9	1.7	1.2
Vegetable, Roasted, Sainsbury's*	½ Pot/151g	103	5.9	68	1.6	6.7	3.9	0.4
PASTA SHAPES								
Alphabetti, in Tomato Sauce, Heinz*	1 Can/200g	118	1	59	1.8	11.7	0.5	1.5
Bob The Builder in Tomato Sauce, Heinz*	1 Can/205g	111	0.6	54	1.7	11.3	0.3	1.5
Cooked, Tesco*	1 Serving/260g	356	2.1	137	5.1	26.3	0.8	1.1
Dried, Tesco*	1 Serving/100g	345	2	345	13.2	68.5	2	2.9
PASTA SHELLS								
Dry, Average	*1 Serving/75g*	*265*	*1.5*	*353*	*11.1*	*71.8*	*2*	*2*
Egg, Fresh, Average	*1 Serving/125g*	*344*	*3.6*	*275*	*11.5*	*49.8*	*2.8*	*3.4*
PASTA TWISTS								
Dry, Average	*1oz/28g*	*99*	*0.4*	*354*	*12.2*	*71.8*	*1.5*	*2.2*
Wheat & GF, Glutafin*	1 Serving/75g	262	1.5	350	8	75	2	0.1
PASTE								
Barbacoa, Tesco*	1 Serving/30g	32	0.8	107	1.9	16.7	2.6	4.5
Beef, Asda*	1 Serving/37g	72	5.2	194	17	0.1	14	0
Beef, Princes*	1 Serving/18g	42	3.1	231	15.2	3.4	17.4	0
Beef, Sainsbury's*	1 Jar/75g	142	9.9	189	16	1.5	13.2	1.4
Chicken, & Ham, Princes*	1 Jar/100g	233	18.6	233	13.6	2.8	18.6	0
Chicken, & Ham, Tesco*	1 Serving/19g	44	3.7	231	12.5	1.4	19.5	0
Chicken, Tesco*	1 Serving/12g	30	2.4	248	14.8	2.3	20	0.1
Chilli, Chipotle, M&S*	¼ Jar/24g	36	1.1	151	2.2	22.8	4.4	5.9
Chilli, Sainsbury's*	1 Tsp/6g	5	0.4	82	1	2.9	5.8	7.3
Crab, Sainsbury's*	1 Spread/5g	6	0.2	115	16.5	1.7	4.7	0.5
Red Pepper, Mild, 1001 Delights, Lidl*	1 Tsp/6g	4	0	70	3	10.5	0.8	0
Salmon, & Haddock, Sainsbury's*	1 Tbsp/17g	21	0.9	123	14.3	4.4	5.1	1.3

	Measure	per Measure		Nutrition Values per 100g / 100ml				
	INFO/WEIGHT	KCAL	FAT	KCAL	PROT	CARB	FAT	FIBRE

PASTE

Salmon, Stockwell & Co., Tesco*	1 Serving/15g	25	1.6	165	12.3	5	10.3	1.6
Salmon, Value, Tesco*	1 Serving/10g	16	1	165	14	4.6	10.1	0.8
Sardine, & Tomato, Asda*	1 Thin Spread/9g	11	0.5	123	14	3.3	6	0
Sardine, & Tomato, Princes*	1 Jar/75g	130	8.1	173	13.9	3.4	10.8	3.2
Sardine, & Tomato, Sainsbury's*	1 Mini Pot/35g	60	3.8	170	16.9	1.2	10.8	1.3
Tamarind, M&S*	¼ Jar/30g	38	0	125	0.9	30.1	0.1	0.5
Tuna, & Mayonnaise, Tesco*	1 Serving/15g	32	2.3	215	15.8	0.7	15.6	2.2

PASTILLES

Fruit, 30% Less Sugar, Rowntree's*	1 Sweet/3g	9	0	325	6.5	68.8	0.1	9.5
Fruit, Average	*1 Tube/33g*	*108*	*0*	*327*	*2.8*	*84.2*	*0*	*0*
Fruit, Rowntree's*	1 Tube/53g	186	0	351	4.4	83.7	0	0
Fruit, Sainsbury's*	4 Sweets/23g	79	0.1	344	4.1	80.6	0.5	0.6

PASTRAMI

Beef, Average	*1 Serving/40g*	*51*	*1.4*	*128*	*23.1*	*1.1*	*3.6*	*0.2*
Turkey, Average	*½ Pack/35g*	*38*	*0.5*	*107*	*21.8*	*1.7*	*1.5*	*0.5*

PASTRY

Apricot, & Custard, Lattice, Bakery, Tesco*	1 Pastry/95g	311	12.9	328	4.8	46.1	13.6	1
Apricot, Danish, Bakery in Store, M&S*	1 Pastry/130g	347	15	267	5.4	34.6	11.5	1.8
Beef, Chilli, Mexican, Slice, Ginsters*	1 Slice/170g	491	32.3	289	8.5	20.2	19	0
Block, GF, Ready to Roll, Sillyyak *	1 Block/325g	1170	73.1	360	0.7	40.1	22.5	2.7
Cannoli, Shells, Hand Rolled, Large, Alessi*	1 Shell/21g	90	4.5	429	4.8	47.6	21.4	0
Case, From Supermarket, Average	*1 Case/230g*	*1081*	*58.9*	*470*	*5.8*	*55.9*	*25.6*	*1.2*
Chicken, & Mushroom, Lattice, Tesco*	1 Lattice/110g	222	6	202	8.4	28.8	5.5	2.1
Chicken, & Mushroom, Slice, Seriously Tasty*	1 Slice/150g	380	18.9	253	8.2	26.2	12.6	1.3
Choux, Cooked, Average	*1oz/28g*	*91*	*5.5*	*325*	*8.5*	*29.8*	*19.8*	*1.2*
Cinnamon Swirls, Bake it Fresh, Jus-Rol*	1 Swirl/45g	162	7.1	360	6.2	47.7	15.7	1.6
Cinnamon Swirls, Danish Selection, Tesco*	1 Swirl/35g	151	8.8	432	6.4	43.5	25.2	2.8
Coronets, Chocolate, & Cherry, Danish Selection, Tesco*	1 Coronet/36g	128	7.1	357	5.5	38.1	19.7	2.7
Croustade, Cups, Mini, Rahms*	1 Cup/2g	10	0.6	520	9.7	49.2	31	2.8
Feta, Herb, & Spinach, Tesco*	2 Pastries/65g	168	8.3	258	7.4	27.2	12.8	2.3
Filo, Average	*1 Sheet/45g*	*137*	*1.2*	*304*	*9*	*61.4*	*2.7*	*0.9*
Flaky, Cooked, Average	*1oz/28g*	*157*	*11.4*	*560*	*5.6*	*45.9*	*40.6*	*1.8*
Horn, Filled with Cream, & Jam, Sainsbury's*	1 Horn/49g	196	10.9	401	4.1	45.4	22.3	1
Onion, & Goat's Cheese, Caramelised, Sainsbury's*	1 Pastry/29g	70	3	244	6.7	29.1	10.7	2.3
Pain Au Chocolat, Bake it Fresh, Jus-Rol*	1 Pain/46g	170	8.7	369	7.4	41	19	2.2
Puff, Cheese, & Pesto, Palmiers, The Best, Morrisons*	1 Palmier/5g	27	1.8	546	15.9	39.7	35.3	2.7
Puff, Cinnamon Sugar, Palmiers, M&S*	2 Palmiers/15g	72	3	477	7.5	64.7	20.2	3.7
Puff, Co-Op*	1 Pack/375g	1462	90	390	5	38	24	2
Puff, Frozen, Average	*1 Serving/47g*	*188*	*12*	*400*	*5*	*29.2*	*25.6*	*0*
Puff, Light, Frozen, Ready Roll Sheets, Jus-Rol*	1/6 Sheet/53g	176	8.7	332	6.4	38.3	16.5	2.3
Puff, Light, Sheet, Jus-Rol*	1 Serving/50g	166	8.2	332	6.4	38.3	16.5	2.3
Puff, Ready Rolled, Chef Select, Lidl*	¼ Sheet/94g	362	22.6	386	5	36	24.1	2.3
Salted Caramel, Mini, Danish Selection, Tesco*	1 Plait/31g	136	8.1	440	5.4	44.6	26.1	2.3
Shortcrust, Cooked, Average	*1oz/28g*	*146*	*9*	*521*	*6.6*	*54.2*	*32.3*	*2.2*
Shortcrust, Raw, Average	*1oz/28g*	*127*	*8.1*	*453*	*5.6*	*44*	*29.1*	*1.3*
Slices, Cream, Cream Cake Selection, Tesco*	1 Slice/65g	249	12.4	383	4	48.3	19	1.2
Spinach, & Feta, Roll, Gail's*	100g	238	15.8	238	8.7	15.3	15.8	0.1
Steak, & Onion, Lattice, Pastry, Tesco*	1 Serving/167g	374	17.9	223	12	18.9	10.7	1.7
Sweet Heart, All Butter, Brompton House*	1 Pastry/11g	59	3.5	539	5.9	56	32	1.6
Twists, Sea Salt, & Pepper, M&S*	1 Twist/9g	44	2.2	491	10.2	56.3	24.2	3.4
Vanilla Slice, Frozen, Tesco*	1 Slice/38g	136	6	359	4.7	48.9	15.8	1.5
Vol-Au-Vents, Jus-Rol*	1 Pastry/17g	67	4.3	392	5	36	25.1	1.1

P

PASTY	Measure INFO/WEIGHT	per Measure KCAL	FAT	Nutrition Values per 100g / 100ml KCAL	PROT	CARB	FAT	FIBRE
Beef, Mini, Asda*	1 Pasty/16g	55	3.3	337	8.1	30	20	2.3
Cauliflower, Curried, Wicked Kitchen, Tesco*	1 Pasty/150g	361	19.5	241	4.1	26.2	13	1.1
Cheese, & Onion, Average	*1 Pasty/150g*	*435*	*27.6*	*290*	*7.3*	*24.5*	*18.4*	*1.4*
Cheese, & Onion, Tesco*	1 Pasty/150g	416	26.4	277	5.9	23.7	17.6	2.2
Chicken, Tikka, Asda*	1 Pasty/30g	103	6	343	8	31	20	2.3
Cornish, Average	*1 Pasty/160g*	*450*	*27.7*	*281*	*7*	*24.2*	*17.3*	*1.6*
Cornish, Crestwood, Aldi*	1 Pasty/130g	358	22.1	275	7.5	22	17	1.5
Cornish, Mini, Sainsbury's*	1 Pasty/70g	280	20.1	400	7.3	28.1	28.7	1.5
Cornish, Morrisons*	1 Pasty/130g	373	25.1	287	7	19.9	19.3	2.9
Cornish, Multi Pack, Ginsters*	1 Pasty/130g	358	24.3	275	6	20.6	18.7	2.6
Cornish, Original, Ginsters*	1 Pasty/227g	549	32.2	242	5.3	23.2	14.2	3.1
Cornish, Tesco*	1 Pasty/150g	466	32.7	311	6.8	21.9	21.8	1.6
Dinky, M&S*	1 Pasty/30g	101	6.5	337	8.3	26	21.7	2
Vegan, Waitrose*	1 Pasty/130g	346	20.3	266	7.7	22.3	15.6	2.6
Vegetable	*1oz/28g*	*77*	*4.2*	*274*	*4.1*	*33.3*	*14.9*	*1.9*
Vegetarian, Cornish Style, Quorn*	1 Pasty/150g	320	15	213	6.9	22.5	10	3
PATE								
Ardennes, BGTY, Sainsbury's*	1 Serving/30g	59	4.5	197	12.3	3.2	15	0.5
Ardennes, Reduced Fat, Waitrose*	¼ Pack/42g	94	7.1	224	15.4	2.6	16.9	0.5
Ardennes, Tesco*	1 Tbsp/15g	53	5	354	13.3	0.5	33.2	1.2
Ardennes, with Bacon, Tesco*	½ Pack/85g	241	20.6	284	11.4	5.1	24.2	1.1
Avocado, & Cashew, Findlater's Fine Foods*	1 Serving/25g	95	9	380	4	8	36	0
Brussels, & Garlic, Tesco*	1 Serving/40g	145	13.5	363	8.7	6	33.8	0
Brussels, 25% Less Fat, Morrisons*	¼ Pack/43g	106	8.8	249	14.2	0.7	20.6	0
Brussels, Co-Op*	1 Serving/15g	51	4.6	340	11	4	31	2
Brussels, M&S*	1 Thin Spread/7g	23	2.1	323	9.9	1.9	30.5	0.5
Brussels, Pate Grand-Mere*	1 Serving/30g	85	6.9	282	13	6	23	0
Brussels, Sainsbury's*	1 Pack/170g	663	64.9	390	10.6	1.1	38.2	0.1
Brussels, Smooth, Eastmans, Tesco*	1 Serving/35g	90	7.5	258	11.2	5	21.4	0.5
Brussels, Smooth, Spreadable, Sainsbury's*	1 Serving/30g	97	8.7	323	10.7	4.7	29	0
Butternut Squash, & Red Pepper, Roasted, Waitrose*	1 Pack/160g	259	16.8	162	2.6	12.9	10.5	2.5
Chicken, Liver, M&S*	½ Pack/85g	173	13.1	204	11	5	15.4	0.5
Chicken, Liver, Organic, Waitrose*	½ Tub/88g	204	16.1	233	12.6	1.8	18.4	1.4
Chicken, Liver, Parfait, Specially Selected, Aldi*	1 Portion/85g	278	26.4	327	11	2.1	31	0.6
Chicken, Liver, Parfait, Waitrose*	1 Pack/100g	258	22.9	258	7.5	4.8	22.9	1.1
Chicken, Liver, with Madeira, Sainsbury's*	1 Serving/30g	84	7.3	279	13.1	1.9	24.3	0
Crab, Waitrose*	1 Pot/113g	218	16.7	193	12.4	2.5	14.8	0.9
De Campagne, Extra Special, Asda*	1 Pate/55g	163	13.2	296	17	2.5	24	0
De Campagne, Sainsbury's*	1 Serving/55g	129	10	235	16.3	1.4	18.2	0
Duck, & Orange, Smooth, Tesco*	1 Serving/50g	188	17.7	377	10.5	4	35.4	0.5
Duck, Liver, Grand Marnier & Orange Jelly, M&S*	½ Pot/75g	218	18.5	291	8.7	8.2	24.7	0.6
Farmhouse, with Mushrooms & Garlic, Tesco*	1 Serving/90g	256	22.8	285	13.8	0.6	25.3	1.3
Farmhouse, with Mushrooms, Sainsbury's*	1 Serving/30g	76	6.8	252	11.3	1.2	22.5	0.5
Garlic, & Herb, Yeast, Tartex*	1 Serving/30g	69	5.4	230	7	10	18	0
Layered, Duck, & Pork, Sainsbury's*	1 Serving/30g	94	8	313	11.3	6.8	26.7	0.5
Mackerel, Smoked	*1oz/28g*	*103*	*9.6*	*368*	*13.4*	*1.3*	*34.4*	*0*
Mackerel, Smoked, Sainsbury's*	½ Pot/57g	176	14.7	308	15	3.7	25.8	0
Mackerel, Smoked, Scottish, M&S*	½ Pot/58g	158	13.3	275	15.9	0.6	23.2	0.1
Mackerel, Tesco*	1 Serving/29g	102	9.5	353	14.3	0.5	32.6	0
Mushroom, Sainsbury's*	½ Pot/58g	85	6.7	147	3.9	5.8	11.6	0
Mushroom, Wild, Yeast, GranoVita*	1oz/28g	60	4.8	213	10	5	17	0
Salmon, Smoked, Tesco*	1 Pack/115g	282	22	245	15	3	19.1	1
Tomato, Lentil, & Basil, Cauldron Foods*	1 Pot/115g	161	7.8	140	6.8	14	6.8	3.2

P

	Measure INFO/WEIGHT	per Measure KCAL	per Measure FAT	Nutrition Values per 100g / 100ml KCAL	PROT	CARB	FAT	FIBRE
PATE								
Trout, Smoked, Waitrose*	1 Serving/34g	59	3.7	176	18.3	0.6	11.1	0
Tuna, Tesco*	1 Pack/115g	332	26.7	289	19.8	0.3	23.2	0.2
Tuna, with Butter & Lemon Juice, Sainsbury's*	½ Pot/58g	145	11.5	251	15.5	2.2	19.9	0.6
Turkey, Pork, & Duck, Liver, Deluxe, Lidl*	1 Pack/125g	366	30.6	293	13.1	4.5	24.5	1
Vegetable	***1oz/28g***	***48***	***3.8***	***173***	***7.5***	***5.9***	***13.4***	***0***
Walnut, & Basil, Organic, GranoVita*	1 Serving/20g	48	4.4	241	8.3	11.5	22	3.6
PATTY								
Beef, Jamaican, Port Royal*	1 Patty/140g	350	17.4	250	6.1	28.1	12.4	1.3
Fish, Salt, Jamaican, Port Royal*	1 Patty/130g	300	13.4	231	6.8	27.8	10.3	0
Jerk, Jamaican, Crust Pattie, Island Delight*	1 Patty/140g	480	29.4	343	7.6	30	21	1
Lamb, Curried, Island Delight*	1 Patty/140g	451	28	322	6.4	28	20	1.4
Lamb, Jamaican, Port Royal*	1 Patty/130g	352	17.4	271	7.2	30.5	13.4	0
Vegetable, Jamaican, Patty, Island Delight*	1 Patty/140g	423	22.4	302	5.2	35	16	0
Vegetarian, Jamaican, Port Royal*	1 Patty/130g	315	13.8	242	12.5	24.1	10.6	0
PAVLOVA								
Maltesers, Mars*	1 Serving/50g	205	8.1	410	3.6	61.7	16.2	0
Raspberry, Individual, M&S*	1 Pavlova/65g	133	1.6	205	4	41.8	2.4	0.2
Raspberry, M&S*	1 Serving/84g	193	8.1	230	2.3	33.3	9.6	0.3
Raspberry, Tesco*	1 Serving/65g	191	8.4	294	2.7	41.8	12.9	1.1
Sticky Toffee, Sainsbury's*	1/6 Pavlova/60g	249	9.8	415	3.7	63.1	16.4	0.9
PAW-PAW								
Raw, Fresh	***1oz/28g***	***10***	***0***	***36***	***0.5***	***8.8***	***0.1***	***2.2***
Raw, Weighed with Skin & Pips	***1oz/28g***	***6***	***0***	***20***	***0.3***	***5***	***0.1***	***1.3***
PEACH								
Dried, Average	***1 Pack/250g***	***472***	***1.6***	***189***	***2.6***	***45***	***0.6***	***6.9***
in Fruit Juice, Average	***1oz/28g***	***13***	***0***	***47***	***0.5***	***11.2***	***0***	***0.7***
in Light Syrup, Canned, As Sold	***1 Serving/100g***	***66***	***0***	***66***	***0.4***	***15.9***	***0***	***1***
Raw, Stoned, Average	***1oz/28g***	***9***	***0***	***33***	***1***	***7.6***	***0.1***	***1.5***
Raw, Weighed with Stone, Average	***1 Peach/125g***	***39***	***0.1***	***31***	***1***	***7.2***	***0.1***	***1.3***
Slices in Fruit Juice, Average	***1 Serving/100g***	***49***	***0***	***49***	***0.6***	***11.6***	***0***	***0.5***
PEANUT BUTTER								
Crunchy, Natural, No Added Sugar or Salt, Average	***1 Tsp/5g***	***30***	***2.4***	***606***	***27.6***	***12.2***	***48.4***	***7***
Crunchy, Rich Roast, 100% Nuts, Meridian Foods*	1 Tsp/5g	31	2.6	622	25	13	51	6.5
Dark, Roasted, Crunchy, Whole Earth*	1 Serving/15g	89	6.9	594	28.9	10.3	46.3	8.3
Marmite, Crunchy, Marmite*	1 Serving/15g	86	6.8	574	28	12	45	7.9
Powder, Peanut Hottie*	1 Tsp/5g	21	0.6	427	45	37	11.3	14.6
Smooth, Average	***1 Serving/20g***	***125***	***10.7***	***623***	***22.6***	***13.1***	***53.7***	***5.4***
Smooth, No Added Sugar, Organic, Whole Earth*	1 Serving/20g	126	10.2	628	25.6	13.7	51.2	4.9
Smooth, No Added Sugar, Sunpat*	1 Serving/30g	183	14.6	610	24.4	14.7	48.8	7.2
Smooth, Unsalted, Biona Organic*	1 Thin Spread/7g	42	3.4	594	25.8	16.1	49.2	8.5
Super Crunchy, Bega*	1 Serving/10g	62	5.1	617	23.7	13.6	51.1	0
Whole Nut, Crunchy, Average	***1 Tsp/10g***	***61***	***5.3***	***606***	***24.9***	***7.7***	***53.1***	***6***
PEANUTS								
Chilli, Average	***½ Pack/50g***	***303***	***25.3***	***605***	***28.2***	***9.3***	***50.6***	***6.8***
Chilli, Spicy, Jumbo, KP Snacks*	1 Serving/30g	183	14.7	609	29	7.5	49	8.5
Chilli, Sweet, Nobby's*	1 Bag/40g	214	13.6	535	15	42	34	3
Chilli, Sweet, Thai, Coated, Sensations, Walkers*	1 Serving/30g	172	11.9	574	14.2	38.7	39.8	2.7
Dry Roasted, Average	***1 Serving/20g***	***117***	***9.8***	***587***	***25.7***	***11.5***	***48.8***	***6.5***
Honey Roasted, Average	***1oz/28g***	***169***	***13.2***	***605***	***26.8***	***23.6***	***47***	***5.5***
Plain, Average	***10 Whole/10g***	***59***	***5***	***592***	***24.7***	***11***	***50***	***6.3***
Roast, Salted, Average	***10 Whole/12g***	***74***	***6.3***	***614***	***27.8***	***7.9***	***52.4***	***4.9***
Salted, Average	***10 Whole/6g***	***37***	***3.1***	***609***	***27***	***8.3***	***52***	***5.4***

P

	Measure INFO/WEIGHT	per Measure KCAL	per Measure FAT	Nutrition Values per 100g / 100ml KCAL	PROT	CARB	FAT	FIBRE
PEARL BARLEY								
Boiled	*1oz/28g*	*34*	*0.1*	*123*	*2.3*	*28.2*	*0.4*	*3.8*
Cooked, Average	*1 Serving/150g*	*184*	*0.7*	*123*	*2.3*	*28.2*	*0.4*	*3.8*
Raw, Average	*1oz/28g*	*99*	*0.3*	*352*	*9.9*	*77.7*	*1.2*	*15.6*
PEARS								
Abate Fetel, Average	*1 Med/133g*	*48*	*0.1*	*36*	*0.4*	*8.3*	*0.1*	*2.2*
Asian, Nashi, Raw, Average	*1 Lge/209g*	*80*	*0.4*	*38*	*0.5*	*9.7*	*0.2*	*3.3*
Blush, Tesco*	1 Pear/133g	62	0.1	47	0.3	10	0.1	2.2
Comice, Raw, Weighed with Core	*1 Med/170g*	*56*	*0*	*33*	*0.3*	*8.5*	*0*	*2*
Conference, Average	*1 Lge/209g*	*88*	*0.2*	*42*	*0.3*	*10.1*	*0.1*	*2*
Dried, Average	*1 Pear Half/16g*	*33*	*0.1*	*204*	*1.9*	*48.4*	*0.5*	*9.7*
in Fruit Juice, Average	*1 Serving/225g*	*102*	*0.1*	*45*	*0.3*	*10.9*	*0*	*1.2*
in Syrup, Average	*1oz/28g*	*16*	*0*	*58*	*0.2*	*14.4*	*0.1*	*1.4*
Prickly, Raw, Fresh	*1oz/28g*	*8*	*0.1*	*30*	*0.4*	*7*	*0.2*	*0*
Raw, Weighed with Core, Average	*1 Med/166g*	*58*	*0.2*	*35*	*0.3*	*8.4*	*0.1*	*1.3*
William, Raw, Average	*1 Med/170g*	*58*	*0.2*	*34*	*0.4*	*8.3*	*0.1*	*2.2*
PEAS								
& Sweetcorn, Frozen, Steam & Serve, Morrisons*	1 Sachet/160g	126	2.1	79	4.6	10.4	1.3	4.1
Courgette, & Leek, Layered, Tesco*	½ Pack/168g	96	3.5	57	2.9	5	2.1	3.3
Dried, Boiled in Unsalted Water, Average	*1oz/28g*	*31*	*0.2*	*109*	*6.9*	*19.9*	*0.8*	*5.5*
Dried, Raw, Average	*1oz/28g*	*85*	*0.7*	*303*	*21.6*	*52*	*2.4*	*13*
Edible Podded, Raw	*1 Cup/63g*	*25*	*0.1*	*39*	*2.6*	*7.1*	*0.2*	*2.4*
Frozen, Average	*1 Serving/85g*	*62*	*0.8*	*73*	*6*	*9.7*	*1*	*4.5*
Frozen, Boiled, Average	*1 Serving/75g*	*51*	*0.7*	*68*	*6*	*9.4*	*0.9*	*5.1*
Garden, Canned with Sugar & Salt, Average	*1 Serving/90g*	*59*	*0.6*	*66*	*5.3*	*9.3*	*0.7*	*5.1*
Garden, Canned, No Sugar Or Salt, Average	*1 Can/80g*	*36*	*0.3*	*45*	*4.4*	*6*	*0.4*	*2.8*
Garden, Frozen, Average	*1 Serving/90g*	*66*	*1*	*74*	*6.3*	*9.8*	*1.1*	*3.3*
Garden, Minted, Average	*1 Serving/80g*	*59*	*0.9*	*74*	*6.3*	*9.7*	*1.1*	*5.9*
Marrowfat, Average	*1 Sm Can/160g*	*134*	*0.9*	*84*	*6.1*	*13.7*	*0.6*	*3.7*
Mushy, Average	*1 Can/200g*	*173*	*1*	*86*	*6.2*	*14.4*	*0.5*	*2.2*
Processed, Canned, Average	*1 Sm Can/220g*	*162*	*1.6*	*74*	*5.6*	*11.3*	*0.7*	*3.4*
Roasted, Paprika, & Chilli, Brave*	1 Pack/35g	132	3.8	378	19	41	11	20
Roasted, Sea Salt, & Vinegar, Brave*	1 Pack/35g	134	3.8	383	19	41	11	19
Roasted, Sea Salt, Classic, Brave*	1 Pack/35g	134	3.8	382	20	41	11	20
Roasted, Sour Cream, & Chive, Brave*	1 Pack/35g	132	3.8	377	20	41	11	20
Sea Salt & Balsamic Vinegar, Snacks, Crunchy, Podberry*	1 Pack/20g	67	0.4	334	22.9	44.8	1.9	22.9
Snow	*1 Serving/80g*	*24*	*0.2*	*29*	*3.3*	*3.9*	*0.2*	*2.1*
Sugar Snap, Average	*1 Serving/80g*	*27*	*0.2*	*33*	*3.2*	*4.8*	*0.2*	*1.4*
Wasabi, Average	*1 Serving/28g*	*114*	*3.8*	*406*	*15.2*	*54*	*13.7*	*8.6*
Wasabi, Ranch, Snapea Crisp, Harvest Snaps, Calbee*	1 Serving/28g	120	5	429	17.9	57.1	17.9	14.3
Wasabi, The Foodie Market, Aldi*	¼ Pack/30g	121	3.9	402	7.1	57	13	15
PEASE PUDDING								
Canned, Re-Heated, Drained	*1oz/28g*	*26*	*0.2*	*93*	*6.8*	*16.1*	*0.6*	*1.8*
PECAN NUTS								
Average	*3 Nuts/6g*	*42*	*4.2*	*692*	*10*	*5.6*	*70.1*	*4.7*
PENNE								
Arrabiata, BGTY, Sainsbury's*	1 Pack/450g	414	7.2	92	2.9	16.5	1.6	1.9
Brown Rice, GF, Pasta, Waitrose*	¼ Pack/125g	250	2.1	200	4.1	41	1.7	1.9
Chickpea, Peaz*	1 Portion/75g	264	4.4	352	26	43	5.8	11
Cooked, Average	*1 Serving/185g*	*244*	*1.3*	*132*	*4.7*	*26.7*	*0.7*	*1.1*
Dry, Average	*1 Serving/100g*	*352*	*1.9*	*352*	*12.4*	*71.3*	*1.9*	*2.7*
Egg, Fresh, Average	*1 Serving/125g*	*352*	*4*	*282*	*11.1*	*52.2*	*3.2*	*2*
Free From, Tesco*	1 Serving/100g	340	2	340	8	72.5	2	2.5
Fresh, Dry, Average	*1 Serving/125g*	*222*	*2.4*	*178*	*7.3*	*32.2*	*1.9*	*1.6*

P

	Measure INFO/WEIGHT	per Measure KCAL	FAT	Nutrition Values per 100g / 100ml KCAL	PROT	CARB	FAT	FIBRE
PENNE								
GF, Cooked, Free From, Morrisons*	1 Serving/170g	287	1	169	3.3	36.7	0.6	1.6
Red Pepper, Roasted, GFY, Asda*	1 Pack/400g	212	2.4	53	1.9	10	0.6	0.8
Rigate, Dry Weight, Average	*1 Serving/90g*	*318*	*1.6*	*353*	*12.3*	*72.1*	*1.8*	*1.8*
Sausage, Tuscan, Spicy Tomato , Meal for One, M&S*	1 Pack/400g	640	36.8	160	4.7	13.9	9.2	1.6
Wholewheat, Asda*	1 Serving/100g	333	2.1	333	12.1	66.3	2.1	6.9
Wholewheat, Authentic, Italiano, Tesco*	1 Portion/75g	244	1.9	325	12.5	62.5	2.5	9
PEPERAMI*								
Hot, Peperami*	1 Stick/23g	112	9.9	497	22	3.2	44	1.2
Lunchbox Minis, 30% Less Fat, Peperami*	1 Stick/10g	40	3.1	400	26	5.5	31	3
Original, Peperami*	1 Stick/25g	126	11	504	24	2.5	44	0.1
PEPPER								
Black, Freshly Ground, Average	*1 Tsp/2g*	*5*	*0.1*	*255*	*11*	*64.8*	*3.3*	*26.5*
Cayenne, Ground	*1 Tsp/2g*	*6*	*0.3*	*318*	*12*	*31.7*	*17.3*	*0*
White	*½ Tsp/1g*	*3*	*0*	*296*	*10.4*	*68.6*	*2.1*	*26.2*
PEPPERCORNS								
Black, Schwartz*	1 Tsp/2g	11	0.4	529	13	68.7	22.5	27
Green, Average	*1 Tsp/10g*	*4*	*0.1*	*44*	*1.6*	*5.3*	*0.8*	*4.7*
PEPPERONI								
Asda*	1 Slice/6g	26	2.2	434	26	1.6	36	0
Sliced, Spicy, Pork, Basics, Sainsbury's*	4 Slices/15g	68	6	453	22	1	40	0.6
Sliced, Tesco*	1 Slice/5g	20	1.7	402	20	2.4	34.7	0
Sliced, Waitrose*	1 Slice/2g	8	0.7	425	23.7	0.1	36.6	0
Slices, Pork, Cured, Chilli & Paprika, Italian, Sainsbury's*	1 Pack/42g	155	12.2	368	26	1	29	0.5
PEPPERS								
Chargrilled, Spirit of Summer, M&S*	1 Pack/105g	45	1.5	43	1	5.6	1.4	2
Chargrilled, Sunflower Oil, Antipasto, Drained, Sainsbury's*	1 Serving/70g	82	5.4	118	1.7	9.5	7.7	1.8
Cherry, Hot, Stuffed with Ricotta, Waitrose*	1 Pack/135g	185	10.3	137	5.4	10.5	7.6	2.7
Chilli, Dried, Flakes, Average	*1 Tsp/3g*	*13*	*0.4*	*425*	*16*	*56*	*15*	*44*
Chilli, Green, Raw, Unprepared, Average	*1 Med/13g*	*4*		*29*	*1.5*	*6.9*	*0.1*	*1.1*
Chilli, Red, Raw, Unprepared, Average	*1 Med/45g*	*13*	*0.1*	*29*	*1.5*	*6.9*	*0.1*	*1.1*
Chilli, Red, Very Lazy, The English Provender Co.*	1 Serving/15g	17	0.6	114	4.2	15.3	4	0.5
Crushed, Hot, Corisca*	1 Tbsp/15g	5	0	33	0	6.7	0	0
Green, Boiled in Salted Water	*1oz/28g*	*5*	*0.1*	*18*	*1*	*2.6*	*0.5*	*1.8*
Green, Raw, Unprepared, Average	*1 Med/160g*	*20*	*0.4*	*13*	*0.7*	*2.2*	*0.3*	*1.3*
Jalapeno, Raw	*1 Pepper/14g*	*4*	*0.1*	*28*	*1.2*	*5.4*	*0.6*	*2.6*
Mixed Bag, From Supermarket, Average	*1oz/28g*	*7*	*0.1*	*25*	*1*	*4.4*	*0.4*	*1.7*
Mixed, Sliced, Frozen, Ocado*	1 Portion/80g	21	0.4	26	0.9	3.9	0.5	1.7
Orange, Sweet, Raw, Average	*1oz/28g*	*8*	*0.1*	*30*	*1.8*	*5*	*0.3*	*1.5*
Red, Boiled in Salted Water	*1oz/28g*	*10*	*0.1*	*34*	*1.1*	*7*	*0.4*	*1.7*
Red, Raw, Unprepared, Average	*½ Med/80g*	*21*	*0.3*	*27*	*0.8*	*5.3*	*0.3*	*1.3*
Red, Sweet Pointed, Organic, Tesco*	1 Serving/100g	33	0.4	33	1	6.4	0.4	1.6
Roasted, in Oil, M&S*	1 Serving/50g	56	4.5	112	0.8	6.2	9	1.5
Stuffed, Cream Cheese, Sweet, Aldi*	1 Serving/60g	92	7.2	154	3.7	6.9	12	2.1
Stuffed, Red, Filled, Halves, Vegetarian, M&S*	1 Pack/295g	239	9.7	81	2.4	9.7	3.3	1.6
Stuffed, with Rice Based Filling, Average	*1oz/28g*	*24*	*0.7*	*85*	*1.5*	*15.4*	*2.4*	*1.3*
Stuffed, with Vegetables, Cheese Topping, Average	*1oz/28g*	*31*	*1.9*	*111*	*3.4*	*9.8*	*6.7*	*1.5*
Sweet, Pointed, Tesco*	1 Pepper/90g	24	0.2	27	0.8	4.3	0.2	2.2
Yellow, Raw, Unprepared, Average	*1 Med/160g*	*35*	*0.3*	*22*	*1*	*4.4*	*0.2*	*1.4*
PERCH								
Raw, Atlantic	*1oz/28g*	*26*	*0.5*	*94*	*18.6*	*0*	*1.6*	*0*
PERNOD*								
Ricard Pastis, Pernod Ricard*	1 Pub Shot/25ml	64	0	257	0	36.7	0	0
'Nduja, No. 16, Sacla*	1 Tsp/5g	17	1.5	331	6.5	8.2	30	1.2

P

	Measure INFO/WEIGHT	per Measure KCAL	per Measure FAT	Nutrition Values per 100g / 100ml KCAL	PROT	CARB	FAT	FIBRE
PESTO								
Basil, Bright & Green, Waitrose*	¼ Jar/48g	217	22.5	453	4.5	2.3	46.9	1.6
Chicken, Pesto, G&B, Asda*	1 Pack/353g	456	9.5	129	7.4	18	2.7	1.8
Chilli, Fiery, Sacla*	1 Tbsp/15g	50	4.8	334	2.8	7.2	32	2.8
Chilli, Sainsbury's*	¼ Jar/48g	110	9.8	231	2.6	7.4	20.5	3.5
Green, Alla Genovese, Finest, Tesco*	¼ Jar/48g	149	14.5	311	5.1	2.9	30.2	3.6
Green, Alla Genovese, Sacla*	1 Serving/30g	116	12.1	388	5.2	0.8	40.4	5.7
Green, Average	*1 Tbsp/20g*	*103*	*9.5*	*517*	*20.4*	*2*	*47.5*	*0*
Green, Classic, Sacla*	1 Serving/40g	185	18.6	462	5.2	7.6	46.5	0
Green, Free From, Asda*	¼ Jar/48g	172	17.1	362	2.9	6	36	1.1
Green, Organic, Sacla*	1 Tbsp/15g	68	6.8	451	4.3	6.4	45	1.8
Green, Reduced Fat, Tesco*	¼ Jar /49g	96	9.5	195	2.6	0.7	19.4	3.4
Green, Sainsbury's*	1 Tsp/5g	17	1.8	347	4.8	1.9	35.1	2
Green, Tesco*	1 Tbsp/15g	50	4.8	331	4.7	4.4	31.9	3.7
Red, Morrisons*	1 Tbsp/15g	47	4.4	311	5.7	6.6	29	5.9
Red, Rosso, Bertolli*	1 Jar/185g	703	64.8	380	6.8	9.5	35	2
Red, Rosso, Sundried Tomato, Finest, Tesco*	¼ Jar/47g	166	16.1	353	4	5.6	34.3	3.2
Rose Harissa, Belazu*	1 Tbsp/15g	50	4.5	333	2.2	10.8	30.3	4.2
Spinach, & Ricotta, Tesco*	1 Tbsp/15g	44	4.2	291	3	3.5	28.2	5
Wild Rocket, Sacla*	1 Serving/30g	128	13	425	5.2	3.2	43.5	4.5
PETIT POIS								
& Baby Carrots, Canned, Drained, Average	*½ Can/122g*	*58*	*0.8*	*47*	*2.9*	*7*	*0.7*	*3.2*
Canned, Drained, Average	*1 Sm Can/200g*	*125*	*1*	*63*	*4.8*	*8.9*	*0.5*	*2.6*
Fresh, Frozen, Average	*1 Serving/80g*	*51*	*0.8*	*63*	*5.4*	*7.1*	*1*	*4.8*
Leeks, & Pancetta, Extra Special, Asda*	½ Pack/120g	163	11.1	136	5.7	4.6	9.3	5.6
PHEASANT								
Meat Only, Roasted	*1oz/28g*	*62*	*3.4*	*220*	*27.9*	*0*	*12*	*0*
Meat Only, Roasted, Weighed with Bone	*1oz/28g*	*32*	*1.7*	*114*	*14.5*	*0*	*6.2*	*0*
Stuffed, Easy Carve, Finest, Tesco*	1 Serving/200g	540	37.4	270	23.2	2.2	18.7	0.9
PHYSALIS								
Raw, without Husk, Average	*5 Fruits/30g*	*16*	*0.2*	*53*	*1.9*	*11.2*	*0.7*	*0.4*
PICCALILLI								
Haywards*	1 Serving/28g	18	0.2	66	0.6	12	0.7	0.7
Heinz*	1 Serving/10g	10	0.1	99	1	20.5	0.6	0.6
Morrisons*	1 Serving/50g	38	0.4	75	1.6	15	0.7	0.6
Sweet & Mild, Haywards*	2 Tbsp/40g	41	0.3	102	0.5	21	0.8	1
PICKLE								
Branston, Original, Crosse & Blackwell*	1 Serving/12g	19	0.1	157	0.5	34	0.7	1.8
Branston, Red Onion & Cranberry, Crosse & Blackwell*	1 Tbsp/14g	13	0.1	92	0.6	21.4	0.4	0.8
Branston, Red Pepper & Tomato, Crosse & Blackwell*	1 Tbsp/14g	12	0	84	1.2	17.7	0.3	1.1
Branston, Sm Chunk, Squeezy, Crosse & Blackwell*	1 Serving/15g	19	0	127	0.9	29.8	0.2	1.1
Branston, Smooth, Squeezy, Crosse & Blackwell*	1 Serving/15g	19	0	127	0.9	29.8	0.2	1.1
Brinjal, Patak's*	1 Tsp/16g	61	4	381	2.1	34.5	24.8	0
Chilli, Patak's*	1 Tsp/16g	52	5.4	325	4.3	1.3	33.7	0
Cornichons, Freshona, Lidl*	1 Serving/50g	18	0.2	35	1.2	5.5	0.3	0
Cornichons, with Mustard Seeds, in Vinegar, Drained, M&S*	¼ Jar/39g	17	0.2	44	1.5	8.1	0.4	1.1
Cucumber, Dill, Krakus*	1 Portion/80g	19	0	24	0	5.4	0	1.2
Dill, No Garlic, Bicks*	1 Pickle/60g	5	0	8	0.3	1.7	0	0
Garlic, Patak's*	1 Tsp/16g	42	3	261	3.6	20	18.5	1.6
Hot Chilli Jam, What A Pickle*	1 Tsp/8g	14	0	178	0.6	44	0.1	1.2
Lime, Hot, Patak's*	1 Tsp/16g	31	3	194	2.2	4	18.7	0.4
Lime, Oily	*1 Serving/39g*	*70*	*6.1*	*178*	*1.9*	*8.3*	*15.5*	*0*
Lime, Sharwood's*	1 Tbsp/20g	28	2	142	1.7	11.5	9.9	1.3
Mango, Mild , Fudco*	1 Tbsp/15g	20	1.5	134	1	10	10	2.5

	Measure INFO/WEIGHT	per Measure KCAL	FAT	Nutrition Values per 100g / 100ml KCAL	PROT	CARB	FAT	FIBRE
PICKLE								
Mild Mustard, Heinz*	1 Tbsp/10g	13	0.1	129	2.2	25.7	1.3	0.9
Mixed, Drained	**1 Serving/100g**	**14**	**0.2**	**14**	**1**	**1.9**	**0.2**	**1**
Mixed, Drained, Haywards*	½ Jar/120g	22	0.4	18	1.4	2.4	0.3	0
Mixed, Patak's*	1 Serving/30g	78	7.7	259	2.3	4.7	25.7	0.8
Red Cabbage, Asda*	1 Serving/50g	16	0	32	1.6	6	0.1	0
Sandwich, Tesco*	1 Tbsp/30g	38	0	126	0.7	29.5	0.1	1.9
Sweet	**1 Tsp/10g**	**14**	**0**	**141**	**0.6**	**36**	**0.1**	**1.2**
Sweet, Batts, Lidl*	1 Serving/15g	17	0.1	114	0.8	26	0.5	1.1
Sweet, Bramwells*	1 Tbsp/15g	20	0.1	130	0.7	30	0.5	1.7
Sweet, Original, Tesco*	1 Tbsp/15g	20	0	135	0.5	31.5	0.1	2.1
Sweet, Savers, Morrisons*	1 Tbsp/15g	18	0	121	0.9	27.2	0.3	1.6
Tangy, Sandwich, Heinz*	1 Tsp/10g	13	0	134	0.7	31.4	0.2	0.9
PICNIC								
Cadbury*	1 Bar/38g	182	8.7	479	7.3	60	23	2.5
PIE								
Admiral's, Ross*	1 Pie/340g	357	15.6	105	4.8	10.9	4.6	0.7
Aloo Gobi, GF, Clive's*	1 Pie/235g	486	29.3	207	3	19.2	12.5	0
Apple, & Blackberry, Co-Op*	1 Serving/138g	338	15.2	245	3	33	11	2
Apple, & Blackberry, Lattice Topped, BGTY, Sainsbury's*	¼ Pie/100g	256	7.5	256	2.8	44.4	7.5	3.1
Apple, & Blackberry, Shortcrust, M&S*	1 Serving/142g	469	17.8	330	4.3	50.2	12.5	1.1
Apple, Bramley, Aunt Bessie's*	¼ Pie/138g	386	15.1	281	2.4	42	11	1.1
Apple, Bramley, Bakery, Tesco*	1/6 Pie/87g	234	9.7	269	3	38.4	11.1	1.5
Apple, Bramley, Free From, Tesco*	1 Serving/67g	173	7.6	260	0.6	37.5	11.4	2.6
Apple, Bramley, Individual, Mr Kipling*	1 Pie/60g	210	7.9	351	3.4	54	13.2	1.4
Apple, Bramley, Individual, Sainsbury's*	1 Pie/54g	165	5	307	3.6	52.2	9.3	1.3
Apple, Bramley, Individual, Tesco*	1 Pie/60g	221	7.6	362	4	57.5	12.5	1.9
Apple, Bramley, Large, Tesco*	1/8 Pie/87g	311	13	358	3.9	51.9	15	1.9
Apple, Commercially Prepared	**1 Slice/125g**	**296**	**13.8**	**237**	**1.9**	**34**	**11**	**1.6**
Apple, Pastry Top & Bottom	**1oz/28g**	**74**	**3.7**	**266**	**2.9**	**35.8**	**13.3**	**1.7**
Apple, Prepared From Recipe, Average	**1oz/28g**	**74**	**3.5**	**265**	**2.4**	**37.1**	**12.5**	**0**
Apple, with Custard	**1 Serving/217g**	**353**	**18.8**	**163**	**2.4**	**25.2**	**8.7**	**1.1**
Banoffee, Mini, Waitrose*	1 Pie/26g	115	5.8	444	3.3	57	22.5	1.2
Beef, & Onion, Minced, Tesco*	1 Pie/150g	454	28.5	303	5.7	27.4	19	1.7
Beef, & Onion, Pukka Pies Ltd*	1 Serving/231g	529	32.6	229	7.6	17.9	14.1	3
Beef, Bourguignon, Deluxe, Lidl*	1 Pie/190g	591	37.6	311	9.6	22.7	19.8	1.8
Beef, Minced, & Onion, Smart Price, Asda*	2 Pies/240g	626	31.2	261	7.4	28	13	1.2
Beef, Minced, Aberdeen Angus, Shortcrust, M&S*	1 Pie/171g	435	26.6	255	9.3	19.3	15.6	3
Chana-Rama, Patties, Pieminister*	1 Patty/60g	161	9	268	6.5	28.4	15	0
Cheese, & Onion, Hollands*	1 Pie/200g	516	24.4	258	6.3	30.9	12.2	0
Cheese, & Onion, Oven Baked, Average	**1 Serving/200g**	**654**	**40**	**327**	**8.2**	**30.4**	**20**	**1.2**
Cheese, & Potato	**1oz/28g**	**39**	**2.3**	**139**	**4.8**	**12.6**	**8.1**	**0.7**
Cheese, & Onion, Fray Bentos*	½ Pie/213g	379	22.6	178	3.8	15.7	10.6	0.7
Cherry, Bakery, Tesco*	1/6 Pie/87g	240	9.7	276	2.6	40.5	11.2	1.3
Chicken, & Asparagus, Tesco*	1 Serving/170g	468	28.7	275	8.3	22.4	16.9	0.8
Chicken, & Bacon, Puff Pastry, Deep Fill, Sainsbury's*	1/3 Pie/200g	532	34	266	9.1	19.1	17	1.3
Chicken, & Beechwood Ham, in Cheese Sauce, Iceland*	1 Pie/210g	614	37	292	10.3	22.3	17.6	1.6
Chicken, & Gravy, Just, Fray Bentos*	½ Pie/215g	267	7.3	124	5.6	17.2	3.4	0.6
Chicken, & Gravy, Roast, Deep Fill, Tesco*	¼ Pie/157g	358	16	228	9.7	23.7	10.2	1.5
Chicken, & Gravy, Shortcrust Pastry, Serves 3, Sainsbury's*	1 Serving/184g	552	33.3	300	10.8	22.7	18.1	1.7
Chicken, & Gravy, Shortcrust Pastry, Tesco*	1 Pie/250g	618	34.5	247	6.8	23.9	13.8	1
Chicken, & Ham, & Leek, Pot, Higgidy*	1 Pie/250g	670	39.8	268	11.1	21.4	15.9	1.2
Chicken, & Ham, Deep Filled, Sainsbury's*	1 Pie/210g	594	37.2	283	8	23	17.7	1

P

PIE

INFO/WEIGHT	Measure	per Measure KCAL	FAT	Nutrition Values per 100g / 100ml KCAL	PROT	CARB	FAT	FIBRE
Chicken, & Leek, & Bacon, Aldi*	1 Pie/210g	601	37.6	286	10.9	19.7	17.9	1
Chicken, & Leek, & Bacon, Deluxe, Lidl*	1/3 Pie/171g	511	30.8	299	11	22	18	2.7
Chicken, & Leek, & Ham, Morrisons*	¼ Pie/137g	393	23.9	286	10.1	21.7	17.4	1
Chicken, & Leek, LC, Tesco*	1 Pie/350g	298	5.6	85	6.6	10.3	1.6	1.3
Chicken, & Leek, M&S*	1oz/28g	70	4.2	250	10.1	18.8	15.1	1.1
Chicken, & Mushroom, Average	*1 Serving/200g*	*540*	*31.7*	*270*	*8*	*23.8*	*15.9*	*1*
Chicken, & Mushroom, Charlie Bigham's*	1 Serving/300g	666	36.9	222	10.5	15.6	12.3	0
Chicken, & Mushroom, Pukka Pies Ltd*	1 Pie/226g	475	29.2	210	7.6	15.7	12.9	3.5
Chicken, & Wiltshire Ham, Finest, Tesco*	1 Pie/250g	688	37.2	275	11.6	22.7	14.9	1.1
Chicken, & Bacon, Lattice, Asda*	1 Pie/468g	1188	56.1	254	11	25	12	0.7
Chicken, & Bacon, Puff Pastry Lid, Tesco*	1 Pie/131g	300	15.7	229	7.6	22	12	1.4
Chicken, & Leek, Filo , COU, M&S*	1 Pack/150g	160	2.8	107	10	12.1	1.9	0.8
Chicken, & Mushroom, COU, M&S*	1 Pack/293g	220	4.1	75	7.7	7.2	1.4	1.2
Chicken, & Mushroom, Serves 1, BGTY, Sainsbury's*	1 Pack/400g	359	9.2	94	7.1	10.5	2.4	1.1
Chicken, & Pancetta, Potato Topped, Finest, Tesco*	½ Pack/385g	539	27.3	140	6.6	11.9	7.1	1
Chicken, & Vegetable, Frozen, Tesco*	1 Pie/129g	282	14.4	219	7.2	21.6	11.2	1.4
Chicken, Creamy, Puff Pastry Topped, Iceland*	1 Pie/135g	400	24.1	296	8.7	24.3	17.8	1.8
Chicken, Deep Filled, Puff Pastry, Sainsbury's*	1 Pie/210g	538	31.9	256	10	19.9	15.2	3.1
Chicken, Ham, & Leek, Charlie Bigham's*	1 Serving/300g	745	46.9	248	11.5	16.3	15.6	0
Chicken, Individual, Ready Made, Average	*1 Pie/155g*	*392*	*22.3*	*253*	*9.5*	*20.9*	*14.4*	*1.6*
Chicken, Leek, Smoked Bacon, Creamy, Gastropub, M&S	½ Pie/250g	693	46.5	277	13	13.5	18.6	1.7
Chicken, Shortcrust, Oven Baked, Birds Eye*	1 Pie/155g	417	23.1	271	8.4	25	15	1.2
Cod, & Haddock, Smoked, COU, M&S*	1 Pack/400g	320	9.6	80	6.1	9	2.4	1.2
Cottage, 1, Waitrose*	1 Pack/400g	580	30.4	145	8.2	10.3	7.6	1.6
Cottage, Aberdeen Angus, Large, Chilled, Finest, Tesco*	½ Pack/400g	420	17.2	105	7.1	8.7	4.3	1.8
Cottage, Aldi*	1 Pack/440g	484	27.3	110	4.1	9.5	6.2	0.2
Cottage, Beef, Delicious, Annabel Karmel*	1 Pack/200g	206	9.6	103	4.7	9.8	4.8	1.1
Cottage, Beef, Extra Special, Asda*	½ Pack/369g	483	22.1	131	7.4	11	6	2.3
Cottage, Calorie Controlled, Love Life, Waitrose*	1 Pack/320g	253	4.5	79	4.5	11.3	1.4	1.6
Cottage, Calorie Counted, Asda*	1 Pack/350g	243	4.9	80	4.1	11	1.6	1.9
Cottage, Cheddar Cheese Crumb, Specially Selected, Aldi*	½ Pack/372g	629	34.2	169	9.6	11	9.2	1.6
Cottage, Chilled, 400g, Quorn*	1 Pack/380g	315	8	83	3.4	11	2.1	3
Cottage, Classic British, Sainsbury's*	1 Pack/450g	414	14.8	92	5.8	9.3	3.3	1
Cottage, Cook*	½ Pack/390g	495	16.4	127	8.3	11.8	4.2	1.4
Cottage, COU, M&S*	1 Pack/400g	340	8	85	6	11	2	1.5
Cottage, Diet Chef Ltd*	1 Pack/270g	235	9.7	87	3.7	9.8	3.6	1.7
Cottage, Finest, Tesco*	1 Pack/400g	447	15.7	114	6.8	12.2	4	0.9
Cottage, for One, Charlie Bigham's*	1 Serving/325g	552	31.2	170	11.1	9.3	9.6	0
Cottage, for Two, Charlie Bigham's*	1 Serving/325g	552	31.2	170	11.1	9.4	9.6	0
Cottage, Frozen, 400g, Quorn*	1 Pack/400g	396	14	99	4.2	11	3.5	4
Cottage, Frozen, Weight Watchers*	1 Pack/320g	252	6.4	79	5.2	9.5	2	1
Cottage, HFC, Tesco*	1 Pack/388g	283	5	73	2.6	12.3	1.3	1.1
Cottage, Lentil & Vegetable, Linda McCartney*	1 Pot/398g	374	10.3	94	2.8	13.5	2.6	2.5
Cottage, Lentil, Co-Op*	1 Pack/400g	300	8.8	75	2.3	10	2.2	2.4
Cottage, Lentil, with Sweet Potato Mash, Sainsbury's*	1 Pack/382g	283	6.1	74	2.6	10.4	1.6	4
Cottage, Little Dish*	1 Pack/200g	188	7.2	94	3.9	10.5	3.6	1.9
Cottage, Low low, Simple Health*	1 Pack/281g	219	4.5	78	3.6	11.8	1.6	1.2
Cottage, Meal for One, M&S*	1 Pack/445g	356	16	80	5.4	6.2	3.6	1.7
Cottage, Meat Free, Morrisons*	1 Pack/337g	239	4.4	71	2.5	10.9	1.3	3
Cottage, Mini Meal, Classic, Sainsbury's*	1 Pack/241g	219	7.5	91	5.5	9.7	3.1	1.1
Cottage, Morrisons*	1 Pack/450g	450	18.4	100	5.2	10.7	4.1	1.2
Cottage, Retail, Average	*1 Pack/400g*	*399*	*15.7*	*100*	*5.5*	*10.5*	*3.9*	*1.3*
Cottage, Savers, Morrisons*	1 Pack/400g	350	13.1	88	4.6	8.2	3.3	3.4

PIE

INFO/WEIGHT	Measure	per Measure KCAL	FAT	Nutrition Values per 100g / 100ml KCAL	PROT	CARB	FAT	FIBRE
Cottage, Serves 1, Basics, Sainsbury's*	1 Pack/286g	269	8.3	94	3.9	12.3	2.9	1.5
Cottage, Tesco*	1 Pack/363g	352	11.6	97	4.7	11.6	3.2	1.6
Cottage, Traditional, Oven Cooked, Morrisons*	1 Pack/331g	348	16.6	105	4.6	9.8	5	1.2
Cottage, with Cheddar Mash, TTD, Sainsbury's*	1 Pack/400g	525	27.2	131	8.6	7.9	6.8	1.8
Cumberland, 530, Oakhouse Foods Ltd*	1 Meal/400g	592	33.6	148	5.4	11.9	8.4	1.6
Cumberland, Asda*	1 Pack/400g	504	22.4	126	6.3	12.7	5.6	1.5
Fish	*1 Serving/250g*	*262*	*7.5*	*105*	*8*	*12.3*	*3*	*0.7*
Fish, 306, Oakhouse Foods Ltd*	1 Meal/400g	420	20.8	105	7.2	7.1	5.2	0.7
Fish, Admirals, Frozen, Oven Baked, Youngs*	1 Pie/291g	338	12.8	116	4.9	13.7	4.4	1
Fish, Calorie Counted, Asda*	1 Pack/388g	318	4.7	82	7.7	10	1.2	0.5
Fish, Classic Kitchen, Tesco*	½ Pack/386g	457	19.8	119	8.7	8.8	5.1	1.3
Fish, Classic, Waitrose*	1 Pack/385g	354	8.5	92	6.3	11.2	2.2	1.2
Fish, Crunchy Topped, Menu, Waitrose*	1 Pack/400g	444	19.2	111	7.5	8.4	4.8	1.8
Fish, Extra Special, Asda*	1 Pack/400g	540	30.8	135	9.8	6.5	7.7	1.1
Fish, for One, As Sold, Charlie Bigham's*	1 Serving/340g	527	31.6	155	8.7	9.5	9.3	0
Fish, for Two, As Sold, Charlie Bigham's*	1 Serving/328g	499	29.9	152	8.4	9.6	9.1	0
Fish, Haddock, Salmon, Pollock, & Prawn, TTD, Sainsbury's	1 Pack/375g	439	17.6	117	7.6	10.7	4.7	1
Fish, HL, Tesco*	1 Pack/384g	311	7.7	81	3.9	11.4	2	0.9
Fish, Little Dish*	1 Pack/200g	206	8.8	103	4.5	10.5	4.4	1.5
Fish, Main for One, The Collection, Gastropub, M&S*	1 Pack/420g	483	20.6	115	8	9.3	4.9	0.8
Fish, Mariner's, Frozen, Oven Baked, Youngs*	1 Pack/340g	444	20.3	140	5.1	15.1	6.4	1
Fish, Meal for One, Oven Baked, Gastro, Youngs*	1 Pie/317g	412	20.3	130	8.5	9.2	6.4	1
Fish, Serves 1, BGTY, Sainsbury's*	1 Pie/450g	369	8.6	90	6.7	10.2	2.1	1.6
Fish, Serves 1, No.1, Waitrose*	1 Pack/334g	457	26	137	6.4	9.4	7.8	1.7
Fisherman's, Youngs*	1 Pack/340g	377	13.6	111	5.6	12.8	4	0.8
Fishermans, Traditional, Morrison's*	1 Pie/327g	425	19.6	130	5.2	13.4	6	0.8
Fruit, Autumn, M&S*	1 Serving/116g	271	7.2	234	1.9	41.8	6.2	1.7
Fruit, Pastry Top & Bottom	*1oz/28g*	*73*	*3.7*	*260*	*3*	*34*	*13.3*	*1.8*
Fruit, Selection, Mr Kipling*	1 Pie/66g	232	9	350	3.5	53.5	13.6	1.3
Holy Chipotle!, Patties, Pieminister*	1 Patty/60g	154	8.1	256	6.1	29.6	13.4	0
Homity, GF, Clive's*	1 Pie/235g	390	22.6	166	4.2	14.4	9.6	0
Lamb, Chunky, & Redcurrant, 247, Oakhouse Foods Ltd*	1 Pie/255g	388	21.2	152	8.8	11	8.3	0.6
Leek, & Potato, Creamy Cheddar Sauce, Pukka Pies Ltd*	1 Pie/226g	596	35	264	6.2	24.2	15.5	1.3
Lemon Meringue	*1 Portion/120g*	*383*	*17.3*	*319*	*4.5*	*45.9*	*14.4*	*0.7*
Lemon Meringue, Sainsbury's*	¼ Pie/110g	351	9.9	319	2.3	57.3	9	0.5
Lemon Meringue, Tesco*	1 Serving/79g	223	6.2	283	3.4	49.1	7.8	1.3
Lentil, & Olive, Greek, Clive's*	1 Pie/235g	477	25.4	203	4.5	20	10.8	0
Macaroni Cheese, Countryside*	1 Serving/144g	282	10.1	196	4.9	28.3	7	1.2
Meat, & Potato, Hollands*	1 Pie/175g	410	19.2	234	6.1	27.5	11	0
Meat, & Potato, Tesco*	1 Serving/150g	414	26.8	276	5.1	23.6	17.9	1.6
Mince, All Butter Pastry, Extra Special, Asda*	1 Pie/70g	278	11.1	400	3.6	59	16	3.2
Mince, All Butter, 1, Waitrose*	1 Pie/61g	238	8.9	391	3.3	60	14.6	3.3
Mince, All Butter, Average	*1 Pie/65g*	*251*	*8.9*	*386*	*4*	*60.2*	*13.8*	*2.4*
Mince, All Butter, Mini, 1, Waitrose*	1 Pie/28g	111	3.8	392	3.1	63.6	13.4	2.5
Mince, All Butter, Mini, Average	*1 Pie/20g*	*78*	*2.8*	*389*	*4.3*	*61.6*	*13.8*	*2.8*
Mince, All Butter, Mini, The Best, Morrisons*	1 Pie/32g	127	4.7	402	4	62	14.9	2
Mince, All Butter, Puff Pastry, Average	*1 Pie60g*	*228*	*10.5*	*381*	*4.3*	*51.1*	*17.4*	*2.2*
Mince, All Butter, Puff Pastry, Extra Special, Asda*	1 Pie/51g	195	10.1	386	3.8	47	20	1.3
Mince, Butter Enriched, Puff Pastry, Bakery, Sainsbury's*	1 Pie/65g	246	9.7	379	4.7	55.4	14.9	2.2
Mince, Christmas, Classic, Asda*	1 Pie/57g	229	9.1	401	3.5	59	16	3.5
Mince, Christmas, Finest, Tesco*	1 Pie/64g	255	9.4	395	4.6	60.3	14.5	1.4
Mince, Christmas, Sainsbury's*	1 Pie/37g	147	6	397	4.5	58	16.3	2.6
Mince, Deep Fill, Holly Lane, Aldi*	1 Pie/61g	235	8.5	386	4	59	14	2.7

P

PIE

INFO/WEIGHT	Measure	per Measure KCAL	FAT	Nutrition Values per 100g / 100ml KCAL	PROT	CARB	FAT	FIBRE
Mince, Deep Filled, All Butter Pastry, Finest, Tesco*	1 Pie/65g	259	10.8	401	5	56.2	16.7	2.7
Mince, Deep, Morrisons*	1 Pie/65g	243	9.1	371	3.7	57.8	13.9	1.5
Mince, Dusted, Mini, Finest, Tesco*	1 Pie/20g	76	2.4	379	7.3	62.9	12.2	5
Mince, Free From, Sainsbury's*	1 Pie/58g	226	7.5	393	2.3	64	13	2.5
Mince, Iced Top, Asda*	1 Pie/55g	220	7.7	399	2.8	63	14	4.7
Mince, Individual, Average	*1 Pie/65g*	*260*	*11*	*400*	*4.2*	*56.3*	*17*	*1.6*
Mince, Individual, Mr Kipling*	1 Pie/66g	253	9.2	381	3.7	59.5	13.8	1.3
Mince, Luxury, Deep Filled, M&S*	1 Pie/65g	234	9	360	4.3	55	13.8	3.8
Mince, Luxury, Extra Special, Asda*	1 Pie/64g	247	8.9	387	4.2	60	14	2.3
Mince, Luxury, Iceland*	1 Pie/60g	230	8.3	383	4.1	59.3	13.8	2.6
Mince, Mini, M&S*	1 Pie/28g	105	4	380	4.3	57.8	14.6	4
Mince, Mini, Specially Selected, Aldi*	1 Pie/29g	111	4.1	382	4	59	14	2.7
Mince, Puff Pastry, Co-Op*	1 Pie/72g	245	11.9	340	5	43.1	16.5	2.6
Mince, Shortcrust, Essential, Waitrose*	1 Pie/53g	226	9.5	423	4	60.1	17.7	3.4
Mince, Tesco*	1 Pie/54g	211	7.5	389	3.8	61.2	13.8	2.6
Mushroom, & Camembert, Puff Pastry Topped, Tesco*	1 Pie/162g	434	26.2	268	5.6	24	16.2	2.1
Mushroom, & Leek, GF, Clive's*	1 Pie/235g	456	26.8	194	3.2	18.3	11.4	0
Mushroom, & Onion, with Parsley Mash, Veggie, M&S*	1 Pack/400g	288	8.4	72	1.7	10.6	2.1	1.9
Mushroom, Country, Fry's*	1 Pie/175g	373	17.3	213	5.4	25.7	9.9	1.5
Mushroom, Creamy, Classic, Clive's*	1 Pie/235g	522	30.8	222	4.8	19.4	13.1	0
Mushroom, Organic, Clive's*	1 Pie/235g	578	37.4	246	4.7	20.1	15.9	0
Mushroom, Tomato, & Red Wine, Kevin, Pieminister*	1 Pie/270g	562	25.7	208	4.4	25	9.5	0
Mushroom, Wild Shroom, Pieminister*	1 Pie/270g	513	26.2	190	5.2	19.5	9.7	2.7
Paneer, Coconut, & Chickpea, Spiced, Higgidy*	1 Pie/260g	700	46.6	269	7.4	20.8	17.9	1.9
Parsnip, Very Merry, Higgidy*	1 Pie/250g	641	37.8	256	4.7	25.2	15.1	2.5
Pork, & Egg, M&S*	¼ Pie/110g	411	31	374	10.9	18.4	28.2	1.5
Pork, & Pickle, Mini, Sainsbury's*	1 Pie/50g	177	11.5	354	9.5	26.2	23	2.1
Pork, & Pickle, Snack, Sainsbury's*	1 Pie/65g	246	15.8	379	8.9	29.9	24.4	2.3
Pork, BBQ, Mini, Tesco*	1 Pie/50g	198	13.2	396	10.7	28.2	26.3	1.9
Pork, Bitesize, Tesco*	1 Pie/25g	98	6.5	393	10.8	28.1	26.1	1.5
Pork, Cheese & Pickle, Mini, Tesco*	1 Pie/49g	191	12.8	389	9.2	29.3	26.1	1.2
Pork, Cheese, & Pickle, Mini, Morrisons*	1 Pie/50g	228	14.9	456	9	36.9	29.8	2
Pork, Cheese, & Pickle, Snack, Morrisons*	1 Pie/75g	326	22.1	435	9.8	31.4	29.5	2.4
Pork, Individual	*1 Pie/75g*	*272*	*19.3*	*363*	*10.8*	*23.7*	*25.7*	*0.9*
Pork, Melton Mowbray, Chef Select, Lidl*	1 Pie/50g	204	14.4	407	10.3	25.9	28.9	1.2
Pork, Melton Mowbray, Cured, Mini, M&S*	1 Pie/50g	192	12.2	385	9.8	32.6	24.4	1
Pork, Melton Mowbray, Individual, Sainsbury's*	½ Pie/70g	234	15.1	334	11.1	22.8	21.6	1.8
Pork, Melton Mowbray, Mini, M&S*	1 Pie/50g	185	12.1	370	11.6	26.1	24.2	1.6
Pork, Melton Mowbray, Mini, Morrisons*	1 Pie/50g	197	12.5	393	10.9	31.3	24.9	0.9
Pork, Melton Mowbray, Mini, Tesco*	1 Pie/50g	192	12.8	383	10.6	26.9	25.6	1.5
Pork, Melton Mowbray, Mini, TTD, Sainsbury's*	1 Pie/50g	204	14.2	407	10.6	26.5	28.4	1.7
Pork, Mini, Retail, Average	*1 Mini/50g*	*198*	*13.7*	*396*	*10.8*	*26.4*	*27.4*	*2.4*
Pork, Mini, Tesco*	1 Pie/45g	162	10.7	359	10.2	25.9	23.8	1
Pork, Sliced	*1 Slice/100g*	*380*	*29.9*	*380*	*10.2*	*18.7*	*29.9*	*0*
Quorn, & Vegetable, 524, Oakhouse Foods Ltd*	1 Meal/420g	391	11.8	93	3.4	10.7	2.8	1.8
Rhubarb, Lattice, Individual, Baked by Us, Morrisons*	1 Pie/135g	433	19.2	321	3.9	43.4	14.2	2
Rhubarb, Shortcrust Pastry, Bakery, Tesco*	1 Slice/87g	219	9.3	251	3.1	34.8	10.7	1.7
Scotch, Co-Op*	1 Pie/132g	408	24.9	309	7.3	27.3	18.9	1.5
Shepherd's, 218, Oakhouse Foods Ltd*	1 Pack/390g	374	15.6	96	5.9	9.4	4	1.5
Shepherd's, Average	*1oz/28g*	*31*	*1.7*	*112*	*6*	*9.3*	*5.9*	*0.7*
Shepherd's, British Classic, Meal For One, Aldi*	1 Pie/450g	614	35.5	142	5.4	11	8.2	1
Shepherd's, Chilled, Finest, Tesco*	½ Pack/400g	414	14	103	6.3	11.1	3.5	1.2
Shepherd's, for Two, Charlie Bigham's*	1 Serving/324g	379	16.5	117	6.8	10.5	5.1	0

	Measure INFO/WEIGHT	per Measure KCAL	FAT	Nutrition Values per 100g / 100ml KCAL	PROT	CARB	FAT	FIBRE
PIE								
Shepherd's, Vegetarian, Average	*1 Serving/400g*	*371*	*14.6*	*93*	*4*	*10.4*	*3.6*	*2.5*
Spinach, Courgette, & Feta Cheese, Vegetarian, Waitrose*	1 Pie/170g	408	25	240	7.4	18.5	14.7	1.8
Steak, & Ale with Chips & Gravy	*1 Serving/400g*	*825*	*42.2*	*206*	*7.2*	*20.5*	*10.6*	*0.5*
Steak, & Ale, Average	*1 Pie/200g*	*507*	*28.7*	*253*	*9.8*	*21.1*	*14.4*	*1.3*
Steak, & Ale, Pub Style, Co-Op*	1 Pie/250g	538	30	215	9	17	12	2
Steak, & Ale, Sainsbury's*	1 Serving/190g	445	23.4	234	8.3	22.6	12.3	0.9
Steak, & Kidney with Puff Pastry, 425g, Fray Bentos*	1 Pie/425g	622	16.6	131	5.6	17.4	3.5	0.6
Steak, & Kidney, Individual	*1 Pie/200g*	*646*	*42.4*	*323*	*9.1*	*25.6*	*21.2*	*0.9*
Steak, & Kidney, Puff Pastry, Sainsbury's*	1 Pie/150g	423	23.6	282	8.2	26.9	15.7	0.9
Steak, & Kidney, Pukka Pies Ltd*	1 Pie/239g	537	28.2	225	9.7	17.7	11.8	4.5
Steak, & Stilton, Charlie Bigham's*	1 Serving/250g	638	12.5	255	10	18	5	0
Steak, & Ale, Charlie Bigham's*	1 Serving/300g	742	39.7	247	13.2	17	13.2	0
Steak, & Ale, Family, Jon Thorners*	1 Serving/250g	610	22.8	244	10	23	9.1	0
Steak, & Ale, Puff Pastry, 550g, Morrisons*	¼ Pie/137g	333	17.3	243	13.3	18.6	12.6	1.1
Steak, & Ale, Puff Pastry, Serves 3, Sainsbury's*	1 Serving/183g	464	24.9	253	9.5	22.7	13.6	0.9
Steak, & Ale, The Best, Morrisons*	1 Pie/208g	545	28.7	262	9.9	23.8	13.8	1.3
Steak, & Ale, with A Rarebit Sauce, Filo, Finest, Tesco*	½ Pie/177g	362	18.8	204	10.1	16.3	10.6	1.4
Steak, & Gravy, Frasers*	1 Pie/130g	335	15.6	258	10	26	12	1.2
Steak, & Red Wine, Shortcrust Topped, Cook*	1 Serving/295g	496	24.2	168	11.6	10.5	8.2	1.2
Steak, & Stilton, Moo & Blue, Pieminister*	1 Pie/270g	637	32.7	236	10.5	21.9	12.1	0
Steak, & Tatties, Frasers*	1 Serving/310g	446	20.2	144	6.7	14	6.5	1
Steak, Aberdeen Angus, Top Crust, Waitrose*	½ Pie/280g	476	24.1	170	10	13.4	8.6	4.1
Steak, All, Pukka Pies Ltd*	1 Pie/233g	495	24.5	212	11.1	17.7	10.5	2.5
Steak, British, Slow Cooked, Extra Special, Asda*	1/3 Pie/186g	494	26.1	265	13	21	14	1.2
Steak, Mini, Asda*	1 Serving/67g	117	5.3	176	9	17	8	0.9
Steak, Puff Pastry Lid, Frozen, Tesco*	1 Pie/131g	304	14.9	232	8.5	23.1	11.4	1.5
Steak, Puff Pastry, Average	*¼ Pie/100g*	*259*	*14.5*	*259*	*9.4*	*21.8*	*14.5*	*1.9*
Steak, Puff Pastry, M&S*	½ Pie/275g	729	41.5	265	12.5	19	15.1	1.6
Steak, Puff Pastry, Serves 3, Sainsbury's*	1 Serving/183g	512	30	280	9.8	22.6	16.4	1.3
Steak, Red Wine, & Mushroom, Higgidy*	1 Pie/250g	601	31.6	240	10.4	21.4	12.6	1.3
Steak, Scotch, Bell's Bakery*	1 Serving/150g	378	20.2	252	13.6	18.6	13.5	0.7
Steak, Shortcrust, Average	*¼ Pie/100g*	*253*	*14.1*	*253*	*9.9*	*21.6*	*14.1*	*1.4*
Steak, Tesco*	1 Pie/150g	408	21.4	272	9.5	25.5	14.3	1.8
Sweet Potato, & Feta, with Pumpkin Seeds, Higgidy*	1 Pie/270g	756	49.4	280	7.2	22.9	18.3	2.1
Vegetable	*1oz/28g*	*42*	*2.1*	*151*	*3*	*18.9*	*7.6*	*1.5*
Vegetable, & Cheese, Asda*	1 Pie/141g	330	16.2	234	5.8	26.9	11.5	1
Vegetable, & Feta, Moroccan, Little, Higgidy*	1 Pie/180g	418	22.5	232	5.1	24.7	12.5	0.6
Vegetable, Retail, Average	*1 Serving/200g*	*348*	*19*	*174*	*3.7*	*18.6*	*9.5*	*1.1*
Vegetarian, Chicken Style, & Mushroom, Quorn*	1 Pie/235g	588	33.2	250	5.5	23.7	14.1	3
Vegetarian, Deep Country, Linda McCartney*	1 Pie/166g	413	23.6	249	5.2	24.9	14.2	2.6
Vegetarian, Mince & Potato, Quorn*	1 Pie/200g	388	16	194	6.5	22.5	8	3
Vegetarian, Mushroom & Ale, Linda McCartney*	1 Pie/200g	439	23.5	219	4.1	25	11.7	1.2
Vegetarian, Shepherd's, Linda McCartney*	1 Pack/340g	286	7.5	84	3.7	12.3	2.2	2.3
Vegetarian, Steak, Meat Free, Quorn*	1 Pie/235g	439	18.8	187	5.6	22	8	2
PIE FILLING								
Apple, Sainsbury's*	1 Serving/75g	67	0.1	89	0.1	22.1	0.1	1
Cherry	*1oz/28g*	*23*	*0*	*82*	*0.4*	*21.5*	*0*	*0.4*
PIGEON								
Meat Only, Roasted, Average	*1 Pigeon/115g*	*215*	*9.1*	*187*	*29*	*0*	*7.9*	*0*
Meat Only, Roasted, Weighed with Bone, Average	*1oz/28g*	*12*	*0.5*	*41*	*6.4*	*0*	*1.7*	*0*
PIKELETS								
Buttermilk, Waitrose*	1 Pikelet/28g	54	0.2	192	7.1	37.7	0.8	2.6
Sainsbury's*	1 Pikelet/24g	55	0.3	230	7.6	45.1	1.4	3.3

P

	Measure INFO/WEIGHT	per Measure KCAL	FAT	Nutrition Values per 100g / 100ml KCAL	PROT	CARB	FAT	FIBRE
PIKELETS								
Tesco*	1 Pikelet/27g	52	0.3	193	6.6	38.1	1	2.4
PILAF								
Bulgur Wheat, Sainsbury's*	1 Pack/381g	347	11.1	91	3.9	12.3	2.9	6.3
Vegetables, with Coconut & Lentil, City Kitchen, Tesco*	1 Pack/385g	474	20.8	123	2.6	14.9	5.4	2.3
with Tomato, Average	*1oz/28g*	*40*	*0.9*	*144*	*2.5*	*28*	*3.3*	*0.4*
PILCHARDS								
Fillets in Tomato Sauce, Average	*1 Can/120g*	*158*	*7.8*	*132*	*16.2*	*2.2*	*6.5*	*0.1*
Fillets in Virgin Olive Oil, Glenryck*	1 Serving/92g	223	14.4	242	23.3	2	15.7	0
PIMMS*								
& Lemonade, Premixed, Canned, Pimms*	1 Can/250ml	160	0	64	0	8.4	0	0
25% Volume, Pimms*	1 Serving/50ml	80	0	160	0	5	0	0
PINE NUTS								
Average	*1 Tbsp/8g*	*56*	*5.5*	*695*	*15.7*	*3.9*	*68.6*	*1.9*
PINEAPPLE								
Chunks, Average	*1 Serving/100g*	*66*	*0.1*	*66*	*0.5*	*15.5*	*0.1*	*0.3*
in Juice, Canned, Average	*1 Can/106g*	*57*	*0*	*53*	*0.3*	*12.9*	*0*	*0.6*
Raw, Flesh Only, Average	*1 Med Slice/80g*	*40*	*0.1*	*50*	*0.5*	*13.1*	*0.1*	*1.4*
PISTACHIO NUTS								
Raw, Average, without Shells	*1 Serving/20g*	*111*	*8.9*	*557*	*20.6*	*28*	*44.4*	*10.3*
Roasted & Salted, without Shells, Average	*1 Serving/25g*	*152*	*13.6*	*608*	*19.6*	*9.9*	*54.5*	*6.1*
Salted, Roasted, Weighed with Shell	*1 Serving/100g*	*331*	*30.5*	*331*	*9.8*	*4.5*	*30.5*	*3.4*
Salted, Roasted, without Shells	*1 Serving/100g*	*601*	*55.4*	*601*	*17.9*	*8.2*	*55.4*	*6.1*
PIZZA								
'Nduja, & Burrata, Sourdough Base, No.1, Waitrose*	¼ Pizza/129g	284	10.6	220	8.9	26.5	8.2	2.1
American, Hot, Thin & Crispy, Stonebaked, Aldi*	½ Pizza/149g	357	16.4	240	9.7	25	11	2.8
American, Supermarket, Pizza Express*	½ Pizza/130g	352	14.5	271	11.3	30.5	11.2	1.5
Bacon, & Mushroom, Thin & Crispy, Sainsbury's*	½ Pizza/150g	396	15.9	264	12.9	29.2	10.6	1.7
Beef, Chilli, Classic Crust, Tex Mex, Tesco*	½ Pizza/260g	655	26.5	252	10.9	27.9	10.2	2.5
Bocconcini, Mozzarella, Sunblush Tomato, TTD,Sainsbury's	1 Pizza/252g	617	20.9	245	11.2	30	8.3	2.5
Cheese & Tomato, Average	*1 Serving/300g*	*711*	*35.4*	*237*	*9.1*	*25.2*	*11.8*	*1.4*
Cheese & Tomato, Baguette, Tesco*	1 Baguette/125g	275	8.5	220	11	28	6.8	2.8
Cheese & Tomato, Deep Pan, Goodfella's*	¼ Pizza/102g	259	10.8	253	11.5	29.6	10.5	3.7
Cheese & Tomato, Everyday Value, Tesco*	1 Pizza/150g	423	9.2	282	9.6	46	6.1	2.2
Cheese & Tomato, Frozen, Sainsbury's*	1 Serving/122g	300	10.7	246	13.7	28	8.8	3
Cheese & Tomato, Meltingly Good, M&S*	½ Pizza/227g	613	22.5	270	10.8	33.5	9.9	2
Cheese & Tomato, Mini, Bruschetta, Iceland*	1 Pizza/34g	63	2.3	188	8	23	7	2.1
Cheese & Tomato, Mini, M&S*	1 Pizza/95g	233	5.5	245	10	38.7	5.8	1.6
Cheese & Tomato, Range, Italiano, Tesco*	1 Pizza/380g	969	35	255	11.4	31.7	9.2	3.3
Cheese & Tomato, Retail, Frozen	*1oz/28g*	*70*	*3*	*250*	*7.5*	*32.9*	*10.7*	*1.4*
Cheese & Tomato, Sainsbury's*	1 Pizza/247g	706	24.5	286	13.7	35.4	9.9	2.4
Cheese & Tomato, Slice, Ross*	1 Slice/77g	148	6.6	192	6.5	22.2	8.6	2
Cheese & Tomato, Slices, CBY, Asda*	1 Slice/14g	62	2.5	453	8.2	63.2	18.1	2.3
Cheese & Tomato, Stonebaked, Thin & Crispy, Tesco*	½ Pizza/161g	388	13.8	241	11.6	29.4	8.6	2.1
Cheese & Tomato, Thin & Crispy, Asda*	1 Pizza/366g	827	36.6	226	11	23	10	2
Cheese & Tomato, Thin & Crispy, Sainsbury's*	1 Serving/135g	344	10	255	14.9	32.2	7.4	5
Cheese & Tomato, Thin & Crispy, Waitrose*	1 Pizza/280g	658	28.3	235	12.3	23.6	10.1	2.3
Cheese & Tomato, Thin, HFC, Tesco*	½ Pizza/144g	361	9.6	250	10.9	35.5	6.7	2.3
Cheese & Tomato, Mini, HFC, Tesco*	1 Pizza/82g	241	9.5	294	11.1	35.1	11.5	3
Cheese & Tomato, Thin & Crispy, M&S*	¼ Pizza/116g	314	12.3	271	12.3	30.7	10.6	1.8
Cheese Feast, Deep Crust, Carlos, Aldi*	1 Pizza/155g	432	14.9	279	9.7	37.3	9.6	2.1
Cheese Feast, Deep Pan, Asda*	½ Pizza/210g	422	18.9	201	13	17	9	2.3
Cheese Feast, Stuffed Crust, Garlic Herb Dip, Sainsbury's*	¼ Pizza/148g	387	13.9	261	12.1	31	9.4	1.8
Cheese Feast, Stuffed Crust, Take Away, Carlos, Aldi*	½ Pizza/238g	650	27	273	11.8	29.4	11.3	2.7

PIZZA

INFO/WEIGHT	Measure	per Measure		Nutrition Values per 100g / 100ml				
		KCAL	FAT	KCAL	PROT	CARB	FAT	FIBRE
Cheese Feast, Thin Crust, Chilled, Tesco*	½ Pizza/175g	467	22.4	267	14.7	23.4	12.8	2.5
Cheese, & Garlic, Tesco*	½ Pizza/102g	304	11.7	298	9.2	38.1	11.5	2.4
Cheese, Four, Deep Dish, Chicago Town*	1 Pizza/148g	433	17.8	292	12	33	12	0
Cheese, Four, Finest, Tesco*	½ Pizza/230g	575	21.2	250	12.1	29.8	9.2	1.3
Cheese, Four, Stonebaked, Thin, Carlos, Aldi*	½ Pizza/176g	498	17.4	283	13	34	9.9	2.8
Cheese, Four, Stuffed Crust, Takeaway, Chicago Town*	¼ Pizza/158g	433	17	275	10.8	33	10.8	1.9
Cheese, Four, Thin & Crispy, Iceland*	½ Pizza/148g	354	12.6	239	10.7	29.1	8.5	1.6
Cheese, Loaded, Stuffed Crust, Takeaway, Chicago Town*	¼ Pizza/150g	436	17.9	292	12	33	12	0
Cheese, Stuffed Crust, Sainsbury's*	1 Pizza/525g	1428	52.5	272	14	31.5	10	2
Cheese, Stuffed Crust, Takeaway, Tesco*	½ Pizza/203g	521	17.7	256	11.5	31.8	8.7	2.5
Cheese, Thick Crust, From Restaurant, Average	**1 Pizza/976g**	**2655**	**107.3**	**272**	**12**	**31.3**	**11**	**1.8**
Cheese, Thin Crust, From Restaurant, Average	**1 Pizza/627g**	**1906**	**98.3**	**304**	**14.2**	**26.5**	**15.7**	**2**
Cheese, Triple, Deep Dish, Chicago Town*	1 Serving/170g	418	18.2	246	9.9	27.6	10.7	0
Cheeseburger, Double, Deep Pan, Oven Baked, Iceland*	1/3 Pizza/103g	272	7.3	264	12.3	36.5	7.1	2.4
Chicken, & Bacon, Loaded, Tesco*	1 Serving/258g	622	25.3	241	12.8	25.4	9.8	1.9
Chicken, & Bacon, Pizzeria, Italian, Sainsbury's*	½ Pizza/170g	508	24.1	300	13.6	29.4	14.2	2.7
Chicken, & Chorizo, 12", TTD, Sainsbury's*	½ Pizza/290g	702	20.9	242	12.2	32.1	7.2	2.6
Chicken, & Chorizo, Sourdough, Carlos, Aldi*	½ Pizza/165g	406	14.2	246	12	29	8.6	4.7
Chicken, & Sweetcorn, Stonebaked, Tesco*	1 Serving/177g	354	9.6	200	11.9	26	5.4	2
Chicken, & Vegetable, Leggera, Pizza Express*	1 Pizza/191g	396	12.8	207	9.9	25.6	6.7	2.5
Chicken, & Vegetable, Stone Baked, GFY, Asda*	½ Pizza/161g	349	3.7	217	13	36	2.3	1.7
Chicken, & Bacon, Large, Takeaway, Chicago Town*	¼ Pizza/123g	355	14.7	289	13	32	12	0
Chicken, Arrabiata, with Nduja, TTD, Sainsbury's*	½ Pizza/163g	408	14.4	250	12.5	28.9	8.8	2.8
Chicken, BBQ, M&S*	½ Pizza/210g	430	11.8	205	11.6	27.5	5.6	1.8
Chicken, BBQ, Stonebaked, Tesco*	½ Pizza/158g	285	9.5	180	10.5	20.9	6	3.9
Chicken, BBQ, Texan, Thin & Crispy, Co-Op*	½ Pizza/190g	418	14.1	220	11	27	7.4	2.1
Chicken, BBQ, Thin & Crispy, Sainsbury's*	½ Pizza/167g	399	12.4	238	11.4	30.4	7.4	2.2
Chicken, Cajun Style, Stonebaked, Tesco*	1 Pizza/561g	1318	55	235	11.9	24.8	9.8	1.4
Chicken, Cajun, & Sweet Red Pepper, The Best, Morrisons*	½ Pizza/196g	451	14.7	230	12.4	26.9	7.5	2.6
Chicken, Cajun, Sainsbury's*	½ Pizza/146g	285	2.6	195	12.9	31.8	1.8	2.6
Chicken, Chargrilled, Iceland*	1 Pizza/381g	804	25.5	211	12.3	25.4	6.7	2
Chicken, Chargrilled, Thin & Crispy, Asda*	1 Pizza/373g	780	18.6	209	9	32	5	1.6
Chicken, Club, Deep Dish, Chicago Town*	1 Pizza/155g	404	14.9	261	11	32	9.6	0
Chicken, Fajita, 10 Inch, CBY, Asda*	½ Pizza/151g	319	9.8	211	10.7	26.3	6.5	2.4
Chicken, Fajita, Thin & Crispy, Iceland*	1 Pizza/361g	729	21.3	202	9.6	26.5	5.9	1.8
Chicken, Garlic, Thin & Crispy, Stonebake, Sainsbury's*	½ Pizza/160g	386	17.3	241	10.7	25.2	10.8	3.5
Chicken, Hot & Spicy, Deep Pan, Morrisons*	½ Pizza/233g	521	13	224	10.5	32.9	5.6	1
Chicken, Hot & Spicy, Deep Pan, Tesco*	½ Pizza/222g	423	7.3	191	10.5	30	3.3	2.1
Chicken, Piri Piri, Classic Crust, Takeaway, Tesco*	1 Pizza/550g	1196	38.4	217	10.3	28.3	7	2.4
Chicken, Romano, Goodfella's*	½ Pizza/189g	447	17.6	236	11	26	9.3	0
Chicken, Smoky BBQ, Stonebaked, M&S*	½ Pizza/230g	513	15.2	223	11.3	28.5	6.6	2.1
Chicken, Sweet Chilli, BGTY, Sainsbury's*	½ Pizza/138g	276	2.3	200	13	33.2	1.7	2.1
Chicken, Sweet Chilli, Extra Thin, Morrison's*	½ Pizza/146g	301	7.9	206	10.7	27.9	5.4	1.7
Chicken, Tandoori, with Garlic & Herb Dip, Gousto*	1 Pizza/475g	902	31.4	190	13.4	19.3	6.6	1.6
Chicken, Tikka, Protein Base, Musclefood*	1 Pizza/200g	380	16	190	16.5	11.8	8	2.4
Falafel, Vegan, Stonebaked, Goodfellas*	½ Pizza/182g	397	12.7	218	6.4	30	7	0
Four Seasons, Stonebaked, Truly Irresistible, Co-Op*	½ Pizza/245g	502	16.2	205	9.5	26.6	6.6	2.6
Funghi, Ristorante, Dr Oetker*	1 Pizza/365g	847	43.4	232	7.6	22.5	11.9	1.8
Goats Cheese, Protein Base, Musclefood*	1 Pizza/200g	386	13.2	193	17.9	17.1	6.6	3.3
Ham, & Cheese, Ultra Thin, Sodebo*	1 Pizza/200g	400	8.6	200	11.3	29.1	4.3	0
Ham, & Mushroom Slices, Farmfoods*	1 Slice/89g	170	2.3	191	8	34	2.6	0.9
Ham, & Mushroom, Average	**1 Serving/250g**	**533**	**16**	**213**	**10.5**	**28.4**	**6.4**	**2.1**
Ham, & Mushroom, Finest, Tesco*	½ Pizza/240g	576	26.4	240	9.5	25.9	11	2.2

PIZZA

INFO/WEIGHT	Measure	per Measure KCAL	FAT	Nutrition Values per 100g / 100ml KCAL	PROT	CARB	FAT	FIBRE
Ham, & Mushroom, Smoked, Thin & Crispy, Co-Op*	1 Pizza/400g	792	18	198	9	30.3	4.5	1.7
Ham, & Mushroom, Thin & Crispy, Asda*	1 Pizza/360g	760	25.2	211	11	26	7	2.4
Ham, & Mushroom, Thin & Crispy, Tesco*	½ Pizza/185g	380	11.1	205	11.2	25.6	6	2.3
Ham, & Pineapple, Average	*1 Serving/250g*	*555*	*16.8*	*222*	*11*	*29.2*	*6.7*	*2.1*
Ham, & Pineapple, Stone Bake, M&S*	1 Pizza/345g	690	19.7	200	10.1	28.3	5.7	1.6
Ham, & Pineapple, Stonebaked, Tesco*	1 Pizza/161g	293	9.2	182	9.2	23.5	5.7	3.5
Ham, & Pineapple, Tesco*	1/6 Pizza/56g	134	4.6	240	10.4	30.9	8.3	2.1
Ham, & Pineapple, Thin & Crispy Italian, Morrisons*	1 Pizza/375g	746	22.9	199	10.2	24.9	6.1	0
Ham, & Pineapple, Thin & Crispy, Sainsbury's*	½ Pizza/165g	371	13.8	226	11.6	24.9	8.4	2
Ham, & Pineapple, Thin Crust, Tesco*	½ Pizza/175g	385	10	220	12.3	29.6	5.7	2.5
Ham, & Vegetable, Beetroot Base, Yes Its Pizza, Dr Oetker*	1 Pizza/315g	743	34.6	236	8.3	25	11	0
Ham, & Cheese, Thin & Crispy, Essential, Waitrose*	½ Pizza/72g	170	4.9	237	12.9	29.7	6.8	2.8
Ham, & Pineapple, Thin Stonebaked, Asda*	1 Slice/52g	111	3.5	213	11	26	6.7	2.2
Ham, Pepperoni & Milano, M&S*	1 Pizza/290g	696	28.4	240	14	23.3	9.8	1.1
Hawaii, Ristorante, Dr Oetker*	¼ Pizza/91g	206	7.7	226	8.8	28	8.5	0
Hawaiian, Stonebaked, Cucina, Aldi*	½ Pizza/165g	326	5.6	198	9.5	32	3.4	1.6
Hawaiian, Thin Crust, Tesco*	½ Pizza/192g	365	9.4	190	10.3	25.6	4.9	1.8
Hog Roast, M&S *	½ Pack/345g	825	33.5	239	12.3	24.9	9.7	1.5
Italian Style, Oumph!*	½ Pizza/200g	362	11.8	181	6.6	24	5.9	2.1
Jackfruit, & Mushroom, BBQ, Vegan, Sainsbury's*	1 Pizza/193g	394	9.5	204	5.4	32.8	4.9	3.6
Jackfruit, Pulled, BBQ, Plant Kitchen, M&S*	1 Pizza/187g	350	10.3	187	5.9	27.3	5.5	2.3
La Reine, Supermarket, Pizza Express*	½ Pizza/153g	322	9.3	211	10.2	27.7	6.1	2.3
Margherita, 12", Finest, Tesco*	½ Pizza/255g	433	9.2	170	8.1	26.4	3.6	2.7
Margherita, Average	*1 Slice/108g*	*239*	*8.6*	*239*	*11*	*30.5*	*8.6*	*1.2*
Margherita, Cheese & Tomato, San Marco*	½ Pizza/200g	454	14.4	227	10.7	29.8	7.2	1.2
Margherita, Classic, Kirstys*	1 Pizza/290g	658	24.9	227	10.3	26.5	8.6	1.4
Margherita, Classic, Supermarket, Pizza Express*	½ Pizza/127g	312	10.8	245	10	31.5	8.5	1.4
Margherita, Classico, Italiano, Tesco*	½ Pizza/191g	414	11.8	217	11.2	29.1	6.2	2.5
Margherita, GF, Free From, Sainsbury's*	½ Pizza/150g	430	18.6	287	8.5	33.3	12.4	3.9
Margherita, GF, Goodfella's*	¼ Pizza/74g	203	8.2	273	11	32	11	0
Margherita, GF, Supermarket, Pizza Express*	½ Pizza/134g	341	13	254	9	31.3	9.7	2.6
Margherita, Lactose Free,, Schar*	1 Pizza/300g	690	27.6	230	7.5	27	9.2	3.8
Margherita, Large, Supermarket, Pizza Express*	½ Pizza/228g	511	17.1	224	10.6	28.6	7.5	2.5
Margherita, Pizzeria, Italian, Sainsbury's*	½ Pizza/169g	426	17.4	253	12.2	27.9	10.3	2.5
Margherita, Speciale, Supermarket, Pizza Express*	½ Pizza/169g	438	17.2	259	11.6	28.5	10.2	3.2
Margherita, Stone Baked, Goodfella's*	1 Slice/36g	95	4.1	263	10.9	31.9	11.4	7.6
Margherita, Stonebaked, 10", Sainsbury's*	½ Pizza/139g	359	11.3	258	12.4	32.2	8.1	3.5
Margherita, Supermarket, Pizza Express*	½ Pizza/127g	312	10.8	245	10	31.5	8.5	1.4
Margherita, The Best, Morrisons*	½ Pizza/216g	569	20.8	263	9.8	32.7	9.6	3.5
Margherita, Thin & Crispy, Iceland*	½ Pizza/170g	391	14.4	230	12.7	25.9	8.5	2.8
Margherita, Thin Crust, Takeaway, Goodfella's*	½ Pizza/206g	594	26.7	289	13	29	13	0
Margherita, Thin Crust, Tesco*	1 Serving/170g	354	13.4	208	10.1	24.1	7.9	3.6
Margherita, Vegan, No Dough Pizza Co*	½ Pizza/157g	316	13	201	5.4	21	8.3	3.7
Meat Feast, Deep & Loaded, Sainsbury's*	½ Pizza/298g	818	30	275	13.2	32.7	10.1	2.6
Meat Feast, Mega, Asda*	½ Pizza/428g	1044	33.8	244	9.5	33.6	7.9	3.2
Meat Feast, Thin & Crispy, Asda*	½ Pizza/183g	410	14.6	224	11	27	8	1.4
Meat Feast, Thin Crust, Tesco*	½ Pizza/178g	430	20.2	242	13.6	21.3	11.4	2.3
Meatball, Marinari, Deep & Loaded, M&S*	¼ Pizza/389g	930	45.1	239	10.2	22.5	11.6	1.7
Meats, Italian, Finest, Tesco*	½ Pizza/217g	449	8.5	207	13.6	29.4	3.9	1.3
Meaty, Mega, Deep Dish, Chicago Town*	1 Pizza/157g	442	18.9	281	11	31	12	0
Mini, Party, Tesco*	1 Pizza/11g	26	1.1	248	11.4	28.6	10.5	1.9
Mozzarella, & Basil, Sourdough, Carlos, Aldi*	¼ Pizza/83g	218	7.8	261	12	31	9.3	2
Mozzarella, & Sunblush Tomato, 12", TTD, Sainsbury's*	½ Pizza/251g	638	17.8	254	12.4	35	7.1	2.6

PIZZA

	Measure INFO/WEIGHT	per Measure KCAL	FAT	Nutrition Values per 100g / 100ml KCAL	PROT	CARB	FAT	FIBRE
Mozzarella, Ristorante, Dr Oetker*	½ Pizza/184g	472	23.9	257	10	25	13	0
Mushroom, & Ricotta, Leggera, Pizza Express*	1 Pizza/170g	371	11.1	218	8.9	29.4	6.5	2.9
Mushroom, Garlic, Thin Crust, Tesco*	½ Pizza/163g	340	14.6	209	11	21.1	9	3.6
Napoletana, Sainsbury's*	½ Pizza/186g	424	14.3	228	9.7	29.9	7.7	3.1
Napoli, Tesco*	½ Pizza/184g	431	11.6	235	11.9	32.6	6.3	1.4
Onion, Caramelised, & Feta, & Rosemary, Bistro, Waitrose*	½ Pizza/230g	607	32	264	8.6	26.1	13.9	2.4
Pancetta, Mushroom, & Mascarpone, Co-Op*	½ Pizza/224g	571	20.6	255	9.5	32	9.2	3.1
Pepperoni, & Cheese, Asda*	½ Pizza/150g	386	13.5	257	10	34	9	2.7
Pepperoni, & Jalapeno Chill, Asda*	1 Pizza/277g	742	22.2	268	10	39	8	1.8
Pepperoni, Aldi*	1 Serving/55g	123	4.3	224	8.7	29.5	7.9	1.4
Pepperoni, Asda*	½ Pizza/150g	386	13.5	257	10	34	9	2.7
Pepperoni, Average	**1 Serving/250g**	**671**	**28.4**	**269**	**11.8**	**29.6**	**11.4**	**2.1**
Pepperoni, Baguette, Ovenbaked, Asda*	1 Baguette/123g	243	7.3	197	9.7	25	5.9	2.4
Pepperoni, Deep & Crispy, Iceland*	1 Serving/175g	490	21	280	11.9	31.1	12	1.8
Pepperoni, Deli, The Pizza Kitchen, Chicago Town*	½ Pizza/174g	544	26.2	312	13	29	15	0
Pepperoni, Double, Thin & Crispy, Loved by Us, Co-Op*	½ Pizza/173g	389	18.9	225	10.5	27.3	10.9	3.4
Pepperoni, Double, Thin & Crispy, Sainsbury's*	½ Pizza/174g	470	20	270	11.2	29.5	11.5	1.9
Pepperoni, Double, Thin, Stonebaked, Carlos, Aldi*	¼ Pizza/76g	198	7.6	259	11	30	9.9	2.4
Pepperoni, Flatbread, Asda*	1 Pizza/237g	670	23.7	283	11	35	10	2.7
Pepperoni, Hot & Spicy, Stuffed Crust, Asda*	1 Pizza/245g	666	30	272	13.9	26.5	12.2	2.4
Pepperoni, Mini, Tesco*	1 Serving/22g	71	3.7	323	11.8	30.5	16.8	2.7
Pepperoni, Mushroom, & Ham, GF, Goodfellas*	½ Pizza/175g	450	17.5	257	10	30	10	0
Pepperoni, Reg Crust, From Restaurant, Average	**1 Pizza/959g**	**2445**	**94**	**255**	**14.3**	**28**	**9.8**	**0**
Pepperoni, Salame, Ristorante, Dr Oetker*	½ Pizza/165g	465	23.2	281	10	28	14	0
Pepperoni, Spicy, Meat'zza, M&S*	½ Pizza/155g	431	34.3	278	12	6.7	22.1	1.9
Pepperoni, Stone Baked, Carlos*	1 Pizza/330g	832	39.6	252	13	23	12	0
Pepperoni, Stonebaked Ciabatta, Goodfella's*	½ Pizza/181g	503	26.1	278	11.9	27.4	14.4	2.4
Pepperoni, Stonebaked, 10", Sainsbury's*	½ Pizza/143g	373	15.1	260	12.2	27.7	10.5	2.7
Pepperoni, Stonebaked, 12", Sainsbury's*	¼ Pizza/103g	301	13.3	292	13.2	29.2	12.9	3.1
Pepperoni, Stonebaked, Chef Select, Lidl*	¼ Pizza/85g	209	7.4	246	11.1	29.5	8.7	2.4
Pepperoni, Takeaway, Fully Loaded, Goodfella's*	½ Pizza/251g	800	47.6	319	11	25	19	0
Pepperoni, Thin & Crispy, Sainsbury's*	½ Pizza/139g	393	18.3	282	12.5	27.6	13.1	1.8
Pepperoni, Thin & Crispy, Cucina, Aldi*	½ Pizza/170g	503	23.8	296	12	29	14	2.4
Pepperoni, Thin & Crispy, Essential, Waitrose*	½ Pizza/133g	380	18	286	12.3	28.8	13.5	1
Pepperoni, Thin & Crispy, HFC, Tesco*	½ Pizza/148g	383	13.2	258	10.6	32.8	8.9	2.4
Pollo, ad Astra, Supermarket, Pizza Express*	½ Pizza/144g	315	8.7	218	11.3	28.9	6	1.8
Pollo, Primavera, Wood Fired, Ultra Thin, M&S*	1 Pizza/185g	414	15.9	224	10.4	25.3	8.6	1.9
Pollo, Ristorante, As Sold, Dr Oetker*	½ Pizza/183g	408	16.5	223	8.8	25.7	9	1.8
Pork, 'n' Pineapple, Punchy, Freshly Prepared, Tesco*	½ Pizza/186g	510	18	274	12.4	32.9	9.7	2.7
Pork, Pulled, BBQ, Fully Loaded, Takeaway, Sainsbury's*	½ Pizza/262g	691	26.7	264	10.5	31.4	10.2	2.2
Prawn, King, Garlic, Wood Fired, Finest, Tesco*	½ Pizza/222g	471	14.7	212	10.4	26.8	6.6	2.1
Prosciutto, Cotto, Mushroom, & Mascarpone, Co-Op*	½ Pizza/239g	600	19.4	251	10	33	8.1	3
Prosciutto, Italian Style, Co-Op*	½ Pizza/183g	421	12.8	230	13	29	7	3
Prosciutto, Ristorante, Dr Oetker*	1 Pizza/330g	752	32.3	228	10.3	24.6	9.8	0
Quattro Formaggi, Ristorante, Dr Oetker*	½ Pizza/170g	457	23.8	269	10.8	24.1	14	1.6
Salame, Ristorante, Dr Oetker*	½ Pizza/160g	455	24.5	285	10.4	26.3	15.3	0
Salami, & Ham, Pizzeria, Waitrose*	½ Pizza/205g	443	13.7	216	10.1	28.7	6.7	1.8
Salami, & Pepperoni, Waitrose*	½ Pizza/190g	578	30.8	304	13.4	23.9	16.2	2.1
Salami, Milano, & 'Nduja, Sourdough, The Best, Morrisons*	½ Pizza/191g	529	24.4	277	11.9	27.2	12.8	2.6
Salami, Napoli Diavolo, Pizza, Wood Fired, M&S*	½ Pizza/244g	549	24.9	225	10.8	21.7	10.2	1.7
Salami, Ultra Thin Italian, Tesco*	1 Serving/263g	692	25.5	263	12	31.9	9.7	1
Salami, Ventricina, Truly Irresistible, Co-Op*	½ Pizza/230g	577	19.6	251	8.5	34	8.5	2.6
Selection, Slices, M&S*	1 Serving/52g	120	4.1	230	9.4	30.3	7.8	1.9

P

	Measure INFO/WEIGHT	per Measure KCAL	FAT	Nutrition Values per 100g / 100ml KCAL	PROT	CARB	FAT	FIBRE
PIZZA								
Sloppy Giuseppe, Supermarket, Pizza Express*	½ Pizza/151g	333	10.9	220	10	28.1	7.2	1.6
Smokin' Vegan, The White Rabbit Pizza Co.*	1 Pizza/340g	741	33.3	218	2.4	31.3	9.8	2.5
Spinach, & Ricotta, Classic Italian, Stonebaked, Tesco*	½ Pizza/190g	460	16.3	240	10.3	29	8.5	1.2
Spinach, & Ricotta, Extra Special, Asda*	1 Pizza/400g	940	28	235	9	34	7	1.9
Spinach, & Ricotta, Italian, Chilled, Sainsbury's*	1 Pizza/361g	859	34.7	238	9.3	28.7	9.6	2.3
Spinach, & Ricotta, Thin Crust, Italian, Tesco*	½ Pizza/190g	365	16.7	192	9.6	18.7	8.8	1.9
Spinach, & Ricotta, Stonebaked, M&S*	½ Pizza/253g	543	17.4	215	8	29.2	6.9	2.1
Supreme, Deep Dish, Individual, Chicago Town*	1 Pizza/170g	456	20.4	268	9.2	30.8	12	1
The Vegan Gardener, The White Rabbit Pizza Co.*	1 Pizza/340g	656	23.8	193	1.7	32.8	7	3.9
The Whole Hog, Deep & Loaded, M&S*	½ Pizza/345g	823	33.4	239	12.3	24.9	9.7	1.5
Truffle, Salsiccia, Truly Irresistible, Co-Op*	½ Pack/97g	296	12.6	305	13	33	13	1.2
Vegetable, & Peppers, Fire Roasted, Waitrose*	½ Pizza/235g	442	16.7	188	9.8	21.3	7.1	2.7
Vegetable, & Pesto, Chargrilled, Specially Selected, Aldi*	½ Pizza/305g	756	29	248	9.2	30	9.5	2.9
Vegetable, Average	*1 Avg Slice/70g*	*133*	*3.7*	*190*	*8.2*	*27.5*	*5.2*	*2.4*
Vegetable, Balsamic Roast, & Mozzarella, Sainsbury's*	½ Pizza/200g	444	15.6	222	8.5	29.4	7.8	2.4
Vegetable, Chargrilled, Frozen, BGTY, Sainsbury's*	1 Pizza/290g	548	13.3	189	10.2	26.7	4.6	3
Vegetable, Deep Pan, Co-Op*	1 Pizza/425g	829	29.8	195	8	25	7	2
Vegetable, Frozen, HL, Tesco*	1 Pizza/400g	604	10.8	151	8.1	23.5	2.7	4.4
Vegetable, GFY, Asda*	¼ Pizza/94g	141	2.7	150	7	24	2.9	3.7
Vegetable, Mediterranean, Pizzeria, Sainsbury's*	1 Serving/211g	397	13.5	188	8	24.7	6.4	3.2
Vegetable, Mediterranean, Stonebaked, Carlos, Aldi*	½ Pizza/173g	323	8.7	187	7.5	26.6	5	2.9
Vegetable, Mediterranean, Stonebaked, Sainsbury's*	½ Pizza/260g	622	16.4	239	9.8	35.7	6.3	3.1
Vegetable, Mediterranean, Thin & Crispy, Tesco*	½ Pizza/179g	350	10.7	195	7.1	27.3	6	2.1
Vegetable, Mediterranean, Thin Crust, Stonebaked, Tesco*	1 Pizza/359g	700	21.5	195	7.1	27.3	6	2.1
Vegetable, Romano, Goodfella's*	½ Pizza/195g	419	15	215	9	26	7.7	0
Vegetable, Salsa, Spicy, Stonebaked, Vegan, Goodfella's*	½ Pizza/181g	385	11.4	213	5.8	32	6.3	2.9
Veggie Feast, Thin Crust, Stonebaked, Asda*	½ Pizza/168g	360	13.6	214	7.9	26	8.1	3.1
Veggie Feast, Vegan, Flatbread, Asda*	1 Pizza/219g	486	15.1	222	5.6	33	6.9	3.1
Veggie Supreme, Takeaway, Tesco*	1 Slice/106g	280	11.8	264	10.4	29.9	11.1	1.4
Veggie, Very, Stonebaked, M&S*	½ Pizza/274g	537	15.9	196	7.9	27	5.8	2.1
PIZZA BASE								
Deep Pan, Italian, Sainsbury's*	1 Base/220g	684	11	311	7	59.5	5	1.4
Deep Pan, Napolina*	1 Base/260g	757	7.8	291	7.9	58	3	0.2
Everyday Value, Tesco*	½ Base/125g	401	2.8	320	9.6	65.2	2.2	0.7
Garlic Bread, Sainsbury's*	¼ Base/59g	109	4.2	186	5.1	25.4	7.1	1.8
Gluten, Wheat & Dairy Free, Free From, Livwell*	1 Base/100g	237	2.6	237	5.2	48.3	2.6	4.7
Italian, Classic, Sainsbury's*	1 Base/150g	452	7.2	301	7.6	57	4.8	1.5
Light & Crispy, Napolina*	1 Base/150g	436	4.5	291	7.9	58	3	0.2
M&S*	1 Base/150g	418	8.1	279	9.2	47.5	5.4	1.9
Mini, Napolina*	1 Base/75g	218	2.2	291	7.9	58	3	0.2
Stone Baked, GF, BFree*	½ Pizza/90g	231	2.6	257	3.5	49.2	2.9	10
Thin & Crispy, Sainsbury's*	1 Base/150g	504	7.8	336	9.9	62.3	5.2	4.3
Wholemeal, Dough, Frozen, The Northern Dough Co*	1 Base/110g	226	1.8	205	9.7	38.9	1.6	0
with Tomato Sauce, Crosta & Mollica*	½ Pizza/135g	282	4.9	209	6	40.7	3.6	3
PIZZA BASE MIX								
Morrisons*	1 Serving/77g	313	3.8	407	12.7	77.9	5	3.6
Sainsbury's*	1 Pack/145g	486	5.5	335	12.8	62.3	3.8	2.9
PLAICE								
Fillets, in Breadcrumbs, Average	*1 Serving/150g*	*331*	*17.9*	*221*	*12.8*	*15.5*	*11.9*	*0.8*
Fillets, Lightly Dusted, Average	*1 Fillet/113g*	*188*	*9.2*	*166*	*12.9*	*10.4*	*8.2*	*0.6*
Fillets, Raw, Average	*1oz/28g*	*24*	*0.4*	*87*	*18.2*	*0*	*1.5*	*0*
Goujons, Baked	*1oz/28g*	*85*	*5.1*	*304*	*8.8*	*27.7*	*18.3*	*0*
Goujons, Fried in Blended Oil	*1oz/28g*	*119*	*9*	*426*	*8.5*	*27*	*32.3*	*0*

	Measure INFO/WEIGHT	per Measure KCAL	FAT	Nutrition Values per 100g / 100ml KCAL	PROT	CARB	FAT	FIBRE
PLAICE								
Grilled	*1oz/28g*	*27*	*0.5*	*96*	*20.1*	*0*	*1.7*	*0*
in Batter, Fried in Blended Oil	*1oz/28g*	*72*	*4.7*	*257*	*15.2*	*12*	*16.8*	*0.5*
Steamed	*1oz/28g*	*26*	*0.5*	*93*	*18.9*	*0*	*1.9*	*0*
PLANTAIN								
Boiled in Unsalted Water	*1oz/28g*	*31*	*0.1*	*112*	*0.8*	*28.5*	*0.2*	*1.2*
Raw, Average	*1 Med/179g*	*218*	*0.7*	*122*	*1.3*	*31.9*	*0.4*	*2.3*
Ripe, Fried in Vegetable Oil	*1oz/28g*	*75*	*2.6*	*267*	*1.5*	*47.5*	*9.2*	*2.3*
PLATTER								
Mediterranean, Tesco*	¼ Pack/58g	119	9.5	206	6.2	5.8	16.4	5
PLUMS								
Average, Stewed without Sugar	*1oz/28g*	*8*	*0*	*30*	*0.5*	*7.3*	*0.1*	*1.3*
Fresh, Raw, Weighed without Stone, Average	*1 Plum/66g*	*24*	*0.1*	*36*	*0.6*	*8.6*	*0.1*	*1.9*
Weighed with Stone, Average	*1 Plum/90g*	*31*	*0.1*	*34*	*0.5*	*8.1*	*0.1*	*1.8*
Yellow, Waitrose*	1 Plum/50g	20	0	39	0.6	8.8	0.1	1.5
POLENTA								
Dry, Merchant Gourmet*	1 Serving/65g	232	0.9	357	7.4	78.8	1.4	1.3
POLLOCK								
Fillets, Breaded, As Prepared, Essential, Waitrose*	1 Fillet/120g	243	9.6	203	14.4	18.3	8	0
Fillets, Breaded, Cooked, Tesco*	1 Fillet/125g	315	12.2	250	15	24.4	9.7	2
Fillets, Breaded, Free From, Morrisons*	1 Fillet/135g	281	14.8	208	12.4	14.2	11	1.3
Fillets, Breaded, HFC, Tesco*	1 Fillet/128g	269	8.2	210	14.6	22.4	6.4	2.1
Fillets, British, Sainsbury's*	1 Pack/218g	157	1.3	72	16.6	0	0.6	0
Fillets, in Batter, Frozen, Chip Shop, Youngs*	1 Fillet/106g	241	14.1	228	11.6	15	13.3	1.1
Fillets, in Breadcrumbs, Boneless, Alaska, Aldi*	1 Fillet/141g	266	12.5	189	12	15	8.9	1.1
POLO								
Fruits, Nestle*	1 Tube/37g	142	0	383	0	96	0	0
Mints, Original, Nestle*	1 Sweet/2g	8	0	402	0	98.2	1	0
Spearmint, Nestle*	1 Tube/35g	141	0.4	402	0	98.2	1.1	0
POMEGRANATE								
Raw, Fresh, Flesh Only, Average	*1 Sm Fruit/86g*	*59*	*0.3*	*68*	*1*	*17.2*	*0.3*	*0.6*
Raw, Weighed with Rind & Skin, Average	*1 Sm Fruit/154g*	*59*	*0.3*	*38*	*0.5*	*9.6*	*0.2*	*0*
POMELO								
Fresh, Raw, Weighed with Skin & Seeds	*100 Grams/100g*	*11*	*0.1*	*11*	*0.2*	*2.5*	*0.1*	*0*
Raw, Flesh Only, Average	*1 Fruit/340g*	*129*	*0.1*	*38*	*0.8*	*9.6*	*0*	*1*
POP TARTS								
Chocolate, Kellogg's*	1 Pastry/50g	198	8.5	396	5	136	17	2
Cookies 'n' Creme, Kellogg's*	1 Pastry/50g	190	5	380	4	70	10	2
Frosted Blueberry, Mini Crisps, Kellogg's*	1 Pouch/23g	100	2.5	435	4.4	78.3	10.9	0
Frosted Brown Sugar Cinnamon, Kellogg's*	1 Tart/50g	210	7	420	6	68	14	2
Frosted Chocolate Fudge, Kellogg's*	1 Pastry/52g	200	5	385	5.8	71.2	9.6	1.9
Frosted Hot Fudge Sundae, Kellogg's*	1 Pastry/48g	190	4.5	396	4.2	70.8	9.4	2.1
Frosted Raspberry, Kellogg's*	1 Pastry/52g	200	5	385	3.8	73.1	9.6	1.9
Strawberry Sensation, Kellogg's*	1 Tart/50g	198	5.5	395	4	70	11	2
POPCORN								
Air Popped, Plain, Average	*1 Sm Bag/17g*	*66*	*0.8*	*387*	*12.9*	*77.9*	*4.5*	*14.5*
Butter, Microwave, Act II*	1 Bag/90g	425	16.2	472	9	69	18	9
Butter, Microwave, Butterkist*	1 Bag/70g	305	12.7	436	8.5	55.2	18.1	9.6
Butter, Microwave, Popz*	1 Serving/100g	480	27.5	480	7.5	51.1	27.5	9.2
Butter, Toffee, Belgian Milk Chocolate Coated, M&S*	1 Pack/100g	505	25	505	6.5	60.4	25	4.1
Butter, Toffee, Tesco*	1 Pack/175g	709	13.5	405	2.2	81.7	7.7	4.3
Caramel, Salted, Bloom's*	1 Bag/28g	135	6.6	483	4.9	60.3	23.4	5.8
Caramel, Salted, Butterkist*	1 Serving/20g	83	1.9	417	3.4	77.7	9.5	3.5
Caramel, Salted, Skinny, Metcalfe's Food Co*	¼ Bag/19g	85	3.6	455	8.9	57	19	10.3

POPCORN

	Measure INFO/WEIGHT	per Measure KCAL	FAT	Nutrition Values per 100g / 100ml KCAL	PROT	CARB	FAT	FIBRE
Chocolate, & Pecan, M&S*	1 Pack/27g	130	5.2	480	3.3	72.9	19.3	3.6
Cookie, Tesco*	1 Serving/25g	113	3.3	452	3.3	79	13.2	1.8
Cotton Candy, American Style, Epic*	1 Pot/150g	766	41.7	511	6.1	59.7	27.8	7
Maize, Unpopped, Love Life, Waitrose*	1 Serving/33g	200	14.1	605	6.2	48.7	42.8	12.7
Maple, Shapers, Boots*	1 Bag/20g	94	3.6	469	12	59	18	10
Peanut Butter, & Almond, Propercorn*	1 Serving/25g	115	5	460	12.9	50.2	20.2	12.9
Peanut, & Almond, Smooth, Propercorn*	1 Serving/25g	120	5.9	481	11.9	49.4	23.5	12.2
Plain, Oil Popped, Average	*1 Bag/74g*	*439*	*31.7*	*593*	*6.2*	*48.7*	*42.8*	*0*
Popping Corn, Average	*1 Serving/30g*	*112*	*1.3*	*375*	*10.9*	*73.1*	*4.3*	*12.7*
Popping Kernels, Golden Tree*	1 Serving/30g	112	1.3	375	10.9	26.8	4.3	12.7
Salt & Vinegar, Snack-A-Jacks, Quaker*	1 Sm Pack/13g	47	1.3	360	12	55	9.9	14
Salted, Blockbuster*	1 Bowl/25g	99	2.9	397	10.6	62.2	11.7	8.6
Salted, Crunch Corn, Propercorn*	1 Serving/30g	140	7.9	468	5	52.1	26.4	12.2
Salted, Diet Chef Ltd*	1 Pack/23g	107	3.8	465	10.5	68.6	16.6	14
Salted, Light, Microwave, Act II*	1 Pack/85g	336	6.5	395	10.6	71	7.6	15.8
Salted, Lightly, Popping Corn, Graze*	1 Punnet/28g	127	7	454	8	44	25	13
Salted, Lightly, Sea Salt, Wholegrain, Sunbites, Walkers*	1 Pack/20g	84	2.6	419	8.6	59.3	12.9	15.7
Salted, Lightly, Sea, Propercorn*	1 Bag/20g	85	3	424	9.3	54	15.1	17.6
Salted, Lightly, Snack-A-Jack, Quaker*	1 Bag/13g	48	1.3	370	12.1	58	9.9	14.6
Salted, Lime & Sea Salt, Captain Theodore's, Ten Acre*	1 Pack/28g	139	7	497	5.3	63.8	25	6.1
Salted, M&S*	1 Pack/25g	132	7.8	530	9.4	50.4	31.1	6.4
Salted, Manhatten Peanuts Limited*	1 Bag/30g	135	4.3	450	10	70	14.3	13.7
Salted, Microwave, Popz*	1 Serving/20g	101	6	504	7	51.5	30	9.2
Salted, Microwave, Sunsnacks*	1 Pack/100g	498	22.9	498	10.7	51.3	22.9	10.8
Salted, Sea Salt, Skinny, Topcorn, Metcalfe's Food Co*	1 Pack/23g	108	5.6	471	6.6	63.7	24.4	15.2
Salted, Simply, Protein, Natural Nutrients*	1 Bag/30g	145	6.4	483	14.7	48.7	21.3	0
Salted, Sold At Cinema, Playtime Popcorn*	1 Sm/74g	384	24.9	519	8.3	45.9	33.6	0
Sour Cream & Black Pepper, Propercorn*	1 Bag/20g	88	3.7	440	10.8	50.1	18.3	15.9
Super, Perri*	1 Pack/30g	139	7	464	8.4	55.5	23.2	8.5
Sweet & Salty, Microwave, Butterkist*	1 Pack/70g	298	14.1	425	8.2	48.5	20.2	8.4
Sweet & Salty, Propercorn*	1 Bag/30g	129	4.7	431	6.5	64.4	15.8	9.9
Sweet & Salted, Regal snacks*	1 Serving/30g	134	5	447	6.7	62	16.7	12
Sweet & Salted, Snackrite, Aldi*	1 Serving/30g	141	6	471	7.1	62	20	7.5
Sweet & Salty, Bloom's*	1 Portion/28g	138	7	492	4	58.6	25	8.5
Sweet & Salty, M&S*	1 Bag/15g	73	3.7	488	7.7	55.4	24.4	7.8
Sweet & Salty, Shapers, Boots*	1 Bag/20g	89	3.2	443	5.8	65	16	10
Sweet & Salty, Skinny Pop*	1 Pack/23g	98	3.4	424	7.2	66.7	14.8	8.9
Sweet Maple, Diet Chef Ltd*	1 Pack/23g	111	3.6	483	9.7	75.2	15.7	13
Sweet, Best-In*	1 Serving/34g	161	5.8	473	7.3	72.6	17	0
Sweet, Butterkist, Butterkist*	1 Pack/120g	612	29.8	510	2.8	68.5	24.8	5.6
Sweet, Cinema Style, Basics, Sainsbury's*	1 Handful/20g	90	4.4	450	5.9	57.5	21.8	11.1
Sweet, Cinema Style, Butterkist*	1 Bag/85g	447	22	526	5.2	65.2	25.9	5.8
Sweet, Coconut & Vanilla, Propercorn*	1 Bag/25g	122	5.5	486	6	61.6	22.1	7.7
Sweet, Deli, Passions, Aldi*	1 Bag/27g	121	4.2	448	7	74.8	15.6	10.7
Sweet, Microwave, Butterkist*	1 Pack/70g	316	15.4	452	7	53	22	7.2
Sweet, Microwave, Cinema, Popz*	1 Bag/85g	420	21.7	494	6	60	25.5	8.2
Sweet, Slightly, Popping Corn, Graze*	1 Punnet/26g	116	5.4	447	7.5	53	21	9.3
Sweet, Snackrite, Aldi*	1 Serving/30g	142	6	474	6	63	20	8.5
Toffee, Butterkist*	1 Sm Bag/50g	212	4.7	424	3.1	80.1	9.4	3.2
Toffee, Chicago Joes*	1 Serving/10g	31	0.5	314	3.1	84.6	4.8	0
Toffee, Sainsbury's*	1 Serving/50g	208	6.4	415	1.8	73.8	12.7	3.3
Toffee, Snack Pack, Butterkist*	1 Bag/25g	106	2.4	424	3.1	80.1	9.4	3.2
Tomato Ketchup, For Kids, Propercorn*	1 Pack/12g	55	2.6	459	7.8	51.7	21.6	13.2

P

	Measure INFO/WEIGHT	per Measure KCAL	FAT	Nutrition Values per 100g / 100ml KCAL	PROT	CARB	FAT	FIBRE
POPCORN								
Tomato, Sun Dried, & Chilli, Propercorn*	1 Bag/20g	88	3.7	439	8.7	50.9	18.6	16.6
Twist of Black Pepper, Graze*	1 Punnet/28g	127	7	452	8	44	25	13
Vanilla, Sweet, Protein, Natural Nutrients*	1 Pack/30g	156	7.9	522	15.7	49.5	26.5	9.7
Wholegrain, Sweet & Salty, Sunbites, Walkers*	1 Pack/30g	127	3.1	424	6.3	67.5	10.4	12.8
POPPADOMS								
Balti, Mini, Vitasia, Lidl*	½ Bag/30g	153	9.5	510	18.4	34.3	31.6	7.4
Fried in Vegetable Oil, Takeaway, Average	*1 Poppadom/13g*	*65*	*5*	*501*	*11.5*	*28.3*	*38.8*	*5.8*
Garlic & Coriander, Ready To Eat, Pappadums, Patak's*	1 Poppadom/10g	45	2.3	453	18.5	37.1	23.4	9.9
Garlic & Coriander, Ready to Eat, Sharwood's*	1 Poppadom/9g	39	1.9	438	18.4	43	21.4	6.5
Indian, Asda*	1 Pack/45g	232	15.7	516	14.5	36.2	34.8	7.8
Mango Chutney Flavour, Mini, M&S*	1 Poppadom/25g	130	8.3	518	13.1	39.9	33	4.5
Mini, Sainsbury's*	½ Pack/50g	249	16.2	498	14.9	36.9	32.3	7.6
Plain, Asda*	1 Poppadom/9g	44	2.5	484	18	40	28	0
Plain, Bilash, Aldi*	1 Poppadom/8g	36	1.8	448	20	38	22	9.7
Plain, Cook to Eat, Sharwood's*	1 Poppadom/12g	32	0.1	273	21.9	45.7	1	10.1
Plain, Indian to Go, Sainsbury's*	1 Poppadom/8g	34	1.5	405	18.4	43.4	17.5	9
Plain, Low Fat, Sharwood's*	1 Poppadom/12g	35	0.1	295	20.7	46.5	0.9	9
Plain, Mini, Cook to Eat, Sharwood's*	1 Poppadom/4g	11	0	273	21.9	45.7	0.3	10.1
Plain, Ready to Eat, Average	*2 Poppadom/16g*	*68*	*2.8*	*427*	*19.8*	*46.6*	*17.3*	*6.6*
Plain, Ready to Eat, Sharwood's*	1 Poppadom/8g	37	1.8	461	19.4	46.3	22	5.6
Plain, Tesco*	1 Serving/9g	41	2	439	17.8	44.4	21.1	4.6
Plain, Waitrose*	1 Serving/9g	37	1.7	408	21	39.3	18.6	9.1
Spicy, Cook to Eat, Sharwood's*	1 Poppadom/12g	30	0.1	257	20.2	43	0.5	13
Spicy, COU, M&S*	1 Pack/26g	84	0.6	325	23.5	51.9	2.4	8.1
Tesco*	1 Poppadom/9g	39	1.9	440	17.8	44.4	21.1	4.6
POPPETS*								
Chocolate Raisins, Poppets*	1 Pack/35g	140	4.7	401	4.9	65.4	13.3	0
Mint Cream, Poppets*	1oz/28g	119	3.6	424	2	75	13	0
Toffee, Milk Chocolate, Poppets*	1 Box/100g	491	23	491	5.3	68	23	0
PORK								
& Stuffing, Sliced, Asda*	1 Slice/53g	79	2.7	148	23	2.2	5.1	0.7
Belly, Fresh, Raw, Weighed with Skin, Average	*1 Serving/100g*	*518*	*53*	*518*	*9.3*	*0*	*53*	*0*
Belly, Hog Roast, Apple Sauce, Crackling, M&S*	½ Pack/240g	785	64.1	327	13.4	8	26.7	0.7
Belly, Roasted, Lean & Fat	*1oz/28g*	*82*	*6*	*293*	*25.1*	*0*	*21.4*	*0*
Belly, Vietnamese Style, with Sticky Caramel Sauce, M&S*	½ Pack/235g	557	40.2	237	16.4	4.4	17.1	0.5
Bites, Smoky BBQ, Fridge Raiders, Mattessons*	1 Pack/80g	196	13.6	245	17	5.7	17	0
Chop, Lean & Fat, Boneless, Raw, Average	*1oz/28g*	*67*	*3.8*	*240*	*29.2*	*0*	*13.7*	*0*
Diced, Lean, Average	*1oz/28g*	*31*	*0.5*	*109*	*22*	*0*	*1.8*	*0*
Escalope, Average	*1 Escalope/75g*	*108*	*1.7*	*144*	*31*	*0*	*2.2*	*0*
Escalope, Lean, Healthy Range, Average	*1 Escalope/75g*	*80*	*1.5*	*106*	*22*	*0*	*2*	*0*
Ham, Hock, Raw, Weighed with Bone, Fat & Skin	*100g*	*124*	*5*	*124*	*18.4*	*0*	*5*	*0*
Joint with Crackling, Ready to Roast, Average	*1 Joint/567g*	*1283*	*80.1*	*226*	*24.2*	*0.8*	*14.1*	*0*
Joint, Ready to Roast, Average	*½ Joint/254g*	*375*	*18*	*148*	*19.2*	*2.3*	*7.1*	*0.2*
Leg, Joint, Healthy Range, Average	*1 Serving/200g*	*206*	*4.4*	*103*	*20*	*0.6*	*2.2*	*0*
Loin, Applewood Smoked, Asda*	1 Slice/15g	18	0.5	122	21.8	0.5	3.6	0
Loin, Chops, Boneless, Grilled, Average	*1oz/28g*	*83*	*4.1*	*298*	*27*	*0*	*14.6*	*0*
Loin, Chops, Grilled, Lean	*1oz/28g*	*52*	*1.8*	*184*	*31.6*	*0*	*6.4*	*0*
Loin, Chops, Raw, Lean & Fat, Weighed with Bone	*1 Chop/130g*	*248*	*19.9*	*191*	*13.2*	*0*	*15.3*	*0*
Loin, Joint, Roast, Lean	*1oz/28g*	*51*	*1.9*	*182*	*30.1*	*0*	*6.8*	*0*
Loin, Joint, Roasted, Lean & Fat	*1oz/28g*	*71*	*4.3*	*253*	*26.3*	*0*	*15.3*	*0*
Loin, Peppered, Roast, Aldi*	1 Slice/20g	26	0.9	132	21	2	4.6	0.5
Loin, Steak, Cajun, Smoky, Cooked, Tesco*	½ Pack/151g	340	22.8	225	19.1	2.7	15.1	1.1
Loin, Steak, Fried, Lean	*1oz/28g*	*53*	*2*	*191*	*31.5*	*0*	*7.2*	*0*

	Measure INFO/WEIGHT	per Measure KCAL	FAT	Nutrition Values per 100g / 100ml KCAL	PROT	CARB	FAT	FIBRE
PORK								
Loin, Steak, Fried, Lean & Fat	**1oz/28g**	**77**	**5.2**	**276**	**27.5**	**0**	**18.4**	**0**
Loin, Steak, Lean, Raw, Average	**1 Serving/175g**	**345**	**19.6**	**197**	**22.7**	**0**	**11.2**	**0.4**
Loin, Steaks, Mediterranean, Grilled, Ashfield Farm, Aldi*	1 Steak/100g	288	17	288	30	3.4	17	0.5
Loin, Steaks, Smokey BBQ, Birchwood Farm, Lidl*	1 Steak/89g	190	11.5	213	19.7	4	12.9	1
Loin, with Rind, Uncooked, Average	**1 Serving/100g**	**246**	**18.8**	**246**	**19.3**	**0**	**18.8**	**0**
Medallions, Average	**1 Medallion/125g**	**140**	**2.6**	**112**	**22.6**	**0**	**2**	**0**
Mince, Lean, Healthy Range, Average	**1 Pack/400g**	**504**	**20.2**	**126**	**19.8**	**0.4**	**5**	**0.3**
Mince, Raw	**1oz/28g**	**46**	**2.7**	**164**	**19.2**	**0**	**9.7**	**0**
Mince, Stewed	**1oz/28g**	**53**	**2.9**	**191**	**24.4**	**0**	**10.4**	**0**
Patties, Breakfast, Frozen, Oakhurst, Aldi*	1 Pattie/45g	132	9.4	293	25	1.6	21	0.5
Pulled, BBQ, Sweet, 585g, Asda*	¼ Pack/107g	247	10.3	231	23	13	9.6	0.5
Pulled, with BBQ Sauce, Boneless, British, Tesco*	1 Serving/150g	256	11.2	171	17.3	8.5	7.5	0
Pulled, with BBQ Sauce, Shoulder, British, Sainsbury's*	1 Serving/120g	290	18.1	242	24.6	1.6	15.1	0.5
Raw, Lean, Average	**1oz/28g**	**42**	**1.2**	**151**	**28.6**	**0**	**4.1**	**0**
Roast, Lean Only, Average	**1oz/28g**	**34**	**0.9**	**121**	**22.7**	**0.3**	**3.3**	**0**
Roast, Slices, Average	**1 Slice/30g**	**40**	**1.4**	**134**	**22.7**	**0.4**	**4.5**	**0**
Saltimbocca, Easy to Cook, Waitrose*	½ Pack/120g	187	5.8	156	28	0.2	4.8	0.1
Schnitzel, Viennese, Aldi*	1 Schnitzel/107g	162	5	151	16.8	9.4	4.7	0
Shoulder, Boneless, Average	**1 Piece/430g**	**127**	**3.4**	**127**	**22.5**	**0**	**3.4**	**0**
Shoulder, Whole, Lean & Fat, Raw, Average	**100g**	**236**	**18**	**236**	**17.2**	**0**	**18**	**0**
Shoulder, Whole, Lean Only, Roasted	**1 Serving/150g**	**345**	**20.3**	**230**	**25.3**	**0**	**13.5**	**0**
Steak, Lean & Fat, Average	**1oz/28g**	**61**	**3.8**	**219**	**23.8**	**0**	**13.7**	**0.1**
Steak, Lean, Stewed	**1oz/28g**	**49**	**1.3**	**176**	**33.6**	**0**	**4.6**	**0**
Steak, Loin, BBQ Chinese, Tesco*	1 Steak/81g	219	14.4	270	21.9	5.3	17.7	1.1
Stir Fry Strips, Lean, Healthy Range, Average	**¼ Pack/113g**	**118**	**2.3**	**104**	**21.3**	**0**	**2**	**0**
Tenderloin, Lean, Boneless, Raw, Average	**1 Serving/100g**	**109**	**2.2**	**109**	**21**	**0**	**2.2**	**0**
PORK DINNER								
Roast, 103, Oakhouse Foods Ltd*	1 Dinner/400g	376	14.8	94	6.7	8.3	3.7	1.4
Roast, Birds Eye*	1 Pack/340g	410	12	121	7.6	14.7	3.5	1.6
PORK IN								
Gravy, & Baby Potatoes, Carrots, & Savoy Cabbage, M&S*	1 Pack395g	288	9.9	73	6.2	5.7	2.5	1.6
Mustard & Cream, Chops	**1oz/28g**	**73**	**6**	**261**	**14.5**	**2.4**	**21.6**	**0.3**
PORK SCRATCHINGS								
Crispy Strips, Mr Porky*	1 Bag/20g	102	5.7	508	62.4	0.6	28.4	0
Crunch, Mr Porky*	1 Pack/25g	129	6.9	515	65.7	0.6	27.7	0
KP Snacks*	1 Pack/20g	125	9.6	624	47.3	0.5	48.1	0.5
Pn, Proteinium*	1 Bag/30g	156	7.9	520	69.7	0.1	26.2	0
Puffs, Spicy BBQ, The Curators*	1 Pack/25g	128	7.1	513	60.3	10	28.4	1
PORT								
Average	**1 Serving/50ml**	**78**	**0**	**157**	**0.1**	**12**	**0**	**0**
White, Average	**1 Glass/125ml**	**182**	**0**	**146**	**0.1**	**11**	**0**	**0**
POT NOODLE*								
Beef & Tomato, King, Made Up, Pot Noodle*	1 Pot/420g	543	19.8	129	3.3	18.5	4.7	1.1
Beef & Tomato, Made Up, Pot Noodle*	1 Pot/320g	426	14.7	133	3.4	19.4	4.6	1.3
Bombay Bad Boy, King, Made Up , Pot Noodle*	1 Pot/420g	542	19.7	129	3.3	18.5	4.7	1.1
Bombay Bad Boy, Made Up, Pot Noodle*	1 Pot/320g	415	15.3	130	3.3	18.4	4.8	1.1
Chicken & Mushroom, King, Made Up, Pot Noodle*	1 Pack/420g	545	19.3	130	3.3	18.8	4.6	1
Chicken & Mushroom, Made Up, Pot Noodle*	1 Pot/305g	430	18	141	3	19	5.9	1
Chilli Beef, Made Up, Pot Noodle*	1 Pot/305g	384	14.6	126	3	17.7	4.8	0.8
Chow Mein Chinese, Made Up, Pot Noodle*	1 Pot/320g	416	14.7	130	3.2	19	4.6	1.3
Curry, Original, King, Made Up, Pot Noodle*	1 Pot/420g	507	18.1	121	2.6	17.9	4.3	1
Curry, Original, Made Up, Pot Noodle*	1 Pot/320g	431	15	135	3.1	20	4.7	1.2
Curry, Spicy, Made Up, Pot Noodle*	1 Pot/300g	393	14.4	131	2.9	19.1	4.8	1.1

	Measure INFO/WEIGHT	per Measure KCAL	FAT	Nutrition Values per 100g / 100ml KCAL	PROT	CARB	FAT	FIBRE
POT NOODLE*								
Piri Piri Chicken, Made Up, Pot Noodle*	1 Pot/307g	430	15.4	140	3	20	5	0
Sweet & Sour, Oriental, Posh, Made Up, Pot Noodle*	1 Pot/300g	375	13.8	125	1.7	19.2	4.6	0.5
POTATO BOMBAY								
Average	*½ Pack/150g*	*176*	*10.2*	*117*	*2*	*13.7*	*6.8*	*1.2*
Indian, Cooked, Sainsbury's*	½ Pack/150g	132	7.4	95	1.6	7.8	5.3	4.9
Indian, Waitrose*	½ Pack/150g	125	5.4	83	1.6	9.7	3.6	3
Tesco*	1 Pack/300g	240	12.6	80	1.3	9.3	4.2	2.1
POTATO CAKES								
Average	*1 Cake/70g*	*127*	*1.2*	*180*	*3.8*	*37.5*	*1.7*	*2.4*
Fried, Average	*1oz/28g*	*66*	*2.5*	*237*	*4.9*	*35*	*9*	*0.8*
POTATO SALAD								
& Egg, with Mayonnaise, Tesco*	½ Tub/150g	115	8.5	77	2.9	3.1	5.7	1.2
& Yoghurt, Meadow Fresh, Lidl*	1 Portion/50g	72	4	144	1.8	15.4	8	1.8
Asda*	¼ Pot/57g	67	4	117	0.9	12.5	7	1.1
Baby, Finest, Tesco*	¼ Pack/69g	143	11.8	206	1.4	11.3	17	0.7
Charlotte, TTD, Sainsbury's*	½ Pack/150g	212	14.1	141	2	11	9.4	2
Creamy, Asda*	½ Tub/150g	226	16	151	1.1	11.3	10.7	2.5
Creamy, Waitrose*	1 Serving/100g	163	11.9	163	1.3	12.7	11.9	1.1
From Restaurant, Average	*1/3 Cup/95g*	*108*	*5.7*	*114*	*1.5*	*13.5*	*6*	*0*
New, Co-Op*	1 Serving/50g	98	8	195	1	10	16	2
Reduced Calorie, Pre Packed	*1oz/28g*	*27*	*1.1*	*97*	*1.3*	*14.8*	*4.1*	*0.8*
Tesco*	1 Serving/50g	90	7.1	179	1	11.1	14.2	1.3
with Mayonnaise, Retail	*1oz/28g*	*80*	*7.4*	*287*	*1.5*	*11.4*	*26.5*	*0.8*
POTATO SKINS								
Cheese & Bacon, Loaded, Asda*	½ Pack/125g	275	15	220	13	15	12	3.3
Cheese & Chive, Sainsbury's*	2 Skins/150g	286	17.8	191	7.7	13.3	11.9	2.8
Cheese, & Jalapeno, Bannisters*	1 Skin/65g	92	4.1	142	5.9	14.1	6.3	2.4
with Sour Cream	*1 Serving/275g*	*541*	*34.6*	*197*	*7.2*	*13.8*	*12.6*	*2.2*
POTATO WAFFLES								
Frozen, Cooked	*1oz/28g*	*56*	*2.3*	*200*	*3.2*	*30.3*	*8.2*	*2.3*
Sweet Potato, Birds Eye*	1 Waffle/59g	150	9.4	255	2.2	24	16	2.9
Uncooked, Average	*1 Waffle/62g*	*113*	*5.1*	*182*	*2.4*	*24.4*	*8.3*	*1.8*
POTATO WEDGES								
Aldi*	1 Serving/100g	150	6.8	150	2.1	20.2	6.8	0
Crispy, M&S*	1 Serving/200g	340	14.2	170	1.3	25.3	7.1	1.7
Fiery & Filthy, Wicked Kitchen, Tesco*	½ Pack/219g	285	7.2	130	2.1	21.5	3.3	3.1
Frozen, Average	*1 Serving/120g*	*145*	*4.1*	*121*	*2*	*20.5*	*3.4*	*2.2*
Harvest Basket, Lidl*	1 Serving/100g	147	5.7	147	2.2	20.5	5.7	2.5
Spicy, Asda*	1 Serving/100g	145	5.7	145	1.8	21.8	5.7	2.1
POTATOES								
Alphabites, Captain Birds Eye, Birds Eye*	9 Bites/56g	75	3	134	2	19.5	5.3	1.4
Anya, Raw, TTD, Sainsbury's*	1 Serving/100g	75	0.3	75	1.5	17.8	0.3	1.1
Baby, Herby, Microwave, Nature's Pick, Aldi*	½ Pack/193g	171	3.5	89	2.2	15	1.8	2.2
Baby, Herby, Microwaved, Growers Selection, Asda*	1 Pack/360g	198	4.7	55	2	7.4	1.3	2.8
Baby, New with Butter, Mint & Parsley, Organic, Asda*	1 Pack/360g	414	10.4	115	1.7	20.4	2.9	2.5
Baby, with Butter & Herbs, Sainsbury's*	¼ Pack/148g	103	0.9	70	1.9	14.2	0.6	2
Baby, with Herbs & Butter, Morrisons*	1 Serving/100g	94	2.3	94	1.9	14.6	2.3	1.9
Baked, & Cheese, Waitrose*	½ Pack/220g	281	8.6	128	3.7	18.1	3.9	2.6
Baked, Chilli Con Carne, COU, M&S*	1 Pack/300g	270	6.3	90	6	11.1	2.1	1.2
Baked, Flesh & Skin, Average	*1 Med/200g*	*218*	*0.2*	*109*	*2.3*	*25.2*	*0.1*	*2.4*
Baked, Flesh Only, Weighed with Skin, Average	*1oz/28g*	*20*	*0*	*72*	*1.5*	*16.6*	*0.1*	*1.2*
Baked, Ham & Cheddar Cheese, Asda*	1 Pack/300g	435	11.1	145	7	21	3.7	1.6
Baked, in Microwave, Flesh & Skin, Average	*1oz/28g*	*29*	*0*	*105*	*2.4*	*24.1*	*0.1*	*2.3*

POTATOES

INFO/WEIGHT	Measure	per Measure KCAL	FAT	Nutrition Values per 100g / 100ml KCAL	PROT	CARB	FAT	FIBRE
Baked, in Microwave, Flesh Only, Average	*1oz/28g*	*28*	*0*	*100*	*2.1*	*23.3*	*0.1*	*1.6*
Baked, in Microwave, Skin Only, Average	*1oz/28g*	*37*	*0*	*132*	*4.4*	*29.6*	*0.1*	*5.5*
Baked, Jacket, with Cheese, Asda*	1 Serving/225g	243	5.8	108	3.9	16	2.6	2.5
Baked, Mature Cheddar Cheese, M&S*	½ Pack/206g	225	6.6	109	3.6	16.9	3.2	1
Baked, Skin Only, Average	*1oz/28g*	*55*	*0*	*198*	*4.3*	*46.1*	*0.1*	*7.9*
Baked, Stuffed, Mini, Tesco*	1 Serving/108g	130	6.3	120	2.3	14.6	5.8	2.3
Baked, Tuna & Sweetcorn, Average	*1 Serving/300g*	*273*	*6.8*	*91*	*5*	*12.6*	*2.2*	*0.9*
Baked, Tuna & Sweetcorn, Morrisons*	1 Serving/300g	243	2.1	81	5.1	13.5	0.7	0
Baked, with Cheese & Butter, Tesco*	1 Potato/214g	212	4.2	99	3	16.4	2	1.9
Baking, Raw, Average	*1 Med/250g*	*198*	*0.2*	*79*	*2.1*	*18*	*0.1*	*1.6*
Boiled with Skin	*1 Potato/125g*	*98*	*0.1*	*78*	*2.9*	*17.2*	*0.1*	*3.3*
Boiled, Average	*1 Serving/120g*	*86*	*0.1*	*72*	*1.8*	*17*	*0.1*	*1.2*
Boulangere, M&S*	½ Pack/225g	180	2	80	2.8	15.9	0.9	0.9
Charlotte, Average	*1 Serving/184g*	*139*	*0.5*	*76*	*1.6*	*17.4*	*0.2*	*3.3*
Chorizo, Ready to Roast, Sainsbury's*	½ Pack/141g	165	8.7	117	3.1	10.9	6.2	2.5
Crispy Slices, M&S*	1 Pack/450g	922	53.1	205	2.5	21.5	11.8	1.4
Crispy, & Seasoned Vegetable Mix, Tesco*	1 Serving/80g	114	6.6	143	1.9	13.5	8.3	3.6
Crispy, Pops, HFC, Tesco*	¼ Pack/111g	215	8.2	194	2.8	27.8	7.4	2.2
Dauphinoise, Average	*1 Serving/200g*	*335*	*23.9*	*168*	*2.2*	*12.8*	*12*	*1.5*
Dauphinoise, Finest, Tesco*	½ Pack/186g	299	18.6	161	2.9	13.9	10	1.5
Dauphinoise, Iceland*	½ Pack/201g	336	23.3	167	3.6	11.2	11.6	1.3
Dauphinoise, Maris Piper, The Best, Morrisons*	½ Pack/190g	375	27.4	197	2.7	13.5	14.4	1.5
Desiree, Average	*1 Serving/200g*	*152*	*0.4*	*76*	*2.2*	*16.4*	*0.2*	*0.6*
Fritters, Crispy, Oven Baked, Birds Eye*	1 Fritter/20g	29	1.6	145	2	16.3	8	1.2
Hasselback, Average	*1 Serving/175g*	*182*	*1.6*	*104*	*1.9*	*22*	*0.9*	*2.9*
Hassleback, Dine in Side, Eat Well, M&S*	½ Pack/175g	195	6	110	2.1	18.3	3.4	1.9
Jacket, Little, Bannisters*	1 Potato/115g	93	0.2	81	3	15.5	0.2	2.6
Jersey Royal, Canned, Average	*1 Can/186g*	*116*	*0.2*	*62*	*1.4*	*14*	*0.1*	*1.2*
Jersey Royal, New, Raw, Average	*1oz/28g*	*21*	*0.1*	*75*	*1.6*	*17.2*	*0.2*	*1.5*
Lattices, Golden, Oven Baked, Asda*	1/6 Pack/91g	180	7.3	198	3	26	8	5.1
Lattices, Tesco*	¼ Pack/103g	221	8.4	215	3	29.8	8.2	5.2
Maris Piper, Raw, Average	*1 Serving/200g*	*151*	*0.4*	*75*	*2*	*16.5*	*0.2*	*1.4*
Mash, Buttery, Creamy, Finest, Tesco*	½ Pack/215g	219	9.5	102	2	13	4.4	1.3
Mash, Creamy, Maris Piper, Extra Special, Asda*	½ Pack/200g	202	10	101	1.3	12	5	2.3
Mash, Creamy, Morrisons*	½ Pack/243g	386	24.3	159	2.1	14.2	10	1.6
Mashed, Buttery, Seasoned, Classic Cuisine, Aldi*	½ Pack/225g	207	8.6	92	1.6	12	3.8	1.3
Mashed, Cheddar, TTD, Sainsbury's*	½ Pack/226g	323	19.7	143	3.8	11.5	8.7	1.9
Mashed, From Restaurant, Average	*1/3 Cup/80g*	*66*	*1*	*83*	*2.3*	*16.1*	*1.2*	*0*
Mashed, From Supermarket, Healthy Range, Average	*1 Serving/200g*	*160*	*3.1*	*80*	*1.8*	*14.6*	*1.6*	*1.3*
Mashed, Home Prepared with Whole Milk	*1 Cup/210g*	*162*	*1.2*	*77*	*1.9*	*17.6*	*0.6*	*2*
Mashed, Instant, Stockwell & Co., Tesco*	1 Serving/201g	135	1.2	67	1.9	12.6	0.6	2.1
Mashed, Jersey Butter & Black Pepper, TTD, Sainsbury's*	½ Pack/225g	243	13.7	108	1.4	11.2	6.1	1.5
Mashed, Made Up with Water, Average	*1 Serving/180g*	*118*	*0.3*	*66*	*1.7*	*14.5*	*0.2*	*1.3*
Mashed, Mash Direct*	½ Pack/200g	190	3.8	95	1.7	17.7	1.9	1.3
Mashed, Original, Dry Weight, Smash*	1 Serving/30g	101	0.3	343	8.3	71.8	1	6.7
Mashed, with Cream & Butter, Ultimate, M&S*	½ Pack/225g	268	13.7	119	2.5	12.8	6.1	1.2
New, & Vegetables, M&S*	1 Pot/170g	76	3.2	45	1.1	4.8	1.9	1.9
New, Average	*1 Serving/100g*	*75*	*0.3*	*75*	*1.5*	*17.8*	*0.3*	*1.1*
New, Baby, Average	*1 Serving/180g*	*135*	*0.5*	*75*	*1.7*	*17*	*0.3*	*1.6*
New, Baby, Canned, Average	*1 Can/120g*	*69*	*0.2*	*58*	*1.4*	*12.9*	*0.2*	*1.4*
New, Easy Steam with Herbs & Butter, Tesco*	1 Serving/125g	94	3.5	75	1.8	9.6	2.8	1.7
New, Garlic, Herb & Parsley Butter, Co-Op*	1 Serving/100g	115	5	115	1	15	5	2
New, with Herbs & Butter, Asda*	½ Pack/170g	146	2.9	86	1.7	16	1.7	1.5

	Measure INFO/WEIGHT	per Measure KCAL	FAT	Nutrition Values per 100g / 100ml KCAL	PROT	CARB	FAT	FIBRE
POTATOES								
Pan Fried, Aldi*	1 Serving/250g	182	2	73	2.7	13.7	0.8	0
Raw, Peeled, Flesh Only	*1 Serving/100g*	*75*	*0.2*	*75*	*2*	*17.3*	*0.2*	*1.4*
Red, Flesh Only, Average	*1 Serving/300g*	*218*	*0.4*	*72*	*2*	*16.4*	*0.2*	*1.2*
Roast, Basted in Beef Dripping, Waitrose*	1 Serving/165g	213	8.9	129	2.2	18	5.4	1.9
Roast, Dry, No Oil, No fat	*1 Serving/100g*	*79*	*0.1*	*79*	*2.7*	*18*	*0.1*	*1.6*
Roast, Frozen, Average	*1 Potato/70g*	*105*	*3.5*	*149*	*2.6*	*23.5*	*5*	*1.4*
Roast, Garlic & Rosemary, Miniature, Tesco*	¼ Pack/125g	85	0.9	68	1.8	12.5	0.7	2.3
Roast, in Lard, Average	*1oz/28g*	*42*	*1.3*	*149*	*2.9*	*25.9*	*4.5*	*1.8*
Roast, in Oil, Average	*1oz/28g*	*42*	*1.3*	*149*	*2.9*	*25.9*	*4.5*	*1.8*
Roast, New, Rosemary, Ainsley Harriott*	1 Serving/150g	133	4	89	2	16	2.7	1.3
Roast, with Goose Fat, TTD, Sainsbury's*	½ Pack/185g	216	4.4	117	2.7	21.1	2.4	3
Roasting, Average	*1 Serving/150g*	*202*	*5.2*	*135*	*2.5*	*23.4*	*3.5*	*1.6*
Saute, with Onion & Bacon, Country Supper, Waitrose*	¼ Pack/100g	112	4.3	112	1.9	16.4	4.3	1.3
Scallops, Battered, Deep Fried, Average	*1 Scallop/67g*	*216*	*14.5*	*323*	*5.4*	*27.3*	*21.6*	*0*
Slices, in Rich Crispy Batter, Crispy, Chilled, Sainsbury's*	¼ Pack/100g	223	10.8	223	2.6	27.3	10.8	2.8
Smiles, Weighed Baked, McCain*	1 Serving/100g	237	10.1	237	3.4	33.4	10.1	3.1
Smiles, Weighed Frozen, McCain*	1 Serving/100g	191	8	191	2.6	27	8	2.7
Vivaldi, Baked with Skin, TTD, Sainsbury's*	1 Potato/180g	248	0.4	138	3.8	28.8	0.2	2.7
White, Raw, Flesh & Skin	*1 Lge/369g*	*284*	*0.3*	*77*	*2*	*17.5*	*0.1*	*2.2*
White, Raw, Weighed with Skin, Flesh Only, Average	*1 Med/213g*	*153*	*0.3*	*72*	*1.9*	*16.1*	*0.2*	*1.2*
POUSSIN								
Meat & Skin, Raw, Average	*1oz/28g*	*57*	*3.9*	*202*	*19.1*	*0*	*13.9*	*0*
Spatchcock, British, Waitrose*	½ Poussin/225g	364	20.2	162	19	1.2	9	0
POWERADE								
Berry & Tropical Fruit, Coca-Cola*	1 Bottle/500ml	90	0	18	0	4.1	0	0
Isotonic, Sports Drink, Coca-Cola*	1 Bottle/500ml	120	0	24	0	5.6	0	0
PRAWN COCKTAIL								
BGTY, Sainsbury's*	½ Pot/85g	119	7.9	140	9.1	4.7	9.3	0.5
Delicious, Boots*	1 Pack/250g	285	6.5	114	5.5	17	2.6	1.2
in Marie Rose Sauce, Rich & Creamy, Waitrose*	½ Pot/100g	338	32.2	338	9.1	2.7	32.2	0.5
International Seafood Co, Morrisons*	½ Pot/90g	316	30.6	351	8.3	3	34	0
King, Extra Special, Asda*	1 Pack/204g	474	22.5	232	8.9	23	11	1.8
LC, Tesco*	1 Pot/140g	210	16	150	7.5	4.3	11.4	1.3
Reduced Fat, M&S*	1 Pack/200g	296	20	148	9.9	4.5	10	0.5
PRAWN CRACKERS								
Asda*	1 Serving/25g	134	8.8	535	2	53	35	0
M&S*	1 Bag/50g	262	15.6	525	2.8	57.4	31.3	0.8
Meal for Two, Meal Box, Tesco*	½ Pack/23g	127	8	554	2	57.3	35	1.1
Ready to Eat, Sharwood's*	1 Bag/60g	316	18.5	527	0.5	62	30.8	1.2
Sainsbury's*	1 Cracker/3g	16	1	537	2.4	60.4	31.7	0.8
Sainsbury's*	1 Serving/25g	134	7.8	534	2.1	60.8	31.3	0.6
Snackrite, Aldi*	1 Pack/25g	136	8	546	2.6	61	32	1.1
PRAWN TOAST								
from Chinese Selection, Ken Hom, Tesco*	1 Toast/14g	50	3.8	364	11	17.1	27.4	2.6
Mini, Oriental Selection, Party, Iceland*	1 Toast/15g	52	3.6	345	10.5	22	23.9	2.1
Oriental Selection, Sainsbury's*	1 Toast/31g	119	9.1	385	10.1	18.8	29.5	2.1
Sesame Prawn, Toasted Triangles, M&S*	1 Pack/220g	616	39.6	280	12.4	17.3	18	2
Sesame, Oriental Snack Selection, Sainsbury's*	1 Toast/12g	40	2.7	335	9.3	23	22.9	5.1
PRAWNS								
Batter Crisp, Lyons*	1 Pack/160g	350	20.3	219	8	18.2	12.7	1.1
Boiled	*1 Prawn/3g*	*3*	*0*	*99*	*22.6*	*0*	*0.9*	*0*
Breaded, Coconut, Oven Baked, Sainsbury's*	½ Pack/84g	214	10.7	255	12.3	22.3	12.7	1.4
Cooked & Peeled, Average	*1oz/28g*	*21*	*0.2*	*77*	*17.6*	*0.2*	*0.6*	*0*

P

	Measure INFO/WEIGHT	per Measure KCAL	FAT	Nutrition Values per 100g / 100ml KCAL	PROT	CARB	FAT	FIBRE
PRAWNS								
Hot & Spicy, Average	*1 Serving/170g*	*461*	*26.9*	*271*	*9.4*	*22.8*	*15.8*	*2.2*
Icelandic, Raw, Average	*1oz/28g*	*30*	*0.4*	*106*	*22.7*	*0*	*1.6*	*0*
King, & Scallops, Lemon & Pink Peppercorn Butter, Youngs	½ Pack/81g	155	10.5	191	17.9	0.6	12.9	0.8
King, Breaded	*1 Prawn/13g*	*33*	*1.8*	*260*	*15.1*	*17.8*	*14*	*1.2*
King, Garlic Marinated, Specially Selected, Aldi*	½ Pack/95g	114	2.8	120	21	1.6	3	0.5
King, Raw, Average	*1 Bag/200g*	*145*	*1.9*	*72*	*15.8*	*0.2*	*1*	*0.1*
King, Tandoori, Average	*1 Prawn/59g*	*33*	*0.6*	*55*	*5.7*	*5.9*	*1.1*	*0.7*
North Atlantic, Peeled, Cooked, Average	*1oz/28g*	*22*	*0.3*	*80*	*17.5*	*0*	*1.1*	*0*
North Atlantic, Raw, Average	*1oz/28g*	*17*	*0.1*	*62*	*14.4*	*0*	*0.4*	*0*
Tiger, Cooked & Peeled, Average	*1 Pack/180g*	*151*	*2*	*84*	*18.4*	*0.1*	*1.1*	*0*
Tiger, Jumbo, Average	*1 Serving/50g*	*39*	*0.2*	*78*	*18.2*	*0.3*	*0.5*	*0*
Tiger, Raw, Average	*1 Prawn/30g*	*19*	*0.2*	*64*	*14.2*	*0*	*0.7*	*0*
Tiger, Tempura, M&S*	1 Prawn/18g	49	3.1	274	8.8	20.1	17.3	1.2
PRAWNS CHILLI								
& Coriander, Cooked & Peeled, Tesco*	1 Pack/160g	144	3.4	90	16.7	0.2	2.1	0.5
Crispy, with Sweet Chilli Dipping Sauce, M&S*	1 Pack/240g	490	20.2	204	8.2	23.6	8.4	0.6
King, Chilli & Coriander Marinated, Just Add, M&S*	1 Pack/80g	82	2.1	102	19	0.1	2.6	0
King, with a Sweet Chilli Sauce, Succulent, Birds Eye*	1 Serving/140g	251	17.2	179	10.5	6.5	12.3	0.1
Skewers, Sweet Chilli, King, BBQ Favourites, Asda*	1 Skewer/48g	48	0.5	100	16.6	5.4	1.1	1
PRAWNS IN								
Creamy Garlic Sauce, Youngs*	1 Serving/158g	261	22.9	165	8.5	0.3	14.5	0
PRAWNS WITH								
Chilli, Coriander & Lime, King, Waitrose*	1 Pack/140g	143	3.2	102	19.9	0.5	2.3	0.6
Ginger & Spring Onion, Sainsbury's*	1 Pack/300g	198	9.3	66	4.7	4.7	3.1	0.3
King, with a Creamy Cocktail Sauce, M&S*	1 Pack/120g	278	23.3	232	12.6	1.3	19.4	1.1
King, with Garlic Butter, M&S*	1 Serving/100g	165	9	165	12.5	9.1	9	0.5
PRESERVE								
Bramble, Seedless, Mackays*	1 Tsp/5g	13	0	269	0.3	66.8	0.1	0
Ginger Shred, Robertsons*	1 Tsp/15g	40	0	267	0.1	66	0	0
Ginger, Asda*	1 Serving/15g	39	0.1	261	0.5	63	0.5	1.7
Rhubarb & Ginger, Mackays Ltd*	1 Serving/10g	27	0	269	0.3	66.7	0	0
PRETZELS								
American Style, Salted, Sainsbury's*	1 Serving/50g	202	2.2	403	10.8	79.7	4.5	1.8
Bavarian, Bakery Instore, Lidl*	1 Pretzel/85g	251	5	295	9.4	50.6	5.9	0
Bites, Rock Salt, Indie bay snacks *	1 Pack/26g	99	1.1	381	13.1	71.2	4.2	3.1
Jumbo, Tesco*	1 Serving/50g	194	3.4	388	9.7	71.9	6.8	5.4
Mini, M&S*	1 Pack/45g	194	6	430	10.4	66.6	13.4	4.9
Pieces, Jalapeno, Snyders*	1 Pack/125g	590	23.3	472	7.1	67.4	18.6	3.2
Plain, Bakery, Tesco*	1 Pretzel/108g	316	5.8	293	9.5	50.3	5.4	2.7
Salted, Average	*1 Serving/30g*	*114*	*0.8*	*380*	*10.3*	*79.8*	*2.6*	*3*
Salted, Mini, M&S*	1 Pack/25g	96	0.5	382	10.9	78	2.1	3.9
Salted, Sainsbury's*	1 Serving/30g	118	1.3	393	10.3	76.7	4.2	3.6
Soft, Cheddar & Red Onion, Knot, New York Bakery Co*	1 Pretzel/59g	168	2.5	284	11.8	46.7	4.3	5.3
Soft, Cinnamon Sugar, Auntie Anne's*	1 Pretzel/112g	380	1	339	7.1	75	0.9	1.8
Soft, Salted, Original, Auntie Anne's*	1 Pretzel/112g	310	1	277	7.1	58	0.9	1.8
Sour Cream & Onion, M&S*	1 Serving/30g	136	4.4	455	11	70.9	14.5	0.7
Sour Cream & Chive, Penn State Pretzels*	1 Serving/25g	111	3.2	443	8.9	71.8	12.9	2
Turkey, Emmental, & Avocado, Finest, Tesco*	1 Pretzel/192g	487	21.9	254	13.1	23.9	11.4	1.6
Wheat, GF, Trufree*	1 Bag/60g	282	12	470	0.5	72	20	0.7
PRINGLES*								
Barbecue, Pringles*	1 Serving/50g	266	18	533	4.9	48	36	5.1
BBQ Spare Rib, Rice Infusions, Pringles*	1 Pack/23g	108	5.3	469	5.1	60	23	2.6
Cheese & Onion, Pringles*	1 Serving/25g	132	8.5	528	4.1	50	34	3.4

	Measure INFO/WEIGHT	per Measure KCAL	FAT	Nutrition Values per 100g / 100ml KCAL	PROT	CARB	FAT	FIBRE
PRINGLES*								
Hot & Spicy, Pringles*	1 Serving/25g	132	8.5	530	4.6	49	34	3.7
Light, Original, Pringles*	1 Serving/25g	121	6.2	484	4.3	59	25	3.6
Light, Sour Cream & Onion, Pringles*	1 Serving/25g	122	6.2	487	4.7	57	25	3.6
Margarita Pizza, Classic Takeaways, Pringles*	1 Serving/25g	134	8	538	3.9	53	32	2.6
Minis, Original, Pringles*	1 Pack/23g	118	6.9	514	5.1	55	30	3.7
Minis, Sour Cream & Onion, Pringles*	1 Pack/23g	118	6.7	511	5.2	56	29	3.5
Original, Pringles*	1 Serving/25g	130	8.5	522	3.8	51	34	2.6
Paprika, Pringles*	1 Serving/25g	132	8.5	529	4.9	49	34	6.5
Peking Duck with Hoisin Sauce, Rice Fusions, Pringles*	1 Serving/30g	146	8.1	485	4.4	55	27	2.5
Prawn Cocktail, Pringles*	1 Serving/25g	130	8	518	4.1	53	32	2.5
Salt & Pepper, Pringles*	1oz/28g	143	9	511	4.4	50	32	2.8
Salt & Vinegar, Pringles*	1 Serving/25g	128	8	512	3.9	52	32	2.4
Sour Cream & Onion, Pringles*	1 Serving/30g	153	9.6	509	3.9	52	32	2.6
Texas BBQ Sauce, Pringles*	1 Serving/25g	132	8.5	527	4.2	50	34	3.5
PROFITEROLES								
12 Chocolate, Waitrose*	3 Profiteroles/65g	284	21.4	437	6	28.7	33	0.4
Asda*	1 Serving/64g	218	17.2	343	5	20	27	0
Black Forest, Tesco*	1 Profiterole/19g	71	4.3	374	4.9	37.4	22.6	0.7
Chocolate, 8 Pack, Co-Op*	¼ Pack/112g	330	17.9	295	6	31	16	2
Chocolate, Sainsbury's*	1/6 Pot/95g	192	8.5	202	5.4	25.1	8.9	0.8
Chocolate, Stack, Sainsbury's*	¼ Pack/76g	311	19.5	409	5.3	39.3	25.6	2
Chocolate, Tesco*	4 Profiteroles/59g	202	16.1	343	5.2	18.5	27.4	1
Choux & Chocolate Sauce, Tesco*	1 Serving/77g	295	22	386	5.1	26.9	28.7	0.5
Classic French, Sainsbury's*	1 Serving/90g	284	15.5	316	6.6	33.7	17.2	0.1
Filled with Cream, Stack, Fresh, M&S*	1 Serving/75g	303	22.8	404	5.6	26.3	30.4	1.5
in a Pot, Waitrose*	1 Pot/80g	207	11.3	259	6.3	25.6	14.1	2.9
Savoury with Cheese & Chive, CBY, Asda*	¼ Pack/15g	95	7.7	634	9.1	32.1	51.3	3.5
Waitrose*	4 Profiteroles/75g	269	17.9	359	4.8	31.1	23.9	0.7
PROSECCO								
12%, Average	*1 Sm/125ml*	*112*	*0*	*89*	*0*	*1.4*	*0*	*0*
PRUNES								
Dried, Average	*1 Prune/7g*	*11*	*0*	*158*	*2.5*	*36.4*	*0.4*	*5.8*
in Apple Juice, Average	*1 Serving/90g*	*76*	*0.1*	*84*	*0.8*	*19.8*	*0.1*	*1.4*
in Fruit Juice, Average	*1oz/28g*	*24*	*0*	*86*	*0.9*	*20.9*	*0.2*	*2.9*
in Syrup, Average	*1oz/28g*	*25*	*0*	*89*	*0.9*	*21.5*	*0.2*	*2.6*
Stewed with Sugar	*1oz/28g*	*29*	*0.1*	*103*	*1.3*	*25.5*	*0.2*	*3.1*
Stewed without Sugar	*1oz/28g*	*23*	*0.1*	*81*	*1.4*	*19.5*	*0.3*	*3.3*
PUDDING								
Apple, & Sultana, Steamed, BGTY, Sainsbury's*	1 Pudding/110g	294	3.2	267	2.9	57.4	2.9	0.8
Beef, & Onion, Minced, Hollands*	1 Pudding/165g	353	19	214	6.5	20.6	11.5	0
Black Forest, Brilliant, Graze*	1 Punnet/37g	97	3.3	262	4	40	9	2
Bread, Retail Average	*1 Slice/120g*	*301*	*8*	*251*	*8.4*	*41.8*	*6.7*	*0.5*
Chocolate, Brownie, Waitrose*	1 Serving/98g	391	24.8	399	4.5	37.7	25.3	1
Chocolate, Fudge, Pot, Pots & Co*	1 Pot/125g	495	30	396	3.8	40	24	2.4
Chocolate, Ganache, Mini Pot, Gu*	1 Pot/45g	199	16.6	442	3.3	26.4	36.8	2.3
Chocolate, M&S*	¼ Pudding/76g	265	12	350	4.1	48	15.8	2.1
Chocolate, Melt in The Middle, Frozen, Waitrose*	1 Pudding/90g	310	14.4	344	6.7	41.4	16	3.5
Chocolate, Melt in The Middle, Mini, Tesco*	1 Pudding/20g	85	5.9	427	7.5	30.2	29.5	5.5
Chocolate, Melting Middle, Hot, Puds, Gu*	1 Pud/100g	409	26.9	409	6	36	26.9	2.7
Chocolate, Melting Middle, M&S*	1 Pudding/155g	510	27.8	330	5.8	36.2	18	3.1
Chocolate, No Moo, Iceland*	1 Pudding/80g	298	18.4	372	5.6	35	23	0.8
Eve's, Average	*1oz/28g*	*67*	*3.7*	*241*	*3.5*	*28.9*	*13.1*	*1.4*
Eves, with Apple Compote, Sainsbury's*	1 Pot/110g	256	9	235	3.2	36.2	8.3	1.2

PUDDING

INFO/WEIGHT	Measure	per Measure KCAL	FAT	Nutrition Values per 100g / 100ml KCAL	PROT	CARB	FAT	FIBRE
Fruit, Corniche, Ace Synergy International Pte Ltd *	1 Pot/80g	67	0	84	0.3	21	0	0
Ginger, Sticky, with Ginger Syrup Sauce, Sainsbury's*	1 Pudding/110g	363	9.5	331	3.2	59.5	8.7	0.9
Gingerbread, & Butterscotch, Melt, Finest, Tesco*	½ Pudding/113g	440	14.6	390	4.9	62.6	12.9	1.7
Golden Syrup, Steamed, Aunty's*	1 Pudding/100g	293	4.1	293	3.3	57.3	4.1	0.8
Jam, Roly Poly, Sainsbury's*	¼ Pack/81g	291	11.5	359	4.4	53.3	14.2	0.5
Queen of Puddings	*1oz/28g*	*60*	*2.2*	*213*	*4.8*	*33.1*	*7.8*	*0.2*
Roly Poly, Jam, Aunt Bessie's*	1 Serving/75g	278	9	370	3.6	62	12	1.4
Souffle, Hot Chocolate, Gu*	1 Pot/65g	298	23.5	458	6	24.1	36.2	2.5
Sponge, Chocolate, with Chocolate Sauce, Sainsbury's*	1 Pudding/107g	382	17.1	356	4.3	48.1	15.9	1.8
Sponge, Spotted Dick, Asda*	1 Pudding/95g	401	21.9	422	4.4	489	23	1.7
Sponge, Winterberry, Individual, Morrisons*	1 Pudding/110g	284	9.5	258	3.7	41	8.6	1
Sponge, with Golden Syrup, Individual, Mr Kipling*	1 Pudding/95g	395	16.7	366	3.1	53.1	15.5	0.6
Sponge, with Raspberry Jam, Individual, Mr Kipling*	1 Pudding/108g	392	16.8	363	3.1	52.4	15.6	0.7
Steak, & Kidney, 407, Oakhouse Foods Ltd*	1 Serving/190g	519	36.1	273	7.1	17.7	19	1.2
Sticky Toffee, Co-Op*	¼ Pudding/100g	355	20	355	3	40	20	0.7
Sticky Toffee, Deluxe, Lidl*	½ Pudding/225g	806	36	358	2.5	50	16	2.1
Sticky Toffee, Extra Special, Asda*	¼ Pudding/100g	378	18	378	1.9	52	18	1.8
Sticky Toffee, Indulgent, Specially Selected, Aldi*	¼ Pudding/112g	387	14.6	344	2.6	54	13	1.5
Sticky Toffee, Puree, Wiltshire Farm Foods*	1 Pack/155g	277	17	179	1.4	19	11	0
Sticky Toffee, Steamed, Aunty's*	1 Pudding/110g	331	5.3	301	2.6	58.4	4.8	1.2
Sticky Toffee, Tesco*	1 Serving/110g	287	14.7	261	3.3	31.8	13.4	0.7
Sticky Toffee, with Toffee Sauce, TTD, Sainsbury's*	¼ Pudding/111g	395	16.8	355	3	50.8	15.1	2
Strawberry, Jelly Pud, with Devon Custard, Ambrosia*	1 Pot/150g	129	1.2	86	0.7	19.4	0.8	0
Suet, Average	*1oz/28g*	*94*	*5.1*	*335*	*4.4*	*40.5*	*18.3*	*0.9*
Summer Fruits, Eat Well, M&S*	1 Pudding/135g	128	0.7	95	1.7	20.8	0.5	3
Summer, Waitrose*	1 Pot/120g	125	0.5	104	2	23.1	0.4	1.4
Syrup, M&S*	1 Serving/105g	370	10.5	352	3.9	61.7	10	0.8
Torte, Cheeky Little Chocolate, Gu*	1 Pud/50g	211	14.6	422	5.7	31.6	29.1	1.8

PUMPKIN

INFO/WEIGHT	Measure	per Measure KCAL	FAT	Nutrition Values per 100g / 100ml KCAL	PROT	CARB	FAT	FIBRE
Boiled in Salted Water	*1oz/28g*	*4*	*0.1*	*13*	*0.6*	*2.1*	*0.3*	*1.1*
Potimarron, Raw, Average	*1 Serving/80g*	*21*	*0.1*	*26*	*1*	*6.5*	*0.1*	*1.9*
Puree, Baking Buddy*	1 Serving/53g	22	0	42	1.7	6.7	0	2.5

	Measure INFO/WEIGHT	per Measure KCAL	FAT	Nutrition Values per 100g / 100ml KCAL	PROT	CARB	FAT	FIBRE
QUAVERS								
Cheese, Walkers*	1 Bag/20g	107	6	534	2.7	62.5	30.1	1.1
Prawn Cocktail, Walkers*	1 Bag/16g	88	5.1	537	2.1	62	31	1.2
QUESADILLA								
Chicken, from Restaurant, Average	*1 Serving/300g*	*867*	*46.7*	*289*	*15.6*	*22.2*	*15.6*	*1.7*
Meal Kit, Toasted Cheese, Old El Paso*	1 Quesadilla/63g	135	2.1	215	6.6	38.4	3.4	2.2
QUICHE								
Asparagus, & Mushroom, Tesco*	½ Quiche/200g	474	32.8	237	5.1	17.2	16.4	1.2
Asparagus, & Vegetable, Herby Summer, Higgidy*	1 Quiche/400g	848	50	212	5.9	18.9	12.5	2.7
Bacon, & Cheese, Sainsbury's*	¼ Quiche/100g	237	15	237	7	18.6	15	0.7
Bacon, & Leek, From Our Deli, As Consumed, Morrisons*	1 Quiche/160g	435	28	272	7.8	20	17.5	1.6
Bacon, Cheese, & Tomato, Asda*	1/3 Pack/133g	345	22.6	259	6.5	20	17	0.7
Bacon, Leek & Mushroom, M&S*	¼ Quiche/100g	245	16.4	245	6.9	17.2	16.4	1.3
Bacon, Smoked & Mature Cheddar, Higgidy*	1 Quiche/400g	1096	74	274	8.4	18.6	18.5	1.5
Broccoli, & Ricotta, Crustless, Gail's*	100g	139	11.5	139	5.2	3.8	11.5	0
Broccoli, Tesco*	1 Serving/100g	249	17.2	249	6	17.6	17.2	1.4
Broccoli, Tomato and Cheese, Classic, Sainsbury's*	1 Serving/100g	223	14.5	223	5.3	17.1	14.5	1.6
Butternut, Kale, & Chilli, Crustless, Tesco*	1 Quiche/160g	345	22.8	216	8.7	12.3	14.3	1.7
Cheddar, & Bacon, Crustless, Crestwood, Aldi*	¼ Quiche/85g	242	16	285	12.9	15.3	18.8	0.6
Cheddar, Somerset, & Tomato, Jon Thorners*	½ Quiche/200g	436	24	218	8.2	14	12	0
Cheese, & Bacon, Crustless, Tesco*	¼ Quiche/85g	196	13.4	230	9.8	11.8	15.7	1.5
Cheese, & Broccoli, Morrisons*	1/3 Quiche/134g	338	22.4	253	7.1	18.4	16.8	1.7
Cheese, & Egg	*1oz/28g*	*88*	*6.2*	*314*	*12.5*	*17.3*	*22.2*	*0.6*
Cheese, & Leek, & Chive, Sainsbury's*	1/3 Quiche/125g	292	20.2	234	7.1	14.9	16.2	1.3
Cheese, & Onion, Caramelised Onion, Finest, Tesco*	¼ Quiche/100g	300	18.6	300	9.4	22.4	18.6	1.7
Cheese, & Onion, Co-Op*	¼ Quiche/88g	262	19.2	300	10	17	22	1
Cheese, & Onion, Crustless, Deli, Morrisons*	1 Quiche/388g	1005	68.3	259	9.7	14.9	17.6	1
Cheese, & Onion, Crustless, Weight Watchers*	1 Quiche/160g	267	12.3	167	11.3	11.1	7.7	4.3
Cheese, & Onion, Finest, Tesco*	1 Serving/130g	346	24.3	266	9.1	15.3	18.7	2.5
Cheese, & Onion, HL, Tesco*	¼ Quiche/100g	180	7.8	180	9.4	17.6	7.8	1.8
Cheese, & Onion, Individual, Sainsbury's*	1 Quiche/170g	434	26	255	7.3	21.7	15.3	1.2
Cheese, & Onion, M&S*	1 Slice/100g	250	17.2	250	8.2	16.1	17.2	1.5
Cheese, & Onion, Mature Cheddar, Crustless, Higgidy*	¼ Quiche/95g	254	16.9	267	7.4	18.7	17.8	1
Cheese, & Onion, Reduced Fat, Eat Smart, Morrisons*	1 Quiche/400g	824	36.8	206	7.7	16.9	9.2	0.7
Cheese, & Onion, Retail, Average	*¼ Quiche/100g*	*262*	*17.8*	*262*	*8.4*	*17.1*	*17.8*	*1.3*
Cheese, & Onion, Value, Tesco*	½ Quiche/200g	526	36.4	263	8.6	16.1	18.2	0.7
Cheese, & Onion, Weight Watchers*	1 Quiche/165g	325	15.3	197	7	21.2	9.3	1.6
Cheese, & Tomato, Retail, Average	*¼ Quiche/100g*	*268*	*17.1*	*268*	*8*	*20.2*	*17.1*	*1.1*
Cheese, & Bacon, Crustless, Ovenbaked, Iceland*	¼ Quiche/85g	178	11.8	209	9.5	11.4	13.9	0.5
Cheese, & Onion, Crustless, Tesco*	¼ Quiche/85g	211	14.4	249	10.8	12.8	16.9	1.2
Cheese, & Onion, Individual, Morrisons*	1 Quiche/170g	502	32.8	295	9.2	20.4	19.3	1.3
Cheese, & Onion, Ovenbaked, Asda*	1/3 Quiche/134g	330	20	247	8.3	19	15	1.3
Cherry Tomato, & Mozzarella, Crustless, Booths*	¼ Quiche/85g	155	9	182	7.8	13.5	10.6	0.9
Goats Cheese, & Caramelised Onion, The Best, Morrisons*	¼ Quiche/113g	420	30.2	373	8.9	23.5	26.8	1.1
Goats Cheese, & Red Pepper, Morrisons*	1 Quiche/160g	450	29.9	281	7	20.7	18.7	1.1
Lorraine , Chef Select, Lidl*	1 Serving/100g	290	18.2	290	12.6	18.3	18.2	1.2
Lorraine, 400g, Morrisons*	¼ Quiche/100g	323	23.7	323	9	17.9	23.7	0.9
Lorraine, Asda*	¼ Quiche/100g	246	16.2	246	6.6	18.5	16.2	4.2
Lorraine, BGTY, Sainsbury's*	1 Serving/128g	273	14	213	10.9	17.7	10.9	0.7
Lorraine, Castle Grove, Lidl*	½ Pie/200g	578	40	289	11	16	20	0.5
Lorraine, Classic , Crestwood, Aldi*	¼ Quiche/100g	283	18	283	13	18	18	0.9
Lorraine, Classics, M&S*	¼ Quiche/100g	251	16.4	251	10.3	15	16.4	0.9
Lorraine, Co-Op*	¼ Quiche/100g	275	20.6	275	8.1	14.9	20.6	2.6
Lorraine, Crustless, Asda*	1 Quiche/160g	259	12.6	162	9.3	13.5	7.9	1.1

	Measure INFO/WEIGHT	per Measure KCAL	FAT	Nutrition Values per 100g / 100ml KCAL	PROT	CARB	FAT	FIBRE
QUICHE								
Lorraine, Crustless, Individual, 150g, Sainsbury's*	1 Quiche/150g	369	23.7	246	10.6	15	15.8	0.7
Lorraine, Crustless, LC, Tesco*	1 Pack/160g	280	13.4	175	12.6	11.8	8.4	2.5
Lorraine, Crustless, You Count, Love Life, Waitrose*	1 Quiche/160g	295	15.4	185	8.9	15.2	9.6	0.9
Lorraine, Extra Special, Asda*	¼ Quiche/100g	270	18	270	8	19	18	2.3
Lorraine, Finest, Tesco*	1 Serving/100g	330	25.1	330	8.4	17.5	25.1	1.5
Lorraine, Individual, Tesco*	1 Quiche/160g	424	27.1	265	10.6	16.9	16.9	1.5
Lorraine, Retail, Average	**¼ Quiche/100g**	**280**	**19.5**	**280**	**9**	**16.8**	**19.5**	**2**
Lorraine, Smoked Bacon & Cheese, M&S*	¼ Quiche/100g	270	18.4	270	9.7	16.4	18.4	1.6
Lorraine, Tesco*	½ Quiche/88g	249	16.6	285	9.3	18.2	19	1.9
Lorraine, TTD, Sainsbury's*	¼ Quiche/100g	286	18.9	286	10.2	18.4	18.9	1.2
Lorraine, West Country Cheddar, Maple Cured Bacon, Aldi*	¼ Quiche/100g	303	20	303	11	19	20	0.9
Mushroom	**1oz/28g**	**80**	**5.5**	**284**	**10**	**18.3**	**19.5**	**0.9**
Mushroom, Medley, Waitrose*	¼ Quiche/100g	222	15.2	222	6.4	15	15.2	2.9
Salmon, & Spinach, Sainsbury's*	1/3 Quiche/125g	318	21.9	254	8.2	15.9	17.5	1
Salmon, & Spinach, Smoked, Little, Higgidy*	1 Quiche/155g	448	31.5	289	8.6	17.5	20.3	0.9
Scotch Egg, Tesco*	1 Quiche/180g	494	31	274	10.7	18.7	17.2	1.2
Spanish, 501, Oakhouse Foods Ltd*	1 Serving/117g	252	14.6	216	7.7	18.2	12.5	0.8
Spinach, & Red Pepper, Goats Cheese, Waitrose*	1 Serving/100g	218	14.3	218	6.5	15.8	14.3	2.6
Spinach, & Ricotta, Tesco*	¼ Quiche/100g	237	14.9	237	5.8	19.9	14.9	1
Spinach, & Roast Red Pepper, Little, Higgidy*	1 Quiche/155g	397	27.3	256	9.1	15.2	17.6	1.2
Spinach, Edamame, & Kale, Crustless, Tesco*	1 Quiche/160g	350	22.2	219	8.7	13.9	13.8	2.2
Spinach, Feta, & Roasted Red Pepper, Higgidy*	½ Quiche/200g	526	35.8	263	8.8	17.4	17.9	1.8
Spinach, Feta, & Roasted Tomato, Higgidy*	1 Quiche/155g	435	29.3	281	10.2	20	18.9	1.8
Swiss Gruyere, & Cheddar, Best Ever, M&S*	¼ Quiche/100g	274	18.2	274	13	13	18.2	1.2
Tomato, & Goats Cheese, Shortcrust, Waitrose*	¼ Quiche/100g	271	18.3	271	5.9	20.1	18.3	1
Tomato, Mozzarella, & Pesto, Crustless, Morrisons*	¼ Quiche/85g	201	13.9	237	8.2	13.6	16.4	1.1
Vegetable, & Sundried Tomato, Tesco*	¼ Quiche/100g	211	12.9	211	6.7	16.4	12.9	1.3
Vegetable, Mediterranean Style, Classic, Sainsbury's*	1 Quiche/400g	868	50.4	217	6.2	19.8	12.6	2.2
QUINCE								
Average	**1 Avg fruit/209g**	**37**	**0.1**	**18**	**0.2**	**4.3**	**0.1**	**1.3**
QUINOA								
Cajun, Good Grains, Worldwide Foods, Aldi*	½ Pack/110g	185	3.5	168	7.7	24	3.2	6.4
Dry Weight, Average	**1 Serving/70g**	**258**	**4.2**	**368**	**14.1**	**64.2**	**6.1**	**7**
Mediterranean, Aldi*	1 Pack/125g	179	5.1	143	4.1	20.8	4.1	3.2
Red	**1 Serving/100g**	**358**	**6**	**358**	**12.9**	**62.2**	**6**	**9.7**
Red & White, Microwaveable, Good Grains, Aldi*	½ Pouch/125g	239	4.6	191	6	32	3.7	2.7
White, Red, & Black, Cooked, Sainsbury's*	1 Serving/120g	176	3.2	147	5.2	23.3	2.7	4.2
Wholegrain, Pilau Style, Express, Quinola, Mothergrain*	½ Pack/125g	179	5.1	143	4.7	19.4	4.1	4.6

Q

	Measure INFO/WEIGHT	per Measure KCAL	FAT	Nutrition Values per 100g / 100ml KCAL	PROT	CARB	FAT	FIBRE
RABBIT								
Meat Only, Raw	*1oz/28g*	*38*	*1.5*	*137*	*21.9*	*0*	*5.5*	*0*
Meat Only, Raw, Weighed with Bone	1 Serving/200g	164	6.6	82	13.1	0	3.3	0
Meat Only, Stewed	*1oz/28g*	*32*	*0.9*	*114*	*21.2*	*0*	*3.2*	*0*
Meat Only, Stewed, Weighed with Bone	*1oz/28g*	*11*	*0.3*	*41*	*7.6*	*0*	*1.1*	*0*
RADISH								
Black, Raw, Average	*1 Lge/9g*	*1*	*0*	*16*	*1*	*3*	*0*	*2*
Mixed, Vibrant & Peppery, Waitrose*	1 Serving/35g	5	0.1	14	0.7	1.9	0.2	0.9
Red, Unprepared, Average	*1 Radish/8g*	*1*	*0*	*11*	*0.6*	*1.7*	*0.2*	*0.8*
White, Mooli, Raw	*1oz/28g*	*4*	*0*	*13*	*0.7*	*2.5*	*0.1*	*0*
RAISINS								
& Sultanas, Jumbo, M&S*	1 Serving/80g	212	0.4	265	2.4	62.4	0.5	2.6
& Sultanas, The Fruit Factory*	1 Box/14g	43	0.1	305	3	72.3	0.5	4
Flame, Tesco*	1 Serving/30g	86	0	288	3.7	66	0	4.2
Lime Infused, Tangy, Nak'd*	1 Pack/25g	68	0	272	2.1	69.3	0	0
Milk Chocolate, Belgian, M&S*	½ Pack/63g	274	9.6	438	4.6	68.9	15.3	2.9
Seedless, Average	*1 Serving/75g*	*215*	*0.4*	*287*	*2.2*	*68.5*	*0.5*	*3.2*
Yoghurt Coated, Fruit Bowl*	1 Pack/25g	114	4.8	455	2	67	19	3
RAITA								
Cucumber & Mint, Patak's*	1oz/28g	18	0.5	64	3.4	8.4	1.8	0
Dip, Indian, Asda*	1 Pot/70g	120	11.5	172	2.6	3.6	16.4	0.5
Plain, Average	*1oz/28g*	*16*	*0.6*	*57*	*4.2*	*5.8*	*2.2*	*0*
RASPBERRIES								
Fresh, Raw, Average	*1 Serving/80g*	*20*	*0.2*	*25*	*1.3*	*4.7*	*0.3*	*6.5*
Frozen, Average	*1 Serving/100g*	*27*	*0.3*	*27*	*1.3*	*4.7*	*0.3*	*5.2*
in Juice, Canned, Morrisons*	½ Can/150g	81	0.3	54	0.4	12	0.2	1.4
RATATOUILLE								
Average	*1oz/28g*	*23*	*2*	*82*	*1.3*	*3.8*	*7*	*1.8*
Provencale, Canned, Cassegrain*	½ Can/188g	156	9.6	83	1.5	5.9	5.1	3.9
RAVIOLI								
Asparagus, & Mozzarella, Dell'ugo*	½ Pack/125g	220	5.4	176	6.8	26.3	4.3	2.8
Asparagus, Waitrose*	1 Serving/150g	303	9	202	10.5	26.4	6	2
Beef	*1 Serving/300g*	*501*	*13.7*	*167*	*6.4*	*25*	*4.6*	*1.4*
Beef, & Red Wine, Italiano, Tesco*	½ Pack/200g	424	13	212	7.3	30	6.5	2.3
Beef, in Tomato Sauce, Heinz*	½ Can/200g	147	3.2	74	2.5	12	1.6	0.8
Butternut Squash, & Marjoram , M&S*	½ Pack/125g	336	15.5	269	8.9	29.2	12.4	2.5
Cheese, & Spinach, G&B, Asda*	1 Pack/368g	302	8.5	82	3.3	11	2.3	1.9
Cheese, & Tomato, Canned, Sainsbury's*	½ Can/200g	170	2	85	3.5	15	1	0.9
Cheese, Four, in Tomato Sauce, COU, M&S*	1 Pack/345g	352	7.6	102	7.5	12.3	2.2	1.5
Cheese, Four, Meal for One, M&S*	1 Pack/375g	668	36.8	178	6.2	15.6	9.8	1.1
Chicken, & Bacon, Cucina, Aldi*	1 Pack/250g	455	14	182	6.9	24.7	5.6	2.7
Crab, & Crayfish, Dell'ugo*	½ Pack/125g	266	10.4	213	12.6	21.5	8.3	0.7
Gorgonzola, & Walnut, M&S*	½ Pack/125g	345	15.8	276	10.6	29.2	12.6	1.5
Mushroom, Porcini, & Spinach, Dell'ugo*	½ Pack/125g	162	1.2	130	3.9	27.1	1	3.1
Spinach, & Ricotta, Waitrose*	1 Serving/125g	309	9	247	10.5	35	7.2	1.9
Spinach, & Ricotta, GF, Made Without Wheat, M&S*	½ Pack/125g	311	12	249	8	29.6	9.6	6
Spinach, GF, Co-Op*	1 Pack/300g	507	18.6	169	5.6	22	6.2	3
Tomato, & Pancetta, Boiled, Tesco*	½ Pack/225g	394	9.7	175	7.5	25.2	4.3	3
RAVIOLINI								
Pumpkin, & Sage, GF, Ugo*	½ Pack/125g	214	3.4	171	2.3	29.8	2.7	9.3
REDCURRANTS								
Raw, Average	*1oz/28g*	*6*	*0*	*20*	*1.1*	*4.3*	*0*	*3.3*
Raw, Stalks Removed	*1 Serving/100g*	*21*	*0*	*21*	*1.1*	*4.4*	*0*	*0*

R

	Measure INFO/WEIGHT	per Measure KCAL	FAT	Nutrition Values per 100g / 100ml KCAL	PROT	CARB	FAT	FIBRE
RELISH								
Barbeque, Sainsbury's*	1 Serving/50g	50	1	100	1	19.3	2.1	1.1
Beetroot, & Horseradish , Tracklements*	2 Tsp/25g	46	0	186	1.7	41.3	0.2	3.1
Corn, Spicy, Stonewall Kitchen*	1 Tbsp/15g	18	0	117	0	26.7	0	0
Onion, Red, Caramelised, Burger, Branston*	1 Squeeze/15g	23	0.2	151	0.8	32	1.4	1.4
Onion, Red, Caramelised, Tesco*	1 Serving/10g	28	0	280	0.6	69.1	0.1	0.7
Onion, Sainsbury's*	1 Serving/15g	23	0.1	151	0.9	36	0.4	0.7
Onion, Sweet, Branston, Crosse & Blackwell*	1 Serving/10g	15	0	153	1	36.3	0.4	0.7
Sweetcorn, American Style, Maryland, Tesco*	1 Serving/15g	15	0	101	1.1	23.9	0.1	0.9
Sweetcorn, Bick's*	1 Tbsp/22g	23	0	103	1.3	24.3	0.2	0
Tomato, Spicy, Bick's*	1 Serving/28g	28	0.1	99	1.3	23.2	0.2	0
Tomato, Sweet, Heinz*	1 Serving/25g	34	0	136	0.9	32.6	0.2	0.9
REVELS								
Mars*	1 Pack/35g	169	7.4	483	5.2	67.6	21	0
RHUBARB								
Chunks, Frozen, Picard*	1 Serving/80g	11	0.4	14	1	1.4	0.5	2.3
In Juice, Canned, Drained, Average	*1 Serving/100g*	*46*	*0*	*46*	*0.5*	*10.8*	*0*	*0.8*
Stewed with Sugar, Average	*1oz/28g*	*32*	*0*	*116*	*0.4*	*31.2*	*0*	*2*
RIBENA*								
Blackcurrant Juice Drink, Ready Made, Ribena*	1 Carton/200ml	82	0	41	0	10.6	0	0
Blackcurrant, Diluted with Water, Ribena*	1 Serving/100ml	46	0	46	0	11.4	0	0
Blackcurrant, Original, Undiluted, Ribena*	1 Serving/50ml	108	0	216	0	53	0	0
Blackcurrant, Really Light, No Added Sugar, Ribena*	1 Carton/250ml	8	0	3	0	0.8	0	0
Light, Ribena*	1 Carton/288ml	26	0	9	0.1	2.1	0	0
Pineapple & Passion Fruit, Juice Drink, Ribena*	½ Bottle/250ml	103	0	41	0	9.9	0	0
Strawberry Juice Drink, Ribena*	1 Carton/288ml	12	0	4	0	0.5	0	0
RIBS								
Beef, Boneless, with Bourbon BBQ Sauce, Asda*	½ Pack/137g	386	23.3	282	26	6.2	17	0.5
Peking, Taste of China, Tesco*	½ Pack/104g	222	12.4	214	16.4	10.1	12	0
Pork, Barbecue, Meat Only, Cooked, Average	*1 Serving/130g*	*360*	*23.4*	*275*	*21.4*	*7.2*	*17.9*	*0.3*
Pork, BBQ, New York, Tesco*	½ Pack/112g	328	22.6	293	22.5	5.1	20.2	0.5
Pork, Chinese Style, Average	*1 Serving/300g*	*736*	*44.7*	*245*	*17.9*	*10*	*14.9*	*0.7*
Pork, Chops, Raw, Lean & Fat, Weighed with Bone	*1 Chop/130g*	*241*	*16.1*	*186*	*18.5*	*0*	*12.4*	*0*
Pork, Full Rack, Sainsbury's*	1 Serving/225g	567	38.7	252	18	6.5	17.2	0.9
Pork, Peking, Rack, Tesco*	4-6 Ribs/108g	228	15.8	211	18.2	1.3	14.6	0.7
Pork, Smokey BBQ, Slow Cooked, Sainsbury's*	½ Pack/165g	455	25.6	276	24.8	8.7	15.5	1
Pork, Smoky BBQ, Rack, Tex Mex, Tesco*	½ Pack/158g	337	21.1	213	17.6	5.6	13.3	0.2
Spare, Barbecue, Chinese Style, Farmfoods*	1 Pack/400g	464	25.2	116	9.3	5.6	6.3	0.1
Spare, Cantonese, Mini, Sainsbury's*	1 Rib/38g	97	5	259	17.2	17.3	13.4	1
Spare, Chinese Style, Summer Eating, Asda*	1 Serving/116g	334	18.6	288	32	4.1	16	0.8
Spare, Sweet, Sticky, Mini, M&S*	½ Pack/75g	215	12.9	286	22.7	9.8	17.2	0.8
Veggie, BBQ, Sweet n Smoky, Ribz, Plant Power*	1 Serving/150g	244	8.8	163	10.4	14.9	5.9	3.2
RICE								
& Lentils, Thai Green Curry Inspired, Twistd*	1 Pot/250g	268	4.5	107	3.9	17.8	1.8	2.3
Arborio, Dry, Average	*1 Serving/80g*	*279*	*0.6*	*348*	*7.1*	*78.3*	*0.8*	*0.8*
Basmati, & Wild, Cooked, Sainsbury's*	½ Pack/125g	150	0.8	120	3.1	25.7	0.6	1.3
Basmati, & Wild, Dry Weight, Tilda*	1 Serving/70g	244	0.3	349	9.4	77	0.5	1
Basmati, Boil in the Bag, Dry, Average	*1 Serving/50g*	*176*	*0.4*	*352*	*8.4*	*77.8*	*0.8*	*0.4*
Basmati, Brown, Dry, Average	*1 Serving/50g*	*177*	*1.5*	*353*	*9.5*	*71.8*	*3*	*2.2*
Basmati, Cooked, Average	*1 Serving/140g*	*190*	*3.9*	*136*	*2.4*	*25.6*	*2.8*	*0.8*
Basmati, Dry Weight, Average	*1 Serving/60g*	*212*	*0.6*	*353*	*8.1*	*77.9*	*1*	*0.6*
Basmati, Indian, Dry, Average	*1 Serving/75g*	*260*	*0.7*	*346*	*8.4*	*76.1*	*0.9*	*0.1*
Basmati, Lemon & Herb, Steamed, Tilda*	1 Serving/125g	172	2.8	137	2.6	26.1	2.2	1.2
Basmati, Microwave, Cooked, Average	*1 Serving/125g*	*182*	*2.3*	*146*	*2.7*	*30*	*1.8*	*0*

R

RICE

INFO/WEIGHT	Measure	per Measure		Nutrition Values per 100g / 100ml				
		KCAL	FAT	KCAL	PROT	CARB	FAT	FIBRE
Basmati, Peri Peri, Tilda*	1 Pack/250g	325	6.2	130	2.5	23.5	2.5	1.8
Basmati, White, Dry, Average	**1 Serving/75g**	**262**	**0.4**	**349**	**8.1**	**77.1**	**0.6**	**2.2**
Basmati, Wholegrain & Wild, Pouch, Tilda*	½ Pack/125g	160	2.6	128	3	23.4	2.1	1.7
Basmati, Wholegrain, Cooked, Tilda*	1 Portion/180g	203	1.6	113	3.3	23	0.9	3.2
Basmati, with Mushroom, Dine In, Veetee*	1 Pack/280g	372	6.4	133	3.3	24.4	2.3	1.2
Basmati, Microwave Pouch, Sainsbury's*	1 Pouch/125g	170	1.5	136	3.2	27.6	1.2	0.9
Brown, Cooked, Average	**1 Serving/140g**	**173**	**1.5**	**123**	**2.6**	**26.6**	**1.1**	**0.9**
Brown, Dry, Average	**1 Serving/75g**	**266**	**2.3**	**355**	**7.5**	**76.2**	**3**	**1.4**
Brown, Long Grain, Dry, Average	**1 Serving/50g**	**182**	**1.4**	**364**	**7.6**	**76.8**	**2.8**	**2**
Brown, Short Grain, Dry, Average	**1 Serving/50g**	**176**	**1.4**	**351**	**6.8**	**77.6**	**2.8**	**1**
Brown, Whole Grain, Cooked, Average	**1 Serving/170g**	**223**	**1.9**	**132**	**2.6**	**27.8**	**1.1**	**1.2**
Brown, Whole Grain, Dry, Average	**1 Serving/40g**	**138**	**1.2**	**344**	**7.4**	**71.6**	**2.9**	**3**
Brown, Whole Grain, Dry, Worldwide Foods, Aldi*	1 Serving/75g	262	2.1	349	8.3	71	2.8	3.6
Brown, with Cauliflower, & Mixed Pulses, Spiced, Waitrose*	½ Pack/150g	203	6.6	135	5.4	15.3	4.4	6.3
Cauliflower, & Parsley, Lets Cook, Aldi*	1 Pack/250g	85	0	34	2.9	2.1	0	2.7
Cauliflower, British, Nature's Pick, Aldi*	½ Pack/150g	58	0.8	39	2.8	4.7	0.5	2
Cauliflower, Frozen, Tesco*	1 Sachet/125g	30	0.2	24	1.8	2.1	0.2	3.2
Cauliflower, Mediterranean, Cauli Rice*	½ Pack100g	46	1.1	46	4	5.8	1.1	2.5
Cauliflower, Microwaved, G&B, Asda*	½ Pack/200g	68	1.8	34	2.9	2.1	0.9	2.7
Cauliflower, Original, Cauli Rice*	1 Serving/100g	34	0.9	34	3.6	3	0.9	1.8
Chicken, & Sweetcorn, Microwave, Sainsbury's*	½ Pack/125g	204	2.6	163	3.9	31.2	2.1	1.9
Chicken, & Sweetcorn, Microwave, Tesco*	½ Pack/125g	204	2.6	163	3.4	31.4	2.1	2.2
Chicken, Savoury, Batchelors*	1 Pack/124g	455	1.9	367	8.9	79.4	1.5	2.6
Chickpea, Harissa & Lemon, Pulses & Rice, Tilda*	1 Pack/140g	139	4.3	99	3.8	11.6	3.1	4.9
Chilli, & Garlic, One Pan, Meal Kit, Old El Paso*	¼ Pack/89g	185	1.1	208	4.7	43.1	1.2	2.8
Chinese Style, Express, Uncle Ben's*	1 Pack/250g	392	5.5	157	3.4	30.9	2.2	0.4
Coconut, & Lime Leaf, Thai, Cook*	1 Serving/160g	228	6.5	143	2.3	24.1	4.1	0.5
Coconut, Chilli, & Lemongrass, Worldwide Foods, Aldi*	½ Pack/125g	218	5.7	174	2.8	29	4.6	2
Curry, Special, Worldwide Foods, Aldi*	½ Pack/125g	194	2	155	3	31	1.6	1.7
Duck, Chicken, & Pork, Fried, Celebration, Sainsbury's*	1 Pack/450g	544	16.2	121	7.9	14.2	3.6	1.5
Egg Fried, Average	**1 Serving/300g**	**624**	**31.8**	**208**	**4.2**	**25.7**	**10.6**	**0.4**
Egg Fried, Chinese Takeaway, Tesco*	1 Serving/250g	462	15.8	185	3.8	27.2	6.3	2.1
Egg Fried, Express, Uncle Ben's*	½ Pack/125g	216	5.2	173	4	29.9	4.2	0.3
Egg Fried, M&S*	1 Pack/300g	543	12	181	4.4	31	4	1.6
Egg Fried, Wholegrain, Pouch, Uncle Ben's*	½ Pouch/125g	194	4.5	155	4.3	25	3.6	1.8
Fried, Chicken, Takeaway, Iceland*	1 Pack/336g	631	18.1	188	7.5	26.5	5.4	1.5
Garlic, Roasted, Express Rice, Uncle Ben's*	½ Pack/125g	190	2.6	152	3.2	30	2.1	0.9
Golden Savoury, Dry Weight, Batchelors*	1 Pack/120g	437	3.4	364	10.1	74.7	2.8	2.4
Golden Vegetable, Special, Worldwide Foods, Aldi*	½ Pack/125g	181	2.1	145	3.7	27	1.7	3
Golden, Savoury, Steam Bags, Iceland*	1 Bag/149g	179	3.1	120	3.1	21.4	2.1	1.6
Indian, Lentil, Spinach, Cauliflower, SteamFresh, Birds Eye*	1 Pack/190g	200	3.2	105	3.5	18	1.7	2
Indonesian Inspired, with Coriander Drizzle, Hello Fresh*	1 Serving/416g	549	16.1	132	3.9	20	3.9	0
Jasmine, Curry Meal Box, Tesco*	½ Pack/194g	250	0.3	129	2.8	28.9	0.1	0.5
Jasmine, Taste of Thailand, Tesco*	1 Pack/242g	312	0.3	129	2.8	28.9	0.1	0.5
Konjac, Zero, Myprotein*	1 Serving/100g	7	0.1	7	0.1	0.1	0.1	3.5
Long Grain, & Wild, Dry, Average	**1 Serving/75g**	**254**	**1.5**	**338**	**7.6**	**72.6**	**2**	**1.7**
Long Grain, & Wild, Microwave, M&S*	1 Pack/130g	212	1.2	163	3.9	34	0.9	1.5
Long Grain, & Wild, Microwave, Uncle Ben's*	½ Pack/125g	188	1.6	150	3.2	30.9	1.3	0.9
Long Grain, American, Cooked, Average	**1 Serving/160g**	**229**	**2.8**	**143**	**3**	**28.8**	**1.8**	**0.2**
Long Grain, American, Dry, Average	**1 Serving/50g**	**175**	**0.5**	**350**	**7.2**	**77.8**	**1.1**	**0.6**
Long Grain, Dry, Average	**1 Serving/50g**	**169**	**0.5**	**337**	**7.4**	**75.5**	**1**	**1.7**
Long Grain, Microwavable, Cooked, Average	**1 Serving/150g**	**180**	**0.9**	**120**	**2.7**	**25.8**	**0.6**	**0.7**
Mexican Inspired, Micro, Tesco*	1 Bag/142g	184	2	130	3.2	25.5	1.4	1.1

R

RICE

INFO/WEIGHT	Measure	per Measure KCAL	FAT	Nutrition Values per 100g / 100ml KCAL	PROT	CARB	FAT	FIBRE
Mexican, Microwave, Morrisons*	½ Pack/125g	185	2.9	148	3.5	27.2	2.3	2
Mexican, Pot, Twistd*	1 Serving/140g	187	2.9	134	3.1	25	2.1	1.1
Mexican, Style, Cooked, Express, Uncle Ben's*	1 Pack/250g	385	4.8	154	3.2	31.1	1.9	0.7
Mushroom, M&S*	1 Pack/300g	417	15	139	3	19.6	5	1.6
Mushroom, Pilau, Bombay Brasserie, Sainsbury's*	1 Pack/400g	672	17.2	168	3.7	28.6	4.3	0.7
Mushroom, Pilau, Indian, Sainsbury's*	1 Serving/100g	119	2.4	119	3	21.3	2.4	1.9
Mushroom, Roasted, Taste of India, Tesco*	½ Pack/135g	177	3.5	131	3.2	23	2.6	1.6
Nasi Goreng, Chef Select, Lidl*	¼ Pack/200g	382	13.6	191	6.8	25.2	6.8	1
Nasi Goreng, Cook*	1 Serving/255g	293	6.4	115	8.3	15.3	2.5	2
Paella, Spanish, Dry, Tesco*	1 Serving/75g	262	0.4	349	6.3	78.9	0.6	1.5
Pilaf, Royal, Microwaved, Mumbai Street Food, Iceland*	1 Meal/158g	463	12.8	293	5.3	48.6	8.1	2.3
Pilau, Cooked, Average	*1 Serving/200g*	*349*	*8.8*	*174*	*3.5*	*30.3*	*4.4*	*0.8*
Pilau, Dry, Average	*1oz/28g*	*101*	*0.7*	*362*	*8.4*	*78.2*	*2.4*	*3.4*
Pilau, Microwavable, Golden Sun, Lidl*	½ Pack/125g	199	3.5	159	3.7	29.3	2.8	1.1
Pudding, Dry Weight, Average	*1 Serving/100g*	*356*	*1.1*	*356*	*6.9*	*82*	*1.1*	*0.4*
Red, Dry, Ingredients, Tesco*	1 Serving/60g	209	1.8	349	8.2	69.8	3	5
Risotto, Dry, Average	*1 Serving/50g*	*174*	*0.6*	*348*	*7.8*	*76.2*	*1.3*	*2.4*
Saffron, Cooked, Average	*1 Serving/150g*	*208*	*4.7*	*139*	*2.6*	*25.3*	*3.2*	*0.5*
Special Fried, Chinese Takeaway, Iceland*	1 Pack/350g	630	17.5	180	5.5	28.2	5	1.2
Special Fried, Chinese, Tesco*	1 Serving/300g	618	33.3	206	6.5	19.9	11.1	0.8
Special Fried, M&S*	½ Pack/150g	300	12.3	200	6.7	24.2	8.2	1.2
Spinach, & Carrot, Pilau, Waitrose*	1 Pack/350g	466	8.4	133	3.1	24.8	2.4	1.2
Sweet & Spicy, Szechuan, Naked Rice, Symingtons*	1 Pot/259g	285	4.1	110	2.3	21.3	1.6	0.9
Thai, Black, Sainsbury's*	1 Serving/180g	205	2	114	3.7	20.4	1.1	3.8
Thai, Cooked, Average	*1 Serving/100g*	*136*	*1.8*	*136*	*2.5*	*27.4*	*1.8*	*0.3*
Thai, Dry, Average	*1 Serving/50g*	*174*	*0.2*	*348*	*7.1*	*78.9*	*0.4*	*0.9*
Thai, Fragrant, Dry, Average	*1 Serving/75g*	*272*	*0.5*	*363*	*7.2*	*82*	*0.7*	*0.3*
Thai, Glutinous, Sticky, White, Dry, Raw	*1 Serving/100g*	*370*	*0.6*	*370*	*6.8*	*81.7*	*0.6*	*2.8*
Tomato, & Basil, Morrisons*	½ Pack/110g	176	2.8	160	4	29.3	2.5	1.8
Vegetable, Golden, Fragrant, Birds Eye*	1 Bag/194g	208	2.7	107	2.7	20	1.4	1.9
Vegetable, Golden, Freshly Frozen, Asda*	1 Sachet/200g	238	2.6	119	3.2	23.6	1.3	1.3
Vegetable, Mediterranean, SteamFresh, Birds Eye*	1 Bag/190g	218	4.9	115	2.4	20	2.6	1.2
Vegetable, Savoury, Mixed, Dry Weight, Tesco*	1 Pack/120g	450	3.2	375	7.8	79.1	2.7	2.9
White, Cooked, Average	*1 Serving/140g*	*182*	*1.1*	*130*	*2.6*	*28.7*	*0.8*	*0.2*
White, Cooked, Frozen, Average	*1 Serving/150g*	*168*	*0.8*	*112*	*2.9*	*23.8*	*0.6*	*1.2*
White, Fried	*1oz/28g*	*37*	*0.9*	*131*	*2.2*	*25*	*3.2*	*0.6*
White, Long Grain, Dry Weight, Average	*1 Serving/50g*	*181*	*1*	*362*	*7.1*	*79.1*	*1.9*	*0.4*
White, Microwave, Cooked, Average	*½ Pack/125g*	*185*	*2.4*	*148*	*3.3*	*29.4*	*1.9*	*1.4*
Whole Grain, Dry, Average	*1 Serving/50g*	*171*	*1.2*	*342*	*8.2*	*72*	*2.3*	*4*
Wholegrain, & Freekeh, Sainsbury's*	½ Pack/125g	206	3.2	165	4.4	29.2	2.6	3.6
Wholegrain, & Quinoa, Sainsbury's*	½ Pack/125g	204	2.1	163	3.8	31.6	1.7	3.2
Wholegrain, & Quinoa, Tomato & Basil, Uncle Ben's*	½ Pack/110g	176	2.5	160	4.3	29.2	2.3	2.5
Wholegrain, & Wild, Sainsbury's*	½ Pack/125g	197	2	157	3.4	30.8	1.6	3.1
Wholegrain, 3, Beans, & Chilli, Uncle Ben's*	½ Pack/110g	176	2.5	160	4.6	28.9	2.3	3
Wholegrain, Cooked, Co-Op*	½ Pack/125g	182	1.4	146	2.9	29	1.1	4
Wholegrain, Micro Rice, Asda*	1 Pack/250g	412	5	165	3.9	31	2	3.4
Wild, Cooked, Average	*1 Cup/164g*	*166*	*0.6*	*101*	*4*	*21.3*	*0.3*	*1.8*
With Red Kidney Beans, Average	*1oz/28g*	*49*	*1*	*175*	*5.6*	*32.4*	*3.5*	*2.5*

RICE CAKES

INFO/WEIGHT	Measure	per Measure KCAL	FAT	Nutrition Values per 100g / 100ml KCAL	PROT	CARB	FAT	FIBRE
Apple, & Cinnamon, Sainsbury's*	2 Cakes/18g	71	0.5	394	8.3	82.8	2.8	2.8
Asda*	1 Cake/8g	31	0.2	386	8.7	81.1	3	2.8
Caramel, Flavour, Kallo*	1 Cake/10g	38	0.5	383	6.2	78.9	4.8	3.9
Caramel, Free From, Tesco*	1 Cake/11g	41	0.3	373	5.9	80.9	2.5	1.8

R

RICE CAKES

INFO/WEIGHT	Measure	per Measure KCAL	FAT	Nutrition Values per 100g / 100ml KCAL	PROT	CARB	FAT	FIBRE
Caramel, Jumbo, Snack-A-Jacks, Quaker*	1 Cake/13g	51	0.3	390	5.5	87	2.1	1.4
Caramel, Jumbo, Tesco*	1 Cake/10g	34	0.3	340	7	74	3	5
Cheese, & Onion, Snack, Snack-A-Jacks, Quaker*	1 Bag/30g	120	2.2	400	6.7	77	7.5	1.5
Chocolate Orange, Tesco*	1 Cake/18g	85	3.6	472	5.1	65.4	20	5.1
Chocolate, Chip, Jumbo, Snack-A-Jacks, Quaker*	1 Cake/15g	62	1	410	6	81	7	1.7
Chocolate, Dark, Kelkin*	1 Cake/17g	83	3.9	486	6.3	61	23	5.2
Chocolate, Dark, Mint, Nature's Store*	1 Cake/17g	82	3.9	485	6.3	61	23.1	5.1
Chocolate, Dark, Organic, Kallo*	1 Cake/12g	57	2.9	471	6.8	57.2	24.1	7.4
Chocolate, Milk, Kelkin*	1 Cake/17g	84	4.1	495	6.7	62	24	2.7
Chocolate, Milk, Mini, Sainsbury's*	1 Pack/30g	138	5	459	7.8	67.9	16.8	2.9
Chocolate, Milk, Minis, Kids, Kallo*	1 Pack/14g	69	3.3	496	6.6	62.6	23.8	0
Chocolate, Milk, Organic, Kallo*	1 Cake/11g	57	3.2	509	6.5	56.2	28.7	3.5
Chocolate, Milk, Sainsbury's*	1 Pack/38g	178	7	469	7.7	66.2	18.5	3.2
Chocolate, Milk, Slices, Morrisons*	1 Slice/11g	53	2.5	469	7.3	58.8	22	3.3
Chocolate, Milk, with Coconut, Sainsbury's*	1 Pack/37g	176	8	480	7.5	61.5	21.7	4.5
Idly, Average	*1 Idly/40g*	*59*	*0.4*	*149*	*4.1*	*30.8*	*1*	*1.3*
Litchi Mochi, World-Wide Co. LTD*	1 Piece/15g	51	0.3	339	1.9	77.7	2.3	0
Low Fat, BGTY, Sainsbury's*	1 Cake/7g	29	0.2	388	8.1	81.5	2.4	3.9
Milk Chocolate, Rivercote, Lidl*	1 Cake/12g	39	1.7	325	4.3	43.1	14.5	1.9
Multigrain, Ryvita*	3 Cakes/11g	43	0.5	384	9.1	76.2	4.7	5.3
Salt & Vinegar, Asda*	1 Cake/8g	30	0.2	353	9.1	72	2.6	3.4
Salt & Vinegar, Tesco*	1 Cake/12g	47	0.7	392	6.3	78	5.7	1.8
Salt, & Vinegar, Balsamic, Sea, Kallo*	1 Cake/9g	33	0.2	364	6.8	78	2.2	2.4
Salt, & Vinegar, Jumbo, Snack-A-Jacks, Quaker*	1 Cake/10g	41	0.6	391	7.4	75.4	5.7	1.6
Salt, & Vinegar, Jumbo, Tesco*	1 Cake/9g	31	0.2	347	8.4	72.7	2.5	6
Salt, & Vinegar, Wholegrain, Tesco*	1 Cake/9g	28	0.2	314	8.4	61.9	2.6	6
Salted, Lightly, Thick Slice, Low Fat, Kallo*	1 Cake/8g	28	0.2	372	8	78.7	2.8	5.1
Salted, Sea, Harvest Morn, Aldi*	1 Cake/7g	27	0.2	379	8.7	78	2.2	5.1
Salted, Slightly, Organic, Thin Slice, Kallo*	1 Cake/5g	17	0.1	372	8	78.7	2.8	5.1
Salted, Slightly, Thick Slice, Organic, Kallo*	1 Cake/8g	28	0.2	372	8	78.7	2.8	5.1
Sesame, No Added Salt, Thick Sliced, Organic, Kallo*	1 Cake/10g	37	0.3	373	8	78	3.2	5.4
Sesame, Toasted, Ryvita*	1 Pack/11g	43	0.5	391	8.4	78.4	4.9	3.5
Sour Cream, & Black Pepper, M&S*	1 Cake/9g	39	1	432	7.1	75.8	10.8	1.6
Sweet Chilli, Harvest Morn, Aldi*	1 Cake/10g	47	1.7	452	7.2	67	16	4.4
Thin Slice, No Added Salt, Organic, Kallo*	1 Cake/5g	19	0.1	372	8	78.7	2.8	5.1
Wholegrain, No Added Salt, BGTY, Sainsbury's*	1 Cake/8g	30	0.2	372	8	78.7	2.8	5.1
Yoghurt, & Orange, Mini, Bunalun Organic*	1 Pack/14g	71	3.5	506	5.9	64	25	1.4

RICE CRACKERS

INFO/WEIGHT	Measure	per Measure KCAL	FAT	Nutrition Values per 100g / 100ml KCAL	PROT	CARB	FAT	FIBRE
Air Baked, Vegetable, Peckish*	¼ Pack/25g	106	1.8	424	6.9	81	7.3	0
Barbecue, Sakata*	½ Pack/50g	204	1.3	407	7.3	85.2	2.6	1.6
Brown, Whole Sesame & Tamari, Organic, Clearspring*	1 Pack/40g	176	5.6	440	14	65	14	11
Cracked Pepper, Sakata*	½ Pack/50g	200	1.5	400	7.3	84.4	3	2
Japanese Style, Mix, Asda*	1 Serving/25g	96	0.2	385	6.8	88	0.6	0.5
Japanese, Philon*	1 Serving/20g	77	0.1	383	0.4	85.8	0.6	8.3
Lightly Salted, The Snack Organisation*	1 Serving/25g	100	0.9	401	6.9	85	3.6	0.9
Sour Cream & Chive, Sakata*	1 Serving/25g	107	2	430	7.8	80.6	7.9	0
Sweet Chilli, The Snack Organisation, Hansells Foods*	1 Serving/25g	106	1.7	424	7.1	83	6.8	1
Teriyaki, The Snack Organisation*	1 Serving/25g	105	1.1	420	6.4	87.2	4.4	2.4
Thai, M&S*	1 Serving/55g	209	1.8	380	7	80.2	3.3	1.2
Thai, Wakama*	1 Cracker/2g	8	0.1	400	6.9	86.9	2.7	0.5

RICE PUDDING

INFO/WEIGHT	Measure	per Measure KCAL	FAT	Nutrition Values per 100g / 100ml KCAL	PROT	CARB	FAT	FIBRE
& Jam, Fat Free, Aunt Bessie's*	¼ Pack/131g	136	0.3	104	2.4	23	0.2	0.6
50% Less Fat, Asda*	½ Can/212g	180	1.7	85	3.3	16.2	0.8	0.2

R

RICE PUDDING

INFO/WEIGHT	Measure per Measure KCAL	FAT	KCAL	PROT	CARB	FAT	FIBRE
Apple Strudel Flavour Sauce, Muller Rice, Muller*	1 Pot/190g	205	4.4	108	3.2	18.6	2.3	0.4
Apple, Ambrosia*	1 Pot/150g	125	2.3	104	2.7	18.8	1.9	0.5
Banana & Toffee (Limited Edition), Muller Rice, Muller*	1 Pot/190g	207	4.2	109	3.1	19.3	2.2	0.4
Canned, Average	*1oz/28g*	*25*	*0.7*	*89*	*3.4*	*14*	*2.5*	*0.2*
Canned, Basics, Sainsbury's*	½ Can/213g	157	1.7	74	3.1	13.7	0.8	1.4
Clotted Cream, Morrisons*	1 Pudding/145g	265	17.3	183	3.1	15.5	11.9	0.7
Cow & Gate*	1 Jar/125g	111	2.5	89	2.5	15.2	2	0.2
Creamed, Canned, Ambrosia*	1 Can/425g	382	8.1	90	3.1	15.2	1.9	0
Creamed, Pot, Ambrosia*	1 Pot/150g	156	3.8	104	3.3	17	2.5	0.1
Creamed, Value, Tesco*	1 Can/425g	348	3.4	82	3.2	15.5	0.8	0
Creamed, with British Milk, Canned, Simply, M&S*	½ Can/200g	230	9.8	115	3.2	13.9	4.9	1.2
Creamy, Tesco*	1 Pudding/190g	278	14.1	146	2.3	17.5	7.4	0.1
Le Riz au Lait, A la Vanille , La Fermiere*	1 Pot/160g	240	9.6	150	2.8	20	6	0
Light, Ambrosia*	1 Pot/150g	120	0.9	80	3.3	15.3	0.6	0.5
Low Fat, Devon, Creamed, Ambrosia*	½ Can/213g	193	2.8	91	3.2	16.5	1.3	0
Low Fat, Muller Rice, Muller*	1 Serving/180g	182	4.7	101	3.4	16.1	2.6	0
Low Fat, Tesco*	1 Can/425g	404	5.5	95	3.2	16.9	1.3	0.1
Original, Muller Rice, Muller*	1 Pot/190g	196	4.9	103	3.6	16.3	2.6	0.3
Pot, Ambrosia*	1 Pot/125g	126	3.1	101	3.3	16.3	2.5	0
Raspberry, Low Fat, Muller Rice, Muller*	1 Pot/180g	189	4	105	3	18.4	2.2	0
Raspberry, Mullerice, Muller*	1 Pot/190g	201	4.4	106	3.2	18.2	2.3	0.5
Riz Au Lait, Bonne Maman*	1 Pot/100g	149	5.3	149	3.3	22	5.3	0.1
Salted Caramel, Divine Rice, Rachel's Organic*	1 Pot/150g	201	6.9	134	3.1	20.1	4.6	0
Stockwell & Co., Tesco*	½ Can/200g	162	1.6	81	3.1	15.3	0.8	0
Strawberry, Milbona, Lidl*	1 Pot/180g	191	3.2	106	2.9	19.3	1.8	0.5
Strawberry, Muller*	1 Pot/180g	191	4	106	3	18.6	2.2	0
Vanilla Custard, Mullerrice, Muller*	1 Pot/200g	230	5	115	3.4	19.8	2.5	0.3

RICE WINE

INFO/WEIGHT	Measure per Measure KCAL	FAT	KCAL	PROT	CARB	FAT	FIBRE
Sake, Average	*1 Tbsp/15ml*	*20*	*0*	*134*	*0.5*	*5*	*0*	*0*

RIGATONI

INFO/WEIGHT	Measure per Measure KCAL	FAT	KCAL	PROT	CARB	FAT	FIBRE
Dry, Average	*1 Serving/80g*	*272*	*1.2*	*340*	*11.4*	*68.4*	*1.5*	*2.7*

RISOTTO

INFO/WEIGHT	Measure per Measure KCAL	FAT	KCAL	PROT	CARB	FAT	FIBRE
Bacon, wiith Mushroom, Oven-Baked, Hello Fresh*	1 Serving/333g	572	18	172	6.6	24.1	5.4	0
Balls, Green Vegetable, & Mozzarella, Sainsbury's*	1 Ball/50g	126	6.4	252	6.8	26	12.7	3
Beetroot, & Goats Cheese, Lovely Vegetables, M&S*	1 Pack/379g	530	17	140	4.4	20.7	4.5	3.6
Butternut Squash, Fresh Ideas, M Kitchen, Morrisons*	1 Pot/350g	371	11.9	106	1.8	16.8	3.4	0.7
Butternut Squash, Italian Style, Aldi*	½ Pack/252g	323	12.6	128	2.6	17	5	1.6
Butternut Squash, Kale, & Spelt, Tesco*	1 Pack/361g	347	8.7	96	3.4	14.1	2.4	2.4
Butternut Squash, Mediterranean, Slim Cook, Tesco*	1 Pack/500g	341	0.9	68	2	13.9	0.2	1.6
Cheese, Onion, & Wine, Rice & Simple, Ainsley Harriott*	1 Pack/140g	253	7	181	3.1	31	5	1.6
Chicken	*1 Serving/380g*	*494*	*17.4*	*130*	*7.2*	*15.2*	*4.6*	*1.3*
Chicken, & Lemon, Weight Watchers*	1 Pack/320g	353	6.3	107	6.3	15.8	1.9	0.7
Chicken, & Mushroom, for Two, Charlie Bigham's*	1 Serving/350g	556	26.2	159	7.2	15.8	7.5	0
Chicken, & Chorizo, Super, Bachelors *	½ Pack/130g	178	2	137	4.2	26.4	1.5	0.7
Chicken, & Mushroom, Finest, Tesco*	1 Pack/387g	472	17	122	7.3	12.7	4.4	1
Chicken, & Mushroom, Meal for One, M&S*	1 Pack/400g	468	13.2	117	8.1	13.3	3.3	0.8
Chicken, & Mushroom, Sainsbury's*	1 Pack/383g	387	11.1	101	6.3	11.9	2.9	1.3
Chicken, Chargrilled, Ready Meal, M&S*	1 Pack/365g	493	25.2	135	6.4	11.6	6.9	0.7
Chicken, Mediterranean, Slimming World*	1 Pack/550g	478	3.3	87	6.9	12.8	0.6	1.4
Courgette, & Pea, Vegan, Waitrose*	½ Pack/187g	172	6.2	92	3.2	11	3.3	2.7
Cremeux, aux Champignons, Danival*	1 Pack/250g	258	13.2	103	2.2	10.8	5.3	1.5
Farro, Tomatoey, Full Of Goodness*	½ Pack/125g	125	1.6	100	4.4	16	1.3	3.6
Green Bean, Asparagus & Pecorino, Finest, Tesco*	1 Pack/400g	460	15.6	115	4.4	15	3.9	1.5

R

	Measure INFO/WEIGHT	per Measure KCAL	FAT	Nutrition Values per 100g / 100ml KCAL	PROT	CARB	FAT	FIBRE
RISOTTO								
Haddock, Smoked, Finest, Tesco*	1 Pack/396g	412	8.7	104	5.6	15.1	2.2	1
Mushroom, HL, Tesco*	1 Pack/366g	339	8.3	93	3.4	14	2.3	1.4
Prawn, COU, M&S*	1 Pack/350g	378	7.7	108	4.3	17.3	2.2	0.8
Prawn, Pea & Mint, King, M&S*	½ Pack/300g	405	18.6	135	3.8	15.9	6.2	0.9
Red Pepper, & Italian Cheese, Roasted, M&S*	1 Pack/400g	500	13.2	125	2.9	20.4	3.3	1
Seafood, Youngs*	1 Pack/350g	424	13	121	4.5	17.4	3.7	0.1
Squash, Orzo, Sumptuous, Orzotto, Jamie Oliver*	½ Pack/125g	169	3.9	135	5	19	3.1	5.6
Vegetable, Average	*1oz/28g*	*41*	*1.8*	*147*	*4.2*	*19.2*	*6.5*	*2.2*
Vegetable, Brown Rice, Average	*1oz/28g*	*40*	*1.8*	*143*	*4.1*	*18.6*	*6.4*	*2.4*
with Mushroom, & Garlic, Cucina, Aldi*	1 Serving/200g	214	3	107	2.6	20	1.5	1
ROCK SALMON								
Raw, Flesh Only, Average	*1oz/28g*	*43*	*2.7*	*154*	*16.6*	*0*	*9.7*	*0*
ROCKET								
Fresh, Raw, Average	*1 Serving/80g*	*12*	*0.4*	*16*	*0.8*	*1.7*	*0.5*	*1.2*
ROE								
Cod, Average	*1 Can/100g*	*96*	*2.8*	*96*	*17.1*	*0.5*	*2.8*	*0*
Cod, Hard, Coated in Batter, Fried	*1oz/28g*	*53*	*3.3*	*189*	*12.4*	*8.9*	*11.8*	*0.2*
Cod, Hard, Fried in Blended Oil	*1oz/28g*	*57*	*3.3*	*202*	*20.9*	*3*	*11.9*	*0.1*
Herring, Soft, Fried in Blended Oil	*1oz/28g*	*74*	*4.4*	*265*	*26.3*	*4.7*	*15.8*	*0.2*
Herring, Soft, Raw	*1oz/28g*	*22*	*0.1*	*78*	*18.2*	*0.5*	*0.4*	*0*
ROGAN JOSH								
Chicken, & Pilau Rice, Morrisons*	1 Pack/419g	528	13.8	126	7.4	15.2	3.3	2.9
Chicken, Breast, Chunks, Hot, Sainsbury's*	½ Pack/114g	143	2	126	23.6	3.9	1.8	1
Chicken, with Pilau Rice, Farmfoods*	1 Pack/325g	354	6.8	109	5.3	17.1	2.1	0.4
Lamb, Indian, Takeaway, CBY, Asda*	½ Pack/200g	218	12	109	8	5.1	6	1.4
Lamb, Sainsbury's*	1 Pack/400g	660	44.4	165	11.3	4.9	11.1	1.9
Lamb, Takeaway, Tesco*	½ Pack/192g	228	14	119	6.3	5.7	7.3	2.5
Prawn, COU, M&S*	1 Pack/400g	360	2.4	90	4.9	16.2	0.6	0.8
ROLL								
Beef, & Roast Onion Mayo, Soft White, M&S*	1 Pack/215g	522	17.6	243	11.5	30	8.2	1.5
Cheese, & Onion, Asda*	1 Serving/67g	199	12	298	7	27	18	2
Cheese, & Onion, Co-Op*	1 Roll/66g	195	11.9	295	7	26	18	2
Cheese, & Onion, Iceland*	1 Roll/67g	222	13.6	332	7.5	29.6	20.4	1.5
Cheese, & Onion, M&S*	1 Roll/25g	80	5.1	320	9.6	24.7	20.5	1.3
Cheese, & Onion, Tesco*	1 Roll/67g	203	12.1	305	7.3	28	18.1	1.9
Cheese, & Pickle, Sainsbury's*	1 Roll/136g	359	13.6	264	10.6	35.1	10	0
Cheese, & Bacon, Snack, Sainsbury's*	1 Roll/30g	95	5.3	318	9.9	28.5	17.8	2.4
Cheese, & Onion, Mini, Sainsbury's*	1 Roll/10g	29	1.5	292	6.9	30.6	15.4	1.9
Cheese, & Onion, Sainsbury's*	1 Roll/66g	190	9.8	288	6.9	30.6	14.8	2.5
Cheese, Tomato & Onion, Sainsbury's*	1 Pack/100g	518	28.1	518	18.4	47.9	28.1	0
Cheese, Tomato, & Pickle, Cheese Topped Roll, M&S*	1 Roll/177g	480	26.4	271	10	22.8	14.9	2.8
Chicken, & Mayonnaise, Roast, Big, Sainsbury's*	1 Pack/185g	479	27.4	259	9.6	21.8	14.8	0
Chicken, & Salad, HE, Tesco*	1 Serving/224g	289	5.8	129	10.3	16	2.6	1.1
Chicken, & Salad, Mini, Selection Pack, British, M&S*	1 Roll/61g	134	4.1	220	11.9	28.1	6.8	2.1
Cornish, in Pastry, Pork Farms*	1 Roll/75g	226	15.1	301	6.6	24.5	20.1	0
Egg Mayo, & Cress, Fullfillers*	1 Roll/125g	266	11.8	213	10	25.7	9.4	0
Egg Mayonnaise, & Cress, Sub, Delicious, Boots*	1 Pack/205g	399	14.1	195	10	23	6.9	2.4
Egg, & Cress, HL, Tesco*	1 Pack/175g	322	6.8	184	9.6	27.7	3.9	1.2
Ham, & Cheese, Leicester, Sub, Waitrose*	1 Pack/206ml	582	31.2	282	12.6	24	15.1	13
Ham, & Egg Mayo, Smoked, Soft White Seeded, M&S*	1 Pack/190g	371	9.5	195	12.7	23.4	5	3
Ham, & Salad, BGTY, Sainsbury's*	1 Roll/178g	292	3.4	164	10.8	25.9	1.9	0
Ham, & Salad, J D Gross, Lidl*	1 Roll/154g	293	9.2	190	7.7	29.1	6	1.9
Ham, & Tomato, Taste!*	1 Serving/112g	211	4.8	188	10.4	27	4.3	0

	Measure INFO/WEIGHT	per Measure KCAL	FAT	Nutrition Values per 100g / 100ml KCAL	PROT	CARB	FAT	FIBRE
ROLL								
Ham, Darwins Deli*	1 Serving/125g	298	7.5	238	11	37.4	6	0
Nems, Mini, Porc, with Sauce, Carrrefour*	1 Roll/32g	66	3.6	204	7	19	11	2.7
Ploughman's, Large, Ginsters*	1 Pack/140g	473	33.5	338	10.2	20.5	23.9	1.8
Pork, Stuffing, & Apple Sauce, Roast, Boots*	1 Roll/218g	602	26.2	276	10	32	12	1.8
Salmon, Oak Smoked, M&S*	1 Roll/55g	139	6.2	252	14.6	23.1	11.3	1.2
Sausage, Lincolnshire, COU, M&S*	1 Roll/175g	280	4.7	160	10	23.2	2.7	2.6
Tuna Mayo, & Cucumber, Taste!*	1 Serving/111g	274	12.5	247	9	27.3	11.3	0
Tuna Mayonnaise, with Cucumber, Yummies*	1 Serving/132g	340	18.6	257	10.4	22.5	14	0
Tuna, & Cucumber, Seasoned Mayo, Soft Sub Roll, M&S*	1 Pack/216g	435	16.4	201	9.4	22.5	7.6	2.3
Tuna, & Sweetcorn, with Mayonnaise, Shell*	1 Pack/180g	536	26.3	298	13.1	28.6	14.6	0
Tuna, Cheese Melt, Boots*	1 Roll/199g	612	35.8	308	13	23	18	1.2
Turkey, Salad, Northern Bites*	1 Roll/231g	323	8.3	140	8.6	19.6	3.6	3
ROLO								
Chocolate, Nestle*	2 Pieces/20g	102	5.3	509	4.1	62.6	26.6	1.3
Little, Nestle*	1 Pack/40g	196	9.4	491	4	65.5	23.5	0.5
Nestle*	1 Sweet/5g	24	1	478	4.4	68.2	20.4	1.1
ROOT BEER								
Average	*1 Can/330ml*	*135*	*0*	*41*	*0*	*10.6*	*0*	*0*
ROSE WATER								
The English Provender Co.*	1 Tsp/5g	0	0	2	0.1	0.6	0.1	0.1
ROSEMARY								
Dried	*1 Tsp/1g*	*3*	*0.2*	*331*	*4.9*	*46.4*	*15.2*	*0*
Fresh	*1 Tsp/0.7g*	*1*	*0*	*99*	*1.4*	*13.5*	*4.4*	*0*
ROSTI								
Cheese, & Onion, Tesco*	1 Rosti/92g	202	10.9	220	5.1	21.6	11.9	3.2
Maris Piper & Onion, M&S*	1 Rosti/35g	77	4.2	219	1.9	24.7	12	2.4
Potato & Root Vegetable, COU, M&S*	1 Rosti/100g	85	2.7	85	1.6	13.3	2.7	1.5
Potato Cakes, Baby, M&S*	1 Rosti/23g	40	1.5	175	3.5	25.1	6.7	1.6
Potato, McCain*	1 Rosti/95g	161	8.6	169	2.2	19.6	9.1	0
Potato, Mini, Party Bites, Sainsbury's*	1 Serving/100g	218	11.5	218	2.5	26.2	11.5	3
Sweet Potato, Tesco*	½ Pack/91g	258	16	283	2.7	26.2	17.6	4.4
ROULADE								
Black Forest, Finest, Tesco*	1/8 Roulade/74g	206	6.5	280	3.2	46.4	8.8	1
Chocolate, Finest, Tesco*	1 Serving/80g	222	4.5	277	3.4	53.2	5.6	2.3
Chocolate, Sainsbury's*	1 Serving/72g	264	15.7	367	5.7	36.9	21.8	1.8
Passion Fruit, M&S*	1oz/28g	83	2.6	295	2.8	50	9.2	0.2
Raspberry, Finest, Tesco*	1/6 Roulade/75g	220	9.2	295	2.7	41.5	12.4	2.7
RUM								
37.5% Volume	*1 Pub Shot/35ml*	*72*	*0*	*207*	*0*	*0*	*0*	*0*
40% Volume	*1 Pub Shot/35ml*	*78*	*0*	*222*	*0*	*0*	*0*	*0*
Captain Morgans & Cola, Premixed, Canned, Diageo*	1 Can/250ml	180	0	72	0	9.1	0	0
Malibu, 21% Volume, Pernod Ricard*	1 Pub shot/25ml	50	0	200	0	29	0	0
White	*1 Pub Shot/35ml*	*72*	*0*	*207*	*0*	*0*	*0*	*0*

R

	Measure INFO/WEIGHT	per Measure KCAL	FAT	Nutrition Values per 100g / 100ml KCAL	PROT	CARB	FAT	FIBRE
SAAG								
Aloo, M&S*	½ Pack/125g	121	7.1	97	1.6	8.7	5.7	2.1
Chicken, Microwaved, Slimming World, Iceland*	1 Pack/500g	395	8	79	11.5	3.9	1.6	1.6
Chicken, Slim Choice, Sainsbury's*	1 Pack/476g	352	5.7	74	11.9	3.7	1.2	0.8
Chicken, with Gunpowder Potatoes, Tesco*	1 Pack/348g	369	15	106	6.7	8.3	4.3	3.9
Paneer, Sainsbury's*	1 Pack/300g	441	32.7	147	7.1	3.9	10.9	2.5
SAFFRON								
Average	*1 Tsp/1g*	*2*	*0*	*310*	*11.4*	*61.5*	*5.9*	*0*
SAGE								
Dried, Ground	*1 Tsp/1g*	*3*	*0.1*	*315*	*10.6*	*42.7*	*12.7*	*0*
Fresh	*1oz/28g*	*33*	*1.3*	*119*	*3.9*	*15.6*	*4.6*	*0*
SALAD								
3 Bean, with Mint Vinaigrette, M&S*	1 Pack/250g	285	4.5	114	6.5	14.8	1.8	6.1
Avocado, & Egg, Nourish Bowl, M&S*	1 Pack/285g	333	15.4	117	6.3	6.6	5.4	8.3
Avocado, & Feta, & Rice, Good to Go, Waitrose*	1 Pack/240g	350	13.4	146	3.4	18.4	5.6	4.1
Avocado, & Feta, Gourmet To Go, M&S*	1 Pack/320g	512	32	160	5.4	12.1	10	3.1
Baby Leaf, & Beetroot, Bistro, M&S*	1 Pack/165g	41	0	25	2	3.6	0	2
Baby Leaf, & Rocket, Florette*	1 Serving/25g	5	0.1	20	2.1	0.9	0.5	2
Baby Leaf, Aldi*	1 Serving/50g	11	0	22	3.5	1	0.1	1.5
Baby Leaf, Italian Style, M&S*	1 Serving/55g	12	0.3	22	1.3	2.3	0.5	1.3
Baby Leaf, Mix, Nature's Pick, Aldi*	½ Bag/55g	15	0.3	27	2.4	2.5	0.5	1.8
Baby Leaf, Seasonal, Morrisons*	½ Pack/50g	10	0.3	21	1.4	1.6	0.6	1.8
Bean, 3, Sainsbury's*	1 Tub/270g	281	6.2	104	7.1	13.6	2.3	5.9
Bean, 3, with Mint Vinaigrette, Spirit of Summer, M&S*	1 Pack/250g	250	6	100	5.9	8.2	2.4	11.1
Bean, Four, Sainsbury's*	½ Pot/125g	121	3.2	107	6.6	11.5	2.8	4.8
Bean, Mixed, in Water, Drained, Essential, Waitrose*	1 Serving/80g	78	0.6	97	6.5	12.9	0.8	6.2
Bean, Salsa, & Quinoa, Mexican, Bol*	1 Pot/270g	260	8.7	87	3	11.3	2.9	1.6
Bean, Three, with Mint Vinaigrette, M&S*	1 Pack/250g	250	6	100	5.9	8.2	2.4	11.1
Beetroot, & Feta, Veggie Pot, Eat Well, M&S*	1 Pot/140g	182	10.5	130	4.4	8.9	7.5	4.7
Beetroot, & Lettuce, Asda*	1 Serving/30g	5	0	16	1.4	2.7	0	2.5
Beetroot, & Tomato, Santini, M&S*	½ Pack/110g	58	1.8	53	1.3	7.8	1.6	1.1
Beetroot, Carrot, & Roasted Lentil, M&S*	1 Pack/230g	109	4.7	47	1.4	4.7	2	2.2
Beetroot, Co-Op*	1 Pack/250g	100	0.8	40	0.9	8	0.3	2
Beetroot, Goats Cheese, & Rocket, Tesco*	1 Pack/120g	72	3.4	60	2.7	5.3	2.8	1.4
Beetroot, Lambs Lettuce, & Red Chard, Bistro, Lidl*	1 Serving/80g	20	0.2	25	1.8	2.9	0.2	2.3
Beetroot, Morrisons*	1 Tsp/10g	4	0	42	1.2	7	0.4	2.7
Beetroot, Roast, & Feta, Truly Irresistible, Co-Op*	1 Pack/216g	320	18.4	148	4.2	13	8.5	1.7
Bistro, Asda*	1 Serving/180g	29	0	16	1.4	2.7	0	2.5
Broccoli, & Peanut, Finest, Tesco*	½ Pack/105g	196	9.2	187	6.9	18.4	8.8	3.3
Bulgur Wheat, Lentil, & Edamame Shaker, Waitrose*	1 Pack/190g	217	10.6	114	4.7	11.1	5.6	4.4
Burrito, BBQ, Bowl, Allplants*	½ Pack/380g	543	12.2	143	4.2	21	3.2	5.3
Caesar	*1 Serving/200g*	*352*	*27.8*	*176*	*4.8*	*8.1*	*13.9*	*0.7*
Caesar, Chicken, Shapers, Boots*	1 Pack/200g	205	5.8	102	8.2	10	2.9	1
Caesar, Kit, Tesco*	1 Pack/262g	404	31.7	154	3.4	7.3	12.1	1.2
Caesar, Kit, Waitrose*	1 Bag/250g	436	36.1	174	4.4	6.1	14.4	1.3
Caesar, Morrisons*	½ Pack/100g	136	10.1	136	4.7	6.1	10.1	1.2
Caesar, Roast Chicken, & Bacon, High Protein, M&S*	1 Pack/220g	187	7	85	11.9	1.9	3.2	0.6
Caesar, with Dressing, Croutons & Parmesan, M&S*	1 Serving/115g	190	15.5	165	4.3	6.4	13.5	1.4
Chicken, & Edamame, & Peanut Drizzle, Protein Pot, M&S*	1 Pot/130g	191	9.8	147	14.2	3.5	7.5	4.5
Chicken, & Noodle, Sweet Chilli, Shapers, Boots*	1 Pack/197g	266	5.1	135	12	16	2.6	0.9
Chicken, & Vegetable, Rice, with Katsu Dressing, Waitrose*	1 Pack/230g	255	7.6	111	6.5	13.4	3.3	0.9
Chicken, & Vegetable, Scratch*	1 Pack/380g	288	9.3	76	7.9	6.6	2.4	2.2
Chicken, Katsu, & Sticky Rice, M&S*	1 Pack/270g	367	11.3	136	6.4	17.7	4.2	0.8
Chicken, Roast, & Coleslaw, M&S*	1 Pack/190g	205	15.2	108	6.5	2	8	0.8

S

SALAD

INFO/WEIGHT	Measure	per Measure		Nutrition Values per 100g / 100ml				
		KCAL	FAT	KCAL	PROT	CARB	FAT	FIBRE
Chicken, Spiced, & Mango, Asda*	1 Pack/225g	133	4	59	4.4	5.1	1.8	2.3
Classic, Asda*	1 Pack/185g	43	1.5	23	1	2.4	0.8	1.1
Cous Cous, & Pepper, Sweety Drop, Asda*	½ Pack/140g	162	0.7	116	4.2	22	0.5	2.8
Cous Cous, & Vegetable, Roasted, Waitrose*	1 Pack/220g	396	13.4	180	5.1	26.1	6.1	1.2
Cous Cous, Veggie, Moroccan Style, Shapers, Boots*	1 Pack/236g	160	3.3	68	2.3	10	1.4	2.2
Crayfish, & Mango, Sainsbury's*	1 Pack/310g	329	6.5	106	4.1	17	2.1	1.2
Crisp, Mixed, Morrisons*	1 Pack/230g	39	0.7	17	1	2.8	0.3	0
Crisp, Mixed, Tesco*	1 Pack/200g	40	0.6	20	1.1	3.2	0.3	2
Crispy, Florette*	1 Portion/100g	22	0.3	22	1.5	3.4	0.3	3
Crunchy, & Crisp, Asda*	1 Pack/250g	55	1.5	22	0.8	3.3	0.6	1.4
Crunchy, Mini, Co-Op*	1 Pack/80g	16	0.4	20	1	2.5	0.5	1.7
Crunchy, Side, Florette*	1 Serving/80g	25	0.4	31	1.1	4	0.5	3.1
Duck, & Herb, Crispy, M&S*	½ Pack/140g	378	25.6	270	20.7	3.7	18.3	1.4
Edamame, & Black Rice, Nourish Bowl, Eat Well, M&S*	1 Pack/295g	395	16.2	134	5.6	12.8	5.5	5.3
Edamame, & Petit Pois, Finest, Tesco*	½ Pack/100g	108	4.3	108	6	9.3	4.3	3.9
Edamame, & Black Rice, Plant Kitchen, M&S*	1 Pack/295g	395	16.2	134	5.6	12.8	5.5	5.3
Edamame, & Butter Bean, TTD, Sainsbury's*	½ Pot/93g	112	4.5	121	6.5	11	4.9	3.5
Edamame, & Feta, High Protein, M&S*	1 Pack/215g	209	9	97	7.5	5.1	4.2	4.3
Edamame, & Pea, with Spinach, & Coriander, M&S*	1 Pot/110g	108	4.3	98	9.7	3.2	3.9	5.4
Edamame, & Sprouting Pea, Finest, Tesco*	1 Serving/100g	136	5.7	136	7.6	11.4	5.7	4.4
Edamame, Asda*	½ Pack/110g	90	3.3	82	5.9	4.8	3	5.9
Egg, & Ham, with Salad Cream Dressing, M&S*	1 Pack/240g	149	7.2	62	4.9	3.2	3	1.2
Egg, & Spinach, Baby, Waitrose*	1 Pack/215g	167	13.5	78	3.5	1.8	6.3	1
Egg, & Avocado, Free Range, M&S*	1 Pack/225g	268	14.4	119	6.9	7.4	6.4	2.3
Egg, & Avocado, Grains, Waitrose*	1 Pack/260g	351	16.1	135	5.3	13.1	6.2	2.9
Egg, & Spinach, High Protein, M&S*	1 Pot/105g	130	8.1	124	11.9	1.7	7.7	0.5
Egg, & Spinach, Protein Pot, Love Life, Waitrose*	1 Pot/90g	102	5.5	113	12.5	1	6.1	1.8
Egg, Avocado, & Quinoa, & Soy Sauce, Protein Pot, M&S*	1 Pot/140g	185	8.1	132	7.2	11.1	5.8	3.5
Egg, Surimi, Daunat*	1 Pack/250g	255	18.8	102	4.1	3.7	7.5	0
English Garden, Tesco*	1 Serving/180g	22	0.4	12	0.7	1.8	0.2	0.7
Falafel, Bulgur Wheat & Houmous, Eat Well, M&S*	1 Pack/300g	375	15.3	125	4.1	13.2	5.1	4.8
Falafel, Squash, & Grain, Mediterranean, Bowl, Waitrose*	1 Pack/250g	312	13.5	125	3.8	13.6	5.4	3.2
Feta, & Sunblushed Tomato, M&S*	1 Serving/190g	361	21.1	190	5.5	17.2	11.1	2.1
Goats Cheese, & Beetroot, with Balsamic Dressing, Tesco*	1 Pack/260g	318	18.2	122	5	8.7	7	2.3
Goats Cheese, & Lentil, M&S*	1 Pack/215g	316	10.3	147	6.9	17.4	4.8	3.3
Greek	*1oz/28g*	*36*	*3.5*	*130*	*2.7*	*1.9*	*12.5*	*0.8*
Greek, Style, Bowl, M&S*	1 Bowl/223g	212	18.3	95	2.5	2.4	8.2	0.7
Greek, Style, Feta, Tip & Mix, M&S*	1 Pack/195g	214	18.3	110	4	2.5	9.4	1.6
Green Bean, Aldi*	½ Pack/80g	62	2.7	77	4.6	5	3.4	3.9
Green, Average	*1oz/28g*	*4*	*0.1*	*13*	*0.8*	*1.8*	*0.3*	*0.9*
Green, Complete, Sainsbury's*	1/3 Pack/55g	92	6.7	168	4.2	10.3	12.2	1.4
Green, Mixed, Average	*1 Serving/100g*	*12*	*0.3*	*12*	*0.7*	*1.8*	*0.3*	*1*
Green, Side, M&S*	1 Serving/200g	30	0.4	15	0.9	2.5	0.2	0
Ham Hock, & Piccalilli, Waitrose*	1 Pack/240g	257	7.4	107	4.7	14	3.1	2.3
Ham Hock, Ploughmans, Waitrose*	1 Pack/185g	170	8.1	92	7.1	5.4	4.4	0.9
Ham, & Egg, Free Range, G&B, Asda*	1 Pack/265g	148	6.3	56	5.3	2.8	2.4	0.9
Ham, & Egg, with Salad Cream, Sainsbury's*	1 Pack/240g	216	14.1	90	4.8	4	5.9	1
Ham, & Egg, Co-Op*	1 Pack/225g	252	14.2	112	8.6	4.8	6.3	0.9
Ham, Egg, & Coleslaw, Tesco*	1 Pack/235g	221	12.2	94	6.8	4.4	5.2	1.1
Ham, Hock, Waitrose*	1 Pack/350g	245	9.5	70	6.6	4.8	2.7	2
Hipster, Wicked Kitchen, Tesco*	½ Pack/100g	146	7.9	146	2.8	14	7.9	3.8
House, Tesco*	½ Pack/60g	18	0.4	30	1.7	3.5	0.6	2.1
Italian, with Pesto Dressing, Teso*	½ Pack/128g	205	14.9	160	6.8	6.1	11.6	1.9

S

SALAD

INFO/WEIGHT	Measure	per Measure		Nutrition Values per 100g / 100ml				
		KCAL	FAT	KCAL	PROT	CARB	FAT	FIBRE
Italian, Strong & Peppery, Sainsbury's*	1 Serving/80g	18	0.4	22	2.5	1	0.5	1.8
Italian, Tomatoes, Balsamic, & Italian Cheese, Sainsbury's*	½ Pack/80g	56	3.6	70	3.3	3.6	4.5	0.8
Italiana, Freshcoolis*	1 Bag/100g	25	0.1	25	1.6	3.4	0.1	1.8
Large, Bowl, Sainsbury's*	1/6 Pack/52g	12	0.2	23	0.9	4.3	0.3	1.1
Lentil, & Sprout, Toppers, Good4U*	1 Serving/30g	44	0.1	146	12	20	0.2	8.9
Lettuce, Lambs, & Pea Shoot, Good Health, Waitrose*	1 Bag/100g	21	0.5	21	1.9	1.3	0.5	1.7
Mediterranean, Bowl, Sainsbury's*	½ Pack/71g	17	0.4	24	1.2	3.9	0.5	1.1
Mediterranean, Style, Asda*	½ Pack/135g	22	0	16	1	3	0	0
Mixed Grains, Chipotle, Tesco*	1 Pack/250g	348	4.5	139	5	22.4	1.8	6.5
Mixed Leaf, Essential, Waitrose*	1 Serving/30g	5	0.2	17	1	2	0.7	1.4
Mixed Leaf, Medley, Waitrose*	1 Serving/25g	4	0.1	15	0.8	1.7	0.5	1.4
Mixed Leaf, Tesco*	1 Serving/20g	3	0.1	14	0.9	1.6	0.4	0.9
Mixed Leaf, Tomato & Olive, Tesco*	1 Serving/170g	150	13.3	88	1	3.4	7.8	2
Mixed Leaf, with Beetroot, Earthy, Waitrose*	1 Bag/140g	34	0.6	24	1.5	3.6	0.4	2.1
Mixed, Bowl, Waitrose*	¼ Pack/64g	9	0.3	14	0.8	1.6	0.5	1.4
Mixed, Crispy, Nightingale, Tesco*	½ Pack/60g	11	0.1	19	1.5	1.7	0.2	2.2
Mixed, Green Leaf, Lasting Leaf*	1 Serving/69g	12	0.3	17	0.8	1.8	0.4	1.5
Mixed, Medley, Bowl, Waitrose*	¼ Pack/60g	9	0.3	15	0.9	1.7	0.5	1
Mixed, Sweet & Crispy, Tesco*	1 Serving/200g	48	0.6	24	1	4.2	0.3	2
Mixed, Sweet & Crunchy, Lasting Leaf*	1 Serving/62g	15	0.2	24	0.8	3.6	0.3	1.9
Moroccan, Mouthwatering, Jamie Oliver*	1 Portion/125g	211	6.5	169	5.5	21.7	5.2	6.6
New Potato, Tomato, & Egg with Salad Cream, M&S*	1 Pack/300g	165	7.2	55	2.9	5.4	2.4	1.3
New Potato, Tuna, & Egg, M&S*	1 Pack/340g	255	12.9	75	3.8	6.7	3.8	0.7
Noodle, Chicken, Hoisin, Well & Good, Co-Op*	1 Pack/244g	288	7.8	118	8.3	13	3.2	1.2
Noodle, Prawn, Sesame, M&S*	1 Pack/220g	242	8.1	110	5.6	12.9	3.7	1.5
Nut, & Grain, Aldi*	½ Pack/100g	138	5.1	138	6	14	5.1	5.9
Octopus, Drained, Medusa*	1 Serving/100g	163	11	163	15	1.6	11	0
Pasta, Mediterranean Orzo, Love Life, Waitrose*	1 Pack/220g	299	10.8	136	3.9	19	4.9	3.2
Pea Shoot, & Baby Leaves, Steve's Leaves*	1 Pack/60g	14	0.4	24	2.7	2	0.6	2
Pea Shoot, Baby Cos & Batavia Lettuce, Bagged, M&S*	1 Bag/120g	24	0.6	20	2.6	0.8	0.5	2.3
Pea Shoot, Mild, Asda*	1 Serving/80g	20	0.4	25	2.5	2.4	0.5	2.1
Potato, Baby, & Free Range Egg, Asda*	1 Pack/270g	159	7.6	59	1.9	5.9	2.8	1.2
Prawn, & Avocado, M&S*	1 Serving/240g	254	16.3	106	3	2	6.8	3.1
Prawn, & Avocado, with Marie Rose Sauce, Waitrose*	1 Pack/240g	334	18.5	139	4.4	11.1	7.7	3.8
Prawn, Cocktail, Tesco*	1 Pack/300g	360	18	120	5.7	10.9	6	0.8
Prawn, King, & Asian Slaw, Aldi*	1 Pack/230g	244	8	106	3.9	14	3.5	0.9
Prawn, Layer, Eat Well, M&S*	1 Pack/220g	205	8.2	93	4.1	10.5	3.7	0.6
Prawn, Layered, Co-Op*	1 Pack/300g	375	18	125	4	14	6	2
Prawn, Layered, M&S*	1 Pack/455g	410	17.7	90	4.5	8.9	3.9	1.2
Prawn, Layered, M&S*	1 Pack/400g	396	17.2	99	4.1	10.4	4.3	1.1
Quinoa, & Avocado, Chipotle, Finest, Tesco*	½ Pack/113g	151	7	135	2.4	16.1	6.3	2
Quinoa, & Kale, Supergreen, Asda*	½ Pot/135g	232	10	172	6.4	16	7.4	8.9
Quinoa, & Supergreen, Eat Well, M&S*	1 Pack/180g	180	10.4	100	4.3	5	5.8	5.3
Quinoa, Tomato, Red Pepper, & Mango, Lidl*	1 Pot/210g	191	4.2	91	2.6	14.1	2	2.5
Rainbow Slaw, Plant Kitchen, M&S*	1 Pack/150g	87	4	58	0.9	5.9	2.7	3
Rainbow, Morrisons*	½ Bowl/72g	20	0.1	27	1.4	3.7	0.2	2.5
Rainbow, Nature's Pick, Aldi*	½ Pack/75g	21	0.4	28	1.1	3.9	0.5	1.5
Ranch, Kit, Morrisons*	¼ Pack/73g	107	7.1	147	4.7	9.2	9.7	1.8
Ribbon, Asda*	1 Pack/115g	33	0.6	29	1.6	4.3	0.5	0.5
Rice, Hoisin, M&S*	1 Pack/200g	312	8.6	156	3.1	25.4	4.3	1.6
Rocket, & Parmesan, Wild, Italian, Sainsbury's*	1 Serving/50g	88	7.4	177	7.5	3.4	14.8	0.5
Salmon, Lime, & Miso, with Sticky Rice, M&S*	1 Pack/285g	396	13.4	139	5.3	18.2	4.7	1.4
Salmon, Moroccan Style, Light Lunch, John West*	1 Pack/220g	299	11.7	136	11.7	8.8	5.3	3.4

SALAD

	Measure INFO/WEIGHT	KCAL	FAT	KCAL	PROT	CARB	FAT	FIBRE
Salmon, Oak Smoked, Aldi*	1 Pack/129g	254	5.8	197	5	8.6	4.5	1.3
Side, Garden, with Cherry Tomatoes, Waitrose*	1 Pack/170g	25	0.7	15	0.8	2	0.4	1.3
Simple, Bowl, Tesco*	1 Bowl/135g	32	0.4	24	1.3	2.9	0.3	2.1
Simple, with Sour Cream, & Chive, Tesco*	1 Pack/165g	139	10.9	84	1.2	4.2	6.6	1.5
Slaw, Rainbow, Wicked Kitchen, Tesco*	½ Pack/75g	60	3.2	80	2	7.3	4.3	2.1
Spicy Mix, Fresh & Naked *	1 Serving/45g	7	0.2	16	2.7	0.4	0.4	1.5
Summer Vegetable, with Basil & Mint Dressing, Waitrose*	1 Pack/165g	196	12.2	119	5.4	3.8	7.4	7.9
Super Grain, with Peanuts, & Zingy Vinaigrette, Morrisons*	1 Serving/50g	82	3.4	163	6.1	17.5	6.8	3.9
Sweet & Crispy, M&S*	1 Serving/140g	49	1.4	35	1.7	4.7	1	1.6
Sweet & Crispy, Side, Sainsbury's*	¼ Bag/93g	23	0.2	25	1.3	4.4	0.2	2.2
Sweet & Crunchy, Bowl, Sainsbury's*	¼ Pack/85g	42	0.6	49	1.6	8.2	0.7	2
Sweet & Crunchy, Side, Eat Well, M&S*	1 Pack/145g	48	0.9	33	1.5	4.3	0.6	2.3
Sweet Leaf, Fully Prepared, Fresh, Sainsbury's*	¼ Pack/75g	12	0.1	16	0.8	3	0.1	2.1
Sweet Leaf, Nightingale Farms, Tesco*	½ Bag/130g	31	0.3	24	1	3.6	0.2	1.8
Sweet Potato, & Red Pepper, Deli, M&S*	1 Serving/250g	113	5.6	45	0.8	5.6	2.2	0.9
Sweet Potato, Skinny, M&S*	1 Serving/70g	69	2.9	99	2	12	4.2	2.6
Sweet, & Crunchy, Co-Op*	1 Pack/160g	43	1.1	27	1	3.7	0.7	0.9
Tabbouleh, & Dill Carrot, Pickled, Waitrose*	1 Pack/299g	266	11.4	89	3	8.7	3.8	3.8
Tomato, & Onion	**1oz/28g**	**20**	**1.7**	**72**	**0.8**	**4**	**6.1**	**1**
Tomato, Cherry, Tesco*	1 Pack/210g	136	9.4	65	0.9	4.2	4.5	1.1
Tomatoes, Santini, Radish, Salad Onion, House, M&S*	1 Bowl/310g	58	1.2	19	1.3	1.9	0.4	1.5
Topper, Mediterranean Inspired, Tesco*	1 Serving/20g	93	6.2	467	24.9	8.8	31.2	25.9
Tuna, & Potato, Tesco*	1 Pack/180g	99	0.9	55	5.5	6.4	0.5	1.4
Tuna, Bowl, Fresh, Asda*	1 Serving/160g	184	11.2	115	8	5	7	0
Tuna, French Style, Light Lunch, John West*	1 Pack/220g	218	6.2	99	7.5	9.8	2.8	2.5
Tuna, Italian Style, Light Lunch, John West*	1 Pack/220g	205	5.7	93	7.3	9.8	2.6	0.5
Tuna, Mediterranean Inspired, Tesco*	1 Pack/220g	200	2	91	8.5	10.5	0.9	3.4
Tuna, Mediterranean Style, Light Lunch, John West*	1 Pack/220g	211	4.2	96	8.5	10	1.9	2.4
Tuna, Mediterranean Style, Lunch On The Go, John West*	1 Serving/100g	96	1.9	96	8.5	10	1.9	2.4
Tuna, Mediterranean Style, Nixe, Lidl*	1 Pack/220g	254	5.5	116	10	12	2.5	2.8
Tuna, Mexican Style, Nixe, Lidl*	1 Tub/220g	293	11	133	11	9.4	5	3
Tuna, Nicoise, No Mayonnaise, Shapers, Boots*	1 Pack/276g	133	3.6	48	4	5	1.3	0.8
Tuna, Nicoise, Tesco*	1 Pack/240g	392	29	163	6.2	6.8	12.1	1.2
Vegetable, Mixed, without Dressing, From Restaurant	**1 ½ Cups/207g**	**33**	**0.1**	**16**	**1.2**	**3.2**	**0.1**	**2.1**
Vitality Mix, Superfood, Florette*	½ Bag/60g	14	0	23	1.8	1.7	0	2.3
Waldorf, Average	**1 Serving/100g**	**193**	**17.7**	**193**	**1.4**	**7.5**	**17.7**	**1.3**
Watercress, Spinach & Rocket, Prepared , Tesco*	½ Bag/40g	10	0.3	26	2.5	1.1	0.8	2
Watercress, Spinach & Rocket, Waitrose*	1 Bag/145g	30	1.2	21	2.2	1.2	0.8	1.5
Wholefood, Super Nutty, M&S*	1 Pack/230g	366	17.5	159	6.8	12.3	7.6	7.1
Wholefood, Super, Creamy Lemon & Mint Dressing, M&S*	1 Pack/290g	371	10.2	128	9.8	9.1	3.5	10.3
Wholegrain, & Edamame, Plant Kitchen, M&S*	1 Pack/290g	505	13.9	174	7.8	20.6	4.8	8.7

SALAD CREAM

	Measure INFO/WEIGHT	KCAL	FAT	KCAL	PROT	CARB	FAT	FIBRE
Average	**1 Tsp/5g**	**17**	**1.4**	**335**	**1.7**	**18.6**	**27.8**	**0.1**
Free From, Tesco*	1 Tbsp/15g	35	2.6	232	0.3	18.8	17.2	0.5
Reduced Calorie, Average	**1 Tsp/5g**	**6**	**0.4**	**130**	**1**	**12.9**	**7.9**	**0.2**

SALAMI

	Measure INFO/WEIGHT	KCAL	FAT	KCAL	PROT	CARB	FAT	FIBRE
Average	**1 Slice/5g**	**18**	**1.3**	**360**	**28.4**	**1.8**	**26.2**	**0**
Danish, Average	**1 Serving/17g**	**89**	**8.8**	**524**	**13.2**	**1.3**	**51.7**	**0**
German, Average	**1 Serving/60g**	**200**	**16.4**	**333**	**20.3**	**1.6**	**27.3**	**0.1**
German, Peppered, Average	**3 Slices/25g**	**86**	**6.8**	**342**	**22.2**	**2.5**	**27.1**	**0.2**
Milano, Average	**1 Serving/70g**	**278**	**22.6**	**397**	**25.9**	**0.9**	**32.2**	**0**
Napoli, Average	**1 Slice/5g**	**17**	**1.3**	**342**	**27.1**	**0.8**	**25.5**	**0**

S

SALMON

	INFO/WEIGHT	KCAL	FAT	KCAL	PROT	CARB	FAT	FIBRE
& Mango, M&S*	1 Pack/306g	370	19	121	6.5	9.1	6.2	1.3
Cooked, Prepacked, Average	*1 Fillet/93g*	*180*	*11.1*	*194*	*21.8*	*0*	*11.9*	*0*
Fillets, Boneless, Scottish, Oven Cooked, Waitrose*	1 Serving/93g	166	8.8	178	23.4	0	9.4	0
Fillets, Boneless, Skin-On, Fresh, Cooked, Average	*1 Sm Fillet/120g*	*265*	*17.1*	*221*	*23.2*	*0.2*	*14.2*	*0.1*
Fillets, Honey Roast, Sainsbury's*	1 Fillet/90g	203	12.1	226	23	3.4	13.4	0
Fillets, Hot Smoked, Sweet Chilli, Lighthouse Bay, Lidl*	1 Fillet/93g	216	13.5	232	21.8	3.2	14.5	0.5
Fillets, Hot Smoked, Sweet Chilli, Waitrose*	1 Fillet/72g	178	9.9	247	26.2	4.5	13.8	0.5
Fillets, Hot Smoked, with Teriyaki, Good Health, Waitrose*	1 Fillet/71g	165	8.9	233	26.2	4	12.5	0
Fillets, in Teriyaki Marinade, Good Health, Waitrose*	1 Fillet/91g	176	9.2	193	23	2.1	10.1	0.9
Fillets, Lemon & Dill Sauce, Pink, Inspirations, Birds Eye*	1 Fillet/225g	349	20.5	155	17.9	0.3	9.1	0.1
Fillets, Lemon Herb, Poached, Skinless, Scottish, Waitrose*	1 Fillet/79g	159	10.1	201	21.4	0.1	12.8	0.1
Fillets, Lighthouse Bay, Lidl*	1 Fillet/115g	245	16	213	21.6	0.1	13.9	0.5
Fillets, Lightly Smoked, Scottish, Waitrose*	1 Serving/175g	382	26.6	218	18.7	1.3	15.2	0.6
Fillets, Orkney, Whole, Organic, Duchy Originals, Waitrose*	1 Serving/140g	224	11.1	160	22.2	0	7.9	0
Fillets, Poached , Sainsbury's*	1 Fillet/90g	218	15.4	242	20.9	0.9	17.1	0.5
Fillets, Prime, Scottish, As Prepared, 1, Waitrose*	1 Serving/107g	222	14	207	22.4	0	13.1	0
Fillets, Raw, Average	*1 Sm Fillet/120g*	*227*	*14*	*189*	*20.9*	*0.1*	*11.7*	*0.1*
Fillets, Raw, Skin-On, Average	*1 Avg Fillet/120g*	*214*	*13.9*	*179*	*18.3*	*0.2*	*11.6*	*0.2*
Fillets, Red Thai Marinade, Infused, Fishmonger, Aldi*	1 Fillet/110g	189	12.1	172	17	1.4	11	0.5
Fillets, Skin On, Boneless, Individual, Sainsbury's*	1 Fillet/97g	259	19.4	267	21.5	0.4	20	0.4
Fillets, Skin On, in Chilli & Tomato Marinade, Waitrose*	1 Fillet/112g	251	16.1	224	21.7	1.8	14.4	0.5
Fillets, Skin On, TTD, Sainsbury's*	1 Fillet/126g	249	14.3	197	23.5	0.2	11.3	0
Fillets, Skinless, Scottish, Prime, As Sold, Waitrose*	1 Serving/100g	212	14.8	212	19.6	0.2	14.8	0.6
Fillets, Sockeye, Wild Pacific, Eat Well, M&S*	1 Fillet/110g	167	5.9	152	22.7	2.9	5.4	0.5
Fillets, Sweet Chilli, Hot Smoked, Ready to Eat, Tesco*	1 Fillet/90g	211	12.4	234	22.7	4.6	13.8	0.4
Fillets, Wild Alaskan, Keta, Sainsbury's*	1 Fillet/115g	178	6.4	155	25.9	0.2	5.6	0.3
Fillets, with Pesto, Scottish, Easy to Cook, Waitrose*	1 Serving/92g	199	12.1	216	23.5	0.5	13.1	0.7
Fillets, with Sweet Chilli Butter, Scottish, Sainsbury's*	½ Pack/125g	271	18.9	216	18.1	1.9	15.1	0.5
Flakes, Honey Roast, Average	*1oz/28g*	*56*	*3*	*198*	*24*	*1.9*	*10.7*	*0.2*
Flakes, Hot Smoked, with Honey, Tesco*	½ Pack/50g	104	5	208	22.8	6.3	10.1	0.5
Flakes, Sweet Chilli, M&S*	½ Pack/70g	143	4.6	204	24.5	11.7	6.6	0.6
Goujons, Average	*1 Pack/150g*	*321*	*16.4*	*214*	*16.4*	*12.4*	*11*	*1.1*
Gravadlax, Cured with Salt, Sugar & Herbs	*1 Serving/100g*	*119*	*3.3*	*119*	*18.3*	*3.1*	*3.3*	*0.4*
Grilled	*1oz/28g*	*60*	*3.7*	*215*	*24.2*	*0*	*13.1*	*0*
Honey Roast, Flakes, Tesco*	½ Pack/60g	147	8.2	244	25.6	4.6	13.6	0.4
Hot Smoked, Average	*1 Serving/62g*	*103*	*4.4*	*166*	*24*	*0.9*	*7.2*	*0.1*
in Watercress Sauce, with Potatoes, Tesco*	1 Pack/399g	342	12.5	86	8.9	5	3.1	0.9
Mild Oak Smoked, Average	*1 Slice/25g*	*46*	*2.5*	*182*	*22.6*	*0.1*	*10.2*	*0*
Oak Smoked, Speybay, M&S*	1 Pack/100g	158	6.5	158	22	2.4	6.5	0.7
Pieces, Scottish, J James*	1 Serving/100g	239	14.9	239	23.5	0.5	14.9	0.6
Pink in Brine, Average	*1 Sm Can/105g*	*129*	*5.5*	*122*	*18.8*	*0*	*5.3*	*0*
Pink, Canned, Average	*1 Serving/125g*	*162*	*7.2*	*130*	*19.5*	*0.1*	*5.8*	*0.1*
Poached, Average	*1 Serving/90g*	*176*	*10.5*	*195*	*22.5*	*0.2*	*11.7*	*0.3*
Portions, Lemon & Pepper, Fish of the Day, Iceland*	1 Portion/130g	281	18.3	216	22.2	0	14.1	0
Red in Brine, Average	*1oz/28g*	*42*	*2.2*	*149*	*19.7*	*0*	*7.8*	*0*
Red, Average	*½ Can/90g*	*141*	*7.4*	*156*	*20.4*	*0.1*	*8.2*	*0.1*
Skewers, Chilli, Lime, & Soy, Morrisons*	1 Skewer/101g	228	14.7	226	18.8	4.6	14.6	0.3
Skewers, Teriyaki, Sweet, M&S*	1 Skewer/48g	96	5.9	201	17.1	5.8	12.2	0
Smoked, Average	*1 Serving/70g*	*126*	*7*	*179*	*21.9*	*0.5*	*10*	*0.1*
Smoked, Lightly, Lemon & Herb, Tesco*	¼ Pack/128g	334	23	261	22.1	2	18	1.2
Smoked, Slices, Fishmonger, Aldi*	½ Pack/100g	158	7.9	158	21	0.5	7.9	0.5
Smoked, Trimmings, Average	*1 Serving/55g*	*101*	*5.7*	*184*	*22.8*	*0.2*	*10.3*	*0*
Steaks	*1 Serving/100g*	*180*	*11*	*180*	*20.2*	*0*	*11*	*0*

	Measure INFO/WEIGHT	per Measure KCAL	FAT	Nutrition Values per 100g / 100ml KCAL	PROT	CARB	FAT	FIBRE
SALMON								
Steamed	*1oz/28g*	*55*	*3.6*	*197*	*20.1*	*0*	*13*	*0*
Sweet Chilli, Bites, Sainsbury's*	½ Pack/50g	135	8	270	25.4	5.7	16.1	0.5
SALMON EN CROUTE								
Charlie Bigham's*	1 Serving/220 g	568	38.5	258	9.3	15.6	17.5	0
Frozen, Tesco*	1 Serving/166g	365	18.4	220	10.1	19.1	11.1	1.1
Retail, Average	*1oz/28g*	*81*	*5.3*	*288*	*11.8*	*18*	*19.1*	*0*
SALMON IN								
Lime & Coriander, Fillets, Good Choice, Iceland*	½ Pack/150g	189	4.4	126	19.8	5.1	2.9	0.8
Tomato & Mascarpone Sauce, Fillets, Asda*	½ Pack/181g	279	19.9	154	13	0.8	11	0.6
White Wine & Cream Sauce, Tesco*	1 Serving/170g	279	19.2	164	13.5	2	11.3	1.2
SALMON WITH								
Garlic & Herb Butter, Tesco*	1 Fillet/112g	291	23.1	260	17.6	0	20.6	0
Giant Cous Cous & Lentils, Creations, John West*	1 Pack/180g	297	15.5	165	7.6	13	8.6	2.5
New Potatoes, Broccoli, Green Beans, BFY, M&S*	1 Pack/385g	331	12.3	86	6.6	7.8	3.2	0.5
SALSA								
Beetroot, Love Beets*	1 Serving/80g	75	0.2	94	1.2	20	0.3	2.9
Chunky, Sainsbury's*	½ Pot/84g	43	1.4	51	1.1	7.8	1.7	1.2
Coconut, & Turmeric, Italian, Organic, Mr Organic*	1 Tbsp/15g	16	1.1	108	1.9	7.8	7.2	0
Cool, Sainsbury's*	¼ Pot/58g	30	1.2	52	1.4	6.3	2.1	1.1
Medium Hot, Discovery*	1 Serving/30g	17	0.1	56	1.4	11.7	0.4	0.8
Medium, Chunky, Newman's Own*	2 Tbsp/32g	10	0	32	3.2	9.7	0	3.2
Mild, Original, Old El Paso*	1 Sachet/144g	60	0.7	42	1.6	9	0.5	0
Original from Dinner Kit, Old El Paso*	1 Jar/226g	71	0.7	32	1.2	6	0.3	0
Red, Medium, M&S*	¼ Jar/49g	34	1.5	69	1.4	8.3	3	1.8
Spicy Mango & Lime, Morrisons*	½ Pot/85g	62	0.3	73	1	15.9	0.4	1.3
Spicy Red Pepper, Fresh, Waitrose*	½ Pot/85g	27	0.8	32	1.9	4.1	0.9	1.6
Tomato, Chunky, Tesco*	1 Pot/170g	68	2.2	40	1.1	5.9	1.3	1.1
Tomato, Cool, Asda*	1 Pot/215g	84	1.1	39	1.4	6.4	0.5	1.5
Tomato, Onion, Coriander & Chilli, Fresh, Waitrose*	1 Tub/170g	110	5.3	65	1.3	8	3.1	1.2
Tomato, Sun Ripened, Tesco*	1 Serving/40g	46	1.7	115	5	14.2	4.2	4.6
SALT								
Alternative, Reduced Sodium, Losalt*	½ Tsp/1g	0	0	0	0	0	0	0
Kosher, Average	*1 Tsp/5g*	*0*	*0*	*0*	*0*	*0*	*0*	*0*
Rock, Average	*¼ Tsp/1g*	*0*	*0*	*0*	*0*	*0*	*0*	*0*
Table, Average	*1 Tsp/5g*	*0*	*0*	*0*	*0*	*0*	*0*	*0*
SAMBUCA								
Average	*1 Pub Shot/35ml*	*122*	*0*	*348*	*0*	*37.2*	*0*	*0*
SAMOSAS								
Chicken, Tikka, Indian, Sainsbury's*	1 Samosa/55g	131	5.5	237	9.4	25	10	4.6
Indian Style Selection, Co-Op*	1 Samosa/21g	50	2.7	240	5	27	13	3
Meat, Takeaway, Average	*1 Samosa/110g*	*299*	*19*	*272*	*11.4*	*18.9*	*17.3*	*2.4*
Vegetable, Average	*1 Samosa/110g*	*258*	*12.8*	*235*	*4.8*	*26.9*	*11.6*	*2.5*
Vegetable, Indian Snack Selection, 12, Sainsbury's*	2 Samosas/45g	114	5.5	253	4.9	28.5	12.3	4.1
Vegetable, Indian Starter Selection, M&S*	1 Samosa/21g	53	2.5	254	5.3	29.3	12.1	3.3
Vegetable, Indian, 4 Pack, Sainsbury's*	1 Samosa/47g	115	5.9	246	4.7	26.3	12.6	4.4
Vegetable, Large, Individual, Sainsbury's*	1 Samosa/110g	254	16.5	231	3.3	20.7	15	2.1
Vegetable, Large, Tesco*	1 Samosa/98g	214	8.9	219	5.3	27.6	9.1	2.8
Vegetable, M&S*	1 Samosa/55g	111	5.5	201	4.5	21.7	9.9	3.6
Vegetable, Mini, Asda*	1 Samosa/23g	52	2	233	6	32	9	2.6
Vegetable, Mini, Indian Snack Selection, Sainsbury's*	1 Samosa/25g	70	4	280	4.7	29.8	15.8	3.2
Vegetable, Mini, Indian Snack Selection, Tesco*	1 Samosa/32g	76	4.2	238	4.7	25.5	13	3.3
Vegetable, On the Go, Sainsbury's*	1 Samosa/50g	124	5.8	248	4.8	29.2	11.5	4.6
Vegetable, Waitrose*	1 Samosa/58g	129	6.6	223	4.5	23.8	11.4	3.8

S

SANDWICH

INFO/WEIGHT	Measure	per Measure KCAL	FAT	Nutrition Values per 100g / 100ml KCAL	PROT	CARB	FAT	FIBRE
All Day Breakfast, One Stop*	1 Sandwich/196g	453	18.2	231	10.5	25.6	9.3	1.4
All Day Breakfast, Tesco Classic*	1 Pack/374g	636	29.9	170	8	14.5	8	3
Avo-Lafel, Urban Eat*	1 Pack/184g	453	18.6	246	7.4	29.5	10.1	4.2
Bacon, & Egg, Co-Op*	1 Pack/188g	536	32	285	13	20	17	2
Bacon, & Egg, Sainsbury's*	1 Pack/160g	384	17.8	240	13	22	11.1	1.8
Bacon, & Egg, Tesco*	1 Pack/213g	494	19.6	232	14.8	21.6	9.2	1.8
Bacon, Lettuce, & Tomato, Loved by Us, Co-Op*	1 Pack/195g	410	14.2	210	10.2	25.1	7.3	2.3
Bacon, Maple Cured, Lettuce, & Tomato, Sainsbury's*	1 Pack/191g	425	19.1	222	9.2	22.3	10	2.8
Bacon, On the Go, Sainsbury's*	1 Pack/163g	454	17.9	279	13.2	30.9	11	1.6
Beef, & Horseradish Mayonnaise, Roast, Rare, Waitrose*	1 Pack/197g	415	15.3	211	12.2	23.1	7.8	2
Beef, & Horseradish, Sainsbury's*	1 Pack/187g	391	12.5	209	12.5	23.8	6.7	1.5
Beef, & Pate, M&S*	1 Pack/188g	310	7.3	165	11.2	21.6	3.9	2.4
Beef, & Salad, Roast, Daily Bread*	1 Pack/202g	319	8.3	158	9	21.4	4.1	0
Beef, & Horseradish Mayo, Soft White Bread, M&S*	1 Pack/200g	398	12.2	199	13	22.4	6.1	1.4
Beef, & Horseradish, Onion Bloomer, Booths*	1 Pack/199g	493	23.9	248	1.4	20	12	1.8
Beef, & Horseradish, Tesco*	1 Pack/175g	364	9.6	208	13.2	25.7	5.5	1.6
Beef, Med Rare, & Stilton, Finest, Tesco*	1 Pack/201g	461	15.3	229	13.5	25.8	7.6	1.9
Beef, Roast, & Horseradish, Specially Selected, Aldi*	1 Pack/192g	394	11	205	13	24	5.7	1.3
Beef, Salt, with Gherkins & Mustard Mayo, Sainsbury's*	1 Pack/242g	486	18.2	201	9.3	24.1	7.5	3.1
BLT, Asda*	1 Pack/172g	325	11.9	189	9.9	21.8	6.9	4.6
BLT, Deep Filled, with Mayonnaise, Eat & Go*	1 Pack/175g	408	15.2	233	13	24	8.7	2.8
BLT, Made Without Wheat, M&S*	1 Pack/206g	476	25.1	231	7.2	21.2	12.2	4
BLT, on Malted Brown Bread, Tesco*	1 Pack/185g	454	21.7	245	10.9	22.9	11.7	2.4
BLT, Waitrose*	1 Pack/184g	398	16.4	216	9.5	24.5	8.9	2.3
BLT, with Mayo, Malted Bread, Just Tasty, Aldi*	1 Pack/186g	437	17.9	235	14	22	9.6	2.4
Brie, & Cranberry, Morrisons*	1 Pack/178g	438	20.3	246	10.4	24.4	11.4	2.2
Brie, & Grape, Finest, Tesco*	1 Pack/209g	527	31.6	252	8.5	20.6	15.1	1.5
Brie, & Wild Cranberry, Delicious, Boots*	1 Pack/168g	413	18.5	246	9.1	27	11	3.3
Brie, & Cranberry, on Malted Brown, Tesco*	1 Pack/159g	387	17.6	244	8.9	25.9	11.1	2.3
Cheddar, & Ham, M&S*	1 Pack/165g	396	18.6	240	15.1	20	11.3	1.7
Cheddar, & Tomato, Red, Tesco*	1 Pack/165g	474	23.8	287	9.2	29.2	14.4	1.9
Cheddar, Oldfields*	1 Pack/121g	384	17.3	317	12.8	33.2	14.3	1.5
Cheese, & Coleslaw, M&S*	1 Pack/186g	498	32.4	268	10.2	17.6	17.4	3.2
Cheese, & Ham, & Pickle, HL, Tesco*	1 Pack/201g	312	4.2	155	13.1	21	2.1	1.7
Cheese, & Ham, & Pickle, Tesco*	1 Pack/215g	497	24.7	231	11.7	20.3	11.5	1.8
Cheese, & Ham, Smoked, Co-Op*	1 Pack/167g	334	8.4	200	15	24	5	2
Cheese, & Marmite, No Mayonnaise, Boots*	1 Pack/156g	420	20	269	12.2	26.3	12.8	1.7
Cheese, & Onion, Eat Smart, Morrisons*	1 Pack/144g	340	10.9	236	13.1	27.8	7.6	2.1
Cheese, & Onion, Essential, Waitrose*	1 Pack/158g	432	21.5	273	11.5	25.2	13.6	2
Cheese, & Onion, Tesco*	1 Pack/172g	505	28.3	294	10.2	24.5	16.5	3.3
Cheese, & Pickle, Tesco*	1 Pack/140g	400	19.3	286	12.7	27.8	13.8	1.4
Cheese, & Pickle, Virgin Trains*	1 Pack/158g	444	19.6	281	11.5	31.1	12.4	0
Cheese, & Salad, & Reduced Fat Mayonnaise, Waitrose*	1 Pack/180g	301	9	167	9.8	20.8	5	3.1
Cheese, & Salad, COU, M&S*	1 Pack/188g	244	3	130	12.1	17	1.6	2.4
Cheese, & Spring Onion, Three, Shell*	1 Pack/168g	672	50.9	400	11.1	20.8	30.3	0
Cheese, & Tomato, Asda*	1 Pack/154g	388	19.7	252	11	23.2	12.8	3.7
Cheese, & Tomato, Co-Op*	1 Pack/155g	365	18.5	235	10.6	21.8	11.9	1.9
Cheese, & Tomato, Organic, M&S*	1 Pack/165g	559	35.3	339	11.8	24.8	21.4	1.9
Cheese, & Apple Slaw, Wholemeal, Nutritious, Boots*	1 Pack/252g	400	14.3	159	8.1	17	5.7	3
Cheese, & Onion, Soft Oatmeal Bread, M&S*	1 Pack/170g	497	30.1	292	10.3	21.9	17.7	2.1
Cheese, Cheddar, & Celery, Malted Brown Bread, M&S*	1 Pack/200g	506	26.4	253	9.6	23.4	13.2	1
Cheese, Cheddar, White Bread, On the Go, Sainsbury's*	1 Pack/131g	417	21.3	319	13.6	28.8	16.3	1.2
Cheese, Simply, Boots*	1 Pack/138g	375	13.9	272	13.8	30.4	10.1	2.2

S

SANDWICH

INFO/WEIGHT	Measure per Measure KCAL	FAT	Nutrition Values per 100g / 100ml KCAL	PROT	CARB	FAT	FIBRE
Cheese, Three, on Oatmeal Bread, Handmade, Spar*	1 Pack/130g	365	19.5	281	14	25	15	2.3
Chicken Mayo, on Malted Bread, Asda*	1 Pack/165g	362	10.6	219	13	26	6.4	1.8
Chicken Mayo, on Malted Bread, On the Go, Sainsbury's*	1 Pack/170g	369	11.4	217	12.6	25.3	6.7	2.6
Chicken Salad, BLT, & Cheese & Tomato, Triple, Tesco*	1 Pack/297g	714	31.5	240	12.1	23	10.6	2.2
Chicken Salad, on Malted Bread, The Tasty Snack Co*	1 Pack/152g	309	9	203	9.6	26.7	5.9	0
Chicken, & Avocado, Black Pepper Mayonnaise, Waitrose*	1 Pack/213g	392	12.4	184	9.8	21.8	5.8	2.5
Chicken, & Avocado, Roast, on Soft Malted Bread, M&S*	1 Pack/200g	412	14.2	206	11.2	23	7.1	2.7
Chicken, & Avocado, Roast, Tesco*	1 Pack/173g	360	13.3	208	12.1	21.4	7.7	2.4
Chicken, & Bacon, & Avocado, M&S*	1 Pack/242g	508	28.3	210	10.7	15.8	11.7	3.2
Chicken, & Bacon, COU, M&S*	1 Pack/179g	250	3.6	140	13.5	15.8	2	3.8
Chicken, & Bacon, Deep Filled, Co-Op*	1 Pack/166g	556	33.2	335	16	23	20	3
Chicken, & Bacon, Tesco*	1 Pack/195g	486	24.2	249	14.3	20	12.4	2.7
Chicken, & Bacon, with Mayo, Malted Grain, Ginsters*	1 Pack/183g	400	14.7	218	12.8	23.4	8	1
Chicken, & Mayo, Simply, Delicious, Boots*	1 Pack/148g	318	8.6	215	14	25	5.8	2.2
Chicken, & Salad, Aldi*	1 Pack/195g	338	4.5	173	11.5	23.8	2.3	2
Chicken, & Salad, Co-Op*	1 Pack/195g	448	21.4	230	10	24	11	2
Chicken, & Salad, Deep Fill, Ginsters*	1 Pack/203g	364	12.4	179	10.3	20.8	6.1	2.1
Chicken, & Salad, M&S*	1 Pack/226g	350	9.3	155	10.6	18.8	4.1	3
Chicken, & Salad, Roast, Waitrose*	1 Pack/217g	482	24.1	222	9.4	21.1	11.1	2
Chicken, & Salad, Sainsbury's*	1 Pack/247g	461	12.6	187	11.8	22.6	5.1	1.6
Chicken, & Stuffing, Co-Op*	1 Pack/208g	420	13	202	13.5	22.6	6.2	2.4
Chicken, & Stuffing, Pork Sage & Onion, Tesco*	1 Pack/136g	376	17	276	12.1	28.1	12.5	1.4
Chicken, & Stuffing, Roast, Soft Malted Brown Bread, M&S*	1 Pack/212g	422	12.3	199	14.5	21.3	5.8	2
Chicken, & Stuffing, Waitrose*	1 Pack/183g	450	18.8	246	12.8	25.6	10.3	1.5
Chicken, & Sweetcorn, British, Eat Well, M&S*	1 Pack/194g	340	10.5	175	11.4	19.6	5.4	3.1
Chicken, & Sweetcorn, Malted Bread, Sainsbury's*	1 Pack/193g	370	9.8	192	12.3	22.9	5.1	2.6
Chicken, & Sweetcorn, Roast, Good to Go, Waitrose*	1 Pack/189g	321	6.2	170	12.1	21.3	3.3	3.3
Chicken, & Sweetcorn, Tesco*	1 Pack/174g	355	11	204	10.8	24.6	6.3	3
Chicken, & Avocado, Limited Edition, Co-Op*	1 Pack/192g	362	11.9	188	10	21	6.2	2.9
Chicken, & Bacon, Maize Topped, Sub, Tesco*	1 Pack/195g	460	15.2	236	13.2	27.5	7.8	1.5
Chicken, & Bacon, on Malted Bread, Co-Op*	1 Pack/194g	449	15.2	231	16	23	7.8	2.5
Chicken, & Mayo, Deli Club, Tesco*	1 Pack/183g	384	10.8	210	15.5	22.8	5.9	2.1
Chicken, & Salad, Roast, Soft Malted Brown Bread, M&S*	1 Pack/256g	440	13.6	172	12	17.6	5.3	2.7
Chicken, & Stuffing, LC, Tesco*	1 Pack/172g	275	4.8	160	14.4	18.7	2.8	6.9
Chicken, Club, The, Tesco*	1 Pack/246g	613	29.8	249	12.9	21.1	12.1	2.1
Chicken, Coronation, M&S*	1 Pack/210g	420	20.4	200	11.2	20.2	9.7	3.1
Chicken, Coronation, on Onion Bread, M&S*	1 Pack/260g	458	16.9	176	10.6	17.7	6.5	2
Chicken, Ham, & Emmental, Club, High Protein, M&S *	1 Pack/149g	289	13.6	194	13.8	13.8	9.1	1.2
Chicken, in White Bread, Tesco*	1 Pack/131g	279	4.6	213	10.8	34.1	3.5	1.1
Chicken, Jerk, & Sunshine Slaw, Boots*	1 Pack/202g	349	7.7	173	10	23	3.8	2
Chicken, Just, No Mayonnaise, Tesco*	1 Pack/146g	298	6.3	204	14.6	25.8	4.3	1.6
Chicken, Mayonnaise, Loved by Us, Co-Op*	1 Pack/151g	352	13.9	233	13	23	9.2	2.1
Chicken, No Mayo, M&S*	1 Pack/142g	248	3.3	175	16.6	20.6	2.3	3.2
Chicken, Pesto, Shapers, Boots*	1 Pack/181g	311	4.2	172	12	26	2.3	1.7
Chicken, Piri Piri, Express Cuisine*	1 Pack/180g	396	12.4	220	10.2	27.6	6.9	2.9
Chicken, Roast, & Mayo, Essential, Waitrose*	1 Pack/150g	329	10.5	219	12.6	25.5	7	1.8
Chicken, Roast, Chorizo, Finest, Tesco*	1 Pack/201g	431	14.1	214	12.6	24.1	7	1.9
Chicken, Soy & Ginger, Sushi, M&S*	1 Pack/241g	292	3.1	121	6.4	20.4	1.3	1.2
Chicken, Tikka, & Mango Chutney, Tesco*	1 Pack/201g	352	4.8	175	11.6	25.4	2.4	2.6
Chicken, Tikka, COU, M&S*	1 Pack/185g	268	3.3	145	12.1	20.5	1.8	3.2
Chicken, Tikka, on Pepper Chilli Bread, Shapers, Boots*	1 Pack/172g	296	4.5	172	13	25	2.6	2.5
Chicken, Triple, On the Go, Sainsbury's*	1 Pack/275g	637	22.2	232	13	23.4	8.1	1.9
Chicken, with Pork, Sage & Onion Stuffing, Sainsbury's*	1 Pack/187g	423	18	226	12	22	9.6	1.9

S

SANDWICH

Measure INFO/WEIGHT	per Measure		Nutrition Values per 100g / 100ml				
	KCAL	FAT	KCAL	PROT	CARB	FAT	FIBRE
SANDWICH							
Club, New York Style, Sainsbury's* — 1 Pack/212g	608	33.5	287	13.3	22.8	15.8	2.7
Corned Beef, on White, Simply, Brambles* — 1 Pack/126g	325	10.8	258	14.2	30.8	8.6	1.4
Corned Beef, Tomato & Onion, Salad Garden* — 1 Pack/137g	338	14.8	247	14.2	23	10.8	0
Crayfish, & Rocket, Finest, Tesco* — 1 Pack/178g	365	10.5	205	9.8	27.5	5.9	2.1
Egg Mayo, & Salad, You Count, Love Life, Waitrose* — 1 Pack/196g	314	10.2	160	8.8	18.5	5.2	2.2
Egg Mayo, Free Range, Asda* — 1 Pack/178g	311	10.1	175	9.3	21.5	5.7	2.1
Egg Mayo, Free Range, on Oatmeal Bread, M&S* — 1 Pack/180g	315	12.2	175	9.4	18.2	6.8	2.8
Egg Mayonnaise, & Cress, Co-Op* — 1 Pack/159g	405	24	255	8.8	20.8	15.1	1.9
Egg Mayonnaise, & Cress, Go Simple, Asda* — 1 Pack/169g	370	18.6	219	10	20	11	1.7
Egg Mayonnaise, & Cress, HL, Tesco* — 1 Pack/149g	271	7.7	182	9	23.5	5.2	2.6
Egg Mayonnaise, Free Range, Soft Oatmeal Bread, M&S* — 1 Pack/176g	345	12.3	196	9.9	21.9	7	3.1
Egg, & Avocado, & Chilli Chutney, M&S* — 1 Pack/209g	368	15.1	176	7.7	18.3	7.2	3.5
Egg, & Bacon, Handmade, Tesco* — 1 Pack/217g	489	20.4	225	13.4	20.8	9.4	2
Egg, & Cress, BGTY, Sainsbury's* — 1 Pack/145g	268	7.5	185	9.1	25.4	5.2	2.7
Egg, & Cress, Co-Op* — 1 Pack/159g	398	23.8	250	9	21	15	2
Egg, & Cress, COU, M&S* — 1 Pack/192g	240	5.2	125	9.8	15.5	2.7	2.8
Egg, & Cress, Free Range, M&S* — 1 Pack/192g	307	9	160	10.7	17.8	4.7	3
Egg, & Cress, Free Range, Sainsbury's* — 1 Pack/183g	346	13	189	9.7	20.5	7.1	2.2
Egg, & Cress, No Mayo, LC, Tesco* — 1 Pack/160g	280	7.2	175	9.4	23.7	4.5	3
Egg, & Ham, Deli Club, Tesco* — 1 Pack/220g	433	15.4	197	11.4	20.5	7	2.7
Egg, & Salad, on Softgrain Bread, HL, Tesco* — 1 Pack/197g	290	4.7	147	7	23.6	2.4	1.7
Egg, & Tomato & Salad Cream, M&S* — 1 Pack/214g	402	14.8	188	7.8	22.6	6.9	2
Egg, & Watercress, Bloomer, Freshly Prepared, M&S* — 1 Pack/221g	465	26.1	210	10.2	15.3	11.8	3
Egg, & Watercress, GF Seeded Bread, Eat Well, M&S* — 1 Pack/192g	382	16.9	199	8	20.6	8.8	2.9
Egg, & Cress, on Oatmeal Bread, Asda* — 1 Pack/162g	323	11.3	200	9.7	23	7	2.1
Egg, & Cress, with Mayonnaise, Eat & Go, Aldi* — 1 Pack/177g	345	13.6	195	9.5	21	7.7	1.7
Egg, & Mayonnaise, Jamie Oliver* — 1 Pack/182g	289	10.2	159	7.3	18.9	5.6	2.2
Egg, & Tomato, with Salad Cream, Delicious, Boots* — 1 Pack/205g	410	16	200	7.8	23.4	7.8	2.6
Egg, & Watercress, Eat Well, M&S* — 1 Pack/190g	355	10.8	187	9.8	22.9	5.7	2.4
Egg, & Watercress, GF, Good to Go, Waitrose* — 1 Pack/174g	376	22.8	216	7.9	15	13.1	3.2
Egg, Free Range, & Farmhouse Cheddar, Salad, M&S* — 1 Pack/172g	260	14.4	151	9.1	12.7	8.4	1.7
Egg, Free Range, & Cheddar, High Protein, M&S * — 1 Pack/253g	319	19.7	126	7.9	5.8	7.8	0.5
Feta Cheese, & Salad, Tastte* — 1 Pack/178g	367	13.4	206	10.6	24	7.5	0
Goat's Cheese, & Cranberry, Shapers, Boots* — 1 Pack/150g	323	6.3	216	8.4	36	4.2	2.6
Green Machine, The Real Wrap Co.* — 1 Pack/163g	385	16.2	236	6.9	29.3	9.9	0
Ham Hock, & Pea Crush, Waitrose* — 1 Pack/200g	394	12.2	197	10.3	24.2	6.1	2.1
Ham Salad, Eat Better, Urban Eat* — 1 Pack/179g	263	5.9	147	9.4	18.3	3.3	3.6
Ham Salad, on Malted Bread, BGTY, Sainsbury's* — 1 Pack/175g	262	4.2	150	9.1	21.8	2.4	2.2
Ham, & Cheese, & Pickle, & Lettuce, No Mayo, Tesco* — 1 Pack/207g	435	16.2	210	12.2	23	7.8	2.7
Ham, & Cheese, & Pickle, Average — ***1 Pack/220g***	***524***	***25.1***	***238***	***12.2***	***21.6***	***11.4***	***2.5***
Ham, & Cheese, Honey Roast, Soft Oatmeal Bread, M&S* — 1 Pack/188g	466	21.6	248	13.9	20.9	11.5	2.7
Ham, & Cheese, on a Croissant, Smoked, M&S* — 1 Croissant/105g	341	22.7	325	13.4	22.2	21.6	3.9
Ham, & Edam, Smoked, Shapers, Boots* — 1 Pack/183g	315	11.9	172	9.3	19	6.5	2.7
Ham, & Egg, Honey Roast, Tesco* — 1 Pack/192g	355	9.8	185	12.8	20.6	5.1	2.5
Ham, & Mustard Mayo, Smoked, Soft Oatmeal Bread, M&S — 1 Pack/150g	282	6.4	188	13.2	23.2	4.3	2
Ham, & Mustard, Ginsters* — 1 Pack/140g	307	9.4	219	11.8	28	6.7	2.5
Ham, & Mustard, Loved by Us, Co-Op* — 1 Pack/162g	310	7.9	191	13.2	22.4	4.9	1.8
Ham, & Mustard, Salad, BGTY, Sainsbury's* — 1 Pack/183g	261	3.8	143	8.7	22.4	2.1	2.6
Ham, & Mustard, Tesco* — 1 Pack/147g	437	27.9	297	10.6	20.8	19	1.2
Ham, & Mustard, Wiltshire, The Ultimate, M&S* — 1 Pack/246g	344	11.8	140	9.8	15	4.8	1.4
Ham, & Salad, Bap, Co-Op* — 1 Bap/164g	295	4.9	180	8	30	3	2
Ham, & Salad, On the Go, Sainsbury's* — 1 Pack/174g	244	3	140	10.1	20	1.7	2
Ham, & Salad, Shapers, Boots* — 1 Pack/195g	269	2.7	138	9.4	22	1.4	1.8

S

SANDWICH

	Measure INFO/WEIGHT	per Measure KCAL	per Measure FAT	Nutrition Values per 100g / 100ml KCAL	PROT	CARB	FAT	FIBRE
Ham, & Soft Cheese, Tesco*	1 Pack/164g	333	12.1	203	11.6	22.5	7.4	2.2
Ham, & Turkey with Salad, Co-Op*	1 Pack/188g	263	5.6	140	9	21	3	2
Ham, & Cheese, Honey Roast, Seeded Bread, GF, M&S*	1 Pack/196g	499	26.6	255	11.9	19.6	13.6	3.1
Ham, & Cheese, Morrisons*	1 Pack/183g	273	4.6	149	12.5	19.2	2.5	4.1
Ham, & Coleslaw, Smoked, Soft Malted Brown Bread, M&S	1 Pack/175g	388	16.3	222	9.2	24.2	9.3	2.5
Ham, & Egg Mayonnaise, Urban Eat*	1 Pack/174g	365	14.4	210	12.4	20.2	8.3	2.6
Ham, & Mature Cheddar, Sub, Tesco*	1 Pack/200g	488	18	244	13.5	26.5	9	1.6
Ham, & Mustard Mayo, Smoked, Good to Go, Waitrose*	1 Pack/160g	309	8	193	12.9	23	5	2.2
Ham, Egg, & Chips, Delicious, Boots*	1 Pack/206g	390	11.8	189	10	23	5.7	2.2
Ham, No Mayo, Just Ham, Tesco*	1 Pack/122g	250	4.9	205	11.6	30.4	4	2.1
Ham, No Mayo, On the Go, Sainsbury's*	1 Pack/131g	256	5.4	195	13.7	24.9	4.1	1.9
Ham, Smoked, & Egg, Club, Delicious, Boots*	1 Pack/268g	472	14.5	176	9.3	21	5.4	2.3
Houmous, & Carrot, Shapers, Boots*	1 Pack/204g	323	10.2	158	7.5	21	5	5.2
Houmous, & Salad, Vegan, Chop Chop*	1 Pack/208g	300	6	144	5.2	21.5	2.9	3.8
Lettuce, Guac, Bacon, Tomato, LGBT, M&S *	1 Pack/250g	443	21	177	8.3	15.6	8.4	2.2
New Yorker, TTD, On the Go, Sainsbury's*	1 Pack/248g	486	17.6	196	10.2	21.8	7.1	2.1
Pastrami, New York Deli, Finest, Tesco*	1 Pack/231g	500	22.7	216	11.9	18.7	9.8	2.9
Ploughman's, Cheese, Cheddar, Deep Fill, Asda*	1 Pack/229g	471	22.9	206	9	20	10	4.3
Ploughman's, Cheese, Deep Fill, Ginsters*	1 Pack/213g	491	24.2	231	8.4	23.8	11.4	2.2
Ploughman's, Red Leicester, On the Go, Sainsbury's*	1 Pack/219g	518	26.3	236	8.8	2	12	2.2
Ploughmans, Cheddar, Tesco*	1 Pack/186g	418	18.6	225	9	23.4	10	2.8
Pork, Roast, Stuffing, & Apple, Roll, Finest, Tesco*	1 Pack/192g	397	8.4	207	8.9	31.9	4.4	1.9
Prawn Cocktail, Free From, Waitrose*	1 Pack/158g	336	17.2	213	6.6	20.8	10.9	2.6
Prawn Mayo, Egg & Cress, CLT, Triple, Waitrose*	1 Pack/262g	557	22.8	213	9.8	22.7	8.7	2.1
Prawn Mayonnaise, Co-Op*	1 Pack/154g	285	6	185	9.7	27.3	3.9	3.2
Prawn Mayonnaise, Morrisons*	1 Pack/157g	234	3.9	149	9	22.7	2.5	3
Prawn Mayonnaise, Oatmeal Bread, Sainsbury's*	1 Pack/174g	357	15.3	205	10.3	20.1	8.8	2.3
Prawn Mayonnaise, Seeded Bread, GF, M&S*	1 Pack/203g	386	16.5	190	9	18.7	8.1	3
Prawn Mayonnaise, Shapers, Boots*	1 Pack/160g	293	7.5	183	9.4	25.6	4.7	2.5
Prawn Mayonnaise, Soft Malted Brown Bread, M&S*	1 Pack/197g	347	8.9	176	11.6	21.1	4.5	2.3
Prawn, King, Sainsbury's*	1 Pack/204g	424	16.3	208	11.6	22.3	8	0
Prawn, Marie Rose, Waitrose*	1 Pack/164g	226	5.6	138	8.8	18	3.4	1.9
Rib, BBQ, Pork, Rustlers*	1 Pack/157g	355	14.1	226	10.2	25.3	9	0
Salami, & Cheese, Migrolino*	1 Pack/140g	486	26.6	347	14	29	19	2
Salmon, & Cream Cheese, Smoked, Morrisons*	1 Pack/160g	342	13.1	214	11	22	8.2	4
Salmon, & Cucumber, M&S*	1 Pack/168g	329	13.9	196	11	19.5	8.3	2.6
Salmon, & Cucumber, Red, Tesco*	1 Pack/144g	284	9.2	197	11.1	23.8	6.4	1.9
Salmon, & Soft Cheese, Smoked, Waitrose*	1 Pack/180g	416	18	231	11.5	22.6	10	2.2
Salmon, & Watercress, Poached, Lochmuir, M&S*	1 Pack/192g	355	11.7	185	10.3	22.3	6.1	1.6
Salmon, & Cream Cheese, Smoked, Sainsbury*	1 Pack/168g	408	17.5	243	11.7	24.5	10.4	2.2
Salmon, & Cucumber, Good to Go, Waitrose*	1 Pack/185g	316	9.2	171	12.1	18	5	2.8
Salmon, Smoked, & Cream Cheese, Finest, Tesco*	1 Pack/200g	483	19.2	242	11.5	26.4	9.6	1.9
Salmon, Smoked, Moray Firth, & Egg, Co-Op*	1 Pack/230g	493	22.1	214	12	19	9.6	1.5
Sausage, Cumberland, & Mustard, On the Go, Sainsbury's*	1 Pack/203g	475	17.5	234	10.3	27.5	8.6	2.5
Sausage, Pigs Under Portionets, Delicious, Boots*	1 Pack/181g	453	16.7	250	11	29	9.2	2.5
Seafood, Medley, M&S*	1 Pack/227g	468	28.1	206	7.2	16.3	12.4	3.5
Steak	*1 Serving/204g*	*459*	*14.1*	*225*	*14.9*	*25.5*	*6.9*	*0*
Sub, Ham, & Tomato Salad, Shapers, Boots*	1 Pack/170g	286	3.9	168	9.2	28	2.3	1.4
Sub, Tuna, & Salad, From Restaurant, Average	*1 Serving/256g*	*584*	*28*	*228*	*11.6*	*21.6*	*10.9*	*0*
Tastes of Christmas, Selection, M&S*	1 Pack/205g	484	21.5	236	12.3	22	10.5	1.9
The Beet Goes On, Roots, Urban Eat*	1 Pack/169g	382	16.2	226	9.7	23.7	9.6	2.7
Tofu, Fiery, & Slaw, Wicked Kitchen, Tesco*	1 Pack/236g	425	11.6	180	6.5	26.4	4.9	2.3

S

SANDWICH

INFO/WEIGHT	Measure	per Measure KCAL	FAT	Nutrition Values per 100g / 100ml KCAL	PROT	CARB	FAT	FIBRE
Tuna Mayo, Essential, Waitrose*	1 Pack/133g	283	7.4	213	13.3	25.9	5.6	2.9
Tuna Mayonnaise, & Cucumber, Finest, Tesco*	1 Pack/183g	387	15	211	10.6	22.5	8.2	2.2
Tuna Mayonnaise, & Salad, Serious About Sandwiches*	1 Pack/192g	305	9	159	8.6	20.5	4.7	2.9
Tuna Mayonnaise, Menu, Boots*	1 Pack/182g	451	20	248	13	23	11	1.1
Tuna Mayonnaise, Sainsbury's*	1 Pack/150g	314	9.9	209	11.4	24.5	6.6	2.8
Tuna, & Cucumber, BGTY, Sainsbury's*	1 Pack/178g	268	3.2	151	11.3	22.3	1.8	3.1
Tuna, & Cucumber, COU, M&S*	1 Pack/204g	294	5.1	144	9.1	20.6	2.5	1.5
Tuna, & Cucumber, Healthy Living, Co-Op*	1 Pack/192g	250	3.5	130	10.9	17.9	1.8	3
Tuna, & Cucumber, NUME, Morrisons*	1 Pack/151g	255	3.5	169	12	23.7	2.3	2.5
Tuna, & Cucumber, On Oatmeal Bread, Ginsters*	1 Pack/175g	290	7.2	166	11.7	20.7	4.1	2.4
Tuna, & Cucumber, On the Go, Sainsbury's*	1 Pack/196g	284	5.5	145	9.6	19.4	2.8	2.1
Tuna, & Cucumber, You Count, Love Life, Waitrose*	1 Pack/195g	321	5.3	165	13	21.4	2.7	1.4
Tuna, & Sweetcorn, Loved by Us, Co-Op*	1 Pack/200g	380	9.2	190	11.7	24.1	4.6	2.4
Tuna, & Sweetcorn, Malted Bread, Asda*	1 Pack/202g	365	10.7	181	11	21	5.3	2.5
Tuna, & Cucumber, Calorie Controlled, Tesco*	1 Pack/180g	268	3.1	149	10.5	22	1.7	1.8
Tuna, & Sweetcorn, BGTY, Sainsbury's*	1 Pack/187g	309	5.1	165	10.8	24.7	2.7	2.8
Tuna, & Sweetcorn, Ginsters*	1 Pack/169g	348	11.4	205	9.6	26.4	6.7	2.4
Tuna, & Sweetcorn, on Malt Bread, Tesco*	1 Pack/170g	425	20.4	250	11.4	22.5	12	3.3
Tuna, Crunch, HL, Tesco*	1 Pack/180g	261	4.3	145	11	19.9	2.4	0.5
Tuna, Crunch, Tesco*	1 Pack/165g	341	8.6	207	8.7	30.3	5.2	1.9
Tuna, Grilled Pepper, & Pea, Nutritious, Boots*	1 Pack/206g	398	7.9	193	11	26	3.8	3
Turkey Feast, Gluten Free, M&S*	1 Pack/242g	520	19.8	215	11.9	21.7	8.2	3.2
Turkey, & Cranberry, COU, M&S*	1 Pack/180g	279	3.1	155	12.1	22.8	1.7	2.9
Turkey, & Pastrami, HL, Tesco*	1 Pack/185g	286	4.8	155	9.6	22.1	2.6	2.6
Turkey, & Salad, Fullfillers*	1 Pack/218g	320	7	147	10.3	18.6	3.2	0
Turkey, & Salad, Healthy Eating, Wild Bean Cafe*	1 Pack/230g	315	2.5	137	10	21.5	1.1	1.8
Turkey, & Trimmings, Christmas, Tesco*	1 Pack/209g	476	16.5	228	12.5	25.5	7.9	2.3
Turkey, & Trimmings, Light Choices, HL, Tesco*	1 Pack/154g	256	4.3	166	10.1	24.1	2.8	2.2
Turkey, Mango, & Houmous, Aldi*	1 Pack/165g	291	8.1	176	9.1	22.4	4.9	3.9

SANDWICH FILLER

INFO/WEIGHT	Measure	per Measure KCAL	FAT	Nutrition Values per 100g / 100ml KCAL	PROT	CARB	FAT	FIBRE
Cheese & Spring Onion, M&S*	1 Serving/56g	199	18.8	355	8.5	5	33.6	0.2
Cheese & Onion, Reduced Fat, Supermarket, Average	*1 Serving/100g*	*227*	*18.1*	*227*	*11.8*	*4.4*	*18.1*	*1.7*
Cheese & Onion, Supermarket, Average	*1 Serving/100g*	*405*	*38.6*	*405*	*10.2*	*4.1*	*38.6*	*1.3*
Cheese & Onion, Tesco*	1 Pack/250g	1060	106.5	424	10	0.2	42.6	1.5
Cheese, Three, & Onion, 35% Less Fat, Asda*	1/5 Pack/50g	120	9.5	240	12	5.3	19	0.5
Chicken & Bacon with Sweetcorn, Sainsbury's*	1 Serving/60g	123	9.4	205	12	4	15.7	0.9
Chicken & Bacon, Asda*	1 Serving/100g	341	29	341	17	3	29	0.5
Chicken Tikka, HE, Tesco*	1 Serving/100g	110	3.6	110	7.1	12.4	3.6	1
Chicken, & Bacon, Creamy, Fresh Ways Food Co*	1 Serving/30g	108	9.6	360	15	2.6	32	0.5
Chicken, Coronation, Deli, Meadow Fresh, Lidl*	1 Serving/30g	78	5.7	261	12	9.8	19	1.2
Chicken, Sweetcorn & Bacon, Tesco*	1 Serving/50g	167	14.8	334	12.3	4.3	29.7	1.6
Coronation Chicken, Sainsbury's*	¼ Tub/60g	183	14.8	305	12.1	8.9	24.6	1.2
Coronation Chicken, Tesco*	1 Tbsp/30g	88	7	293	11.4	9.2	23.2	0.7
Egg & Bacon, Fresh, Tesco*	1 Serving/45g	112	9	248	12.7	4.2	20.1	0.6
Egg & Bacon, Free Range, Deli, Essential, Waitrose*	½ Pot/85g	267	23.6	314	12.7	3.3	27.8	0.5
Egg Mayonnaise, BGTY, Sainsbury's*	1 Serving/63g	71	4.1	113	10.2	3.4	6.5	0.1
Egg Mayonnaise, Country Fresh, Aldi*	¼ Pack/50g	106	8.9	211	9.8	2.9	17.8	0
Egg Mayonnaise, Free Range, Co-Op*	1 Pack/200g	260	17.6	130	10.1	2.4	8.8	0.5
Egg Mayonnaise, Tesco*	1 Serving/50g	100	7.8	199	10.9	3.5	15.6	0.5
Prawn Marie Rose, Sainsbury's*	1 Serving/60g	121	10.6	201	8.1	2.5	17.6	0.9
Prawn Mayonnaise, Deli, Asda*	1 Serving/50g	170	16.5	339	9	1.6	33	0.4
Prawn Mayonnaise, Morrisons*	1 Serving50g	122	10.8	244	7.7	4.3	21.7	0.5
Seafood Cocktail, Asda*	1 Serving/50g	104	8.5	207	4.8	9	17	0.5

S

	Measure INFO/WEIGHT	per Measure KCAL	FAT	Nutrition Values per 100g / 100ml KCAL	PROT	CARB	FAT	FIBRE
SANDWICH FILLER								
Seafood Cocktail, Sainsbury's*	1 Serving/55g	99	6.9	180	5.9	10.6	12.6	0.5
Smoked Salmon & Soft Cheese, M&S*	1 Pack/170g	450	40.6	265	11.1	4.9	23.9	0
Tuna & Sweetcorn, Reduced Fat, Supermarket	*1 Serving/100g*	*119*	*5.4*	*119*	*11.5*	*5.8*	*5.4*	*1.2*
Tuna & Sweetcorn, Tesco*	1 Serving/54g	127	9.8	235	8.6	8.1	18.1	0.6
Tuna Mayonnaise & Cucumber, Choice, Tesco*	1 Serving/200g	463	22.8	232	12.8	23.2	11.4	1.6
Tuna Mayonnaise, BGTY, Sainsbury's*	1 Serving/100g	114	3.4	114	17.6	3.5	3.4	0.1
SANDWICH SPREAD								
Beef, Classic, Shippam's Foods*	1 Pot/75g	133	8.8	177	15.5	2.2	11.8	0
Chicken, Classic, Shippam's Foods*	1 Serving/35g	64	4.4	182	15.5	1.8	12.5	0
Heinz*	1 Tbsp/10ml	22	1.3	220	1	24	13	1
Light, Heinz*	1 Tbsp/10g	16	0.9	161	1.1	18.2	9.2	0.9
SARDINES								
A La Antigua, Tinned, in Olive Oil, Ortiz, Brindisa*	1 Tin/140g	267	15.4	191	23	0	11	0
Canned, in Tomato Sauce, Nixe, Lidl*	1 Can/120g	229	14.4	191	19	1.6	12	0.5
Grilled	*1oz/28g*	*55*	*2.9*	*195*	*25.3*	*0*	*10.4*	*0*
in Brine, Canned, Drained	*1oz/28g*	*38*	*2.1*	*136*	*17*	*0*	*7.6*	*0*
in Oil, Canned, Drained	*1oz/28g*	*51*	*3.2*	*180*	*19.1*	*0*	*11.6*	*0*
in Spring Water, Portuguese, Sainsbury's*	1 Can/90g	176	10.5	195	21.3	1.2	11.6	0.5
in Tomato Sauce, Canned	*1oz/28g*	*45*	*2.8*	*162*	*17*	*1.4*	*9.9*	*0*
Raw, Whole with Head	*1oz/28g*	*22*	*1.2*	*78*	*9.7*	*0*	*4.3*	*0*
SATAY								
Chicken with Peanut Sauce, Waitrose*	1 Pack/250g	492	27	197	18.9	6	10.8	0.5
Chicken, 12 Mini, Taste Original*	½ Pack/60g	102	3.9	170	23.3	4.4	6.5	0.7
Chicken, Indonesian, Mini, Sainsbury's*	1 Stick/10g	17	0.7	171	23	4	7	0.7
Chicken, Sticks, Asda*	1 Stick/20g	43	2.8	216	18	4.5	14	0
Chicken, with Peanut Dip, Sainsbury's*	1 Pack/90g	171	10	190	15.4	6.3	11.1	1.5
Satay, Spicy, with Noodles, G&B, Asda*	1 Pack/365g	336	9.1	92	6.5	10	2.5	1.3
Spicy Chicken & Noodles, Microwaved, Asda*	1 Portion/380g	361	10.3	95	6.4	10	2.7	1.4
SATSUMAS								
Fresh, Raw, Flesh Only, Average	*1 Sm/56g*	*21*	*0*	*37*	*0.9*	*8.6*	*0.1*	*1.3*
Weighed with Peel, Average	*1 Sm/60g*	*16*	*0*	*26*	*0.6*	*6.1*	*0.1*	*0.6*
SAUCE								
Apple, Bramley, Colman's*	1 Tbsp/15ml	17	0.1	111	0.5	28	0.5	0
Apple, Bramley, Sainsbury's*	1 Tsp/15g	17	0	111	0.2	27.2	0.1	1.8
Apple, Everyday Value, Tesco*	1 Tbsp/15g	15	0	105	0.1	24.8	0.1	0.5
Arrabiata, Italian, Tesco*	½ Pot/175g	74	0.9	42	1.1	7.9	0.5	1
Bacon & Tomato, Smoked, Stir in, Dolmio*	½ Tub/75g	74	4.2	98	4.6	7.2	5.6	1.3
Balti, Cooking, Sharwood's*	¼ Jar/140g	120	8.3	86	1.2	7.1	5.9	1.4
Balti, Curry, Tesco*	1 Serving/200g	126	9.2	63	1.7	4.3	4.6	1.7
Balti, Loyd Grossman*	½ Jar/175g	180	11.7	103	1.3	8.4	6.7	1.7
Barbecue, Sweet, Heinz*	1 Tbsp/15g	27	0	181	0.9	44	0.2	0
Barbeque, Cook in, Homepride*	1 Can/500g	375	7.5	75	0.7	14.6	1.5	0.6
BBQ, 50% Less Sugar, Dr Will's Ltd*	1 Tbsp 15g	10	0	69	2.1	13.2	0.3	0
BBQ, Bold Spicy Texas, Bulls-Eye*	1 Serving/20g	27	0	135	1.1	31	0	0
BBQ, Heinz*	1 Serving/20g	28	0.1	139	1.1	31.7	0.3	0.5
BBQ, Jerk, Reggae Reggae, Levi Roots*	1 Jar/310g	375	0.3	121	1.1	28.8	0.1	0.5
BBQ, Sticky, Spread & Bake, Heinz*	¼ Jar/78g	131	0.5	168	1	39.6	0.6	1.2
Bearnaise, Sainsbury's*	1 Tbsp/15g	59	6.2	393	0.6	5	41	0
Bechamel, M&S*	1 Jar/425g	480	34.8	113	2.1	7	8.2	1.6
Bhuna, Cooking, Sharwood's*	¼ Jar/105g	83	4.9	79	1.1	7.1	4.7	1.9
Biryani, Med & Aromati, Oven Bake, Patak's*	½ Jar/175g	140	9.3	80	1.1	6.1	5.3	0
Biryani, Reduced Fat, Waitrose*	1 Serving/115g	55	1.8	48	1.8	5.7	1.6	1.9
Black Bean, & Red Pepper, Sharwood's*	½ Jar/213g	132	3	62	1.9	10.5	1.4	1.2

S

SAUCE	Measure INFO/WEIGHT	per Measure KCAL	FAT	Nutrition Values per 100g / 100ml KCAL	PROT	CARB	FAT	FIBRE
Black Bean, Asda*	1 Serving/55g	55	0.8	100	2.9	19	1.4	0
Black Bean, Canton, Stir Fry, Blue Dragon*	½ Pack/60g	53	1.2	88	2.8	14.8	2	1.5
Black Bean, M&S*	½ Jar/140g	130	3.8	93	2.9	14.1	2.7	0.5
Black Bean, Stir Fry, Sharwood's*	1 Jar/195g	127	0.6	65	2.3	12.9	0.3	0
Bolognese, Dolmio*	1 Serving/100g	33	0.2	33	1.5	6.3	0.2	1.3
Bolognese, Lentil, & Mushroom, Waitrose*	½ Pot/175g	124	6.5	71	2.9	4.7	3.7	3.6
Bolognese, Loyd Grossman*	¼ Jar/106g	80	3.1	75	2	10.2	2.9	1.4
Bolognese, No Added Sugar, Dolmio*	½ Jar/175g	67	1.1	38	1.3	6.2	0.6	1.3
Bolognese, No Added Sugar, Tesco*	¼ Jar/125g	43	0.9	34	1.3	5.4	0.7	0.6
Bolognese, Smart Price, Asda*	¼ Jar/110g	44	1	40	0.1	7.6	0.9	0.5
Bouillabaisse, M&S*	½ Pouch/100g	132	11.8	132	1.8	4.3	11.8	0.7
Bread, Christmas, Tesco*	1 Serving/60g	64	3.2	107	3.3	11.8	5.3	0.5
Bread, Made with Semi-Skimmed Milk	*1 Serving/45g*	*42*	*1.4*	*93*	*4.3*	*12.8*	*3.1*	*0.3*
Brown, Bottled	*1 Tsp/6g*	*6*	*0*	*99*	*1.1*	*25.2*	*0*	*0.7*
Brown, Bramwells, Aldi*	1 Tbsp/15g	17	0.1	115	0.5	27	0.5	1
Brown, Original, HP*	1 Tbsp/15g	18	0	122	0.9	28.3	0.1	0.4
Brown, Reduced Salt & Sugar, HP*	1 Tbsp/15g	13	0	87	0.7	20	0.1	0.3
Brown, Reduced Sugar & Salt, Tesco*	1 Tbsp/15g	13	0.1	88	0.7	17.1	0.5	0.8
Brown, Tesco*	1 Tsp/10g	10	0	104	0.7	25.1	0.1	0.6
Brown, Value, Value, Tesco*	1 Serving/15g	13	0	86	0.7	18.8	0.1	0.5
Burger, Heinz*	1 Tbsp/15g	56	5.3	372	0.9	12	35.5	0
Burger, Hellmann's*	1 Tbsp/15g	36	3.2	240	1.1	12	21	0
Butter & Tarragon, Chicken Tonight, Knorr*	¼ Jar/125g	132	13	106	1	2.1	10.4	0.7
Butter Chicken, Classic, The Spice Tailor*	1 Pack/300g	363	23.1	121	3.3	8.9	7.7	1.7
Butter Chicken, Patak's*	1 Jar/500g	645	49	129	1.2	8.2	9.8	0
Butter Chicken, Tesco*	¼ Jar/125g	134	10.4	107	0.8	6.9	8.3	0.8
Butterscotch, Tate & Lyle*	1 Tbsp/15ml	46	0	309	0.5	77.3	0	0
Caesar, Dressing, Florette*	1 Tbsp/15g	45	4.6	302	1.4	2.8	31	0.3
Caramel, Salted, Finest, Tesco*	¼ Pot/65g	266	8.5	409	3.2	69	13.1	1.2
Carbonara, TTD, Sainsbury's*	½ Pot/175g	347	31	198	5.2	4.5	17.7	0.5
Cheese, Cornish Cruncher, M&S*	½ Pouch/100g	159	12.9	159	4.8	5.7	12.9	0.5
Cheese, Four, for Pasta, Waitrose*	1 Pot/350g	546	41	156	6.7	5.8	11.7	0.1
Cheese, Fresh, Waitrose*	1 Pot/350g	458	34.3	131	5.1	5.7	9.8	0
Cheese, Made with Semi-Skimmed Milk	*1 Serving/60g*	*107*	*7.6*	*179*	*8.1*	*9.1*	*12.6*	*0.2*
Cheese, Made with Whole Milk	*1 Serving/60g*	*118*	*8.8*	*197*	*8*	*9*	*14.6*	*0.2*
Cheese, Sainsbury's*	1 Serving/125g	140	9.4	112	5	6.1	7.5	1.2
Chilli & Garlic, Blue Dragon*	1 Serving/30ml	26	0.1	85	1.1	19.7	0.2	0
Chilli Con Carne, Homepride*	½ Jar/250g	145	1.2	58	1.6	11.1	0.5	1.6
Chilli Con Carne, Hot, Uncle Ben's*	1 Jar/500g	295	3	59	2.3	10.9	0.6	1.7
Chilli, & Lime, Cuban, Capsicana*	½ Pack/50g	102	2.2	204	1.8	39.5	4.4	0
Chilli, Barbeque, Encona*	1 Tbsp/15ml	19	0	129	1.3	30.7	0.1	0
Chilli, Cooking, Medium, Fiesta, Aldi*	¼ Jar/125g	60	0.6	48	2.3	7.3	0.5	2.7
Chilli, Hot, Mexican, Morrisons*	¼ Jar/125g	72	0.6	58	2.2	11.2	0.5	2
Chilli, Korean, Yogiyo*	½ Pack/50g	107	0.2	213	2.2	49.1	0.4	0
Chilli, Mild, Tesco*	1 Jar/550g	302	1.6	55	2.3	10	0.3	3.4
Chilli, Sriracha, Uni eagle*	1 Tbsp/15ml	14	0.3	95	1.3	18	1.7	1.4
Chilli, Sweet, Thai, Dipping, Original, Blue Dragon*	1 Serving/30ml	69	0.2	230	0.6	55.1	0.7	1.6
Chilli, Tesco*	1 Tsp/5ml	4	0.2	90	1.3	14	3.2	1.1
Chilli, Tomato Based, Bottled, Average	*1 Tbsp/15g*	*16*	*0*	*104*	*2.5*	*19.8*	*0.3*	*5.9*
Chinese Stir Fry, Sainsbury's*	½ Sachet/75g	61	1.9	81	0.4	14.1	2.5	1
Chocolate, Dessert, M&S*	1 Dtsp/11g	35	1	330	2.1	59.3	9.4	1.9
Chow Mein, Stir Fry, Asda*	½ Pack/85g	101	6.3	119	0.8	12	7.4	0.6
Chow Mein, Stir Fry, Blue Dragon*	1 Sachet/120g	127	1.3	106	0.9	23	1.1	0.4

SAUCE

INFO/WEIGHT	Measure	per Measure		Nutrition Values per 100g / 100ml				
		KCAL	FAT	KCAL	PROT	CARB	FAT	FIBRE
Chow Mein, Stir Fry, Straight to Wok, Amoy*	1 Pack/120g	172	7	143	0.9	21.9	5.8	0.5
Coconut, & Lemon Grass, Tesco*	½ Pack/90g	74	5.3	82	1.3	5.4	5.9	1.2
Country French, Chicken Tonight, Knorr*	¼ Jar/125g	110	8.8	89	0.4	5.3	7.1	0.8
Cranberry Jelly, Morrisons*	1 Tsp/12g	23	0	189	0.2	47	0	0.1
Cranberry, Sainsbury's*	1 Tsp/15g	26	0.1	170	0.5	41.5	0.5	0.5
Cranberry, Tesco*	1 Tsp/15g	23	0	156	0.1	38.8	0	0.9
Cream, GraddsÃƒÂ¥s, Ikea*	1 Serving/60ml	72	6.6	120	1	4	11	0
Creamy, Vegan, Waitrose*	½ Pot/175g	159	10.8	91	1.6	7	6.2	2.3
Curry, Asda*	1 Tbsp/15g	62	2.1	414	13	59	14	1.3
Curry, Basics, Sainsbury's*	¼ Jar/110g	70	2.8	64	0.7	9.7	2.5	0.9
Curry, Chinese Style, Tesco*	¼ Jar/125g	59	0.5	47	0.4	10.3	0.4	0.5
Curry, Chip Shop, Knorr*	1 Sachet/150ml	146	6.9	97	1.7	12.4	4.6	0.7
Curry, Chip Shop, Prepared, CBY, Asda*	1 Serving/62ml	50	3	80	0.5	8.6	4.8	0.2
Curry, Cook in, Homepride*	½ Can/250g	170	6.2	68	0.8	10.5	2.5	0.7
Curry, Green Thai, Finest, Tesco*	1 Serving/350g	420	37.1	120	1.4	4.8	10.6	0.7
Curry, HFC, Tesco*	¼ Jar/110g	57	1.3	52	0.5	9.2	1.2	1.1
Curry, Medium, Uncle Ben's*	1 Jar/500g	330	10	66	0.9	10.9	2	0
Curry, Red Thai, Finest, Tesco*	1 Jar/350g	388	31.5	111	1.3	6.2	9	0.9
Curry, Thai Coconut, Uncle Ben's*	1 Serving/125g	128	6	102	1.4	13.2	4.8	0
Damson, Fruity, Jelly, Tracklements*	1 Tsp/10g	28	0	281	0.2	70.2	0	0
Dhansak, Sharwood's*	1 Jar/445g	668	34.7	150	4.7	15.2	7.8	1.4
Dill & Lemon, Delicate for Fish, Schwartz*	1 Pack/300g	387	34.2	129	1.1	5.6	11.4	0.5
Fajita, Asda*	¼ Jar/125g	79	5.4	63	1	5	4.3	1
Fruity, HP*	1 Tbsp/15g	20	0	135	0.9	31.5	0	0.3
Garlic & Chive, Table & Dip, Heinz*	1 Serving/10ml	32	3	323	1	12.1	29.9	0.2
Garlic, & Tomato, Peruvian, Santa Maria*	½ Pack/100g	60	2.8	60	1.4	6.2	2.8	2.3
Garlic, Creamy, Sainsbury's*	1 Tbsp/15g	44	4.3	296	0.5	7.6	29	1.5
Garlic, Heinz*	1 Tbsp/15g	60	5.4	398	2.2	15	36	0.3
Hoi Sin, Yau's*	1 Tsp/5g	11	0.4	223	3.8	34	7	0
Hoisin, & Garlic, Blue Dragon*	1 Serving/60g	80	1.6	133	1.2	26.1	2.6	0
Hoisin, & Plum, Stir Fry, HL, Tesco*	1 Serving/250g	148	3.2	59	2.1	9.7	1.3	1.3
Hoisin, & Spring Onion, Stir Fry, Sharwood's*	1 Jar/165g	196	1.5	119	1.3	26.5	0.9	0.8
Hoisin, & Plum, Deliciously Versatile, M&S*	½ Bottle/75g	112	1.1	149	2.7	29.3	1.5	2.4
Hoisin, Rich & Fruity, Tesco*	1 Serving/29g	48	0.4	166	1.7	36.4	1.3	0.8
Hoisin, Sharwood's*	1 Tbsp/15g	32	0	211	2.7	49.5	0.3	0.1
Hoisin, Stir Fry, Amoy*	½ Pouch/60g	66	1.4	110	2.1	20.3	2.3	0.1
Hoisin, Stir Fry, Asda*	½ Pack/63g	54	0.4	86	0.6	18	0.6	3.1
Hollandaise, Cook with, M&S*	1oz/28g	76	7.8	271	0.7	4.3	27.8	0.4
Hollandaise, Finest, Tesco*	1 Serving/98g	473	44.5	485	1.4	17.2	45.6	0.3
Hollandaise, Fresh, Average	**1 Pack/150g**	**342**	**32.4**	**228**	**2.4**	**6.1**	**21.6**	**0**
Hollandaise, M&S*	½ Pouch/100g	327	34	327	1	4	34	0.5
Hollandaise, Style, Inspired Vegan*	1 Tsp/5g	27	2.8	531	1.7	6.9	55.1	0.2
Hollandaise, Waitrose*	½ Pack/90g	267	26.7	297	1.3	6	29.7	0
Honey & Mustard, Chicken Tonight, Knorr*	¼ Jar/125g	132	6.6	106	1	12.6	5.3	1.8
Horseradish, Colman's*	1 Tbsp/15ml	17	0.9	112	1.9	9.8	6.2	2.6
Horseradish, Creamed, M&S*	1 Tsp/5g	16	1.5	325	2.4	12.1	29.3	2.5
Horseradish, Creamed, Waitrose*	1 Tbsp/16g	30	1.6	185	2.4	19.6	9.9	2.3
Horseradish, Creamy, Sainsbury's*	1 Tsp/5g	11	0.6	223	2.8	28.9	11.8	1.6
Horseradish, Hot, Morrisons*	1 Serving/20g	31	1.5	157	2.2	19.1	7.7	1.7
Horseradish, Hot, Tesco*	1 Tsp/5g	12	0.8	233	1.8	17.4	16.9	2.1
Hot Pepper, Encona*	1 Tsp/5ml	3	0.1	52	0.5	10.5	1.2	0
Hot, Original, Cholula Hot Sauce*	1 Tsp/5ml	1	0	19	0.9	0.4	0.9	2.8
Hot, Pineapple, Barnfathers*	1 Serving/10ml	4	0	43	0.6	7.8	0	0

SAUCE

INFO/WEIGHT	Measure	per Measure KCAL	FAT	Nutrition Values per 100g / 100ml KCAL	PROT	CARB	FAT	FIBRE
Hunters Chicken, Taste of*	¼ Jar/133g	131	0.1	99	1.4	22.5	0.1	1.4
Hunters Chicken, Cooking, Tesco*	1/3 Jar/163g	155	0.3	95	1.2	20.6	0.2	0.8
Jalfrezi, Average	*1 Sm Jar/350g*	*326*	*23.7*	*93*	*1.3*	*6.7*	*6.8*	*1.6*
Jalfrezi, Slimming World*	1 Tub/350g	119	1.8	34	1.7	4.5	0.5	2.2
Jalfrezi, Specially Selected, Aldi*	½ Jar/180g	171	8.1	95	1.7	5.8	4.5	0
Kashmiri, Creamy, Sharwood's*	½ Pouch/125g	151	10.6	121	1.2	9.1	8.5	1.6
Katsu, Spice & Simmer, Taste of Japan, Asda*	1/3 Jar/115g	142	9.1	123	1.3	11	7.9	1
Kicap Manis, Malay Taste*	1 Tbsp/15ml	36	0.1	237	1.3	55.9	0.9	0
Korean BBQ, Skewers, Street Food, Kit, Blue Dragon*	½ Pack/71g	134	1.4	190	2	41	2	0
Korma, 30% Less Fat, Sharwoods*	¼ Jar/105g	101	6.2	96	1.1	9.2	5.9	0.9
Korma, Coconut & Cream, Mild, in Glass Jar, Patak's*	½ Jar/225g	326	25	145	1.2	9.4	11.1	0
Korma, Cooking Sauce, Waitrose*	1 Jar/350g	696	51.8	199	3.4	12.2	14.8	1.8
Korma, Curry, Loyd Grossman*	½ Jar/175g	224	14.5	128	1.5	11.3	8.3	0.8
Korma, Curry, Uncle Ben's*	1 Jar/500g	630	42	126	1.4	11.1	8.4	0
Korma, Deluxe, Lidl*	1 Jar/350g	640	40.2	183	2.7	16.4	11.5	1.5
Korma, Mild Curry, BFY, Morrisons*	¼ Jar/118g	150	7.2	127	1.3	16.8	6.1	1.5
Korma, Tesco*	¼ Jar/125g	192	14.6	154	2.4	9.9	11.7	1.3
Madeira, & Wild Mushroom, Atkins & Potts*	½ Pack/175g	136	4.6	78	1	7.5	2.6	1.1
Madras, Aldi*	1 Serving/113g	68	2.3	60	1.5	9	2	0
Madras, Cooking, Sharwood's*	1 Tsp/2g	2	0.1	86	1.5	6.9	5.8	1.3
Makhani, Butter, M&S*	½ Jar/170g	291	22.6	171	1.9	10	13.3	1.9
Mango, & Yoghurt, Dipping, Bilash, Aldi*	1 Serving/10g	6	0.1	56	2.4	9.4	0.7	1.7
Mint, Bramwells, Aldi*	1 Serving/30g	28	0.2	93	0.5	21	0.5	0
Mint, Mezita*	1 Tsp/5g	1	0	17	0.9	3.4	0.3	1.4
Mint, Reduced Sugar, Tesco*	1 Tbsp/15g	12	0.1	81	1.8	16.2	0.5	2.1
Mint, Sainsbury's*	1 Dtsp/10g	13	0	126	2.5	28.7	0.1	4
Mint, Smart Price, Asda*	1 Serving/15g	6	0.1	39	0.5	7.2	0.5	1.6
Mint, Value, Tesco*	1 Serving/10g	4	0	41	1.1	9	0.1	1.8
Mushroom, Creamy, Asda*	¼ Jar/121g	126	9.8	104	0.8	6.7	8.1	0.5
Mushroom, Creamy, Chicken Tonight, Knorr*	¼ Jar/125g	100	7.4	80	0.8	5.7	5.9	0.6
Oyster & Spring Onion, Stir Fry, Blue Dragon*	1 Sachet/120g	134	0	112	1.5	26.3	0	0
Oyster, Blue Dragon*	1 Tsp/5ml	6	0	121	3.4	26.9	0	0
Pad Thai, Stir Fry, Morrisons*	1 Pack/120g	142	5.2	118	2.2	17.4	4.3	0.4
Parsley, Fresh, Microwaved, Sainsbury's*	1/3 Pot/100g	78	5.4	78	1.7	5.3	5.4	0.5
Parsley, Ready To Cook, Market Street, Morrisons*	½ Pack/90g	112	8.9	124	2.1	6.2	9.9	0.9
Parsley, Tesco*	½ Pack/89g	85	5.1	95	2.8	8.1	5.7	1.1
Pasta Bake, Tuna, Homepride*	½ Jar/250g	208	13	83	1.4	7.6	5.2	0.9
Peanut, Sainsbury's*	1 Sachet/70g	185	9.2	264	1.9	34.7	13.1	1.6
Pepper, As Prepared, Colman's*	1 Portion/75ml	89	4.7	119	4.7	11	6.3	0
Pepper, Creamy, Tesco*	1 Serving/85ml	128	11.4	151	1.2	6.4	13.4	0.5
Pepper, Southern, Curry, The Spice Tailor*	1 Serving/100g	167	13	167	2.4	8.4	13	3.8
Peppercorn, with a Dash of Brandy, M&S*	½ Pouch/100g	100	7.9	100	1.5	5.4	7.9	0.5
Peri Peri, Medium, Nando's*	1 Serving/20g	14	0.7	69	0.5	8.4	3.7	0.8
Perinaise, Mild, Squeezy Bottle, Nando's*	1 Serving/15g	46	4.2	309	0.3	13	28	0
Pesto, with Basil, Buitoni*	1 Serving/62g	290	27	467	11.3	8.1	43.5	0
Plum, Dipping, M&S*	1 Tbsp/15g	34	0	228	0.1	56.2	0.2	0.3
Plum, Sticky, Stir Fry, Blue Dragon*	1 Serving/60g	145	0.2	242	0.1	35.6	0.3	0
Poke, Kikkoman*	1 Tbsp/15ml	28	0.3	184	4.8	35	2	0
Pomodoro, TTD, Sainsbury's*	½ Pot/175g	152	10.7	87	1.8	5.3	6.1	1.8
Prawn Cocktail, Frank Cooper*	1 Tbsp/15g	47	4	316	0.8	18.3	26.7	0.1
Prawn Cocktail, Morrisons*	1 Portion/15ml	81	8.5	540	1.4	5.5	56.9	1.1
Ranch, American, Morrisons*	1 Tbsp/15g	72	7.2	479	2.4	9.8	47.7	0.2
Raspberry, Dessert, M&S*	1 Serving/20g	24	0.1	120	0.5	28.7	0.3	2.6

S

SAUCE

	Measure INFO/WEIGHT	per Measure KCAL	FAT	Nutrition Values per 100g / 100ml KCAL	PROT	CARB	FAT	FIBRE
Red Hot, Buffalo Wings, Bramwells, Aldi*	1 Tbsp/15g	8	0.4	53	1.5	4.6	2.6	2.5
Red Hot, Wings, Buffalo, Franks*	1 Tbsp/15g	4	0.2	30	0.8	2	1.5	2.5
Red Pepper, Roasted, & Chorizo, Waitrose*	1 Serving/50g	125	11.2	250	3.2	7	22.5	3.1
Redcurrant, Colman's*	1 Tsp/12g	44	0	368	0.7	90	0	0
Rogan Josh, Deluxe, Lidl*	1/3 Jar/116g	122	7.3	105	2.3	8.8	6.3	1.9
Rogan Josh, Low Fat, Tesco*	¼ Jar/125g	38	0.6	31	0.9	4.9	0.5	1.4
Rogan Josh, Medium, Sharwood's*	½ Jar/210g	151	7.6	72	1.4	8.6	3.6	0.5
Rogan Josh, Slimming World*	1 Pot/350g	133	2.1	38	1.7	5.3	0.6	2.4
Rogan Josh, Spice & Simmer, Asda*	1/3 Jar/120g	101	5.6	84	1.3	8.3	4.7	1.5
Rouille , Benedicta*	1 Serving/50g	276	29.9	552	0.6	2.7	59.8	0
Salted Caramel, Dipping, Waitrose*	1 Tsp/5g	21	1.2	425	2.4	46.4	24.5	4.4
Satay, Marinade, Skeeters, Aldi*	1 Tbsp/15g	28	1.6	188	5	17	11	15
Satay, Peanut, Roast, Stir Fry, Straight to Wok, Amoy*	½ Pack/60g	106	6.4	176	4	16.3	10.6	1.3
Satay, Peanut, Roasted, Stir Fry Sensations, Amoy*	1 Pouch/160g	354	19.8	221	4.7	21.9	12.4	1
Satay, Tesco*	1 Jar/180g	265	14	147	4.7	10.9	7.8	7.1
Sausage Casserole, Cook in, Homepride*	½ Jar/250g	92	0.5	37	0.7	8	0.2	0.6
Seafood, Average	*1 Tsp/5g*	*20*	*1.9*	*410*	*1.4*	*15.4*	*38*	*0.2*
Seafood, Colman's*	1 Tbsp/15g	44	3.4	296	0.9	21.5	22.9	0.4
Seafood, Sainsbury's*	1 Tbsp/15g	53	4.5	356	1.2	20.1	30	0.5
Soy, & Garlic, Stir Fry, Fresh Tastes, Asda*	1 Pack/180g	175	6.7	97	1.7	14.1	3.7	0.5
Soy, & Plum, Stir Fry Additions, COOK!, M&S*	½ Sachet/60g	48	0.2	80	1.5	17.5	0.3	1.5
Soy, & Chilli, M&S*	½ Pack/75g	70	0.1	93	0.9	21.9	0.1	0.5
Soy, & Garlic, Spiced, Deliciously Vesatile, M&S*	¼ Bottle/38g	156	14.8	415	2.3	10.3	39.5	4.6
Soy, & Garlic, Stir Fry, Asda*	½ Pack/85g	89	3	105	0.9	17	3.5	0.5
Soy, Average	*1 Tsp/5ml*	*3*	*0*	*64*	*8.7*	*8.3*	*0*	*0*
Soy, Dark, Average	*1 Tsp/5g*	*4*	*0*	*84*	*4*	*16.7*	*0.1*	*0.2*
Soy, Light, Amoy*	1 Tsp/5ml	3	0	52	2.5	10.5	0	0
Soy, Reduced Salt, Amoy*	1 Tsp/5ml	3	0	56	4	10	0	0
Spanish Chicken, Batts, Lidl*	½ Jar/250g	122	4.8	49	1.3	5.9	1.9	1.4
Spanish Chicken, Chicken Tonight, Knorr*	¼ Jar/125g	68	2	55	1.6	7.3	1.6	2.3
Spare Rib, Lee Kum Kee*	2 Tbsp/38g	80	1	211	2.6	39.5	2.6	2.6
Sriracha, Huy Fong*	1 Tbsp/15g	15	0.2	100	2	16	1	0
Sriracha, M&S*	1 Tsp/5g	6	0	125	1.4	25.4	1	4.2
Sriracha, Thai Style, Oh So Delish, Aldi*	1 Pack/26g	109	3.4	420	11	60	13	9.3
Stir Fry, Vegetarian, Lee Kum Kee*	1 Serving/40g	53	0.2	133	1.3	32	0.5	0
Stroganoff, Cooking, Loyd Grossman*	½ Pack/165g	203	14.8	123	1.6	8.6	9	0.7
Stroganoff, Creamy, M&S*	1 Pouch/200g	190	15.2	95	0.6	4.6	7.6	1.8
Sweet & Sour, Chinese, Sainsbury's*	½ Jar/150g	222	0.2	148	0.2	36.6	0.1	0.1
Sweet & Sour, Cook In, Glass Jar, Homepride*	1 Jar/500g	335	0.5	67	0.3	16.2	0.1	0.5
Sweet & Sour, Cooking, Chinese, Sainsbury's*	¼ Jar/125g	155	0.1	124	0.6	30.1	0.1	0.7
Sweet & Sour, Spicy, Sharwood's*	1 Serving/138g	142	0.7	103	0.7	23.8	0.5	0.4
Sweet & Sour, Spicy, Uncle Ben's*	1 Jar/400g	364	0.4	91	0.6	22.1	0.1	0
Sweet & Sour, Stir Fry Additions, Tesco*	1 Sachet/50g	84	0.5	167	0.8	38.7	1	0.5
Sweet & Sour, Stir Fry, Asda*	1 Serving/63g	146	3.2	232	0.8	46	5	0
Sweet & Sour, Stir Fry, Sharwood's*	1 Jar 160g	168	0.8	105	0.6	24.5	0.5	0.8
Sweet & Sour, Stir Fry, Tesco*	½ Jar/222g	164	0.4	74	0.6	17	0.2	0.4
Sweet & Sour, Take-Away	*1oz/28g*	*44*	*1*	*157*	*0.2*	*32.8*	*3.4*	*0*
Sweet & Sour, Aromatic, Flavour Burst, Uncle Ben's*	1 Serving/50g	62	1	125	0.7	26	2	0.5
Sweet & Sour, Cooking, HL, Tesco*	½ Jar/250g	98	1	39	0.2	8.3	0.4	0.6
Sweet & Sour, Extra Pineapple, Uncle Ben's*	1 Serving/165g	147	0.3	89	0.3	21.2	0.2	0.7
Sweet & Sour, Light, Uncle Ben's*	¼ Jar/125g	71	0.1	57	0.4	12.6	0.1	0.9
Sweet & Sour, M&S*	½ Jar/145g	144	1	99	1.1	22	0.7	0.5
Sweet & Sour, No Added Sugar, Uncle Ben's*	1 Jar/440g	123	0.4	28	0.4	5.5	0.1	0.8

SAUCE

INFO/WEIGHT	Measure	per Measure KCAL	FAT	Nutrition Values per 100g / 100ml KCAL	PROT	CARB	FAT	FIBRE
Sweet & Sour, Stir Fry, Pouch, Average	**1 Pouch/120g**	**148**	**2.3**	**124**	**0.8**	**25.7**	**1.9**	**1**
Sweet & Sour, Stir Fry, Sachet, Blue Dragon*	1 Sachet/120g	145	0.1	122	0.2	29.7	0.1	0.3
Sweet Chilli & Garlic, Stir Fry & Dipping, Tesco*	½ Jar/95ml	78	0	82	0.3	20.1	0	0.1
Sweet Chilli, Dipping, M&S*	1 Tbsp/15g	34	0.1	225	0.9	53.2	0.7	0.6
Sweet Chilli, Dipping, Morrisons*	1 fl oz/30ml	64	0.6	212	0.4	47.3	2.1	1
Sweet Chilli, Heinz*	1 Serving/25g	38	0.1	150	0.3	36.5	0.4	6.4
Sweet Chilli, M&S*	½ Pack/75g	72	0.3	96	0.8	21.9	0.4	0.8
Sweet Chilli, Stir Fry, Additions, Tesco*	1 Serving/50g	106	3.8	211	0.3	35.2	7.6	0.6
Sweet Chilli, Thai, Blue Dragon*	1 Serving/15g	28	0.1	188	0.5	45.5	0.6	0
Sweet Curry, Eazy Squirt, Heinz*	1 Serving/10ml	12	0	124	0.7	29	0.3	0.5
Sweet Pepper, Stir in, Dolmio*	½ Pot/75g	77	4.6	103	1.4	9.6	6.2	1.6
Sweet Thai Chilli, Flavour Burst, Uncle Ben's*	1 Serving/75g	83	0.4	110	0.5	27	0.5	0.5
Szechuan Style, Stir Fry, Fresh Ideas, Tesco*	1 Sachet/50g	114	4.8	228	1.9	33.4	9.7	0.1
Szechuan, Spicy Tomato, Stir Fry, Blue Dragon*	½ Sachet/60g	59	1.8	98	1.3	15.8	3	0.9
Szechuan, Tomato, Spicy, Stir Fry, Sharwoods*	½ Jar/98g	56	0.3	57	1.1	12	0.3	0.8
Tamari, Soya, Clearspring*	1oz/28g	55	0.1	196	14	34	0.2	0
Tamarind & Lime, Stir Fry, Sainsbury's*	1 Serving/75g	88	5.6	117	1.1	11.4	7.4	0.8
Tartare	**1oz/28g**	**84**	**6.9**	**299**	**1.3**	**17.9**	**24.6**	**0**
Tartare, Colman's*	1 Tbsp/15g	45	3.7	290	1.5	17	24	0.6
Tartare, Finest, Tesco*	1 Tbsp/15g	47	4.7	312	1.3	5.7	31.1	2.1
Tartare, Mild & Creamy, Heinz*	1 Tbsp/15g	47	4.2	312	0.9	13.4	28.3	0.1
Tartare, Rich, Colman's*	1 Tsp/5ml	14	1.2	284	1.2	17	23	0.6
Tartare, Sainsbury's*	1 Tbsp/15ml	42	3.6	281	1.4	15.4	23.7	0.5
Tartare, Tesco*	1 Tbsp/15g	47	3.9	312	0.7	18.7	25.8	1.1
Teriyaki Chicken, Stir Fry, Celebrate Health*	1 Serving/100g	30	1	30	0.8	6.6	1	0
Teriyaki, Asda*	1 Serving/98g	99	0.1	101	2.1	23	0.1	0
Teriyaki, Deliciously Versatile, M&S*	1 Tbsp/15g	19	0.2	127	2.6	25.7	1.3	0
Teriyaki, Japanese Grill, Kikkoman*	1 Serving/15ml	24	0	158	4.5	30.8	0.1	0
Teriyaki, Lee Kum Kee*	1 Serving/15g	27	0	178	2.2	42.4	0	0.5
Teriyaki, Stir Fry, Blue Dragon*	1 Pack/120g	131	0.2	109	0.9	25.9	0.2	0
Teriyaki, Stir Fry, Fresh Ideas, Tesco*	1 Serving/25g	33	0.6	133	1.1	26.9	2.3	0
Tikka Masala, Cooking, HL, Tesco*	¼ Jar/125g	78	3.1	62	0.4	9	2.5	0.7
Tikka Masala, Cooking, Sainsbury's*	¼ Jar/125g	131	7.6	105	1.5	10.1	6.1	1.6
Tikka Masala, Deluxe, Lidl*	1/3 Jar/116g	126	7.2	109	2.7	10	6.2	1.3
Tikka Masala, GFY, Asda*	½ Jar/250g	190	8	76	2.9	9	3.2	0.5
Tikka Masala, Low Fat, Tesco*	¼ Jar/125g	60	2.5	48	0.5	6.7	2	0.7
Tikka Masala, M&S*	½ Jar/170g	309	26.9	182	1.8	7.2	15.8	2
Tikka Masala, Medium, Cooking, Sharwood's*	1/3 Jar/140g	150	9.7	107	1.3	9.7	6.9	0.5
Tikka Masala, Mild, Low Fat, Morrisons*	¼ Jar/112g	73	2.5	65	1.3	9.3	2.2	1.4
Tikka Masala, Ready Made, Average	**1 Sm Jar/350g**	**422**	**28.8**	**121**	**2**	**9.6**	**8.2**	**1.2**
Tikka Masala, Sizzle & Spice, Pataks*	½ Jar/180g	220	13.7	122	1.5	11	7.6	0
Toffee, GFY, Asda*	1 Serving/5g	15	0.1	306	2.2	68	2.8	0
Toffee, Luxury, Rowse*	1 Serving/20g	67	0.7	336	1.9	73.9	3.7	0.4
Tomato & Cheese, Pasta Bake, Dolmio*	¼ Jar/125g	70	1.5	56	2.1	9.1	1.2	1.2
Tomato & Herb, Creamy, Pasta Bake, Homepride*	1 Serving/125g	128	8.8	102	1.5	8.3	7	0.9
Tomato & Marscapone, Finest, Tesco*	1 Serving/350g	270	17.5	77	2.7	5.4	5	0.8
Tomato & Mushroom, Pasta, Cucina, Aldi*	¼ Jar/125g	59	0.6	47	2	8.2	0.5	1.4
Tomato & Basil Sauce, Fresh, Tesco*	1 Pot/500g	245	9	49	1.5	6.8	1.8	0.8
Tomato & Basil, for Meatballs, Dolmio*	¼ Jar/125g	48	0.2	38	1.5	6.9	0.2	1.3
Tomato & Basil, Italian, Fresh, Asda*	½ Tub/175g	107	5.7	60	1.5	6.1	3.2	0.6
Tomato & Basil, Italian, Sainsbury's*	½ Pot/175g	88	3	50	1.9	6.2	1.7	1
Tomato & Garlic, for Meatballs, Dolmio*	1 Portion/125g	46	0.1	37	1.6	6.5	0.1	0
Tomato, & Bacon, Pasta Bake, Aldi*	¼ Jar/123g	107	6.8	87	1.5	7.4	5.5	0.9

S

SAUCE	Measure INFO/WEIGHT	per Measure KCAL	per Measure FAT	Nutrition Values per 100g / 100ml KCAL	PROT	CARB	FAT	FIBRE
Tomato, & Red Pepper, Extra Special, Asda*	½ Pot/175g	96	2.3	55	1.3	8.6	1.3	1.6
Tomato, Heinz*	1 Tbsp/17g	18	0	103	0.9	24.1	0.1	0.7
Tomato, Heirloom, Pressed, Odysea *	1 Jar/300g	75	0.3	25	0.8	4.5	0.1	1.2
Tomato, Pizza Topping, Napolina*	1 Serving/70g	34	1.5	49	0.9	6.3	2.2	0.6
Tomato, Pomodorini, Finest, Tesco*	½ Pot/125g	79	3.9	63	1.2	5.8	3.1	3.7
Vegetable, Chargrilled, with Olives, Waitrose*	100g	75	4.6	75	1.3	6.6	4.6	1.1
Vindaloo, Hot, Patak's*	1 Jar/540g	518	34.6	96	1.5	6.4	6.4	0
Watercress, & Stilton, Creamy for Fish, Schwartz*	1 Pack/300g	141	12.3	47	0.6	2	4.1	0.7
Watercress, Sainsbury's*	1 Serving/100g	87	6.4	87	2.8	4.2	6.4	0.5
White Wine, & Cream, Cook in, Classic, Homepride*	¼ Can/125g	101	5.1	81	1	8	4.1	0.4
White Wine, & Mushroom, BGTY, Sainsbury's*	¼ Jar/125g	81	2.5	65	2.8	9	2	0.3
White Wine, & Parsley, Pour Over, Loyd Grossman*	½ Sachet/85g	94	7.9	111	1	5.6	9.3	0.5
White, Savoury, Made with Semi-Skimmed Milk	*1oz/28g*	*36*	*2.2*	*128*	*4.2*	*11.1*	*7.8*	*0.2*
White, Savoury, Made with Whole Milk	*1oz/28g*	*42*	*2.9*	*150*	*4.1*	*10.9*	*10.3*	*0.2*
Worcestershire Sauce, Sainsbury's*	1 Tbsp/15ml	16	0	107	0.7	23.3	0.1	0.3
Worcestershire, Average	*1 Tsp/5g*	*3*	*0*	*65*	*1.4*	*15.5*	*0.1*	*0*
Worcestershire, Lea & Perrins*	1 Tsp/5ml	5	0	96	0.8	21	0.9	0
Yuzu, & Soy, Waitrose*	½ Pack/60g	68	0.3	113	1.9	25.1	0.5	0.9
SAUCE MIX								
Beef Bourguignon, Colman's*	1 Pack/40g	136	0.8	340	7	72	2	3
Beef Stroganoff, Colman's*	1 Pack/40g	140	3.6	350	11.6	56.1	8.9	2.7
Bread, As Sold, M&S*	¼ Pack/18g	64	1.2	368	11.4	62.4	6.9	5.5
Bread, Made Up, Colman's*	1 Serving/75ml	70	1.5	95	5	14	2	0.6
Cheddar Cheese, Colman's*	1 Pack/40g	164	6	410	19	51	15	2
Cheddar Cheese, Dry Mix, Schwartz*	1 Pack/40g	144	3	361	18.4	55.1	7.4	2.3
Cheese Flavour, Dairy Free, Free & Easy*	4 Tsp/15g	4	0.1	26	0.6	4.9	0.4	0.3
Cheese, Made Up with Skimmed Milk	*1 Serving/60g*	*47*	*1.4*	*78*	*5.4*	*9.5*	*2.3*	*0*
Chicken Chasseur, Schwartz*	1 Pack/40g	126	1.8	316	9.6	59.1	4.6	6.8
Chilli Con Carne, Asda*	1 Sachet/50g	157	0.8	314	7	68	1.6	2.5
Chilli Con Carne, Recipe Mix, Schwartz*	1 Pack/41g	133	1.5	324	8.2	60.8	3.6	0
Chip Shop Curry, Dry Weight, Bisto*	1 Dtsp/9g	38	1.6	427	3.4	63.5	17.7	1.3
Cream, for Meatballs, Ikea*	1 Pack/40g	179	9.4	448	9.6	49.2	23.6	0
Dauphinoise Potato Bake, Schwartz*	1 Pack/40g	161	10.5	402	6.8	34.7	26.3	15.8
Four Cheese, Colman's*	1 Pack/35g	127	3.9	362	17.1	48.4	11.1	1.8
Hollandaise, Colman's*	1 Pack/28g	104	3.1	372	6.4	61.6	11.1	1.8
Hollandaise, Made Up, Schwartz*	1 Serving/79g	58	2	73	3.9	8.7	2.5	0
Lemon Butter for Fish, Schwartz*	1 Pack/38g	136	3	357	6.1	65.3	8	5.8
Mixed Herbs for Chicken, So Juicy, Maggi*	1 Pack/34g	97	1	285	8.3	53.8	2.8	5.5
Paprika For Chicken, So Juicy, Maggi*	1 Pack/34g	91	1.4	267	8.8	45.5	4	7.1
Parsley & Chive for Fish, Schwartz*	1 Pack/38g	150	4.3	394	9.4	61.8	11.4	3.5
Parsley, Creamy, Made Up, Schwartz*	1 Serving/79g	59	2	75	4.2	8.7	2.5	0.3
Parsley, Made Up, Bisto*	1 Serving/50ml	43	2.5	86	1	9.6	5	1
Pepper, Creamy, Schwartz*	1 Pack/25g	86	1.7	342	17.9	52	6.9	7
Peppercorn, Made Up with Water, CBY, Asda*	1 Serving/63ml	52	3.9	84	0.7	5.4	6.2	1.7
Peppercorn, Mild, Creamy, Schwartz*	1 Pack/25g	88	2.2	352	13.8	55	8.6	5
Savoury Mince, Schwartz*	1 Pack/35g	108	0.7	310	14.6	58.3	2	1.8
Shepherd's Pie, Schwartz*	1 Pack/38g	118	0.9	311	8.2	60.3	2.3	11.1
Shepherds Pie, Bramwells*	1 Pack/50g	168	3	336	8.6	62	6	6.9
Spaghetti Bolognese, Colman's*	1 Pack/40g	120	0.4	300	8.9	64.1	0.9	5.2
Spaghetti Bolognese, Schwartz*	1 Pack/40g	114	0.6	285	9.2	59	1.6	7
Spaghetti Carbonara, Schwartz*	1 Pack/32g	135	6.4	421	10.4	49.4	20.1	7.2
Stroganoff, Beef, Schwartz*	1 Pack/35g	125	3.6	358	15.6	50.8	10.3	4.4
Stroganoff, Mushroom, Schwartz*	1 Pack/35g	121	3.1	345	10.9	52.4	8.9	5.9

	Measure INFO/WEIGHT	per Measure		Nutrition Values per 100g / 100ml				
		KCAL	FAT	KCAL	PROT	CARB	FAT	FIBRE
SAUCE MIX								
Sweet, & Sour, So Juicy, Maggi*	¼ Pack/12g	42	0.3	354	3.7	78.7	2.2	2.2
Thickening Granules, McDougalls*	1 Tbsp/10g	46	1.9	463	0	73.7	18.7	0
Tuna Napolitana, Schwartz*	1 Pack/30g	107	3.9	357	10.3	49.6	13.1	0.5
White, Dry Weight, Bisto*	1 Dtsp/9g	45	2.5	496	3.2	57.4	28.2	0.4
White, Instant, Made Up, Sainsbury's*	1 Serving/90ml	65	2.5	72	0.8	10.9	2.8	0.1
White, Made Up with Semi-Skimmed Milk	*1oz/28g*	**20**	**0.7**	*73*	*4*	*9.6*	*2.4*	*0*
White, Made Up with Skimmed Milk	*1oz/28g*	**17**	**0.3**	*59*	*4*	*9.6*	*0.9*	*0*
White, Savoury, Colman's*	1 Pack/25g	105	3.8	420	9	63	15	2
SAUERKRAUT								
Average	*1oz/28g*	**3**	**0**	*11*	*1.1*	*1.6*	*0*	*0.9*
SAUSAGE								
Beef, Average	*1 Sausage/60g*	**151**	**11.1**	*252*	*14.5*	*7*	*18.5*	*0.6*
Beetroot, The Beet Goes On, Vegetarian, Heck*	2 Sausages/80g	138	6.9	173	5.5	10.8	8.6	15.1
Best Of British, Quorn*	1 Sausage/56g	115	5.8	206	15	10.4	10.4	5.4
Bockwurst, Average	*1 Sausage/45g*	**114**	**10.4**	*253*	*10.8*	*0.8*	*23*	*0*
Bollywood Bangers, Indian Style, Vegetarian, Heck*	2 Sausages/76g	123	4.8	162	6.9	13.2	6.3	12.4
Braai Flavour, Fry's Special Vegetarian*	1 Sausage/63g	86	4.4	138	16.5	10	7	4
Bratwurst, German, Morrisons*	1 Sausage/90g	279	25.5	310	12.7	0.8	28.3	0.5
Bratwurst, Nuremberg, Dulano, Lidl*	1 Sausage/22g	77	7	349	14	1	32	0.5
Cauliflower, Masala, Roast, The Deli, Aldi*	1 Sausage/41g	42	0.6	103	2.6	18	1.4	3.8
Chicken, & Sweetcorn, Oven Baked, Slimming World*	1 Sausage/60g	83	1.9	139	23.9	1.9	3.2	3.1
Chicken, British, Tesco*	1 Sausage/57g	99	4.4	175	17.2	8.4	7.8	1.1
Chicken, Chipolata, Italian, Grilled, Heck*	2 Chipolatas/68g	99	1.8	145	28.5	2.4	2.6	0
Chicken, Chipolatas, Italian, Warren & Sons, Lidl*	1 Sausage/34g	50	2.8	148	17	0.7	8.2	1.6
Chicken, Italia, Grilled, Heck*	1 Sausage/34g	49	0.9	145	28.5	2.4	2.6	0
Chicken, Morliny*	1 Sausage/200g	374	26	187	17	0.6	13	0
Chicken, Organic, Free Range, Daylesford*	1 Sausage/57g	71	1.7	125	18.6	6	2.9	0
Chipolata, Average	*1 Sausage/28g*	**81**	**6.5**	*291*	*12.1*	*8.7*	*23.1*	*0.7*
Chipolata, Chicken, Smoky Paprika, Grilled, Heck*	2 Chipolatas/68g	109	1.7	159	27.3	5.8	2.5	0
Chipolata, Pork, Black Pepper & Nutmeg, Waitrose*	1 Sausage/22g	50	2.4	229	20	12.7	10.9	0.5
Chipolata, Pork, Classic, Extra Special, Asda*	2 Sausages/50g	128	11	255	13	1.3	22	0
Chipolata, Premium, Average	*1 Serving/80g*	**187**	**13.8**	*234*	*14.8*	*4.7*	*17.3*	*1.2*
Chorizo, Average	*1 Serving/80g*	**250**	**19.4**	*313*	*21.1*	*2.6*	*24.2*	*0.2*
Chorizo, Diced, Cooks' Ingredients, Waitrose*	1 Serving/60g	285	24.5	475	25.9	0.7	40.8	0.8
Chorizo, Lean, Average	*1 Sausage/67g*	**131**	**9.2**	*195*	*15.7*	*2.3*	*13.7*	*0.8*
Chorizo, Spanish, Sliced, Morrisons*	1 Slice/3g	10	0.8	328	23.1	0.8	25.8	0.2
Cocktail, Average	*1 Sausage/7g*	**23**	**1.9**	*323*	*12.1*	*8.6*	*26.7*	*0.9*
Cumberland, Average	*1 Sausage/57g*	**167**	**13**	*293*	*13.8*	*8.6*	*22.8*	*0.8*
Cumberland, Cauldron Foods*	1 Sausage/46g	75	4	163	14	6.5	8.6	2
Cumberland, Meat Free, Quorn*	1 Sausage/47g	105	4.7	222	17.9	12.5	9.9	5.9
Cumberland, Naked, Finnebrogue*	3 Sausages/200g	532	44	266	15	0.5	22	1.5
Free From, Wheat & Gulten, Sainsbury's*	2 Sausages/104g	268	20	257	13.3	7.2	19.2	1
Garlic, Average	*1 Slice/11g*	**25**	**2**	*227*	*15.7*	*0.8*	*18.2*	*0*
GF, Quorn*	2 Sausages/100g	172	7.2	172	13	11.1	7.2	5.6
Irish, Average	*1 Sausage/40g*	**119**	**8.3**	*298*	*10.7*	*17.2*	*20.7*	*0.7*
Italian, Cooked, Johnsonville*	2oz/56g	170	13	304	17.9	1.8	23.2	0
Kabanos, Klansyczny , Tarczynski*	½ Pack/100g	469	38	469	23	7.8	38	0
Kindziuk, with Garlic, Kuljanka*	1 Pack/100g	254	14	254	30	1.7	14	0.5
Lamb, & Mint, M&S*	1oz/28g	63	4.6	225	13.3	6.6	16.3	1.7
Lincolnshire, Average	*1 Sausage/42g*	**122**	**9.1**	*291*	*14.6*	*9.2*	*21.8*	*0.6*
Lincolnshire, Cauldron Foods*	1 Sausage/46g	84	4.5	182	16.1	5.5	9.8	3.6
Lincolnshire, Meat Free, Quorn*	1 Sausage/41g	60	2.7	146	13.5	7.2	6.6	5.2
Lincolnshire, Vegetarian, Grilled, Linda McCartney*	1 Sausage/50g	104	5.8	209	13.6	10.2	11.5	5

SAUSAGE

INFO/WEIGHT	Measure	per Measure KCAL	per Measure FAT	Nutrition Values per 100g / 100ml KCAL	PROT	CARB	FAT	FIBRE
Lorne, Average	1 Sausage/25g	78	5.8	312	10.8	16	23.1	0.6
Merguez	1 Merguez/55g	165	14.3	300	16	0.6	26	0
Mushroom, & Leek, Bangers, Vegan, Waitrose*	2 Sausages/86g	95	2.1	111	6.8	13.3	2.4	4.4
Outrageously Succulent, Grilled, Linda Mccartney's*	2 Sausages/88g	141	4.8	160	17.9	7.5	5.4	5
Patties, Quorn*	1 Pattie/42g	53	2	127	12.8	5.8	4.9	4.7
Pigs in Portionets, Cooked, Morrisons*	1 Roll/22g	52	2.9	235	22.9	5.2	13.3	1.5
Pigs In Portionets, Cooked, Sainsbury's*	1 Roll/15g	42	2.8	280	3.1	11.2	18.5	1
Polish Kabanos, Sainsbury's*	1 Sausage/25g	92	7.6	366	23	0.1	30.4	0.1
Pork & Beef, Average	1 Sausage/45g	133	10.2	295	8.7	13.6	22.7	0.5
Pork & Herb, Average	1 Sausage/75g	231	19.5	308	13.2	5.4	26	0.4
Pork & Tomato, Grilled, Average	1 Sausage/47g	127	9.7	273	13.9	7.5	20.8	0.4
Pork & Apple, Average	1 Sausage/57g	146	10.7	256	14.5	7.5	18.8	1.9
Pork, & Caramelised Onion, Thick, Cooked, Morrisons*	1 Sausage/45g	125	8.3	279	20.1	7.1	18.6	0.9
Pork, & Leek, Thick, Signature, Morrisons*	1 Sausage/55g	127	8.6	231	20.5	1.5	15.6	1.4
Pork, & Herb, in Onion, & Red Wine Gravy, Parsley Box*	1 Pack/300g	324	12	108	8.7	9.2	4	0.6
Pork, 3% Fat, Bakery in Store, M&S*	1 Sausage/66g	79	1.8	119	16.6	6.4	2.7	1.2
Pork, Average	1 Sausage/45g	139	11.2	309	11.9	9.8	25	0.8
Pork, Battered, Thick, Average	1oz/28g	126	10.2	448	17.3	21.7	36.3	2
Pork, Chickpea, & Spinach, Spanish Style, Waitrose*	2 Sausages/119g	218	14.3	183	12.4	4.8	12	3.1
Pork, Chipolata, Finest, Tesco*	1 Chipolata/22g	74	6	336	19.1	2.6	27.5	1
Pork, Chipolata, Reduced Fat, Grilled, Heck*	2 Chipolatas/53g	85	2.2	160	20	11.2	4.1	0
Pork, Chorizo, Mini, Sainsbury's*	2 Sausages/36g	166	14.4	458	19.7	4.5	39.8	1.6
Pork, Cumberland, Reduced Fat, Grilled, Asda*	1 Sausage/40g	65	3.1	163	16	6.7	7.7	1.3
Pork, Cumberland, Reduced Fat, Tesco*	1 Sausage/50g	104	5.6	209	12.4	14.4	11.1	1.2
Pork, Extra Lean, Average	1 Sausage/54g	84	3.7	155	17.3	6.1	6.8	0.8
Pork, Frozen, Fried	1oz/28g	88	6.9	316	13.8	10	24.8	0
Pork, Frozen, Grilled	1oz/28g	81	5.9	289	14.8	10.5	21.2	0
Pork, Garlic & Herb, Average	1 Sausage/76g	203	16.5	268	12	6	21.8	1.2
Pork, GF, Finest, Tesco*	2 Sausages/102g	320	26.5	314	18.5	1.5	26	0.5
Pork, Premium, Average	1 Sausage/74g	191	13.6	258	14.9	8.3	18.4	1
Pork, Reduced Fat, Chilled, Grilled	1 Sausage/45g	104	6.2	230	16.2	10.8	13.8	1.5
Pork, Reduced Fat, Healthy Range, Average	1 Sausage/57g	86	3.4	151	15.6	9	6	0.9
Pork, Silesian, Dulano, Lidl*	1 Sausage/83g	198	14.9	239	16	3	18	0.5
Pork, Skinless, Average	1oz/28g	81	6.6	291	11.7	8.2	23.6	0.6
Pork, Skinny, Aldi*	1 Sausage/60g	74	1.7	124	17	6.5	2.9	1.6
Pork, Thick, Average	1 Sausage/39g	115	8.7	296	13.3	10	22.4	1
Pork, Thick, Reduced Salt & Fat, Grilled, Richmond*	1 Sausage/38g	78	3.8	204	14	12	10	0
Pork. Cumberland, British, M&S*	1 Sausage/67g	166	13.5	248	13.9	2.4	20.2	0.7
Premium, Chilled, Fried	1oz/28g	77	5.8	275	15.8	6.7	20.7	0
Premium, Chilled, Grilled	1oz/28g	82	6.3	292	16.8	6.3	22.4	0
Red Pepper, & Butternut Squash, The Deli, Aldi*	1 Sausage/42g	50	0.6	118	4.8	18	1.4	6.8
Saveloy, Unbattered, Takeaway, Average	1 Saveloy/65g	192	14.5	296	13.8	10.8	22.3	0.8
Shroomdogs, Chorizo, Love Your Veg!, Sainsbury's*	2 Sausages/70g	111	4.6	158	6	16	6.6	5.3
Shroomdogs, Red Pepper, Love Your Veg!, Sainsbury's*	2 Sausages/100g	109	2.5	109	4.7	14.3	2.5	4.9
Smoked Pork, Reduced Fat, Mattessons*	1 Serving/50g	120	10	240	16	0	20	0
Smoked, Average	1 Sausage/174g	588	52.2	338	13	4	30	0
Sweet Fusions, Veggie, Heck*	2 Sausages/83g	120	3.8	144	3.1	18.2	4.6	8.9
Toulouse, with Bacon, Red Wine, & Garlic, Waitrose*	2 Sausages/106g	275	19.4	260	20.8	2.4	18.3	1
Turkey & Chicken, Average	1 Sausage/57g	126	8.2	222	14.4	8.2	14.6	1.8
Turkey, Average	1 Sausage/57g	90	4.6	157	15.7	6.3	8	0
Vegan, Breakfast, Grilled, Heck*	2 Sausages/77g	112	6	146	5.5	8.1	7.8	10.3
Vegetarian, Bangers, Quorn*	1 Sausage/50g	58	2.4	116	11.7	6.6	4.8	3
Vegetarian, Cocktail, Quorn*	1 Sausage/15g	31	1.7	206	12.4	11.6	11.3	4.3

	Measure INFO/WEIGHT	per Measure KCAL	FAT	Nutrition Values per 100g / 100ml KCAL	PROT	CARB	FAT	FIBRE
SAUSAGE								
Vegetarian, Quorn*	1 Sausage/40g	79	4.5	198	11.2	10.6	11.1	5.5
Venison & Pork, Waitrose*	1 Sausage/64g	93	4	146	16.5	5.3	6.3	1.1
Wiejska, Polish, Sainsbury's*	1/8 Pack/50g	78	4.5	157	18.7	0.4	9	0.5
Wild Boar	*1 Sausage/85g*	*220*	*17*	*259*	*16.5*	*1.2*	*20*	*0*
SAUSAGE & MASH								
2 British Pork & Rich Onion Gravy, M&S*	1 Pack/400g	340	6.8	85	5.7	12.2	1.7	1.3
Classic Kitchen, Tesco*	1 Pack/450g	510	23.2	113	4	12	5.1	1.3
Frozen, HFC, Tesco*	1 Pack/380g	371	8.4	98	3.3	15.5	2.2	1.4
LC, Tesco*	1 Pack/400g	360	8.8	90	4.4	11.8	2.2	1.4
Lincolnshire, & Root Vegetable Mash, Weight Watchers*	1 Pack/380g	285	6.5	75	4.4	9.3	1.7	2.6
One Stop*	1 Pack/450g	507	23.1	113	4	12	5.1	1.3
with Ale Gravy, & Champ Potato, Pork, Gastropub, M&S*	1 Pack/400g	728	50.8	182	8.1	8.1	12.7	1.3
with Beans, Little Dish*	1 Pack/200g	204	7.4	102	4.7	11.4	3.7	2.1
with Onion Gravy, Bangers, British Classic, Sainsbury's*	1 Pack/450g	562	30.6	125	4.8	9.9	6.8	2.6
SAUSAGE MEAT								
Pork, Average	*1oz/28g*	*96*	*8.2*	*344*	*9.9*	*10.2*	*29.4*	*0.6*
SAUSAGE ROLL								
Bacon, & Cheddar, Smoked, M&S*	1 Roll/45g	167	10.7	372	13.8	24.9	23.8	1.4
Bacon, & Cheddar, Smoked, Vintage, Finest, Tesco*	1 Roll/47g	199	15.1	423	12.6	20.2	32.1	1.3
Buffet, HE, Tesco*	1 Roll/30g	83	3.8	278	9.6	31.2	12.8	1.5
Cocktail, Average	*1 Roll/15g*	*57*	*3.7*	*378*	*8.9*	*29.4*	*24.9*	*1.9*
Frozen, Greggs Iceland Exclusive*	1 Roll /103g	349	24.7	339	8	22	24	1.5
GF, Genius*	1 Roll/100g	281	17.5	281	8.2	21.8	17.5	1.7
Jumbo, Sainsbury's*	1 Roll/145g	456	26.3	314	9.5	27.2	18.1	2.3
Kingsize, Pork Farms*	½ Roll/50g	241	15.9	483	10.5	39.9	31.8	0
Lincolnshire, Snack, Chef Select, Lidl*	1 Roll/30g	110	7.4	368	8.9	27.2	24.6	1.2
Linda McCartney*	1 Roll/51g	145	8.2	287	10.9	22.7	16.2	3.8
Mini, Linda McCartney*	1 Roll/14g	41	2.2	293	11.3	23.7	15.8	5.2
Mini, Oven Baked, Greggs, Iceland*	1 Roll/25g	76	6	303	7.9	21	24	0
Mini, Waitrose*	1 Roll/35g	124	9.2	353	13	16.1	26.3	1
Pork, Cocktail, Mini, M&S*	1 Roll/42g	152	9.9	361	11.1	25.5	23.5	1.6
Pork, Finest, Tesco*	1 Roll/47g	174	11.5	371	12.2	24.9	24.4	1.5
Pork, Mini, Tesco*	1 Roll/11g	35	2	322	9	29.9	17.9	2.3
Pork, Morrisons*	1 Roll/70g	195	9	278	9.6	31.2	12.8	1.5
Pork, TTD, Sainsbury's*	1 Roll/65g	242	16.8	372	11.5	22.9	25.8	1.1
Puff Pastry	*1 Med/60g*	*230*	*16.6*	*383*	*9.9*	*25.4*	*27.6*	*1*
TTD, Sainsbury's*	1 Roll/27g	103	7	383	12.3	23.9	26.1	1.4
Vegan, Mae's Kitchen, Aldi*	1 Roll/90g	284	17.1	316	8.2	27	19	3.9
Vegetarian, Chilled, Quorn*	1 Roll/70g	181	8.8	259	10.1	24.5	12.5	3.9
Vegetarian, Chilled, Single Pack, Quorn*	1 Roll/130g	292	12.1	225	12.3	21.2	9.3	3.8
SCALLOPS								
Raw, Bay or Sea with Roe, Average	*1 Scallop/15g*	*13*	*0.1*	*88*	*16.8*	*2.4*	*0.8*	*0*
Steamed, Average	*1oz/28g*	*33*	*0.4*	*118*	*23.2*	*3.4*	*1.4*	*0*
SCAMPI								
& Chips, Chunky, Finest, Tesco*	1 Pack/280g	420	15.4	150	5.9	18.3	5.5	1.4
& Chips, with Peas	*1 Serving/490g*	*822*	*43.6*	*168*	*10.1*	*11.3*	*8.9*	*1.2*
Bites, Everyday, Value, Tesco*	½ Pack/125g	262	10	210	9.4	23.4	8	1.2
Bites, Vegetarian, Linda McCartney*	½ Pack/125g	279	11.5	223	14.7	18.3	9.2	3.7
Breaded, Baked, Average	*½ Pack/255g*	*565*	*27.4*	*222*	*10.7*	*20.5*	*10.7*	*1*
Breaded, Co-Op*	1 Pack/200g	428	18.4	214	8.2	24	9.2	0.9
Breaded, Free From, Tesco*	½ Pack/101g	192	7.2	190	15.6	15.1	7.1	1.6
Breaded, Fried in Oil, Average	*1 Serving/100g*	*237*	*13.6*	*237*	*9.4*	*20.5*	*13.6*	*0*
Breaded, Oven Baked, Whitby Seafoods*	1 Pack/220g	447	15.4	203	9.3	24.5	7	0

S

	Measure INFO/WEIGHT	per Measure KCAL	FAT	Nutrition Values per 100g / 100ml KCAL	PROT	CARB	FAT	FIBRE
SCAMPI								
White Tail, Aldi*	½ Pack/125g	256	9.6	205	10	23	7.7	2.4
Wholetail, Breaded, Fresh, Waitrose*	1 Serving/81g	176	7.9	217	13.6	17.9	9.7	1.7
Wholetail, Crispy, in Breadcrumbs, Ocean Trader, Lidl*	½ Pack/125g	270	10.8	216	11.9	22.2	8.6	1.1
Wholetail, in Breadcrumb Coating, Morrisons*	½ Pack/113g	244	8.7	216	11	24.5	7.7	2.5
Wholetail, Jumbo, Oven Baked, Gastro, Youngs*	1 Serving/103g	228	10.1	221	9.4	23	9.8	1.6
SCHNAPPS								
Vodkat, Intercontinental Brands Ltd*	1 Serving/25ml	31	0	124	0	0.8	0	0
SCONE								
All Butter, & Cherry, Finest, Tesco*	1 Scone/70g	245	7.2	349	7.1	56	10.3	1.9
All Butter, Finest, Tesco*	1 Scone/70g	258	10.5	369	7.5	50.1	15	1.8
All Butter, Sultana, TTD, Sainsbury's*	1 Scone/70g	241	7	344	7.7	54	10	3.7
All Butter, Tesco*	1 Scone/60g	222	7.6	371	6.4	56.7	12.7	2
Apricot, Blueberry, & Ginger Drop, Gail's*	100g	329	14.1	329	5.3	25.2	14.1	2.3
Cheddar, Cheese, Farmhouse, TTD, Sainsbury's*	1 Scone/70g	235	9.7	335	12	39.4	13.8	2.8
Cheese & Black Pepper, Mini, M&S*	1 Scone/18g	67	3.3	370	10.2	41.1	18.3	1.7
Cheese, Average	*1 Scone/40g*	*145*	*7.1*	*363*	*10.1*	*43.2*	*17.8*	*1.6*
Cherry, Double Butter, Genesis Crafty*	1 Scone/63g	198	4.8	314	6.8	54.5	7.6	1.4
Cherry, Genesis Crafty*	1 Scone/81g	226	5.8	279	4.9	50.5	7.1	0
Cherry, M&S*	1 Scone/60g	202	7.3	337	6.9	49.7	12.2	1.9
Clotted Cream, Cornish, TTD, Sainsbury's*	1 Scone/70g	269	12.7	384	8.4	46.6	18.2	2.1
Cream, Mini, Co-Op*	1 Scone/24g	86	4.1	360	6.8	44	17	1.1
Devon, M&S*	1 Scone/59g	225	9.6	380	7.1	50.8	16.2	1.5
Devon, M&S*	1 Scone/70g	258	10.8	368	7.4	49.1	15.4	1.9
Fresh Cream with Strawberry Jam, Tesco*	1 Scone/88g	299	12.9	340	6.3	44.7	14.7	1.8
Fruit, Aldi*	1 Scone/65g	239	5.8	367	6.3	64.4	9	1.6
Fruit, Average	*1 Scone/40g*	*126*	*3.9*	*316*	*7.3*	*52.9*	*9.8*	*0*
Fruit, Gail's*	100g	377	15.8	377	7.8	51.1	15.8	2.6
Fruit, Smart Price, Asda*	1 Scone/41g	139	4.1	338	7	55	10	3
Fruit, Waitrose*	1 Scone/59g	190	4.8	325	6.3	56.5	8.2	2.2
Gruyere, & Chive, Gail's*	100g	346	21.7	346	11.6	27.4	21.7	1.4
Maple, & Pecan Drop, Gail's*	100g	478	28.5	478	6.1	47.9	28.5	2.8
Plain, All Butter, Sainsbury's*	1 Scone/58g	213	7.4	366	8.1	54.1	12.7	1.6
Plain, Average	*1 Scone/40g*	*145*	*5.8*	*362*	*7.2*	*53.8*	*14.6*	*1.9*
Plain, Butter Enriched, Tesco*	1 Scone/90g	317	8	352	7.7	59.8	8.9	1.2
Plain, Genesis Crafty*	1 Scone/74g	227	7.4	307	6.8	49.1	10	0
Potato, Average	*1 Scone/40g*	*118*	*5.7*	*296*	*5.1*	*39.1*	*14.3*	*1.6*
Potato, Mother's Pride*	1 Scone/37g	77	0.8	207	4.7	42	2.2	4.3
Red Berry, Mixed, Finest, Tesco*	1 Scone/110g	344	9.5	313	7.8	50.1	8.6	1.9
Sour Cherry, & Dark Chocolate Drop, Gail's*	100g	409	22.6	409	6.3	45.1	22.6	2.7
Strawberry, Fresh Cream, BGTY, Sainsbury's*	1 Scone/50g	154	5.6	309	5.1	47	11.2	1.1
Sultana, All Butter, Tesco*	1 Scone/60g	216	6.5	360	4.6	59.1	10.9	3.5
Sultana, All Butter, The Best, Morrisons*	1 Scone/67g	222	6.4	332	7.4	52.5	9.5	3.5
Sultana, Finest, Tesco*	1 Scone/70g	238	7.6	340	8.9	50.9	10.9	2.1
Sultana, H.W. Nevill's*	1 Scone/41g	136	3.1	334	6.8	58.6	7.5	2.3
Sultana, M&S*	1 Scone/66g	231	8.2	350	6.5	53	12.5	2
Sultana, Rowan Hill Bakery, Lidl*	1 Scone/60g	220	7.2	367	7.1	57	12	1.1
Sultana, Tesco*	1 Scone/90g	304	6.8	338	7.2	59.5	7.6	1.6
Sultana, Value, Tesco*	1 Scone/40g	134	4	335	6.5	53.8	10.1	2.7
Tattie, Scottish, Nick Nairn's*	1 Scone/21g	42	0.3	199	4	34.7	1.6	0.7
Wholemeal	*1 Scone/40g*	*130*	*5.8*	*326*	*8.7*	*43.1*	*14.4*	*5.2*
Wholemeal, Fruit	*1 Scone/40g*	*130*	*5.1*	*324*	*8.1*	*47.2*	*12.8*	*4.9*
SEA BASS								
Cooked, Dry Heat, Average	*1 Fillet/100g*	*124*	*2.6*	*124*	*23.6*	*0*	*2.6*	*0*

S

	Measure INFO/WEIGHT	per Measure KCAL	FAT	Nutrition Values per 100g / 100ml KCAL	PROT	CARB	FAT	FIBRE
SEA BASS								
Fillets, Caramelised Ginger & Lime Butter, Sainsbury's*	1 Fillet/115g	258	18.1	224	19.9	0.5	15.7	0.5
Fillets, with Butter, Cooked, Tesco*	1 Fillet/86g	189	13	220	19.4	1	15.1	1.7
Fillets, with Cheddar, Lemon & Parsley Crumb, M&S*	½ Pack/115g	222	13.3	193	17.1	4.8	11.6	0.5
Fillets, With Rocket Pesto Butter, Waitrose*	½ Pack/95g	220	15.4	232	20.1	1.2	16.2	0.5
Raw, Fillet, Average	*1 Fillet/95g*	*108*	*3.4*	*113*	*20.3*	*0*	*3.5*	*0.1*
SEA BREAM								
Fillet, Cooked, Dry Heat, Average	*1 Serving/100g*	*124*	*3*	*124*	*24*	*0*	*3*	*0*
Fillets, Raw, Average	*1oz/28g*	*27*	*0.8*	*96*	*17.5*	*0*	*2.9*	*0*
Fillets, with Rocket Pesto Butter, Waitrose*	1 Fillet/87g	220	15.4	253	22.7	0.5	17.7	0.5
SEAFOOD								
Cocktail, Average	*1oz/28g*	*24*	*0.4*	*87*	*15.6*	*2.9*	*1.5*	*0*
Mussels, Clams, & Prawns, in Tomato & Herb, Iceland*	½ Pack/139g	236	18.9	170	8.2	3.1	13.6	1.3
Selection, Fresh, Tesco*	1 Pack/234g	187	2.3	80	17.7	0.1	1	0
Selection, Sainsbury's*	½ Pack/100g	75	1	75	15.2	1.3	1	0.5
SEAFOOD STICKS								
Average	*1 Stick/15g*	*16*	*0*	*106*	*8*	*18.4*	*0.2*	*0.2*
Chilled, or Frozen, Youngs*	1 Stick/14g	16	0.2	114	6.4	20	1.4	0
SEASONING MIX								
Cajun, Perfect Shake, As Sold, Schwartz*	1 Tbsp/1g	2	0.1	249	9.9	27.2	7	19
Cajun, Tesco*	1 Tsp/5g	16	0.3	314	10.9	45.9	6.5	14
Chicken, Lemon & Herb, Tray Bake, Schwartz*	1 Serving/110g	352	3.1	320	7.7	60.9	2.8	10.1
Chicken, Provencal Herb, Tray Bake, Schwartz*	1 Pack/30g	89	0.6	296	9.3	55.3	2	9.9
Dukkah, Cooks' Ingredients, Waitrose*	1 Serving/5g	19	0.8	388	18.3	30.7	17	19.6
Dukkah, Cooks' Ingredients, Waitrose*	1 Serving/5g	19	0.8	388	18.3	30.7	17	19.6
Fajita, Mild, M&S*	1 Pack/35g	112	2.2	319	10.2	44.7	6.2	21.9
Fajita, Original, Mild, Latin American Kitchen, Santa Maria*	¼ Sachet/7g	20	0.4	283	8.6	46	5	11
Garlic, For Chicken, So Juicy, Maggi*	1 Pack/30g	95	0.8	316	9.4	58.9	2.8	8.7
Garlic, Papyrus Sheets, SoTender, Maggi*	1 Sheet/6g	25	1.9	438	6.3	24.4	32.5	11.4
Italian Herb, Schwartz*	1 Tsp/1g	3	0	338	11	64.5	4	0
Italian Herbs, Papyrus Sheets, SoTender, Maggi*	1 Sheet/6g	26	2	440	7.3	22.1	34.1	7.7
Jamaican Jerk Chicken, Recipe, Schwartz*	1 Pack/27g	75	0.8	276	9.8	69.8	3	17.2
Jerk, Dunns River*	1 Tbsp/15g	31	0.9	209	4.5	24	5.9	0
Lamb Hot Pot, Colman's*	¼ Pack/10g	32	0.2	320	12	61	1.5	4
Lemon & Herb, for Chicken, Cook in Bag, Average	*1 Bag/34g*	*121*	*1.9*	*356*	*10.8*	*63.7*	*5.5*	*4.1*
Mediterranean Chicken, Season & Shake, Colman's*	1 Pack/33g	99	0.7	300	10.3	56.8	2.1	5.9
Mediterranean, for Chicken, Cook in Bag, Average	*1 Bag/33g*	*99*	*0.7*	*302*	*10.6*	*56.6*	*2*	*7*
Mexican Chicken, As Sold, So Juicy, Maggi*	1 Pack/40g	123	1.7	308	7.4	57.2	4.2	6
Paprika, for Chicken, Cook in Bag, Average	*1 Bag/34g*	*96*	*1.3*	*283*	*12.3*	*45.8*	*4*	*8.1*
Paprika, Papyrus Sheets, SoTender, Maggi*	1 Sheet/6g	25	2	431	9.1	12.2	35.2	14.5
Plri Piri, Smoky & Aromatic, Maggi*	1 Pack/27g	87	1.4	324	6.9	58	5	9.7
Pork, Sage & Onion, Schwartz*	1 Tsp/5g	15	0.3	300	10.6	44.5	5.3	15.8
Potato Wedges, Garlic & Herb, Schwartz*	1 Pack/38g	106	1.9	278	11.4	47.1	4.9	11.7
Shepherd's Pie, Colman's*	1 Pack/50g	170	1	340	13	60	2	5
Smoked Paprika Chicken, As Sold, Schwartz*	1 Pack/28g	87	1.6	309	10.3	44.4	5.7	0
Spaghetti Bolognaise, Naturally Tasty, As Sold, Knorr*	1 Pack/43g	132	1.8	306	8.5	54	4.3	12
Taco, Old El Paso*	¼ Pack/9g	30	0.4	334	5.5	69	4	0
Takeaway, Classic Flavour, Spice Bag, McDonnell's*	1 Tbsp/15g	29	1	192	18.2	9.1	7	0
SEAWEED								
Crispy, Average	*1oz/28g*	*182*	*17.3*	*651*	*7.5*	*15.6*	*61.9*	*7*
Mixed, Trimmed, Sea Vegetables, Waitrose*	1 Pack/80g	15	0.2	19	2.1	1	0.3	1.8
Nori, Dried, Raw	*1oz/28g*	*38*	*0.4*	*136*	*30.7*	*0*	*1.5*	*44.4*
Spaghetti, Dry Weight, Tesco*	½ Pack/40g	89	0.2	223	10	29	0.5	31
Wakame, Dried, Raw	*1oz/28g*	*20*	*0.7*	*71*	*12.4*	*0*	*2.4*	*47.1*

S

	Measure INFO/WEIGHT	per Measure KCAL	FAT	Nutrition Values per 100g / 100ml KCAL	PROT	CARB	FAT	FIBRE
SEED MIX								
3, Toasted, Tesco*	1 Serving/25g	141	11.5	562	26	1.4	45.9	19.8
Chia & Flaxseed, Sprinkles, Tesco*	1 Serving/26g	135	9.2	518	24.2	15.9	35.3	20.2
Four, Whitworths*	1 Serving/25g	141	11.8	565	26.8	1.4	47.2	14.5
Omega, Morrisons*	¼ Pack/25g	138	11.4	554	20.9	15	45.6	6.4
Omega, Munchy Seeds*	1 Bag/30g	184	14.9	613	28.4	13.1	49.7	2.2
Original, The Food Doctor*	1 Serving/30g	157	13.3	522	28.2	3.7	44.4	17.7
Roasted Sunflower & Pumpkin, Salad Sprinkles, Tesco*	1 Serving/20g	112	8.5	561	30	9.4	42.6	10.2
Super Seeds, Food Doctor*	1 Serving/30g	168	13.5	560	26	3	45	18.7
Super Seeds, Salad Topper, Good4U*	1 Serving/25g	144	11.2	575	30	7	45	10
SEEDS								
Chia, Black, The Chia Co*	1 Tbsp/15g	67	5.2	447	20	45	35	37
Chia, Organic, BuyWholeFoodsOnline*	1 Tsp/5g	22	1.6	436	20	2	31	37.9
Chia, Organic, Sevenhills Wholefoods*	1 Tbsp/15g	66	4.3	437	22.1	6.7	28.8	31.3
Chia, Sainsbury's*	1 Serving/15g	62	3.8	414	21.8	8.6	25	33.6
Chia, Tesco*	1 Serving/15g	64	4.3	428	22.3	2.6	28.8	34.7
Chia, White, Organic, KoRo*	1 Tbsp/15g	59	3.8	395	22	2.9	25.1	37.9
Chia, White, The Chia Co*	1 Tbsp/15g	67	4.7	447	20.7	4.7	31.3	37.3
Chironji, Raw, Average	*1 Serving/10g*	*7*	*0.6*	*66*	*1.9*	*1.2*	*5.9*	*0.4*
Fiery, Graze*	1 Pack/34g	173	14.8	510	21.8	17.3	43.5	7.9
Flaxseed, Sunflower & Pumpkin, Milled, Linwoods*	1 Scoop/10g	54	4.9	542	22.7	2.4	49.1	16.2
Hemp, Shelled, Linwoods*	2 Tbsps/30g	178	14.8	593	35.1	7.6	49.5	5.9
Mixed, Wholesome, Love Life, Waitrose*	1 Serving/30g	166	13.6	554	21.3	15.5	45.2	8
Mustard, Average	*1 Tsp/3.3g*	*15*	*0.9*	*469*	*34.9*	*34.9*	*28.8*	*14.7*
Nigella, Average	*1 Tsp/5g*	*20*	*1.7*	*392*	*21.3*	*1.9*	*33.3*	*8.4*
Phool Makhana, Raw, Average	*1 Serving/10g*	*35*	*0*	*350*	*9.7*	*77*	*0.1*	*7.6*
Poppy, Average	*1 Tbsp/9g*	*47*	*3.9*	*533*	*18*	*23.7*	*44.7*	*10*
Pumpkin, & Sunflower, Toasted, Sainsbury's*	1 Serving/10g	64	5.6	643	28	1.9	56	9.8
Pumpkin, Alesto, Lidl*	1 Serving/25g	128	9	511	34.5	4.2	36.2	15.2
Pumpkin, Average	*1 Tbsp/10g*	*57*	*4.6*	*568*	*27.9*	*13*	*45.9*	*3.8*
Sesame, Average	*1 Tsp/2g*	*12*	*1.1*	*610*	*22.3*	*3.6*	*56.4*	*7.8*
Sesame, Tesco*	1 Tsp/4g	24	2.3	598	18.2	0.9	58	7.9
Sunflower, Average	*1 Tbsp/10g*	*59*	*4.9*	*585*	*23.4*	*15*	*48.7*	*5.7*
SEMOLINA								
Average	*1oz/28g*	*98*	*0.5*	*348*	*11*	*75.2*	*1.8*	*2.1*
Pudding, Creamed, Ambrosia*	1 Can/425g	344	7.2	81	3.3	13.1	1.7	0.2
Pudding, Creamed, Co-Op*	1 Can/425g	382	8.5	90	4	15	2	0
SHALLOTS								
Pickled in Hot & Spicy Vinegar, Tesco*	1 Onion/18g	14	0	77	1	18	0.1	1.9
Raw, Average	*1 Serving/80g*	*16*	*0.2*	*20*	*1.5*	*3.3*	*0.2*	*1.4*
SHANDY								
Bitter, Original, Ben Shaws*	1 Can/330ml	89	0	27	0	6	0	0
Canned, Morrisons*	1 Can/330ml	36	0	11	0	1.8	0	0
Homemade, Average	*1 Pint/568ml*	*148*	*0*	*26*	*0.2*	*2.9*	*0*	*0*
Lager, 0.9%, Bavaria*	1 Can/330ml	76	0	23	0.1	5	0	0
Lemonade, Traditional Style, Tesco*	1 Can/330ml	63	0	19	0	4.7	0	0
SHARK								
Raw	*1oz/28g*	*29*	*0.3*	*102*	*23*	*0*	*1.1*	*0*
SHARON FRUIT								
Average	*1oz/28g*	*19*	*0*	*68*	*0.7*	*17.3*	*0*	*1.5*
SHERRY								
Dry, Average	*1 Glass/120ml*	*139*	*0*	*116*	*0.2*	*1.4*	*0*	*0*
Medium	*1 Serving/50ml*	*58*	*0*	*116*	*0.1*	*5.9*	*0*	*0*
Sweet	*1 Serving/50ml*	*68*	*0*	*136*	*0.3*	*6.9*	*0*	*0*

S

	Measure INFO/WEIGHT	per Measure KCAL	FAT	Nutrition Values per 100g / 100ml KCAL	PROT	CARB	FAT	FIBRE
SHORTBREAD								
All Butter, Deans*	1 Biscuit/15g	77	3.8	511	4.9	65.7	25.4	1.2
All Butter, Finger, Highland, TTD, Sainsbury's*	1 Biscuit/20g	103	5.5	515	4.6	61.8	27.4	1.2
All Butter, Fingers, Highland, Sainsbury's*	2 Biscuits/40g	208	11.5	521	4.8	59.4	28.8	2.7
All Butter, Fingers, Scottish, M&S*	1 Finger/18g	90	4.9	510	5.7	58.9	27.8	4.7
All Butter, Giant, Fingers, Higland, Sainsbury's*	1 Biscuit/35g	182	10.1	520	4.8	59.4	28.8	1.8
All Butter, Petticoat Tails, Co-Op*	1 Biscuit/13g	68	3.8	520	5	60	29	2
All Butter, Round, Luxury, M&S*	1 Biscuit/20g	105	5.8	525	6.2	60	29	2
All Butter, Selection, Waitrose*	1 Biscuit/18g	95	11	527	5.3	58.3	61.1	3
All Butter, Trufree*	1 Biscuit/11g	58	3.1	524	2	66	28	0.9
All Butter, with Toffee, Scottish, M&S*	1 Biscuit/6g	32	1.7	515	5.7	61.9	26.9	1.2
Average	***1oz/28g***	***139***	***7.3***	***498***	***5.9***	***63.9***	***26.1***	***1.9***
Belgian Chocolate Chunk, Asda*	1 Biscuit/20g	106	6.2	531	7	56	31	1.8
Butter Enriched, Bites, Bakery, Sainsbury's*	1 Bite/16g	84	4.7	527	6	58	29.8	1.4
Butter, with Real Lemons, Mini, Deluxe, Lidl*	3 Biscuits/24g	125	7	521	5.6	57.6	29.1	3.2
Caramel, Millionaires, Fox's*	1 Serving/16g	75	3.9	483	6.1	57.9	25.3	0.1
Choc Chip, Fair Trade, Co-Op*	1 Biscuit/19g	100	6	526	5.3	57.9	31.6	2.6
Chocolate Chip, Jacob's*	1 Biscuit/17g	87	4.7	513	5.2	61.2	27.5	1.8
Chocolate Chip, Tesco*	1 Serving/20g	105	6.1	525	7.5	55	30.6	3
Chocolate, Belgian, Chunky, TTD, Sainsbury's*	1 Piece/70g	353	19	505	5.5	58.8	27.2	1.4
Chocolate, Triple, Finest, Tesco*	1 Square/63g	325	18.5	516	5.8	56.3	29.4	1.5
Clotted Cream, Finest, Tesco*	1 Biscuit/20g	109	6.4	543	5.2	58	32.2	1.7
Clotted Cream, with Chocolate Pieces, Cornish, Furniss*	1 Biscuit/20g	107	5.7	534	5.8	61.6	28.4	0
Demerara, Rounds, TTD, Sainsbury's*	1 Biscuit/22g	113	5.9	508	5.1	62.2	26.5	1.8
Double Choc Chip, Petit Four, Scottish, Tesco*	1 Serving/50g	266	15	531	5.1	60.4	30	1.7
Fingers, Asda*	1 Finger/18g	93	5.1	519	5.8	60.3	28.3	18
Fingers, Scottish, Finest, Tesco*	1 Biscuit/21g	104	5	498	5.1	65.5	23.9	2
Millionaire, Squares, Free From, Asda*	1 Square/30g	153	8.4	510	2.9	60	28	1.7
Mini Bites, Co-Op*	1 Biscuit/10g	53	3	530	7	59	30	2
Mini, Bites, Tesco*	1 Bite/12g	63	3.5	528	7.2	58.1	29.3	1.3
Pecan All Butter, Sainsbury's*	1 Biscuit/18g	99	6.5	548	5.3	49.9	36.3	2.5
Petticoat Tails, All Butter, Highland, Sainsbury's*	1 Biscuit/12g	65	3.6	521	6.3	58	28.8	2.2
Rings, Handbaked, Border*	1 Biscuit/17g	86	4.9	520	6.2	61.2	29.5	0
Rose Petal, & Chinese Tea, 1, Waitrose*	1 Biscuit/10g	53	2.9	527	5.8	59.6	29	2.1
Spotty Scottie Dogs, with Chocolate Chips, Sainsbury's*	1 Biscuit/12g	62	3.3	515	5.1	60.5	27.5	2.5
Wheat & GF, Free From Range, Tesco*	1 Shortbread/18g	93	4.9	521	5.4	61.7	27.6	1.9
SHORTCAKE								
Caramel, Baked in the Tray, Tesco*	1 Slice/49g	247	13.2	504	3.4	61.6	26.9	1.1
Caramel, Mini, Thorntons*	1 Piece/14g	69	4.1	491	5	50.6	29.5	0
SHRIMP								
Boiled, Average	***1 Serving/60g***	***70***	***1.4***	***117***	***23.8***	***0***	***2.4***	***0***
Frozen, Average	***1oz/28g***	***20***	***0.2***	***73***	***16.5***	***0***	***0.8***	***0***
SKATE								
Grilled	***1oz/28g***	***22***	***0.1***	***79***	***18.9***	***0***	***0.5***	***0***
in Batter, Fried in Blended Oil	***1oz/28g***	***47***	***2.8***	***168***	***14.7***	***4.9***	***10.1***	***0.2***
Raw, Edible Portion	***1oz/28g***	***18***	***0.1***	***64***	***15.1***	***0***	***0.4***	***0***
SKIPS								
Cheesy, KP Snacks*	1 Bag/17g	89	5	524	6.2	58.5	29.5	1
Prawn Cocktail, KP Snacks*	1 Bag/17g	92	5.4	544	4.9	58	32	0.7
SKITTLES								
Mars*	1 Pack/55g	223	2.4	406	0	90.6	4.4	0
Sweet Heat, Mars*	¼ Pack/49g	196	2.1	399	0	89.8	4.2	0
SLICES								
Bacon & Cheese, Pastry, Tesco*	1 Slice/165g	480	32	291	7.4	21.7	19.4	1

S

	Measure INFO/WEIGHT	per Measure KCAL	FAT	Nutrition Values per 100g / 100ml KCAL	PROT	CARB	FAT	FIBRE
SLICES								
Beef, Minced Steak & Onion, Tesco*	1 Slice/150g	424	27.2	283	8.7	21.3	18.1	1.6
Cheese & Onion, Pastry, Tesco*	1 Slice/150g	502	37	335	8	20.1	24.7	1.4
Chicken & Mushroom, Tesco*	1 Slice/165g	457	28.9	277	9.2	20.6	17.5	0.9
Chicken & Bacon, Wall's*	1 Slice/225g	576	33.5	256	10.5	19.9	14.9	0
Chicken & Mushroom, Ginsters*	1 Slice/180g	439	26.8	244	8.3	19.1	14.9	1.8
Chicken & Mushroom, Sainsbury's*	1 Slice/164g	427	26.5	259	7.3	21.3	16.1	1
Chicken Fajita, Puff Pastry, Sainsbury's*	1 Pack/180g	452	23	251	9.1	23.6	12.8	2.5
Chicken, & Bacon, Asda*	1 Slice/156g	416	21.9	266	10	24	14	1.4
Chicken, Spicy, Ginsters*	1 Pack/170g	466	28.7	274	8.5	21.1	16.9	0
Custard, Pastry, Tesco*	1 Slice/94g	266	10.7	283	3.2	41.6	11.3	0.9
Fresh Cream, Tesco*	1 Slice/75g	311	21	414	3.5	37.4	27.9	1
Goats Cheese & Spinach, Crisp & Creamy, Waitrose*	1 Slice/100g	351	22.7	351	7.6	28.3	22.7	1.8
Ham & Cheese, Ginsters*	1 Pack/180g	511	33.7	284	8.5	20.4	18.7	2.5
Minced Steak & Onion, Sainsbury's*	1 Slice/165g	475	29.9	288	15.2	16	18.1	2.5
Raisin, Crispy, LC, Tesco*	1 Biscuit/15g	56	0.6	370	6	76.6	3.9	5.5
Steak, Peppered, Ginsters*	1 Slice/180g	457	27	254	8.4	21.3	15	1.6
SLIM FAST*								
Bars, Chocolate Caramel Treat, Snack, Slim Fast*	1 Bar/26g	95	2.6	360	3.5	63	10	1.5
Bars, Chocolate, Nutty, Nougat, Snack, Slim Fast*	1 Bar/25g	95	3	380	4	63	12	1.5
Bars, Heavenly Chocolate Delight, Snack, Slim Fast*	1 Bar/24g	95	3.2	390	5	58	13	7
Bars, Heavenly Chocolate, Crunch Snack, Slim Fast*	1 Bar/24g	95	3.2	390	5	58	13	7
Bars, Nutty Salted Caramel, Meal, Slim Fast*	1 Bar/60g	218	6.8	364	25.4	26.9	11.3	18.7
Bars, Summer Berry, Meal, Slim Fast*	1 Bar/60g	210	5	350	23.3	51.7	8.3	5.8
Chunky Chocolate, Shake, Ready to Drink, Slimfast*	1 Shake/325ml	204	5.2	63	4.6	6.6	1.6	1.5
Crackers, Cheddar Flavour Bites, Snack Bag, Slim Fast*	1 Pack/22g	92	2	417	9.6	72.8	9.2	2.5
Milk Shake, Blissful Banana, Powder, Dry, Slim Fast*	2 Scoops/37g	131	2.4	359	13.4	60.2	6.7	11
Milk Shake, Chunky Chocolate, Powder, Dry, Slim Fast*	2 Scoops/37g	132	2.7	363	13.9	59	7.5	10.9
Milk Shake, Simply Vanilla, Powder, Dry, Slim Fast*	2 Scoops/37g	131	2.4	360	13.4	60.9	6.5	11
Milk Shake, Summer Strawberry, Powder, Dry, Slim Fast*	2 Scoops/37g	139	2.4	380	13.5	60.1	6.6	11.1
Milk Shake,Caramel Temptation, Powder, Dry, Slim Fast*	1 Serving/37g	139	2.2	380	14	62	6	11
Noodles, Chicken Tikka Masala, Box, Slim Fast*	1 Box/250g	81	2.2	33	2.3	2.7	0.9	2.5
Noodles, Spicy Thai, Slim Fast*	1 Box/240g	70	3.1	29	0.9	2.4	1.3	2.4
Pretzels, Sour Cream & Chive, Snack Bag, Slim Fast*	1 Pack/23g	99	2.2	432	9.7	74.9	9.5	4.1
Tortillas, Barbecue Flavour, Snack Bag, Slim Fast*	1 Bag/22g	96	2.6	435	6.5	73.9	11.8	3.6
SLUSH PUPPY								
Raspberry, Blue, Manchester Drinks Co.*	1 Serving/250ml	95	0	38	0.5	8.3	0	0
SMARTIES								
Mini Eggs, Nestle*	5 Eggs/17g	85	3.5	499	3.9	73.5	20.4	2.8
Mini, Treat Size, Smarties, Nestle*	1 Carton/14g	68	2.8	471	5	68.1	19.6	1
Nestle*	1 Tube/40g	188	7.1	469	3.9	72.5	17.7	2.4
Tree Decoration, Nestle*	1 Chocolate/18g	95	5.4	529	5.6	58.9	30.1	0.8
SMOOTHIE								
Apples & Blackcurrants for Kids, Innocent*	1 Carton/180ml	104	0.2	58	0.3	14.1	0.1	0.1
Berry Set Go, Innocent*	1 Bottle/330ml	142	0	43	0	11	0	0
Berry, & Beetroot, Sachet, M&S*	1 Sachet/110g	65	0.2	59	1.2	12.1	0.2	2.2
Blackberries & Blueberries, Innocent*	1 Bottle/250ml	120	0.2	48	0.5	12	0.1	2.1
Breakfast Oats, Mindful Chef*	1 Pack/140g	158	2.8	113	2.5	19.1	2	3
Cherries & Strawberries, Innocent*	1 Bottle/250ml	122	0.2	49	0.6	12.6	0.1	0
Cherries, & Strawberries,, Just For Kids, Innocent*	1 Carton/180ml	92	0	51	0.4	11	0	1.3
Coconut, Pineapple & Banana, Coldpress*	1 Serving/150ml	96	1.2	64	0.7	12.7	0.8	0
Cucumber, Avocado, & Lime, M&S*	1 Bottle/250ml	148	3.5	59	0.4	10.4	1.4	1.4
Fruit, & Cereal, Forest Fruits, Morning Boost , Tropicana*	1 Serving/250ml	152	0	61	0.7	13	0	2.4
Grape Escape, Love Smoothies*	1 Serving/120ml	74	0.4	62	0.7	13	0.3	2.3

S

	Measure INFO/WEIGHT	per Measure KCAL	FAT	Nutrition Values per 100g / 100ml KCAL	PROT	CARB	FAT	FIBRE
SMOOTHIE								
Green, Lean, Mindful Chef*	1 Pack/140g	78	0.8	56	1.3	10	0.6	2.5
Kefir, Cacao, Bio-tiful Dairy*	1 Bottle/250ml	162	6.8	65	3.1	6.8	2.7	0
Kefir, Raspberry, Bio-tiful Dairy*	1 Bottle/250ml	162	6.8	65	3	7.2	2.7	0
Magnificent Mango, Innocent*	1 Bottle/250ml	136	0	54	0.4	12	0	1.4
Mango, Pineapple, & Passion Fruit, Eat Well, M&S*	1 Bottle/250g	170	1.2	68	0.5	14.9	0.5	0.9
Mangoes & Passion Fruits, Pure Fruit, Innocent*	1 Bottle/250ml	135	0	54	0.4	12	0	1.4
Mixed Berry, CBY, Asda*	1 Glass/250ml	143	0	57	0.6	12.6	0	1.6
Orange, Banana, Mango, Morning Boost, Tropicana*	1 Serving/250ml	125	0	50	0.1	9.2	0	2.3
Orange, Mango, & Passionfruit, On the Go, Sainsbury's*	1 Serving/150g	84	0.8	56	0.5	12.8	0.5	0.7
Oranges, Mangoes & Pineapples For Kids, Innocent*	1 Carton/180ml	94	0.2	52	0.7	11.7	0.1	0.9
Peaches & Passionfruit, for Kids, Innocent*	1 Carton/180ml	95	0	53	0.6	14.7	0	0.9
Peaches, Bananas & Passionfruit, PJ Smoothies*	1 Bottle/250g	128	0.2	51	0.4	12.1	0.1	0
Pear, Kiwi, Kale, & Fennel, Waitrose*	1 Serving/150ml	64	0	43	0.5	9.8	0	0.9
Pineapple, Apple, & Carrot, Innocent*	1 Carton/180ml	94	0	52	0.6	12	0	0.3
Pineapple, Banana & Coconut, CBY, Asda*	1 Glass/250ml	178	2.8	71	0.7	13.6	1.1	1
Pineapples, Bananas & Coconuts, Innocent*	1 Bottle/250ml	172	2.8	69	0.7	13.6	1.1	1
Pomegranates, Blueberries & Acai, Special, Innocent*	1 Serving/250ml	170	0.5	68	0.6	15.6	0.2	0.8
Protein Superfood, Mango & Banana, PhD Nutrition*	1 Serving/130g	175	7.7	135	15.4	4.2	5.9	1.4
Raspberry & Blueberry, Plus, Tesco*	1 Serving/100ml	59	0.3	59	2.6	11.6	0.3	0.5
Strawberries & Bananas, Pure Fruit, Innocent*	1 Bottle/250ml	132	0.2	53	0.7	13.1	0.1	1.3
Strawberries, Blackberries, Raspberries, Kids, Innocent*	1 Carton/180ml	81	0.2	45	0.5	9.9	0.1	1.3
Strawberry & Banana, Tesco*	1 Bottle/250ml	112	0.5	45	0.6	10.1	0.2	0.8
Summer Sunrise, Mindful Chef*	1 Pack/140g	78	0.3	56	0.9	11.6	0.2	1.8
Super Orange, Cold Pressed, Raw Fruit & Veg, Savse*	1 Bottle/250ml	110	0.2	44	0.9	9.8	0.1	0.7
Super Red, Cold Pressed, Raw Fruit & Veg, Savse*	1 Bottle/250ml	98	0.2	39	0.8	8.4	0.1	0.7
Super, Power, M&S*	1 Bottle/250ml	388	2.8	155	2.2	10.5	1.1	0.7
Super, Protect, M&S*	1 Bottle/250ml	190	7	76	0.8	11.4	2.8	0.8
Superfruits, Pomegranates, Blueberries & Acai, Innocent*	1 Serving/250ml	170	0.5	68	0.5	15.6	0.2	0.8
Vanilla Bean, M&S*	1 Bottle/500ml	450	13	90	3.3	13.9	2.6	0
Watermelon, & Raspberry, Lean, Naked Juice Co*	1 Bottle/360ml	97	0	27	0.2	6.6	0	0
SMOOTHIE MIX								
Banana, Kale & Mango, As Sold, Iceland*	1 Sachet/150g	90	0.4	60	1.1	12.2	0.3	2.3
Beautiful Berries, My Goodness, Sainsbury's*	1 Serving/80g	39	0.4	49	1	8.9	0.5	3.7
Berry, Banana, Frozen, Sainsbury's*	1 Serving/80g	43	0.4	54	0.8	10.3	0.5	3.1
Berry, Frozen, Love Life, Waitrose*	1 Serving/80g	31	0	39	1.1	7.2	0	2.9
Greens, Glowing, My Goodness, Sainsbury's*	1 Serving/80g	47	2.1	59	2.1	5.5	2.6	2.6
Kale, Spinach, & Mango, Kale Kick, Love Smoothies*	1 Pouch/120g	50	0	42	1.7	7	0	0
Mango & Pineapple, CBY, Asda*	1 Portion/80g	48	0.4	59	0.6	12	0.5	1.9
Strawberry & Banana, Frozen, Love Life, Waitrose*	1 Serving/80g	37	0.3	46	0.7	8.2	0.4	3.4
Strawberry, Blueberry, & Banana, Lidl*	1 Pack/150g	82	0.6	55	1	9.9	0.4	2.6
Tropical, Frozen, Love Life, Waitrose*	1 Serving/80g	45	0.2	57	0.7	11.8	0.3	1.9
Tropical, Lidl*	1 Serving/75g	39	0.2	52	0.5	11.4	0.2	0.8
Yellow Frozen, Morrisons*	1 Portion/80g	41	0.2	51	0.5	10.9	0.2	1.9
SNACKS								
Box, Smokehouse BBQ, Crunch, Graze*	1 Pack/31g	137	4.6	441	9.9	60	15	7.3
Corn, Original, Mister Corn*	1 Serving/30g	145	6.3	482	7.6	63	21	5.5
Grilled Cheese Crunch, Graze*	1 Punnet/27g	150	10.5	555	18	35	39	7.4
Mild Green Curry, Baked Pea Sticks, Yushoi *	1 Serving/21g	87	3	415	19.1	45.7	14.2	14.3
Mini C's, Cheese, GF, Schar*	1 Serving/30g	137	5.1	457	7.3	67	17	3.5
Mix, Sweet & Salty, Reese's*	½ Pack/28g	139	7.6	496	12.4	54.7	27.1	0
Mumbai Mix, streetmix, Sensations, Walkers*	1 Serving/30g	176	11.8	585	14	42.1	39.3	4.1
Nut Butter Cups, Almond, Nature Valley*	2 Cups/35g	176	9	503	8.4	56.3	25.8	6
Pea, Chorizo, & Red Pepper, Snackrite, Aldi*	1 Pack/21g	86	2.9	411	20	43	14	16

S

INFO/WEIGHT	Measure	per Measure		Nutrition Values per 100g / 100ml				
		KCAL	FAT	KCAL	PROT	CARB	FAT	FIBRE
SNACKS								
Pea, Malaysian Sweet Curry Flavour, Passions, Aldi*	1 Pack/21g	89	3.2	422	19	47	15	13
Pea, Thai Red Curry Flavour, Passions, Aldi*	1 Pack/21g	88	2.9	421	19	48	14	12
Protein Power, Veggie, Alesto, Lidl*	1 Serving/28g	134	7.3	479	30.3	25.5	26	10.7
Rancher Mix, Smokin' Joe's, Natural Selection, Aldi*	1 Snack Box/31g	141	5.6	455	8.8	62	18	6.3
Salt & Pepper, Combo Mix, Sainsbury's*	1 Serving/30g	143	6.4	476	4.3	65.5	21.2	3.1
Slightly Salted, Baked Pea Sticks, Yushoi *	1 Pack/21g	88	3.2	419	19.4	43.1	15.4	15.5
Smoky Barbecue, Crunch, Retail, Graze*	1 Pack/31g	137	5	443	11	57	16	7.9
Smoky Salt & Pepper, Baked Pea Sticks, Yushoi *	1 Serving/21g	86	2.7	409	19.3	46.5	13	14.3
Sour Cream & Onion, Lentil Curls, Passions Deli, Aldi*	1 Pack/20g	91	3.4	454	11	63	17	3.6
Soy & Balsamic Vinegar, Baked Pea Sticks, Yushoi *	1 Serving/21g	88	2.9	417	18.6	47.9	13.7	13.5
Sweet Chilli, Crunch, Graze*	1 Punnet/31g	139	5.3	448	15	55	17	9.9
Sweet Chilli, with Lemon, Baked Pea Sticks, Yushoi *	1 Pack/21g	90	3.2	428	17.4	48.1	15.3	13.1
Teddy Faces, Snackrite, Aldi*	1 Bag/19g	96	5.1	505	3.4	61	27	2.7
Thai Sriracha Mix, Natural Selection*	1 Pack/26g	109	3.4	420	11	60	13	9.3
Veggie Caesar, Graze*	1 Punnet/24g	115	4.6	478	17	52	19	9.4
SNAILS								
in Garlic Butter, Average	**6 Snails/50g**	**219**	**20.8**	**438**	**9.7**	**8**	**41.5**	**1**
Raw, Average	**1 Snail/5g**	**4**	**0.1**	**90**	**16.1**	**2**	**1.4**	**0**
SNAPPER								
Red, Fried in Blended Oil	**1oz/28g**	**35**	**0.9**	**126**	**24.5**	**0**	**3.1**	**0**
Red, Weighed with Bone, Raw	**1oz/28g**	**12**	**0.2**	**42**	**9.2**	**0**	**0.6**	**0**
SNICKERS								
Crispy, Mars*	1 Serving/20g	97	4.6	483	7.1	61	23	0
Mars*	1 Single/48g	245	13.4	510	9.5	54.3	27.9	1.3
Protein, Mars*	1 Bar/51g	199	7.1	391	35.6	36.1	13.9	0
White, Mars*	1 Bar/49g	241	11.8	491	9	59	24	0
SOLE								
Dover, on the Bone, Pan Fried, Sainsbury's*	1 Fillet/200g	190	2.2	95	19.4	1.5	1.1	0.5
Fillet, Yellowfin, Lightly Dusted, Northern Catch, Aldi*	1 Fillet/114g	171	4.6	150	20	7.6	4	2.5
Yellow Fin, Fillets, Lemon & Parsley, Tasty Catch, Aldi*	1 Fillet/115g	193	8.3	168	15	10	7.2	1
Yellow, Fillet, Lightly Dusted, As Consumed, Morrisons*	1 Fillet/124g	218	8.5	176	14	13.9	6.9	1
SOPOCKA								
Sliced, Cured, Pork Loin	**1 Serving/100g**	**101**	**2.9**	**101**	**17.8**	**0.8**	**2.9**	**0**
SORBET								
Blackcurrant, Yorvale Ltd*	1 Serving/100g	120	0.2	120	0	28.8	0.2	0
Exotic Fruit, Sainsbury's*	1 Serving/75g	90	1.5	120	1.2	24.1	2	0
Jamaican Me Crazy, Ben & Jerry's*	1 Serving/100g	130	0	130	0.2	32	0	0.4
Lemon	**1 Scoop/60g**	**79**	**0**	**131**	**0.9**	**34.2**	**0**	**0**
Lemon, Sainsbury's*	¼ Pot/89g	100	0	112	0	28.1	0	0.1
Lemon, Tesco*	1 Scoop/68g	81	0.2	120	0.1	28.8	0.3	0.5
Lemon, Zesty, Morrisons*	1 Scoop/50ml	40	0	79	0.2	19.1	0.1	0.3
Mandarin Orange, Yorvale Ltd*	1 Serving/100g	125	0.2	125	0.1	30.5	0.2	0
Mango, Tesco*	1 Scoop/50g	57	0.4	113	0.5	25.6	0.8	0.8
Mango, Waitrose*	1 Pot/100g	90	0	90	0.1	22.1	0	0.6
Orange, Del Monte*	1 Sorbet/500g	625	0.5	125	0.2	32.1	0.1	0
Passion Fruit, & Mango, Yellow, Truly Irresistible, Co-Op*	1 Scoop/50g	54	0.2	109	0.7	25	0.5	0.6
Passion Fruit, Yorvale Ltd*	1 Serving/100g	109	0.2	109	0.1	26.6	0.2	0
Raspberry & Blackberry, Fat Free, M&S*	1 Sorbet/125g	140	0	112	0.4	27.5	0	0.6
Raspberry, Haagen-Dazs*	½ Cup/105g	120	0	114	0	28.6	0	1.9
Raspberry, Tesco*	1 Scoop/70ml	79	0.4	114	0.2	26.8	0.5	0.5
SOUFFLE								
Cheese	**1oz/28g**	**71**	**5.4**	**253**	**11.4**	**9.3**	**19.2**	**0.3**
Cheese, Alizonne*	1 Serving/33g	129	3.4	392	60.5	14.5	10.2	0.2

	Measure INFO/WEIGHT	per Measure KCAL	FAT	Nutrition Values per 100g / 100ml KCAL	PROT	CARB	FAT	FIBRE
SOUFFLE								
Cheese, Mini, Waitrose*	1 Souffle/14g	32	2.4	232	16	2.9	17.4	2.4
Lemon, Finest, Tesco*	1 Pot/80g	270	20.5	338	2.9	24.1	25.6	0.2
Raspberry & Amaretto, M&S*	1oz/28g	83	4.7	298	2.8	33.1	16.7	0.1
Ricotta & Spinach, M&S*	1 Serving/120g	186	13.3	155	8	6.2	11.1	2.1
Strawberry, M&S*	1 Serving/95g	171	10.1	180	1.6	19.5	10.6	0.9
SOUP								
Asparagus, Cream of, Canned, M&S*	½ Can/200g	108	7.2	54	0.9	4.3	3.6	0.2
Asparagus, New Covent Garden Food Co*	1 Carton/600g	264	14.4	44	1.5	4.1	2.4	0.9
Asparagus, with Croutons, Aldi*	1 Sachet/229ml	96	3.7	42	0.5	6.5	1.6	0.5
Bacon, & Bean, Smoked, Diet Chef Ltd*	1 Pack/300g	162	3.3	54	2.8	8.2	1.1	2.1
Bacon, & Bean, Three, Smoked, Chunky, Baxters*	1 Can/400g	232	4.8	58	2.9	8.8	1.2	1.8
Bacon, & Lentil, CBY, Asda*	½ Pot/300g	177	4.2	59	3.8	7.2	1.4	1.2
Bacon, & Bean, Smoked, Parsley Box*	1 Pack/300g	159	3.6	53	2.4	8.1	1.2	0.6
Bean, & Sweet Potato, Mexican, Super, Glorious!*	½ Pot/300g	137	0.6	46	2.3	6.9	0.2	3.4
Bean, & Vegetable, Three, HL, Tesco*	1 Portion/200g	90	0.6	45	2.1	7.5	0.3	1.9
Bean, & Vegetable, Three, LC, Tesco*	½ Can/200g	110	0.6	55	2.6	9.7	0.3	1.9
Bean, & Veg, Stew, Mighty, Big Soup, Heinz*	1 Can/500g	355	4.5	71	3	11.8	0.9	3
Bean, & Vegetable, Chunky, Sainsbury's*	1 Can/400g	268	4	67	3.5	9.3	1	3.6
Bean, Broad, Gammon, & Parsley, Crosse & Blackwell*	1 Can/400g	212	7.6	53	2.6	5.6	1.9	1.4
Bean, Butter, & Chorizo, Meal, Sainsbury's*	1 Pot/400g	257	9.6	64	3.9	5.6	2.4	2.3
Bean, Chilli, Mexican, Tesco*	1 Carton/600g	270	6.6	45	2.2	6.4	1.1	1.9
Bean, Chilli, Three, Fresh, Tesco*	½ Pot/300g	129	0.3	43	3.3	6	0.1	2.2
Bean, Hearty, Italian Inspired, Love Life, Waitrose*	½ Pot/300g	151	6.6	50	1.5	5.2	2.2	1.8
Bean, Italian Style, Tesco*	1 Can/300g	153	3.6	51	2.8	7.3	1.2	1.1
Bean, Mexican, Fresh, Morrisons*	½ Pot/300g	171	3.9	57	2.1	8.3	1.3	1.9
Bean, Smoky Chipotle, with Quinoa, Meal, Sainsbury's*	1 Pot/400g	369	12.8	92	3.5	10.5	3.2	3.7
Bean, Tuscan, Canned, HL, Tesco*	½ Can/200ml	140	3.6	70	3.5	10.3	1.8	1.3
Bean, Tuscan, Chunky, Love Life, Waitrose*	½ Can/200g	101	1	50	2.6	7.6	0.5	2.3
Bean, Tuscan, Slimming World, Iceland*	½ Pot/250g	100	0.5	40	2.6	5.1	0.2	3.7
Bean, Tuscan, Tesco*	1 Can/400g	248	3.2	62	3.4	8.1	0.8	4.3
Bean, Tuscan, with Roasted Garlic & Tomatoes, Heinz*	1 Can/400g	188	3.6	47	1.3	7.7	0.9	1.1
Beef, & Bean, Chilli, Mexican, Soups of the World, Heinz*	1 Can/515g	360	9.3	70	4.5	9	1.8	1.6
Beef, & Mushroom, Big Soup, Heinz*	1 Can/515g	216	2.6	42	2.3	7	0.5	0.7
Beef, & Tomato, Cup a Soup, Made Up, Batchelors*	1 Serving/252g	83	1.6	33	0.6	6.3	0.6	0.4
Beef, & Vegetable, Big Soup, Heinz*	1 Can/400g	212	4	53	3.5	7.5	1	0.9
Beef, & Vegetables, Chunky, Newgate, Lidl*	1 Tin/400g	232	3.2	58	3.6	8.2	0.8	1.8
Beef, Broth, Big Soup, Heinz*	1 Can/400g	184	2.8	46	2.5	7	0.7	0.9
Beef, Broth, Classic, Heinz*	1 Can/400g	180	2	45	1.9	7.6	0.5	0.8
Beef, Broth, Rich, with Smoky Paprika, Heinz*	½ Can/200g	82	1	41	1.8	6.9	0.5	0.7
Beef, Chilli, Bean, & Rice, M&S*	½ Pot/300g	159	2.4	53	2.7	7.8	0.8	1.9
Beef, Chilli, Chunky, Asda*	1 Can/400g	212	4	53	4.2	5.7	1	2.4
Beef, Fiery, Pho, Vietnamese, Naked Soup*	1 Pack/300g	108	2.1	36	0.9	6.5	0.7	0
Beetroot, Apple, & Grains, Super Soups, Glorious!*	½ Pot/300g	132	2.7	44	1.8	6.2	0.9	1.7
Beetroot, Curly Kale, with Quinoa, Tideford Organics*	½ Pack/300g	87	2.1	29	0.8	4.2	0.7	1.1
Black Bean, Mexican, Extra Special, Asda*	½ Pot/263g	194	10.8	74	2.3	7	4.1	1.7
Broccoli, & Stilton, Canned, Sainsbury's*	½ Can/200g	84	4	42	1.5	4.2	2	0.6
Broccoli, & Stilton, Canned, Tesco*	1 Can/400g	240	14	60	1.7	5	3.5	0.4
Broccoli, & Stilton, Classics, Fresh, Tesco*	½ Pot/300g	156	10.8	52	2.4	1.8	3.6	1.5
Broccoli, & Stilton, Cup Soup, Ainsley Harriott*	1 Sachet/230g	99	2.1	43	0.9	7.8	0.9	0.2
Broccoli, & Stilton, Fresh, Sainsbury's*	½ Pot/300ml	141	9.9	47	2.7	1.8	3.3	1.5
Broccoli, & Stilton, New Covent Garden Food Co*	1 Carton/600ml	240	14.4	40	2.2	1.9	2.4	1.1
Broccoli, & Stilton, Tesco*	1 Can/400g	192	10.4	48	1.9	4.2	2.6	1.2
Broccoli, & Zucinni, Cream Of, Canned, Italiamo*	½ Can/195ml	84	5.1	43	0.9	3.8	2.6	0.5

SOUP

INFO/WEIGHT	Measure	per Measure		Nutrition Values per 100g / 100ml				
		KCAL	FAT	KCAL	PROT	CARB	FAT	FIBRE
Broccoli, Pea & Pesto, New Covent Garden Food Co*	½ Carton/350g	182	7.4	52	2.3	5.2	2.1	1.4
Broccoli, Salmon & Watercress, Stay Full, Baxters*	1 Can/400g	244	8.8	61	3.3	5.8	2.2	2.4
Broccoli, Spinach & Pea, Super, M&S*	1 Serving/300g	102	3.9	34	2.1	2.7	1.3	1.6
Broccoli, with Kale, & Watercress, Naked Locals*	½ Pack/250ml	130	6.8	52	1.7	3.9	2.7	2.8
Brown Rice Miso, with Mushroom, Kale, & Tamari, Tideford*	1 Pot/600g	216	4.8	36	1.7	4.9	0.8	0.7
Butternut Squash, & Chilli, Sainsbury's*	½ Pot/300g	112	7.2	37	0.7	3.1	2.4	0.2
Butternut Squash, & Lentil, Curried, Seeds of Change*	1 Pack/400g	164	1.2	41	2.3	7.2	0.3	1.9
Butternut Squash, & Red Pepper, Canned, Sainsbury's*	½ Can/195g	99	4.3	51	1	6.6	2.2	3.6
Butternut Squash, & Red Pepper, Vegetarian, Baxters*	1 Can/415g	149	2.5	36	0.9	6.6	0.6	0.5
Butternut Squash, & Sage, New Covent Garden Food Co*	½ Carton/300g	153	6.9	51	0.9	6.6	2.3	0.7
Butternut Squash, & Tarragon, Waitrose*	½ Pot/300g	123	6.6	41	0.8	4.5	2.2	1
Butternut Squash, & Chickpea, Spiced, Heinz*	½ Can/200g	69	1	35	1.1	6.3	0.5	1.2
Butternut Squash, Fresh, Waitrose*	½ Pot/300g	153	8.7	51	0.5	5.8	2.9	0.8
Butternut Squash, M&S*	1 Serving/400g	132	3.2	33	0.6	5.3	0.8	1
Butternut Squash, New England, Skinnylicious, Glorious!*	½ Pot/300g	87	2.1	29	0.5	4.5	0.7	1.4
Butternut Squash, Soupreme, Aldi*	½ Pot/300g	60	3.3	20	0.5	1.5	1.1	1.5
Butternut Squash, Tesco*	½ Pot/300g	82	4.3	27	0.4	2.5	1.4	1.5
Carrot, & Butter Bean, Vegetarian, Baxters*	1 Can/415g	237	7.9	57	1.5	7.2	1.9	2.2
Carrot, & Coriander, Average	**1 Can/400g**	**167**	**8.6**	**42**	**0.6**	**4.8**	**2.2**	**1**
Carrot, & Coriander, Blended, Heinz*	½ Can/200g	104	5.4	52	0.7	6.2	2.7	0.6
Carrot, & Coriander, Canned, BGTY, Sainsbury's*	½ Can/200g	62	2	31	0.8	4.8	1	0.9
Carrot, & Coriander, Canned, M&S*	½ Can/210g	94	5	45	0.4	5.9	2.4	0.9
Carrot, & Coriander, Canned, Tesco*	1 Can/400g	220	11.6	55	0.7	5.7	2.9	0.8
Carrot, & Coriander, Classic Homestyle, M&S*	1 Can/425g	170	8.5	40	0.6	5.6	2	0.7
Carrot, & Coriander, Classic, Classic, Heinz*	1 Can/400g	164	6.4	41	0.4	5.8	1.6	0.9
Carrot, & Coriander, Fresh, New Covent Garden Food Co*	½ Carton/300g	129	6	43	0.5	5.2	2	1.1
Carrot, & Coriander, Fresh, Organic, Simply Organic*	1 Pot/600g	276	18	46	0.5	4.5	3	1.3
Carrot, & Coriander, Fresh, Tesco*	½ Pot /300g	99	4.8	33	0.6	2.9	1.6	2.2
Carrot, & Ginger, Fresh, Sainsbury's*	1 Pot/600g	150	5.4	25	0.4	3.9	0.9	1
Carrot, & Lentil, Weight Watchers*	1 Can/295g	87	0.3	29	1.3	5.5	0.1	0.7
Carrot, & Parsnip, Chantenay, Fresh, Extra Special, Asda*	½ Pot/300g	153	8.4	51	1.2	4.8	2.8	0.8
Carrot, & Coconut, Thai, Fragrant, Soup of the Day, Heinz*	½ Carton/200g	104	5.6	52	0.9	5.5	2.8	1.8
Carrot, & Coriander, Fresh, Asda*	½ Pot/300g	117	7.5	39	0.5	3.1	2.5	1.2
Carrot, & Lentil, Farmers Market, Heinz*	1 Serving/200g	84	0.3	42	1.7	7.8	0.2	0.9
Carrot, Butternut, & Ginger, Bol*	1 Pack/500g	175	8	35	0.5	3.8	1.6	1.4
Carrot, Red Lentil & Cumin, Organic, Waitrose*	1 Pack/350g	175	8.8	50	0.2	6.7	2.5	0.5
Carrot, Thai, Skinny, Aldi*	½ Pot/300g	90	4.8	30	0.5	3.3	1.6	0.6
Cauliflower, & Celeriac, Love Life, Waitrose*	1 Pot/350g	79	3.1	23	1.6	1.4	0.9	1.3
Cauliflower, Chicken, & Turmeric, Waitrose*	1 Pot/400g	221	7.6	55	3	5.8	1.9	1.4
Cauliflower, Chickpea, & Turmeric, Indian, Glorious!*	½ Pot/300g	114	2.4	38	2	4.4	0.8	2.7
Cauliflower, Gail's*	100g	85	6.1	85	2.3	4.7	6.1	1.2
Cauliflower, Onion, & Potato, Soup of the Day, Heinz*	½ Carton/200g	76	3.2	38	1.4	4.4	1.6	1
Celeriac, Velvety, Waitrose*	½ Pot/300g	151	11.5	50	0.8	2.8	3.8	0.9
Chicken Noodle, Canned, Sainsbury's*	½ Can/217g	78	0.7	36	1.7	7.4	0.3	0.7
Chicken Noodle, Classic, Heinz*	1 Can/400g	124	1.2	31	1.2	6	0.3	0.2
Chicken Noodle, Clear, Weight Watchers*	1 Can/295g	51	0.6	17	0.8	3.1	0.2	0.2
Chicken Noodle, Cup Soup, Dry, Heinz*	1 Sachet/20g	48	0.5	240	8	46	2.5	1.5
Chicken Noodle, Cup Soup, Made Up, Heinz*	1 Serving/218ml	48	0.4	22	0.7	4.3	0.2	0.1
Chicken Noodle, Dry, Nissin*	1 Pack/85g	364	14.1	428	9.5	62	16.6	3.3
Chicken Noodle, Fresh, CBY, Asda*	½ Pot/297g	98	1.2	33	2.5	4.3	0.4	0.9
Chicken Noodle, In a Cup, BGTY, Sainsbury's*	1 Sachet/219ml	59	1.1	27	1.7	4.9	0.5	0.5
Chicken Noodle, in a Cup, You Count, Love Life, Waitrose*	1 Cup/205ml	43	0.2	21	0.7	4.5	0.1	0.1
Chicken Noodle, Soup in a Cup, Made Up, Sainsbury's*	1 Serving/200ml	44	0.2	22	0.7	4.7	0.1	0.2

S

SOUP

	Measure INFO/WEIGHT	per Measure KCAL	FAT	Nutrition Values per 100g / 100ml KCAL	PROT	CARB	FAT	FIBRE
Chicken Noodle, Super Good, Baxters*	1 Can/400g	200	5.2	50	3.1	6.6	1.3	0.5
Chicken Noodle, Super, Dry, Knorr*	1 Pack/56g	182	2.7	325	14.3	56	4.9	1.8
Chicken Noodle, Teriyaki, Musclefood*	1 Serving/400g	140	6.8	35	4.6	0.2	1.7	0.1
Chicken Noodle, Thai Green, Yorkshire Provender*	½ Pot/300g	159	6	53	2.9	5.6	2	0
Chicken Noodle, with Sweetcorn, Canned, M&S*	1 Can/400g	184	3.2	46	2.8	6.8	0.8	0.4
Chicken, & Bean, Mexican Spiced, Eat Smart, Morrisons*	1 Can/400g	200	2	50	2.9	7.3	0.5	1.9
Chicken, & Black Eyed Pea, Gumbo, Hearty, Baxters*	1 Can/400g	184	2	46	2.6	6.7	0.5	1.5
Chicken, & Chorizo, New Covent Garden Food Co*	½ Carton/300g	132	4.5	44	1.9	5.3	1.5	0.9
Chicken, & Leek, Cup a Soup, Made Up, Batchelors*	1 Serving/259g	96	4.7	37	0.5	4.7	1.8	0.7
Chicken, & Lentil, Spinach, & Cumin, Yorkshire Provender*	½ Pot/300g	117	4.2	39	3.9	5.2	1.4	0.4
Chicken, & Multigrain, Finest, Tesco*	½ Pot/298g	125	3.6	42	3.2	3.9	1.2	1.3
Chicken, & Mushroom, Grain Soup , Sainsbury's*	1 Pot/600g	332	14.5	55	3.8	4.4	2.4	0.5
Chicken, & Orzo, Tuscan, Glorious!*	½ Pot/300g	120	1.2	40	2.8	6.2	0.4	0.7
Chicken, & Sweetcorn, Canned, HL, Tesco*	½ Can/200g	74	0.6	37	1.7	6.3	0.3	1.2
Chicken, & Sweetcorn, Cup Soup, Asda*	1 Sachet/200ml	109	3.9	54	0.7	8.5	2	0.3
Chicken, & Sweetcorn, Fresh, Average	*1 Serving/300g*	*146*	*3.1*	*48*	*2.4*	*7.3*	*1*	*0.6*
Chicken, & Vegetable Broth, Fresh, M Kitchen, Morrisons*	½ Pot/298g	131	4.5	44	2.8	4	1.5	1.6
Chicken, & Vegetable, Big Soup, Heinz*	½ Can/200g	110	2.4	55	3.3	7.2	1.2	0.8
Chicken, & Vegetable, Canned, Average	*1 Can/400g*	*192*	*8.5*	*48*	*2.5*	*4.6*	*2.1*	*0.8*
Chicken, & Vegetable, Chunky, Canned, Soupreme, Aldi*	1 Can/400g	184	2.4	46	3	6.4	0.6	1.3
Chicken, & Vegetable, Chunky, Meal Soup, Tesco*	1 Can/400g	184	7.2	46	2.5	4.6	1.8	1
Chicken, & Vegetable, Fresh, Tesco*	½ Pack/300g	118	3.3	39	3.6	3.2	1.1	1.1
Chicken, & Vegetable, Healthy, Baxters*	1 Can/415g	170	2.1	41	1.9	6.3	0.5	1.8
Chicken, & Vegetable, Mighty, Asda*	1 Can/410g	176	5.3	43	2.5	6.8	1.3	0.7
Chicken, & Vegetable, Moroccan, Love Life, Waitrose*	½ Pot/300g	192	5.7	64	3.7	7.9	1.9	1.9
Chicken, & Vegetable, with Pasta, Select, Campbell's*	1 Can/480ml	220	1	46	2.9	7.9	0.2	0.8
Chicken, & Barley, Broth, Heinz*	1 Can/400g	128	1.2	32	1.3	5.9	0.3	0.8
Chicken, & Chorizo, Smoky, Waitrose*	½ Pot/300g	123	4.2	41	2.5	3.9	1.4	1.2
Chicken, & Chorizo, Spanish, Extra Special, Asda*	½ Pot/300ml	150	7.5	50	2.5	4.2	2.5	0.5
Chicken, & Spelt, Broth, Deluxe, Lidl*	½ Pot/300g	141	3.3	47	3	5.6	1.1	1.5
Chicken, & Sweetcorn, Musclefood*	1 Serving/400g	176	5.2	44	4.5	3.8	1.3	0.3
Chicken, & Vegetable, Chunky, Canned, Asda*	½ Can/200g	90	2	45	4.3	4.3	1	0.8
Chicken, & Vegetable, Chunky, Morrisons*	1 Can/400g	184	4.4	46	3.8	4.8	1.1	1
Chicken, & Vegetable, Creamy, Sainsbury's*	1 Pot/400g	220	7.6	55	1.7	6.6	1.9	2.1
Chicken, & Vegetable, Meal Soup, Sainsbury's*	1 Pot/400g	268	9.6	67	3.8	7	2.4	1.3
Chicken, & Vegetable, Slimming World*	1 Carton/500g	170	2	34	3.7	3.3	0.4	1.1
Chicken, Balti, Meal, Sainsbury's*	1 Pack/400g	242	7.1	61	3.9	6.3	1.8	1.8
Chicken, Broth, Favourites, Baxters*	1 Can/400g	140	1.2	35	1.7	5.9	0.3	1
Chicken, Chardonnay Wine & Tarragon, Finest, Tesco*	½ Pot/300g	171	9.6	57	3.1	3.7	3.2	0.3
Chicken, Chorizo, & Rice, M&S*	½ Pot/300g	162	5.7	54	2.7	6.3	1.9	0.6
Chicken, Classic, New Covent Garden*	½ Carton/300g	204	7.5	68	1.9	9.3	2.5	0.2
Chicken, Courgette & Orzo Pasta, Meal Soup, Glorious!*	½ Pot/300g	141	4.2	47	3.5	5.1	1.4	0.8
Chicken, Cream Of, Bramwells, Aldi*	1 Can/400g	208	12	52	1.5	4.7	3	0.5
Chicken, Cream of, Canned, Tesco*	1 Can/400g	192	12	48	2.5	2.8	3	0.1
Chicken, Cream Of, No Added Sugar, Heinz*	½ Can/200g	106	6	53	1.6	4.9	3	0.1
Chicken, Cream of, Reduced Salt, Heinz*	1 Can/400g	216	12	54	1.7	4.9	3	0.1
Chicken, Cream of, Soupreme, Aldi*	1 Can/400g	228	15.2	57	1.8	3.8	3.8	0.4
Chicken, Golden, Instant, Vifon*	1 Pack/70g	50	2.3	72	1.3	9.1	3.3	0
Chicken, Green Thai, Spiced, M&S*	½ Pot/300g	195	11.4	65	2	6.3	3.8	0.6
Chicken, Green Thai, Waitrose*	1 Pot/600g	462	30	77	4.4	3.5	5	1.6
Chicken, Hotpot, Chunky, Big Soup, Heinz*	½ Can/258g	126	3.1	49	2.3	7.4	1.2	0.8
Chicken, Jamaican Jerk, TTD, Sainsbury's*	½ Carton/300g	198	5.1	66	3.9	7.6	1.7	2.6
Chicken, Katsu, Naked, Hearty, Sainsbury's*	1 Pot/397g	258	11.9	65	2.1	6.5	3	1.6

SOUP

INFO/WEIGHT	Measure	per Measure KCAL	FAT	Nutrition Values per 100g / 100ml KCAL	PROT	CARB	FAT	FIBRE
Chicken, Keralan, Sainsburys*	½ Carton/300g	252	15.3	84	3.5	5.5	5.1	1.1
Chicken, Miso, Noodle, Waitrose*	1 Pot/400g	268	8.8	67	5.9	5.9	2.2	0.9
Chicken, Moroccan Inspired, Love Life, Waitrose*	½ Pot/300g	136	2.4	45	2.7	6.1	0.8	1.4
Chicken, Moroccan, Finest, Tesco*	½ Pot/300g	201	5.1	67	4.2	8.1	1.7	1.2
Chicken, Moroccan, Harira, Hearty, Baxters*	1 Can/400g	236	2.8	59	3.2	9.5	0.7	1.9
Chicken, Mulligatawny, Finest, Tesco*	½ Pot/300g	237	9.9	79	5	6.7	3.3	1
Chicken, Multigrain, Hearty, Waitrose*	½ Pot/300g	141	3	47	3.6	4.9	1	2.1
Chicken, Mushroom & Rice, M&S*	1 Pack/350g	206	7.7	59	2.7	6.6	2.2	0.9
Chicken, Mushroom, & Potato, Big Soup, Heinz*	½ Can/200g	132	4.6	66	3.4	8.1	2.3	0.4
Chicken, Peri Peri, Asda*	½ Can/197g	77	1.8	39	1.8	5.5	0.9	0.6
Chicken, Potato & Bacon, Big Soup, Heinz*	1 Can/515g	294	11.3	57	3	6.1	2.2	0.5
Chicken, Potato & Leek, Weight Watchers*	1 Can/295g	97	2.4	33	1.1	5.1	0.8	0.3
Chicken, Potato, & Bacon, Chunky, Tesco*	½ Can/200g	100	2.6	50	3.6	5.7	1.3	0.7
Chicken, Spicy Thai, Nupo*	1 Serving/32g	114	2.4	356	38	39	7.6	9.3
Chicken, Thai Style, Canned, Soupreme, Aldi*	1 Can/400g	200	10.8	50	2.5	3.8	2.7	1.1
Chicken, Thai Style, Thick & Creamy, in a Mug, Tesco*	1 Sachet/28g	107	4	390	3.7	61.3	14.5	5.1
Chicken, Thai, Fresh, Finest, Tesco*	½ Tub/300g	176	9.9	59	3.2	3.4	3.3	1.3
Chicken, Tomato & Red Pepper, Italian, Big Soup, Heinz*	½ Can/200g	78	1.8	39	1.6	6.2	0.9	0.7
Chicken, Tomato, & Grains, Tuscan, Glorious!*	½ Pack/300g	111	2.1	37	2	4.9	0.7	1.5
Chicken, Weight Watchers*	1 Can/295g	97	3	33	1.6	4.4	1	0
Chilli, Tomato, & Pasta, COU, M&S*	1 Serving/300g	150	5.7	50	1.3	7.2	1.9	0.9
Chilli, Vegan, New Covent Garden Food Co*	½ Carton/300g	121	0.9	40	2	6.7	0.3	1.5
Chorizo, & Butter Bean, Chunky, Sainsbury's*	½ Can/200g	150	5.6	75	3.4	7.8	2.8	2.7
Chowder, Corn, Spicy, New Covent Garden Food Co*	½ Carton/300g	132	5.4	44	1.6	4.3	1.8	2.2
Chowder, Ham & Sweetcorn, Diet Chef Ltd*	1 Pack/300g	165	3.6	55	1.9	9.2	1.2	0.9
Chowder, Seafood, Waitrose*	1 Can/404g	226	11.3	56	2.2	5.6	2.8	0.6
Chowder, Smoked Haddock & Salmon, Cully & Sully*	1 Pack/400g	232	9.2	58	2.6	6.2	2.3	0.9
Chowder, Sweetcorn, Microwaved, Slimming World*	1 Pot/500g	160	2.5	32	1.1	5.3	0.5	0.7
Cock-A-Leekie, Favourites, Baxters*	1 Can/400g	116	2.4	29	1.1	4.7	0.6	0.3
Coconut, Corn, & Sweet Potato, Creamy, Bol*	1 Pot/500g	280	6	56	1.7	7.8	1.2	3.5
Coconut, Lime, & Chilli, Glorious!*	½ Tub/300g	168	2.4	56	3.4	6.7	0.8	4.1
Country Garden, Canned, Vegetarian, Baxters*	1 Can/400g	144	2	36	1	6.2	0.5	1
Country Vegetable, Chunky, Canned, Sainsbury's*	1 Can/400g	152	2.4	38	1	6.5	0.6	1.2
Courgette, & Parmesan, Fresh, Sainsbury's*	1 Pack/300ml	198	16.8	66	1.5	2.5	5.6	0.4
Cucumber, Gazpacho, Innocent*	1 Bowl/200ml	70	3.6	35	0.7	3	1.8	2.1
Daal, Lentil, Bangalore, Glorious!*	1 Pot/600g	294	8.4	49	2	6.1	1.4	2.2
Dahl, Indian Spiced, Asda*	½ Pot/300g	138	3	46	2.2	5.8	1	2.6
Dahl, Lentil, Bangalore, Sainsbury's*	1 Serving/300g	117	2.7	39	1.7	4.7	0.9	2.3
Fish, Bouillabaise, Bistro, M&S*	1 Pack/820g	2665	18	325	10	4.3	2.2	1.3
Game, Royal, Favourites, Baxters*	1 Can/400g	152	0.8	38	1.8	6.9	0.2	0.3
Garden Vegetable, Fresh, Tesco*	½ Pot/300g	117	0.6	39	1.4	7.2	0.2	1.4
Golden Vegetable, Cup-A-Soup, Made Up, Golden Wonder	1 Sachet/215ml	68	1.7	32	0.4	5.5	0.8	0.5
Golden Vegetable, Made Up, Cup a Soup, Batchelors*	1 Sachet/250ml	80	2.3	32	0.3	5.5	0.9	0.4
Green Vegetable, & Kale, British, Crosse & Blackwell*	1 Can/394g	130	1.2	33	1.6	5.1	0.3	1.8
Haddock, Smoked, Chowder, M&S*	½ Pot/300g	141	6.6	47	2.1	4.3	2.2	0.6
Ham Hock, & Vegetable, Broth, Crosse & Blackwell*	1 Can/400g	158	2	40	2.7	5.7	0.5	0.8
Ham Hock, Leek & Potato, Chunky, Soup Pot, Tesco*	1 Pot/350g	174	6.3	50	2.5	5.5	1.8	1
Highlander's Broth, Favourites, Baxters*	1 Can/400g	192	5.6	48	1.7	6.3	1.4	0.9
Hot & Sour	*1 Serving/233g*	*90*	*2.8*	*39*	*2.6*	*4.3*	*1.2*	*0.5*
Kotosoupa, with Noodles, Greek, Knorr*	½ Pack/505ml	106	2.5	21	0.8	4.2	0.5	0.5
Lamb, & Vegetable, Big Soup, Heinz*	½ Can/200g	120	2.6	60	3	9.1	1.3	1.3
Lamb, Minted, Hot Pot, Big Soup, Heinz*	1 Can/500g	295	6.5	59	2.8	8.5	1.3	1
Leek, & Chicken, Knorr*	1 Serving/300ml	82	5.2	27	0.6	2.4	1.7	0.1

SOUP

Measure INFO/WEIGHT		per Measure		Nutrition Values per 100g / 100ml				
		KCAL	FAT	KCAL	PROT	CARB	FAT	FIBRE
Leek, & Maris Piper Potato, Chilled, M&S*	1 Serving/300g	165	11.4	55	0.6	4.5	3.8	0.9
Leek, & Potato	*1oz/28g*	*15*	*0.7*	*52*	*1.5*	*6.2*	*2.6*	*0.8*
Leek, & Potato, Canned, Asda*	1 Can/400g	160	3.6	40	0.9	6.5	0.9	1
Leek, & Potato, Canned, Sainsbury's*	½ Can/200g	92	3.2	46	1	6.7	1.6	0.3
Leek, & Potato, Classics, Canned, Heinz*	1 Can/400g	184	7.2	46	0.8	6.7	1.8	0.6
Leek, & Potato, Cup a Soup, Batchelors*	1 Sachet/28g	115	4.9	411	7.5	53.9	17.5	3.6
Leek, & Potato, Favourites, Baxters*	1 Can/400g	192	7.2	48	1	6.6	1.8	0.9
Leek, & Potato, Fresh with Cream, Tesco*	½ Tub/300g	146	8.4	49	0.7	4.6	2.8	1.2
Leek, & Potato, Fresh, Sainsbury's*	½ Pot/300ml	141	7.2	47	1	5.3	2.4	0.4
Leek, & Potato, Fresh, Waitrose*	½ Pot/300g	108	5.1	36	0.7	4.6	1.7	0.9
Leek, & Potato, Soup in a Mug, HL, Tesco*	1 Serving/16g	54	0.9	336	4.3	67.1	5.6	7.4
Leek, & Potato, Fresh, Soupreme, Aldi*	½ Pot/300g	192	11.1	64	0.8	6.4	3.7	0.8
Lentil & Vegetable, Vegan, Gail's*	100g	91	3.2	91	2.1	12	3.2	1.9
Lentil, & Bacon, Canned, Sainsbury's*	½ Can/200g	102	1.4	51	4.1	6.6	0.7	1
Lentil, & Bacon, Canned, Tesco*	1 Serving/200g	96	1.4	48	3.2	7.2	0.7	0.5
Lentil, & Bacon, Chunky, Canned, M&S*	1 Can/400g	204	2.4	51	3.3	7.2	0.6	1.8
Lentil, & Bacon, Classic, Heinz*	1 Can/400g	232	5.6	58	2.7	8.4	1.4	0.7
Lentil, & Bacon, Favourites, Baxters*	1 Can/400g	208	2.8	52	3.4	7.3	0.7	0.8
Lentil, & Barley, Superbean, M&S*	1 Pack /600g	270	9	45	1.8	5.1	1.5	2.1
Lentil, & Chick Pea, Fresh, Organic, Tesco*	1 Serving/300ml	117	2.4	39	1.9	6.1	0.8	0.5
Lentil, & Ham, Red, Waitrose*	½ Pot/300g	147	3.3	49	3.9	5.8	1.1	2
Lentil, & Smoked Bacon, Fresh, Tesco*	1 Pack/600g	420	11.4	70	3.9	8.5	1.9	1.6
Lentil, & Tomato, New Covent Garden Food Co*	½ Carton/300g	171	3.3	57	3.6	8.1	1.1	0.7
Lentil, & Tomato, Spicy, Chunky, Fresh, Tesco*	½ Pot/300g	195	5.4	65	2.6	9.7	1.8	1.3
Lentil, & Vegetable Soup, Healthy, Baxters*	1 Can/415g	174	1.2	42	1.9	7.4	0.3	1.2
Lentil, & Vegetable, LC, Tesco*	1 Can/400g	188	0.8	47	2.5	8.8	0.2	1.1
Lentil, & Vegetable, Spicy, Chilled, M&S*	½ Serving/300g	150	2.4	50	2.7	8	0.8	1.1
Lentil, & Bacon, Smoked, New Covent Garden Food Co*	1 Carton/600g	306	6	51	3.7	8.9	1	4.3
Lentil, & Vegetable, Spiced, Protein Boosting, Bol*	1 Serving/500g	200	3	40	3.3	7.2	0.6	3.8
Lentil, & Vegetable, Vegetarian, Baxters*	½ Can/200g	86	0.6	43	2.1	7.4	0.3	1.3
Lentil, Asda*	½ Can/202g	89	0.4	44	2.6	8	0.2	0.7
Lentil, Bacon & Mixed Bean, Low Fat, Aldi*	1 Serving/400g	260	3.6	65	4.7	9.5	0.9	1.6
Lentil, Classic, Heinz*	1 Can/400g	180	0.8	45	2.4	8.5	0.2	0.8
Lentil, Dahl, Co-Op*	1 Pot/600g	228	9	38	1.1	4.5	1.5	0.8
Lentil, Red, with Carrots, Potato & Onion, Asda*	1 Can/400g	192	0.8	48	1.4	10.2	0.2	1.2
Lentil, Scotty Brand*	1 Pot/550g	374	1.6	68	3.9	10.4	0.3	3.8
Lentil, Spiced, High Protein, Cup a Soup, Batchelors*	1 Pack/255g	97	1.5	38	1.9	6	0.6	0.5
Lentil, Spicy, M&S*	1 Serving/100g	50	1.1	50	2.6	6.3	1.1	2.1
Lobster, Bisque, Waitrose*	½ Carton/300g	201	13.8	67	0.9	5.5	4.6	0.6
Lobster, Bisque, with Brandy & Fresh Cream, Baxters*	½ Can/200g	150	8.6	75	3.3	4.2	4.3	0.2
Massaman, Sweet Potato, Thai, Street Food, Glorious!*	1 Pot/400g	220	8.8	55	1.3	7	2.2	1.3
Minestrone, Canned, Average	*1 Can/400g*	*252*	*12*	*63*	*1.8*	*7.6*	*3*	*0.9*
Minestrone, Chunky, Fresh, Sainsbury's*	½ Pot/300g	93	0.6	31	1.4	6.1	0.2	2.3
Minestrone, Chunky, Love Life, Waitrose*	1 Can/400g	166	0.4	42	1.3	8.7	0.1	1.9
Minestrone, Classic, Heinz*	1 Can/400g	128	0.8	32	1	6.2	0.2	0.8
Minestrone, Diet Chef Ltd*	1 Pack/300g	123	1.8	41	1.4	7.5	0.6	1.2
Minestrone, Favourites, Baxters*	1 Can/400g	168	2.4	42	1.6	7	0.6	1.2
Minestrone, Fresh, Asda*	½ Pot/300g	138	2.1	46	1.8	8.2	0.7	1.2
Minestrone, Fresh, Average	*1 Carton/600g*	*244*	*4.9*	*41*	*1.7*	*6.8*	*0.8*	*1.2*
Minestrone, Fresh, Co-Op*	1 Pot/600g	260	8.4	43	1	6.2	1.4	1.3
Minestrone, Fresh, Morrisons*	½ Pot/300g	147	3	49	1.6	7.6	1	1.6
Minestrone, Fresh, Tesco*	½ Carton/300g	132	3	44	1.8	6.3	1	1.4
Minestrone, Fresh, Waitrose*	1 Pack/600g	240	8.4	40	1.1	5.8	1.4	0.8

S

SOUP

INFO/WEIGHT	Measure	per Measure KCAL	FAT	Nutrition Values per 100g / 100ml KCAL	PROT	CARB	FAT	FIBRE
Minestrone, Loved by Us, Co-Op*	½ Pot/300g	135	4.2	45	1	6.2	1.4	1.3
Minestrone, Pack, Dry, Knorr*	1 Pack/61g	204	2.4	335	12	58.8	4	6.9
Minestrone, Parsley Box*	1 Pack/300g	126	2.4	42	1.6	7	0.8	0.6
Minestrone, Sainsbury's*	½ Can/200g	66	0.8	33	1.1	6.3	0.4	0.9
Minestrone, Slimming World*	½ Pot/250g	90	0.5	36	1.7	5.9	0.2	2.1
Minestrone, Soupreme, Aldi*	½ Pot/300g	162	2.7	54	1.9	8.5	0.9	2.2
Minestrone, with Croutons in a Cup, Sainsbury's*	1 Sachet/225ml	72	0.9	32	0.9	6.3	0.4	0.5
Minestrone, with Croutons in a Mug, Tesco*	1 Sachet/23g	83	1.9	360	9	62.6	8.1	2.7
Minestrone, with Croutons, Dry, Soupreme, Aldi*	1 Serving/27g	94	1.7	349	7.6	65.3	6.4	4.4
Minestrone, with GF Pasta, Tideford*	1 Pot/600g	180	4.8	30	1.3	3.9	0.8	1.4
Minestrone, with Pasta, Chunky, Co-Op*	1 Pack/400g	140	2.4	35	1	6	0.6	0.7
Miso, Barley, Mugi, Miso Tasty*	1 Sachet/20g	45	1.5	223	8.7	26	7.4	5.1
Miso, Japanese, Made Up, Yutaka*	1 Serving/250ml	24	0.7	10	0.6	1.1	0.3	0
Miso, Paste, Wakame, Sachets, Yutaka*	1 Sachet/18g	18	0.6	100	7.1	16	3.6	0
Miso, Wakama*	1 Sachet/8g	27	0.6	336	18.7	48.6	7.6	0
Miso, with Tofu, Instant, Kikkoman*	1 Sachet/10g	35	1	350	30	30	10	0
More Bangalore, Skinnylicious, Skinny Soup, Glorious!*	½ Pot/300g	147	4.2	49	2	6.1	1.4	2.2
Moroccan Bean, Very Special, Wattie's*	1 Serving/265g	176	0.8	66	3.2	11.4	0.3	2
Moroccan, Inspired, Pot, Tesco*	½ Pack/266g	146	2.4	55	1.9	8.9	0.9	1.9
Moroccan, with Vegan Pieces, Quorn*	½ Pot/283g	136	1.7	48	4.2	4.4	0.6	3.7
Mulligatawny	*1 Serving/220g*	*213*	*15*	*97*	*1.4*	*8.2*	*6.8*	*0.9*
Mulligatawny, Canned, Morrisons*	1 Can/400g	196	6.4	49	1.8	6.5	1.6	0.8
Mulligatawny, Canned, Tesco*	1 Can/400g	188	4	47	1.3	8.1	1	0.3
Mulligatawny, Classic, Heinz*	1 Can/400g	232	7.6	58	1.9	8	1.9	0.5
Mulligatawny, Slimming World*	1 Serving/200ml	82	0.6	41	2.3	6.5	0.3	1.6
Mushroom, & Chestnut, Fresh, Finest, Tesco*	1 Serving/250g	130	8.2	52	1.1	4.7	3.3	0.7
Mushroom, & Roasted Garlic, Soup of the Day, Heinz*	½ Carton/200g	75	3	38	0.8	5.5	1.5	0.4
Mushroom, Canned, HL, Tesco*	1 Can/400g	132	5.6	33	0.5	4.4	1.4	0.2
Mushroom, Cream of, Canned, Tesco*	½ Can/200g	94	5.8	47	0.7	4.8	2.9	0.2
Mushroom, Cream of, Classics, Heinz*	1 Can/400g	208	11.2	52	1.5	5.2	2.8	0.1
Mushroom, Cream of, Condensed, Batchelors*	1 Can/295g	330	25.1	112	1.3	7.5	8.5	0.2
Mushroom, Cream of, Fresh, Finest, Tesco*	½ Pot/300g	238	19	79	1.9	3.5	6.3	0.5
Mushroom, Cream Of, Tesco*	½ Can/200g	116	7.2	58	1.3	5	3.6	0.4
Mushroom, Diet Chef Ltd*	1 Pack/300g	105	5.1	35	1.9	3.2	1.7	0.9
Mushroom, for One, Heinz*	1 Can/290g	148	7.8	51	1.4	5.1	2.7	0.1
Mushroom, Fresh, Average	*1 Serving/300g*	*146*	*9.3*	*49*	*1.3*	*4*	*3.1*	*0.8*
Mushroom, Fresh, M&S*	½ Pack/300g	165	11.7	55	1.8	3.5	3.9	0.9
Mushroom, Fresh, The Best, Morrisons*	½ Pot/300g	177	14.1	59	0.8	3.1	4.7	0.6
Mushroom, Potage, Woodland Mushrooms, Baxters*	1 Can/415g	328	20.8	79	1.6	6.9	5	0.3
Mushroom, Risotto, Grain, Meal Soup, Sainsbury's*	1 Pack/400g	257	11.2	64	2	7	2.8	1.5
Mushroom, Three, Broth, Soupologie*	1 Serving/300g	48	0.6	16	0.7	2.4	0.2	0.7
Mushroom, Wild, & Tarragon, TTD, Sainsbury's*	½ Can/200g	109	6.1	54	1.3	5.3	3	0.5
Mushroom, Wild, New Covent Garden Food Co*	1 Carton/600g	162	8.4	27	1	1.9	1.4	1.5
Mushroom, with Croutons in a Cup, Waitrose*	1 Sachet/212g	102	4.2	48	0.6	6.8	2	0.5
Mushroom, with Croutons, Soup in a Mug, Tesco*	1 Serving/226ml	115	4.7	51	1	6.8	2.1	0.4
Noodle, Cantonese Hot & Sour, Baxters*	1 Serving/215g	133	2.8	62	1.4	11.1	1.3	0.5
Noodle, Cup, Shin, Nongshim*	1 Cup/75g	326	11.2	435	7	68	15	0
Noodle, Ramen, Instant, Nissin*	1 Pack/100g	87	3.7	87	2.1	10.8	3.7	0
Noodle, Sweet & Spicy, Cup Soup, Made Up, Tesco*	1 Sachet/220g	77	0.2	35	0.7	7.5	0.1	0.6
Onion, French	*1oz/28g*	*11*	*0.6*	*40*	*0.2*	*5.7*	*2.1*	*1*
Onion, French, & Cider, Waitrose*	1 Can/425g	94	0.4	22	0.5	4.8	0.1	0.4
Onion, French, & Gruyere Cheese, Fresh, Finest, Tesco*	½ Pot/300g	210	15.3	70	1.4	4.7	5.1	0.5
Onion, French, Chilled, M&S*	½ Pot/300g	150	4.5	50	2	7.2	1.5	1

SOUP

INFO/WEIGHT	Measure	per Measure		Nutrition Values per 100g / 100ml				
		KCAL	FAT	KCAL	PROT	CARB	FAT	FIBRE
Onion, French, Favourites, Baxters*	½ Can/200g	66	1.2	33	0.7	5.8	0.6	0.6
Oxtail, Average	*1 Can/400g*	*163*	*4.5*	*41*	*2*	*5.8*	*1.1*	*0.4*
Oxtail, Canned	*1 Serving/220g*	*97*	*3.7*	*44*	*2.4*	*5.1*	*1.7*	*0.1*
Oxtail, Classic, Heinz*	1 Can/400g	168	2	42	1.9	7.3	0.5	0.3
Oxtail, Favourites, Baxters*	1 Can/400g	152	2.8	38	1.9	5.7	0.7	0.5
Oxtail, For One, Heinz*	1 Can/300g	126	1.5	42	1.9	7.3	0.5	0.3
Oxtail, Soupreme, Aldi*	1 Can/400g	152	2	38	2.2	6	0.5	0.5
Pad Thai, Ramen, Made Up, Naked Noodle, Symingtons*	1 Pack/224g	83	0.2	37	1.1	7.2	0.1	0.3
Pancetta, Barley, & Kale, Finest, Tesco*	½ Pot/302g	148	5.4	49	2.6	4.4	1.8	2.6
Parsnip, & Honey, Festive, New Covent Garden Food Co*	½ Carton/350g	217	7	62	0.9	9.2	2	1.9
Parsnip, & Honey, Fresh, Sainsbury's*	½ Carton/300g	192	12.6	64	1.1	5.4	4.2	1.5
Parsnip, Pilaf, Warming, Super, Meal Soup, Glorious!*	½ Pot/300g	153	4.2	51	1.3	7	1.4	2.6
Parsnip, Silky, with Yorkshire Honey, Yorkshire Provender*	½ Pot/300g	132	5.1	44	0.9	5.4	1.7	1.8
Parsnip, Spicy, Aldi*	1 Serving/250g	132	8.5	53	0.6	4.9	3.4	1.4
Parsnip, Spicy, Average	*1 Serving/400g*	*212*	*11.2*	*53*	*0.9*	*6*	*2.8*	*1.6*
Parsnip, Spicy, Vegetarian, Baxters*	1 Can/425g	212	10.6	50	0.7	5.3	2.5	1.7
Pea, & Ham	*1 Serving/220g*	*154*	*4.6*	*70*	*4*	*9.2*	*2.1*	*1.4*
Pea, & Ham, Canned, Favourites, Baxters*	1 Can/400g	218	4	55	3.3	7.1	1	2
Pea, & Ham, Canned, Tesco*	1 Can/400g	184	2	46	3.1	6.1	0.5	2.1
Pea, & Ham, CBY, Asda*	1 Pot/600g	282	6.6	47	2.9	5.6	1.1	1.4
Pea, & Ham, Classic, Heinz*	1 Can/400g	252	3.2	63	2.8	10.1	0.8	1.1
Pea, & Ham, Diet Chef Ltd*	1 Pack/300g	138	3.3	46	3.2	5.8	1.1	2.6
Pea, & Ham, Fresh, Sainsbury's*	½ Pack/300ml	120	1.5	40	1.9	7	0.5	0.3
Pea, & Ham, Fresh, Waitrose*	1 Serving/300g	196	10	65	2.9	6.2	3.3	1.6
Pea, & Ham, Petit Pois, Fresh, TTD, Sainsbury's*	½ Pot/300g	201	7.8	67	3.8	6.1	2.6	2.2
Pea, & Ham, Split, Asda*	1 Serving/300g	129	0.6	43	3.5	6.9	0.2	0.7
Pea, & Mint, Best of British, Crosse & Blackwell*	1 Can/400g	192	8.4	48	1.7	4.6	2.1	1.9
Pea, & Mint, Canned, M&S*	½ Can/200g	96	4.2	48	1.7	4.6	2.1	1.9
Pea, & Mint, Fresh, Co-Op*	½ Tub/300g	105	1.7	35	1.7	4.8	0.6	1.8
Pea, & Mint, Fresh, Finest, Tesco*	1 Serving/300g	165	7.2	55	1.3	6	2.4	1.5
Pea, & Mint, Fresh, M&S*	1 Serving/164g	49	0.2	30	1.8	6.3	0.1	1.5
Pea, & Mint, Fresh, Sainsbury's*	½ Pot/300g	102	2.7	34	1.4	5	0.9	1.9
Pea, & Mint, Fresh, Tesco*	½ Pot/300g	145	3.3	48	2.4	6	1.1	2.4
Pea, & Mint, Garden, Vegetarian, Baxters*	½ Can/200g	100	1.6	50	2.5	7.3	0.8	1.9
Pea, & Mint, Slimming World, Iceland*	1 Tub/500g	205	2	41	2.5	5.6	0.4	2.7
Pea, & Mint, with Leek, Fresh, Waitrose*	1 Serving/300g	123	4.5	41	1.7	4.4	1.5	1.5
Pea, & Ham, Rustic, Newgate, Lidl*	1 Can/400g	204	2.8	51	3	6.8	0.7	2.6
Pea, & Mint, Cup, Waitrose*	1 Cup/215ml	103	2.2	48	1.1	8.3	1	0.5
Pea, Hearty, & Wiltshire Cured Ham Hock, Waitrose*	½ Carton/300g	165	4.2	55	3.1	6.6	1.4	1.8
Pea, Split, Yellow, Simply Organic*	1 Pot/600g	354	3	59	4.3	10.4	0.5	2.6
Pepper, & Chorizo, Canned, Sainsbury's*	1 Can/400ml	172	4	43	2	1		0
Pepper, with Chilli, Italiamo, Lidl*	1 Can/390ml	222	9.4	57	0.6	7.6	2.4	1.3
Prawn, King, & Glass Noodles, Pho, pot	*1 Pot/642g*	*212*	*2.6*	*33*	*1.8*	*5.4*	*0.4*	*0.5*
Prawn, Tom Yum, Cook*	1 Portion/335g	231	3	69	3.5	10.8	0.9	0
Pumpkin, & Chestnut, Cream of, Organic, Bio, La Potagere*	1 Pack/300ml	114	3.3	38	0.8	5.5	1.1	1.5
Pumpkin, & Ginger, New Covent Garden Food Co*	½ Carton/300g	129	4.8	43	0.7	5.7	1.6	1.5
Pumpkin, Creamy, Very Special, Heinz*	1 Sm Can/290g	188	5.5	65	1.3	9.9	1.9	1.1
Pumpkin, Spiced, Spooky, New Covent Garden Food Co*	½ Carton/350g	168	5.2	48	1.8	6	1.5	1.6
Pumpkin, Spicy, Fresh, Sainsbury's*	½ Pot/300g	87	3	29	0.9	4.2	1	1.3
Pumpkin, Sweet Potato & Red Pepper, SO, Sainsbury's*	½ Pot/300g	111	3.9	37	0.8	5.6	1.3	0.8
Red Pepper, & Wensleydale, Asda*	1 Carton /600g	306	12.6	51	2.5	5	2.1	0.8
Red Pepper, Roasted, & Tomato, Canned, Sainsbury's*	1 Can/400g	196	6	49	1	7.5	1.5	0.9
Red Pepper, Roasted, & Tomato, M&S*	1 Serving/150g	105	7.4	70	1.4	5	4.9	0.6

S

SOUP

INFO/WEIGHT	Measure	per Measure KCAL	FAT	Nutrition Values per 100g / 100ml KCAL	PROT	CARB	FAT	FIBRE
Red Pepper, Roasted, Fresh, Waitrose*	1 Pack/600g	172	9	29	0.8	3	1.5	1
Scotch Broth, Canned, Tesco*	½ Can/200g	85	2.6	42	1.3	5.9	1.3	0.8
Scotch Broth, Classic, Heinz*	1 Can/400g	156	2.4	39	1.4	6.7	0.6	0.6
Scotch Broth, Favourites, Baxters*	1 Can/400g	168	4	42	1.8	6.8	1	1.4
Scotch Broth, Scotty Brand*	½ Pot/275g	72	0.8	26	1.1	5.8	0.3	2.2
Seafood Chowder, Canned, TTD, Sainsbury's*	½ Can/200g	114	5.6	57	1.9	5.9	2.8	0.5
Spinach, & Green Lentil, Spiced, Asda*	½ Pot/250g	122	5	49	2.7	5	2	0
Spinach, & Watercress, New Covent Garden Food Co*	½ Carton/300g	60	1.2	20	1.3	2.8	0.4	0.8
Spinach, Creme Fraiche, & Nutmeg, Organic, Waitrose*	½ Pot/300g	243	22.8	81	0.9	2.3	7.6	1.1
Steak, & Potato, Angus, Big Soup, Heinz*	½ Can/250g	120	2	48	3.1	6.8	0.8	0.6
Steak, & Ale, Chunky, Asda*	1 Can/400g	188	4.4	47	3	5.9	1.1	0.6
Stilton, Celery & Watercress, Morrisons*	1 Serving/250g	272	23	109	3.9	3.1	9.2	0.3
Super Grain, Brazilian, Glorious!*	½ Pot/300g	163	4.2	54	2.6	6.6	1.4	2.3
Sweet Potato, & Cauliflower, Super Soup, Bol*	½ Pot/250g	142	3.2	57	3.4	10	1.3	3.9
Sweet Potato, & Lentil, Dahl, Yorkshire Provender*	1 Pot/600g	330	16.2	55	2.6	6.9	2.7	0
Sweet Potato, & Red Chilli, Asda*	½ Pot/300g	144	5.4	48	0.5	7.1	1.8	0.8
Sweet Potato, & Split Pea, Curry, Hearty, Bowl, Sainsbury's*	1 Bowl/400g	316	7.6	79	3.4	10.4	1.9	3.2
Sweet Potato, Coconut & Chilli, TTD, Sainsbury's*	½ Pot/300g	176	5.7	59	0.9	8.5	1.9	1.8
Sweet Potato, Coconut, & Chilli, Finest, Tesco*	½ Pot/300g	216	13.5	72	1.1	6.5	4.5	0.6
Sweet Potato, with Coconut, & Coriander, Soulful Food Co*	½ Pot/300g	159	9	53	1	6.4	3	1.6
Sweetcorn, & Yellow Pepper, Blended, Heinz*	½ Can/200g	98	4.2	49	0.9	6.6	2.1	0.6
Texan BBQ Bean, & Corn, Hearty, Bowl, Sainsbury's*	1 Pack/400g	300	8	75	2.9	9.4	2	3.7
Thai Chicken, & Lemongrass, Cup Soup, Ainsley Harriott*	1 Sachet/224g	101	3.4	45	0.6	7.3	1.5	0.1
Thai Green, Vegetable, Naked, Hearty, Sainsbury's*	1 Pot/400g	256	10.8	64	0.8	8.3	2.7	1.6
The Big Broth, Yorkshire Provender*	½ Pot/300g	159	6	53	2.9	5.6	2	0
Tomato, & Balsamic, Sicilian, Skinny Soup, Glorious!*	1 Carton/600g	216	11.4	36	1	3.3	1.9	0.7
Tomato, & Basil, CBY, Asda*	½ Pot/297g	89	2.4	30	1	4.3	0.8	0.7
Tomato, & Basil, Creamy, Cully & Sully*	1 Pack/400g	216	18.5	54	0.8	2.5	4.6	0.5
Tomato, & Basil, Cup a Soup, Made Up, GFY, Asda*	1 Serving/250ml	50	0.2	20	0.4	4.4	0.1	0.2
Tomato, & Basil, Cup, Co-Op*	1 Sachet/45g	158	1.8	350	2	76	4	4
Tomato, & Basil, Flavoured, CWP*	1 Sachet/54g	200	4.9	370	33.2	35.7	9.1	4.6
Tomato, & Basil, Fresh, Finest, Tesco*	½ Pot/300g	219	14.7	73	1	6.3	4.9	0.6
Tomato, & Basil, Fresh, Low Fat, Sainsbury's*	½ Carton/300ml	75	1.8	25	1.1	4.1	0.6	0.7
Tomato, & Basil, Fresh, M Kitchen, Morrisons*	½ Pot/300g	115	3.6	38	1	5.5	1.2	0.7
Tomato, & Basil, Fresh, M&S*	½ Pot/300g	120	5.1	40	1	5	1.7	1.3
Tomato, & Basil, Italian Plum, Finest, Tesco*	1 Pot/600g	360	13.8	60	1.3	7.2	2.3	0.6
Tomato, & Basil, Italian Plum, PB, Waitrose*	½ Pot/300g	69	1.5	23	0.9	3.8	0.5	0.9
Tomato, & Basil, Italian Style, Co-Op*	1 Pack/500g	200	10	40	1	4	2	0.6
Tomato, & Basil, Italian, Vegetarian, Baxters*	1 Can/415g	170	3.7	41	1.4	5.7	0.9	0.6
Tomato, & Basil, M&S*	½ Pot/300g	105	4.2	35	0.7	4.5	1.4	1
Tomato, & Basil, Plum, New Covent Garden Food Co*	½ Carton/300g	132	6	44	1.3	5.2	2	1.3
Tomato, & Basil, Rich, Waitrose*	1 Serving/130g	53	1.3	41	1.3	6.3	1	0.7
Tomato, & Basil, Sun Dried, Heinz*	1 Serving/275ml	124	5.2	45	0.6	6.5	1.9	0.1
Tomato, & Basil, Weight Watchers*	1 Serving/295g	114	1.8	39	0.6	7.5	0.6	0.6
Tomato, & Brown Lentil, Healthy, Baxters*	1 Can/415g	199	0.8	48	2.6	9	0.2	2.7
Tomato, & Butter Bean, Classic, Heinz*	½ Can/200g	92	1.4	46	1.3	8.1	0.7	0.8
Tomato, & Lentil, Organic, Tideford*	1 Carton/300g	120	2.7	40	2.3	8.1	0.9	0.9
Tomato, & Lentil, Truly Irresistible, Co-Op*	½ Pot/300g	165	2.1	55	3.1	8	0.7	1.2
Tomato, & Red Pepper, Fire Roasted, Asda*	½ Tub/265g	114	6.9	43	0.7	4.1	2.6	1
Tomato, & Rice, with Sweetcorn, Spicy, Healthy, Baxters*	1 Can/414g	219	1.2	53	1.8	9.4	0.3	0.9
Tomato, & Roasted Red Pepper, COU, M&S*	1 Serving/415g	145	0.4	35	1	7.6	0.1	0.9
Tomato, & Three Bean, Canned, BGTY, Sainsbury's*	½ Can/200g	120	2.2	60	2.8	8.4	1.1	2.4
Tomato, & Three Bean, Co-Op*	½ Can/200g	130	1.8	65	3.7	10.2	0.9	2

S

SOUP

INFO/WEIGHT	Measure	per Measure KCAL	per Measure FAT	Nutrition Values per 100g / 100ml KCAL	PROT	CARB	FAT	FIBRE
Tomato, & Three Bean, Eat Smart, Morrisons*	1 Can/400g	228	4	57	2.8	8.2	1	2.2
Tomato, & Thyme, Organic, Duchy, Waitrose*	½ Pot/300g	140	8.9	47	1.2	3.3	3	1
Tomato, & Vegetable, Cup a Soup, Batchelors*	1 Serving/218g	107	2.6	49	1.1	8.5	1.2	0.6
Tomato, & Vegetable, Spicy, Healthy Living, Co-Op*	1 Can/400g	180	3.2	45	2	8	0.8	2
Tomato, & Vegetable, Mediterranean, Fresh, Tesco*	½ Pot/300g	105	2.1	35	1	6.2	0.7	0.7
Tomato, & Balsamic, Finest, Tesco*	½ Pot/300g	116	4.2	38	1.2	4.9	1.4	0.7
Tomato, Bean, & Chipotle, New Covent Garden Food Co*	½ Carton/300g	138	1.5	46	2.7	6.5	0.5	2.2
Tomato, Big Red, Heinz*	½ Can/210g	63	0.8	30	0.5	6.4	0.4	0
Tomato, Borlotti Bean & Kale, Fresh, M&S*	1 Pot/600g	318	10.2	53	2	6.3	1.7	2.1
Tomato, Canned, LC, Tesco*	½ Can/200g	90	3.8	45	0.9	5.9	1.9	0.4
Tomato, Cannellini Beans, & Garlic, Heinz*	½ Can/200g	110	2.2	55	2.4	9.1	1.1	2.4
Tomato, Cherry, Roasted, Mascarpone, TTD, Sainsbury's*	1 Pot/400g	212	11.2	53	1.5	4.2	2.8	2.4
Tomato, Chunky, Organic, Canned, Amy's Kitchen*	1 Can/400g	212	5.6	53	1.2	8.6	1.4	1.2
Tomato, Cream of, Asda*	½ Can/200g	122	6.4	61	0.7	7.3	3.2	0.7
Tomato, Cream of, Canned, Average	*1 Can/400g*	*208*	*12*	*52*	*0.8*	*5.9*	*3*	*0.7*
Tomato, Cream of, Canned, Crosse & Blackwell*	1 Can/400g	228	10	57	0.9	7.4	2.5	0.8
Tomato, Cream of, Canned, Tesco*	½ Can/192g	115	4.8	60	0.9	7.4	2.5	0.8
Tomato, Cream of, Classic, Heinz*	½ Can/200g	102	4.2	51	0.8	6.8	2.1	0.6
Tomato, Cream of, Classics, Soupreme, Aldi*	1 Can/400g	192	8	48	0.8	6.4	2	0.8
Tomato, Cream of, Eat Well, M&S*	½ Pot/300g	189	9.9	63	0.8	7.1	3.3	0.6
Tomato, Cream of, Favourites, Baxters*	½ Can/200g	132	5.4	66	1.1	6.9	2.7	0.4
Tomato, Cream of, for One, Heinz*	1 Can/300g	189	10.8	63	0.8	6.9	3.6	0.4
Tomato, Cream of, Fresh, Sainsbury's*	1 Pot/600g	318	19.2	53	0.8	5.2	3.2	1.3
Tomato, Cream Of, Pot, Heinz*	1 Pot/280g	135	3.1	48	1.2	8	1.1	0.8
Tomato, Cream of, Sainsbury's*	1 Can/400g	244	12.8	61	0.7	7.3	3.2	0.7
Tomato, Cream Of, with a Hint of Basil, Heinz*	½ Can/200g	114	6	57	0.9	6.6	3	0.4
Tomato, Cream of, with Spanish Chorizo, Heinz*	1 Can/400g	244	12	61	1.4	6.9	3	0.4
Tomato, Fresh, Mediterranean, Organic, Sainsbury's*	1 Serving/250ml	78	3.5	31	1.3	3.3	1.4	1
Tomato, Gazpacho, Innocent*	1 Bowl/200g	80	4.6	40	0.6	2.8	2.3	2.4
Tomato, Herb Roasted, & Wheatberry, Waitrose*	1 Pot/400g	222	9.9	56	1.1	6.4	2.5	1.5
Tomato, Kale, & Borlotti Bean, Italian, Asda*	½ Tub/300g	144	3.9	48	1.9	6.1	1.3	2.2
Tomato, Original, Cup a Soup, Batchelors*	1 Sachet/254g	104	2.3	41	0.6	7.3	0.9	0.5
Tomato, Red Lentil & Pepper, CBY, Asda*	½ Pot/300g	177	3.3	59	3	8.8	1.1	0.9
Tomato, Red Pepper, & Lentil, Morrisons*	1 Pot/600g	372	12.6	62	2.2	7.4	2.1	2.3
Tomato, Roasted Garlic, & Black Pepper, Heinz*	½ Carton/200g	98	3.8	49	1.2	6.7	1.9	1.1
Tomato, Singapore Crushed, Skinny Soup, Glorious!*	½ Pot/300g	117	4.8	39	0.9	4.8	1.6	1
Tomato, Slow Roast, New Covent Garden Food Co*	½ Carton/300g	84	1.2	28	0.9	4.4	0.4	1.5
Tomato, Smart Price, Asda*	1 Can/400g	184	7.6	46	0.6	6.5	1.9	0.9
Tomato, Spicy, Lentil, & Red Pepper, Fresh, Sainsbury's*	1 Pot/600g	390	7.8	65	3.7	8.8	1.3	1.8
Tomato, Spinach, & Lentil, Heinz*	½ Can/200g	85	1.4	43	1.7	7.7	0.7	1.1
Tomato, Weight Watchers*	1 Can/295g	76	1.5	26	0.7	4.6	0.5	0.3
Tomato, Mediterranean, Slim a Soup, Cup, Batchelors*	1 Serving/208g	56	1.2	27	0.5	4.8	0.6	0.4
Tomato, Mediterranean, Vegetarian, Baxters*	1 Can/400g	126	0.4	32	0.9	5.6	0.1	0.8
Turkey, Broth, Canned, Baxters*	½ Can/208g	79	1.5	38	1.3	6.5	0.7	0.7
Vegetable Tagine, Slimming World*	1 Tub/500g	215	2	43	2.6	5.6	0.4	3.1
Vegetable, & Three Bean, Chunky, M&S*	1 Can/400g	228	3.6	57	3	7.7	0.9	3.1
Vegetable, & Barley, Ready to Serve, Wattie's*	½ Can/262g	97	0.5	37	1.6	6.4	0.2	1.6
Vegetable, Barley, Amy's Kitchen*	1 Can/400g	152	4.8	38	0.8	5.3	1.2	1.2
Vegetable, Broth, Best of British, Crosse & Blackwell*	1 Can/400g	135	1.6	34	1.1	5.9	0.4	1.1
Vegetable, Broth, Hearty, Weight Watchers*	1 Can/295g	135	0.6	46	2	8.2	0.2	1.4
Vegetable, Canned	*1oz/28g*	*13*	*0.2*	*48*	*1.4*	*9.9*	*0.6*	*1.5*
Vegetable, Canned, Essential, Waitrose*	½ Can/200g	103	1	52	1.9	9.2	0.5	1.4
Vegetable, Canned, Tesco*	½ Can/200g	70	1	35	1.1	5.9	0.5	1

SOUP

Item	INFO/WEIGHT	KCAL	FAT	KCAL	PROT	CARB	FAT	FIBRE
Vegetable, Canned, Tesco*	½ Can/200g	100	2	50	1.4	8.1	1	1.3
Vegetable, Chunky, Canned, Sainsbury's*	1 Can/400g	184	2.8	46	1.5	8.3	0.7	1.2
Vegetable, Chunky, Canned, Soupreme, Aldi*	1 Can/400g	172	4	43	1.1	6.4	1	2.3
Vegetable, Chunky, Diet Chef Ltd*	1 Pack/300g	114	0.9	38	1.4	7.4	0.3	1.3
Vegetable, Chunky, Fresh, CBY, Asda*	½ Pot/300g	117	2.1	39	1.6	5.9	0.7	1.1
Vegetable, Chunky, Fresh, Tesco*	½ Pot/300g	138	4.8	46	1.4	5.7	1.6	1.6
Vegetable, Chunky, Fresh, Waitrose*	½ Pot/300g	132	5.4	44	1.3	4.5	1.8	2.1
Vegetable, Chunky, Parsley Box*	1 Pack/300g	108	0.6	36	1.5	7.4	0.2	0.6
Vegetable, Classic, Heinz*	1 Can/400g	188	3.2	47	1.1	8.3	0.8	0.9
Vegetable, Country, Canned, Heinz, Weight Watchers*	1 Can/295g	97	0.6	33	1.2	5.9	0.2	1
Vegetable, Country, Chunky, Baxters*	1 Can/400g	188	2.4	47	1.6	7.2	0.6	2
Vegetable, Country, Fresh, Soupreme, Aldi*	1 Tub/600g	204	3.6	34	1.1	5.1	0.6	1.7
Vegetable, Country, Hearty, Canned, Baxters*	1 Can/400g	192	2.4	48	1.9	7.5	0.6	1.9
Vegetable, Country, Knorr*	1 Pack/500ml	160	3.5	32	0.9	5.5	0.7	1.2
Vegetable, Country, Weight Watchers*	1 Can/295g	97	0.3	33	1.2	6.3	0.1	1
Vegetable, Cully & Sully*	1 Pack/400g	204	14.4	51	0.6	4.2	3.6	0.9
Vegetable, Cup Soup, Dry, Heinz*	1 Sachet/16g	54	1.1	348	5.8	64.5	7.1	3.2
Vegetable, Cup Soup, Made Up, Heinz*	1 Cup/200g	62	0.6	31	0.5	6.3	0.3	0.3
Vegetable, Farmhouse, Thick, Co-Op*	1 Can/400g	140	1.6	35	1	7	0.4	0.3
Vegetable, Fresh, Average	**1 Serving/300g**	**118**	**4.1**	**40**	**1.4**	**5.4**	**1.4**	**1.3**
Vegetable, Fresh, Co-Op*	1 Pack/600g	150	6	25	0.6	4	1	1
Vegetable, Golden, Cup, GFY, Asda*	1 Sachet/217ml	52	1.1	24	0.5	4.4	0.5	0.2
Vegetable, Golden, Slim a Soup, Batchelors*	1 Sachet/207g	58	1.7	28	0.5	4.7	0.8	0.7
Vegetable, Golden, with Croutons Cup Soup, Co-Op*	1 Sachet/25g	120	6.5	480	4	56	26	2
Vegetable, Green, & Grains, Vegan, Waitrose*	1 Pot/400g	248	12	62	3.1	3.8	3	3.6
Vegetable, Gyoza, with Miso Broth, Everdine*	1 Serving/450g	369	5	82	2.9	13.3	1.1	3.6
Vegetable, in a Cup, HL, Tesco*	1 Sachet/18g	66	1.4	367	7.2	66.1	7.8	2.8
Vegetable, Instant, Cup, Average	**1 Pack/19g**	**69**	**2**	**362**	**8.7**	**57.1**	**10.5**	**5.5**
Vegetable, Moroccan, Tagine, Yorkshire Provender*	½ Pot/300g	171	5.1	57	2.3	7.2	1.7	0.7
Vegetable, No Added Sugar, Canned, Heinz*	½ Can/200g	84	1.4	42	1.2	7.2	0.7	1.2
Vegetable, Pot, Classic, Heinz*	1 Pot/355g	142	3.2	40	1	7.8	0.9	1
Vegetable, Root, & Turmeric, Baxters*	1 Can/400g	164	5.6	41	0.8	6.3	1.4	0.5
Vegetable, Scotty Brand*	½ Pot/275g	118	1	43	2.3	9.2	0.4	3.3
Vegetable, Spring, Classic, Heinz*	1 Can/400g	148	1.6	37	0.8	7	0.4	0.8
Vegetable, Spring, Florida, Dry, Knorr*	1 Pack/36g	104	2	290	7.8	52.2	5.6	5.2
Vegetable, Spring, Sainsbury's*	½ Can/200g	72	0.8	36	0.8	7.4	0.4	0.6
Vegetable, Ten, Broth, Morrisons*	1 Pot/600g	240	7.8	40	1.7	5.8	1.3	1.1
Vegetable, Winter, & Lentils, Mouline, Bio, La Potagere*	1 Pack/300ml	111	5.1	37	0.9	3.5	1.7	2.2
Vegetable, Winter, New Covent Garden Food Co*	½ Carton/300g	117	2.1	39	2	5.1	0.7	2.3
Vegetable, Roasted, Fresh, Sainsbury's*	½ Pot/300ml	78	1.5	26	0.5	4.8	0.5	1.2
Watercress, M&S*	½ Pot/300g	75	5.1	25	1.3	1.5	1.7	0.6

SOUP MIX

Item	INFO/WEIGHT	KCAL	FAT	KCAL	PROT	CARB	FAT	FIBRE
Broth, Pearl Barley, Peas, & Lentils, Made Up, G&B, Asda*	1 Serving/100g	88	0.6	88	3.4	15	0.6	4.6
Butternut Squash, Sainsbury's*	¼ Pack/147g	47	1	32	0.8	5.3	0.7	0.5
Country, Morrisons*	1 Serving/80g	82	0.6	102	6	13.7	0.8	7.8
Leek & Potato, As Sold, G&B, Asda*	¼ Pack/125g	69	0.4	55	1.7	10.5	0.3	1.7
Minestrone & Bean, Cooks' Ingredients, Waitrose*	½ Pack/200g	118	1	59	2.7	9	0.5	3.6
Potato, & Leek, Sainsbury's*	1 Serving/100g	31	0.5	31	1.4	5.5	0.5	1
Red Pepper, & Carrot, Nature's Pick, Aldi*	1 Serving/100g	16	0.5	16	1.4	1.8	0.5	0.8
Soup & Broth Mix, Dry, Wholefoods, Tesco*	¼ Pack/125g	456	2.4	365	14.7	71.4	1.9	7.3
Sweet Potato, Nature's Pick, Aldi*	1 Serving/100g	24	0.5	24	0.8	4.1	0.5	1.2
Vegetable, & Lentil, Scotty Brand*	1 Pack/500g	265	2	53	2.3	8.8	0.4	2.6
Vegetable, Kit, Morrisons*	1 Pack/500g	220	3.5	44	1.2	6.6	0.7	3

	Measure INFO/WEIGHT	per Measure KCAL	FAT	Nutrition Values per 100g / 100ml KCAL	PROT	CARB	FAT	FIBRE
SOUTHERN COMFORT								
37.5% Volume	*1 Pub Shot/35ml*	*72*	*0*	*207*	*0*	*0*	*0*	*0*
SOUVLAKI								
Chicken, World Deli, Waitrose*	1 Skewer/28g	38	0.8	138	27.5	0.2	3	0
SOYA								
Chicken, Bites, Organic, Like, Like meat*	1 Pack/180g	259	4	144	18	1.4	2.2	6.1
Chunks, Dried, Cooked, Sainsbury's*	1oz/28g	27	0.1	98	14	9.8	0.3	1.1
Chunks, Protein, Natural, Nature's Harvest*	1 Serving/50g	172	0.5	345	50	35	1	4
Chunks, with Chilli, Coriander, & Soy Marinade, M&S*	1 Pack/175g	180	1.6	103	18.6	1.7	0.9	6.8
Mince, Dry Weight, Sainsbury's*	1 Serving/50g	164	0.4	328	47.2	33.2	0.8	3.6
SPAGHETTI								
50/50, Dry, Napolina*	1 Serving/75g	257	1.4	343	11.2	67	1.8	7.2
Bare Naked, Barenaked*	1 Serving/100g	17	0.1	17	0.3	0.9	0.1	3.4
Black Bean, Cooked, The Foodie Market, Aldi*	1 Serving/125g	125	2.9	100	15	1.6	2.3	7.9
Black Bean, Organic, Dry, Aldi*	1 Serving/50g	162	2.6	325	46	13	5.3	21
Black Bean, Organic, Dry, Explore Asian*	1 Serving/56g	198	2	353	44	15	3.6	21
Cooked, Average	*1oz/28g*	*33*	*0.2*	*119*	*4.1*	*24.8*	*0.6*	*1.1*
Dry, Average	*1oz/28g*	*98*	*0.4*	*350*	*12.1*	*72.1*	*1.5*	*2.4*
Durum Wheat, Dry, Average	*1oz/28g*	*97*	*0.1*	*348*	*12.4*	*71.8*	*0.4*	*1.4*
Edamame, Organic, Dry, Explore Asian*	1 Serving/56g	204	2	365	45	18	3.6	20
Fresh, Cooked, Average	*1 Serving/125g*	*182*	*2.2*	*146*	*6.1*	*26.9*	*1.7*	*1.8*
Fresh, Dry, Average	*1 Serving/100g*	*278*	*3*	*278*	*10.8*	*53*	*3*	*2.2*
GF, Cooked, Free From, Morrisons*	1 Portion/75g	129	0.4	172	2.8	38.6	0.6	0.9
GF, Free From, Tesco*	1 Serving/75g	266	0.8	355	7	78.4	1	2
Hoops, Canned, Smart Price, Asda*	½ Can/205g	127	0.6	62	1.7	13	0.3	0.4
Hoops, in Tomato Sauce, Heinz*	½ Can/200g	106	0.4	53	1.7	11.1	0.2	0.5
Hoops, in Tomato Sauce, Snap Pot, Heinz*	1 Pot/190g	115	0.4	61	1.7	12.6	0.2	0.6
in Rich Tomato Sauce, Canned, Corale, Aldi*	½ Can/200g	114	1	57	2.1	10	0.5	2.6
in Tomato Sauce with Parsley, Weight Watchers*	1 Sm Can/200g	100	0.4	50	1.8	9.9	0.2	0.6
In Tomato Sauce, Basics, Sainsbury's*	1 Can/410g	197	1.2	48	1.4	10	0.3	0.7
in Tomato Sauce, Canned	*1oz/28g*	*18*	*0.1*	*64*	*1.9*	*14.1*	*0.4*	*0.7*
in Tomato Sauce, Canned, Alphabetti, Heinz*	½ Can/200g	118	0.8	59	1.9	11.7	0.4	0.7
in Tomato Sauce, Canned, Smedley's*	½ Can/195g	125	0.8	64	1.5	13.2	0.4	0.6
in Tomato Sauce, Heinz*	½ Can/200g	120	0.6	60	1.7	12.7	0.3	2.4
Lentil, & Mushroom, Italian, Good Health, Waitrose*	1 Pack/373g	433	14.6	116	3.4	14	3.9	5.5
Loops, in Tomato Sauce, Savers, Morrisons*	½ Can/205g	115	0.8	56	1.3	11.4	0.4	0.7
Marinara	*1 Serving/450g*	*675*	*18.9*	*150*	*8*	*19*	*4.2*	*0.9*
Pancetta, Smoked, & Mushroom, Creamy Sauce, Tesco*	1 Serving/350g	590	33.3	168	7	13	9.5	1.3
Tomato, & Basil, Sainsbury's*	1 Pack/395g	367	7.9	93	3.1	14.6	2	2
Whole Wheat, Cooked, Average	*1oz/28g*	*32*	*0.3*	*113*	*4.7*	*23.2*	*0.9*	*3.5*
Whole Wheat, Dry, Average	*1 Serving/100g*	*324*	*2.6*	*324*	*13.5*	*62.2*	*2.6*	*8*
with Sausages, in Tomato Sauce, Heinz*	1 Can/400g	352	14	88	3.4	10.8	3.5	0.5
SPAGHETTI & MEATBALLS								
Beef & Pork, Calorie Controlled, Love Life, Waitrose*	1 Pack/356g	342	9.3	96	5.5	11.9	2.6	1.3
Frozen, Tesco*	1 Serving/368g	488	19	133	5.6	15	5.2	2
GFY, Asda*	1 Pack/400g	344	6	86	7	11	1.5	1.5
Italian Cuisine, Tesco*	1 Pack/413g	516	18.2	125	7.4	13	4.4	1.4
Low Fat, Co-Op*	1 Pack/390g	355	9	91	5.2	11	2.3	2
Meal for One, Microwaved, Iceland*	1 Meal/453g	421	4.5	93	4.4	15.7	1	1.8
Meatballs, Italian, As Prepared, Waitrose*	1 Pack/400g	520	23.8	131	6.1	12.8	6	0.8
Pork & Beef, in Tomato Sauce, Prepared, Sainsbury's*	1 Pack/401g	566	27.3	141	7.3	11.9	6.8	1.6
Spicy Meat & Vegetable, My Goodness, Sainsbury's*	1 Pack/380g	357	9.5	94	5.7	10.9	2.5	2.7
SPAGHETTI WITH								
King Prawn, Italian, Cooked, Finest, Tesco*	1 Pack/390g	485	22.9	125	5	12.2	5.9	1.3

S

	Measure INFO/WEIGHT	per Measure KCAL	FAT	Nutrition Values per 100g / 100ml KCAL	PROT	CARB	FAT	FIBRE
SPAGHETTI WITH								
Tomato, & Basil, Parsley & Parmesan Cheese, M&S*	1 Pack/400g	584	29.2	146	3.8	15.1	7.3	2.2
SPAM*								
Pork & Ham, Chopped, Spam*	1 Serving/100g	289	24.3	289	15	3.2	24.3	0
SPELT								
Bulgur, Organic, Garofalo*	1 Serving/50g	170	1.1	341	13	64	2.2	7.1
Canned, in Water, Drained, Napolina*	½ Can/120g	71	1	59	2.7	9.2	0.8	2.1
SPICE								
Paprika, Sumptuously Smokey, Maggi*	1 Serving/6g	27	2.1	446	8.9	18.9	35.4	8.2
SPICE MIX								
Chilli Con Carne, Bramwells, Aldi*	¼ Sachet/13g	41	0.5	318	9.7	55	3.7	13
Chilli Con Carne, Tex Mex, Recipe Mix, Schwartz*	1 Sachet/35g	97	2.3	277	12.9	66.6	6.6	24.6
Creole, Seasoned Pioneers*	1 Tbsp/15g	47	0.8	313	8.3	43.2	5.2	15.1
for Burritos, Old El Paso*	½ Pack/23g	68	0.9	304	13	54	4	0
for Fajitas, Old El Paso*	1 Pack/35g	107	2.1	306	9	54	6	0
for Mexican Fajitas, Discovery*	½ Pack/15g	34	1	230	8	35	6.5	17.5
Madras, South Indian, Meal Kit, Patak's*	1 Pack/156g	228	16.4	146	1.8	9.2	10.5	0
Moroccan, Rub, Schwartz*	1 Serving/3g	9	0.3	309	15	36.4	11.4	19.5
Napoli, Spaghetti, Kania*	1 Serving/22g	68	0.3	311	7.1	63.5	1.4	0
Ras El Hanout, Al'fez*	1 Tsp/2g	4	0.2	217	9.8	25.7	8.3	17.5
Ras El Hanout, Blend, Finest, Tesco*	1 Tsp/5g	16	0.5	320	9.4	37.1	9.2	23.6
Rogan Josh, Authentic, Schwartz*	1 Pack/35g	108	3.5	309	11.1	30.3	10	26.7
Smokehouse BBQ, Wrap It, Schwartz*	¼ Pack/8g	24	0.2	317	8.1	59.2	3.2	9.5
Zaatar, Waitrose*	1 Serving/10g	42	3	416	14.7	8.2	30.2	26.1
SPICE PASTE								
Ajika, Kortava's*	1 Tsp/5g	1	0.1	29	2.9	5.2	1.5	0
Laksa, for Malay Curry, Cooks' Ingredients, Waitrose*	1 Serving/45g	58	3	128	2.9	13.2	6.6	2.2
SPINACH								
Baby Leaf, Whole, Frozen, Sainsbury's*	1 Serving/80g	18	0.6	22	3.2	0.5	0.7	1.2
Baby, Average	*1 Serving/90g*	*22*	*0.7*	*25*	*2.8*	*1.6*	*0.8*	*2.1*
Boiled or Steamed, Average	*1 Serving/80g*	*17*	*0.6*	*21*	*2.6*	*0.9*	*0.8*	*2.1*
Canned, Average	*1 Serving/80g*	*16*	*0.4*	*20*	*2.8*	*1.3*	*0.5*	*2.7*
Chopped, Heritage*	1 Serving/80g	21	0.6	26	3.1	0.5	0.8	2.1
Leaf, Frozen, Lidl*	1 Serving/80g	37	0.6	46	3.9	4.3	0.8	0
Mornay, Waitrose*	½ Pack/125g	112	8.6	90	3.3	3.6	6.9	1.6
Raw, Average	*1 Serving/80g*	*19*	*0.6*	*24*	*2.9*	*1.4*	*0.7*	*2.2*
SPIRALI								
Dry, Average	*1 Serving/50g*	*176*	*0.8*	*352*	*12.2*	*72.6*	*1.6*	*2.8*
SPIRITS								
40% Volume	*1 Shot/35ml*	*78*	*0*	*222*	*0*	*0*	*0*	*0*
Juniper, & Inca Berry, Non Alcoholic, Caleno*	1 Serving/50ml	20	0	39	0	9	0	0
Non Alcoholic, Garden, Seedlip Ltd*	1 Serving/50ml	0	0	0	0	0	0	0
Non Alcoholic, Spice 94, Botanical, Seedlip Ltd*	1 Serving/50ml	0	0	0	0	0	0	0
Spiced Citrus, Ultra Low Alcohol, Atopia*	1 Single/25ml	6	0	23	0	5	0	0
Three Spirit, Non Alcoholic, Elixir, Three Spirit*	1 Serve/50ml	26	0	52	0	0	0	0
SPLIT PEAS								
Dried, Average	*1oz/28g*	*89*	*0.5*	*319*	*22.1*	*57.4*	*1.7*	*3.2*
Green, Dried, Average	*1 Serving/80g*	*261*	*1.3*	*326*	*22.5*	*45*	*1.6*	*20*
SPONGE FINGERS								
Almond Fingers, Tesco*	1 Finger/46g	174	6.1	379	5.3	58.8	13.2	1.7
Boudoir, Sainsbury's*	1 Finger/5g	20	0.2	396	8.1	82.8	3.6	0.4
Tesco*	1 Finger/5g	19	0.2	386	7.6	80.6	3.7	1
Trifle, Average	*1 Sponge/24g*	*77*	*0.5*	*319*	*5.2*	*69.9*	*2.2*	*0.8*

S

SPONGE PUDDING	Measure INFO/WEIGHT	per Measure KCAL	FAT	Nutrition Values per 100g / 100ml KCAL	PROT	CARB	FAT	FIBRE
Average	1 Portion/170g	578	27.7	340	5.8	45.3	16.3	1.1
Blackberry & Apple, HE, Tesco*	1 Pot/103g	159	1.4	155	3.1	32.6	1.4	0.7
Cherry & Almond Flavour, Sainsbury's*	¼ Pudding/110g	334	15.7	304	3.5	40.3	14.3	0.7
Chocolate & Sauce, Co-Op*	1 Pack/225g	608	29.2	270	5	34	13	0.6
Chocolate, Less Than 3% Fat, BGTY, Sainsbury's*	1 Pudding/105g	180	2	171	4.5	34	1.9	0.9
Chocolate, M&S*	1 Pudding/105g	401	24.3	382	5.7	36	23.1	3.5
Chocolate, Sainsbury's*	¼ Pudding/110g	464	28.3	422	5.4	42.3	25.7	0.8
Chocolate, Tesco*	1 Serving/115g	430	19.2	374	3.7	50.8	16.7	2.7
Chocolate, Trufree*	1 Serving/115g	374	17.2	325	2.5	44	15	2
Chocolate, Waitrose*	1 Pudding/110g	400	22.5	363	3.6	41.4	20.4	1.7
Golden Syrup, Co-Op*	1 Can/300g	945	39	315	2	47	13	0.6
Honey& Fig, M&S*	¼ Pudding/73g	225	12	310	3.6	34.8	16.6	3.4
Lemon Curd, Heinz*	¼ Can/78g	236	9.1	302	2.6	46.7	11.7	0.6
Lemon, M&S*	1 Pudding/105g	326	16	310	4.3	39.4	15.2	2.3
Lemon, Waitrose*	1 Serving/105g	212	2.5	202	3.4	41.7	2.4	1.4
Milk Chocolate, Sticky Puds, Cadbury*	1 Pudding/95g	390	17.3	360	4.2	48.9	16	0.8
Mixed Berry, BGTY, Sainsbury's*	1 Pudding/110g	189	2.6	172	2.4	33.3	2.4	3.8
Pear & Ginger, COU, M&S*	1 Pudding/100g	175	0.7	175	1.9	39.8	0.7	1.1
Raspberry, Tesco*	1 Serving/100g	377	14.5	377	3.2	58.2	14.5	0.7
Salted Caramel, Specially Selected, Aldi*	1 Pudding/115g	459	20.7	399	3.6	54	18	1
Salted Caramel, Tesco*	1 Pudding/115g	464	21.6	404	3.2	55.2	18.8	0.6
Sticky Ginger, Really Good Puds, M Kitchen, Morrisons*	1 Pudding/110g	372	12	338	3.5	56.2	10.9	0.5
Strawberry Jam, Heinz*	¼ Can/82g	230	6.2	281	2.6	50.4	7.6	0.6
Sultana with Toffee Sauce, HL, Tesco*	1 Serving/80g	280	2.2	350	3.2	60.2	2.8	1
Syrup, BGTY, Sainsbury's*	1 Pudding/110g	338	4.5	307	2.8	64.6	4.1	0.4
Syrup, Finest, Tesco*	1 Pudding/115g	330	9	287	3.1	51.2	7.8	0.6
Syrup, GFY, Asda*	1 Sponge/105g	207	4.3	197	2	38	4.1	2.6
Syrup, Individual, Tesco*	1 Pudding/110g	390	14.5	355	3.1	55.6	13.2	0.5
Syrup, Sainsbury's*	¼ Pudding/110g	408	13	371	2.7	63.5	11.8	0.4
Syrup, Value, Tesco*	1 Serving/100g	307	10.2	307	2.1	51.7	10.2	0.6
Toffee & Pecan	½ Pudding/100g	395	18.4	395	4.3	52.3	18.4	1.4
Toffee, & Pecan, Finest, Tesco*	½ Sponge/100g	395	18.4	395	4.3	52.3	18.4	1.4
Treacle with Custard, Farmfoods*	1 Serving/145g	539	33.1	372	3.2	38.4	22.8	0.8
Treacle, Heinz*	1 Serving/160g	445	13	278	2.5	48.9	8.1	0.6
Treacle, Waitrose*	1 Pudding/105g	385	13.8	367	2.8	59.5	13.1	0.5
with Custard	1 Serving/200g	521	24.9	261	4.8	34.1	12.4	0.9
with Jam or Treacle	1oz/28g	93	4	333	5.1	48.7	14.4	1
SPOTTED DICK								
Average	1 Serving/105g	343	17.5	327	4.2	42.7	16.7	1
Individual, Tesco*	1 Pudding/121g	417	14.5	345	3.2	55.2	12	1.2
with Custard	1 Serving/210g	438	15.6	209	3.4	31.5	7.4	1.3
SPRATS								
Fried	1oz/28g	116	9.8	415	24.9	0	35	0
Raw	1oz/28g	33	2.1	117	12.4	0	7.5	0
SPREAD								
Average	1 Thin Spread/7g	51	5.7	726	0.1	0.5	81	0
Butter Me Up, Light, Tesco*	1 Thin Spread/7g	24	2.7	350	0.3	0.5	38	0
Butter Me Up, Tesco*	1 Thin Spread/7g	35	3.8	503	0.7	1	55	0.5
Butter Style, Average	1 Thin Spread/7g	44	4.8	627	0.7	1.1	68.9	0
Butterlicious, Vegetable, Sainsbury's*	1 Thin Spread/7g	44	4.8	628	0.6	1.1	69	0
Butterlicious, Vegetable, Sainsbury's*	1 Serving/10g	41	4.5	414	0.5	1.5	45	1
Buttersoft, Light, Reduced Fat, Sainsbury's*	1 Thin Spread/7g	38	4.2	544	0.4	0.5	60	0
Buttery Taste, Benecol*	1 Thin Spread/7g	40	4.4	575	0	0.8	63.3	0

S

	Measure	per Measure		Nutrition Values per 100g / 100ml				
	INFO/WEIGHT	KCAL	FAT	KCAL	PROT	CARB	FAT	FIBRE

SPREAD

	Measure	KCAL	FAT	KCAL	PROT	CARB	FAT	FIBRE
Buttery, ProActiv, Flora *	1 Thin Spread/7g	38	4.1	542	0.5	0.5	59	0
Clover, Light, Dairy Crest Ltd*	1 Serving/7g	32	3.4	455	0.7	2.9	49	0
Cocoa, & Hazelnut, Butter, Nature's Energy, Meridian*	1 Tsp/5g	33	3	661	13.2	14.5	59.9	5.6
Dairy Free, Organic, Pure Spreads*	1 Thin Spread/7g	37	4.1	533	0.5	0	59	0
Enriched Olive, Tesco*	1 Thin Spread/7g	38	4.1	540	0.2	1.2	59	0
Fruit, Strawberry, Organic, Nature's Energy, Meridian*	1 Tsp/5g	6	0	129	0.6	29.6	0.3	1.4
Gold, Made with Buttermilk, Low Low, Kerry*	1 Spread/10g	48	5.3	483	0.6	0.8	53	0
Heart, Cholesterol Reducing, Dairygold	*1 Thin Spread/7g*	*24*	*2.5*	*338*	*0.7*	*2.8*	*36*	*0*
Irish Gold, Light, Tesco*	1 Thin Spread/7g	24	2.7	344	0.2	0.3	38	0
Lactofree Spreadable, Lactofree, Arla*	1 Serving/10g	68	7.5	679	0.5	0.5	75	0
Light, Benecol*	1 Thin Spread/7g	23	2.4	333	2.5	0	35	0
Light, Flora*	1 Thin Spread/7g	28	3.2	398	0.5	0.5	45	0
Low Fat, Average	*1 Thin Spread/7g*	*27*	*2.8*	*390*	*5.8*	*0.5*	*40.5*	*0*
Nut Butter, Macadamia, Nature's Energy, Meridian Foods*	1 Tbsp/15g	119	12	792	8.9	7.4	79.9	3.8
Olive Oil, 55% Reduced Fat, Benecol*	1 Thin Spread/7g	35	3.8	498	0.3	0.5	55	0
Olive Oil, Bertolli*	1 Serving/10g	53	5.9	532	0.5	0.5	59	0
Olive, Light, Tesco*	1 Spread/10g	28	3	278	0.1	0.6	30.5	0.5
Olive, Low Fat, Morrisons*	1 Thin Spread/7g	24	2.7	346	0.9	0	38	0
Olive, Reduced Fat, Asda*	1 Thin Spread/7g	38	4.1	536	0.2	1.1	59	0
Olive, Sainsbury's*	1 Thin Spread/7g	29	3.2	410	0.5	1	45	0.5
Olive, Tesco*	1 Thin Spread/7g	29	3.2	415	0.2	2	45	0.7
Olive, Waitrose*	1 Thin Spread/7g	29	3.2	409	0.5	0.6	45	0.5
Orange, Thick Cut, St Dalfour*	1 Spread/11g	23	0	211	0.6	52	0.1	1.6
Original, Made with Buttermilk, Low Low, Kerry*	1 Spread/10g	39	4.2	394	0.2	3	42	0
Pro Activ with Olive Oil, Flora*	1 Thin Spread/7g	22	2.4	320	0.5	0.5	35	0
Pro Activ, Light, Flora*	1 Thin Spread/7g	22	2.4	320	0.5	0.5	35	0
Pro Active, Becel*	1 Serving/7g	22	1.8	320	0	0	25	0
Reduced Fat, Average	*1 Thin Spread/7g*	*25*	*2.7*	*356*	*0.6*	*3*	*38*	*0*
Seed Butter, 3, Daylesford*	1 Thick Spread/12g	73	5.8	609	34.7	5.8	48.1	7
Slightly Salted, M&S*	1 Thick Spread/12g	87	9.6	725	0.6	0.6	80	0.3
Soft, Reduced Fat, Smart Price, Asda*	1 Thin Spread/7g	32	3.5	455	0.2	1	50	0
Soft, Value, Tesco*	1 Thin Spread/7g	30	3.4	433	0	0	48.1	0
Spreadable, with Real Butter, Reduced Fat, Asda*	1 Thick Spread/12g	62	6.8	513	0.5	0.6	57	0
Sunflower, Average	*1 Thin Spread/7g*	*42*	*4.6*	*595*	*0.1*	*0.4*	*65.9*	*0.4*
Sunflower, Dairy Free, Free From, Asda*	1 Thin Spread/7g	36	3.9	510	0.5	0.5	56	0.5
Sunflower, Enriched, Tesco*	1 Thin Spread/7g	37	4.1	535	0.1	0.2	59	0
Sunflower, Light, BFY, Morrisons*	1 Thin Spread/7g	24	2.7	342	0	0	38	0
Sunflower, Light, Greenvale, Aldi*	1 Thin Spread/7g	20	2.1	290	5	5	30	5
Sunflower, Light, Reduced Fat, Asda*	1 Thin Spread/7g	24	2.7	347	0.3	1	38	0.1
Sunflower, Low Fat, Aldi*	1 Thin Spread/7g	26	2.7	366	0.2	5.7	38	0
Sunflower, M&S*	1 Thin Spread/7g	44	4.9	630	0	0	70	3
Sunflower, Sainsbury's*	1 Thin Spread/7g	37	4.1	532	0.1	0.2	59	0
Utterly Butterly*	1 Thin Spread/7g	32	3.4	452	0.3	2.5	49	0
Vegan Block, Organic, Naturli*	1 Thin Spread/7g	47	5.2	670	0.5	0.5	75	0
Vegan, Spreadable, Organic, Naturli*	1 Thin Spread /7g	48	5.2	681	0.5	0.5	75	0
Vegetable, Soft, Tesco*	1 Thin Spread/7g	46	5.1	661	0.1	1	73	0
Vitalite, Dairy Free, Dairy Crest Ltd*	1 Thin Spread/7g	35	3.9	503	0	0	56	0
with Soya, Dairy Free, Pure Spreads*	1 Thin Spread/7g	34	3.8	490	0.5	1	54	0
with Sunflower, Dairy Free, Organic, Pure Spreads*	1 Thin Spread/7g	38	4.1	537	0.5	1	59	0

SPRING ROLLS

	Measure	KCAL	FAT	KCAL	PROT	CARB	FAT	FIBRE
Chicken, Asda*	1 Roll/58g	115	5.2	199	4.6	25	9	3.4
Chicken, Oriental Snack Selection, Sainsbury's*	1 Roll/15g	38	1.5	256	11.5	30.3	9.9	1.7
Duck, Hoisin , Sainsbury's*	1 Roll/20g	57	3	287	5.9	30.6	15.3	1.8

	Measure INFO/WEIGHT	per Measure KCAL	FAT	Nutrition Values per 100g / 100ml KCAL	PROT	CARB	FAT	FIBRE
SPRING ROLLS								
Duck, Mini, Asda*	1 Roll/18g	47	1.9	259	8.7	32.8	10.3	1.9
Duck, Party Bites, Sainsbury's*	1 Roll/20g	49	1.8	245	10.1	31.4	8.8	1
Duck, Party, Asda*	1 Roll/18g	47	2	259	7.1	32	11	3.1
Duck, Sainsbury's*	1 Roll/50g	138	7.4	275	9.8	22.8	14.8	5.9
From Restaurant, Average	*1 Roll/140g*	*344*	*14.8*	*246*	*11.1*	*23.2*	*10.6*	*0*
M&S*	1 Roll/36g	66	2.3	183	4.6	25.6	6.4	2.2
Mini Vegetable, Co-Op*	1 Roll/18g	40	1.6	220	4.1	30.9	9.1	2.7
Mini, Asda*	1 Roll/20g	35	0.6	175	3.5	33.6	3	1.9
Mini, Sainsbury's*	1 Roll/12g	27	1.2	221	4.2	28.7	9.9	1.6
Oriental Vegetable, Tesco*	1 Roll/60g	148	7.4	248	3.6	29.7	12.4	1.4
Pork & Vegetable, Mini, Taste Thailand, Banquet Box, M&S*	½ Pack/51g	122	5.5	240	6.3	28.9	10.7	1.6
Prawn, Crispy, M&S*	1 Roll/34g	75	3.4	220	10	22.2	9.9	1.3
Thai, Sainsbury's*	1 Roll/30g	69	3.4	229	2.9	28.8	11.3	3.5
Vegetable, Asda*	1 Roll/62g	126	5.6	203	3.5	27	9	2.7
Vegetable, Cantonese, Large, Sainsbury's*	1 Roll/63g	130	6.3	205	3.6	25.3	9.9	1.5
Vegetable, Chilled, Tesco*	1 Roll/68g	149	7.6	221	4	25.9	11.3	1.6
Vegetable, Chinese Favourites Box, M&S*	½ Pack/70g	128	4.5	183	4.6	25.6	6.4	2.2
Vegetable, Chinese Selection, Frozen, Tesco*	1 Roll/17g	42	2	251	5.2	29	12.2	2.4
Vegetable, Chinese Takeaway, Sainsbury's*	1 Roll/59g	100	3.7	170	4	24.4	6.3	2.8
Vegetable, M&S*	1 Roll/37g	80	3.6	215	4.3	27.8	9.6	2
Vegetable, Meal for Two, Meal Box, Tesco*	2 Rolls/36g	94	4.1	264	5.5	33	11.4	3.5
Vegetable, Mini, Nirvana*	1 Roll/26g	54	2.7	208	3.5	25.1	10.4	1.7
Vegetable, Mini, Occasions, Sainsbury's*	1 Roll/24g	52	2.3	216	4.1	28.2	9.6	2.9
Vegetable, Mini, Party Food, M&S*	1 Roll/20g	40	1.6	200	3.7	26.2	8.1	2.7
Vegetable, Mini, Tesco*	1 Roll/16g	33	1.3	208	4	28.3	8.1	3
Vegetable, Oriental Selection, Party, Iceland*	1 Roll/15g	36	1.4	241	4.3	34.1	9.7	2.1
Vegetable, Oriental, Waitrose*	1 Roll/36g	90	4.3	249	5.7	27.1	12	4.8
Vegetable, Parcels, Snack Selection, Oriental, Waitrose*	1 Parcel/18g	48	2	267	4.5	34.6	11.3	4.6
Vegetable, Sainsbury's*	2 Rolls/84g	239	13.1	284	6	28.8	15.6	2.1
Vegetable, Tempura, M&S*	1 Pack/140g	280	12	200	2.8	27.9	8.6	1.8
SPRITE*								
Sprite*	1 Bottle/500ml	70	0	14	0	3.3	0	0
Zero, Lemon & Lime, Sprite*	1 Bottle/500ml	6	0	1	0	0	0	0
Zero, Sprite*	1 Can/330ml	3	0	1	0	0	0	0
SPRITZER								
Red Grape, Non-Alcoholic, Extra Special, Asda*	1 Bottle/750ml	330	0	44	0	11	0	0
Rose & Grape, Non Alcoholic, Extra Special, Asda*	1 Bottle/750ml	90	0	12	0	3	0	0
White Wine, Echo Falls*	1 Serving/125ml	78	0	39	0	0	0	0
with White Zinfadel, Echo Falls*	1 Serving/200ml	216	0	108	0	0	0	0
SQUASH								
Apple & Blackcurrant, No Added Sugar, Tesco*	1 Serving/30ml	4	0	15	0.2	2	0	0
Apple & Blackcurrant, Special R, Diluted, Robinson's*	1 Serving/30ml	2	0	8	0.1	1.1	0.1	0
Apple & Elderflower, High Juice, No Added Sugar, Co-Op*	1 Serving/250ml	12	1.2	5	0.5	1	0.5	0
Apple & Mango, High Juice, Diluted, Sainsbury's*	1 Serving/250ml	88	0	35	0	8.5	0	0.2
Apple, & Mango, High Juice, Diluted , Tesco*	1 Glass/250ml	50	0	20	0	4.8	0	0.1
Apple, Blackcurrant, Low Sugar, Diluted, Sainsbury's*	1 Glass/250ml	5	0.2	2	0.1	0.2	0.1	0.1
Apple, Cherry & Raspberry, High Juice, Robinson's*	1 Serving/25ml	49	0	196	0.2	47.6	0.1	0
Blackcurrant, High Juice, Tesco*	1 Serving/75ml	215	0	287	0.3	70	0	0
Blackcurrant, No Added Sugar, Tesco*	1 Serving/25ml	4	0	14	0.4	1.7	0	0
Cherries & Berries, Tesco*	1 Serving/25ml	5	0	21	0.2	3.2	0	0
Cherries & Berries, Sugar Free, Diluted, Tesco*	1 Glass/250ml	5	0	2	0	0.3	0	0
Cranberry, Light, Classic, Undiluted, Ocean Spray*	1 Serving/50ml	32	0	63	0.2	14.1	0	0
Elderflower, 0%, No Added Sugar, Undiluted, Teisseire*	1 Serving/20ml	5	0	23	0.1	0.5	0.1	0

S

	Measure	per Measure		Nutrition Values per 100g / 100ml				
	INFO/WEIGHT	KCAL	FAT	KCAL	PROT	CARB	FAT	FIBRE
SQUASH								
Fruit & Barley Orange, Diluted, Robinson's*	1 Serving/50ml	6	0	12	0.2	1.7	0	0.1
Fruit & Barley, No Added Sugar, Robinson's*	1 fl oz/30ml	4	0	14	0.3	2	0	0
Fruit & Barley, Tropical, No Added Sugar, Robinson's*	1 Serving/60ml	7	0	12	0.2	1.6	0	0
Lemon & Lime, Double Strength, No Added Sugar, Asda*	1 Glass/200ml	4	0	2	0	0	0	0
Lemon Barley Water, Made Up, Robinson's*	1 Serving/250ml	48	0	19	0.1	4.4	0	0
Lemon, Double Concentrate, Value, Tesco*	1 Serving/25ml	3	0	11	0.2	0.3	0	0
Lemon, High Juice, Diluted, Sainsbury's*	1 Glass /250ml	98	0.2	39	0.1	9.1	0.1	0.1
Lemon, No Added Sugar, Double Concentrate, Tesco*	1 Serving/25ml	4	0	16	0.3	0.7	0	0
Lemon, Real Fruit, Diluted, Robinson's*	1 Serving/250ml	12	0	5	0	0	0	0
Orange & Mango, Low Sugar, Sainsbury's*	1 Serving/250ml	5	0.2	2	0.1	0.2	0.1	0.1
Orange & Mango, Special R, Diluted, Robinson's*	1 Serving/250ml	20	0	8	0.2	0.9	0	0
Orange & Pineapple, Original, Undiluted, Robinson's*	1 Serving/250ml	138	0	55	1	13	0	0
Orange & Mango, No Added Sugar, Robinson's*	1 Serving/25ml	2	0	8	0.2	0.9	0	0
Orange & Pineapple, No Sugar Added, Robinson's*	1 Serving/25ml	2	0	8	0.2	0.7	0	0.2
Orange, Light, Harboe*	1 Serving/200ml	6	0	3	0	0	0	0
Orange, No Added Sugar, High Juice, Sainsbury's*	1 Serving/100ml	6	0.1	6	0.1	1.1	0.1	0.1
Orange, Special R, Diluted, Robinson's*	1fl oz/30ml	2	0	8	0.2	0.7	0.1	0
Pear Drop Flavour, Diluted, Tesco*	1 Serving/50ml	3	0	6	0.1	0.5	0	0
Pink Grapefruit, High Juice, Low Sugar, Tesco*	1 Serving/75ml	12	0.1	16	0.2	3.7	0.1	0
Spaghetti, Baked	*1oz/28g*	*6*	*0.1*	*23*	*0.7*	*4.3*	*0.3*	*2.1*
Spaghetti, Including Pips & Rind, Raw	*1oz/28g*	*5*	*0.1*	*20*	*0.4*	*3.4*	*0.4*	*1.7*
Strawberry, & Kiwi, Creations, Diluted, Robinson's*	1 Serving/200ml	6	0	3	0	0.6	0	0
Summer Fruit, No Added Sugar, Sainsbury's*	1 Serving/250ml	5	0.2	2	0.1	0.2	0.1	0.1
Summer Fruits & Barley, no Added Sugar, Tesco*	1 Serving/50ml	6	0	11	0.2	1.7	0	0
Summer Fruits, High Juice, Undiluted, Robinson's*	1fl oz/30ml	61	0	203	0.1	49	0.1	0
Summer Fruits, No Added Sugar, Double Strength, Asda*	1 Serving/50ml	1	0	2	0	0.2	0	0
Summer Fruits, No Added Sugar, Made Up, Morrisons*	1 Glass/200ml	3	0	2	0	0.2	0	0
Summer Fruits, No Added Sugar, Sun Quench, Aldi*	1 Serving/25ml	5	0.1	21	0.5	2.9	0.5	0.5
Summer Fruits, Robinson's*	1 Measure/25ml	14	0	56	0.1	13	0	0
Summer, All Varieties	*1 Sm/118g*	*19*	*0.2*	*16*	*1.2*	*3.4*	*0.2*	*1.1*
Tropical, Double Strength, No Added Sugar, CBY, Asda*	1 Serving/100ml	2	0	2	0	0.2	0	0
Winter, Acorn, Baked, Average	*1oz/28g*	*16*	*0*	*56*	*1.1*	*12.6*	*0.1*	*3.2*
Winter, Acorn, Raw, Average	*1oz/28g*	*9*	*0*	*30*	*0.6*	*6.8*	*0.1*	*1.7*
Winter, All Varieties, Flesh Only, Raw, Average	*1oz/28g*	*10*	*0*	*34*	*1*	*8.6*	*0.1*	*1.5*
SQUID								
in Batter, Fried in Blended Oil, Average	*1oz/28g*	*55*	*2.8*	*195*	*11.5*	*15.7*	*10*	*0.5*
Raw, Average	*1oz/28g*	*23*	*0.5*	*81*	*15.4*	*1.2*	*1.7*	*0*
Salt & Pepper Chargrilled, Cooked, Tesco*	1 Pack/80g	78	2.3	98	17.9	0	2.9	0.1
STAR FRUIT								
Average, Tesco*	1oz/28g	9	0.1	31	0.5	7.1	0.3	1.3
STARBAR								
Cadbury*	1 Bar/53g	260	14.8	491	10.7	49	27.9	0
STARBURST								
Fruit Chews, Tropical, Mars*	1 Tube/45g	168	3.3	373	0	76.9	7.3	0
Mars*	1 Pack/45g	182	3.3	405	0	83.9	7.3	0
STEAK & KIDNEY PUDDING								
M&S*	1 Pudding/121g	260	13.4	215	9.2	19.4	11.1	3.2
Tesco*	1 Serving/190g	437	22.6	230	10	20.7	11.9	1.2
Waitrose*	1 Pudding/223g	497	26.1	223	8.9	20.4	11.7	1.2
STEW								
Bean, Moroccan, V Taste, Morrisons*	1 Pack/301g	256	5.1	85	4	11.6	1.7	3.8
Beef & Dumplings, British Classics, Tesco*	1 Pack/450g	563	29.7	125	7.9	8.6	6.6	0.5
Beef & Dumplings	*1 Serving/652g*	*766*	*32.7*	*117*	*7.4*	*10.7*	*5*	*0.8*

S

	Measure INFO/WEIGHT	per Measure		Nutrition Values per 100g / 100ml				
		KCAL	FAT	KCAL	PROT	CARB	FAT	FIBRE
STEW								
Beef with Dumplings, Classic British, Sainsbury's*	1 Pack/450g	657	29.2	146	8.4	12.9	6.5	1.2
Beef with Dumplings, COU, M&S*	1 Pack/454g	431	11.8	95	8.9	9.1	2.6	0.8
Beef, & Dumplings, Aldi*	1 Pack/450g	567	27.9	126	8	8.6	6.2	2
Beef, & Dumplings, Frozen, Tesco*	1 Serving/400g	380	12.8	95	5.7	10.5	3.2	1.5
Beef, & Dumplings, HFC, Tesco*	1 Pack/384g	347	7.7	90	7.1	9.6	2	2.6
Beef, Asda*	½ Can/196g	178	4.9	91	10	7	2.5	1.5
Beef, Canned, Asda*	1 Can/392g	353	13.7	90	8.9	5.3	3.5	0.9
Beef, Classic, Puree, Wiltshire Farm Foods*	1 Serving/480g	523	25	109	4.5	10	5.2	0
Beef, Diet Chef Ltd*	1 Pack/270g	200	3.5	74	7.3	7.8	1.3	1.1
Beef, Meal for One, M&S*	1 Pack/440g	350	8.4	80	7	8.7	1.9	2
Beef, Minced, & Onion, Tesco*	1 Pack/300g	219	7.2	73	3.6	8.8	2.4	0.9
Beef, Moroccan, with Couscous, & Courgette, Hello Fresh*	1 Serving/703g	682	21	97	6.5	10.8	3	0
Beef, Value, Tesco*	1 Serving/200g	170	9.8	85	4	6.2	4.9	1
Chicken & Dumplings, Birds Eye*	1 Pack/320g	282	8.6	88	7	8.9	2.7	0.5
Chicken & Dumplings, Tesco*	1 Serving/450g	567	29.7	126	7.6	9.1	6.6	0.7
Chicken, Morrisons*	1 Pack/400g	492	7.6	123	17.6	8.9	1.9	0.5
Chickpea, Moroccan, Allplants*	½ Pack/380g	551	20.1	145	4.8	17	5.3	3.9
Chickpea, Roast Sweet Potato, & Feta, Stewed!*	½ Pot/250g	188	7.2	75	3.3	8.8	2.9	2.7
Haddock, Harissa, with Yoghurt, Gousto*	1 Serving/408g	595	12.2	146	9.6	19	3	2.9
Irish, Tesco*	1 Can/400g	308	11.2	77	7	5.9	2.8	0.8
Lamb, with Basmati Rice, Hello Fresh*	1 Serving/369g	336	1	91	3	19	0.3	0
Lentil & Vegetable, Organic, Simply Organic*	1 Pack/400g	284	6	71	3.5	11	1.5	1.3
Moroccan, Vegetable, Slimfree, Aldi*	1 Pack/500g	155	2.5	31	1.2	4.7	0.5	1.9
Roots, Hearty, Allplants*	½ Pack/380g	433	19.8	114	4.2	11	5.2	3
Sweet Potato, & Bean, Vegan, Waitrose*	½ Pack/220g	152	2.9	69	2.2	9.3	1.3	5.8
Tuscan Bean, Tasty Veg Pot, Innocent*	1 Pot/400g	320	7.6	80	3.1	12.5	1.9	3.6
Vegetable, Rainbow, & Dumplings, Sainsbury's*	1 Pack/385g	354	14.6	92	2.7	9.9	3.8	4
STIR FRY								
Bean Sprout & Vegetable with Red Peppers, Asda*	1 Pack/350g	126	3.9	36	1.8	4.7	1.1	2.3
Beef, BGTY, Sainsbury's*	½ Pack/125g	156	5.1	125	22	0.1	4.1	0
Beef, Chilli, Spicy, Musclefood*	1 Serving/353g	314	8.8	89	13.4	2.5	2.5	1.6
Beef, Steak, The Juicy Meat Co.*	½ Pack/140g	277	9.9	198	31.6	1.6	7.1	0.5
Beef, Teriyaki, M&Ss*	1 Pack/500g	375	3.5	75	10	7.1	0.7	0.1
Butternut Squash, & Edamame, Waitrose*	½ Pack/151g	74	1.5	49	3.1	6.2	1	1.6
Cabbage, Carrot, Broccoli & Onion, Vegetable, Tesco*	1 Serving/100g	31	0.4	31	1.9	4.9	0.4	2.6
Chicken Chow Mein, Fresh, HL, Tesco*	1 Pack/400g	312	4.8	78	5.7	11.4	1.2	1.3
Chicken, 387, Oakhouse Foods Ltd*	1 Pack/430g	404	2.6	94	8.4	12.9	0.6	1.8
Chicken, Chinese, Meal Kit, Aldi*	½ Pack/210g	277	8.6	132	16	7.6	4.1	1.2
Chicken, Fajita, Kit, Tesco*	½ Pack/230g	288	10.6	122	14.8	4.4	4.5	2.2
Chicken, Fajita, Musclefood*	1 Serving/358g	301	10.4	84	11.4	2	2.9	2.3
Chicken, Hoisin, with Red Pepper, & Noodles, Hello Fresh*	1 Serving/379g	572	13	151	13.2	17.2	3.4	0
Chicken, Naked, Musclefood*	1 Serving/350g	217	4.2	62	9.9	2.5	1.2	1
Chicken, Thai, Musclefood*	1 Serving/336g	279	8.7	83	11.8	1.9	2.6	2.4
Chinese Chicken, As Consumed, Iceland*	½ Pack/371g	353	2.6	95	6.5	15.2	0.7	1
Chinese Prawn, Iceland*	1 Pack/340g	235	4.4	69	3.1	11.1	1.3	2.1
Chinese Style Rice with Vegetables, Tesco*	1 Serving/550g	495	13.8	90	2.2	14.8	2.5	0.3
Edamame Bean, Oaklands, Lidl*	½ Pack/150g	70	2.4	47	3.5	3	1.6	3.3
Family Pack, Vegetables & Beansprouts, Fresh, Tesco*	1 Pack/600g	108	0.6	18	2	2.2	0.1	2.1
Green Vegetable, M&S*	1 Pack/220g	165	13	75	3.1	2.5	5.9	2.2
Hot & Spicy, Mixed Vegetables, Cooked, Sainsbury's*	½ Pack/149g	85	4.6	57	1.2	4.9	3.1	2.2
Mixed Pepper, Sainsbury's*	1 Pack/300g	188	12.9	70	1.5	4.6	4.8	1.2
Mixed Vegetable & Beansprout, Tesco*	1 Bag/320g	170	6.1	53	2.5	5.1	1.9	2.5
Mushroom, Morrisons*	¼ Pack/80g	25	0.4	31	2.1	3.5	0.5	2.1

S

	Measure INFO/WEIGHT	per Measure KCAL	FAT	Nutrition Values per 100g / 100ml KCAL	PROT	CARB	FAT	FIBRE
STIR FRY								
Noodles & Bean Sprouts, Tesco*	½ Pack/125g	131	2.6	105	4.2	16.1	2.1	0.7
Oriental Style Pak Choi, M&S*	1 Pack/220g	165	12.5	75	2.2	3.5	5.7	2.4
Oriental Style, Vegetables, Sainsbury's*	1 Pack/300g	195	14.4	65	1.5	4.1	4.8	2.1
Pork, Chinese Style, Musclefood*	1 Serving/328g	282	8.9	86	11.6	2.7	2.7	1.9
Pork, with Mangetout, & Coriander, Thai Style, Hello Fresh*	1 Serving/372g	595	13	160	9.7	22.3	3.5	0
Rice, Quinoa & Vegetable, Waitrose*	½ Pack/134g	199	7.8	148	5.4	15.6	5.8	6
Singapore, Noodle, Iceland*	½ Pack/346g	294	10.7	85	5.4	8.2	3.1	1.5
Steak, with Peppers, & Mange Tout, Hello Fresh*	1 Serving/292g	347	3	119	4.4	22.6	1	0
Sweet Mixed Pepper, Waitrose*	½ Pack/150g	111	6.1	74	2.1	4.2	4.1	5.8
Tenderstem Broccoli, & Mangetout, Waitrose*	½ Pack/142g	44	0.7	31	2.3	3.6	0.5	1.5
Vegetable & Mushroom, Asda*	½ Pack/160g	59	2.4	37	2.4	3.4	1.5	3.4
Vegetable Mix, As Consumed, Tesco*	½ Pack/128g	72	3	56	1.9	5.5	2.3	3
Vegetable, Chop Suey, Chinese, Sharwood's*	1 Pack/310g	223	3.4	72	1.5	13.9	1.1	0.6
Vegetable, Oriental Mix, Tesco*	½ Pack/126g	88	4.4	70	2.6	5.7	3.5	2.7
Vegetable, Rainbow, Fresh Tastes, Asda*	½ Pack/225g	119	5	53	1.8	4.6	2.2	3.8
Vegetable, Ready Prepared, M&S*	½ Pack/150g	38	0.4	25	2.2	3.5	0.3	2.2
Vegetable, Thai Style, Tesco*	½ Pack/135g	42	0.7	31	2.3	4.2	0.5	2.1
Vegetables, Co-Op*	1 Serving/80g	29	0.4	36	1.8	5	0.5	2.7
Vegetables, Frozen, Farm Foods*	1 Pack/650g	208	3.2	32	1.9	4.9	0.5	2.2
Vegetables, Mixed with Slices of Pepper, Cooked, Tesco*	½ Pack/125g	58	1.6	47	2.4	5.6	1.3	2.4
Vegetables, Superbright, Waitrose*	½ Pack/150g	129	7.2	86	3.5	4.3	4.8	5.6
STOCK								
Beef Bone, Broth, Ossa*	1 Cup/250ml	45	1.2	18	3.6	0.8	0.5	0.5
Beef, Cooks' Ingredients, Waitrose*	1 Jar/500g	110	2.5	22	3.2	0.9	0.5	0.5
Beef, Fresh, Sainsbury's*	¼ Pot/113g	27	0.6	24	5.1	0.5	0.5	0.5
Beef, Fresh, Tesco*	1 Serving/300ml	54	0.9	18	2.1	1.6	0.3	0.5
Beef, Made Up, Stock Pot, Knorr*	1 Serving/100ml	10	0.4	10	0.2	1	0.4	0
Beef, Pots, Unprepared, Sainsbury's*	1 Pot/28g	31	1.7	112	4.1	8.5	6.2	2.9
Beef, Rich, Stock Pot, Knorr*	1 Pot/28g	42	1.1	150	3	27	4	0.8
Beef, Slow Cooked, Finest, Tesco*	¼ Pouch/113ml	18	0.2	16	2	1.6	0.2	0
Chicken, As Sold, Stock Pot, Knorr*	1 Pot/28g	45	1.1	160	4	26	4	0.8
Chicken, Bone, Broth, Ossa*	1 Cup/250ml	28	1.2	11	2.6	0.2	0.5	0.5
Chicken, Concentrated, Liquid, Knorr*	1 Portion/100ml	4	0.5	4	0.5	0.5	0.5	0.5
Chicken, Concentrated, M&S*	1 Tsp/5g	16	0.9	315	25.6	12.2	18.1	0.8
Chicken, COOK!, M&S*	¼ Pack/125ml	10	0.2	8	1.4	0.1	0.2	0
Chicken, Cooks' Ingredients, Waitrose*	1 Pack/500ml	75	0.5	15	3.2	0.3	0.1	0.2
Chicken, Fresh, Sainsbury's*	½ Pot/142ml	23	0.1	16	3.7	0.1	0.1	0.3
Chicken, Fresh, Tesco*	1 Serving/300ml	27	0.3	9	1.6	0.5	0.1	0.5
Chicken, Granules, Knorr*	1 Tsp/4.5g	10	0.2	232	13.1	36.5	3.7	0.4
Chicken, Home Prepared, Average	*1fl oz/30ml*	*7*	*0.3*	*24*	*3.8*	*0.7*	*0.9*	*0.3*
Chicken, Made Up, Stock Pot, Knorr*	1 Serving/125ml	15	0.3	12	0.2	1.6	0.2	0
Chicken, Rich & Savoury, Pot, As Sold, Tesco*	1 Pot/28g	48	1.6	171	7.1	22.8	5.7	1.4
Chicken, Slow Roasted, Fresh, Extra Special, Asda*	1 Serving/100g	21	0.5	21	4.2	0.5	0.5	0.5
Fish, Home Prepared, Average	*1 Serving/250ml*	*42*	*2*	*17*	*2.3*	*0*	*0.8*	*0*
Mushroom, Pot, As Sold, Knorr*	1 Pot/28g	41	0.8	148	2.8	28	2.7	1.6
Vegetable, As Sold, Stock Pot, Knorr*	1 Serving/5g	5	0.3	100	6.2	6.4	5.3	1.3
Vegetable, Cooks Ingredients, Waitrose*	1 Pouch/500ml	15	0.5	3	0.2	0.4	0.1	0.5
Vegetable, Fresh, COOK!, M&S*	¼ Pouch/125ml	15	0.1	12	0.3	2.5	0.1	0.1
Vegetable, Granules, Knorr*	2 Tsp/9g	18	0.1	199	8.5	39.9	0.6	0.9
Vegetable, Made Up, Stock Pot, Knorr*	1 Serving/125ml	8	0.6	6	0.5	0.5	0.5	0.5
STOCK CUBES								
Beef, Dry Weight, Bovril*	1 Cube/6g	12	0.2	197	10.8	29.3	4.1	0
Beef, Dry Weight, Oxo*	1 Cube/6g	15	0.3	265	17.4	38.4	4.9	4.2

S

	Measure INFO/WEIGHT	per Measure KCAL	FAT	Nutrition Values per 100g / 100ml KCAL	PROT	CARB	FAT	FIBRE
STOCK CUBES								
Beef, Knorr*	1 Cube/10g	31	2.3	310	5	19	23	0
Beef, Knorr*	1 Cube/11ml	1	0.1	7	0.5	0.5	0.5	0.5
Beef, Made Up, Oxo*	1 Cube/189ml	17	0.4	9	0.6	1.3	0.2	0.1
Beef, Organic, Kallo*	1 Cube/12g	25	1	208	16.7	16.7	8.3	0
Beef, Reduced Salt, Made Up, Oxo*	1 Cube/500ml	45	2.5	9	0.6	1.3	0.5	0.5
Beef, Tesco*	1 Cube/7g	17	0.2	260	9.7	48.9	2.8	1.3
Chicken	*1 Cube/6g*	*14*	*0.9*	*237*	*15.4*	*9.9*	*15.4*	*0*
Chicken, Dry, Average	*1 Cube/10g*	*29*	*1.8*	*293*	*7.3*	*25.5*	*18*	*0.4*
Chicken, Dry, Oxo*	1 Cube/7g	17	0.2	249	10.9	44	3.3	0.9
Chicken, Just Bouillon, Kallo*	1 Cube/12g	30	1.3	247	11.8	26.1	10.6	1
Chicken, Knorr*	1 Cube/10g	31	2	310	4	29	20	0
Chicken, Made Up, Average	*1 Pint/568ml*	*43*	*1*	*8*	*0.4*	*1.1*	*0.2*	*0.1*
Chicken, Made Up, Sainsbury's*	1 Cube/200ml	16	0.2	8	0.3	1.4	0.1	0.1
Chicken, Organic, As Sold, Kallo*	1 Stock Cube/11g	35	2	318	4.6	36.4	18.2	4.6
Chicken, Prepared, Oxo*	1 Cube/100ml	9	0.1	9	0.4	1.5	0.1	0.1
Chicken, Reduced Salt, Dry, Oxo*	1 Cube/7g	22	0.3	321	14.6	54.9	3.9	2.8
Chicken, Reduced Salt, Prepared, Oxo*	1 Cube/500ml	50	2.5	10	0.5	1.7	0.5	0.5
Chicken, Tesco*	1 Cube/11g	32	2.5	290	10.5	11.1	22.6	0.7
Chicken, Value, Tesco*	1 Cube/10g	15	0.6	150	9.4	14.3	5.9	0.8
Fish, Knorr*	1 Cube/10g	32	2.4	321	8	18	24	1
Fish, Sainsbury's*	1 Cube/11g	31	2.2	282	19.1	7.3	20	0.9
Ham, Knorr*	1 Cube/10g	31	1.9	313	11.8	24.4	18.7	0
Lamb, Made Up, Knorr*	1 Serving/100ml	5	0.6	5	0.3	0.3	0.6	0.1
Vegetable, Average	*1 Cube/7g*	*18*	*1.2*	*253*	*13.5*	*11.6*	*17.3*	*0*
Vegetable, Bouillon, Vegetarian, Amoy*	1 Cube/10g	30	2	300	0	20	20	0
Vegetable, Bouillon, Yeast Free, Made Up, Marigold*	1 Serving/250ml	19	1.6	8	0	0.5	0.6	0
Vegetable, Dry, Oxo*	1 Cube/6g	17	0.3	251	10.4	41.4	4.9	1.4
Vegetable, Knorr*	1 Cube/10g	33	2.4	330	10	25	24	1
Vegetable, Low Salt, Organic, Made Up, Kallo*	1 Serving/500ml	50	3.5	10	0.3	0.7	0.7	0.2
Vegetable, Made Up, Organic, Kallo*	2 Cubes/100ml	7	0.4	7	0.1	0.5	0.4	0.1
Vegetable, Made up, Oxo*	1 Cube/500ml	40	2.5	8	0.5	1.3	0.5	0.5
Vegetable, Organic, Yeast Free, Dry, Kallo*	1 Cube/11g	37	3.1	334	11.4	8.2	27.8	2.3
Vegetable, Value, Tesco*	1 Cube/10g	14	0.3	145	10.6	17.4	3.3	3.6
STOLLEN								
Bites, Marzipan, Holly Lane, Aldi*	1 Bite/27g	111	4.8	412	5.9	55	18	1.9
Bites, with Jamaican Rum, Aldi*	1 Bite/23g	92	4.4	400	6.2	51	19	2.4
STOVIES								
Chef Select, Lidl*	1 Pack/412g	346	3.7	84	4.6	13	0.9	2.9
STRAWBERRIES								
Dried, Urban Fresh Fruit*	1 Pack/35g	111	0.1	318	1.6	77	0.4	5.9
Fresh, Raw, Average	*1 Berry/12g*	*3*	*0*	*28*	*0.8*	*6*	*0.1*	*1.4*
Frozen, Average	*1 Serving/100g*	*30*	*0.2*	*30*	*0.8*	*6.3*	*0.2*	*1*
in Fruit Juice, Canned, Average	*1/3 Can/127g*	*58*	*0*	*46*	*0.4*	*11*	*0*	*1*
in Syrup, Canned, Average	*1 Serving/100g*	*63*	*0*	*63*	*0.4*	*15.2*	*0*	*0.6*
STROGANOFF								
Beef, & Rice, Charlie Bigham's*	1 Serving/395 g	675	34.8	171	8.5	13.1	8.8	0
Beef, & Rice, TTD, Sainsbury's*	1 Pack/410g	595	20.9	145	9.6	15.2	5.1	1.7
Beef, 604, Wiltshire Farm Foods*	1 Serving/360g	466	22	129	6	11	6.1	0
Beef, Asda*	1 Serving/120g	276	20.4	230	16	3.3	17	0.6
Beef, Creamy, COOK!, M&S*	½ Pack/250g	292	17	117	10.3	3.5	6.8	0
Beef, Finest, Tesco*	½ Pack/200g	330	13.4	165	9.4	16.2	6.7	0.7
Beef, Slow Cooked, Cream & Brandy Sauce, Sainsbury's*	½ Pack/239g	320	14.3	134	17.2	2.4	6	0.8
Beef, Steak, & Wild Rice, Slow Cooked, TTD, Sainsbury's*	1 Pack/450g	662	32.8	147	6.3	13.2	7.3	1.5

S

	Measure INFO/WEIGHT	per Measure KCAL	FAT	Nutrition Values per 100g / 100ml KCAL	PROT	CARB	FAT	FIBRE
STROGANOFF								
Beef, with White & Wild Rice, Heated, Finest, Tesco*	1 Pack/426g	591	21.3	139	10.3	12	5	2.2
Chicken, with Rice, BGTY, Sainsbury's*	1 Pack/415g	448	5.4	108	7	17.1	1.3	1.1
Mushroom, Co-Op*	1 Pack/350g	444	15.4	127	3.3	18	4.4	1.6
Mushroom, Eat Smart, Morrisons*	1 Pack/400g	312	4.4	78	2.6	14.3	1.1	1
Mushroom, Portobello, Charred, Finest, Tesco*	½ Pack/164g	207	14.9	126	3.9	6.1	9.1	2.2
Mushroom, Roasted, Plant Kitchen, M&S*	1 Pack/350g	252	14.3	72	2.9	5.4	4.1	0.5
Mushroom, with Rice, BGTY, Sainsbury's*	1 Serving/450g	418	6.8	93	3.3	16.6	1.5	1
Pork, Classic Kitchen, Tesco*	½ Pack/222g	284	13.5	128	12.9	4.6	6.1	1.2
STRUDEL								
Apple & Mincemeat, Tesco*	1 Serving/100g	322	16.7	322	3.3	39.6	16.7	2
Apple with Sultanas, Tesco*	1/6 Strudel/100g	245	12	245	2.9	30.9	12	0.7
Apple, Co-Op*	1 Slice/100g	225	12	225	3	28	12	3
Apple, Ovenbaked, CBY, Asda*	1 Slice/100g	249	12	249	2.7	31.6	12	1.7
Apple, Plum & Custard, Heavenly Desserts, Aldi*	1/6 Strudel/94g	265	13.2	282	4	35	14	2
Apple, Sainsbury's*	1 Serving/90g	233	11.7	259	2.8	31.6	13	1.9
Apple, Tesco*	1 Serving/94g	226	11.6	241	2.6	28.9	12.4	1.7
Berry, Frozen, Tesco*	1 Serving/94g	220	9.9	234	2.7	31.2	10.5	1.9
STUFFING								
Olde English Chestnut, Sainsbury's*	1 Serving/110g	216	12.8	196	9.4	13.5	11.6	2.1
Pork, Chestnut & Onion, Cooked, Finest, Tesco*	1/8 Pack/41g	108	6.9	263	12.9	13.6	16.8	2.4
Pork, Cranberry, Sage & Onion, Tesco*	2 Balls/82g	140	4.2	170	11.3	18.5	5.1	2.3
Pork, with Chestnuts & Leek, Waitrose*	1 Serving/100g	192	8.8	192	12.5	14.9	8.8	1.3
Sage & Onion with Lemon, Paxo*	1 Serving/50g	61	0.6	122	3.4	24.2	1.2	1.9
Sage & Onion, for Chicken, Paxo*	1 Serving/50g	60	0.6	120	3.4	22.8	1.3	1.7
Sausagemeat, Pork, Gourmet, British, Cooked, Waitrose*	1 Serving/59g	134	6.4	229	20	12.7	10.9	0.5
Sausagemeat, Sainsbury's*	1 Serving/100g	175	4.2	175	7	27	4.2	2.3
STUFFING BALLS								
British Pork, Sage & Onion, Cooked, Finest, Tesco*	2 Balls/49g	110	5	224	13.9	17.4	10.2	2.2
Pork, Sage, & Onion, Sainsbury's*	1 Ball/24g	63	4.4	258	12	11	18	2.2
Pork, Sausagemeat, Aunt Bessie's*	1 Ball/26g	55	2.1	212	7.2	27.3	8.2	3
Sage & Onion, Aunt Bessie's*	1 Ball/26g	60	1.6	229	5.5	39	6.3	3.1
STUFFING MIX								
Apple & Herb, Special Recipe, Sainsbury's*	1 Serving/41g	68	0.9	165	3.8	32.4	2.2	2.2
Apple, & Herb, Made Up, Tesco*	1 Serving/50g	87	0.8	173	3.6	34.7	1.5	3.3
Apricot & Walnut, Made Up, Celebrations, Paxo*	1 Serving/50g	80	1.8	161	4.3	28	3.5	2.8
Chestnut & Cranberry, Celebration, Paxo*	1 Serving/25g	35	0.5	141	4	26.7	2	2.4
Chestnut, Morrisons*	1 Serving/20g	33	0.7	165	4.6	29.1	3.4	3.7
Dry, Average	*1 Serving/25g*	*84*	*1*	*338*	*9.6*	*70.1*	*3.8*	*5.3*
Garlic, & Herb, Tesco*	1 Serving/50g	90	1.3	179	4.7	32.8	2.6	2.8
Parsley, Thyme & Lemon, Sainsbury's*	1 Pack/170g	240	2.2	141	4.2	28.2	1.3	1.3
Sage & Onion, Asda*	1 Ball/30g	56	0.7	187	5.3	35	2.2	3.4
Sage & Onion, Co-Op*	1 Serving/28g	94	0.6	335	10	68	2	6
Sage & Onion, Prepared, Tesco*	1 Serving/100g	50	0.4	50	1.5	10.1	0.4	0.9
Sage & Onion, Dry Weight, Tesco*	1 Std Pack/170g	578	4.1	340	10.3	69.3	2.4	6.3
Sage & Onion, Dry, Asda*	1 Serving/11g	56	0.7	527	15.1	94.1	6.6	9.4
Sage & Onion, M&S*	1 Serving/30g	108	1	359	11.4	67.8	3.4	6
Sage & Onion, with Apple, Made Up, Paxo*	1 Serving/50g	69	0.8	138	3.8	26	1.6	2.2
Sausage Meat, Morrisons*	1 Serving/20g	35	0.5	174	6.8	30.8	2.6	2.9
SUBS								
Chicken Salad, Tesco*	1 Pack/205g	367	12.5	179	10.5	18.8	6.1	3.4
Pizza, Cheese, & Tomato, Iceland*	1 Sub/135g	302	10.4	224	10.8	26.3	7.7	3.2
SUET								
Beef, Tesco*	1 Serving/100g	854	91.9	854	0.6	6.2	91.9	0.1

S

	Measure INFO/WEIGHT	per Measure KCAL	FAT	Nutrition Values per 100g / 100ml KCAL	PROT	CARB	FAT	FIBRE
SUET								
Vegetable, Average	*1oz/28g*	*234*	*24.6*	*836*	*1.2*	*10.1*	*87.9*	*0*
SUGAR								
Brown, Soft, Average	*1 Tsp/4g*	*15*	*0*	*382*	*0*	*96.5*	*0*	*0*
Brown, Soft, Light, Average	*1 Tsp/5g*	*20*	*0*	*393*	*0.2*	*97.8*	*0.1*	*0*
Caster, Average	*1 Tsp/5g*	*20*	*0*	*399*	*0*	*99.8*	*0*	*0*
Dark Brown, Muscovado, Average	*1 Tsp/7g*	*27*	*0*	*380*	*0.2*	*94.8*	*0*	*0*
Dark Brown, Soft, Average	*1 Tsp/5g*	*18*	*0*	*369*	*0.1*	*92*	*0*	*0*
Demerara, Average	*1 Tsp/5g*	*18*	*0*	*368*	*0.2*	*99.2*	*0*	*0*
Golden, Unrefined, Average	*1 Tsp/4g*	*16*	*0*	*399*	*0*	*99.8*	*0*	*0*
Granulated, Organic, Average	*1 Tsp/4g*	*16*	*0*	*398*	*0.2*	*99.7*	*0*	*0*
Icing, Average	*1 Tsp/4g*	*16*	*0*	*394*	*0*	*102.2*	*0*	*0*
Light Or Diet, Average	*1 Tsp/4g*	*16*	*0*	*394*	*0*	*98.5*	*0*	*0*
Muscovado, Light, Average	*1 Tsp/5g*	*19*	*0*	*384*	*0*	*96*	*0*	*0*
White Plus Stevia Blend, Light at Heart, Tate & Lyle*	1 Serving/2g	8	0	398	0	99.6	0	0
White, Granulated, Average	*1 Tsp/5g*	*20*	*0*	*398*	*0*	*100*	*0*	*0*
SULTANAS								
Average	*1oz/28g*	*82*	*0.1*	*291*	*2.8*	*69.2*	*0.4*	*2*
SUNDAE								
Blackcurrant, M&S*	1 Sundae/53g	212	10.2	400	3	54.2	19.2	1.9
Caramel, From Restaurant, Average	*1 Sundae/155g*	*304*	*9.3*	*196*	*4.7*	*31.8*	*6*	*0*
Chocolate & Vanilla, HL, Tesco*	1 Sundae/120g	193	3.1	161	2.8	31.5	2.6	0.6
Chocolate & Vanilla, Tesco*	1 Sundae/70g	140	6	199	2.8	27.5	8.6	0.5
Chocolate Brownie, Tesco*	1 Pot/136g	271	15	199	5.2	18.8	11	1.9
Chocolate Mint, COU, M&S*	1 Pot/90g	108	2.3	120	5.4	17.8	2.6	0.5
Chocolate Nut	*1 Serving/70g*	*195*	*10.7*	*278*	*3*	*34.2*	*15.3*	*0.1*
Chocolate, Double, Belgian, COU, M&S*	1 Pot/130g	170	3.2	131	3.6	23.1	2.5	0.8
Chocolate, Sainsbury's*	1 Pot/140g	393	29.8	281	2.5	19.3	21.3	0.6
Hot Fudge, Two Scoop, Baskin Robbins*	1 Serving/203g	530	29	261	3.9	30.5	14.3	0
Ice Cream	*1 Serving/170g*	*482*	*15.4*	*284*	*5.9*	*45.3*	*9.1*	*0.3*
Strawberry & Vanilla, Tesco*	1 Serving/68g	120	3.9	177	2	29.5	5.7	0.1
Strawberry, M&S*	1 Sundae/45g	173	8	385	3.4	53.3	17.8	1
Toffee & Vanilla, Tesco*	1 Serving/70g	133	4.5	189	2.1	30.7	6.4	0.1
Toffee, Asda*	1 Serving/120g	322	19.2	268	2.1	29	16	0
Toffee, Good Puds, M Kitchen, Morrisons*	1 Pot/138g	268	13.4	194	3.6	22.9	9.7	0.4
Toffee, Sainsbury's*	1 Sundae/140g	378	27.2	270	3.1	20.2	19.4	0.9
Vanilla Caramel, Aldi*	1 Sundae/72g	159	7.4	221	2.6	29.2	10.3	0.7
SUPPLEMENT								
6 Protein Blend, Ultra Premium, Hexapro*	1 Serving/44g	180	4	409	56.8	22.7	9.1	9.1
Apple Fibre, 100%, Myprotein*	2 Sm Scoops/5g	22	0	440	0	90	0	40
Blackcurrant, Flaxseed, & Cacao, Ceres Organic*	1 Serving/30g	146	11	485	17.5	9.4	36.8	26.1
Chocolate, Forever Lite, Ultra, Powder, Forever Living*	1 Scoop/25g	90	1	360	68	16	4	4
Drink, Daily Biobasics, Life Plus*	2 Scoops/26g	66	0	252	50	0	0	61
Drink, Protein, Recovery, Strawberries & Cream, Torq*	4 Scoops/100g	358	0.2	358	22	66.4	0.2	0
Fibre Force, Holland & Barrett*	1 Capsule/1g	2	0	250	0	50	0	70
Fibre, Powder, Benefibre*	1 Tsp/3.2g	6	0	200	0.5	15	0	85
Flavdrops, All Flavours, Myprotein*	1 Drop/1ml	0	0	0	0	0	0	0
Go Hydro, Lemon Flavour, Science in Sport*	1 Tablet/4g	9	0	200	0	19	0	4.4
Green Apple, Vitamin Drink, Low Calorie, Vit Hit*	1 Serving/100ml	8	0.1	8	0.1	1.4	0.1	0.1
GU Energy Gel, Chocolate Outrage, TCL Sports*	1 Pack/32g	100	2	312	0	62.5	6.2	0
GU Energy Gel, Vanilla Bean, TCL Sports*	1 Pack/32g	100	0	312	0	78.1	0	0
High Protein Powder, Sanatogen*	2 Tsp/7g	25	0.1	360	81	5.8	1.2	0
Hypotonic Electrolyte Drink, Tangerine , Torq*	1 Stick/18g	62	0	342	0	85	0	0
Inulin, Powder, Bulk Powders*	1 Serving/5g	10	0	210	0	8	0	89

S

SUPPLEMENT	Measure INFO/WEIGHT	per Measure KCAL	FAT	Nutrition Values per 100g / 100ml KCAL	PROT	CARB	FAT	FIBRE
Inulin, Powder, Pure, SimplyGo*	1 Scoop/5g	10	0	210	0	8	0	89
Lupin, Flakes, Lupin*	1 Serving/40g	129	2.6	323	42	4	6.4	37
Powder, Energy Elixir, Alchemy*	1 Serving/10g	33	0.4	330	31	32	3.5	21
Protein Powder, Vegan, Neat Nutrition *	1 Sachet/35g	131	2.2	374	70.6	6	6.3	4.6
Protein Shake, Coconut, Purition*	1 Serving/40g	192	12.8	480	41	7.8	32	17.2
Protein Shake, Macadamia & Vanilla, Purition*	1 Serving/40g	198	14	495	39.1	8.6	35	15.6
Protein Shake, Protein Haus*	1 Bottle/330ml	275	8	83	7.2	5.7	2.4	0
Protein Shake, Pumpkin Spice, Puriton*	1 Serving/40g	187	12.4	467	41.2	7.7	31	15.7
Protein Shake, Vegan Hemp, Chocolate, Purition*	1 Serving/40g	194	12.1	484	35.4	11.3	30.3	27.3
Protein, Rice, Pulsin*	1 Serving/10g	43	1	435	80.6	4.4	9.9	2.8
Protein, Total Gainer, Myprotein*	1 Serving/100g	411	9.8	411	34.7	46	9.8	3.3
Protein, Vanilla, Multitasker, Missfits*	1 Sachet/25g	76	0.1	304	61.2	13.2	0.3	2
Protein, Vanilla, Powder, Vivo alkaline complete *	1 Scoop/40g	165	4	412	73	7.5	10	0
Psyllium Husk, Average	**1 Tsp/5g**	**19**	**0**	**377**	**0.4**	**89**	**0.4**	**58**
Psyllium Husk, Capsules, Solgar*	1 Capsule/1g	2	0	200	0	50	0	50
Psyllium Husk, NaturaleBio*	1 Serving/10g	19	0	191	1	2.2	0.2	88.3
Psyllium Husk, Organic, Planete Au Naturel*	1 Tsp/5g	0	0	10	0.9	0.2	0.6	85
Psyllium Husk, Organic, Powder, Sevenhills Wholefoods*	1 Tsp/5g	15	0.3	301	0.2	34.8	6	53.5
Psyllium Husk, Raw, Nutriseed*	1 Tsp/5g	9	0	189	1.5	0.1	0.6	89
Shake, Chocolate, Low Carb, Atkins*	1 Serving/33g	137	5.2	411	54.5	9.3	15.6	9
Shake, Protein, Diet, Slimzest*	1 Scoop/30g	114	1.2	380	80	6	4	0
Shake, Strawberry, Dairy Free, Powder, Purition*	1 Serving/40g	156	11.2	391	36.5	16.1	28	17.2
Shake, Triple Protein, Vanilla, Life Plus*	1 Scoop/27g	91	0.8	336	73.8	3.7	3	0.7
Soya Protein Isolate Powder, Holland & Barrett*	1 Scoop/28g	109	1.3	391	86.6	1	4.5	0
Superfood, Fibre Blend, Organic, Cleanse, Neal's Yard*	1 Scoop/5g	12	0.2	236	7	41	4	50
Tablet, Berocca*	1 Tablet/4.5g	5	0	109	0	5.7	0.1	0
Total Superfood, Powder, Nutriseed*	1 Serving/10g	40	1.7	405	22.2	29.2	17.1	18.3
Vegan, Superfood Blend, Myprotein*	1 Serving/38g	135	2.7	354	41	22	7	19
Whey Protein, Chocolate, Mo protein*	2 Scoops/45g	177	2.7	393	75.6	6.9	6	1.6
Whey protein, Holland & Barrett*	1 Serving/24g	94	1.9	392	73.3	7.1	7.9	0
Whey Protein, Select, Rebuild, USN*	1 Scoop/28g	115	2.6	411	71.4	11.8	9.3	0.4
Whey, Chocolate, White, Diet, PhD Nutrition*	1 Serving/50g	195	2.5	390	70	12.5	5	3.7
Whey, High Protein, Cookies & Cream, Whey Box*	1 Serving/20g	82	1.7	411	70	13	8.7	3.3
SUSHI								
California Roll, Selection, M&S*	1 Pack/159g	234	5.6	147	5.4	22.6	3.5	1.6
California Rolls 8 Pack	**1 Pack/206g**	**354**	**9.3**	**172**	**5.1**	**27.5**	**4.5**	**1.4**
California Set, Waitrose*	1 Pack/120g	223	9.1	186	3.8	25.2	7.6	1.7
Californian Roll & Nigiri, Selection, M&S*	1 Pack/215g	355	5.8	165	7.1	28	2.7	1.1
Chicken & Duck, Asian Inspired, Selection, Tesco*	1 Pack/205g	333	6.3	163	4.4	28.9	3.1	0.7
Chicken, & Duck, Hoisin, Selection, Asda*	1 Pack/167g	278	4.5	166	5	30	2.7	1.3
Chicken, Katsu, Tesco*	1 Pack/76g	122	2.6	161	4.4	27.4	3.4	1.5
Classic, My Sushi, Lidl*	1 Pack/200g	328	42	164	4.7	31.5	21	0
Dragon Roll, Firecracker Prawn, M&S*	1 Pack/166g	224	4.5	135	4.2	22.9	2.7	0.9
Duck, & Chicken, Eat & Go, Aldi*	1 Pack/125g	178	0.9	142	4.3	29	0.7	1
Fish Roll, Nigiri & Maki Selection, M&S*	1 Pack/210g	315	4.8	150	6.5	25.8	2.3	1
Fish Selection, Large, Tesco*	1 Pack/218g	365	6.8	167	5.3	29	3.1	0.9
Fish, Selection, Asda*	1 Pack/153g	242	2.6	158	5.3	30	1.7	0.6
Fish, Snack Pack, On the Go, Sainsbury's*	1 Pack/96g	150	2.4	156	5.5	27.3	2.5	1.2
Fish, Snack, Tesco*	1 Pack/104g	159	2.6	153	4.5	28	2.5	1.5
Hosomaki, Vegan, Morrisons*	1 Pack/140g	220	1.7	158	3	33	1.2	1.5
Komachi Set with Salmon, Whiting & Handroll, Waitrose*	1 Pack/257g	447	13.9	174	5.3	25.8	5.4	1.2
Naniwa, Box, Lidl*	1 Pack/190g	262	3.8	138	4.6	25	2	0.6
Nigiri Set, Taiko, Salmon & Tuna, Waitrose*	1 Pack/113g	174	2.3	154	6.3	26	2	0.6

S

	Measure INFO/WEIGHT	per Measure KCAL	FAT	Nutrition Values per 100g / 100ml KCAL	PROT	CARB	FAT	FIBRE
SUSHI								
Rolls, Veggie, Snack, Shapers, Boots*	1 Pack/66g	93	0.6	141	3.5	28.8	0.9	1.4
Salmon & Roll Set, Sainsbury's*	1 Serving/101g	167	2.6	165	4.9	30.4	2.6	0.8
Salmon & Avocado Roll, with Edamame Salad, Tanpopo*	1 Pack/160g	286	9.9	179	6.9	26.3	6.2	1.5
Salmon & Prawn, Nigiri, M&S*	1 Pack/125g	186	1.4	149	7	27.2	1.1	1
Salmon & Tuna, Tesco*	1 Pack/151g	248	5.6	164	6.9	25.6	3.7	0.5
Salmon Wrap, Taiko Foods*	1 Pack/200g	284	4.6	142	5.1	24.8	2.3	0
Salmon, Smoked, Snack Pack, Tesco*	1 Pack/69g	114	1.9	165	5	29.1	2.7	0.9
Snack Box, with Soy Sauce, Eat Well, M&S*	1 Box/78g	115	1.1	147	4.5	28.8	1.4	0.6
Taiko, California, Waitrose*	1 Pack/140g	246	10.1	176	4.1	22	7.2	4.1
Taiko, Fuji Set, Waitrose*	1 Pack /332g	515	10	155	5	28	3	1
Tuna, to Snack Selection, Food to Go, M&S*	1 Serving/150g	225	3.9	150	5.2	26.4	2.6	2.3
Vegetable Selection Pack, M&S*	1 Pack/154g	215	2.8	140	2.8	28.1	1.8	1.3
Vegetable, Box, Select & Go*	1 Serving/210g	212	9.4	101	3.8	25.4	4.5	1.6
Vegetable, Mixed, Pick & Mix, Snack Pack, Tesco*	1 Pack/85g	132	2	155	3.7	28.6	2.4	1.4
Vegetable, Morrisons*	1 Pack/75g	126	2.9	168	3.4	29.2	3.9	1.4
Vegetable, Selection, Aldi*	1 Pack/149g	238	5.1	160	3.1	29	3.4	1.1
Vegetable, Taster, Co-Op*	1 Pack/68g	118	3.5	174	3.8	27.9	5.2	1
Vegetarian with Pickled Vegetables, Waitrose*	1 Pack/135g	244	4.9	181	5	27.8	3.6	1.7
Vegetarian, Snack Selection, Tesco*	1 Pack/85g	106	2.8	125	3.7	20.1	3.3	0.6
Yo!, Bento Box, Sainsbury's*	1 Pack/208g	530	6.2	255	8.4	48.7	3	0.9
SWEDE								
Boiled, Average	*1oz/28g*	*3*	*0*	*11*	*0.3*	*2.3*	*0.1*	*0.7*
Raw, Flesh Only, Peeled	*1 Serving/100g*	*24*	*0.3*	*24*	*0.7*	*5*	*0.3*	*1.6*
Raw, Unprepared, Average	*1oz/28g*	*5*	*0.1*	*18*	*0.7*	*3.8*	*0.3*	*1.6*
SWEET & SOUR								
Chicken, & Noodles, Chinese Takeaway, Tesco*	1 Pack/350g	350	0.7	100	5.7	18.8	0.2	0.2
Chicken, Balls, Chinese Takeaway, Iceland*	1 Pack/255g	311	3.3	122	9.9	17.5	1.3	6
Chicken, Breaded, Fried, From Restaurant, Average	*6 Pieces/130g*	*346*	*18*	*266*	*13*	*22.3*	*13.8*	*0*
Chicken, Chinese Favourites Box, M&S*	½ Pack/125g	146	0.8	117	8.1	19.3	0.6	1.1
Chicken, Chinese Takeaway, Sainsbury's*	1 Pack/264g	515	16.9	195	13.1	21.3	6.4	1
Chicken, Crispy, with Sweet & Sour Sauce, Tesco*	½ Pack/165g	354	16.7	214	11.1	19.3	10.1	1
Chicken, in Batter, Cantonese, Chilled, Sainsbury's*	1 Pack/350g	560	21	160	8.9	22.4	6	0.9
Chicken, M&S*	1 Pack/300g	465	10.8	155	6.6	24.4	3.6	0.8
Chicken, with Egg Fried Rice, Chilled, HL, Tesco*	1 Pack/400g	388	4	103	6.9	15.5	1.1	1.9
Chicken, with Noodles, Steamed, HE, Tesco*	1 Pack/370g	289	0.7	78	8.3	10.8	0.2	0.6
Chicken, with Rice, 233, Oakhouse Foods Ltd*	1 Meal/400g	544	12	136	6.3	20.7	3	0.6
Chicken, with Rice, Chilled, BGTY, Sainsbury's*	1 Pack/400g	344	3.6	86	6	13.5	0.9	1
Chicken, with Rice, Weight Watchers, Heinz*	1 Pack/310g	360	3.1	116	5.2	21.2	1	0.4
Chicken, without Batter, Cantonese, Chilled, Sainsbury's*	1 Pack/350g	410	4.9	117	8.5	17.6	1.4	1
Pork	*1oz/28g*	*48*	*2.5*	*172*	*12.7*	*11.3*	*8.8*	*0.6*
Pork, Battered, Sainsbury's*	½ Pack/175g	306	8.8	175	7.3	25.1	5	0.6
Sweet & Sour, Stir Fry, Aldi*	½ Pack/199g	310	10.5	156	13	13	5.3	1.2
Sweet & Sour, with Rice, Counted, Morrisons*	1 Pack/303g	358	2.1	118	6.7	20.4	0.7	1.4
Sweet & Sour, with Rice, Oh So Lean*	1 Pack/400g	106	0.8	27	0.8	5.8	0.2	0.5
with Long Grain Rice, Rice Time, Uncle Ben's*	1 Pot/300g	393	2.4	131	1.9	28.4	0.8	0.7
SWEET POTATO								
Baked, Flesh Only, Average	*1 Med/130g*	*150*	*0.5*	*115*	*1.6*	*27.9*	*0.4*	*2.8*
Boiled in Salted Water, Average	*1 Med/200g*	*168*	*0.6*	*84*	*1.1*	*20.5*	*0.3*	*2.3*
Mash, Frozen, As Consumed, Aunt Bessie's*	1 Serving/80g	70	1.1	88	0.8	17	1.4	2.3
Mash, Tesco*	½ Pack/200g	181	3.6	90	1.4	16	1.8	2.2
Puffs, Frozen, Alexia*	1 Serving/84g	140	4.5	167	1.2	27.4	5.4	3.5
Raw, Peeled, Average	*1 Sm/130g*	*112*	*0.1*	*86*	*1.6*	*20.1*	*0*	*2.1*
Raw, Unprepared, Average	*1 Potato/200g*	*174*	*0.6*	*87*	*1.2*	*21.3*	*0.3*	*3*

	Measure INFO/WEIGHT	per Measure KCAL	FAT	Nutrition Values per 100g / 100ml KCAL	PROT	CARB	FAT	FIBRE
SWEET POTATO								
Steamed, Average	*1 Med/200g*	*168*	*0.6*	*84*	*1.1*	*20.4*	*0.3*	*2.3*
Wedges, Chilled, Cooked, Sainsbury's*	½ Pack/150g	150	3	100	1.7	17.1	2	3.4
Wedges, Eat Well, M&S*	½ Pack/150g	123	2.2	82	1.4	14.5	1.5	2.6
Wedges, Sainsbury's*	1 Serving/125g	186	6.2	149	2.2	21.8	5	3.9
Wedges, Spicy & Zesty Chilli & Lime, Waitrose*	½ Pack/195g	205	7	105	1.3	15.2	3.6	3.5
SWEETBREAD								
Lamb, Fried	*1oz/28g*	*61*	*3.2*	*217*	*28.7*	*0*	*11.4*	*0*
SWEETCORN								
Baby, Frozen, Average	*1oz/28g*	*7*	*0.1*	*24*	*2.5*	*2.7*	*0.4*	*1.7*
Boiled, Average	*1oz/28g*	*31*	*0.6*	*111*	*4.2*	*19.6*	*2.3*	*2.2*
Canned with Sugar & Salt, Average	*1 Lge Can/340g*	*369*	*4*	*108*	*3.2*	*21.5*	*1.2*	*1.9*
Frozen, Average	*1 Serving/80g*	*84*	*1.7*	*105*	*3.8*	*17.9*	*2.1*	*1.8*
No Sugar & Salt, Canned, Average	*½ Can/125g*	*99*	*1.3*	*79*	*2.7*	*15*	*1.1*	*1.6*
with Peppers, Canned, Average	*1 Serving/50g*	*40*	*0.2*	*79*	*2.6*	*16.4*	*0.3*	*0.6*
SWEETENER								
Calorie Free, Truvia*	1 Sachet/1.5g	0	0	0	0	99	0	0
Canderel*	1 Tbsp/2g	8	0	379	24.7	7	0	5.3
Canderel, Spoonful, Canderel*	1 Tsp/0.5g	2	0	384	2.9	93	0	0
Erythritol, 100%, Pure Via*	1 Tsp/5g	0	0	0	0	100	0	0
Granulated, Low Calorie, Splenda*	1 Tsp/0.5g	2	0	391	0	97.7	0	0
Granulated, Silver Spoon*	1 Tsp/0.5g	2	0	387	1	96.8	0	0
Granulated, Tesco*	1 Tsp/1g	4	0	383	1.8	94	0	0
Lucuma Powder, Navitas*	1 Tbsp/15g	60	0	400	6.7	86.7	0	0
Natural Syrup, Fruit, Dark, Sweet Freedom*	1 Tsp/5g	13	0	292	0	79	0	0
Silver Spoon*	1 Tablet/0.1g	0	0	325	10	71	0	0
Stevia Leaf, Granules, Pure Via*	1 Tsp/5g	0	0	2	0	99	0.5	0
Stevia, & Erythritol, Nkd Living*	1 Tsp/5g	0	0	0	0	99.5	0	0
Stevia, Sweet, Crystal, Stevia Sweet*	1 Tsp/5g	0	0	1	0	0	0	0
Sukrin:1, Sukrin*	1 Tbsp/15g	0	0	0	0	0	0	0
Sweet' N Low*	1 Sachet/1g	3	0	368	0	92	0	0
Tablet, Average	*1 Tablet/0.1g*	*0*	*0*	*355*	*8.7*	*73*	*0*	*0.8*
Tablets, Low Calorie, Canderel*	1 Tablet/0.1g	0	0	342	13	72.4	0	0
Tablets, Splenda*	1 Tablet/0.1g	0	0	345	10	76.2	0	1.6
Tablets, Tesco*	1 Tablet/1g	0	0	20	2	2	0.5	0
The Pantry, Aldi*	1 Tsp1g	4	0	376	0.5	94	0.5	0.5
Xylosweet, Xylitol*	1 Serving/4g	10	0	240	0	100	0	0
SWEETS								
Almonds, Sugared, Dragee*	1 Sweet/4g	17	0.6	472	10	68.3	17.9	2.5
Balla Stixx, Strawberry, Haribo*	1 Stick/25g	93	0.9	373	2.7	82	3.6	0
Banana Split Eclairs, Walker's Nonsuch Ltd*	1 Serving/40g	200	8.9	501	2.7	72.4	22.2	0
Banana, Baby Foam, M&S*	1/3 Pack/34g	131	0	385	4.1	92.7	0	0
Big Purple One, Quality Street, Nestle*	1 Sweet/39g	191	9.9	490	4.7	60.5	25.5	0.7
Black Jacks & Fruit Salad, Bassett's*	1 Serving/190g	760	11.8	400	0.7	84.9	6.2	0
Blackcurrant & Liquorice, M&S*	1 Sweet/8g	32	0.3	400	0.6	89	4.3	0
Blackcurrant Liquorice, Dark, Glacier, Fox's*	1 Sweet/5g	18	0	360	0	90.1	0	0
Blueberry, Bliss, Candy Kittens*	1 Sweet/6g	20	0	335	0.8	81	0.1	0
Boiled, Spiced Pumpkin, Uncle Joe's*	1 Sweet/6g	23	0	387	0	96.4	0.2	0.1
Bon Bons, Raspberry, Tesco*	1 Serving/25g	103	1.5	411	0.1	89.3	5.9	0.5
Bon Bons, Strawberry, Classic Favourites, Asda*	1 Sweet/5g	20	0.3	402	0	88	5.6	0
Butter Candies, Original, Werther's*	1 Sweet/5g	21	0.4	424	0.1	85.7	8.9	0.1
Butter Mintoes, Dominion, Aldi*	3 Sweets/22g	93	1.7	418	0.5	87	7.8	0.5
Candy Cane, Average	*1 Cane/13g*	*50*	*0*	*386*	*0*	*96*	*0*	*0.2*
Candy Cane, Peppermint, Sainsbury's*	1 Cane/12g	48	0	386	0	96.5	0	0

S

SWEETS

INFO/WEIGHT	Measure	per Measure KCAL	FAT	Nutrition Values per 100g / 100ml KCAL	PROT	CARB	FAT	FIBRE
Candy Corn, Brachs*	19 Pieces/39g	140	0	359	0	92.3	0	0
Candy Floss, Asda*	1 Tub/75g	292	0	390	0	100	0	0
Candy Foam Shapes, Fun Fruits, Value, Tesco*	1 Serving/25g	94	0	374	3.1	90.3	0.1	0.5
Cherry Lips, Chewits*	1 Serving/100g	319	0.2	319	5.6	72.1	0.2	0
Chew	*1oz/28g*	*107*	*1.6*	*381*	*1*	*87*	*5.6*	*1*
Chewits, Blackcurrant, Leaf*	1 Chew/3g	12	0.1	385	0.2	87.5	3	0
Chewits, Cola, Leaf*	1 Chew/3g	12	0.1	385	0.2	87.5	3	0
Chewits, Fruit Salad, Leaf*	1 Chew/3g	12	0.1	385	0.2	87.5	3	0
Chewits, Strawberry, Leaf*	1 Chew/3g	12	0.1	385	0.2	87.5	3	0
Chewitts, Blackcurrant	*1 Pack/33g*	*125*	*0.9*	*378*	*0.3*	*86.9*	*2.7*	*0*
Chews, Just Fruit, Fruit-tella*	1 Serving/43g	170	2.8	400	0.9	79.5	6.5	0
Chews, Spearmint, Victoria, Aldi*	1 Sweet/10g	40	0.8	405	0.3	83.8	7.6	0
Chews, Strawberry Mix, Starburst*	1 Sweet/4g	15	0.3	401	0	83.9	7.3	0
Chewy, Vimto*	1 Pack/30g	115	0.9	384	0	88	3	0
Choco & Mint, Mentos*	1 Pack/38g	156	3.2	410	2.8	79	8.5	0
Chocolate Caramels, Milk, Tesco*	1 Sweet/3g	15	0.5	444	2.7	72.1	16.1	0.1
Chocolate Eclairs, Cadbury*	1 Sweet/8g	36	1.4	455	4.5	68.9	17.9	0
Chocolate Eclairs, Co-Op*	1 Sweet/8g	38	1.6	480	3	71	20	0.6
Chocolate Eclairs, Holland & Barrett*	1 Sweet/6g	18	0.7	306	1.8	81.9	11.3	1.4
Chocolate Limes, Pascall*	1 Sweet/8g	27	0.2	333	0.3	77.2	2.5	0
Chocolate Limes, Poundland*	1 Sweet/5g	21	0.2	414	0.5	95.5	3.3	0
Citrus Mix, Fruit Drops, Fruit-tella*	5 Sweets/12g	29	0	235	0	89	0.1	0
Cocoa & Orange, Super Bites, Truffles, Good 4u*	1 Bag/40g	153	6.1	383	10.8	46.9	15.2	7.7
Cola Bottles, Asda*	1 Serving/100g	329	0.2	329	9	73	0.2	0
Cola Bottles, Barratt*	1 Sweet/10g	34	0	337	1.3	82	0.4	0.1
Cola Bottles, Fizzy, M&S*	1 Pack/200g	650	0	325	6.4	75	0	0
Cola Bottles, Giant, Morrisons*	1 Pack/140g	469	0.1	335	8.9	74.3	0.1	0.6
Cola Sherbets, Sugar Free, Dominion, Aldi*	2 Sweets/10g	23	0	238	0.5	96	0.5	0.5
Cream Caramel, Sula*	1 Sweet/3g	10	0	297	0.4	86.1	0	0
Creamy Strawberry, Sugar Free, Dominion, Aldi*	1 Sweet/4g	11	0.2	266	0.5	87	6.2	0
Dolly Mix, Bassett's*	1 Bag/45g	171	1.4	380	3	85.1	3.1	0.4
Dolly Mixtures, M&S*	1 Pack/115g	431	1.6	375	1.8	89.2	1.4	0
Dolly Mixtures, Sainsbury's*	1 Serving/10g	40	0.2	401	1.4	94.4	1.9	0.1
Dolly Mixtures, Smart Price, Asda*	1 Sweet/3g	11	0	380	0.5	91	1.6	0
Dolly Mixtures, Tesco*	1 Pack/100g	376	1.5	376	1.6	88.9	1.5	0
Double Lolly, Swizzels Matlow*	1 Lolly/10g	41	0.3	407	0	92.4	3.4	0
Drops, Lemon & Orange, M&S*	1 Pack42g	97	0	230	0	61	0	0
Drumstick, Matlow's*	1 Pack/40g	164	2.2	409	0.4	88.3	5.5	0
Drumstick, Squashies, Swizzels*	1 Bag/160g	568	0.2	355	3.4	83.5	0.1	0
Edinburgh Rock, Gardiners of Scotland*	1 Piece/2g	8	0	380	0.1	94.4	0.3	0.8
Eton Mess, Candy Kittens*	1 Sweet/6g	20	0	340	1.4	82	0.2	0
Fizzy Belts, Multi Coloured, Dominion, Aldi*	1/3 Pack/25g	24	0.1	94	0.9	28.7	0.5	0.5
Fizzy Fish, Maynards*	4 Sweets/26g	92	0	352	0.1	87	0.1	0
Fizzy Mix, Tesco*	½ Bag/50g	166	0	332	5.2	75.2	0	0
Fizzy Pop, M&S*	1 Sweet/4g	14	0	352	0.1	88.7	0.5	0.5
Flumps, Bassett's*	1 Serving/5g	16	0	325	4	77	0	0
Flumps, Fluffy Mallow Twists, Fat Free, Bassett's*	1 Twist/13g	30	0	230	4.1	77.1	0	0
Flying Saucers, Tesco*	½ Pack/9g	34	0.1	380	1.3	90.8	1	1.2
Foamy Mushrooms, Chewy, Asda*	1 Sweet/2.6g	9	0	347	4.2	82	0.2	0
Fruit Gums & Jellies	*1 Tube/33g*	*107*	*0*	*324*	*6.5*	*79.5*	*0*	*0*
Fruit, Mentos*	1 Sweet/3g	10	0	333	0	100	0	0
Fruity Chews, Starburst*	1 Sweet/8g	34	0.6	404	0	83.4	7.4	0
Fruity Frogs, Rowntree's*	1 Serving/40g	128	0.1	321	4.7	74.5	0.2	0

S

SWEETS

INFO/WEIGHT	Measure	per Measure KCAL	per Measure FAT	Nutrition Values per 100g / 100ml KCAL	PROT	CARB	FAT	FIBRE
Fudge, Clotted Cream, Spar*	3 Sweets/30g	134	4.2	447	2	78.2	14	0.1
Go Bananas, & Monkeys, M&S*	1 Bag/70g	264	0.1	377	2.9	91.3	0.1	0.5
Gobstoppers, Everlasting, Wonka*	9 Pieces/15g	60	0	400	0	93.3	0	0
Gummy Bears	**10 Bears/25g**	**80**	**0**	**320**	**8**	**76**	**0**	**0**
Gummy Mix, Tesco*	1 Pack/100g	327	0.1	327	5.9	75.7	0.1	0
Gummy Worms	**10 Worms/74g**	**286**	**0**	**386**	**0**	**98.9**	**0**	**98.9**
Gummy Zingy Fruits, Bassett's*	1 Sm Bag/40g	135	0	337	5.1	79.2	0	0
Ice Cream Sundae, Asda*	1 Sweet/2g	9	0	387	4.9	70	0.5	0.5
Jellies, Fruit, Ringtons*	4 Jellies/44g	150	0.2	341	0.1	84	0.4	0.7
Jellies, Very Berry, Rowntrees*	1 Sweet/4g	12	0	326	5	74.8	0.2	0.1
Jelly Beans, Lucozade*	1 Pack/30g	111	0	370	0	92	0	0
Jelly Beans, Tesco*	¼ Bag/63g	243	0.2	385	0.1	94.5	0.3	0.3
Jelly Bunnies, Bassetts, Maynards*	4 Sweets/26g	87	0	330	3.5	78	0.1	0
Jelly Tots, Rowntree's*	1 Pack/42g	145	0	346	0.1	86.5	0	0
Kisses, Hershey*	1 Sweet/5g	28	1.6	561	7	59	32	0
Laces, Apple Flavour, Tesco*	5 Laces/15g	52	0.5	347	3.6	74.8	3.2	2.1
Laces, Strawberry, Sainsbury's*	1 Serving/25g	94	1.2	377	3.3	76.3	4.6	0.1
Laces, Strawberry, Tesco*	1 Serving/75g	260	2.4	347	3.6	74.8	3.2	2.1
Lances, Strawberry & Cream Flavour, Tesco*	1 Bag/75g	276	0.9	368	3.2	86.1	1.2	2.1
Lances, Strawberry Flavour, Fizzy, Tesco*	½ Pack/50g	177	1.3	354	2.8	79.8	2.6	1.8
Lemon Mint Flavour, Herb Drops, Sugar Free, Ricola*	1 Sweet/3g	7	0	235	0	96	0	0
Licorice, Sugar Free, Dominion, Aldi*	1 Serving/25g	56	0.1	224	0.5	77	0.5	1.6
Liquorice, Boiled, Sugar Free, Sula*	1 Sweet/3g	7	0	227	0.2	93	0	0.2
Liquorice, Gums, Lion*	1 Sweet/4g	14	0	351	8.5	77.7	0.6	0.7
Lovehearts, Swizzels*	1 Sweet/2g	7	0	359	0.7	88.2	0	0
Maynards Sours, Bassett's*	1 Pack/52g	169	0	325	6.1	75	0	0
Midget Gems, Co-Op*	12 Sweets/28g	100	0.1	356	0.5	89	0.5	0.5
Midget Gems, Free From Fellows*	1 Sweet/2g	4	0	217	0	81	0.3	0
Midget Gems, Maynards*	1 Sweet/1g	3	0	340	8.7	76.2	0	0
Midget Gems, Value, Tesco*	1 Serving/40g	130	0.1	324	4.5	76.1	0.2	0
Milk Chocolate Eclairs, Sainsbury's*	1 Sweet/8g	33	1.1	442	2.1	75.7	14.5	0.5
Milk Chocolate Eclairs, Value, Tesco*	1 Bag/200g	918	32.6	459	2.6	75.2	16.3	1
Milk Duds, Hershey*	13 Pieces/33g	170	6	510	3	84	18	0
Mini Gums, Sugar Free, Dominion, Aldi*	1 Serving/25g	53	0.1	213	0.5	80	0.5	0.5
Mini Macs, CBY, Asda*	1 Pack/200g	437	13.1	218	1	38.8	6.6	0
Mini Marti, Mushrooms, Asda*	1 Sweet/3g	10	0	340	3.8	81.1	0.1	0
Minions, Haribo*	½ Pack/35g	120	0.2	342	6.6	77	0.5	0
Mint Balls, Uncle Joe's*	1 Sweet/6g	24	0	393	0	97	0.5	0
Mint Humbugs, Sugar Free, Morrisons*	1 Sweet/3g	9	0.2	287	0.3	92.5	7	0
Mint, Assortment, Happy Shopper*	½ Bag/40g	138	0.6	344	0.5	82	1.6	0
Original, Chocolate Soft Caramel, Speciality, Werther's*	1 Piece/6g	30	1.5	480	5.1	61.5	23.5	1
Paradise Fruits, Dominion, Aldi*	1 Sweet/6g	23	0	382	0	95.5	0	0
Parma Violets, Swizzlers*	1 Sm Tube/10g	41	0.3	414	0	94.9	3.3	0
Pear Drops, Free From Fellows*	1 Sweet/4g	11	0	273	0	97	0	0
Pencils, Strawberry, Co-Op*	2 Pencils/16g	59	0.5	369	3.1	87.5	3.1	3.1
Percy Pig & Pals, Soft, M&S*	1 Sweet/8g	30	0	344	5.8	80	0.1	0
Pic 'n' Mix, Woolworths*	1 Serving/180g	750	6	417	0	96.7	3.3	0
Pizza, Gummi, Gummy zone*	1 Pack/23g	80	0.1	347	5.8	81	0.5	0.5
Randoms, 30% Less Sugar, Rowntree's*	9 Sweets/35g	106	0	299	5	63	0.1	13
Randoms, Rowntree's*	1 Pack/50g	164	0.2	328	4.9	75.7	0.3	0.6
Refreshers, Candyland, Barratt*	1 Tube/34g	129	0.5	380	0	89.1	1.4	0
Refreshers, Softies, Mini, Barratt*	1 Bag/30g	107	0.2	358	3.2	85	0.6	0.5
Rhubarb & Custard, Sainsbury's*	1 Sweet/8g	28	0	351	0.1	87.7	0	0

	Measure INFO/WEIGHT	per Measure		Nutrition Values per 100g / 100ml				
		KCAL	FAT	KCAL	PROT	CARB	FAT	FIBRE
SWEETS								
Rhubarb & Custards, Tesco*	1 Sweet/8g	32	0	395	0.1	98.2	0.1	0.5
Scary Sours, Rowntree's*	1 Serving/100g	321	0	321	3.5	74.7	0	0
Sherbert Dib Dab with Strawberry Lolly, Barratt*	1 Pack/23g	90	0	385	0.1	95.6	0.1	0
Sherbert Lemons, M&S*	1 Serving/20g	76	0	380	0	93.9	0	0
Sherbet Lemons, Bassett's*	1 Sweet/7g	25	0	375	0	93.9	0	0
Shrimps & Bananas, Sainsbury's*	½ Pack/50g	188	0	376	2.5	91.3	0.1	0.5
Soft Fruits, Trebor*	1 Roll/45g	165	0	367	0	90.9	0	0
Soft Jellies, Scary Jellies, Maynards*	1 Pack/17g	54	0	321	3.1	76	0.2	0
Sour Apple Sticks, Fizzy Wizzy, Woolworths*	1 Sweet/5g	18	0.1	358	2.8	79.8	2.7	0
Sour Snakes, Organic, Biona Organic*	1 Pack/75g	257	0.1	343	0.3	84	0.1	0.3
Spogs, Average	*1 Sweet/4g*	*13*	*0*	*332*	*3.9*	*79*	*0.1*	*0*
Squidglets, Haribo*	1 Sweet/3g	11	0	339	4.5	79	0.5	0
Squidgy Babies, Haribo*	1 Serving/25g	86	0.1	346	5.7	80	0.5	0
Strawberry & Cream, Sugar Free, Diablo*	1 Sweet/4g	12	0.4	292	0.1	86.9	9.1	0
Strawberry & Cream, Sugar Free, Sula*	1 Sweet/3g	9	0.2	267	0.2	90.5	5.4	0
Strawberry Straws, Fizzy, Sainsburys*	1 Straw/8g	30	0.2	373	2.8	85	2.2	1.2
Strawberry Trunks, Bebito*	1 Stick/15g	57	0.2	381	2.1	90	1.4	0
Strawberry, Wild, Candy Kittens*	1 Sweet/6g	20	0	334	0.8	81	0.1	0
Sugar Free, Sula*	1 Sweet/3g	7	0	231	0	96.1	0	0
Tangfastics, Mini, Haribo*	1 Pack/16g	55	0.1	346	6.6	80	0.5	0
Tangfastics, Stixx, Haribo*	1 Stick/25g	95	0.8	381	1.3	87	3.3	0
Throat Pastilles, Original, Vocalzone*	1 Pastille/1g	2	0	374	0.3	92.6	0.2	0.1
Tic Tac, Cool Cherry, Ferrero*	1 Pack/18g	69	0.1	382	0.2	92.2	0.7	0
Tootsie Roll, Sm Midgees, Tootsie*	1 Sweet/7g	23	0.5	350	2.5	70	7.5	0
Tooty Frooties, Rowntree's*	1 Bag/28g	111	1	397	0.1	91.5	3.5	0
Wine Gummies, Matlow, Swizzels*	1 Pack/16g	52	0	324	0	58.7	0	0
Yo Yo's, All Flavours, 100% Fruit, We Are Bear*	1 Roll/10g	28	0	275	1.9	63.4	0.2	12
Yo Yo's, Strawberry 100% Fruit, We Are Bear*	1 Roll/10g	28	0	275	1.9	63.4	0.2	12
SWORDFISH								
Grilled, Average	*1oz/28g*	*39*	*1.5*	*139*	*22.9*	*0*	*5.2*	*0*
Raw, Average	*1oz/28g*	*42*	*2*	*149*	*21.1*	*0*	*7.2*	*0*
SYRUP								
Artificial Maple Flavour, Sugar Free, Cary's*	1 Serving/60ml	30	0	50	0	20	0	0.5
Black Forest, Premium, Monin*	1 Serving/30ml	100	0	334	0	82	0	0
Blueberry, Blackberry Patch*	1 Tbsp/15g	22	0.1	150	0.3	38.2	0.4	0
Butterscotch, Monin*	1 Serving/30ml	100	0	333	0	80	0	0
Caramel, for Coffee, Lyle's*	2 Tsps/10ml	33	0	329	0	83	0	0
Caramel, Sugar Free, Monin*	1 Serving/30ml	0	0	0	0	13.3	0	0
Chocolate Mint, Monin*	1 Serving/30ml	100	0	333	0	80	0	0
Chocolate, Smooth, The Skinny Food Co.*	1 Serving/15ml	1	0	4	0.1	0.3	0	1.2
Cinnamon, Monin*	1 Serving/30ml	100	0	333	0	80	0	0
Fire, Gold, Sukrin*	1 Serving	600	0	2000	0	8	0	69
Gingerbread, Monin*	1 Serving/30ml	90	0	300	0	76.7	0	0
Golden, Average	*1 Tbsp/20g*	*61*	*0*	*304*	*0.4*	*78.2*	*0*	*0*
Golden, Zero Calorie, The Skinny Food Co.*	1 Tbsp/15ml	1	0	4	0	0.2	0	1.1
Hazelnut, Monin*	1 Serving/30ml	90	0	300	0	73.3	0	0
Maple, Average	*1 Tbsp/20g*	*52*	*0*	*262*	*0*	*67.2*	*0.2*	*0*
Maple, Canadian, Pure, Deluxe, Lidl*	1 Tbsp/15ml	52	0	350	0.1	87.2	0.1	0
Maple, Pure, Vermont, 100%, Butternut Mountain Farm*	1 Tbsp/15ml	50	0	334	0	88	0	0
Maple, Red, Pure, Clarks*	1 Tbsp/15ml	58	0	386	0.4	95.5	0	0
Organic Rice Malt, Clearspring*	2 Tbsp/42g	133	0.2	316	1.5	76.8	0.4	0
Passion Fruit, Premium, Monin*	1 Serving/30ml	103	0	343	0	84.9	0	0
Stem Ginger, Average	*1 Tbsp/15ml*	*45*	*0*	*300*	*0*	*76.7*	*0*	*0*

S

	Measure INFO/WEIGHT	per Measure KCAL	FAT	Nutrition Values per 100g / 100ml KCAL	PROT	CARB	FAT	FIBRE

SYRUP

	Measure INFO/WEIGHT	per Measure KCAL	FAT	KCAL	PROT	CARB	FAT	FIBRE
Strawberry, Aardbeien Siroop, Plein Sud, Lidl*	1 Serving/20ml	56	0	280	0	71	0	0
Sugar	*1 Tbsp/20g*	*64*	*0*	*319*	*0*	*83.9*	*0*	*0*
Vanilla, Monin*	1 Shot/35ml	119	0	340	0	84.4	0	0
Vanilla, Sugar Free, Monin*	1 Serving/30ml	0	0	0	0	13.3	0	0
Yacon, Alovitox*	1 Tsp/5ml	7	0	140	0	80	0	0

S

	Measure INFO/WEIGHT	per Measure KCAL	FAT	Nutrition Values per 100g / 100ml KCAL	PROT	CARB	FAT	FIBRE
TABOULEH								
Average	*1oz/28g*	*33*	*1.3*	*119*	*2.6*	*17.2*	*4.6*	*0*
TACO KIT								
Crispy Chicken, Soft, Stand 'N' Stuff, Old El Paso*	1 Taco/44g	100	1.5	227	7	41.1	3.4	2.5
Enchilada, Open, Stand 'N' Stuff, Old El Paso *	1 Enchilada/50g	102	2	204	5.5	34.7	4	3.4
Garlic & Paprika, Crunchy, As Sold, Old El Paso *	1 Taco/26g	77	3.6	296	3.8	37.3	13.8	2.7
TACO SHELLS								
Corn, Crunchy, Old El Paso*	1 Taco/13g	66	3.5	509	5.4	59.2	27	3.6
Old El Paso*	1 Taco/12g	57	2.7	478	7.4	60.8	22.8	0
TAGINE								
Aubergine, Spiced, Allplants*	1 Pack/380g	429	9.5	113	3.8	17	2.5	3.1
Beef, Slow Cooked, Cook*	1 Serving/325g	462	15.6	142	13.5	11.2	4.8	1.3
Chicken, & Chickpeas, Men's Health *	1 Pack/422g	394	5.5	93	9	10.2	1.3	2.5
Chicken, Moroccan, for Two, Charlie Bigham's*	1 Serving/299 g	395	18	132	11.2	8.2	6	1.3
Chickpea, & Vegetable, Everdine*	1 Serving/450g	351	9	78	1.9	10.9	2	3.9
Chickpea, Creationz, Heinz*	½ Can/196g	176	5.1	90	4	11	2.6	3.4
Chickpea, Moroccan, Geo Organics*	½ Can/200g	172	5.2	86	3.5	10.9	2.6	2.5
Lamb, & Couscous, Finest, Tesco*	1 Pack/422g	570	16	135	7.2	17.1	3.8	1.8
Lamb, Frozen, Giraffe*	1 Pack/373g	421	8.6	113	7.1	15	2.3	1.6
Lamb, Moroccan Style with Couscous, COU, M&S*	1 Pack/400g	340	5.6	85	8.9	8.3	1.4	1.6
Lamb, Slow Cooked, M&S*	½ Pack/234g	290	9.1	124	15.6	5.8	3.9	1.6
Lamb, Spiced, with Bulgur Wheat, Weight Watchers, Heinz*	1 Pack/399g	295	6.8	74	4	9.5	1.7	2.1
Moroccan, Quorn*	1 Pack/376g	361	4.1	96	4.7	15.2	1.1	3.3
Moroccan, Veggie Bowl, Birds Eye*	1 Serving/380g	433	11.4	114	4.9	15	3	3.3
Seitan, Moroccan, with Spelt, One Pot, Soulful Food Co*	1 Pot/380g	319	4.9	84	4.5	14.7	1.3	2.5
Squash, Apricot, & Chickpeas, Sunset, Allplants*	½ Pack/380g	353	11	93	3.8	11	2.9	3.5
TAGLIATELLE								
Beef Ragu, Musclefood*	1 Pack/320g	342	7.7	107	7.2	13.3	2.4	1.9
Cooked, Co-Op*	1 Serving/150g	214	2.1	143	3.8	27	1.4	3.3
Dry, Average	*1 Serving/100g*	*356*	*1.8*	*356*	*12.6*	*72.4*	*1.8*	*1*
Egg, Dry, Average	*1 Serving/75g*	*272*	*2.5*	*362*	*14.2*	*68.8*	*3.3*	*2.3*
Egg, Fresh, Dry, Average	*1 Serving/125g*	*345*	*3.5*	*276*	*10.6*	*53*	*2.8*	*2.1*
Fresh, Dry, Average	*1 Serving/75g*	*211*	*2*	*281*	*11.4*	*53.3*	*2.6*	*2.6*
Ham & Mushroom, BGTY, Sainsbury's*	1 Pack/400g	371	7.4	95	5.1	13.8	1.9	1.2
Ham & Mushroom, Italian, Waitrose*	1 Pack/400g	585	24	151	7.1	16.3	6.2	1
Ham, & Mushroom, Creamy, Meal for One, M&S*	1 Pack/400g	636	26.8	159	7.5	16.7	6.7	0.9
Ham, & Mushroom, Sainsbury's*	1 Pack/396g	570	20.2	144	6.6	17.4	5.1	1.1
Ham, & Mushroom, Taste of Italy, Tesco*	1 Pack/450g	460	15.5	110	6.5	11.5	3.7	2.1
Lamb Ragu, Slow Cooked, Finest, Tesco*	1 Pack/400g	560	19.2	140	8.5	14.9	4.8	1.1
Verdi, Fresh, Average	*1 Serving/125g*	*171*	*1.8*	*137*	*5.5*	*25.5*	*1.5*	*1.8*
Wholewheat, Cooked, Co-Op*	1 Serving/100g	138	1.1	138	5.1	24	1.1	5.9
Wholewheat, Cooked, Morrisons*	1 Serving/150g	242	3	161	5.4	28.2	2	4.4
with Mushrooms, in Creamy Sauce, Inspirations, Birds Eye*	1 Pack/346g	613	28.1	177	4.8	20	8.1	2.5
TAHINI PASTE								
Average	*1 Tbsp/15g*	*97*	*8.9*	*649*	*23*	*8.1*	*59.3*	*8.1*
TANGERINES								
Fresh, Raw	*1 Sm/50g*	*18*	*0*	*35*	*0.9*	*8*	*0.1*	*1.3*
Fresh, Raw, Weighed with Peel, Average	*1 Med/70g*	*13*	*0.1*	*18*	*0.5*	*4.2*	*0.1*	*0.7*
TANGO*								
Cherry, Britvic*	1 Bottle/500ml	55	0	11	0	2.4	0	0
Orange, Britvic*	1 Can/330ml	63	0	19	0.1	4.4	0	0
Orange, Sugar Free, Britvic*	1 Can/330ml	13	0	4	0	0	0	0
TAPAS								
Basque Beef, Estofado Vasco, Tapas at, Tesco*	½ Pack/80g	80	3.1	100	9.5	6.4	3.9	1.5

T

	Measure INFO/WEIGHT	per Measure KCAL	FAT	Nutrition Values per 100g / 100ml KCAL	PROT	CARB	FAT	FIBRE
TAPAS								
Champinones Al Ajillo, Tapas at, Tesco*	½ Pack/85g	123	11.6	145	2.3	2.5	13.6	1.5
Chorizo & Cheese Croquettes, Tapas at, Tesco*	½ Pack/117g	263	11.1	225	5.4	28.6	9.5	2.6
TAPENADE								
Black Olive, M&S*	¼ Jar/33g	122	12.8	374	1.2	0.1	39.5	6.8
Black Olive, Specially Selected, Aldi*	1 Tbsp/20g	46	4.6	231	1.4	2.7	23	4.4
TAPIOCA								
Creamed, Ambrosia*	½ Can/213g	159	3.4	75	2.6	12.6	1.6	0.2
Raw	*1oz/28g*	*101*	*0*	*359*	*0.4*	*95*	*0.1*	*0.4*
TARAMASALATA								
Average	*1 Tbsp/30g*	*143*	*14.4*	*478*	*4.2*	*7.9*	*47.9*	*1.1*
Reduced Fat, Waitrose*	1 Pack/170g	522	48.3	307	4	8.9	28.4	1.5
TARRAGON								
Dried, Ground	*1 Tsp/2g*	*5*	*0.1*	*295*	*22.8*	*42.8*	*7.2*	*0*
Fresh, Average	*1 Tbsp/3.8g*	*2*	*0*	*49*	*3.4*	*6.3*	*1.1*	*0*
TART								
Apple & Custard, Asda*	1 Tart/84g	227	11	270	3.1	35	13.1	0.1
Apple, & Salted Caramel, Tesco*	1 Slice/83g	222	7.9	267	3.1	41.5	9.5	1.9
Bacon, Maple, & Extra Mature Cheddar, Finest, Tesco*	½ Pack/200g	642	42.8	321	10.5	21	21.4	1.4
Bakewell, Average	*1 Tart/50g*	*228*	*14.8*	*456*	*6.3*	*43.5*	*29.7*	*1.9*
Bakewell, Individual, Bakery, Tesco*	1 Tart/78g	319	13.6	409	6.3	55.5	17.5	2
Bakewell, Lemon, Average	*1 Tart/46g*	*206*	*9.7*	*447*	*3.7*	*60.9*	*21.1*	*0.9*
Blackcurrant, Sundae, Tesco*	1 Tart/55g	240	11	436	3	60	19.9	2.2
Caramel, Salted, & Chocolate, Waitrose*	1/12 Tart/79g	349	18.5	443	5.1	52.2	23.5	1.2
Chocolate, Co-Op*	1 Tart/22g	102	6.8	465	4	42	31	0.7
Chocolate, Dark, Cherry, & Pecans, Graze*	1 Pack/40g	184	10	459	4.8	57	25	6.9
Courgette, & Pecorino, Finest, Tesco*	¼ Tart/100g	302	21.6	302	5.8	20.5	21.6	1.3
Custard, Individual, Average	*1 Tart/94g*	*260*	*13.6*	*277*	*6.3*	*32.4*	*14.5*	*1.2*
Custard, Portuguese, Tesco*	1 Tart/55g	157	6	286	3.6	42.8	10.8	1.3
Date, Pecan & Almond, Sticky, Sainsbury's*	1/8 Tart/75g	298	10.3	397	5	63.5	13.7	1.7
Egg Custard, Asda*	1 Tart/80g	215	10.4	269	9	29	13	1.2
Egg Custard, Free Range, Sainsbury's*	1 Tart/85g	232	10	273	6.3	35	11.8	0.9
Egg Custard, Twin Pack, Tesco*	1 Tart/85g	229	10.5	270	6.1	33.1	12.4	0.8
Feta Cheese & Spinach, Puff Pastry, Tesco*	1 Tart/108g	306	19.2	283	7.1	23.5	17.8	0.9
Gruyere Pancetta & Balsamic Onion, Finest, Tesco*	¼ Tart/106g	320	21.9	301	7.7	21.3	20.6	3.3
Jam, Average	*1 Slice/90g*	*342*	*13.4*	*380*	*3.3*	*62*	*14.9*	*1.6*
Jam, Real Fruit, Mr Kipling*	1 Tart/35g	139	4.7	396	3.5	64.5	13.4	1.5
Jam, Real Fruit, Sainsbury's*	1 Tart/37g	142	5.2	383	3.4	60.9	14	1.4
Lemon Curd, Asda*	1 Tart/30g	121	4.5	402	2.8	64	15	2.2
Lemon Curd, Tesco*	1 Tart/30g	128	4.7	428	3.4	67	15.8	2
Lemon, & Raspberry, Finest, Tesco*	1 Tart/120g	360	16.8	300	5.2	38.4	14	2.9
Lemon, M&S*	1/6 Tart/50g	208	14.6	415	5	32.7	29.3	0.9
Lemon, Sainsbury's*	1/8 Tart/56g	258	15.8	459	4.4	47	28.1	0.6
Lemon, Zesty, Tesco*	1/6 Tart/64g	260	15.5	405	5.3	41	24.2	0.7
Mixed Fruit, Fresh, Waitrose*	1 Tart/129g	351	17.4	272	4.2	32.8	13.5	1.5
Pecan, Free From, Sainsbury's*	1 Tart/50g	239	13.2	477	4.7	54.4	26.4	1.7
Pineapple, Individual, Waitrose*	1 Tart/54g	216	6.1	400	2.2	77.2	11.3	0.5
Plum, Seriously Fruity, Waitrose*	1/6 Tart/95g	183	5.9	192	2.9	30.2	6.2	1.9
Raspberry, & Blueberry, Tesco*	1 Serving/85g	168	7.5	198	2.7	27	8.8	2.8
Spinach, & Ricotta, Individual, TTD, Sainsbury's*	1 Tart/170g	466	33.7	274	7.5	16.5	19.8	1.4
Strawberry, & Fresh Cream, Finest, Tesco*	1 Tart/129g	350	19.1	271	3.3	31.1	14.8	1.2
Strawberry, Custard, Asda*	1 Tart/100g	335	15	335	3.1	47	15	0
Strawberry, Fresh, M&S*	1 Tart/120g	305	18.4	255	3.1	26.4	15.4	2.4
Tomato, & Mascarpone, Cherry, Asda*	1 Tart/160g	290	18	181	4.4	15.6	11.2	1.1

T

	Measure INFO/WEIGHT	per Measure KCAL	FAT	Nutrition Values per 100g / 100ml KCAL	PROT	CARB	FAT	FIBRE
TART								
Tomato, & Olive, Provencale, GF, Clive's*	1 Tart/190g	361	25.1	190	2.8	13.8	13.2	0
Treacle, Average	*1 Serving/125g*	*460*	*17.6*	*368*	*3.7*	*60.4*	*14.1*	*1.1*
Treacle, with Custard	*1 Serving/251g*	*586*	*23.5*	*233*	*3.1*	*36.1*	*9.4*	*0.8*
Vegetable & Feta, Deli, M&S*	½ Tart/115g	315	18.4	274	5	20	16	6
Vegetable, Roasted, Finest, Tesco*	¼ Tart/113g	213	10.4	188	2.9	22.5	9.2	2.1
Vegetables, Bombay, with Daal, GF, Clive's*	1 Tart/191g	416	22.5	218	6	19.9	11.8	0
TARTE								
Au Chocolat, Seriously Chocolatey, Waitrose*	1/6 Tarte/70g	348	22.8	497	6	43.8	32.6	2.6
Au Citron, Frozen, TTD, Sainsbury's*	1/6 Tarte/80g	232	13.4	290	4.7	40.7	16.8	7.7
Au Citron, Waitrose*	1 Tarte/100g	325	18.1	325	4.9	35.7	18.1	1
Bacon, Leek & Roquefort, Bistro, Waitrose*	¼ Tarte/100g	277	18.2	277	8.4	19.8	18.2	0.6
Mixed Berry, Crumble, Frozen, Waitrose*	1/6 Tarte/76g	224	8.3	296	3.3	44.8	11	2.2
Tatin, 1, Waitrose*	1 Serving/50g	106	4.6	212	1.9	29.9	9.1	1.6
TARTLETS								
All Butter, Sweet, TTD, Sainsbury's*	1 Tartlet/23g	116	5.5	504	6.3	64.8	24.1	1.7
Bacon, & Cheese, Wheat Free, Made Without Wheat, M&S*	1 Serving/160g	450	31.9	281	6.6	18.2	19.9	1.3
Brie & Cranberry, Filo, Waitrose*	1 Tartlet/16g	44	2.2	275	8.9	26.9	13.9	3.5
Brie, & Cranberry, Party Food, M&S*	1 Tartlet/19g	56	3.2	295	7.8	26.9	17.1	1.3
Butternut Squash, & Goats Cheese, Linda McCartney*	1 Tartlet/150g	405	25	270	6.3	24.2	16.7	1.2
Cheese, Goats, & Caramelised Onion, Aldi*	1 Tartlet/150g	402	26	268	7.3	20.7	17.3	1.2
Framboise, Bonne Maman*	1 Tartlet/15g	62	1.7	411	3	73	11.5	0
Lemon, Petit, Bonne Maman*	1 Tartlet/14g	61	2.4	439	5	66	17	0
Raspberry, Mini, M&S*	1 Tartlet/27g	90	5.4	330	4.3	34.4	19.6	0.5
Tomato, & Goats Cheese, Waitrose*	1 Tartlet/130g	295	19	227	6.6	17.4	14.6	2
TEA								
Apple & Cinnamon, Made Up, Heath And Heather*	1 Mug/250ml	8	0	3	0.1	0.7	0	0
Assam, Blended, TTD, Sainsbury's*	1 Serving/2g	0	0	0	0	0	0	0
Beetroot, with Ginger, & Orange, Superblends, Twinings*	1 Mug/200ml	2	0	1	0	0.5	0	0
Blackberry & Nettle, Twinings*	1 Mug/250ml	5	0	2	0	0.3	0	0
Blackcurrant, Fruit Creations, Typhoo*	1 Sm Cup/100ml	5	0	5	0.2	0.8	0	0.2
Camomile, Pure, Classic Herbal, Twinings*	1 Serving/200ml	4	0	2	0	0.3	0	0
Chai Latte, Skinny Blend, Drink Me Chai*	1 Serving/15g	62	1.2	415	7.5	77.7	8	1.3
Chai, Latte, Spiced, Drink Me*	1 Sachet/15g	68	2.3	452	7.6	70.5	15.3	1.2
Chai, Twinings*	1 Mug/200ml	2	0	1	0.1	0	0	0
Chamomile & Spiced Apple, Warming, Twinings*	1 Mug/100ml	2	0	2	0	0.3	0	0
Choco, Yogi Tea*	1 Mug/200ml	8	0	4	0	1	0	0
Cranberry & Elderflower, Boost, Tetley*	1 Mug/225ml	5	0	2	0.1	0.6	0	0
Damask, Rose, Chinese, Choi Time*	1 Mug/500ml	0	0.3	0	0	0	0.1	0
Darjeeling Infusion, with Raspberry Juice, M&S*	1 Bottle/500ml	170	0	34	0	8.5	0	0
Decaf, Tetley*	1 Mug/100ml	1	0	1	0	0.3	0	0
Earl Grey, Infusion with Water, Average	*1 Mug/250ml*	*2*	*0*	*1*	*0*	*0.2*	*0*	*0*
Fruit Or Herbal, Made with Water, Twinings*	1 Mug/200ml	8	0	4	0	1	0	0
Fruit, Twinings*	1 Mug/227ml	4	0	2	0	0.4	0	0
Ginger, Herbal, Brit & Tang*	1 Tea Bag/2g	5	0	278	0	55.6	0	0
Green, Matcha, Twinings*	1 Mug/250ml	2	0	1	0	0	0	0
Green, Pure, Tetley*	1 Mug/250ml	2	0	1	0	0.3	0	0
Green, Rooibos, Naturally Caffeine Free, Tick Tock*	1 Mug/250ml	0	0	0	0	0	0	0
Green, with Jasmine, Twinings*	1 Mug/100ml	1	0	1	0	0.2	0	0
Green, with Mint, Whittards of Chelsea*	1 Mug/100ml	1	0	1	0.2	0.1	0	0
Green, with Pomegranate, Twinings*	1 Mug/200ml	2	0	1	0	0.2	0	0
Green, with Yerba Mate & Honey, Herbal Mist*	1 Mug/240ml	80	0	33	0	8.3	0	0
Ice, with Lemon, Lipton*	1 Bottle/325ml	91	0	28	0	6.9	0	0
Ice, with Mango, Lipton*	1 Bottle/500ml	165	0	33	0	8.1	0	0

T

TEA	Measure INFO/WEIGHT	per Measure KCAL	FAT	Nutrition Values per 100g / 100ml KCAL	PROT	CARB	FAT	FIBRE
TEA								
Ice, with Peach, Lipton*	1 Bottle/500ml	140	0	28	0	6.8	0	0
Iced, No Sugar Peach Flavour, Nestle*	1 Glass/100ml	1	0	1	0	0.1	0	0
Iced, Peach, Low Calories, Lipton*	1 Bottle/505ml	96	2.5	19	0.5	4.7	0.5	0
Iced, Peach, Sparkling, Organic, San Pellegrino*	1 Can/250ml	50	0	20	0	4.6	0	0
Iced, Peach, Twinings*	1 Mug/200ml	60	0.2	30	0.1	7.3	0.1	0
Iced, Raspberry, Bottle, Lipton*	1 Mug/250ml	48	1.3	19	0.5	4.6	0.5	0
Lemon, & Earl Grey Flavour, Sainsbury's*	1 Mug/250ml	7	1.2	3	0.5	0.7	0.5	0.5
Lemon, & Ginger, Lipton*	1 Cup/200ml	8	0	4	0.5	0.5	0	0
Lemon, & Ginger, Lazy Days, Tea Pigs*	1 Mug/200ml	2	0	1	0	0	0	0
Lemon, Ginger, & Manuka Honey, Pukka Herbs*	1 Mug/200ml	6	0	3	0	0	0	0
Lemon, Iced, Diet, Nestea*	1 Glass/250ml	3	0	1	0	0	0	0
Lemon, Instant, Original, Lift*	2 Tsp/7g	23	0	324	1.4	79.6	0	0
Lemon, Instant, Tesco*	1 Serving/7g	23	0	326	1	80.5	0	0
Lemon, Orange, & Ginger, Cold Infuse, Twinings*	1 Mug/200ml	4	0	2	0	0	0	0
Light & Delicate, Green with Lemon, Twinings*	1 Mug/100ml	1	0.1	1	0.1	0.2	0.1	0.1
Made with 1% Milk, Average	**1 Mug/250ml**	**12**	**0.2**	**5**	**0.4**	**0.8**	**0.1**	**0**
Made with Water	**1 Mug/227ml**	**0**	**0**	**0**	**0.1**	**0**	**0**	**0**
Made with Water with Semi-Skimmed Milk, Average	**1 Mug/200ml**	**14**	**0.4**	**7**	**0.5**	**0.7**	**0.2**	**0**
Made with Water with Skimmed Milk, Average	**1 Mug/270ml**	**16**	**0.5**	**6**	**0.5**	**0.7**	**0.2**	**0**
Made with Water with Whole Milk, Average	**1 Mug/200ml**	**16**	**0.8**	**8**	**0.4**	**0.5**	**0.4**	**0**
Mango, with Yerba Mate, Herbal Mist*	1 Mug/240ml	70	0	29	0	7.5	0	0
Mint, Lemon, & Cucumber, Cold Infusion, Tetley*	1 Mug/200ml	4	0	2	0.1	0.6	0	0
Morning Detox, Twinings*	1 Mug/200ml	5	0	2	0	0.3	0	0
Nettle & Peppermint, Twinings*	1 Mug/200ml	2	0	1	0	0.2	0	0
Nettle & Sweet Fennel, Twinings*	1 Mug/200ml	4	0	2	0	0.3	0	0
Oolong, Average	**1 Mug/200ml**	**5**	**0.2**	**2**	**0.1**	**0.2**	**0.1**	**0.2**
Orange & Mango, Herbal, Organic, Honest, Coca-Cola*	1 Bottle/500ml	96	0	19	0	4.7	0	0
Passionfruit, Mango, Blood Orange, Cold Infuse, Twinings*	1 Mug/200ml	4	0	2	0	0	0	0
Peppermint, Made with Water, Average	**1 Mug/200ml**	**3**	**0**	**2**	**0**	**0.2**	**0**	**0**
Raspberry & Cranberry, T of Life, Tetley*	1 Mug/100ml	36	0	36	0	9	0	0
Red Berries, Brewed, PG Tips*	1 Mug/200ml	5	0	2	0	0.6	0	0
Red Bush, Made with Water, Tetley*	1 Mug/250ml	2	0	1	0	0.1	0	0
Red, ChariTea*	1 Bottle/330ml	53	0	16	0	3.4	0	0
Sleep, Herbal Infusion, Brewed, Twinings*	1 Mug/200ml	4	0	2	0	0.3	0	0
Strawberry Lemonade, Cold Infuse, Twinings*	1 Mug/200ml	4	0	2	0	0	0	0
Super Fruits, Multi Vitamin, Tetley*	1 Mug/200ml	4	0	2	0.1	0.6	0	0
Turmeric, Orange, & Star Anise, Superblends, Twinings*	1 Mug/200ml	2	0	1	0	0.5	0	0
Turmeric, Spiced, Infusions, Sainsbury's*	1 Teabag/2g	1	0.1	65	5	0	5	0
White Milk, Sachets, Old Town*	1 Sachet/40g	178	5.2	444	5.5	76.3	13	0
TEACAKES								
Average	**1 Teacake/60g**	**178**	**4.5**	**296**	**8**	**52.5**	**7.5**	**0**
Black Forest, Co-Op*	1 Teacake/22g	94	3.6	427	4.6	63.6	16.4	2.3
Caramel, Highlights, Mallows, Cadbury*	1 Teacake/15g	61	1.9	408	6.2	69.1	12.4	3.6
Cinnamon, & Raisin, Irish, Rankin Selection*	1 Teacake/60g	172	3.5	287	5.8	68.5	5.8	2.5
Fruity, Warburton's*	1 Teacake/63g	164	1.9	262	8.7	48	3	3.2
Large, Sainsbury's*	1 Teacake/73g	212	3.6	291	7.6	52.4	4.9	3.4
Marshmallow, Milk Chocolate, Tunnock's*	1 Teacake/24g	106	4.6	440	4.9	61.9	19.2	2.4
Mini Bites, M&S*	1 Bite/6g	29	1.2	484	3.2	72.6	20.3	2.1
Richly Fruited, Waitrose*	1 Teacake/72g	205	2.7	285	7.8	55	3.7	2.2
Salted Caramel, M&S*	1 Teacake/18g	80	3.2	448	5.3	65.3	17.9	1.4
Toasted, Average	**1 Teacake/60g**	**197**	**5**	**329**	**8.9**	**58.3**	**8.3**	**0**
with Orange Filling, M&S*	1 Teacake/20g	80	2.8	410	4.5	66.6	14.2	0.9

	Measure INFO/WEIGHT	per Measure KCAL	per Measure FAT	Nutrition Values per 100g / 100ml KCAL	PROT	CARB	FAT	FIBRE
TEMPEH								
Average	*1oz/28g*	*46*	*1.8*	*166*	*20.7*	*6.4*	*6.4*	*4.3*
Barbecue, Slices, Oasis*	1 Serving/30g	58	4.2	193	12.4	2.9	14	0
Curry Flavoured, Pieces, Plant Power*	½ Pack/90g	331	27	368	21	3.5	30	7.7
Original, Organic, Plant Power*	½ Pack/200g	368	19.4	184	19	2	9.7	6.5
TEQUILA								
Average	*1 Pub Shot/35ml*	*78*	*0*	*224*	*0*	*0*	*0*	*0*
TERRINE								
Crab, & King Prawn, M&S*	1 Pack/120g	244	17.6	203	8.9	8.6	14.7	0.1
Ham Hock, M&S*	1 Slice/70g	98	4.1	140	22.5	0.1	5.8	0.5
Salmon & King Prawn, Waitrose*	1 Serving/75g	98	4	130	19.3	1.3	5.3	0
Salmon, Pate, Sainsbury's*	1 Terrine/50g	116	9.7	233	11.8	2.5	19.4	0.5
Salmon, Three, M&S*	1 Serving/80g	168	12.2	210	17.6	0.8	15.3	0.9
Vegetable, Waitrose *	1 Serving/60g	86	5.1	143	3.5	11.7	8.4	3.7
THYME								
Dried, Average	*1 Tsp/1g*	*3*	*0.1*	*276*	*9.1*	*45.3*	*7.4*	*0*
Fresh, Average	*1 Tsp/1g*	*1*	*0*	*95*	*3*	*15.1*	*2.5*	*0*
TIA MARIA								
Original	*1 Pub Shot/35ml*	*105*	*0*	*300*	*0*	*0*	*0*	*0*
TIC TAC								
Extra Strong Mint, Ferrero*	2 Tic Tacs/1g	4	0	381	0	95.2	0	0
Fresh Mint, Ferrero*	2 Tic Tacs/1g	4	0	390	0	97.5	0	0
Lime & Orange, Ferrero*	2 Tic Tacs/1g	4	0	386	0	95.5	0	0
TIKKA MASALA								
Cauliflower, Fire Roasted, Bol*	1 Serving/405g	413	15	102	3.5	12.3	3.7	2.5
Chicken, & Pilau Basmati Rice, Frozen, Patak's*	1 Pack/400g	580	20	145	9.9	15.1	5	0.2
Chicken, & Pilau Rice, Charlie Bigham's*	1 Serving/403 g	737	43.9	183	6.9	15.3	10.9	0
Chicken, & Pilau Rice, Waitrose*	1 Pack/400g	644	32.4	161	6.8	13.4	8.1	3.8
Chicken, & Rice, Ready Meal, Healthy Range, Average	**1 Serving/400g**	**390**	**6.4**	**98**	**6.6**	**14.3**	**1.6**	**1.1**
Chicken, & Pilau Rice, BGTY, Sainsbury's*	1 Pack/364g	400	6.5	110	6.8	15.2	1.8	2.5
Chicken, & Pilau Rice, Meal for One, M&S*	1 Pack/400g	592	20.4	148	8.9	15.3	5.1	2.7
Chicken, & Rice, Finest, Tesco*	1 Pack/450g	637	18.6	154	8.6	19.1	4.5	1.2
Chicken, & Rice, Pot, Musclefood*	1 Serving/309g	334	5.6	108	12.5	9.4	1.8	1.7
Chicken, Asda*	1 Pack/400g	584	35.6	146	12	3.6	8.9	1.5
Chicken, Calorie Counted, Asda*	1 Pack/399g	395	6	99	6.7	15	1.5	0.5
Chicken, Chef Select, Lidl*	1 Pack/450g	707	31	157	8.7	13.1	6.9	4
Chicken, Curry Kit, Musclefood*	1 Serving/385g	285	6.9	74	11.3	3.2	1.8	0.1
Chicken, Dinner For Two, Co-Op*	1 Serving/380g	471	16	124	1.9	3.7	4.2	0.5
Chicken, Hot, Sainsbury's*	1 Pack/400g	604	37.2	151	13.2	3.6	9.3	1.5
Chicken, Hot, Takeaway, Tesco*	½ Pack/194g	244	13.9	126	9	5.3	7.2	2
Chicken, Indian Takeaway, Iceland*	1 Pack/400g	484	28.4	121	8.9	6	7.1	1.9
Chicken, Indian, Medium, Sainsbury's*	1 Pack/400g	848	61.2	212	13.2	5.3	15.3	0.1
Chicken, M&S*	½ Pack/200g	288	15.6	144	13.5	4.7	7.8	0.7
Chicken, Parsley Box*	1 Pack/270g	319	12.7	118	12	6.7	4.7	0.7
Chicken, Slow Cooked, British, Sainsburys*	½ Pack/225g	367	20	163	17.6	3	8.9	0.6
Chicken, Tikka Masala, Meal For Two, Tesco*	½ Pack/155g	231	14	149	11.4	4.7	9	1.9
Chicken, with Pilau Rice, Frozen, Waitrose*	1 Pack/400g	676	32.4	169	9.3	14.6	8.1	2.1
Chicken, with Pilau Rice, Serves 1, Sainsbury's*	1 Pack/450g	724	24.8	161	7.5	18.7	5.5	3.3
Chicken, with Rice, Free From, Sainsbury's*	1 Pack/375g	435	12.8	116	7.2	12.5	3.4	3.1
Vegetarian, Chef's Selection, Quorn*	½ Pack/170g	274	17	161	6	10	10	3.5
TILAPIA								
Raw, Average	*100g*	*95*	*1*	*95*	*20*	*0*	*1*	*0*
Roasted, Spiced, with Tomatoes, & Lentils, Hello Fresh*	1 Serving/483g	261	3	54	7	4.3	0.6	0

T

	Measure INFO/WEIGHT	per Measure KCAL FAT		Nutrition Values per 100g / 100ml KCAL PROT CARB FAT FIBRE				

TIME OUT

	Measure INFO/WEIGHT	per Measure KCAL	FAT	KCAL	PROT	CARB	FAT	FIBRE
TIME OUT								
Break Pack, Cadbury*	1 Serving/20g	108	6.3	530	6.2	58.3	30.7	0
Chocolate Fingers, Cadbury*	2 Fingers/35g	186	10.6	530	7.1	57.3	30.3	1.1
TIRAMISU								
Asda*	1 Pot/100g	252	11	252	4.3	34	11	0.5
Classic, Sainsbury's*	1 Serving/84g	209	8.5	250	4.2	31.7	10.2	1.1
Dine in Dessert, M&S*	½ Dessert/145g	515	36.7	355	2.6	28.8	25.3	0.7
Family Size, Tesco*	1 Serving/125g	356	18.1	285	4.3	34.5	14.5	4.3
Morrisons*	1 Pot/90g	248	9.9	276	4	38	11	0
Single Size, Tesco*	1 Pot/100g	290	12.9	290	3.8	35.1	12.9	4.5
Waitrose*	1 Pot/90g	221	11.2	246	6.4	27.2	12.4	0
TOAD IN THE HOLE								
Average	*1 Serving/231g*	*640*	*40.2*	*277*	*11.9*	*19.5*	*17.4*	*1.1*
Classic Kitchen, Tesco*	1 Pack/340g	859	49.3	268	12.2	19	15.4	2.4
Frozen, Cooked, CBY, Asda*	1 Slice/72g	168	7.5	232	9.2	24.2	10.4	2.6
HFC, Tesco*	1 Pack/223g	463	18.3	208	9.5	23.3	8.2	1.4
Large, Great Value, Asda*	¼ Pack/81g	238	13.8	293	10	25	17	2.3
Mini, Aunt Bessie's*	1 Serving/62g	118	6.8	191	11	12	11	3.6
with Three Sausages, Asda*	1 Pack/150g	435	27	290	10	22	18	1
TOAST								
Melba, Co-Op*	1 Pack/20g	76	0.5	380	11.1	75.3	2.6	5.9
Olive, Walnut, & Pimenton, Kent & Fraser*	1 Slice/7g	26	1.1	373	7.1	51.2	15.5	3
TOASTIE								
All Day Breakfast, M&S*	1 Serving/174g	375	13.8	215	11.2	25	7.9	1.7
Cheese & Pickle, M&S*	1 Toastie/136g	320	9.1	235	10.4	33.5	6.7	2.6
Cheese & Onion, Ginsters*	1 Toastie/122g	330	12.3	269	10.9	33.1	10	1.5
Cheese, Tomato, & Spinach, Frozen, Tesco*	1 Pack/134g	291	6.6	218	9.4	32.4	4.9	3.1
Ham & Cheddar, British, M&S*	1 Pack/128g	269	8.6	210	15.5	22.3	6.7	1.3
Ham & Cheese, Tesco*	1 Pack/124g	349	10.4	282	13.2	37.2	8.4	2.4
Ham & Cheese, White Bread	*1 Toastie/150g*	*409*	*14.9*	*273*	*14.5*	*31.3*	*9.9*	*0.9*
TOFFEE APPLE								
Average	*1 Apple/141g*	*188*	*3*	*133*	*1.2*	*29.2*	*2.1*	*2.3*
TOFFEE CRISP								
Biscuit, Nestle*	1 Biscuit/19g	99	5.3	519	3.9	62.3	27.8	1.4
Bitesize, Nestle*	1 Serving/20g	101	5.4	518	3.8	63	27.6	1.3
TOFFEES								
Assorted, Bassett's*	1 Toffee/8g	35	1.1	434	3.8	73.1	14	0
Assorted, Sainsbury's*	1 Toffee/8g	37	1.3	457	2.2	76.5	15.8	0.2
Butter, Smart Price, Asda*	1 Toffee/8g	37	1.3	440	1.3	75	15	0
Chewy, Werther's*	1 Toffee/5g	22	0.8	436	3.5	71.3	15.2	0.1
Chocolate Covered, Emotionali, Lidl*	3 Toffees/28g	132	5.7	472	3	68	20.2	3.1
Dairy, Waitrose*	1 Toffee/8g	37	1.1	458	2	80.2	14.3	0.5
Devon Butter, Thorntons*	1 Toffee/9g	40	1.5	444	1.7	72.2	16.7	0
English Butter, Co-Op*	1 Toffee/8g	38	1.6	470	2	71	20	0
Everyday Value, Tesco*	3 Toffees/23g	101	3.3	450	2.1	77.3	14.8	0.3
Liquorice, Thorntons*	1 Bag/100g	506	29.4	506	1.9	58.8	29.4	0
Milk Chocolate Covered, Thorntons*	1 Bag/215g	1120	66	521	4.1	57.2	30.7	0.9
Milk Chocolate Smothered, Thorntons*	1 Pack/125g	655	38.5	524	4.3	57.5	30.8	1.1
Mixed, Average	*1oz/28g*	*119*	*5.2*	*426*	*2.2*	*66.7*	*18.6*	*0*
Original, Thorntons*	1 Bag/100g	514	30.1	514	1.8	59.3	30.1	0
TOFU								
Average	*1 Pack/250g*	*297*	*16.5*	*119*	*13.4*	*1.4*	*6.6*	*0.1*
Beech Smoked, Organic, Cauldron Foods*	½ Pack/110g	124	7.8	113	10.9	1	7.1	0.5
Crispy, Wholemeal, Chunkies, The Tofoo Co.*	½ Pack/113g	269	14.2	238	12.7	22.5	12.6	3.8

	Measure INFO/WEIGHT	per Measure KCAL	FAT	Nutrition Values per 100g / 100ml KCAL	PROT	CARB	FAT	FIBRE
TOFU								
Fried, Average	*1oz/28g*	*75*	*4*	*268*	*28.6*	*9.3*	*14.1*	*0*
Original, Cauldron Foods*	1 Pack/396g	467	28.1	118	12.6	1	7.1	1.9
Pieces, Marinated, Organic, Cauldron Foods*	1 Pack/160g	363	27.2	227	17.5	1	17	2.7
Southern Fried, Crispy, Bites, The Tofoo Co.*	½ Pack/113g	272	16	241	12.4	23.5	14.2	4.1
Teriyaki, Organic, Cauldron Foods*	½ Pack/80g	168	12	210	16	2.8	15	2.1
TOMATILLOS								
Raw	*1 Med/34g*	*11*	*0.3*	*32*	*1*	*5.8*	*1*	*1.9*
TOMATO PASTE								
Average	*1 Tbsp/20g*	*19*	*0*	*96*	*5*	*19.2*	*0.2*	*1.5*
Sun Dried, Average	*1 Hpd Tsp/10g*	*38*	*3.5*	*385*	*3.2*	*13.8*	*35.2*	*0*
TOMATO PUREE								
Average	*1 Tsp/5g*	*4*	*0*	*76*	*4.5*	*14.1*	*0.2*	*2.3*
Double Concentrate, Average	*1 Tbsp/15g*	*13*	*0*	*85*	*4.9*	*14.9*	*0.2*	*3.6*
Garlic, Double Concentrate, Morrisons*	1 Tbsp/15g	13	0	86	3.9	14.9	0.3	3.8
Sun Dried, & Olive Oil & Herbs, GIA*	1 Tsp/5g	10	1.1	204	2.6	0.5	21.6	0
TOMATOES								
Cherry, Average	*1 Tomato/15g*	*3*	*0*	*18*	*0.7*	*3*	*0.3*	*0.5*
Cherry, on the Vine, Average	*1 Serving/80g*	*15*	*0.3*	*18*	*0.7*	*3.1*	*0.3*	*1.2*
Chopped, Canned, Branded Average	*1 Serving/130g*	*27*	*0.2*	*21*	*1.1*	*3.8*	*0.1*	*0.8*
Chopped, Canned, Organic, Valfrutta*	1 Can/400g	108	0.8	27	1.1	44	0.2	0.8
Chopped, Italian, Average	*½ Can/200g*	*47*	*0.2*	*23*	*1.3*	*4.4*	*0.1*	*0.9*
Chopped, with Garlic, Average	*½ Can/200g*	*43*	*0.3*	*21*	*1.2*	*3.8*	*0.1*	*0.8*
Chopped, with Herbs, Average	*½ Can/200g*	*42*	*0.3*	*21*	*1.1*	*3.8*	*0.1*	*0.8*
Chopped, with Olive Oil & Roasted Garlic, Sainsbury's*	1 Pack/390g	187	8.2	48	1.3	5.9	2.1	1
Diced, Fire Roasted, Hunt's*	½ Can/123g	30	0	24	0.8	4.9	0	1.6
Fresh, Raw, Average	*1 Med/123g*	*22*	*0.2*	*18*	*0.9*	*3.9*	*0.2*	*1.2*
Fried in Blended Oil	*1 Med/85g*	*77*	*6.5*	*91*	*0.7*	*5*	*7.7*	*1.3*
Grilled, Average	*1 Med/85g*	*17*	*0.3*	*20*	*0.8*	*3.5*	*0.3*	*1.5*
Heritage, Jewel, TTD, Sainsbury's*	1 Pack/250g	62	1.2	25	1.1	3.4	0.5	1.2
Marinated, with Garlic & Oregano, The Deli, Aldi*	½ Pack/75g	68	3.5	90	2.8	7.8	4.7	2.7
Marmonde, Raw, Waitrose*	1 Tomato/120g	24	0.4	20	0.7	3.1	0.3	1
Mix, Summer Selection, Eat Well, M&S*	¼ Pack/70g	15	0.4	22	1.1	3.6	0.5	1.3
Plum, Baby, Average	*1 Serving/50g*	*9*	*0.2*	*18*	*1.5*	*2.3*	*0.3*	*1*
Plum, Baby, Mixed, Gold, Ocado*	1 Serving/80g	21	0.4	26	1.1	3.6	0.5	1.3
Plum, in Tomato Juice, Average	*1 Can/400g*	*71*	*0.4*	*18*	*1*	*3.3*	*0.1*	*0.7*
Plum, in Tomato Juice, Premium, Average	*1 Can/400g*	*93*	*1.2*	*23*	*1.3*	*3.8*	*0.3*	*0.7*
Pome Dei Moro, Waitrose*	1 Serving/80g	16	0.2	20	0.7	3.1	0.3	1.2
Pomodorino, TTD, Sainsbury's*	1 Tomato/8g	2	0	25	1.1	3.4	0.5	1.2
Ripened on the Vine, Average	*1 Med/123g*	*22*	*0.4*	*18*	*0.7*	*3.1*	*0.3*	*0.7*
Ruby Jewel, Raw, Sainsbury's*	1 Tomato/45g	9	0.2	20	0.7	3.1	0.5	1
Santini, M&S*	1 Serving/80g	16	0.2	20	0.7	3.1	0.3	1
Slicing, Essential, Waitrose*	1 Tomato/250g	50	0.1	20	0.7	3.1	0	1
Stuffed with Rice Based Filling, Average	*1oz/28g*	*59*	*3.8*	*212*	*2.1*	*22.2*	*13.4*	*1.1*
Sugardrop, Finest, Tesco*	1 Tomato/14g	3	0	20	0.7	3.1	0.3	1
Sun Dried in Oil	*100g*	*301*	*24.8*	*301*	*5.8*	*13.5*	*24.8*	*7*
Sun Dried, Average	*3 Pieces/20g*	*43*	*3.2*	*214*	*4.7*	*13*	*15.9*	*3.3*
Sun Dried, Zero Oil, Drained, Ponti*	1 Serving/100g	108	1.8	108	3.9	15	1.8	8.3
Sweet, Baby, Mixed, Finest, Tesco*	½ Pack/125g	25	0.4	20	0.7	3.1	0.3	1
Tri-Colour, On the Vine, Finest, Tesco*	8 Tomatoes/80g	21	0.4	26	1.1	3.6	0.5	1.2
TONGUE								
Lunch, Average	*1oz/28g*	*51*	*3*	*181*	*20.1*	*1.8*	*10.6*	*0*
Ox, Deli Counter, Sainsbury's*	1 Serving/100g	195	13.3	195	18.3	0.5	13.3	0.1
Slices, Average	*1oz/28g*	*56*	*3.9*	*201*	*18.7*	*0*	*14*	*0*

T

	Measure INFO/WEIGHT	per Measure KCAL	FAT	Nutrition Values per 100g / 100ml KCAL	PROT	CARB	FAT	FIBRE
TONIC WATER								
Average	*1 Glass/250ml*	*82*	*0*	*33*	*0*	*8.8*	*0*	*0*
Diet, Asda*	1 Glass/200ml	2	0	1	0	0	0	0
Hibiscus, Merchant's Heart*	1 Bottle/200ml	66	0	33	0	7.4	0	0
Indian with Lime, Low Calorie, Tesco*	1 Glass/250ml	5	0	2	0	0	0	0
Indian, Britvic*	1 Mini Can/150ml	39	0.2	26	0.1	6.2	0.1	0.1
Indian, Diet, Schweppes*	1 Glass/100ml	1	0	1	0	0	0	0
Indian, Fever-Tree*	1 Bottle/200ml	72	0	36	0	8.9	0	0
Indian, Low Calorie, Vive, Aldi*	1 Glass/250ml	3	0	1	0	0	0	0
Indian, Schweppes*	1 Glass/250ml	55	0	22	0	5.1	0	0
Indian, Slimline, Schweppes*	1 Serving/188ml	3	0	2	0.4	0	0	0
Low Calorie, Tesco*	1 Glass/200ml	4	0	2	0	0.5	0	0
Pink Grapefruit, Fentiman's*	1 Bottle/500ml	175	0	35	0	7.7	0	0
Quinine, Schweppes*	1 Glass/125ml	46	0	37	0	9	0	0
Rhubarb, & Ginger, Lixir*	1 Bottle/200ml	70	0	35	0	8	0	0
with Quinine, Lidl*	1 Glass/200ml	36	0	18	0	4.2	0	0
TOPIC								
Mars*	1 Bar/47g	234	12.3	498	6.2	59.6	26.2	1.7
TORTE								
Chocolate & Pecan Brownie, Gu*	1/6 Torte/67g	292	17.7	436	5.3	45.1	26.4	3.1
Chocolate Brownie, Belgian, TTD, Sainsbury's*	1 Slice/90g	360	24.6	400	5.6	32.5	27.3	0.8
Chocolate Fondant, Gu*	1/8 Torte/62g	264	18.9	423	5.7	32	30.2	1.8
Chocolate Orange & Almond, Gu*	1 Serving/65g	273	19.8	420	5	28.2	30.5	2.7
Chocolate Truffle, Waitrose*	1 Serving/116g	359	20.1	309	4.6	30.1	17.3	1.4
Chocolate, Tesco*	1 Serving/50g	126	6	251	3.6	32.3	11.9	1
Lemon & Mango, Waitrose*	1 Serving/80g	142	2.4	177	3.9	33.6	3	0.6
Salted Caramel & Chocolate, Weight Watchers, Heinz*	1 Dessert/65g	164	3.8	252	4.1	45	5.8	1.8
TORTELLINI								
Beef, & Red Wine, Italian, Asda*	½ Pack/150g	242	4.2	161	9	25	2.8	0
Cheese, & Ham, Italiano, Tesco*	½ Pack/150g	396	12.3	264	12.8	34.8	8.2	3
Cheese, Tomato & Basil, Cooked, Tesco*	1 Serving/270g	551	15.1	204	6.7	30.5	5.6	2.5
Ham, & Cheese, Fresh, Asda*	½ Pack/150g	255	9	170	6	23	6	1.7
Meat, Italian, Tesco*	1 Serving/125g	332	9.5	266	10.6	38.9	7.6	2.3
Mushroom, Asda*	1 Serving/125g	218	5.2	174	6	28	4.2	2.3
Pepperoni, Spicy, Asda*	½ Pack/150g	252	6	168	7	26	4	0
Pesto, & Goats Cheese, Fresh, Sainsbury's*	½ Pack/150g	310	12.2	207	8.9	24.6	8.1	2.6
Ricotta, & Spinach, Giovanni Rana*	½ Pack/125g	319	10	255	9	35.5	8	10
Sausage, & Ham, Italiano, Tesco*	1 Pack/300g	816	27.9	272	13.1	34	9.3	3.7
Spinach, & Ricotta, Italian, Asda*	½ Pack/150g	189	3.6	126	5	21	2.4	0.6
Spinach, & Ricotta, Filled, Aldi*	½ Pack/150g	252	3	168	7.5	29	2	2.3
Tomato, & Mozzarella, Fresh, Sainsbury's*	½ Pack/150g	291	12	194	7.5	23	8	3.4
TORTELLONI								
Arrabiata, Sainsbury's*	½ Pack/210g	407	11.8	194	7.1	28.8	5.6	2.6
Beef, & Red Wine, Sainsbury's*	½ Pack/150g	256	5.8	171	7.4	25.9	3.9	1.7
Bolognese, Italian, Fresh, As Consumed, Morrisons*	1 Pack/210g	482	14.5	230	8.9	32.1	6.9	1.8
Cheese, & Smoked Ham, As Consumed, Tesco*	½ Pack/270g	535	17.3	198	8.4	25.8	6.4	1.8
Cheese, & Tomato, Italian, Cooked, Asda*	½ Pack/209g	454	13.4	217	7.9	31	6.4	2.1
Chicken & Bacon, As Consumed, Italiano, Tesco*	½ Pack/280g	567	14	202	6.8	30.7	5	3.7
Chicken, & Chorizo, Italian, As Prepared, Morrisons*	½ Pack/210g	406	11.1	193	7.2	28.6	5.3	1.3
Chicken, & Mushroom, Italian, Cooked, Asda*	½ Pack/209g	427	8.6	204	7.5	33	4.1	2.3
Chicken, & Prosciutto, Buitoni*	1 Serving/109g	330	9	302	14.7	42.2	8.2	1.8
Chorizo, Smoky, Fresh, Sainsbury's*	½ Pack/203g	398	12.8	196	8.5	25.6	6.3	1.5
Cream Cheese, Garlic & Herb, Fresh, Morrisons*	1 Serving/150g	400	9	267	10.3	46.1	6	3.2
Ham & Cheese, Italian Cuisine, Aldi*	½ Pack/150g	340	10.2	227	9.3	31	6.8	1.6

T

	Measure INFO/WEIGHT	per Measure KCAL	per Measure FAT	Nutrition Values per 100g / 100ml KCAL	PROT	CARB	FAT	FIBRE
TORTELLONI								
Mushroom, Fresh, Sainsbury's*	1 Pack/400g	656	10.8	164	5.9	27.9	2.7	2.3
Sausage, & Ham, As Consumed, Italiano, Tesco*	1/3 Pack/180g	355	12.6	197	8.6	23.8	7	2
Spinach, & Ricotta Cheese, Co-Op*	½ Pack/126g	315	6.3	250	10	41	5	4
Spinach, & Ricotta, Fresh, Waitrose*	½ Pack/150g	239	5.3	159	6.3	24.4	3.5	2.5
Spinach, & Ricotta, Sainsbury's*	½ Pack/150g	326	10.8	217	7.8	30.2	7.2	2.4
Spinach, & Ricotta, Chef Select, Lidl*	1 Serving/125g	288	11.9	230	9.5	24.4	9.5	4.6
Spinach, & Ricotta, Rana La Famiglia*	1 Serving/125g	355	15	284	10	33	12	0
Tomato, & Mozzarella, Sainsbury's*	1 Serving/175g	340	14	194	7.5	23	8	3.4
Wild Mushroom, Italian, Sainsbury's*	½ Pack/150g	309	12.3	206	7.7	25.4	8.2	2.3
TORTIGLIONI								
Dry, Average	*1 Serving/75g*	*266*	*1.4*	*355*	*12.5*	*72.2*	*1.9*	*2.1*
TORTILLA								
Chorizo, & Roasted Vegetables, Morrisons*	1 Tortilla/130g	238	15.2	183	9.1	10	11.7	1
Mozzarella, & Cherry Tomato, M&S*	¼ Serving/90g	151	9.8	168	6.6	9.7	10.9	2.5
Onion, Caramelised, & Potato, Eat Well, M&S*	½ Pack/110g	148	6	135	5.9	13.5	5.5	3.7
Potato & Caramelised Onion, Good Life, Co-Op*	1 Slice/112g	175	9.9	156	5.8	12	8.8	2.2
Red Pepper & Chorizo, Slices, Waitrose*	1 Slice/113g	180	10.3	160	10	8.6	9.2	1.6
Vegetable, Roasted, Mediterranean, M&S*	½ Pack/110g	138	5.9	125	6.9	11.1	5.4	2.3
TORTILLA CHIPS								
Aldi*	¼ Pack/50g	234	9.5	469	6.3	66	19	4.2
Chilli, with Chopped Jalapeno, Tyrrells*	1 Serving/30g	154	8.3	512	5.9	57.3	27.5	0
Chorizo & Red Pepper, M&S*	1 Serving/25g	122	5	487	5.9	68.2	20.2	4.3
Cool Flavour, BGTY, Sainsbury's*	1 Pack/22g	94	2.7	425	7.1	71.4	12.3	4.5
Cool Flavour, Sainsbury's*	1 Serving/50g	232	9.4	463	5.7	68.1	18.7	3.7
Cool Original, Snaktastic, Lidl*	1 Serving/25g	116	5.3	466	5.9	60.6	21.2	4.5
Cool, Tesco*	1 Serving/40g	190	9.9	474	6.3	56.7	24.7	7.8
Jalapeno, Food Should Taste Good*	12 Chips/28g	130	6	464	7.1	64.3	21.4	7.1
Lightly Salted, M&S*	1 Serving/20g	98	4.8	490	7.2	61.5	24.1	4.5
Lightly Salted, Tesco*	1 Serving/50g	248	13.8	495	4.8	56.8	27.6	7.5
Lightly Salted, Waitrose*	1 Serving/40g	187	8.6	468	7.1	61.2	21.6	6.5
Lighty Salted, Basics, Sainsbury's*	½ Pack/50g	242	11.9	483	6.5	60.7	23.8	5.3
Multiseed, & Bean, The Foodie Market, Aldi*	1 Serving/40g	192	9.6	480	12	47	24	14
Nachips, Original, Old El Paso*	1 Serving/50g	250	13.4	500	6.2	56.4	26.7	4.7
Plain	*1 Serving/100g*	*486*	*21.1*	*486*	*6.8*	*62*	*21.1*	*4.2*
Rainbow, Sainsbury's*	1 Pack/20g	96	4.3	479	5.5	62.1	21.5	7.6
Salsa, M&S*	½ Bag/75g	364	18.8	485	5.7	59.1	25.1	6.1
Sweet Potato, Food Should Taste Good*	12 Chips/28g	140	7	500	7.1	64.3	25	3.6
Tortilla Rolls, Texan Barbecue, The Best, Morrisons*	1 Serving/25g	127	6.2	508	5.2	63.6	24.9	4.5
Tortillas, Nacho Cheese Flavour, Weight Watchers*	1 Pack/18g	78	2.9	433	6.1	66.7	16.1	3.9
Tortillas, Sour Cream, & Lime, TTD, Sainsbury's*	1 Serving/30g	148	6.9	495	5.7	63.9	23.1	4.4
Veggie, Lightly Salted, Co-Op*	1 Serving/33g	165	8.3	499	5.9	60	25	4.8
with Guacamole	*1 Serving/100g*	*515*	*30.8*	*515*	*6*	*53*	*30.8*	*6.3*
TREACLE								
Black, Average	*1 Tbsp/20g*	*51*	*0*	*257*	*1.2*	*67.2*	*0*	*0*
TRIFLE								
Average	*1 Serving/170g*	*272*	*10.7*	*160*	*3.6*	*22.3*	*6.3*	*0.5*
Berry, Mixed, Waitrose*	1 Pot/120g	200	13	167	2.2	15	10.8	0.7
Chocolate , Tesco*	1 Pot/120g	238	13	198	3.2	21.7	10.8	0.7
Fruit Cocktail, Individual, M&S*	1 Pot/135g	205	9.2	150	2.7	19.3	6.7	0.7
Fruit Cocktail, Individual, Tesco*	1 Pot/113g	175	8.8	155	1.7	19.6	7.8	0.6
Fruit, Cocktail, Morrisons*	1 Pot/135g	167	7.2	124	1.7	17	5.3	0.8
Peach & Zabaglione, COU, M&S*	1 Glass/130g	150	3	115	2.8	20.6	2.3	0.8
Raspberry & Sherry, Waitrose*	1 Pot/120g	223	14.3	186	2.5	16.9	11.9	0.7

T

	Measure INFO/WEIGHT	per Measure KCAL	per Measure FAT	KCAL	PROT	CARB	FAT	FIBRE
				Nutrition Values per 100g / 100ml				

TRIFLE

	Measure INFO/WEIGHT	KCAL	FAT	KCAL	PROT	CARB	FAT	FIBRE
Raspberry, Co-Op*	1 Trifle/125g	206	10	165	2	22	8	0.3
Raspberry, Large, Tesco*	¼ Pack/150g	207	10.2	138	1.8	17.1	6.8	0.6
Raspberry, Pot, Sainsbury's*	1 Pot/125g	181	7.6	145	2.1	19.9	6.1	1.3
Raspberry, Tesco*	1 Pot/145g	188	8.8	130	1.7	16.8	6.1	0.6
Sherry, 742, Oakhouse Foods Ltd*	1 Trifle/175g	385	22.8	220	2.9	22.2	13	0.8
Strawberry, Aldi*	1/3 Trifle/153g	193	8	126	1.9	18	5.2	0.7
Strawberry, Co-Op*	1 Serving/120g	175	9.1	146	1.7	16.7	7.6	1.4
Strawberry, Everyday Value, Tesco*	¼ Trifle/118g	157	6.4	133	1.4	18.5	5.4	2.4
Strawberry, Individual, Pots, Tesco*	1 Pot/135g	174	6.1	129	1.8	20	4.5	0.6
Strawberry, Individual, Waitrose*	1 Pot/150g	206	8.6	137	1.8	19.7	5.7	1
Strawberry, Low Fat, COU, M&S*	1 Pot/140g	148	3.5	106	2.9	17.6	2.5	0.8
Strawberry, Milbona, Lidl*	1 Trifle/125g	196	11.2	157	1.9	16.8	9	0
Strawberry, Tesco*	1 Trifle/605g	998	55.7	165	1.5	19.1	9.2	0.8

TRIPE

& Onions, Stewed	**1oz/28g**	**26**	**0.8**	**93**	**8.3**	**9.5**	**2.7**	**0.7**
Ox, Real Lancashire*	1 Serving/100g	36	0.7	36	7.2	0.1	0.7	0

TROUT

Brown, Steamed, Average	**1 Serving/120g**	**162**	**5.4**	**135**	**23.5**	**0**	**4.5**	**0**
Fillets, Loch, Scottish, M&S*	1 Fillet/110g	226	13.2	205	24.2	0	12	0
Fillets, Smoked, The Port of Lancaster Smokehouse Ltd*	1 Fillet/64g	96	3.9	150	23.3	0	6.1	0.6
Fillets, with Juniper Berries, Ocean Sea, Lidl*	1 Serving/63g	87	3.5	138	22	0	5.5	0
Grilled, Weighed with Bones & Skin	**1 Serving/100g**	**98**	**3.9**	**98**	**15.7**	**0**	**3.9**	**0**
Rainbow, Grilled, Average	**1 Serving/120g**	**162**	**6.5**	**135**	**21.5**	**0**	**5.4**	**0**
Rainbow, Raw, Average	**1oz/28g**	**33**	**1.3**	**118**	**19.1**	**0**	**4.7**	**0**
Rainbow, Smoked, Average	**1 Pack/135g**	**190**	**7.6**	**140**	**21.7**	**0.8**	**5.6**	**0**
Raw, Average	**1 Serving/120g**	**159**	**6.5**	**132**	**20.6**	**0**	**5.4**	**0**
Smoked, Average	**2 Fillets/135g**	**187**	**7.1**	**138**	**22.7**	**0.3**	**5.2**	**0.1**

TUMS

Reg, Tums*	1 Tablet/2g	2	0	125	0	25	0	0

TUNA

Bluefin, Cooked, Dry Heat, Average	**1 Serving/100g**	**184**	**6.3**	**184**	**29.9**	**0**	**6.3**	**0**
Chilli, & Garlic, Fusions, Fishmonger, Aldi*	1 Can/80g	142	7.4	177	21	2	9.2	0.5
Chipotle, No Drain, Infusions, John West*	1 Pot/80g	165	8.4	206	24.4	3.3	10.5	0
Chunks, Canned in Spring Water, Drained, John West*	½ Can/51g	50	0.3	99	23.5	0.1	0.5	0.1
Chunks, in Brine, Average, Drained	**1 Can/130g**	**141**	**0.7**	**108**	**25.9**	**0**	**0.5**	**0**
Chunks, in Brine, Drained, Average	**1 Can/130g**	**141**	**0.7**	**108**	**25.9**	**0**	**0.5**	**0**
Chunks, in Spring Water, Average, Drained	**1 Sm Can/56g**	**60**	**0.4**	**108**	**25.4**	**0**	**0.6**	**0.1**
Chunks, in Sunflower Oil, Average, Drained	**1 Can/138g**	**260**	**12.6**	**188**	**26.5**	**0**	**9.2**	**0**
Chunks, Skipjack, in Brine, Average	**1 Can/138g**	**141**	**0.8**	**102**	**24.3**	**0**	**0.6**	**0**
Chunks, Skipjack, in Springwater, Drained, Asda*	½ Can/50g	55	0.5	109	25	0	1	0
Flakes, in Brine, Average	**1oz/28g**	**29**	**0.2**	**104**	**24.8**	**0**	**0.6**	**0**
Flakes, in Lime & Black Pepper, Canned, Sainsbury's*	1 Can/80g	103	2.4	128	22	2.2	3	2.2
in a Light Mayonnaise, Slimming World, Princes*	1 Can/80g	96	3.3	120	17.3	3.6	4.1	0
in a Tomato & Herb Dressing, Weight Watchers*	1 Can/80g	79	2.9	99	11.6	5.1	3.6	0.5
in Coronation Style Dressing, Weight Watchers*	1 Can/80g	75	2	94	9.3	8.7	2.5	0.4
in Water, Average	**1 Serving/120g**	**126**	**1**	**105**	**24**	**0.1**	**0.8**	**0**
Jalapeno, & Spicy Couscous, Infusions, John West*	1 Serving/285g	390	7.7	137	9.9	17.7	2.7	1.7
Jalapeno, Infusions, John West*	1 Can/80g	142	6.1	177	24.1	3	7.6	0
Lime & Black Pepper, John West*	1 Serving/85g	134	7	158	18	2	8.2	2.1
Mexican Style, Spreadables, John West*	1 Can/80g	149	9.8	186	13.1	5.6	12.3	1.3
Mexican, Filler, Princes*	1 Pot/85g	134	8.2	158	13.9	3.7	9.7	0.2
Soy, & Ginger, Fusions, Fishmonger, Aldi*	1 Can/80g	152	8	190	17	3.2	10	0.5
Steaks, Canned, in Water, Drained, Essential, Waitrose*	1 Can/151g	178	1.7	118	27.1	0	1.1	0

T

	Measure INFO/WEIGHT	per Measure KCAL	per Measure FAT	Nutrition Values per 100g / 100ml KCAL	PROT	CARB	FAT	FIBRE
TUNA								
Steaks, in Brine, Average	*1 Sm Can/99g*	*106*	*0.5*	*107*	*25.6*	*0*	*0.6*	*0*
Steaks, in Olive Oil, Average	*1 Serving/111g*	*211*	*10.7*	*190*	*25.8*	*0*	*9.6*	*0*
Steaks, in Sunflower Oil, Average	*1 Can/150g*	*269*	*12.6*	*179*	*26*	*0*	*8.4*	*0*
Steaks, Raw, Average	*1 Serving/140g*	*179*	*2.7*	*128*	*27.6*	*0.1*	*1.9*	*0.2*
Steaks, Skipjack, in Brine, Average	*½ Can/75g*	*73*	*0.4*	*98*	*23.2*	*0*	*0.6*	*0*
Steaks, with a Little Springwater, No Drain, John West*	1 Can/120g	151	1.2	126	29	0	1	0
with Basil, & Sun-Dried Couscous, John West*	1 Pot/285g	430	13.4	151	9.7	16.9	4.7	0
with Lemon & Black Pepper, Tesco*	1 Can/85g	144	6.5	170	21.2	4	7.6	0.5
with Soy, Ginger, & Mushroom, Couscous, John West*	1 Pot/285g	413	10	145	10	17.9	3.5	0
Yellowfin, Cooked, Dry Heat, Average	*1 Serving/100g*	*139*	*1.2*	*139*	*30*	*0*	*1.2*	*0*
TUNA MAYONNAISE								
Mayo, & Sweetcorn, Fillers, Princes*	1 Pot/85g	121	5.1	142	13.2	8.6	6	0.3
with Sweetcorn, Spreadable, John West*	1 Serving/20g	45	3.5	227	12.7	4.6	17.4	0.5
TURBOT								
Grilled	*1oz/28g*	*34*	*1*	*122*	*22.7*	*0*	*3.5*	*0*
Raw	*1oz/28g*	*27*	*0.8*	*95*	*17.7*	*0*	*2.7*	*0*
TURKEY								
BBQ Smoked, Slices, Fire & Smoke, Henry Denny's*	1 Slice/25g	32	0.4	127	28	1.1	1.6	0
Breast, Butter Basted, Average	*1 Serving/75g*	*110*	*3.6*	*146*	*23.7*	*1.9*	*4.9*	*0.4*
Breast, Butter Basted, Joint, with Stuffing, Roasted, Tesco*	¼ Joint/150g	294	15	196	24.3	2.1	10	0.2
Breast, Diced, Healthy Range, Average	*1oz/28g*	*30*	*0.4*	*108*	*23.8*	*0*	*1.3*	*0*
Breast, Honey Roast, Sliced, Average	*1 Serving/50g*	*57*	*0.7*	*114*	*24*	*1.6*	*1.4*	*0.2*
Breast, Joint, Raw, Average	*1 Serving/125g*	*134*	*2.6*	*108*	*21.3*	*0.7*	*2.1*	*0.6*
Breast, Raw, Average	*1oz/28g*	*33*	*0.6*	*117*	*24.1*	*0.5*	*2*	*0.1*
Breast, Roasted, Average	*1oz/28g*	*37*	*0.9*	*131*	*24.6*	*0.7*	*3.3*	*0.1*
Breast, Roll, Cooked, Average	*1 Slice/10g*	*9*	*0.1*	*92*	*17.6*	*3.5*	*0.8*	*0*
Breast, Slices, Cooked, Average	*1 Slice/20g*	*23*	*0.3*	*114*	*24*	*1.2*	*1.4*	*0.3*
Breast, Smoked, Sliced, Average	*1 Slice/20g*	*23*	*0.4*	*113*	*23.4*	*0.7*	*2*	*0*
Breast, Steaks, in Crumbs, Average	*1 Steak/76g*	*217*	*14.1*	*286*	*13.7*	*16.4*	*18.5*	*0.2*
Breast, Steaks, Raw, Average	*1oz/28g*	*30*	*0.3*	*107*	*24.3*	*0*	*1.1*	*0*
Breast, Strips, for Stir Fry, Average	*1 Serving/175g*	*205*	*2.7*	*117*	*25.6*	*0.1*	*1.6*	*0*
Dark Meat, Raw, Average	*1oz/28g*	*29*	*0.7*	*104*	*20.4*	*0*	*2.5*	*0*
Leg, Dark Meat, Raw , Average, Weighed with Bone	*1 Serving/100g*	*73*	*1.8*	*73*	*14.3*	*0*	*1.8*	*0*
Light Meat, Raw, Average	*1oz/28g*	*29*	*0.2*	*105*	*24.4*	*0*	*0.8*	*0*
Light Meat, Roasted	*1 Cup/140g*	*163*	*3.3*	*116*	*22.1*	*0*	*2.4*	*0*
Mince, Average	*1oz/28g*	*45*	*2*	*161*	*23.9*	*0*	*7.2*	*0*
Mince, Lean, Healthy Range, Average	*1oz/28g*	*33*	*1.1*	*118*	*20.3*	*0*	*4.1*	*0*
Rashers, Average	*1 Rasher/26g*	*26*	*0.4*	*101*	*19.1*	*2.3*	*1.6*	*0*
Rashers, Smoked, Average	*1 Serving/75g*	*76*	*1.4*	*101*	*19.8*	*1.5*	*1.8*	*0*
Rashers, Unsmoked, Grilled, Freshcure, Aldi*	2 Rashers/46g	71	0.6	155	33	2.2	1.4	0.5
Roast, Meat & Skin, Average	*1oz/28g*	*48*	*1.8*	*171*	*28*	*0*	*6.5*	*0*
Roast, Meat Only, Average	*1 Serving/100g*	*157*	*3.2*	*157*	*29.9*	*0*	*3.2*	*0*
Smoked, Applewood, 1, Waitrose*	½ Pack/40g	48	0.4	121	27.3	0.5	1.1	0.1
Steak, Cajun, with Crushed Beans, & Slaw, Hello Fresh*	1 Serving/507g	416	8	82	10.3	6.1	1.6	0
Steak, Golden Breaded, Cooked, Bernard Matthews*	1 Steak/100g	296	17.5	296	13.4	19.9	17.5	3.1
Steak, Pan Fried, with Mushroom Sauce, Hello Fresh*	1 Serving/584g	561	22.9	96	7	8.2	3.9	0
Steak, Spiced, with Sweet Potato, & Avocado, Hello Fresh*	1 Serving/621g	602	24.1	97	7.9	7.9	3.9	0
Strips, Stir-Fried, Average	*1oz/28g*	*46*	*1.3*	*164*	*31*	*0*	*4.5*	*0*
Thigh, Diced, Average	*1oz/28g*	*33*	*1.2*	*117*	*19.6*	*0*	*4.3*	*0*
Thigh, Mince, Cooked, Tesco*	¼ Pack/100g	145	5.5	145	23.7	0.1	5.5	0.1
Thigh, Mince, Raw, Tesco*	¼ Pack/125g	145	5.5	116	19	0.1	4.4	0.1
Vegetarian, Slices, Deli, with Stuffing, Quorn*	½ Pack/50g	60	1.2	120	16	8.9	2.3	4
Vegetarian, Slices, with Sage, Meat Free, Quorn*	¼ Pack/25g	32	0.6	128	16	8.9	2.3	4

T

	Measure INFO/WEIGHT	per Measure KCAL	FAT	Nutrition Values per 100g / 100ml KCAL	PROT	CARB	FAT	FIBRE
TURKEY								
Wafer Thin, Honey Roast, Average	*1 Slice/10g*	*11*	*0.2*	*109*	*19.2*	*4.2*	*1.7*	*0.2*
TURKEY DINNER								
& Ham, Irish Classics, Tesco*	1 Pack/500g	481	12.5	96	7.3	10.4	2.5	1.6
Roast Dinner, 105, Oakhouse Foods Ltd*	1 Serving/430g	331	9	77	5.4	8.5	2.1	1.6
Roast, Asda*	1 Pack/400g	344	6.4	86	7	11	1.6	2
Roast, Meal for One, M&S*	1 Pack/370g	462	16.3	125	9.1	12.4	4.4	2.7
Roast, Sainsbury's*	1 Pack/450g	354	9	79	6.8	8.4	2	1.9
Traditional, Birds Eye*	1 Pack/340g	292	7.8	86	6.1	10.3	2.3	1.7
TURKEY HAM								
Average	*1 Serving/75g*	*81*	*2.9*	*108*	*15.6*	*2.8*	*3.9*	*0*
TURKISH DELIGHT								
Fry's*	1 Bar/51g	185	3.4	363	1.2	74	6.7	1.2
Milk Chocolate, M&S*	1 Pack/55g	220	4.7	400	1.6	79	8.5	0
with Rose, Hazer Baba*	1 Square/18g	70	0.3	389	1.6	88.6	1.7	0
TURMERIC								
Powder	*1 Tsp/3g*	*11*	*0.3*	*354*	*7.8*	*58.2*	*9.9*	*0*
TURNIP								
Boiled, Average	*1oz/28g*	*3*	*0.1*	*12*	*0.6*	*2*	*0.2*	*1.9*
Mashed, Mash Direct*	½ Pack/200g	84	0.8	42	0.8	7.4	0.4	3.1
Mashed, McKinlays*	1 Serving/100g	55	2	55	1	7	2	2.3
Raw, Unprepared, Average	*1oz/28g*	*5*	*0.1*	*17*	*0.7*	*3.5*	*0.2*	*1.8*
TURNOVER								
Apple, Bramley & Cream, Sainsbury's*	1 Turnover/78g	243	13.6	312	3.9	34.3	17.4	1.3
Apple, Bramley, & Cream, Waitrose*	1 Turnover/82g	254	15	309	4.1	31	18.3	2.3
Apple, Co-Op*	1 Turnover/77g	308	20.8	400	4	35	27	1
Apple, Puff Pastry, Bakery, Tesco*	1 Turnover/83g	263	13	317	4.3	38.6	15.7	1.8
Raspberry, Fresh Cream, Asda*	1 Turnover/100g	411	23	411	6	45	23	2.1
Raspberry, Fresh Cream, Tesco*	1 Turnover/74g	244	15.6	330	4.4	29.9	21.1	1.6
TWIGLETS								
Original, Jacob's*	1 Sm Bag/25g	104	3	414	13.3	57.3	12	11.5
TWIRL								
Cadbury*	1 Finger/22g	118	6.8	535	7.6	56	30.9	0.8
Treat Size, Cadbury*	1 Bar/21g	115	6.6	535	7.6	56	30.9	0.8
TWIX								
'Xtra, Mars*	1 Pack/85g	416	20.1	490	4.7	65.5	23.7	1.5
Fun Size, Mars*	1 Bar/20g	99	4.8	495	4.5	64.6	24	1.5
Standard, Mars*	1 Pack/58g	284	13.7	490	4.7	65.5	23.7	1.5
Top, Mars*	1 Bar/28g	143	7.8	511	5.2	60.2	27.7	0
White, Fingers, Mars*	1 Bar/23g	115	5.8	502	4.8	64	25	0
White, Mars*	1 Pack/46g	231	11.5	502	4.8	64	25	0
TZATZIKI								
Average	*1 Tbsp/15g*	*11*	*0.8*	*76*	*3.4*	*3.4*	*5.5*	*0.2*

T

INFO/WEIGHT	Measure	per Measure		Nutrition Values per 100g / 100ml				
		KCAL	FAT	KCAL	PROT	CARB	FAT	FIBRE
VANILLA EXTRACT								
Average	*1 Tbsp/13g*	*37*	*0*	*288*	*0.1*	*12.6*	*0.1*	*0*
VEAL								
Chop, Loin, Raw, Weighed with Bone, Average	*1 Chop/195g*	*317*	*17.8*	*163*	*18.9*	*0*	*9.1*	*0*
Escalope, Breaded, M&S*	1 Escalope/130g	292	13.9	225	13.6	18.7	10.7	0.4
Escalope, Fried, Average	*1oz/28g*	*55*	*1.9*	*196*	*33.7*	*0*	*6.8*	*0*
Mince, Raw, Average	*1oz/28g*	*40*	*2*	*144*	*20.3*	*0*	*7*	*0*
Shoulder, Lean Only, Roasted, Average	*1oz/28g*	*35*	*1.3*	*125*	*19.9*	*0*	*4.4*	*0*
Sirloin, Lean & Fat, Roasted, Average	*1oz/28g*	*43*	*2.2*	*152*	*18.9*	*0*	*7.8*	*0*
Sirloin, Lean Only, Roasted, Average	*1oz/28g*	*33*	*1.2*	*118*	*18.4*	*0*	*4.4*	*0*
VEGAN								
Fillets, Quorn*	1 Fillet/63g	58	0.4	92	14.2	3.5	0.6	7.8
Mexican, Ready Meal, Lazy Vegan*	1 Pack/350g	434	15	124	7.7	12	4.3	3.3
Pieces, Vegan, Quorn*	¼ Pack/70g	79	2	113	15.3	3.9	2.8	5.3
VEGEMITE								
Australian, Kraft*	1 Tsp/5g	9	0	173	23.5	19.7	0	0
VEGETABLE CHIPS								
As Sold, Aunt Bessie's*	1 Serving/125g	189	11	151	2.1	13	8.8	5.3
Cassava, Average	*1oz/28g*	*99*	*0.1*	*353*	*1.8*	*91.4*	*0.4*	*4*
Oven Cooked, Aunt Bessie's*	1 Serving/125g	205	11.9	164	2.2	14	9.5	5.8
VEGETABLE FINGERS								
Crispy, Birds Eye*	2 Fingers/60g	107	4.8	179	3.2	23.5	8	2.3
Sainsbury's*	3 Fingers/79g	191	8.4	243	4.6	30	10.7	4.1
Tesco*	1 Finger/25g	52	2.2	206	4.1	26.4	8.6	3.3
VEGETABLE MEDLEY								
Carrots, Sweetcorn, Peas, Broccoli, Four, Tesco*	¼Pack/84g	51	0.9	61	3.6	7.2	1.1	3.9
Chargrilled, Waitrose*	1 Serving/100g	77	3	77	2.5	8.3	3	3.3
Four Seasons, Aldi*	1 Serving/80g	38	0.7	48	3.1	5.6	0.9	2.6
Frozen, M&S*	1 Pack/500g	175	4	35	3.4	3.9	0.8	3.1
Green Grocers, Lidl*	1 Serving/80g	22	0.4	28	1.6	2.8	0.5	2.7
Green, Frozen, Morrisons*	1 Serving/80g	45	1	56	4.6	4.9	1.2	3.5
Green, Peas, Broccoli, Beans & Leek, Mint Butter, Co-Op*	½ Pack/130g	99	5.8	76	2.9	4.2	4.5	3.7
Green, with Bouillon Butter, Co-Op*	1 Serving/80g	54	2.4	67	3.5	4.8	3	3.2
Mange Tout, Corn, Broccoli, Spring Onion, Chilli, Tesco*	½ Pack/110g	38	0.3	35	2.7	4.4	0.3	2.1
Medley, Tender, Green, Sainsbury's*	1 Pack/160g	62	0.8	39	2.9	4.3	0.5	3.6
Mixed, Tesco*	½ Pack/112g	46	0.6	41	2.3	4.9	0.5	3.8
Roasted, Waitrose*	½ Pack/200g	282	15.6	141	1.2	16.4	7.8	3.7
VEGETABLES								
& Bean, Stew Mix, Cooks' Ingredients, Waitrose*	½ Pack /200g	166	3.8	83	4.2	10.2	1.9	4.3
Asparagus, & Tenderstem Broccoli, Tesco*	½ Pack/95g	29	0.4	31	3.1	2.8	0.4	1.8
Balls, Mushroom, & Lentil, Vegetarian, Tesco*	½ Pack/131g	173	4.5	132	7.2	15	3.4	6.4
Carrots, & Peas, Chilled, Fresh Tastes, Asda*	1 Serving/200g	76	0.8	38	2.4	4.8	0.4	2.9
Casserole, Cooks' Ingredients, Waitrose*	¼ Pack/138g	48	0.4	35	0.9	6	0.3	2.5
Collard Greens, Raw, Average*	1 Serving/80g	26	0.5	32	3	5	0.6	4
Green, Petit Pois & Beans, Parsley, Mint & Butter, Tesco*	½ Pack/129g	106	6.6	82	3.4	2.6	5.1	6.1
Grilled Mix, Frozen, Essential, Waitrose*	1 Serving/80g	34	0.2	42	1.8	8.1	0.3	2.4
Grilled, Frozen, Sainsbury's*	1 Serving/80g	42	2.9	52	1.2	3.8	3.6	1.5
Indian Spiced, HL, Tesco*	1 Pack/347g	267	5.5	77	3	11.5	1.6	2.7
Layered, Super Green, with Minted Butter, M&S*	1 Serving/80g	51	2.2	64	3.6	4.4	2.7	3.6
Layered, with Butter, Waitrose*	1 Pack/280g	207	16.2	74	1.7	3.6	5.8	2.4
Mediterranean Style, Roast, Nature's Pick, Aldi*	½ Pack/200g	114	6.4	57	1.2	5.2	3.2	1.5
Mediterranean, Chunky, Cooked, Sainsbury's*	¼ Pack/119g	56	2	47	1.1	5.9	1.7	2
Mediterranean, Ready to Roast, Waitrose*	1 Serving/200g	128	8	64	1.3	5.6	4	1.6
Peas, Spinach, Spring Greens, & Samphire, M&S*	½ Pack/105g	85	4.4	81	3.8	4.7	4.2	4.6

V

	Measure INFO/WEIGHT	KCAL	FAT	KCAL	PROT	CARB	FAT	FIBRE
VEGETABLES								
Pepper, Red, & Carrot, Mash, Smoky, M&S*	1 Pack/300g	162	9.3	54	0.5	4.4	3.1	3.2
Peppers, Mixed, Stir Fry, Tesco*	1 Pack/320g	173	9	54	1.6	4.4	2.8	2.4
Roasted, & Goats Cheese, 837, Oakhouse Foods Ltd*	1 Meal/400g	348	20.8	87	4.5	6.1	5.2	1.5
Roasted, Italian, M&S*	1 Serving/95g	218	20	230	1.8	7.1	21	1.7
Roasted, Summer, Tesco*	1 Serving/80g	46	1.7	58	1.5	7.5	2.1	1.6
Roasting, with Rosemary, & Thyme, Tesco*	1 Serving/100g	119	3.1	119	1.3	18	3.1	7
Root, for Mashing, Eat Fresh, Tesco*	1 Pack/720g	238	2.9	33	0.7	5.4	0.4	2.7
Root, Mashed, Microwaved, Growers Selection, Asda*	½ Pack/200g	116	4.4	58	0.7	7.2	2.2	2.7
Root, Parmentier, Cooked, Sainsbury's*	½ Pack/117g	122	3.7	104	1.6	15.5	3.2	3.4
Root, Rainbow, Collection, M&S*	½ Pack/176g	67	2.5	38	0.7	3.9	1.4	3.6
Root, Roasted, Extra Special, Asda*	½ Pack/205g	160	3.1	78	1.1	15	1.5	6
Root, Roasted, Ready to Roast, Mash Direct*	1 Pack/350g	200	7.4	57	0.8	5.8	2.1	5.9
Selection, Lightly Buttered & Seasoned, M&S*	½ Pack/150g	122	7.5	81	1.5	6.2	5	2.6
Selection, Roasted, COU, M&S*	1 Pack/250g	88	2	35	1.2	6.1	0.8	0.6
Soup Mix, Winter, Sainsbury's*	1 Serving/149g	61	0.3	41	1.1	7.9	0.2	1.7
Stir Fry, Colourful, Ribbon, Waitrose*	½ Pack/116g	57	2.4	49	1.3	5	2.1	2.3
Stir Fry, Frozen, Sainsbury's*	1 Serving/80g	19	0.2	24	1.3	3.9	0.3	2
Stir Fry, Hot, & Spicy, Natures Pick, Aldi*	1 Serving/100g	37	0.5	37	1.6	5.3	0.5	2.3
Stir Fry, Oriental, Oaklands*	1 Pack/300g	60	1.5	20	1.1	3	0.5	1.8
Stir Fry, Tesco*	1 Serving/150g	38	0.2	25	0.9	5	0.1	1.4
Stir Fry, Water Chestnut, & Bamboo Shoot, Spicy, Waitrose*	½ Pack/133g	98	5.9	74	1.9	4	4.4	5.6
Swede, & Carrot, Cubed, Ready to Cook, M&S*	¼ Pack/120g	40	0.5	33	0.7	5.4	0.4	2.7
Thai Style, Frozen, Four Seasons, Aldi*	1 Serving/100g	57	2.2	57	1.9	6.1	2.2	2.4
VEGETABLES MIXED								
Broccoli & Cauliflower Florets, Baby Carrots, Mixed, Asda*	1 Serving/113g	28	0.7	25	2.2	2.6	0.6	2.4
Broccoli, Cauliflower & Carrots, Farmhouse, Birds Eye*	1 Bag/135g	46	0.8	34	1.8	3.3	0.6	2.2
Broccoli, Peas & Green Beans, Mixed, Co-Op*	1 Serving/80g	36	0.3	45	4.8	3.8	0.4	3.6
Broccoli, Sweet Potato, Beetroot, Kale, Steam Bags, Tesco*	1 Bag/160g	93	0.3	58	1.9	10.5	0.2	3.2
Carrot, Broccoli, & Sweetcorn, Iceland*	1 Pack/300g	150	3	50	2.5	6.1	1	3.6
Carrot, Cauliflower & Broccoli, Prepared, Mixed, Co-Op*	1 Pack/250g	100	1.5	40	2.4	5	0.6	2.7
Carrot, Cauliflower, & Broccoli, Fresh, Mixed, Tesco*	1 Serving/80g	26	0.2	32	2.6	3.9	0.2	2.8
Carrot, Cauliflower, & Broccoli, Meadow Fresh, Lidl*	1 Serving/80g	213	2.7	266	13.3	38	3.3	14
Carrots, Broccoli & Sweetcorn, Mixed, Sainsbury's*	1 Pack/120g	67	1.4	56	2.6	8.7	1.2	2
Carrots, Cauliflower & Broccoli, Mixed, Waitrose*	1 Serving/80g	32	0.5	40	2.4	4.9	0.6	2.9
Carrots, Peas, Cauliflower, & Broccoli, Frozen, Tesco*	1 Serving/80g	36	0.6	45	2.4	5.4	0.8	3.1
Carrots, Peas, Green Beans & Sweetcorn, Mixed, Tesco*	1 Serving/80g	47	0.8	58	3.3	6.9	1	4.3
Casserole with Baby Potatoes, Fresh, Mixed, M&S*	½ Pack/350g	140	1	40	1.2	7.8	0.3	2.1
Casserole, Mixed, Tesco*	1 Serving/80g	35	0.2	44	1	7.9	0.3	2.6
Casserole, Nature's Pick, Aldi*	¼ Pack/150g	62	0.8	41	1.1	7.8	0.5	2
Coleslaw, Crunchy, Kit, Morrisons*	½ Pack/150g	217	2.1	145	0.7	2	1.4	3.6
Fajita, Ready to Cook, Tesco*	½ Pack/139g	82	2.4	59	1.1	8.5	1.7	2.4
Farmhouse, Mixed, Frozen, Boiled in Salted Water, Tesco*	1 Serving/80g	41	0.7	51	3.2	5.7	0.9	3.5
Fine Cut, Steamers, Waitrose*	1 Pouch/160g	77	1	48	3.2	5.5	0.6	4.1
Frozen, Organic, Duchy, Waitrose*	1 Serving/80g	41	0.7	51	3	6	0.9	3.6
Greens, & Corn, Mixed, Steam Bags, Tesco*	1 Bag/160g	90	1.9	56	3.9	5.4	1.2	4
Mediterranean, & Potatoes, Morrisons*	1 Serving/125g	176	7.1	141	2.3	18.1	5.7	4
Mediterranean, Chargrilled, Frozen, Sainsbury's*	1 Serving/80g	73	4.3	91	1.5	8	5.3	2.7
Mediterranean, Oven Baked, Asda*	½ Pack/200g	126	7	63	0.7	6.2	3.5	1.7
Mediterranean, Roasting, Cooked, Tesco*	¼ Pack/100g	28	0.2	28	1.1	4.7	0.2	1.5
Melange De Legumes, Grilled, Picard*	1 Serving/200g	78	0.8	39	1.6	6	0.4	2.8
Mix, Steamer, Love Life, Waitrose*	1 Bag/160g	83	1.8	52	2.8	7.7	1.1	2.8
Mixed, Baby, Steam, Fresh, Tesco*	1 Pack/160g	72	1.3	45	2.7	6.7	0.8	3.8
Mixed, Bag, M&S*	1 Serving/200g	70	0.4	35	2.9	5.6	0.2	0

	Measure INFO/WEIGHT	per Measure KCAL	FAT	Nutrition Values per 100g / 100ml KCAL	PROT	CARB	FAT	FIBRE
VEGETABLES MIXED								
Mixed, Freshly Frozen, Asda*	1 Serving/80g	42	0.6	52	3.2	8	0.8	3
Mixed, Freshly Frozen, Iceland*	1 Serving/100g	54	0.8	54	3.3	8.3	0.8	3.7
Mixed, Frozen, Cooked, Sainsbury's*	1 Serving/80g	45	0.6	56	2.9	7.5	0.7	4
Mixed, Layered, Classics, M&S*	½ Pack/160g	112	6.2	70	1.2	7.3	3.9	1.2
Mixed, Roast, Four Seasons*	1 Serving/187g	79	0.4	42	1.2	8.8	0.2	0
Mixed, Special, Sainsbury's*	1 Serving/120g	68	1.2	57	3.2	8.9	1	2.9
Peas & Carrots, Buttery & Tender, Mixed, Tesco*	½ Pack/150g	138	6.1	92	3.7	7.9	4.1	4.5
Peas, Cabbage, & Tenderstem, Layers, Waitrose*	1/3 Pack/83g	85	4.2	103	6.2	6.2	5	4
Peas, Carrots, & Sweetcorn, Black Pepper & Butter, Tesco*	½ Pack/178g	128	4.4	72	2.8	7.6	2.5	3.9
Peas, Courgette, & Spring Greens Selection, Tesco*	½ Pack/122g	78	3.7	64	3.4	3.3	3	5.1
Peas, Sweetcorn, Broccoli, Spinach, Steam Bags, Ocado*	1 Bag/153g	121	1.1	79	3.5	13	0.7	3.2
Red Pepper, Butternut, Courgette, & Red Onion, M&S*	½ Pack/143g	48	0.3	34	1.2	5.9	0.2	1.9
Roasting Tray, Quick Cook, Tesco*	½ Pack/200g	144	5	72	2.5	8.6	2.5	2.5
Roasting, in Herb, & Honey Glaze, Farmfoods*	1 Serving/80g	52	1.5	65	1.2	9.3	1.9	0
Roasting, Selection, Sweet & Colourful, Waitrose*	½ Pack/300g	147	3	49	1	7.5	1	2.8
Root, Diced, Tesco*	1/3 Pack/240g	120	0.7	50	0.6	9.3	0.3	3.6
Tenderstem, & Mixed Vegetables, Tesco*	1 Serving/80g	54	0.6	34	2.1	4.2	0.4	2.6
Winter, Maple Roasted, Waitrose*	½ Pack/168g	294	11.3	175	2.1	24.1	6.7	5.1
VEGETARIAN								
Roast, Nut & Date, with Gravy, Asda*	1 Serving/196g	300	12.7	153	4.7	16.1	6.5	5.5
Schnitzel, Breaded, Tivall*	1 Schnitzel/100g	202	9.5	202	16	11	9.5	4
Slices, Sage & Onion, Vegi Deli, The Redwood Co*	1 Slice/10g	23	1.4	233	21.4	5	14.1	0.5
Steak, Beef Style, Quorn*	1 Steak/86g	126	4.5	146	16	5.3	5.2	6.9
Steak, Vivera*	1 Steak/100g	222	13	222	17	7.8	13	3.6
Strips, BBQ, Quorn*	½ Pack/140g	183	4.1	131	14.3	8.4	2.9	6.8
Strips, Sweet, & Smoky, Quorn*	3 Strips/92g	171	3.3	186	10.6	25.1	3.6	5.5
VEGETARIAN MINCE								
Meat Free, Improved Recipe, Frozen Sainsbury's*	1 Serving/77g	131	3.9	170	18.6	11.7	5	2
Meat Free, The Meatless Farm Co *	¼ Pack/100g	199	10.2	199	21.1	3.2	10.2	5.2
Simply, Garden Gourmet*	1 Serving/80g	119	2.4	149	19.3	6.9	3	8.8
Sunflower, Organic, Dry, Just Wholefoods*	1 Serving/18g	55	0.4	305	51	9	2	20
Vegan, Meat Free, Ocado*	¼ Pack/128g	115	0.6	90	15	3.7	0.5	5.8
Vegemince, Realeat*	1 Serving/125g	218	12.5	174	18	3	10	3
Vegetarian, Mince, Frozen & Chilled, Quorn*	1 Serving/87g	91	1.7	105	14.5	4.5	2	5.5
Vivera*	1 Pack/220g	240	0.2	109	21	3.3	0.1	5.9
VENISON								
Grill Steak, Average	*1 Steak/150g*	*178*	*3.8*	*119*	*19*	*5*	*2.5*	*1*
in Red Wine & Port, Average	*1oz/28g*	*21*	*0.7*	*76*	*9.8*	*3.5*	*2.6*	*0.4*
Minced, Cooked, Average	*1 Serving/100g*	*187*	*8.2*	*187*	*26.4*	*0*	*8.2*	*0*
Minced, Raw, Average	*1 Serving/100g*	*157*	*7.1*	*157*	*21.8*	*0*	*7.1*	*0*
Raw, Haunch, Meat Only, Average	*1 Serving/100g*	*103*	*1.6*	*103*	*22.2*	*0*	*1.6*	*0*
Roasted, Average	*1oz/28g*	*46*	*0.7*	*165*	*35.6*	*0*	*2.5*	*0*
Steak, Raw, Average	*1oz/28g*	*30*	*0.5*	*108*	*22.8*	*0*	*1.9*	*0*
VERMICELLI								
Dry	*1oz/28g*	*99*	*0.1*	*355*	*8.7*	*78.3*	*0.4*	*0*
Egg, Cooked, Average	*1 Serving/185g*	*239*	*2.6*	*129*	*5*	*24*	*1.4*	*1*
VERMOUTH								
Dry	*1 Shot/50ml*	*54*	*0*	*109*	*0.1*	*3*	*0*	*0*
Sweet	*1 Shot/50ml*	*76*	*0*	*151*	*0*	*15.9*	*0*	*0*
VIMTO*								
Cordial, No Added Sugar, Diluted, Vimto*	1 Serving/250ml	6	0.2	2	0.1	0.4	0.1	0
Cordial, No Added Sugar, Undiluted, Vimto*	1 Serving/50ml	2	0	4	0	0.7	0	0
Cordial, Original, Diluted, Vimto*	1 Serving/200ml	60	0	30	0	7.4	0	0

V

	Measure INFO/WEIGHT	per Measure KCAL	FAT	Nutrition Values per 100g / 100ml KCAL	PROT	CARB	FAT	FIBRE
VIMTO*								
Cordial, Original, Undiluted, Vimto*	1 Serving/50ml	49	0	98	0	23.6	0	0
Grape, Blackcurrant & Raspberry Drink, Fizzy, Vimto*	1 Can/330ml	147	0	44	0	11	0	0
Mango, Strawberry & Pineapple, Remix, Diluted, Vimto*	1 Serving/200ml	4	0	2	0	0.2	0	0
Raspberry, Orange & Passionfruit, Remix, Vimto*	1 Serving/200ml	4	0	2	0	0.2	0	0
VINAIGRETTE								
Balsamic Vinegar & Pistachio, Finest, Tesco*	1 Tbsp/15ml	56	5.9	370	0.2	2.8	39.2	0
Balsamic, Hellmann's*	1 Tbsp/15ml	12	0.4	82	0.1	9.6	2.7	0.6
Cider Vinegar, Maille*	1 Tsp/5ml	20	2	400	0.5	7	40	0
Fat Free, Hellmann's*	1 Tbsp/15ml	8	0.1	48	0.5	11	0.5	0
French Style, Finest, Tesco*	1 Tbsp/15ml	93	9.8	620	0.6	6.3	65.3	0.2
French, Real, Briannas*	2 Tbsp/30ml	150	17	500	0	0	56.7	0
Luxury French, Hellmann's*	1 Tsp/5ml	15	1.3	305	0.8	16	26.1	0.4
Olive Oil & Lemon, Amoy*	½ Sachet/15ml	38	3.6	250	0.3	3	24	0
PB, Waitrose*	1 Tsp/5ml	4	0	89	0.4	20.9	0.4	0.5
Rhubarb, & Vinegar, The Little Herb Farm*	1 Tbsp/15ml	21	0	139	0.3	33.9	0	0.5
VINDALOO								
Chicken, Average	**1 Serving/410g**	**787**	**51.2**	**192**	**18.5**	**2.6**	**12.5**	**0.3**
Chicken, Sainsbury's*	1 Pack/400g	460	16.8	115	14.6	4.8	4.2	0.6
Chicken, Waitrose*	1 Pack/340g	398	18.4	117	10.6	6.4	5.4	1.6
Volcanic, Takeaway, Morrisons*	½ Pack/175g	205	9.8	117	10.7	5.1	5.6	2
VINE LEAVES								
Stuffed with Rice	**1oz/28g**	**73**	**5**	**262**	**2.8**	**23.8**	**18**	**0**
VINEGAR								
Balsamic, Average	**1 Tsp/5ml**	**6**	**0**	**115**	**0.9**	**26**	**0**	**0**
Cider	**1 Tbsp/15ml**	**2**	**0**	**14**	**0**	**5.9**	**0**	**0**
Malt, Average	**1 Tbsp/15g**	**1**	**0**	**4**	**0.4**	**0.6**	**0**	**0**
Red Wine, Average	**1 Tbsp/15ml**	**3**	**0**	**19**	**0**	**0.3**	**0**	**0**
VODKA								
& Diet Coke, Average	**1 Serving/150ml**	**68**	**0**	**45**	**0**	**0**	**0**	**0**
& Tonic, Ready Mixed, M&S*	1 Can/250ml	202	0	81	0	6.3	0	0
37.5% Volume	**1 Pub Shot/35ml**	**72**	**0**	**207**	**0**	**0**	**0**	**0**
40% Volume	**1 Pub Shot/35ml**	**78**	**0**	**222**	**0**	**0**	**0**	**0**
Cookies & Cream, Sidekick, Halewood International Ltd*	1 Serving/30ml	48	0.5	160	0.3	7.7	1.6	0
Rhubarb, Average	**1 Single/25ml**	**57**	**0**	**229**	**0**	**0**	**0**	**0**
Smirnoff & Cranberry, Premixed, Canned, Diageo*	1 Can/250ml	175	0	70	0	8.5	0	0
Smirnoff & Diet Cola, Premixed, Canned, Diageo*	1 Can/250ml	100	0	40	0	0	0	0
Smirnoff & Schweppes Tonic, Premixed, Canned, Diageo*	1 Can/250ml	158	0	63	0	6.4	0	0
VOL AU VENTS								
Deluxe, Lidl*	1 Pastry/7g	40	2.8	567	7.8	41.5	40.7	1.5
Mushroom, Sainsbury's*	1 Serving/14g	49	3.1	350	6.9	30.8	22.1	1.4
Seafood, Party, Youngs*	1 Serving/17g	60	4.2	354	8.3	26	24.8	1

	Measure INFO/WEIGHT	per Measure KCAL	FAT	Nutrition Values per 100g / 100ml KCAL	PROT	CARB	FAT	FIBRE
WAFERS								
Cafe Curls, Rolled, Askeys*	1 Wafer/5g	21	0.4	422	5.8	80.3	8.6	0
Caramel, Dark Chocolate, Tunnock's*	1 Wafer/30g	148	7.6	492	5.2	60.7	25.4	0
Caramel, Log, Tunnock's*	1 Wafer/32g	150	6.7	468	4.2	65.7	21	3.4
Caramel, Tunnock's*	1 Wafer/30g	134	5.2	448	3.6	69.2	17.4	2.5
Coconut, with Milk Chocolate, Free From, Morrisons*	1 Bar/25g	132	7	528	3.4	64.7	28	2
for Ice Cream, Askeys*	1 Wafer/2g	6	0	388	11.4	79	2.9	0
Hazelnut, Milky, Slices, Sondey, Lidl*	1 Slice/25g	135	8.3	539	6.3	52	33	3.7
Timeout, Cadbury*	1 Bar/21g	111	6	524	6.7	60	28.3	2.1
WAFFLES								
Belgian, Sugar, Aldi*	1 Waffle/55g	249	12.6	452	5.7	54	23	2
Belgian, TTD, Sainsbury's*	1 Waffle/25g	122	7.3	490	6	50.6	29.3	1.2
Caramel, Asda*	1 Waffle/8g	37	1.8	459	3.3	62	22	1.1
Classic, Frozen, Hello Morning, Birds Eye*	1 Waffle/30g	97	4.3	319	7	40	14	2.6
GF, Schar*	1 Waffle/25g	120	7	478	4.8	52	28	1.1
Stroopwafel, Caramel, Daelmans*	1 Wafel/29g	131	6.1	452	3	62	21	1.5
Sweet, American Style, Sainsbury's*	1 Waffle/35g	160	8.9	457	7.2	50.6	25.3	1.1
Toasting, McVitie's*	1 Waffle/25g	115	6.3	461	5.7	52.6	25.5	0.8
Toffee, Tregroes, Aldi*	1 Waffle/35g	160	6.2	463	3.5	71.7	18	2.2
WAGON WHEEL								
Chocolate, Original, Epic Inside, Burton's*	1 Biscuit/39g	172	5.7	441	5.1	68.7	14.5	2.1
Jammie, Burton's*	1 Biscuit/40g	168	5.6	420	5.1	67.7	14.1	1.9
WALNUT WHIP								
Classic, M&S*	1 Whip/28g	144	8.1	515	6.8	55.8	28.9	2
Nestle*	1 Whip/35g	173	8.8	494	5.3	61.3	25.2	0.7
WALNUTS								
Average	*1 Nut/7g*	*48*	*4.8*	*688*	*14.7*	*3.3*	*68.5*	*3.5*
Halves, Average	*1 Half/3g*	*23*	*2.3*	*669*	*17.4*	*6.3*	*65*	*4.7*
Pickled, in Malt Vinegar, Drained, Opies*	1 Walnut/25g	23	0	92	0.8	23	0	3.4
WASABI								
Paste, Ready Mixed, Japanese, Yutaka*	1 Tsp/5g	14	0.4	286	2.7	53	7	0
WATER								
Apple, & Raspberry, Flavoured, Sparkling, Spar*	1 Glass/250ml	2	0	1	0	0	0	0
Apple, & Raspberry, Sparkling, Spring, Tesco*	1 Glass/330ml	7	0	2	0	0.5	0	0
Apple, & Strawberry, Flavoured, Morrisons*	1 Serving/200ml	3	0	2	0.2	0.1	0	0
Blackcurrant, & Apple, Juicy Spring, Drench*	1 Serving/250ml	98	0	39	0	9.2	0	0
Cactus, Truenopal*	1 Serving/330ml	30	0	9	0	2.2	0	0
Cherry, & Plum, Flavoured, Asda*	1 Serving/250ml	2	0	1	0	0.5	0	0
Coconut, Not From Concentrate, Coco Loco, Aldi*	1 Serving/250ml	48	1.2	19	0.5	4.5	0.5	0.5
Cranberry, & Raspberry, Flavoured, Morrisons*	1 Serving/200ml	3	0	2	0.2	0.1	0	0
Cranberry, & Raspberry, Spring, Drench*	1 Bottle/440ml	146	0.4	33	0.1	7.7	0.1	0
Elderflower, & Pear, Detox, V Water*	1 Bottle/500ml	40	0	8	0	1.9	0	0
Elderflower, Presse, Bottle Green*	1 Serving/250ml	88	0	35	0	8.9	0	0
Elderflower, Presse, Sparkling, M&S*	1 Bottle/330ml	99	0.3	30	0.1	7.4	0.1	0.5
Lemon & Lime, Flavour Sparkling Spring, Co-Op*	1 Serving/200ml	2	0	1	0	0	0	0
Lemon & Lime, Flavoured, Sparkling, Spring, Sainsbury's*	1 Glass/250ml	4	0.2	2	0.1	0.1	0.1	0.1
Lemon & Lime, Flavoured, Strathmore*	1 Bottle/500g	85	0	17	0	4	0	0
Lemon & Lime, Spring Water, This Juicy Water*	1 Bottle/420ml	164	0	39	0	9.7	0	0
Lemon & Lime, Sugar Free, Touch of Fruit, Volvic*	1 Bottle/150ml	2	0	1	0	0	0	0
Lemon & Lime, Sparkling, M&S*	1 Bottle/500ml	15	0	3	0	0.4	0	0
Lemon & Lime, Still, M&S*	1 Bottle/500ml	5	0	1	0	0.2	0	0
Lemon, Cloudy, Sparkling, Sparkling Ice*	1 Bottle/500ml	12	0	2	0	0.5	0	0
Mineral Or Tap	*1 Glass/200ml*	*0*	*0*	*0*	*0*	*0*	*0*	*0*
Orange, & Passionfruit, Spring, Drench*	1 Serving/250ml	95	0.5	38	0.1	9	0.2	0

W

	Measure INFO/WEIGHT	per Measure KCAL	FAT	Nutrition Values per 100g / 100ml KCAL	PROT	CARB	FAT	FIBRE
WATER								
Orange, & Passionfruit, Still, Refresh'd, Robinson's*	1 Bottle/500ml	35	0	7	0	1.3	0	0
Peach, & Orange, Flavoured, Morrisons*	1 Serving/200ml	3	0	2	0.2	0.1	0	0
Peach, & Raspberry, Still, M&S*	1 Bottle/500ml	10	0	2	0	0	0	0
Peach, & Passion Fruit, Sparkling, Tesco*	1 Glass/250ml	5	0	2	0	0.3	0	0
Peach, Slightly Sparkling, Tesco*	1 Serving/200ml	4	0	2	0	0.2	0	0
Raspberries, & Blackcurrants, Spring Water, Juicy Water*	1 Bottle/420ml	155	0	37	0	9.3	0	0
Raspberry, & Apple, Still, Shapers, Boots*	1 Serving/250ml	10	0	4	0	0.8	0	0
Sparkling, San Pellegrino*	1 Glass/200ml	0	0	0	0	0	0	0
Sparkling, Smart Price, Asda*	1 Glass/300ml	0	0	0	0	0	0	0
Still, Highland Spring*	1 Bottle/750ml	0	0	0	0	0	0	0
Strawberry, & Guava, Still, M&S*	1 Glass/250ml	5	0	2	0	0.1	0	0
Strawberry, & Kiwi, Flavoured, Loved by Us, Co-Op*	1 Serving/250ml	2	0	1	0	0	0	0
Strawberry, & Kiwi, Sparkling, Sugar Free, Perfectly Clear*	1 Glass/250ml	2	0	1	0	0	0	0
Strawberry, & Kiwi, Still, Shapers, Boots*	1 Glass/250ml	2	0	1	0	0.1	0	0.9
Strawberry, & Kiwi, Still, Sainsbury's*	1 Serving/200ml	8	0	4	1	0	0	0
Strawberry, Flavoured, Sparkling, Spring, Tesco*	1 Serving/250ml	4	0	2	0	0.2	0	0
Strawberry, Original, Touch of Fruit, Volvic*	1 Bottle/500ml	99	0	20	0	4.8	0	0
Strawberry, Sparkling, Spring, Tesco*	1 Bottle/1000g	20	0	2	0	0.2	0	0
Strawberry, Sugar Free, Touch of Fruit, Volvic*	1 Bottle/500ml	7	0	1	0	0.1	0	0
Vitamin, XXX, Triple Berry, Glaceau, Coca-Cola*	1 Bottle/500ml	65	0	13	0	3	0	0
Vitamineral, Power, Ale Coq*	1 Bottle/750ml	150	0	20	0	4.8	0	0
Watermelon, Sugar Free, Touch of Fruit, Volvic*	1 Serving/250ml	2	0	1	0	0	0	0
WATER CHESTNUTS								
Raw, Average	*1oz/28g*	*8*	*0*	*29*	*0.8*	*6.6*	*0*	*0.1*
with Bamboo Shoots, Sainsbury's*	1 Serving/50g	29	0.1	58	2	12	0.2	1.1
WATERCRESS								
Raw, Trimmed, Average	*1 Sprig/2.5g*	*1*	*0*	*22*	*3*	*0.4*	*1*	*1.5*
WATERMELON								
Flesh Only, Average	*1 Serving/250g*	*75*	*0.8*	*30*	*0.4*	*7*	*0.3*	*0.4*
Raw	*1 Wedge/286g*	*48*	*0.6*	*17*	*0.3*	*3.7*	*0.2*	*0.3*
Raw, Weighed with Skin, Average	*1 Wedge/286g*	*49*	*0.5*	*17*	*0.2*	*4*	*0.2*	*0.2*
WELLINGTON								
Beetroot, Vegan, Waitrose*	1 Wellington/187g	411	23.2	220	4.2	21.5	12.4	2.6
Portabello Mushroom, Vegetarian, Tesco*	¼ Pack/117g	268	12.2	229	5.1	27.6	10.4	2
Salmon, Chapman's*	1 Wellington/205g	517	30.8	252	10	18	15	0
WHEAT BRAN								
Average	*1 Tbsp/7g*	*14*	*0.4*	*206*	*14.1*	*26.8*	*5.5*	*36.4*
WHEATGRASS								
& Kale, Shot, M&S*	1 Bottle/100ml	39	0	39	0.3	9.4	0	0.1
WHISKY								
37.5% Volume	*1 Pub Shot/35ml*	*72*	*0*	*207*	*0*	*0*	*0*	*0*
40% Volume	*1 Pub Shot/35ml*	*78*	*0*	*222*	*0*	*0*	*0*	*0*
Scots, 37.5% Volume	*1 Pub Shot/35ml*	*72*	*0*	*207*	*0*	*0*	*0*	*0*
Scots, 40% Volume	*1 Pub Shot/35ml*	*78*	*0*	*224*	*0*	*0*	*0*	*0*
WHITE PUDDING								
Average	*1oz/28g*	*126*	*8.9*	*450*	*7*	*36.3*	*31.8*	*0*
Denny*	1 Slice/25g	50	2.8	198	12	13	11	0
WHITEBAIT								
in Flour, Fried	*1oz/28g*	*147*	*13.3*	*525*	*19.5*	*5.3*	*47.5*	*0.2*
Raw, Average	*1 Serving/100g*	*172*	*11*	*172*	*18.3*	*0*	*11*	*0*
WHITING								
in Crumbs, Fried in Blended Oil	*1 Serving/180g*	*344*	*18.5*	*191*	*18.1*	*7*	*10.3*	*0.2*
Raw	*1oz/28g*	*23*	*0.2*	*81*	*18.7*	*0*	*0.7*	*0*

W

	Measure INFO/WEIGHT	per Measure KCAL	FAT	Nutrition Values per 100g / 100ml KCAL	PROT	CARB	FAT	FIBRE
WHITING								
Steamed	*1 Serving/85g*	*78*	*0.8*	*92*	*20.9*	*0*	*0.9*	*0*
WIENER SCHNITZEL								
Average	*1oz/28g*	*62*	*2.8*	*223*	*20.9*	*13.1*	*10*	*0.4*
WINE								
Diet, Lambrini*	1 Glass/125ml	29	0	23	0	0	0	0
Fruit, Average	*1 Glass/125ml*	*115*	*0*	*92*	*0*	*5.5*	*0*	*0*
Light, made with Italian Pinot Grigio, First Cape*	1 Glass/125ml	51	0	41	0	0	0	0
Madeira, Henriques & Henriques*	1 Glass/125ml	162	0	130	0	0	0	0
Mead, Average	*1 Glass/125ml*	*193*	*0*	*155*	*0*	*17.4*	*0*	*0*
Mulled, Homemade, Average	*1 Glass/125ml*	*245*	*0*	*196*	*0.1*	*25.2*	*0*	*0*
Mulled, Sainsbury's*	1 Glass/125ml	112	0	90	0	8.6	0	0
Mulled, Tesco*	1 Glass/125ml	120	0	96	0	0	0	0
Mulled, Vinglogg, Average*	1 Glass/125ml	162	0	130	0	14	0	0
Nosecco , Alcohol Free, Asda*	1 Glass/125ml	35	0.6	28	0.5	7	0.5	0
Original, Lambrini*	1 Glass/125ml	88	0	70	0	0	0	0
Red, Alcohol Free, Winemakers' Selection, Sainsbury's*	1 Glass/125ml	32	0	26	0.5	6	0	0.5
*Red, Amarone, Average**	*1 Glass/125ml*	*120*	*0*	*96*	*0.1*	*3*	*0*	*0*
Red, Average	*1 Glass/125ml*	*104*	*0*	*83*	*0*	*2*	*0*	*0*
Red, Beaujolais Villages, Louis Jadot*	1 Glass/125ml	156	0	125	0	4	0	0
Red, Burgundy, 12.9% Abv, Average	*1 Glass/125ml*	*110*	*0*	*88*	*0.1*	*3.7*	*0*	*0*
Red, Cabernet Sauvignon, 13.1% Abv, Average	*1 Glass/125ml*	*105*	*0*	*84*	*0.1*	*2.6*	*0*	*0*
Red, Cabernet Sauvignon, Non Alcoholic, Eisberg*	1 Glass/125ml	26	0	21	0	4.5	0	0
Red, Cabernet Tempranillo, Low Alcohol, Tesco*	1 Glass/125ml	78	0	62	0	14.7	0	0
Red, California, Blossom Hill*	1 Glass/125ml	94	0	75	0	0.9	0	0
Red, Claret, 12.8% Abv, Average	*1 Glass/125ml*	*105*	*0*	*84*	*0.1*	*3*	*0*	*0*
Red, Gamay, 12.3% Abv, Average	*1 Glass/125ml*	*99*	*0*	*79*	*0.1*	*2.4*	*0*	*0*
Red, Garnacha Syrah, De-Alcoholised, Natureo, Torres*	1 Glass/125ml	29	0	23	0	3.5	0	0
Red, Merlot, 13.3% Abv, Average	*1 Glass/125ml*	*105*	*0*	*84*	*0.1*	*2.5*	*0*	*0*
Red, Merlot, Alcohol Free, Vintense*	1 Glass/125ml	21	0	17	0	3.9	0	0
Red, Merlot, Cabernet Sauvignon, 13.5%, Church Road*	1 Glass/125ml	138	0	110	0.1	3.9	0	0
Red, Merlot, House, Sainsbury's*	1 Glass/125ml	89	0	71	0	0	0	0
Red, Merlot, Maipo, TTD, Sainsbury's*	1 Glass/125ml	97	0	78	0	0	0	0
Red, Merlot, Red Grape, Alcohol Free, M&S*	1 Glass/125ml	55	0.1	44	0.2	10.7	0.1	0.1
Red, Non Alcoholic, Ame*	1 Glass/125ml	42	0	34	0	5.7	0	0
Red, Petit Sirah, 13.5% Abv, Average	*1 Glass/125ml*	*108*	*0*	*86*	*0.1*	*2.7*	*0*	*0*
Red, Pinot Noir, 13% Abv, Average	*1 Glass/125ml*	*104*	*0*	*83*	*0.1*	*2.3*	*0*	*0*
Red, Sangiovese, 13.6% Abv, Average	*1 Glass/125ml*	*109*	*0*	*87*	*0.1*	*2.6*	*0*	*0*
Red, Shiraz, Burra Brook*	1 Glass/125ml	120	0	96	0	0	0	0
Red, Syrah, 13.1% Abv, Average	*1 Glass/125ml*	*105*	*0*	*84*	*0.1*	*2.6*	*0*	*0*
Red, Willow & Stone*	1 Glass/125ml	79	0	63	0	1.7	0	0
Red, Zinfandel, 13.9% Abv, Average	*1 Glass/125ml*	*111*	*0*	*89*	*0.1*	*2.9*	*0*	*0*
Rose, Alcohol Free, Eisberg*	1 Glass/125ml	32	0	26	0	5.9	0	0
Rose, Baron Saint Jean, Aldi*	1 Glass/125ml	106	0	85	0	0	0	0
Rose, Dealcoholised, Delight, McGuigan*	1 Glass/125ml	34	0.1	27	0.2	6	0.1	0
Rose, Garnacha, Low Alcohol, Tesco*	1 Glass/125ml	78	0	62	0	14.7	0	0
Rose, Medium, Average	*1 Glass/125ml*	*98*	*0*	*79*	*0*	*2.1*	*0*	*0*
Rose, Muscat, Non Alcoholic, Co-Op*	1 Glass/125ml	55	0	44	0	11	0	0
Rose, Pinot, Sparkling, TTD, Sainsbury's*	1 Glass/125ml	82	0	66	0	0	0	0
Rose, Sparkling, Average	*1 Glass/125ml*	*102*	*0*	*82*	*0*	*2.5*	*0*	*0*
Rose, Syrah Cabernet Sauvignon, De-Alcoholised, Torres*	1 Glass/125ml	20	0	16	0	2.6	0	0
Rose, The Pink Chill, Co-Op*	1 Glass/125ml	85	0	68	0	0	0	0
Rose, White Grenache, Blossom Hill*	1 Glass/125ml	105	0	84	0	3.2	0	0
Rose, White Zinfandel, Barefoot*	1 Glass/125ml	74	0	60	0	0	0	0

W

	Measure INFO/WEIGHT	per Measure KCAL	per Measure FAT	Nutrition Values per 100g / 100ml KCAL	PROT	CARB	FAT	FIBRE
WINE								
Rose, White Zinfandel, Ernest & Julio Gallo*	1 Glass/125ml	101	0	81	0.2	2.7	0	0
Sangria, Average	*1 Glass/125ml*	*95*	*0*	*76*	*0.1*	*9.9*	*0*	*0.1*
Vie, Rose, Low Alcohol, Blossom Hill*	1 Glass/125ml	66	0	53	0	3.9	0	0
White, Average	*1 Glass/125ml*	*95*	*0*	*76*	*0*	*2.4*	*0*	*0*
White, Cava, Zero, Codorniu*	1 Glass/125ml	39	0	31	0	7	0	0
White, Chardonnay, Alcohol Free, Vintense*	1 Glass/125ml	22	0	18	0	4.1	0	0
White, Chardonnay, Alcohol Removed, Fre*	1 Glass/125ml	33	0	26	0	7.5	0	0
White, Chardonnay, Southern Australia, Kissing Tree*	1 Bottle/185ml	85	0	46	0	0	0	0
White, Chenin Blanc, 12% Abv, Average	*1 Glass/125ml*	*101*	*0*	*81*	*0.1*	*3.3*	*0*	*0*
White, Dry, Average	*1 Glass/125ml*	*88*	*0*	*70*	*0.1*	*0.6*	*0*	*0*
White, Dry, House, Sainsbury's*	1 Glass/125ml	89	0	71	0	0	0	0
White, Fume Blanc, 13.1% Abv, Average	*1 Glass/125ml*	*104*	*0*	*83*	*0.1*	*2.3*	*0*	*0*
White, Gewurztraminer, 12.6% Abv, Average	*1 Glass/125ml*	*102*	*0*	*82*	*0.1*	*2.6*	*0*	*0*
White, Hock, House, Sainsbury's*	1 Glass/125ml	82	0	66	0	0	0	0
White, Late Harvest, 10.6% Abv, Average	*1 Glass/125ml*	*141*	*0*	*113*	*0.1*	*13.4*	*0*	*0*
White, Medium, Average	*1 Glass/125ml*	*92*	*0*	*74*	*0.1*	*3*	*0*	*0*
White, Muller-Thurgau, 11.3% Abv, Average	*1 Glass/125ml*	*96*	*0*	*77*	*0.1*	*3.5*	*0*	*0*
White, Muscat, 11% Abv, Average	*1 Glass/125ml*	*104*	*0*	*83*	*0.1*	*5.2*	*0*	*0*
White, Pinot Blanc, 13.3% Abv, Average	*1 Glass/125ml*	*102*	*0*	*82*	*0.1*	*0*	*0*	*0*
White, Pinot Grigio, 12.5%, Morrisons*	1 Glass/125ml	90	0	72	0	0	0	0
White, Pinot Grigio, 13.4% Abv, Average	*1 Glass/125ml*	*105*	*0*	*84*	*0.1*	*2.1*	*0*	*0*
White, Pinot Grigio, Wave Break, 12% Abv, M&S*	1 Glass/125ml	89	0	71	0	0	0	0
White, Riesling, 11.9% Abv, Average	*1 Glass/125ml*	*101*	*0*	*81*	*0.1*	*3.7*	*0*	*0*
White, Sauvignon Blanc, 13.1% Abv, Average	*1 Glass/125ml*	*102*	*0*	*82*	*0.1*	*2*	*0*	*0*
White, Sauvignon Blanc, Alcohol Free, Vintense*	1 Glass/125ml	20	0	16	0	4.5	0	0
White, Sauvignon Blanc, Low Alcohol, Tesco*	1 Glass/125ml	66	0	53	0	12.6	0	0
White, Sauvignon Blanc, Low Alcohol, TTD, Sainsbury's*	1 Glass/125ml	26	0	21	0	0	0	0
White, Sauvignon, Alcohol Free, Eisberg*	1 Glass/125ml	28	0	22	0	4.9	0	0
White, Semillon, 12.5% Abv, Average	*1 Glass/125ml*	*104*	*0*	*83*	*0.1*	*3.1*	*0*	*0*
White, Sparkling, Average	*1 Glass/125ml*	*92*	*0*	*74*	*0.3*	*5.1*	*0*	*0*
White, Sparkling, Low Alcohol, Tesco*	1 Glass/125ml	66	0	53	0	12.6	0	0
White, Sweet, Average	*1 Glass/125ml*	*118*	*0*	*94*	*0.2*	*5.9*	*0*	*0*
WINE GUMS								
Average	*1 Sweet/6g*	*19*	*0*	*315*	*5*	*73.4*	*0.2*	*0.1*
Haribo*	1 Pack/175g	609	0.4	348	0.1	86.4	0.2	0.4
Sour, Bassett's*	¼ Bag/50g	160	0	319	3.7	78	0	0
WISPA								
Cadbury*	1 Bar/40g	220	13.6	550	7.3	52.5	34	1
Gold, Cadbury*	1 Bar/52g	265	15.1	510	5.3	56	29	0.7
WONTON								
Prawn, Crispy from Selection, Modern Asian, M&S*	1 Wonton/25g	65	3.3	250	9.5	23.4	12.7	2
Prawn, Dim Sum Selection, Sainsbury's*	1 Wonton/10g	26	1.2	259	11.3	26.8	11.8	1.3
Prawn, Oriental Selection, Waitrose*	1 Wonton/18g	45	2	252	9.1	29.2	11	1.1
Prawn, Oriental Snack Selection, Sainsbury's*	1 Wonton/20g	53	2.7	265	10.6	25.6	13.4	2
Vegetable, Sweet & Sour, Tesco*	1 Wonton/14g	39	1.9	281	4.5	33.6	13.5	3.6
WOTSITS								
Baked, Really Cheesy, Walkers*	1 Bag/23g	123	7.4	546	5.5	56	33	1.1
Really Cheesy, Big Eat, Walkers*	1 Bag/36g	197	11.9	547	5.5	56	33	1.1
WRAP								
BBQ Chicken, One Stop*	1 Pack/154g	339	7.2	220	12	31.6	4.7	1.7
Bean, Spicy, with Cheese, Tesco*	1 Pack/198g	423	15.8	213	7.6	25.8	8	3.9
Caesar, Wicked Kitchen, Tesco*	1 Pack/240g	602	28.5	251	7.2	27.5	11.9	2.5
Chicken, & Bacon, Caesar, Just Tasty, Aldi*	1 Pack/196g	459	18	234	12.8	24	9.2	1.5

W

WRAP

INFO/WEIGHT	Measure	per Measure KCAL	FAT	Nutrition Values per 100g / 100ml KCAL	PROT	CARB	FAT	FIBRE
Chicken, & Bacon, Caesar, Co-Op*	1 Pack/205g	484	20.5	236	12	24	10	1.1
Chicken, & Bacon, Caesar, COU, M&S*	1 Pack/205g	607	31	296	13.3	26	15.1	1.3
Chicken, BBQ, No Mayo, Tesco*	1 Pack/154g	353	8.6	229	12.2	31.7	5.6	1.7
Chicken, BBQ, Shapers, Boots*	1 Pack/156g	278	4.5	178	11	26	2.9	1.8
Chicken, Caesar, One Stop*	1 Pack/174g	444	20.9	255	9.7	26.6	12	1.1
Chicken, Cajun, Sandwich King*	1 Pack/138g	386	19.9	279	12.3	25	14.4	0
Chicken, Cajun, Tesco*	1 Pack/175g	310	10	177	6.3	24.6	5.7	1.1
Chicken, Coronation , Waitrose*	1 Pack/164g	283	8.3	173	10.1	21.3	5.1	2.2
Chicken, Curry, Thai Green, Tesco*	1 Pack/175g	390	14.9	223	9.3	26.5	8.5	1.9
Chicken, Fajita, M&S*	1 Pack/213g	394	15.1	185	8.8	20.1	7.1	2.5
Chicken, Fajita, Morrisons*	1 Pack/214g	430	16.5	201	9.5	22.5	7.7	1.9
Chicken, Fajita, Omelette, Tesco*	1 Pack/161g	289	16.6	179	16.7	4	10.3	1.5
Chicken, Fajita, PB, Waitrose*	1 Pack/218g	368	5.7	169	10.5	26	2.6	1.9
Chicken, Fillets, with Cheese, & Bacon, Asda*	1 Pack/164g	366	21.3	223	25	1.4	13	0
Chicken, Harissa, Eat Better, Urban Eat*	1 Pack/167g	322	8.7	193	9.2	23.6	5.2	7.5
Chicken, Jerk, Tesco*	1 Pack/218g	473	16.1	217	9.4	26.2	7.4	4
Chicken, Korma, Rainbow, Co-Op*	1 Pack/198g	348	8.5	176	8.6	24	4.3	2.4
Chicken, Lemon, & Garlic, Tesco*	1 Pack/185g	411	14.6	222	10.1	27.2	7.9	1.1
Chicken, M&S*	1 Pack/247g	530	24.9	215	8.2	23.4	10.1	1.6
Chicken, Mexican Style, Co-Op*	1 Pack/163g	367	14.7	225	11	26	9	3
Chicken, Piri Piri, No Mayonnaise, Tesco*	1 Pack/185g	352	9.3	190	8.6	26.6	5	2.1
Chicken, Salad, Roast, Sainsbury's*	1 Pack/214g	443	19.9	207	10	20.9	9.3	2.5
Chicken, Southern Fried, CBY, Asda*	1 Pack/210g	452	17	215	7.1	27	8.1	2.7
Chicken, Sweet Chilli , Sainsbury's*	1 Pack/209g	434	11.5	208	8.5	30.1	5.5	1.8
Chicken, Sweet Chilli, Shapers, Boots*	1 Pack/195g	302	3.7	155	10	24	1.9	3
Chicken, Tikka, Average	*1 Wrap/200g*	*403*	*15.1*	*202*	*9.5*	*23.6*	*7.6*	*4.4*
Duck, Hoisin, Delicious, Boots*	1 Pack/160g	295	4.3	184	11	28	2.7	2
Duck, Hoisin, GF, M&S*	1 Pack/183g	285	6	156	10.2	17.5	3.3	7.6
Duck, Hoisin, M&S*	1 Pack/225g	405	8.3	180	8.4	27.7	3.7	1.5
Duck, Hoisin, No Mayo, Tesco*	1 Pack/178g	361	10	203	9.8	27.7	5.6	1.2
Falafel, & Houmous, GF, Chop Chop*	1 Pack/195g	392	11.3	201	3.8	29.4	5.8	7.6
Falafel, & Spinach, Aldi*	1 Pack/207g	486	24.8	235	6.7	25	12	2.9
Feta, Beetroot, & Spiced Butternut Squash, Co-Op*	1 Pack/232g	421	17	181	5.6	22.4	7.3	1.9
Feta, Salad, Greek , Shapers, Boots*	1 Pack/158g	241	5.7	153	6.4	24	3.6	1.2
Frijoles, Spicy, Wicked Kitchen, Tesco*	1 Pack/238g	431	14	181	4.3	26.2	5.9	2.8
Ham, & Mozzarella, Smoked, Soft Olive Oil Wrap, M&S*	1 Pack/203g	465	14	229	10.3	30.4	6.9	1.9
Hoisin, No Duck, Plant Kitchen, M&S*	1 Pack/200g	418	9.6	209	9.9	30	4.8	3.3
Lamb, Minted, Darwins Deli*	1 Pack/250g	287	6.3	115	3.2	19.9	2.5	0
Pork, Mexican, Tesco*	1 Pack/237g	448	17.3	189	7.9	22	7.3	1.6
Pork, Pulled, Mexican Spiced, Good to Go, Waitrose*	1 Pack/189g	339	14.2	179	7.2	19.8	7.5	1.8
Prawn, Sweet Chilli, King, M&S*	1 Pack/155g	225	3.1	145	8	24.2	2	2.1
Soft Cheese, & Spinach, to Go*	1 Pack/250g	278	6.7	111	4.5	17.4	2.7	0
Sushi Rice, & Vegetables, Japanese, Vegan, Morrisons*	1 Pack/189g	401	9.8	212	5.1	32.5	5.2	2.2
Tuna, Sweetcorn, & Red Pepper, BGTY, Sainsbury's*	1 Pack/178g	306	8.2	172	11.5	21.2	4.6	2.1
Turkey, Bacon, & Cranberry, COU, M&S*	1 Pack/144g	230	2.2	160	9.6	27.1	1.5	2.3
Turkey, Feast, Sainsbury's*	1 Pack/212g	502	18.2	237	11.3	27.6	8.6	1.8
Turkey, Ranch, & Bacon, Roast, Arby's*	1 Pack/279g	620	31	222	13.3	14	11.1	1.4

W

INFO/WEIGHT	Measure	per Measure		Nutrition Values per 100g / 100ml				
		KCAL	FAT	KCAL	PROT	CARB	FAT	FIBRE
YAM								
Baked	**1oz/28g**	**43**	**0.1**	**153**	**2.1**	**37.5**	**0.4**	**1.7**
Boiled, Average	**1oz/28g**	**37**	**0.1**	**133**	**1.7**	**33**	**0.3**	**1.4**
YEAST								
Extract	**1 Tsp/9g**	**16**	**0**	**180**	**40.7**	**3.5**	**0.4**	**0**
Extract, Reduced Salt, Sainsbury's*	1 Tsp/4g	10	0	246	41.2	17.6	0.5	4.3
Flakes, Nutritional, Whole Food Earth*	1 Tbsp/5g	17	0.2	341	53	34.8	5	21
Quick, Doves Farm*	1 Serving/8g	28	0.5	355	43.5	19	5.7	27
YOGHURT								
0% Fat, Active, Brooklea, Aldi*	1 Pot/125g	59	0.6	47	4.2	7.3	0.5	0.5
Activia, Danone*	1 Pot/132g	125	4.2	94	3.5	12.8	3.2	2
After Dinner Mint, Limited Edition, Mullerlight, Muller*	1 Pot/165g	91	0.8	55	4.3	7.6	0.5	0
Apple, & Berry Pie, Dessert Recipe, Weight Watchers*	1 Pot/120g	58	0.1	49	4.1	6.8	0.1	0.3
Apple, & Peach, Bircher Muesli, Moma Foods*	1 Pot/170g	224	4.1	132	4.3	24.3	2.4	1.7
Apple, & Pear, Low Fat, Sainsbury's*	1 Pot/125g	115	1.9	92	4.3	15.2	1.5	0.2
Apple, Cinnamon, Light & Fruity, 0% Fat, Onken*	1 Serving/150g	75	0	50	4.6	6.2	0	1.3
Apricot, Bio Activia, Danone*	1 Pot/125g	121	4	97	3.7	13.3	3.2	1.7
Apricot, Fat Free, Weight Watchers*	1 Pot/110g	45	0.1	41	4	5	0.1	0.2
Apricot, Low Fat, Brooklea, Aldi*	1 Pot/125g	99	1	79	2.8	15.1	0.8	0
Apricot, Low Fat, Sainsbury's*	1 Pot/124g	108	1.6	87	4.2	14.3	1.3	0.5
Apricot, Low Fat, Tesco*	1 Pot/125g	112	2.2	90	4.3	14.1	1.8	0
Banana, & Custard, Smooth, Mullerlight, Muller*	1 Pot/175g	94	0.2	54	4.1	8.6	0.1	0.6
Banana, & Custard, Yeo Valley*	1 Serving/100g	109	4.3	109	4.6	13	4.3	0
Banana, Choco Flakes, Crunch Corner, Muller*	1 Pot/135g	193	6.9	143	4.3	19.3	5.1	0.3
Banana, Low Fat, Average	**1 Serving/100g**	**98**	**1.4**	**98**	**4.6**	**16.7**	**1.4**	**0.1**
Banoffee, Left Yeo-Vers, Yeo Valley*	1 Serving/150g	162	6	108	4.5	13.5	4	0
Banoffee, Snackpot, Activia, Danone*	1 Pot/155g	116	0.2	75	5	13.3	0.1	0.3
Banoffee, Thick & Creamy, Specially Selected, Aldi*	1 Pot/150g	191	10	127	2.8	14	6.7	0
Berry, & Apple, Low Fat, Breakfast Pot, Tesco*	1 Pot/215g	233	2.6	108	0	14.5	1.2	2.4
Berry, & Granola, Simply Lunch*	1 Pot/239g	370	22.2	155	4.5	20.8	9.3	2.3
Bio, Low Fat, Spelga*	1 Pot/125g	125	2.1	100	3.9	17	1.7	0
Blackberry, & Raspberry, Fruit Corner, Muller*	1 Pot/150g	158	5.8	105	3.8	13.1	3.9	0.9
Blackberry, Soya, Alpro*	1 Pot/125g	94	2.4	75	3.6	9.7	1.9	1.1
Blackcurrant, & Elderflower, Soya, Alpro*	1 Pot/125g	92	2.4	74	3.6	9.5	1.9	1.1
Blackcurrant, Garden Fruits, Low Fat, Tesco*	1 Pot/125g	120	2.4	95	3.8	15.1	1.9	0.3
Blackcurrant, Probiotic, Organic, Yeo Valley*	1 Pot/150g	152	5.8	101	4.1	12.4	3.9	0.2
Blackcurrant, Soya, Go On, Alpro*	1 Pot/150g	122	4.2	81	5.1	7.5	2.8	2
Blueberry, Blast, Skyr, Icelandic, Light & Free, Danone*	1 Pot/150g	81	0.8	54	9.1	3.8	0.5	0.5
Blueberry, Bursting, Intensely Creamy, Activia, Danone*	1 Pot/110g	112	3.3	102	5	13.4	3	0.5
Blueberry, Fruit Corner, Muller*	1 Pot/150g	156	5.7	104	3.8	12.9	3.8	0.4
Blueberry, Greek Style, Alpro*	1 Pot/150g	123	4	82	4.7	8.6	2.7	1.7
Blueberry, Icelandic Style, Isey Skyr*	1 Pot/180g	157	0.4	87	9.7	12	0.2	0
Blueberry, Icelandic Style, Skyr, Brooklea, Aldi*	1 Pot/150g	122	0.8	81	7.7	12	0.5	0.5
Blueberry, Protein, Arla*	1 Pot/200g	140	0.4	70	10	6.5	0.2	0
Blueberry, Soya, Alpro*	1 Pot/125g	91	2.5	73	3.6	9.4	2	1.2
Blueberry, with Crunchy Granola, Organic, Yeo Valley*	1 Pot/135g	217	7.7	161	5.6	21.1	5.7	0
Bramble, & Apple, Virtually Fat Free, Longley Farm*	1 Pot/150g	118	0.2	79	5.5	13.9	0.1	0
Caramel, Indulgent Layered, Specially Selected, Aldi*	1 Pot/150g	276	16.5	184	2.3	19	11	1.4
Caramel, Salted, Cheesecake, Greek, Whipped, Muller*	1 Pot/100g	180	7.9	180	4.2	21.8	7.9	0
Caramel, Salted, Greek Style, Luxury, Oykos, Danone*	1 Pot/110g	172	9.2	157	2.7	17.6	8.4	0
Cereals, Fibre, Bio Activia, Danone*	1 Pot/120g	119	4.1	99	3.7	13.5	3.4	3
Cherry Bakewell, Bio Live, Llaeth Y Llan, Village Dairy*	1 Pot/150g	121	6.4	81	2.3	8.2	4.3	0.1
Cherry, Biopot, Onken*	1 Serving/150g	153	4	102	3.8	14	2.7	0
Cherry, Black, & Cream, The Best, Morrisons*	1 Pot/150g	218	9.4	146	3.2	19	6.3	0

Y

YOGHURT

INFO/WEIGHT	Measure	per Measure		Nutrition Values per 100g / 100ml				
		KCAL	FAT	KCAL	PROT	CARB	FAT	FIBRE
Cherry, Black, 0%, Greek Style, Yeo Valley*	1 Serving/150g	108	0	72	6.6	10.7	0	0
Cherry, Black, Average	*1 Serving/100g*	*96*	*2.2*	*96*	*3.4*	*16.5*	*2.2*	*0.1*
Cherry, Black, Excellence, Liberte*	1 Serving/110g	150	8.5	136	2.8	13	7.7	0.1
Cherry, Black, Extremely Fruity, Bio, M&S*	1 Pot/150g	165	2.2	110	4.9	18.4	1.5	0.2
Cherry, Black, Garden Fruits, Fat Free, Benecol*	1 Pot/125g	79	0.6	63	3	11	0.5	2.1
Cherry, Black, Greek Style, Corner, Muller*	1 Pot/150g	172	4.5	115	5	16.2	3	0.1
Cherry, Black, Low Fat, Average	*1 Serving/100g*	*69*	*0.6*	*69*	*3.8*	*12.2*	*0.6*	*0.3*
Cherry, Black, Organic, Yeo Valley*	¼ Pot/125g	122	5	98	4.5	11	4	0
Cherry, Black, Swiss, Finest, Tesco*	1 Pot/150g	195	8.8	130	3.5	15.7	5.9	0.5
Cherry, Black, Thick & Creamy, Waitrose*	1 Pot/125g	139	3.1	111	3.7	18.3	2.5	0.4
Cherry, Charmer, Greek Style, Light & Free, Danone*	1 Pot/115g	59	0.1	51	4.7	7.7	0.1	0.1
Cherry, Fat Free, Activia, Danone*	1 Pot/125g	64	0.1	51	4.7	7.7	0.1	0.1
Cherry, Fruity, Mullerlight, Muller*	1 Pot/175g	86	0.2	49	4.3	7	0.1	0.2
Cherry, Greek Style, Fruitopolis, Mullerlight, Muller*	1 Pot/130g	65	0.1	50	4.7	7.2	0.1	0
Cherry, Greek Style, Layered, Brooklea, Aldi*	1 Pot/125g	89	0.6	71	5.7	11	0.5	0.5
Cherry, Light, Fat Free, Muller*	1 Pot/175g	88	0.2	50	3.9	7.9	0.1	0.2
Cherry, Low Fat, CBY, Asda*	1 Pot/125g	90	1.6	72	3.6	11.4	1.3	0.3
Cherry, Luscious, Intensely Creamy, Activia, Danone*	1 Pot/110g	109	3.3	99	5	12.8	3	0.2
Cherry, Morello, Specially Selected, Aldi*	1 Pot/150g	171	7.5	114	2.5	15	5	0.5
Cherry, Red, Fruit Corner, Muller*	1 Pot/150g	158	5.8	105	3.8	13	3.9	0.5
Cherry, Red, Summer Fruits, Benecol*	1 Pot/120g	90	2	75	0.2	9.7	1.7	3.7
Cherry, Soya, Alpro*	1 Pot/125g	91	2.5	73	3.6	9.4	2	1.2
Coconut, & Lemon, Dairy Free, Koko*	1 Pot/125g	141	6.9	113	0.7	15.1	5.5	0.3
Coconut, & Vanilla, Greek Style, Fat Free, Brooklea, Aldi*	1 Pot/125g	74	0.6	59	5.9	7.6	0.5	0.5
Coconut, Greek Style, Brooklea, Aldi*	1 Serving/150g	212	12.9	141	3.7	12	8.6	0.5
Coconut, Greek Style, Milbona, Lidl*	1 Pot/150g	236	14.7	157	3.9	13	9.8	0.5
Coconut, Low Fat, Tesco*	1 Serving/150g	150	4	100	5	13.8	2.7	0.1
Coconut, Protein, Arla*	1 Pot/200g	144	1	72	10	6.2	0.5	0
Cranberry, Bio Activia, Danone*	1 Pot/125g	115	4	92	3.6	12.3	3.2	1.7
Fat Free, Smooth, Milbona, Lidl*	1 Pot/175g	88	0.2	50	4.4	7.3	0.1	0.1
Fig, & Honey, Greek Style, Light & Free, Danone*	1 Pot/115g	60	0.6	52	4.8	7.7	0.5	0
Fig, Bio, Activia, Danone*	1 Pot/125g	124	4.2	99	3.6	13.4	3.4	0.2
Forest Fruits, Soya, Dairy Free, Alpro*	1 Serving/100g	79	2.2	79	3.8	10.1	2.2	1.2
French, Set, Low Fat, Iceland*	1 Pot/125g	100	1.5	80	3.6	13.6	1.2	0
Fruit, Low Fat, Average	*1 Pot/125g*	*112*	*0.9*	*90*	*4.1*	*17.9*	*0.7*	*0*
Fruity, Favourites, Organic, Yeo Valley*	1 Pot/125g	126	4.9	101	4.1	12.4	3.9	0.2
Fudge, Devonshire Style, Finest, Tesco*	1 Pot/150g	206	9.2	137	4	16.4	6.1	0.4
Fudge, Gourmet, Moo!, Aldi*	¼ Pot/113g	143	6.4	127	4.2	15	5.7	0.5
Full Cream, Fresh, Al Rawabi*	1 Serving/100g	72	3.2	72	4.2	6.4	3.2	0
Gin & Tonic, Inspired, Mullerlight, Muller*	1 Pot/160g	72	0.7	45	4.4	6	0.5	0
Ginger, Greek Style, Bio, Live, Rachel's Organic*	1 Serving/100g	137	7.4	137	3.2	14.4	7.4	0
Goat's Milk, Natural, Fat Free, St Helen's Farm*	1 Serving/150g	63	0.2	42	6	4.3	0.1	0
Goat's Milk, Natural, St Helen's Farm*	1 Serving/150g	158	11	105	5.5	4.3	7.3	0
Goats Whole Milk	*1 Carton/150g*	*94*	*5.7*	*63*	*3.5*	*3.9*	*3.8*	*0*
Gooseberry, & Elderflower, Fragrant, Creamy, Waitrose*	1 Pot/150g	188	9.9	125	2.6	13.8	6.6	0.5
Gooseberry, Garden Fruits, Low Fat, Tesco*	1 Pot/125g	115	2.4	90	3.3	14.9	1.9	0.3
Gooseberry, Low Fat, Average	*1 Serving/100g*	*90*	*1.4*	*90*	*4.5*	*14.5*	*1.4*	*0.2*
Gooseberry, Virtually Fat Free, Longley Farm*	1 Pot/150g	122	0.2	81	4.2	15.7	0.1	0.5
Gourmet, Live, Deluxe, Lidl*	1 Serving/150g	206	8.4	137	5	16.4	5.6	0.5
Greek Style, Fat Free, Counted, Eat Smart, Morrisons*	¼ Pot/125g	95	0.6	76	7	10.9	0.5	0
Greek Style, Fat Free, Morrisons*	¼ Pot/125g	59	0.2	47	5.8	5.4	0.2	0
Greek Style, Fat Free, Berry Compote, Granola, M&S*	1 Pot/205g	260	6.2	127	6	18	3	1.8
Greek Style, Low Fat, M&S*	1 Serving/100g	71	2.6	71	5.2	6.6	2.6	0.5

YOGHURT

INFO/WEIGHT	Measure KCAL	FAT	Nutrition Values per 100g / 100ml KCAL	PROT	CARB	FAT	FIBRE
Greek Style, Strained, 0%, Glenisk Organic Dairy Co* — 1 Pot/150g	84	0	56	10	4	0	0
Greek Style, Unsweetened, Lite, Hansells Foods* — 1 Serving/125g	84	1.6	67	5.7	8.2	1.3	0
Greek Style, Unsweetened, Thick, Hansells Foods* — 1/5 Pot/200g	212	11.8	106	5.6	7.8	5.9	0
Greek Style, with Banana, M&S * — 1 Pack/171g	220	7.2	129	5.5	16.8	4.2	1.2
Greek Style, with Blueberry Layer, Luxury, Oykos, Danone* — 1 Pot/110g	152	9.4	138	2.7	12.5	8.5	0.4
Greek Style, with Honey, Brooklea, Aldi* — 1/3 Pot/150g	206	11	137	3.3	15	7.3	0.5
Greek Style, with Honey, Tesco* — 1 Pot/100g	144	8	144	4.2	13.7	8	0
Greek Style, with Passion Fruit, Carrefour* — 1 Pot/150g	178	13.6	119	2.4	14	9.1	0
Greek Style, with Peach, Carrefour* — 1 Pot/150g	177	9	118	2.4	13.3	6	0
Greek, 0% Fat, Strained, Authentic, Total, Fage* — 1 Sm Pot/170g	92	0	54	10.3	3	0	0
Greek, 0%, Mevgal* — 1 Serving/100g	52	0	52	8	5	0	0
Greek, 2% Fat, Strained, Authentic, Total, Fage* — 1 Pot/170g	119	3.4	70	9.9	3	2	0
Greek, 5% Fat, Brooklea, Aldi* — 1 Serving/200g	208	11.2	104	8.7	4.8	5.6	0.5
Greek, Authentic, 10% Fat, Morrisons* — ¼ Pot/125g	164	12.5	131	6	4.3	10	0
Greek, Authentic, Fat Free, TTD, Sainsbury's* — ¼ Pot/125g	81	0.6	65	9.9	6	0.5	0.5
Greek, Authentic, Natural, Strained, Waitrose* — 1 Serving/125g	164	12.8	131	5.9	3.7	10.2	0.3
Greek, Authentic, TTD, Sainsbury's* — 1 Serving/100g	137	10.7	137	6	4.1	10.7	0
Greek, Creamy, Authentic, Milbona, Lidl* — 1 Serving/100g	132	10	132	6	4.5	10	0
Greek, with Blueberries, Total 0%, Total, Fage* — 1 Serving/150g	123	0	82	8.3	12.3	0	0
Greek, with Espresso, Finest, Tesco* — 1 Pot/150g	133	0.2	88	8.6	13.1	0.2	0
Hazelnut, Irish, Coolree Creamery* — 1 Pot/48g	50	1.6	105	4.1	14	3.4	0.8
Hazelnut, Light, Amore, Muller* — 1 Pot/130g	82	0.6	63	8	6.7	0.5	0
Hazelnut, Longley Farm* — 1 Pot/150g	201	8.5	134	5.5	16	5.7	0
Hazelnut, Low Fat, Deliciously Nutty, Waitrose* — 1 Pot/150g	153	4.2	102	6.1	12.9	2.8	0.5
Hazelnut, Sainsbury's* — 1 Serving/150g	183	3.4	122	5	20.3	2.3	0.2
Honey, & Ginger, West Country, Luxury, M&S* — 1 Pot/150g	219	11.6	146	3.6	15.6	7.7	0
Honey, Breakfast Pot, Activia, Danone* — 1 Pot/160g	192	4.2	120	4.9	18.8	2.6	0.7
Honey, Golden, Greek Style, Activia, Danone* — 1 Pack/126g	122	3.5	97	5	13	2.8	0.1
Honey, Greek Style, 0% Fat, Tesco* — 1/3 Pot/150g	122	0.3	81	6.8	13.1	0.2	0
Honey, Greek Style, Milbona, Lidl* — 1 Pot/100g	145	8.3	145	3.8	13.5	8.3	0.5
Honey, Greek Style, Morrisons* — 1/3 Pot/150g	236	14.3	157	4.1	13.5	9.5	0.7
Honey, Greek Style, Strained, 0% Fat, Liberte, Yoplait* — 1 Pot/100g	92	0.1	92	7.7	14.1	0.1	0.1
Honey, Icelandic Style, Strained, Fat Free, Skyr, Arla* — 1 Serving/150g	110	0.2	73	9.4	7.8	0.1	0
Kefir, Blueberry Hemp, The Great Dairy Collective* — 1 Serving/150ml	139	5.6	93	4.4	9.5	3.7	2.1
Kefir, Coconut, & Honey, The Great Dairy Collective* — 1 Serving/250g	143	6.5	57	3	8.2	2.6	0
Kefir, Mango & Turmeric, The Great Dairy Collective* — 1 Serving/150ml	138	5.4	92	4.3	9.7	3.6	2.2
Kefir, Natural, Organic, Yeo Valley* — 1 Pot/350g	224	7.4	64	4.7	6.4	2.1	0
Kefir, Natural, The Great Dairy Collective* — 1 Serving/150g	155	8.3	103	5	8.7	5.5	0
Kefir, Nature, Coop Naturaplan* — 1 Pot/150g	117	5.2	79	4.5	6	3.5	0
Kefir, Strawberry, Organic, Yeo Valley* — ½ Pot/175g	138	3.3	79	4.2	11.1	1.9	0
Kefir, Vanilla, The Great Dairy Collective* — 1 Serving/150g	154	7.5	103	5.6	9.6	5	0
Kiwi, Bio, Activia, Danone* — 1 Pot/125g	122	4.2	98	3.6	12.9	3.4	0.3
Kiwi, Mixed Fruit, Activia, Danone* — 1 Pot/120g	109	3.5	91	3.9	12.2	2.9	0
Latte, Skinny, Fat Free, Mullerlight, Muller* — 1 Pot/165g	84	0.2	51	4.1	7.7	0.1	0
Lemon Curd, West Country, Extra Special, Asda* — 1 Pot/150g	252	13	168	3.2	19	8.7	0
Lemon Curd, West Country, TTD, Sainsbury's* — 1 Pot/150g	243	10	162	3.7	21.6	6.7	0.5
Lemon Curd, Whole Milk, Yeo Valley* — 1 Pot/120g	149	5.3	124	4.7	16.3	4.4	0
Lemon Meringue, Inspired, Goodies, Mullerlight, Muller* — 1 Pot/107g	82	0.1	77	3.6	14.8	0.1	0
Lemon, Greek Style, Fat Free, Brooklea, Aldi* — 1 Pot/125g	71	0.6	57	5.8	8	0.5	0.5
Lemon, Greek Style, Whipped, Bliss Corner, Muller* — 1 Pot/110g	177	6.5	161	4	22.2	5.9	0
Lemon, Lavish, Greek Style, Light & Free, Danone* — 1 Pot/115g	56	0.1	49	4.9	7.1	0.1	0.1
Lemon, Longley Farm* — 1 Pot/150g	159	5.6	106	5	13.4	3.7	0
Lemon, Luscious, Greek Style, Mullerlight, Muller* — 1 Pot/125g	75	0.2	60	6.3	7.5	0.2	0

YOGHURT

	Measure INFO/WEIGHT	per Measure KCAL	FAT	Nutrition Values per 100g / 100ml KCAL	PROT	CARB	FAT	FIBRE
Lemon, Sicilian, The Best, Morrisons*	1 Pot/150g	235	12.1	157	3.4	17.5	8.1	0
Lime, Cheesecake, Greek Style, Bliss, Corner, Muller*	1 Pot/100g	179	7.9	179	4.7	21.5	7.9	0
Mandarin, Fat Free, Mullerlight, Muller*	1 Pot/175g	95	0.2	54	4.2	8.5	0.1	0
Mandarin, Llaeth Y Llan, Village Dairy*	1 Pot/125g	130	3.5	104	5.6	14.3	2.8	0.1
Mandarin, Longley Farm*	1 Pot/150g	141	5.7	94	4.9	13.3	3.8	0
Mango, & Passion Fruit, Low Fat, Sainsbury's*	1 Pot/125g	105	1.6	84	4.2	13.5	1.3	0.5
Mango, & Honey, Kefir, M&S*	1 Pack/140g	98	2.4	70	3.8	9.9	1.7	0.5
Mango, & Passion Fruit, Finest, Tesco*	1 Pot/150g	166	7.6	111	3.8	12.3	5.1	0.2
Mango, & Passion Fruit, Natural, Live, Glenilen Farm*	1 Pot/140g	115	4.1	82	3.6	8.5	2.9	0
Mango, Bio, Activia, Danone*	1 Pot/125g	124	4.2	99	3.5	13.5	3.4	0.2
Mango, Papaya, & Passion Fruit, Bio, Morrisons*	1 Serving/150g	156	5.1	104	3.1	14.9	3.4	0.5
Mango, Passionfruit, & Granola, Greek Style, Asda*	1 Pot/135g	189	4.9	140	5	21	3.6	1.2
Mango, Soya, Go On, Alpro*	1 Pot/150g	129	4.2	86	5	9.1	2.8	1.3
Muesli, Bircher Style, M&S*	1 Pot/190g	230	5.9	121	5.4	17	3.1	1.6
Muesli, Bircher, Summer Berry, M&S*	1 Pot/195g	277	13.1	142	3.7	15	6.7	3.4
Myrtille, Bon. App*	1 Pot/180g	167	6.1	93	3.4	12	3.4	0
Natural, Almond Milk, Dairy Free, Nush Foods*	1 Pot/125g	165	10	132	4	3	8	0
Natural, Bio Activia, Individual Pots, Danone*	1 Pot/125g	86	4.2	69	4.2	5.5	3.4	0
Natural, Bio Live, Low Fat, Organic, Waitrose*	¼ Pot/125g	81	1.2	65	5.8	8.3	1	0
Natural, Bio Set, Low Fat, Sainsbury's*	1 Pot/150g	78	2.2	52	3.9	5.7	1.5	0
Natural, Bio, Lancashire Farm*	3 Dstsps/40g	32	1.4	80	5.2	7	3.5	0.5
Natural, Biopot, Onken*	1 Serving/125g	82	4.4	66	4.5	4.1	3.5	0
Natural, Cal Frutos*	1 Serving/125g	71	4.2	57	4.1	2.6	3.4	0
Natural, Fat Free, Eat Smart, Morrisons*	1 Pot/150g	88	0.3	59	7	7.2	0.2	0
Natural, Fat Free, Lancashire Farm Dairies*	1 Serving/100g	48	0.1	48	5	7.3	0.1	0.9
Natural, Fat Free, Llaeth Y Llan, Village Dairy*	1 Serving/100g	57	0.2	57	5.7	7.9	0.2	0.1
Natural, Fat Free, Onken*	1 Serving/150g	63	0	42	5.6	3.1	0	0
Natural, Greek Style, 0% Fat, Mullerlight, Muller*	1 Serving/150g	102	0.8	68	7.5	8.5	0.5	0
Natural, Greek Style, Average	*1 Serving/100g*	*138*	*10.6*	*138*	*4.7*	*6.1*	*10.6*	*0*
Natural, Greek Style, Bio Live, Rachel's Organic*	1 Pot/450g	518	40.5	115	3.6	4.9	9	0
Natural, Greek Style, Bio Live, Tims Dairy*	1 Serving/50g	65	5	130	5.7	4.9	10	0
Natural, Greek Style, Fat Free, CBY, Asda*	1 Serving/30g	16	0.2	55	7.4	5.3	0.5	0
Natural, Greek Style, Fat Free, Essential, Waitrose*	1 Serving/125g	68	0.5	54	7.8	4.8	0.4	0
Natural, Greek Style, Fat Free, Tesco*	1 Pot/100g	55	0.2	55	7.5	4.8	0.2	0.4
Natural, Greek Style, Llaeth Y Llan, Village Dairy*	½ Pot/225g	209	8.3	93	6.3	8.7	3.7	0.1
Natural, Greek Style, Low Fat, Average	*1 Serving/100g*	*77*	*2.7*	*77*	*6.1*	*7.3*	*2.7*	*0.2*
Natural, Greek Style, Low Fat, Tesco*	1 Serving/100g	77	3	77	5.5	7	3	0
Natural, Greek Style, Milbona, Lidl*	1 Serving/150g	183	15	122	4.6	3.2	10	0
Natural, Greek Style, Milbona, Lidl*	1 Pot/125g	135	10.6	108	3.2	4.3	8.5	0.5
Natural, Greek Style, Organic, M&S*	1 Pot/150g	186	13.8	124	4.6	5.6	9.2	0.5
Natural, Greek Style, Strained, 0% Fat, Liberte, Yoplait*	¼ Pot/125g	70	0.1	56	9.6	3.2	0.1	0.1
Natural, Icelandic Style, Strained, Fat Free, Skyr, Arla*	1 Serving/150g	98	0.3	65	11	4	0.2	0
Natural, Icelandic Style, Strained, Fat Free, Skyr, Arla*	1 Serving/150g	98	0.3	65	11	4	0.2	0
Natural, Light, Mullerlight, Muller*	1 Pot/175g	93	0.2	53	5.6	6.7	0.1	0
Natural, Longley Farm*	1 Pot/150g	118	5.2	79	4.8	7	3.5	0
Natural, Low Fat, 6 Grain Cereal, Live, Irish Yogurts*	1 Serving/150g	102	2.6	68	5	8.2	1.7	0.5
Natural, Low Fat, Average	*1 Med Pot/125g*	*75*	*1.6*	*60*	*5.4*	*7*	*1.3*	*0*
Natural, Low Fat, Creamfields*	1 Serving/125g	71	2	57	4.9	5.5	1.6	0.5
Natural, Low Fat, Everyday Value, Tesco*	1 Pot/125g	78	1.9	62	5	7.2	1.5	0
Natural, Low Fat, Live, Waitrose*	1 Pot/175g	114	1.8	65	5.8	8.2	1	0
Natural, Pouring, Icelandic Style, Skyr, Arla*	1 Serving/150g	70	0.8	47	6.8	3.8	0.5	0
Natural, Probiotic, Fat Free, Organic, Yeo Valley*	1 Pot/150g	87	0.2	58	5.9	8.4	0.1	0
Natural, Probiotic, Organic, Yeo Valley*	1 Pot/120g	98	5.4	82	5.1	5.6	4.5	0

YOGHURT

INFO/WEIGHT	Measure	per Measure		Nutrition Values per 100g / 100ml				
		KCAL	FAT	KCAL	PROT	CARB	FAT	FIBRE
Natural, Scottish, Mccallums*	1 Serving/150g	116	4.8	78	4.9	7.2	3.2	0
Natural, Whole Milk, Set, Biopot, Onken*	1 Serving/125g	85	4.4	68	4.5	4.1	3.5	0
Natural, Wholemilk, Live Bio, Organic, Waitrose*	1 Serving/100g	88	4.4	88	5.1	7.1	4.4	0
Natural, with Honey, Greek Style, Sainsbury's*	1 Sm Pot/125g	174	9.8	139	3.7	13.4	7.8	0.5
Natural, with Oat Clusters, & Chocolate, Nomadic*	1 Pot/169g	326	12.5	193	4.9	25.5	7.4	2.2
Nectarine, Fat Free, Weight Watchers*	1 Pot/110g	45	0.1	41	4.1	4.8	0.1	0.3
Nectarine, Juicy, Weight Watchers*	1 Serving/110g	45	0.1	41	4.1	4.8	0.1	0.3
Oats, & Wheat, Whole Grain, Bio Live, Activia, Danone*	1 Pot/120g	122	3.8	102	3.6	13.5	3.2	2.1
Orange, Sprinkled with Dark Chocolate, Brooklea, Aldi*	1 Pot/165g	73	0.8	44	3.5	6.9	0.5	0.5
Orange, Sprinkled with Dark Chocolate, Light, Muller*	1 Pot/165g	91	0.8	55	4.3	7.4	0.5	0.1
Orange, with Chocolate Flakes, Fat Free, Brooklea, Aldi*	1 Pot/165g	84	0.8	51	3.5	8.3	0.5	0.5
Original, Dairy Free, Koko*	1 Serving/100g	79	4.9	79	0.6	8	4.9	0.2
Passion Fruit, Gourmet, Live, The Great Dairy Collective*	1 Pot/150g	190	8.2	127	5.1	14.2	5.5	0
Passion Fruit, Greek Style, Luxury, Oykos, Danone*	1 Pot/110g	163	9.1	148	2.9	15.4	8.3	0.1
Passion Fruit, Light & Fruity, 0% Fat, Onken*	1 Serving/150g	76	0	51	4.9	6.3	0	0
Passion Fruit, Soya, Go On, Alpro*	1 Pot/150g	126	4.4	84	5.2	8.5	2.9	1.4
Peach, & Apricot, Fruit Corner, Muller*	1 Pot/150g	160	5.7	107	3.9	13.5	3.8	0.5
Peach, & Apricot, HL, Tesco*	1 Bottle/100g	70	1.2	70	2.3	12.4	1.2	0.2
Peach, & Cream, Intensely Creamy, Activia, Danone*	1 Pot/120g	118	3.6	98	4.8	13	3	0.3
Peach, & Mango, Thick & Creamy, Waitrose*	1 Pot/125g	136	3.1	109	3.7	17.8	2.5	0.3
Peach, & Pineapple, Fat Free, Mullerlight, Muller*	1 Pot/175g	89	0.2	51	4.3	7.7	0.1	0.2
Peach, & Pear, Soya, No Bits, Alpro*	1 Pot/125g	99	2.5	79	3.7	10.7	2	1
Peach, Bio, Activia, Fat Free, Danone*	1 Sm Pot/125g	71	0.1	57	4.7	9.3	0.1	1
Peach, Greek Style, Luxury, Oykos, Danone*	1 Pot/110g	154	8.9	140	3.1	13.4	8.1	0.3
Peach, Greek Style, Yeo Valley*	1 Pot/100g	65	0.2	65	6.4	9.4	0.2	0
Peach, Low Fat, Average	*1 Serving/100g*	*86*	*1.1*	*86*	*4.5*	*14.6*	*1.1*	*0.2*
Peach, Melba, Low Fat, Average	*1 Serving/100g*	*75*	*0.7*	*75*	*2.6*	*14.5*	*0.7*	*0*
Peach, Summer Fruits, Weight Watchers*	1 Pot/120g	58	0.1	48	4.1	6.8	0.1	0.2
Pineapple, & Peach, Fruity, Mullerlight, Muller*	1 Pot/175g	89	0.2	51	4.2	7.7	0.1	0.2
Pink Grapefruit, Mullerlight, Muller*	1 Serving/121g	74	0.2	61	6.3	7.8	0.2	0
Plain, Coconut, Dairy Free, Just Free, Lidl*	1 Pot/125g	85	4.4	68	0.5	8.4	3.5	0.2
Plain, Go On, Alpro*	1 Serving/100g	71	3.6	71	6.2	2.5	3.6	1.5
Plain, Greek Style, Alpro*	1 Serving/50g	34	1.6	68	5.8	2.6	3.3	1.5
Plain, High Protein, Alpro*	1 Serving/100g	68	3.3	68	5.8	2.6	3.3	1.5
Plain, Low Fat, Average	*1 Serving/100g*	*63*	*1.6*	*63*	*5.2*	*7*	*1.6*	*0*
Plain, Soya, Average	*1oz/28g*	*20*	*1.2*	*72*	*5*	*3.9*	*4.2*	*0*
Plain, Soya, Simply, Alpro*	1 Tbsp/20g	10	0.5	50	4	2.1	2.3	1
Plain, Whole Milk, Average	*1oz/28g*	*22*	*0.8*	*79*	*5.7*	*7.8*	*3*	*0*
Plain, with Almond, Soya, Alpro*	1 Tbsp/20g	11	0.6	54	3.9	2.3	2.8	1.1
Plain, with Coconut, Soya, Alpro*	1 Tbsp/20g	11	0.6	55	3.9	2.3	3	0.8
Plum, & Custard, Greek Style, 0% Fat, COU, M&S*	1 Pot/141g	83	0.3	59	6.4	8	0.2	0.5
Pomegranate, Soya, Alpro*	1 Pot/125g	92	2.4	74	3.6	9.5	1.9	1.1
Protein Greens, Mango, Kale, & Lime, 20g, Arla*	1 Pot /200g	155	1.2	77	10.1	8	0.6	0
Prune, Bio, Activia, Danone*	1 Pot/125g	122	4.1	98	3.6	13.1	3.3	0.8
Prune, Live, M&S*	1 Pack/159g	254	6.5	160	5.4	24.4	4.1	1.7
Quark, Plain, Muller*	1 Pot/150g	176	9.2	117	7.1	8.3	6.1	0
Quark, Strawberry, Muller*	1 Pot/150g	186	7.2	124	5.5	13.7	4.8	0
Quark, Vanilla, Muller*	1 Pot/150g	186	7.4	124	6.4	13.4	4.9	0
Raspberry, & Blueberry, High Protein, Breakfast, Fuel 10K*	1 Pouch/150g	111	1.4	74	5.5	10.8	0.9	1.1
Raspberry, & Cranberry, Fat Free, Milbona, Lidl*	1 Pot/174g	87	0.2	50	4.2	7.8	0.1	0.5
Raspberry, & Cranberry, Fat Free, Mullerlight, Muller*	1 Pot/175g	91	0.2	52	4.3	7.8	0.1	0.5
Raspberry, & Cream, The Best, Morrisons*	1 Pot/150g	205	9.7	137	3.2	16.2	6.5	0.3
Raspberry, & Cranberry, Skyr, Arla*	1/3 Pot/150g	118	0.8	79	9.2	8.1	0.5	0.3

Y

YOGHURT

INFO/WEIGHT	Measure	per Measure KCAL	FAT	Nutrition Values per 100g / 100ml KCAL	PROT	CARB	FAT	FIBRE
Raspberry, & Cranberry, Soya, Alpro*	1 Pot/125g	94	2.4	75	3.6	9.7	1.9	1.1
Raspberry, Bio Live, Low Fat, Rachel's Organic*	1 Pot/125g	114	2	91	4.1	15.1	1.6	0.1
Raspberry, Bio, Activia, Fat Free, Danone*	1 Pot/125g	68	0.1	54	4.7	7.2	0.1	2.6
Raspberry, Biopot, Onken*	1 Serving/150g	150	3.9	100	3.8	14	2.6	0
Raspberry, Fat Free, Average	*1 Serving/100g*	*64*	*0.1*	*64*	*4.9*	*11*	*0.1*	*1.7*
Raspberry, Fat Free, Probiotic, Organic, Yeo Valley*	1 Pot/125g	98	0.1	78	5.2	14	0.1	0.4
Raspberry, Greek Style, Bio-Live, Rachel's Organic*	1 Serving/150g	194	10.6	129	3.1	13.1	7.1	0
Raspberry, Greek Style, Light, Fat Free, Brooklea, Aldi*	1 Pot/125g	72	0.6	58	5.8	8.2	0.5	0.5
Raspberry, High Protein, Fat Free, Milbona, Lidl*	1 Pot/180g	223	0.7	124	12.6	3.4	0.4	0.5
Raspberry, Intensely Creamy, Juicy, Activia, Danone*	1 Pot/110g	109	3.3	99	4.8	12.7	3	0.6
Raspberry, Lactose Free, Lactofree, Arla*	1 Pot/125g	130	3.4	104	3.3	16.5	2.7	0.7
Raspberry, Low Fat, Average	*1 Serving/100g*	*83*	*1.1*	*83*	*4.1*	*14.1*	*1.1*	*0.8*
Raspberry, Low Fat, Deliciously Fruity, Waitrose*	1 Pot/125g	99	1.4	79	4.5	12.6	1.1	0.5
Raspberry, Low Fat, Stapleton*	1 Serving/150g	105	0.8	70	3.3	13.6	0.5	2
Raspberry, or Strawberry, Smooth (No Bits), Ski, Nestle*	1 Pot/120g	118	3.2	98	3.9	13.6	2.7	0
Raspberry, Organic, Yeo Valley*	1 Pot/150g	152	5.8	101	4.2	12.3	3.9	0.4
Raspberry, Pouring, Icelandic Style, Skyr, Arla*	1 Serving/150g	96	0.8	64	6	9.1	0.5	0.1
Raspberry, Protein, Arla*	1 Pot/200g	140	0.4	70	10	6.5	0.2	0
Raspberry, Razzle, Greek Style, Light & Free, Danone*	1 Pot/115g	61	0.1	53	4.7	7.8	0.1	1.1
Raspberry, Skyr, Icelandic, Siggi's*	1 Pot/150g	108	0	72	10	7.7	0	0
Raspberry, Skyr, Milbona, Lidl*	½ Pot/175g	100	0.4	57	8.9	4.6	0.2	0.5
Raspberry, Squidgy Pouches, Brooklea, Aldi*	1 Pouch/80g	67	2.3	84	3.4	11	2.9	0.5
Raspberry, Summer Fruits, Benecol*	1 Pot/120g	90	2	75	0.2	9.7	1.7	3.7
Raspberry, Summer, Biopot, Onken*	1/5 Pot/90g	91	2.4	101	3.8	15	2.7	0.6
Red Berry, Vitality, Low Fat, with Omega 3, Muller*	1 Pot/150g	138	2.8	92	4.3	13.8	1.9	0.7
Rhubarb, & Beetroot, Icelandic Style, Skyr, Arla*	1 Pot/149g	103	0.3	69	9.4	7.1	0.2	0.6
Rhubarb, & Champagne, Finest, Tesco*	1 Pot/150g	212	11.6	141	3.4	14.1	7.7	0.7
Rhubarb, & Fiery Ginger, Greek Style , Brooklea, Aldi*	1/3 Pot/150g	207	11	138	3	15	7.3	0.5
Rhubarb, & Vanilla, Gourmet, The Collective Dairy*	1 Bowl/100g	124	5	124	4.9	14.7	5	0
Rhubarb, Bio Live, Low Fat, Luscious, Rachel's Organic*	1 Pot/125g	104	2	83	4	13.1	1.6	0.1
Rhubarb, Champagne, Scottish, Deluxe, Lidl*	1 Pot/150g	198	9.3	132	4	14.7	6.2	0.5
Rhubarb, Crumble, Inspired, Mullerlight, Muller*	1 Pot/172g	86	0.2	50	4.1	7.5	0.1	0
Rhubarb, Fruity, Mullerlight, Muller*	1 Pot/175g	91	0.2	52	4.2	7.9	0.1	0
Rhubarb, Layer, Bonne Maman*	1 Pot/125g	134	5.1	107	2.3	15	4.1	0.6
Rhubarb, Live, Thick & Creamy, Manor Farm*	1 Pot/128g	166	9.3	130	5	13.4	7.3	0
Rhubarb, Longley Farm*	1 Pot/150g	165	5.6	110	4.9	14.3	3.7	0
Rhubarb, Low Fat, Average	*1 Serving/100g*	*83*	*1.2*	*83*	*4.6*	*13.3*	*1.2*	*0.2*
Rhubarb, Low Fat, Garden Fruits, Tesco*	1 Pot/125g	119	2.4	95	3	15.5	1.9	0.3
Rhubarb, Spiced, Thick & Creamy, COU, M&S*	1 Pot/170g	68	0.2	40	4.3	5.8	0.1	0.5
Rhubarb, Timperley, TTD, Sainsbury's*	1 Pot/150g	170	9.9	113	3.2	10.1	6.6	0.5
Salted Caramel, Thick & Creamy, Live, Nomadic*	1 Pot/160g	181	6.7	113	5.4	13.4	4.2	0.5
Sheep's, Organic, Vrai*	¼ Pot/100g	101	6.8	101	5.3	4.7	6.8	0
Strawberry, & Cream, 0.06% Fat, TTD, Sainsbury's*	1 Pot/150g	183	8.2	122	3.5	14.7	5.5	0.4
Strawberry, & Cream, Finest, Tesco*	1 Pot/150g	206	10.4	137	3.4	15.4	6.9	0.5
Strawberry, & Cream, Scottish, Deluxe, Lidl*	1 Pot/150g	198	9	132	4.1	15.1	6	0.5
Strawberry, & Raspberry, High In Protein , Go On, Alpro*	1 Pot/150g	128	4.2	85	5.1	8.8	2.8	1.2
Strawberry, & Rhubarb, Greek Style, Brooklea, Aldi*	1/3 Pot/150g	202	11.7	135	3	13	7.8	0.5
Strawberry, & Banana, Bircher Muesli, Moma Foods*	1 Pot/220g	295	4.8	134	4.2	23.4	2.2	2.1
Strawberry, & Banana, Soya, No Bits, Alpro*	1 Pot/125g	99	2.5	79	3.7	10.7	2	1
Strawberry, Active, Fat Free, Optifit, Aldi*	1 Pot/125g	54	0.5	43	3	7.1	0.4	0.4
Strawberry, Bio Live, Llaeth Y Llan, Village Dairy*	1 Pot/125g	130	3.5	104	5.5	14	2.8	0.1
Strawberry, Bio, Activia, Danone*	1 Pot/125g	124	4.1	99	3.6	13.6	3.3	0.2
Strawberry, Breakfast Crunch, Corner, Muller*	1 Pot/135g	163	3.5	121	5.5	0	2.6	0

YOGHURT

INFO/WEIGHT	Measure	per Measure KCAL	per Measure FAT	Nutrition Values per 100g / 100ml KCAL	PROT	CARB	FAT	FIBRE
Strawberry, Everyday Low Fat, Co-Op*	1 Pot/125g	88	0.9	70	3	13	0.7	0
Strawberry, Fat Free, Average	**1 Serving/100g**	**66**	**0.1**	**66**	**4.9**	**11.1**	**0.1**	**0.6**
Strawberry, Greek Style, 0% Fat, Liberte, Yoplait*	1 Pot/100g	79	0.2	79	8	11	0.2	0.4
Strawberry, Greek Style, Bio Live, Activia, Danone*	1 Pot/110g	109	3.3	99	5	12.9	3	0.2
Strawberry, Greek Style, Fat Free, Brooklea, Aldi*	1 Pot/125g	72	0.3	57	4.9	8.8	0.2	0.2
Strawberry, Greek Style, Fruitopolis, Mullerlight, Muller*	1 Pot/130g	84	0.1	65	4.8	10.8	0.1	0
Strawberry, Greek Style, Luxury, Oykos, Danone*	1 Pot/110g	159	8.9	145	3.2	14.6	8.1	0.3
Strawberry, Greek Style, Milbona, Lidl*	1 Pot/125g	160	7.8	128	2.4	15.5	6.2	0.5
Strawberry, Greek Style, Whipped, Bliss, Corner, Muller*	1 Pot/110g	142	6.5	129	4.1	14.3	5.9	0
Strawberry, Icelandic Style, Strained, Fat Free, Skyr, Arla*	1 Pot/150g	109	0.7	73	9.6	7.4	0.5	0.1
Strawberry, Lactose Free, Lactofree, Arla*	1 Pot/125g	126	3.2	101	3.5	15.9	2.6	0.4
Strawberry, Layer, Bonne Maman*	1 Pot/125g	139	5.1	111	2.3	16	4.1	0.4
Strawberry, Light & Free, Skyr, Danone*	1 Pot/150g	81	0.8	54	9.1	3.8	0.5	0.5
Strawberry, Light, Brooklea, Aldi*	1 Pot/200g	154	0.2	77	6.1	12.9	0.1	0.4
Strawberry, Low Fat, Average	**1 Serving/100g**	**81**	**1**	**81**	**4.5**	**13.6**	**1**	**0.2**
Strawberry, Milbona, Lidl*	1 Pot/175g	175	5.2	100	3	15	3	0
Strawberry, Organic, Yeo Valley*	1 Pot/120g	114	40.6	95	4.5	10.5	33.8	0
Strawberry, Probiotic, Organic, Yeo Valley*	1 Pot/125g	125	5	100	4.4	11.7	4	0.1
Strawberry, Protein 20g, Arla*	1 Pot/200g	140	0.4	70	10	6.5	0.2	0
Strawberry, Rice, Low Fat, Muller*	1 Pot/180g	193	4.1	107	3.2	18.4	2.3	0.4
Strawberry, Shortcake, Crunch Corner, Muller*	1 Pot/130g	192	7.3	148	4.5	19.3	5.6	0.1
Strawberry, Soya, Alpro*	¼ Pot/125g	92	2.4	74	3.6	9.4	1.9	1
Strawberry, Suckies, The Great Dairy Collective*	1 Pack/100g	77	3.1	77	3.2	9.2	3.1	0
Strawberry, Summer Fruits, Benecol*	1 Pot/120g	90	2	75	0.2	9.7	1.7	3.7
Strawberry, Super, Kefir, Kids, The Great Dairy Collective*	1 Pot/85g	92	3.3	108	4.7	12.7	3.9	0
Strawberry, Thick & Creamy, Golden Acre*	1 Pot/150g	219	11.7	146	2.3	16.5	7.8	0.5
Strawberry, Totally, Low Fat, CBY, Asda*	1 Pot/125g	104	1.2	83	4.1	14.2	1	0.4
Strawberry, Yoplait*	1 Pot/125g	61	0.2	49	4.2	7.6	0.2	0.9
Tiramisu, Greek Style, Luxury, Oykos, Danone*	1 Pot/110g	177	9.2	161	2.9	18	8.4	0
Toffee, & Vanilla, Fat Free, Multipack, Weight Watchers*	1 Pot/110g	50	0.1	45	4.1	6	0.1	0.1
Toffee, Cheesecake, Inspired, Goodies, Mullerlight, Muller*	1 Pot/107g	97	2	91	4.5	13.4	1.9	0
Toffee, Low Fat, Deliciously Silky, Waitrose*	1 Pot/151g	143	3	95	4.6	14.5	2	0.5
Toffee, Smooth, Fat Free, Mullerlight, Muller*	1 Pot/175g	89	0.2	51	4.1	7.9	0.1	0
Toffee, Smooth, Milbona, Lidl*	1 Pot/175g	105	0.4	60	4.5	9.7	0.2	0.5
Toffee, Tempting, Greek Style, Muller Light *	1 Pot/120g	84	0.1	70	6.3	10.1	0.1	0
Toffee, with Chocolate Hoops, Crunch Corner, Muller*	1 Pot/135g	209	7.8	155	4.2	20.8	5.8	0.2
Tropical, Granola, Duo, Brooklea, Aldi*	1 Pot/135g	177	6.2	131	3.6	18.5	4.6	0.8
Tropical, Papaye, Goyave, & Passion, Mamie Nova*	1 Pot/150g	132	3.6	88	3.4	13	2.4	0
Turkish Cream, Yayla*	1 Serving/100g	83	6	83	3.6	3.7	6	0
Turkish Delight, Mullerlight, Muller*	1 Pot/165g	91	0.8	55	4.5	7.4	0.5	0
Vanilla, & Chocolate Sprinkles, Fat Free, Milbona, Lidl*	1 Pot/175g	93	0.9	53	3.9	7.6	0.5	0.1
Vanilla, & Granola, Low Fat, Activia, Danone*	1 Pot/165g	185	3.3	112	5.3	18.2	2	1.8
Vanilla, Average	**1 Serving/120g**	**100**	**5.4**	**83**	**4.5**	**12.4**	**4.5**	**0.8**
Vanilla, Breakfast Topper, Activia, Danone*	1 Pot/160g	165	4	103	4.9	15.1	2.5	0
Vanilla, Cashew Milk, Dairy Free, Nush Foods*	1 Pot/125g	88	5.2	70	2	3	4.2	0
Vanilla, Choco Balls, Crunch Corner, Snack Size, Muller*	1 Pot/85g	118	4.1	139	3.8	20.2	4.8	0
Vanilla, Creamy, with Mini Smarties, Nestle*	1 Pot/120g	182	6.5	152	3.6	21.5	5.4	0
Vanilla, Fat Free, Onken*	½ Pot/225g	166	0.2	74	4.4	12.6	0.1	0.3
Vanilla, Greek Style, 0% Fat, COU, M&S*	1 Pot/140g	81	0.3	58	6.8	7.2	0.2	0.5
Vanilla, Intensely Creamy, Velvety, Activia, Danone*	1 Pot/120g	116	3.6	97	4.8	12.7	3	0.1
Vanilla, Low Fat, Probiotic, Organic, M&S*	1 Serving/100g	85	1.8	85	6.2	10.9	1.8	0
Vanilla, Madagascan, West Country, TTD, Sainsbury's*	1 Pot/150g	197	11.8	132	3.1	11.9	7.9	0.5
Vanilla, Non Dairy, The Coconut Collaborative*	1 Pot/350g	508	42	145	1.4	7.9	12	0

Y

	Measure INFO/WEIGHT	per Measure KCAL	FAT	Nutrition Values per 100g / 100ml KCAL	PROT	CARB	FAT	FIBRE
YOGHURT								
Vanilla, Organic, Probiotic, Fat Free, Yeo Valley*	1 Pot/500g	400	0.5	80	5.4	14.2	0.1	0
Vanilla, Smooth, Light, Fat Free, Mullerlight, Muller*	1 Pot/175g	88	0.2	50	4.3	7.2	0.1	0
Vanilla, Soya, Alpro*	1 Pot/125g	106	2.4	85	3.2	13.6	1.9	0.5
Vanilla, SoYummy, Aldi*	1 Serving/150g	106	2	71	3.5	10.9	1.3	0
Vanilla, Sprinkled with Dark Chocolate, Brooklea, Aldi*	1 Pot/165g	82	0.8	50	3.5	8.2	0.5	0.5
Vanilla, Thick & Creamy, Channel Island, M&S*	1 Pot/150g	188	6.6	125	4.5	17.5	4.4	1
Vanilla, Vibe, Light & Free, Danone*	1 Pot/115g	61	0.1	53	4.9	7.1	0.1	0
Vanilla, Virtually Fat Free, Yeo Valley*	1 Pot/150g	122	0.2	81	5.1	15	0.1	0
Vanilla, with Oreo Pieces, Muller*	1 Pot/120g	186	7.1	155	3.5	21.3	5.9	0
with Raspberry Layer, Bonne Maman*	1 Pot/125g	136	5.1	109	2.4	15	4.1	1
YOGHURT DRINK								
Actimel, Blueberry, Danone*	1 Bottle/100g	74	1.5	74	2.6	11.8	1.5	0.5
Average	*1fl oz/30ml*	*19*	*0*	*62*	*3.1*	*13.1*	*0*	*0*
Blueberry, & Blackcurrant, Skyr, Arla*	1 Bottle/350ml	214	0.7	61	5.8	8.1	0.2	0
Blueberry, Cholesterol Lowering, Tesco*	1 Bottle/100g	49	1.5	49	2.5	6.2	1.5	0.1
Cholesterol Lowering, Asda*	1 Bottle/100g	76	1.4	76	2.9	13	1.4	1
Fruit, Mixed, Actimel, Danone*	1 Bottle/100ml	88	1.5	88	2.7	16	1.5	0
Light, Benecol*	1 Bottle/68g	40	1.4	60	2.8	7.3	2.1	0.1
Light, Yakult*	1 Bottle/65ml	27	0	42	1.4	10.2	0	1.8
Multi Fruit, Actimel, Danone*	1 Bottle/100g	85	1.5	85	2.7	14.4	1.5	0.1
Original, 0.1% Fat, Actimel, Danone*	1 Bottle/100g	27	0.1	27	2.7	3	0.1	0.2
Original, Cholesterol Lowering, Pro Activ, Flora*	1 Bottle/100ml	44	1.5	44	3	4.5	1.5	1.1
Original, Cholesterol Lowering, Sainsbury's*	1 Bottle/100g	36	1.1	36	2.7	3.4	1.1	0.5
Original, No Added Sugar, Benecol*	1 Bottle/68g	32	1.4	47	2.8	4.3	2	0
Peach, & Apricot, Benecol*	1 Bottle/68g	33	1.4	49	2.9	4.8	2	0
Strawberry, Actimel, Danone*	1 Bottle/100g	74	1.5	74	2.9	11.5	1.5	0
Strawberry, Benecol*	1 Bottle/68g	38	1.4	56	3.2	6.2	2	0
Strawberry, Cholesterol Lowering, Brooklea, Aldi*	1 Bottle/100g	38	1.3	38	0	0	1.3	0
Strawberry, Cholesterol Reducing, Pro Activ, Flora*	1 Bottle/100ml	42	1.5	42	2.9	4.4	1.5	0
Strawberry, Cholesterol Reducing, Tesco*	1 Bottle/100g	46	1.7	46	2.7	4.7	1.7	0.8
Strawberry, Fat Free, Actimel, Danone*	1 Bottle/100ml	27	0.1	27	2.6	3.2	0.1	0.2
Yakult*	1 Bottle/65ml	43	0.1	66	1.3	14.7	0.1	0
YORKIE								
Original, Nestle*	1 Bar/55g	302	17.4	546	6.2	57.9	31.5	1.9
Raisin & Biscuit, Nestle*	1 Bar/67g	338	16.9	508	5.3	61.9	25.4	1.7
YORKSHIRE PUDDING								
3", Baked, Aunt Bessie's*	1 Pudding/36g	91	2.8	252	9	36.4	7.9	1.7
Average	*1 Pudding/30g*	*62*	*3*	*208*	*6.6*	*24.7*	*9.9*	*0.9*
Baked, Frozen, 4 Pack, Morrisons*	1 Pudding/34g	82	2.3	241	8.4	36.7	6.7	1.6
Batters, in Foils, Ready to Bake, Frozen, Aunt Bessie's*	1 Pudding/17g	47	1.8	276	9.1	32.6	10.8	1.4
Beef Dripping, Cooked, Specially Selected, Aldi*	1 Pudding/44g	129	5.7	293	9.4	32	13	3
Beef, Mini, Waitrose*	1 Pudding/14g	33	1.3	234	13.5	23.2	9.4	1.3
Carvery, Aunt Bessie's*	1 Pudding/57g	140	4.2	244	9.1	34	7.3	3.3
Frozen, Ovenbaked, Iceland*	1 Pudding/20g	53	1.8	262	7.4	36.8	8.8	3.1
Fully Prepared, M&S*	1 Pudding/22g	63	2.9	285	9.4	31.6	13.2	1.2
Giant, Aunt Bessie's*	1 Pudding/97g	260	7.5	269	8.6	42	7.8	2.6
Home Bake, Aunt Bessie's*	1 Pudding/47g	78	2.1	165	6.1	25	4.4	1
Home Bake, Rise in 20 Minutes, Baked, Aunt Bessie's*	1 Pudding/25g	43	1.7	174	6	20	7	3.1
Mini, Co-Op*	1 Pudding/16g	50	2	312	6.2	43.8	12.5	2.5
Mini, Farmfoods*	1 Pudding/3g	8	0.2	281	9.6	43.2	7.7	1.9
Ready to Bake, Baked, Aunt Bessie's*	1 Pudding/17g	42	1.4	246	8.5	35.1	8	1.7
Ready to Bake, Sainsbury's*	1 Pudding/18g	48	1.6	263	9.9	35.9	8.9	1.3
with Chicken, & Pigs in Portionets, Filled, Morrisons*	1 Pack/375g	578	21	154	8.1	16.8	5.6	1.7

Y

YULE LOG

INFO/WEIGHT	Measure	per Measure		Nutrition Values per 100g / 100ml				
		KCAL	FAT	KCAL	PROT	CARB	FAT	FIBRE
Chocolate, Belgian, Finest, Tesco*	1 Slice/93g	294	14.6	316	4.7	38.2	15.7	1.8
Chocolate, Frozen, Tesco*	1 Slice/80g	251	14.6	315	7.5	28.8	18.3	2.3
Chocolate, Iceland*	1 Slice/75g	243	14.4	324	7.1	29.7	19.2	2.3
Chocolate, Sainsbury's*	1 Slice/35g	153	7.7	432	5	51.6	21.8	4.6
Chocolate, Tesco*	1 Slice/30g	133	6.7	439	5.3	52.6	22.2	3.6
Christmas Range, Tesco*	1 Slice/30g	131	6.4	442	4.9	56.8	21.7	2.8
Mini, M&S*	1 Cake/36g	165	8.4	460	5.7	56.9	23.3	1.1

ALL BAR ONE

BEEF
Steak, & Frites	1089
Steak, Ribeye, 8oz, with Peppercorn Sauce, & Fries	1069

BEETROOT
Carpaccio	313

BREAD
Rustic, with Olive Oil	711

BREAKFAST
Vegan	745
Vegetarian	801
Vegetarian, Sm Appetites	499

BREAKFAST - FULL ENGLISH
& Toasted Sourdough	1098
with Spinach & Potato Hash, & Toasted Sourdough	1419
Sausage, Egg, Beans, & Toast, Sm Appetites	629

BREAKFAST - POT
Chorizo, Egg	610
Egg, Protein	725

BREAKFAST - PROTEIN POWER UP
Salmon, Egg, Avocado, & Grapefruit, with Salad	372

BREAKFAST - SHAKSHUKA
Standard	589
with Avocado	1017
with Halloumi	1017
with Sourdough	748
with Streaky Bacon	702

BREAKFAST CEREAL
Bircher, Blueberry	528

BROWNIES
Chocolate, with Bourbon Vanilla Ice Cream	582
Chocolate, with Vanilla Ice Cream, Sm Appetites	389

BRUSCHETTA
Avocado, & Tomato, Crushed	545

BURGERS
Beef, Bacon & Cheese	921
Beef, Classic	543
Beef, Dirty	914
Beef, Sliders, Sm Appetites	445
Beef, The Californian	1267
Beef, The French	1166
Beef, The Hipster	1243
Beef, The Skinny	549
Beef, The Smoky	1399
Beef, The Spanish	1205
Beef, The Wagyu	1403
Chicken, Grilled, Classic	496
Vegan, Plant Based	755

BURGERS VEGETARIAN
Tomato, Beetroot, & Mozzarella	905
Tomato, Beetroot, & Mozzarella, The Californian	1205
Tomato, Beetroot, & Mozzarella, The French	1104
Tomato, Beetroot, & Mozzarella, The Hipster	1181
Tomato, Beetroot, & Mozzarella, The Skinny	487

ALL BAR ONE

BURGERS VEGETARIAN
Tomato, Beetroot, & Mozzarella, The Smoky	1337
Tomato, Beetroot, & Mozzarella, The Spanish	1144

BURRITO
Chicken	776
Chicken, with Fries	1179
Chicken, with House Salad	967

CAKE
Chocolate, Mascarpone, & Orange, Mousse	250
Raspberry, & Pistachio, Traybake	150

CHEESECAKE
Biscoff, with Banana, & Caramel	849
Lemon, Sicilian, with Blueberry Compote, Baked	558

CHICKEN
Karaage, Sticky, Bites	477
Schnitzel, with Fries, & Garlic Cream	694
Skewers, Teriyaki, Ginger	335
Wings, BBq	586
Wings, Buttermilk	657

CHICKEN KATSU
Main	702

CHICKEN PIRI PIRI
Half	450
Half, with Fries	853
Half, with House Salad	641

CROISSANT
with Butter, & Jam	661

DOUGHNUTS
Churros	582

DUMPLINGS
Duck, Crispy	400

EGGS - BENEDICT
Standard	750
with Avocado	1178

EGGS - FLORENTINE
Standard	748
with Avocado	1176

EGGS - POACHED
with Mushrooms, on Toasted Sourdough	461

EGGS - ROYALE
Standard	824
with Avocado	1252

EGGS - SCRAMBLED ON TOAST
with Smoked Salmon, on Toasted Sourdough	722

FISH & CHIPS
Main	758

FISH - BATTERED COD
with Mushy Peas, & Tartare Sauce, Sm Appetites	301

FISH - GOUJONS
with Aioli	349
with Tartare Sauce, Sm Appetites	278

FISH CAKES
Haddock, Smoked, & Mustard	291

ALL BAR ONE

FISH CAKES
Haddock, Smoked, & Mustard, with Fries	694
Haddock, Smoked, & Mustard, with House Salad	482

FLATBREAD
Garlic, Stonebaked	1054
Houmous, & Kale	615

FRIES - HALLOUMI
Standard	460

FRIES - POTATO
Standard	399
Sm Appetites	177
with Parmesan, Truffle Oil, & Rosemary, Side	482
with Smoked Paprika & Saffron Aioli, Side	482

FRIES - TRIO
Standard	1125

FRUIT
Strawberries, & Bananas, Fresh, Sm Appetites	253

HASH
Potato, Spinach, & Onion, Pan Fried	582

HOUMOUS
Duo	715

ICE CREAM
Trio	318
Vanilla, 2 Scoops, Sm Appetites	244

KEBAB
Chorizo, & Halloumi, Skewers	601

LAMB
Kibbeh	553

LASAGNE
Plant Based	747

MACARONI CHEESE
Portion	430

MEATBALLS
Lamb, Spiced	499

MELT
Chicken, BBQ, Bacon, & Cheese	774

MEZZE
Little, Sm Appetites	738

MUFFIN
Blueberry	547
Blueberry Cheesecake	463
Carrot Cake	459
Chocolate, Triple	505
Lemon, & White Chocolate	462

NACHOS
Original	997
Vegan	831
with BBQ Pulled Pork	1425

NOODLES
Pad Thai	606
Pad Thai, Little, Sm Appetites	313
Pad Thai, with Chicken Breast	808
Pad Thai, with Pan Fried King Prawns	703

ALL BAR ONE

NOODLES
Pad Thai, with Sliced Beef Fillet	775

PAIN AU CHOCOLAT
Pastry	425

PANCAKES - BUTTERMILK
with Maple Syrup, Banana, & Berries	491
withÃ‚Â Maple Syrup, & Smoked Bacon	568

PASTRY
Spinach & Feta, Bourek	303

PIE
Pecan, Bourbon, with Cinnamon Ice Cream	540

PLATTER
Brunch Board, for Two, Breakfast, Ã‚Â½ Board	1137
Deli Board, Sharing, Whole Board	1826
Grazing Board, Sharing, Whole Board	2170
Mezze Board, Sharing, Whole Board	2016

POTATOES
Patatas Bravas	283

PRAWN CRACKERS
Portion	58

PRAWNS
King, Pan Fried, Add On	104
King, Pan Fried	292

QUESADILLA
Chicken	514
Lentil, & Chickpea	460

RIBS
BBQ, Smoked	1494

RICE
Miso, Bowl	474
Miso, Bowl, with Chicken Breast	670
Miso, Bowl, with Pan Fried King Prawns	585
Miso, Bowl, with Sliced Beef Fillet	726
Steamed, Sm Appetites	179

ROLL
Bacon, Sour Cream, Chilli Tomato Jam, & Coriander	716

SALAD
Chicken, & Avocado, Chargrilled	905
Chicken, & Avocado, Chargrilled, Sm Appetites	427
Duck, Crispy	568
Feta, Beetroot, & Walnut	509
Feta, Carrot, & Quinoa	626
House	202
Rocket, & Parmesan	234
Side	202
Small Appetites	96
Superfood	440
Superfood, with Chicken Breast	634
Superfood, with Garlic & Lemon Marinated Halloumi	634
Superfood, with Pan Fried King Prawns	654

SANDWICH
Bacon, with Sliced Tomatoes, & Tomato Sauce	670
Chicken, Grilled, Focaccia	610

	KCAL		KCAL

ALL BAR ONE

SANDWICH

Club	1454
Sausage	939
Sausage, Veggie	685
Steak, Fillet	606

SAUCE

Katsu Curry	156

SAUSAGE

Cocktail, Maple Glazed	572

SORBET

Raspberry, 2 Scoops, Sm Appetites	255
Raspberry	546

SOUP

Tomato, Vegetable, & Quinoa	122

SQUID

Calamari, Salt & Pepper	404

TACO

Chilli Non Carne	503

TOAST

Sourdough, with Avocado, & Feta	732

TORTE

Chocolate, Salted Caramel, with Hazelnut Ice Cream	535

TORTILLA

Huevos Rancheros	585

VEGETABLES

Tempura	351

WAFFLES

Belgian, with Maple Syrup, Fruit, & Yoghurt	1028

WRAP

Fish Finger	534

ASK ITALIAN

ARANCINI

Pumpkin, Risotto, with Tomato Dip	285
Spinach & Ricotta, with Tomato Dip	387

AUBERGINE

Melanzane Al Forno, Main	578
Melanzane Al Forno, Starter	301

BOLOGNESE

Spaghetti, Vegan	849

BREADS / NIBBLES

Fonduta, with Dough Sticks	771
Garlic Bread	588
Garlic Bread Speciale - with Balsamic Onions	838
Garlic Bread Speciale - with Purple Pesto	801
Garlic Bread with Mozzarella	784
Italian Olives	204
Rosemary, & Sea Salt	499

BREADSTICKS

& Tomato, Dip, Tiny Tums, Kids Menu	159

BROWNIES

Chocolate, & Banana, Kids Menu	183

CAKE

Pistachio, & Olive Oil, Vanilla Gelato	452

CALZONE

Con Carne Piccante	970
Goats Cheese, & Spinach	991
Pollo	899

CANNELLONI

Sausage, Ragu, Baked, with Creme Fraiche	658

CARBONARA

Tagliatelle	882
Asparagus & Pancetta, Light, with Salad	541
Linguine	814

CHEESECAKE

Honeycomb. with Vanilla Gelato	719
Passion Fruit, & Raspberry	556

CHICKEN

Goujons, with Chips, Kids Menu	183
Goujons, with Roast Potatoes, Kids Menu	413
Pollo, Milanese	1009
Pollo, Milanese, with Chips	753

COURGETTE

Zucchine Fritti	281

DESSERTS

Fruity Ice Lolly - Apple, & Raspberry, Kids Menu	43
Chocolate, Eton Mess, Melting	472
Chocolate Etna	767
Frutti, Kids Menu	14
Fruity Ice Lolly - Orange & Apple, Kids Menu	45
Panna Cotta	191
Chocolate Pizza, Kids Menu	195
Tiramisu	419

DESSERTS - GELATO

Chocolate, 2 Scoops	225

ASK ITALIAN

DESSERTS - GELATO

Hazelnut	283
Pistachio, 2 Scoops	273
Salted Caramel	252
Strawberry	266
Vanilla	242
Warm Cookie, & Salted Caramel	929
Gelato Gondola, Chocolate, & Nut	628
Gelato Gondola, Salted Caramel	536

DESSERTS - MAKE YOUR OWN SUNDAE

Grapes, Topping, Kids Menu	8
Ice Cream, Chocolate, Kids Menu	109
Sauce, Chocolate, Kids Menu	325
Ice Cream, Strawberry, Kids Menu	102
Ice Cream, Vanilla, Kids Menu	117
Sauce, Choconut, Kids Menu	57
Sauce, Strawberry, Kids Menu	22
White Chocolate Swirl, Topping, Kids Menu	55

DESSERTS - SORBET

Mango	179
Rasperry	166

FETTUCCINE

Bolognese	692

FETTUCCINE

Con Melanzane, Vegan	843
Con Verdure, Vegan	1042

FRIES

Sweet Potato, Rosemary	300

GIRASOLE

Spinach, & Ricotta	743

GNOCCHI

Chocolate, Baked	473

LASAGNE

Beef, & Pork, Ragu	717

LINGUINE

Seafood, Con Frutti Di Mare	828

MOUSSE

White Chocolate Swirl	342

NUTS

Chilli, Nuts	291

PASTA

Cartwheel, Dip & Dunk, Kids Menu	459
with Tomato Sauce, & Cheese, Dip, & Dunk	459
Crab & Ricotta, Half Moon	692
in Tomato Sauce, Tiny Tums, Kids Menu	201
with Butter, Tiny Tums, Kids Menu	245

PASTA CARTWHEELS

in Bolognese Sauce, Kids Menu	424
in Cheese Sauce, Kids Menu	504
in Tomato Sauce, Kids Menu	396

PENNE

Arrabiata	759
Arrabiata, with Chicken	869

ASK ITALIAN

PENNE

Chicken, Al Pollo Della Casa	842
in Bolognese Sauce, Kids Menu	457
in Cheese Sauce, Kids Menu	537
in Tomato Sauce, Kids Menu	429

PIZZA

Beef, & Gorgonzola, Prima	948
Black Olives, & Chicken, Kids Menu	401
Black Olives, & Ham, Kids Menu	391
Black Olives, & Mushrooms, Kids Menu	371
Black Olives, & Pepperoni, Kids Menu	450
Black Olives, & Roasted Red Peppers, Kids Menu	434
Black Olives, & Spinach, Kids Menu	361
Black Olives, Kids Menu	357
Caprina, Light, Prima (Pizza Only)	382
Caprina, Prima	863
Chicken, & Ham, Kids Menu	422
Chicken, & Mushrooms, Kids Menu	402
Chicken, & Pepperoni, Kids Menu	481
Chicken, & Roasted Red Pepper, Kids Menu	465
Chicken, & Spinach, Kids Menu	392
Chicken, Kids Menu	388
Fiorentina, Two Egg, Prima	903
Ham, & Roasted Red Peppers, Kids Menu	455

PIZZA

Ham, & Smoked Scarmorza Cheese, Prima	1082
Ham, & Spinach, Kids Menu	382
Ham, Kids Menu	378
Lamb, Slow Cooked, Prima	1043
Margherita, Classic	802
Margherita, Four Cheese	738
Margherita, No Topping, Kids Menu	344
Margherita, Speciale, Alto Base	1137
Margherita, Vegan, Prima	535
Mushrooms, & Ham, Kids Menu	392
Mushrooms, & Roasted Red Pepper, Kids Menu	435
Mushrooms, & Spinach, Kids Menu	362
Mushrooms, Kids Menu	358
Pepperoni, & Ham, Kids Menu	471
Pepperoni, & Mushrooms, Kids Menu	451
Pepperoni, & Roasted Red Pepper, Kids Menu	514
Pepperoni, & Spinach, Kids Menu	441
Pepperoni, Alto Base	1338
Pepperoni, Kids Menu	437
Pollo E Funghi	764
Pollo Picante Con Pancetta, Light, Prima (Pizza Only)	435
Pollo Picante Con Pancetta, Prima	914
Roasted Red Peppers, Kids Menu	421
Salami, Misti, Prima	1011
Salsiccia, Sausage, Spicy, Prima	1116
Spinach, & Roasted Red Pepper, Kids Menu	425
Spinach, Kids Menu	348
Stromboli, Classic	881

ASK ITALIAN

PIZZA
Super Green, Prima	691
Verdure, Classic	793

PORK
Belly, Porchetta	1143

PRAWNS
King, Butterfly, Light	114

RAVIOLI
Beef, & Chianti	728

RIGATONI
Meatballs, Ragu, Mozzarella, Al Manzo Piccante	718

RISOTTO
Con Pollo E Funghi	818
Pea, & Asparagus	646
Pea, & Prosciutto	694

SALAD
Caesar, Chicken	571
Caesar, Kale, Side	187
Cheese, Burrata, Tomatoes, Rocket, Caprese	303
Goats Cheese, Mediterranean	604
Insalata Di Pollo E Pancetta	743
Mediterranean, Vegan	286
Mozzarella, & Mixed Grain	501
Rainbow, Side	66
Rainbow, Vegan	243

SALAD
Salmon, Roast, & Mixed Grain	624

SALMON
Fillet, Roast, Wrapped	694

SEA BASS
Al Forno	465

SEAFOOD
Calamari, Breaded	476

SIDES
Baked Broccoli with Chilli Cheese Crumb	147
Chips Garlic & Cheese	892
Mixed Salad	18
Plum Tomatoes, Kids Menu	4
Broccoli, Kids Menu	13
Side Salad, Kids Menu	44
Courgette Sticks, Battered	281

SNACKS
Nibbles, Spicy	167

SORBET
Lemon	144
Prosecco	103

SOUFFLE
Pea, & Ricotta	405

SOUP
Super Green	127

SPAGHETTI
Al Pomodoro, Vegan	765
Al Pomodoro, with Mozzarella	672

ASK ITALIAN

SPAGHETTI
in Bolognese Sauce, Kids Menu	483
in Cheese Sauce, Kids Menu	563
in Tomato Sauce, Kids Menu	455
Lentil, Ragu, Vegan	849

STARTERS & SHARES
Mushrooms Al Forno	540
Chicken Lecca-Lecca	675
Bruschetta, Marinated Tomatoes, Basil, & Ricotta	365
Baked Dough Ball - Fontal Cheese and Chilli	711
Antipasti - Fritto	1196
Butterfly King Prawns	416
Plain	550
Meatballs Picante	718
Antipasti - Classico, The Mixed One	1310
Tuscan Bean Soup	433

TAGLIATELLE
Beef, Brisket, Rago	630
Lobster, & Prawn, Aragosta E Gamberoni	652
Pesto, Genovese, Purple	926
Pesto, Genovese, Purple, Light, with Salad	486

TART
Chocolate, & Blood Orange	322
Pear, with Raspberries, & Cream	342

TORTELLINI
Cheese, & Vegetable, Dip & Tip	263

VEGETABLES
Vegetable Sticks with Bread Soldiers, Kids Menu	175

WHITEBAIT
Breaded	683

BEEFEATER RESTAURANT

BEANS

Baked, in Tomato Sauce, Side, Kids Menu	51
BBQ, Spiced, Side	157

BEEF

Duo	1437
Slow Cooked, Kids, Sunday Lunch Menu	697
Slow Cooked, Sunday Lunch Menu	1351

BEEF - STEAK

& Frites	686
& Frites, Daytime Saver Menu	629
Fillet, 8oz, with Chips	813
Fillet, 8oz, with Chips & Salad	831
Fillet, 8oz, with Side Salad	461
Fillet, 8oz, with Veg Medley	505
Flat Iron, 6oz, with Chips	747
Flat Iron, 6oz, with Chips & Salad	765
Flat Iron, 6oz, with Side Salad	395
Flat Iron, 6oz, with Veg Medley	439
Porterhouse, 18oz, with Chips	1503
Porterhouse, 18oz, with Chips & Salad	1521
Porterhouse, 18oz, with Side Salad	1151
Porterhouse, 18oz, with Veg Medley	1197
Rib-eye, 10oz, with Chips	988
Rib-eye, 10oz, with Chips & Salad	993
Rib-eye, 10oz, with Side Salad	624
Rib-eye, 10oz, with Veg Medley	668
Ribs, & Prawn, Combo	1720
Rump, 10oz, with Chips	941
Rump, 10oz, Daytime Saver Menu	844
Rump, 10oz, with Chips & Salad	966
Rump, 10oz, Daytime Saver Menu	832
Rump, 10oz, with Veg Medley	651
Rump. 10oz, with Side Salad	595
Sirloin, 8oz, with Chips	802
Sirloin, 8oz, with Chips & Peas, Daytime Saver Menu	705
Sirloin, 8oz, with Chips & Salad	808
Sirloin, 8oz, Daytime Saver Menu	693
Sirloin, 8oz, with Salad	437
Sirloin, 8oz, with Veg Medley	482
with Chips, Kids Menu	461

BREAD

Brown, Buttered, Extra	257
Flatbread, Garlic, & Dips	912
Flatbread, Garlic, Strips	1013
Garlic	218
Garlic, Kids Menu	112
White, Buttered, Extra	254

BROWNIES

Chocolate	555
Chocolate, Daytime Saver Menu	555

BURGERS

Beef, Bacon & Cheese, Triple	1697
Beef, Kids Menu	587

BEEFEATER RESTAURANT

BURGERS

Steak, Daytime Saver Menu	863
Steak, Double, Daytime Saver Menu	1152
Steak, with Cheese & Bacon, Daytime Saver Menu	1080
Beef, Bacon & Cheese, Double	1530
Steak, with Cheese & Bacon	1187
Chicken, Tabasco, Crispy	1059
Steak, Smoky BBQ, Summer BBQ Specials	1463
Vegan, with BBQ Pulled Soya	938

BURGERS VEGETARIAN

Main	910

CAKE

Trio of Sponges, with Custard	695

CAULIFLOWER CHEESE

Sunday Lunch Menu	283

CHEESE

Halloumi, Battered, & Chips, Daytime Saver Menu	983

CHEESECAKE

Vanilla, Baked	675

CHICKEN

BBQ, with Half Rack Of Ribs	1025
BBQ, with Whole Rack Of Ribs	1432
Breast, Kids, Sunday Lunch Menu	453
Breast, Plain	693
Breast, Smoky Paprika, Grilled	729
Breast, Smoky Paprika, Grilled, Daytime Saver Menu	578
Escalope, Breast, Breaded	1309
Goujons, Buttermilk, Summer BBQ Specials	742
Half, Roasted, Sunday Lunch Menu	1486
Melt, BBQ Sauce, Grilled	858
Poppin, with Chips, & Beans, Kids Menu	400
Wings, with BBQ, Spicy, 3, Side	160
Wings, with BBQ, Crispy, 5	260
Wings, with BBQ, Crispy, 8	401
Wings, with Piri Piri, Crispy, 5	252
Wings, with Piri Piri, Crispy, 8	394
Wings, with Piri Piri, Spicy, 3, Side	153

CHIPS

Cheesy, & Gravy	726
Side, Kids Menu	187
Triple Cooked, Side	418
Triple Cooked, Spicy, Side	420

COD

Bites, Breaded, Kids Menu	517

CORN

Cob, Mini, Side	61
Cob, Mini, Side, Kids Menu	29

CRUMBLE

Apple, Toffee, Salted	596

DESSERT

Caramel Apple Betty, with Custard	496
Caramel Apple Betty, with Ice Cream	462
Caramel Apple Betty, with Pouring Cream	531

BEEFEATER RESTAURANT

	KCAL
DESSERT	
Caramel Apple Betty, with Whipped Cream	455
Chocolate Challenge, Mini, Kids Menu	342
Mississippi Mud Pie	991
DOUGHNUTS	
Mini, Kids Menu	249
FISH & CHIPS	
Beer Battered, Daytime Saver Menu	886
FRIES	
Skinny, Side	328
Skinny, Spicy, Side	329
FROZEN YOGHURT	
Strawberry	235
Strawberry, Kids Menu	197
FRUIT SALAD	
Mixed, Kids Menu	49
GAMMON	
Blackened, with Egg, Daytime Saver Menu	751
Blackened, with Pineapple, Daytime Saver Menu	729
Steak, Blackened, in Spicy Rub	1034
Steak, Chargrilled, with Egg & Pineapple	1026
Steak, with Egg, Daytime Saver Menu	746
Steak, with Pineapple, Daytime Saver Menu	723
HADDOCK - BEER BATTERED	
with Chips, Ultimate, Daytime Saver Menu	920
with Chips & Mushy Peas	958
with Chips & Peas	920
ICE CREAM	
Vanilla, with Caramel Sauce, Kids Menu	254
Vanilla, with Chocolate Sauce, Kids Menu	253
Vanilla, with Raspberry Sauce, Kids Menu	253
with Chocolate Sauce	279
with Chocolate Sauce, Sunday Lunch Menu	275
KEBAB	
Pork & Beef, Kofta, Grilled	444
LAMB	
Rump, Minted, Grilled	720
Rump, Sunday Lunch Menu	1270
LASAGNE - BEEF & PORK	
with Chips, Daytime Saver Menu	872
with Salad, Daytime Saver Menu	595
LASAGNE - SWEET POTATO & FETA	
with Chips	975
with Chips, Daytime Saver Menu	937
with Salad	697
with Salad, Daytime Saver Menu	659
LINGUINE	
Roast Vegetable, in Tomato Sauce	563
LINGUINE	
Roast Vegetable, In Tomato Sauce, with Chicken	718
Roast Vegetable, in Tomato Sauce, with Salmon	1010
MACARONI CHEESE	
Daytime Saver Menu	888

BEEFEATER RESTAURANT

	KCAL
MAKHANI	
Chicken, Daytime Saver Menu	998
MEATBALLS	
Arrabiata, Linguine	821
MIXED GRILL	
Rump Steak, Chicken Breast, Gammon, Sausage	1741
Flat Iron Steak, Chicken Breast, Gammon, Sausage	1498
Sirloin Steak, Chicken Breast, Gammon, Sausage	1583
MUSHROOMS	
Crispy, Flat Cap, in Breadcrumbs	489
NACHOS	
with Cheesy Yoghurt Dip, Kids Menu	235
ONION RINGS	
Beer Battered, Crispy, Side	221
PASTA	
Penne, in Tomato Sauce, Kids Menu	347
PATE	
Duck, with Ciabatta	430
PEAS	
Side, Kids Menu	47
PIE	
Banoffee	701
Beef, & Cheddar, with Mash & Gravy	1397
Chicken & Ham, Daytime Saver Menu	1114
PLATTER	
The Beefeater, Sharing	700
The Beefeater, with Ribs, Sharing	904
POTATO MASH	
Side, Kids Menu	131
POTATOES	
Crushed, Garlic, Side	344
Dauphinoise, Sunday Lunch Menu	320
Dippers, With Cheese, & Bacon, Loaded	587
Dippers, with Cheese, Loaded	492
Dippers, with Cheese, Sharing	1262
Dippers, with Cheese & Spring Onion, Loaded	517
Jacket, Side	438
PRAWN COCKTAIL	
Classic, with Ciabatta	340
PRAWNS	
Garlic, with Ciabatta	371
King, Garlic, 3, Side	151
PROFITEROLES	
Main Menu	465
Daytime Saver Menu	465
PUDDING	
Apple Crisp	299
RIBS - BBQ	
Sticky, Summer BBQ Specials	451
Half Rack, & Chips, & Coleslaw, Daytime Saver Menu	946
Sticky Bourbon, Grill	1320
RISOTTO	
Chicken, & Mushroom, Creamy	833

BEEFEATER RESTAURANT

RISOTTO

Chicken, & Mushroom, Daytime Saver Menu	831
Mushroom, Creamy	678
Mushroom, Daytime Saver Menu	676

SALAD

BLT, with Egg, Daytime Saver Menu	328
Caesar, Chicken, Goujons, Summer BBQ Specials	986
Caesar, Chicken, Grilled, Daytime Saver Menu	463
Caesar, Salmon, Blackened, Summer BBQ Specials	1076
Caesar, Summer BBQ Specials	421
Chicken, Jerk, Mango, Summer BBQ Specials	323
Chunky Slaw, Side	149
Greek, Crunchy, Side	173
Halloumi, Jerk, Mango, Summer BBQ Specials	421
Mixed, Large, Side	68
Mixed Bean	604
Salmon, Jerk, Mango, Summer BBQ Specials	621
Side, Kids Menu	6
Steak, with Pear	778

SALMON

Grilled	1014

SANDWICH

Chicken Goujons, Buttermilk, Daytime Saver Menu	1054
Steak, Open, with Fries, Daytime Saver Menu	986

SAUCE

Bearnaise, Steak Sauces	135
Beef, Rich, Steak Sauces	42
Cheddar, Pulled Ham, & Mushroom, Steak Sauces	98
Peppercorn, Triple, Steak Sauces	41
Prawn & Lobster, Steak Sauces	67

SAUSAGE & MASH

Bangers, Kids Menu	391
Portion	902
Quorn	729
Vegetarian, Bangers, Kids Menu	361

SEA BASS

Oven Baked, with Crunchy Greek Salad	451

SORBET

Lemon Curd	242

SOUP

Tomato	351

SPAGHETTI BOLOGNESE

Kids Menu	345

SPINACH

Creamy, Side	123

SUNDAE

Cookie Dough	694
Funny Face, Kids Menu	265

SUNDAE

Rocky Road	688

TRIFLE

Strawberry, Pimms, Summer BBQ Specials	699

BEEFEATER RESTAURANT

VEGETABLE MEDLEY

Side	112

VEGETABLES

Sticks, Side, Kids Menu	28
Sticks, with Yoghurt Dip	51

WAFFLES

Apple, Salted, Toffee, Summer BBQ Specials	881

WELLINGTON

Vegetable, Sunday Lunch Menu	1646

WRAP

Chicken Breast, Cheese, Vegetables, Kids Menu	540
Quorn Sausage, Cheese, Vegetables, Kids Menu	540
Salmon, Cheese, Vegetables, Kids Menu	605

YOGHURT

Strawberry, Kids Menu	127

BILL'S

ASPARAGUS
& Baby Spinach, Side	154

BEEF
Steak, Flat Iron	694
Steak, Minute, with Chips, & Egg, & Garlic Butter	968
Steak, no Chips, Kids	359
Steak, Ribeye, 14oz	650
Steak, Sirloin, 10oz	617
Steak, with Chips, Kids	534

BREAD
& Houmous, For 2	392
Basket, with Butters, Ã,Â½ Basket	730
Basket, without Butters, Whole Basket	956
Flatbread, Smoky, Italian, Ã,Â½ Bread	333
Focaccia, for Soup	130
Focaccia, with Houmous, & Olives	392
Garlic, & Herb, Flatbread, Ã,Â½ Bread	290
Sourdough, Rosemary, Pea Houmous, & Garlic	632
Sourdough, Rosemary & Garlic, Grilled, & Eggs	960
Stone Baked, with Balsamic, & Olive Oil, For 2	264
Tortilla, Corn, Spiced, with Guacamole	516
Tortilla, Corn, Spiced, without Guacamole	441

BREAKFAST
Kids	558

BREAKFAST - BAKED EGGS
with Spicy Beans, & Chorizo	444
with Spicy Beans, & Chorizo, & Flatbread	564

BREAKFAST - FULL ENGLISH
Brunch, with Toast	1317
with Toast	887
Veggie, with Toast	807

BREAKFAST - GARDEN
No Hollandaise	707
Plate, No Hollandaise	951

BREAKFAST - VEGAN
Full	626

BREAKFAST CEREAL
Porridge, Oat	600

BROCCOLI
Long Stem	179

BROWNIES
Chocolate, Warm, no Ice Cream	569
Chocolate, Warm, no Ice Cream, Kids	218
Chocolate, Warm, with Ice Cream	676
Chocolate, Warm, with Ice Cream, Kids	325

BUNS
Bacon, Breakfast	667
Sausage, Cumberland, Breakfast	563

BURGERS
Chicken, Buttermilk, no Chipotle Mayo	592
Chicken, Buttermilk, with Chipotle Mayo	822
Chicken, Fillet, Kids	365
Halloumi, with Lime Mayo	939

BILL'S

BURGERS
Halloumi	684
Hamburger	696
Hamburger, with Mayo, Kids	372
Lamb, no Tzatziki	804
Lamb, with Tzatziki	833
Naked, with Salad, & Tzatziki, no Bun	525

CAKE
Carrot, no Whipped Cream	198
Carrot, with Whipped Cream	312
Victoria Sponge	598

CAULIFLOWER CHEESE
for Two, Ã,Â½ Portion	119

CHEESE
Halloumi, Sticks, Crispy, no Lemon Garlic Mayo	578

CHEESECAKE
Banana, & Honeycomb	827

CHICKEN
Half, Paprika, Garlic, & Chilli, with Fries	1302
Milanese, with Salad	738
Paillard	596
Pan Fried, with Wild Mushrooms	705

CHICKEN - SKEWERS
Dakkochi	452
Mojo Marinated, with Dressed Salad	1057
Mojo Marinated, with Dressed Salad, & Flatbread	1154

CHOCOLATES
Truffles, Salted Caramel, 3 Truffles	168

COD - BEER BATTERED
with Pea Puree, Tartare Sauce, & Fries	1123

CRAB CAKES
Baked, with Tartare Sauce	567
Baked, without Tartare Sauce	417

CRAB CAKES
with Egg, & Asparagus	655

CREME BRULEE
Coconut, & Orange Rice	344

CRUMBLE
Apple, & Salted Caramel	613

CURRY
Chicken, Thai Green, with Rice	734
Chicken, Thai Green, without Rice	507

DESSERT
Chocolate Bombe, Meltin	937
Eton Mess, Mango, & Passion Fruit	477

DHAL - AUBERGINE
Lentil, & Chickpea, Roasted	543
Lentil, & Chickpea, Roasted, with Flatbread	695

DOUGHNUTS
Strawberry Dusted, Warm	711

DOUGHNUTS - CINNAMON
Mini, Warm, no Sauce	483
Mini, Warm, Salted Caramel & Chocolate Sauce	649

BILL'S

DUMPLINGS

Chicken, Sesame, with Chutney	336
Pork, Sesame, Golden Fried, with Dipping Sauce	451

EGGS

Benedict, with Hollandaise	468
Benedict, without Hollandaise	244
Florentine, with Hollandaise	680
Florentine, without Hollandaise	456
on Toast, Kids	337
Royale, with Hollandaise	534
Royale, without Hollandaise	310
Scrambled, on Toast	731
Scrambled, on Toast, with Bacon	745
Scrambled, on Toast, with Salmon	698

FISH FINGERS

Cod, Kids	271

FRIES

Potato, Kids	175
Potato	349
Sweet Potato	510

FRUIT

Strawberries, & Banana, no Sauce, Kids	93
Strawberries, & Banana, Chocolate Sauce, Kids	198

GNOCCHI

Diablo	928

ICE CREAM

Vanilla, Kids	107

KALE

Sauteed	104

MACARONI

Kids	429

MACARONI CHEESE

with Focaccia	1290
with Mushroom, & Leek	1167
with Side Salad, & Dressing	1269
with Side Salad, No Dressing	1172
without Sides	1160

MASH

Potato, Side	194

MAYONNAISE

Chipotle	216
Truffle, Side	347

MERINGUE

Eton Mess, Lemon	847

MEZZE

Halloumi, & Houmous, for 4	377
Sharing, for 4, ¼ Mezze	429
Veggie, Sharing, for 4, ¼ Mezze	343

MOUSSE

Chocolate, & Hazelnut, Kids	202

MUSHROOMS

Garlic, Sauteed, Chestnut	180

BILL'S

NUTS

Spiced, & Roasted Corn, For 2	303

OLIVES

Green, Giant, Gordal	161

OMELETTE

Summer	488

PANCAKES - BUTTERMILK

Kids	375
with Bacon, & Syrup, 3 Stack	803
with Bacon, & Syrup, 5 Stack	1271
with Banana, Berries, with Syrup, 3 Stack	542
with Banana, Berries, with Syrup, 5 Stack	845

PATE

Chicken Liver, Oak Smoked, Parfait, with Toast	809
Chicken Liver, Oak Smoked, Parfait, without Toast	528

PIE

Fish	794

PRAWN COCKTAIL

Portion	356

RIBS

BBQ, Kids	305
Main	791

RISOTTO

Crab, & Courgette	620

SALAD

Caesar, Chicken, without Dressing	627
Chicken, with Turmeric, & Freekeh	1292
Feta, Crispy, & Watermelon	425
Glow Bowl	1133
Halloumi, Grilled, & Pesto Toast, with Dressing	706
Halloumi, Grilled, with Dressing	548
Halloumi, Grilled, no Dressing	356
Halloumi, Grilled, & Pesto Toast, no Dressing	514
Kale, Chickpea, & Miso, Houmous	755
Mixed, no Dressing	24
Mixed, with Dressing	121
Rainbow, Side	137
Salmon, Seared	728
Summer	695
Summer, with Flatbread	815

SANDWICH

Bacon, Kids	512
Fish Finger	884
Sausage, Kids	482

SAUCE

Bearnaise, for Steak	158
Garlic Butter, for Steak	193
Hollandaise	224
Mushroom, for Steak	69
Peppercorn, for Steak	46

SAUSAGE

Cumberland, Kids	427
Cumberland, Mini, Glazed	294

BILL'S

SCONE

	KCAL
Cream Tea, No Clotted Cream	552
Cream Tea, with Clotted Cream	728
with Jam, & Clotted Cream, Warm	709
with Jam, Warm	562

SEA BASS

Pan Fried, with Rosti	523

SOUP

Pea, & Watercress, without Focaccia	161
Salad, & Half Sandwich	676
Tomato, Roasted, with Cream	209
Tomato, Roasted, with Cream & Pesto Toast	367
Tomato, Roasted, with Pesto Toast	250
Tomato, Roasted, without Cream & Pesto Toast	92

SQUID

Calamari, Crispy, with lemon Garlic Mayonnaise	624
Calamari, Crispy, without lemon Garlic Mayonnaise	369

SUNDAE

Granola, Breakfast	467
Banoffee, Melting	658
Ice Cream, Vanilla, Kids	292

TART

Ricotta, Red Pepper, & Cheddar, no Dressing	664
Ricotta, Red Pepper, & Cheddar, with Dressing	761

TEACAKES

Toasted, no Butter	267
Toasted, with Butter	527

TOAST

& Butter, Bloomer	356
with Avocado, & Bacon	687
with Avocado, & Poached Eggs	426
with Avocado, & Salmon	640
with Avocado	497
with Beans, Kids	219
with Butter, Kids	180

TOASTIE

Ham, & Cheese, Kids	478

TORTILLA CHIPS

Corn, Crispy, Kids	247
Spiced, For 2	258

WELLINGTON

Carrot, & Cashew Nut	715

YOGHURT

Strawberries, Banana, & Honey, Kids	108

BREWERS FAYRE

BACON

	KCAL
Back, Rasher, Breakfast	165

BEANS

Baked, Breakfast	91
Baked, in Tomato Sauce, Side, Kids Menu	51

BEEF

Steak, Rib-eye, with Hollandaise Sauce	1250
Steak, Rib-eye, with Peppercorn Sauce	1199
Steak, Rump, Grilled	874
Steak, Sirloin, Grilled	886
Steak & Eggs	1041
Yorkshire, Wrap, with Chips, & Gravy	1129

BHAJI

Sweet Potato	58

BITES

Hog Roast, with Apple Sauce	263
Mac 'N' Cheese	442

BREAD

Flatbread, Garlic	312
Flatbread, Garlic, with Cheese	379
Garlic, Kids Menu	110
Garlic, Side, Kids Menu	106
Garlic, with Cheese, Side	318

BROWNIES

Chocolate, with Ice Cream	755

BUBBLE & SQUEAK

Side	348

BURGERS

Chicken, Breaded, The South Western	925
Beef, Bash Street, Kids Menu	697
Beef, Black & Blue, with Chips	1328
Beef, Cheese, & Mushroom	988
Beef, Cheese, & Mushroom, Double	1308
Beef, Extra	327
Beef, Ultimate, with Chips	1741
Chicken, Extra	211
Cluck 'N' Ale, with Chips	1517
Cluck 'N' Ale, with Sweet Potato Fries	1564
Halloumi, Heaven, with Chips	1136
Halloumi Heaven, with Sweet Potato Fries	1069
The New Yorker	1139
Vegan, with Chips	899

BURRITO

Bowl, with Salad	555
Chicken, Bowl	710

CAKE

Chocolate, & Orange, Mousse, Mini	220
Chocolate, Fudge, Luxury	810

CAULIFLOWER CHEESE

Side	281

CHEESE

& Bacon, Extra	115
Brie, Breaded, Bites	326

BREWERS FAYRE

CHEESE

Halloumi, & Chips, with Mushy Peas	1035
Halloumi, & Chips, with Peas	997
Mozzarella, Sticks, Side	330

CHEESECAKE

Raspberry, & Prosecco	502
Vanilla, with Blackcurrant & Prosecco Compote	375

CHICKEN & RIBS COMBO

Full Rack Ribs, with Chips, Coleslaw, & Salad	1628
Half Rack Ribs, with Chips, Coleslaw, & Salad	1248

CHICKEN - BITES

Breaded, Kids Menu	525
Buffalo, Poppin	246

CHICKEN - BREAST

Garlic, Breaded	1326
Smoky Paprika, Grilled	430

CHICKEN - BUTTERMILK

& Cheesy Nachos	750

CHICKEN - COMBO

Combo	1344

CHICKEN - FORESTIERE

with Crushed Potatoes, & Green Beans	441

CHICKEN - GOUJONS

Combo Feast	1849
with Chicken Wings, Combo Feast	2269
Southern Fried	406

CHICKEN - HALF, ROASTED

Lemon & Thyme, with Chips	1600
with Chips	799
BBQ, with Chips	436

CHICKEN - SKEWERS

Honey & Mustard	212
Jerk	292

CHICKEN - SMOTHERED

BBQ Sauce,	914
BBQ Sauce, Double Up	1271
BBQ Sauce, with Mac 'N' Cheese	1213

CHICKEN - STUFFED, MOZZARELLA

with Bacon, & Chips	886
with Bacon, & Roast Potatoes	746

CHICKEN - WINGS

Buffalo	463

CHICKEN KATSU

Curry	1037

CHICKEN TIKKA

with Rice	851

CHILLI

Bean, Three, with Rice, & Tortilla Chips	537
Beef, Mexican, with Rice	716

CHIPS

Side	363
Smothered, Creamy Cheese Sauce, Side	551
Smothered, Curry Sauce, Side	467

BREWERS FAYRE

CHIPS

Smothered, Gravy, Side	436

COD

Bites, Breaded, Kids Menu	642
Loin, Baked, with Ratatouille, & Roast Potatoes	447

COLESLAW

Side	138
Side, Kids Menu	40

CORN

Cob, Mini, Side, Kids Menu	29

CRUMBLE

Apple, Toffee, Salted	670

DESSERT

Caramel Apple Betty	496
Chocolate, Mini, Mash Up, Kids Menu	344
Dirty Mud Pie	995
Fondue, Chocolate Fudge, Sharing	854

DIP

Dessicated Coconut	158

DOUGHNUTS

Cinnamon	547

EGGS

Breakfast	311

EMPANADAS

Cheese	401

FISH & CHIPS

with Mushy Peas	939
with Peas	901

FISH CAKES

Single	126

FRIES

Furious, Side	409
Tiger, Side	381

FROZEN YOGHURT

Strawberry	274

FRUIT SALAD

Kids Menu	49

GAMMON

Steak, With Egg, Grilled	903
Steak, with Egg & Pineapple, Grilled	833
Steak, with Pineapple, Grilled	764

GRILLS

Mixed, Mediterranean	1355
Mixed, Mediterranean, with Rice	1199
Ultimate, Summer	1781
Ultimate, Summer, with Prawns	1983

HADDOCK

Battered, with Chips & Mushy Peas, Atlantic, Giant	1093
Battered, with Chips & Peas, Atlantic, Giant	1055

HOT DOG

The Big Bad Dog, Kids Menu	612

ICE CREAM

Vanilla, with Caramel Sauce, Kids Menu	259

BREWERS FAYRE

ICE CREAM
Vanilla, with Chocolate Sauce, Kids Menu	256
Vanilla, with Raspberry Sauce, Kids Menu	256

LAMB
Shank, Slow Cooked, in Gravy	760

LASAGNE
Beef, & Pork	580
Beef, & Pork, with Side Salad	713
Sweet Potato & Feta, with Side Salad	744

MEATBALLS
Chicken, Tikka	261

MIXED GRILL - FLAT ITRON STEAK
Gammon, Chicken Breast, & Sausage	1412

MIXED GRILL - RUMP STEAK
Gammon, Chicken Breast, & Sausage, Ultimate	1485

MOUSSE
Lemon	730
Lemon, Mini	151

MUSHROOMS
Closed Cup, Breakfast, Brewers Fayre*	169
Garlic, & Herb, Breaded	303

NACHOS
with Cheesy Yoghurt Dip, Kids Menu	230

ONION RINGS
Battered, Side	467

PASTA
in Tomato Sauce, Kids Menu	344
Mac 'N' Cheese, Side	301
Mac 'N' Cheese, with Garlic Bread, & Salad	896
Penne, Tomato, & Roasted Vegetable, with Chicken	731

PATE
Chicken Liver, with Toast	388

PEAS
Side, Kids Menu	47

PEPPERS
Jalapeno, Cheesy, Poppers, Side	378

PIE
Apple, with Custard	316
Beef, & Stout, with Mash, Beans, & Gravy	1171
Chicken, & Chorizo, Creamy Sauce	516
Fish	747
Lemon Meringue, with Cream	606

PIZZA
Chocolate, Kids Menu	375

PLATTER
Chip Shop	1327

POPPADOMS
Single	32

POTATOES
Dippers, Crispy	483
Dippers, Loaded, Sharing	526
Dippers, Spicy Cheese Sauce, Loaded, Sharing	494

BREWERS FAYRE

PRAWN COCKTAIL
Starter	369

PRAWNS
Crispy, with Garlic Mayo	488
King, Tempura, with Sweet Chilli	475

PROFITEROLES
with Salted Caramel Sauce	422

PUDDING
Beef, & Doom Bar Ale	1300
Bread & Butter, Summer Berry	587
Jaffa, Sharing	1034
Sticky Toffee, with Custard	753
Sticky Toffee	719

QUICHE
Cheese, Three, Crustless	572

RIBS
Full Rack, BBQ	1297
Pork, Full Rack, in Whisky Glaze	1160

SALAD
Caesar, Chicken & Bacon	536
Chicken, & Bacon, Grilled	434
Chicken, Coronation	549
Cobb, Brewers	567
Mixed, Side	51
Ploughmans	480
Prawn, Sweet Chilli, Battered	718
Salmon	384

SALMON
Baked, with Hollandaise Sauce	727

SAMOSAS
Vegetable	191

SANDWICH
Chicken, Strip, Spicy, Brown Bread	688
Chicken, Strip, Spicy, White Bread	682
Fish, Goujons, Brown Bread	682
Fish, Goujons, White Bread	676
Ham, & Cheese, Brown Bread	630
Ham, & Cheese, White Bread	624
Prawn, Brown Bread	589
Prawn, White Bread	583

SAUCE
Blue Cheese	39
Hollandaise	81
Peppercorn	29
Tennessee Whisky Glaze, Jack Daniels	89

SAUSAGE
Egg, & Chips	1012
Pork, Battered	159
Premium, Breakfast	137
Vegetarian, Egg, & Chips	858

SAUSAGES & MASH
Bangers, Kids Menu	391
Vegetarian, Bangers, Kids Menu	364

	KCAL
BREWERS FAYRE	
SCAMPI	
Wholetail, Breaded, with Mushy Peas	868
Wholetail, Breaded, with Peas	830
SOUP	
Tomato	251
SPAGHETTI BOLOGNESE	
Beano-ese, Kids Menu	320
SUNDAE	
Choc-A-Block, Caramel, Cadbury	583
Choc-a-block, Cadbury	639
Funny Face, Kids Menu	268
Oreo	919
Salted Caramel, Brownie, & Popcorn	714
TOAST	
with Creamy Mushrooms	210
TOMATOES	
Grilled, Halved, Breakfast	28
TRIFLE	
Strawberry Pimms	634
VEGETABLES	
Green, Medley, Side	112
Sticks, & Cucumber Yoghurt Dip, Kids Menu	49
Sticks, Side, Kids Menu	28
WAFFLES	
Belgian, with Chocolate Honeycomb Ice Cream	497
Belgian, with Salted Caramel Ice Cream	468
WRAP	
Chicken, Build Your Own, Kids Menu	491
Salmon, Build Your Own, Kids Menu	495
Sausage, Quorn, Build Your Own, Kids Menu	491
YORKSHIRE PUDDING	
with Sausage & Mash, Giant	1329
with Sausage & Mash, Vegetarian, Ultimate	1093

	KCAL
BURGER KING	
BITES	
Cheese, Chilli, 4 Bites	180
Cheese, Chilli, 4	240
Cheese, Chilli, 6	370
BROWNIES	
Chocolate, Hottie, with Real Ice Cream	450
BURGERS	
Bacon, Double Cheese, XL	930
Bacon King	1040
Bacon King, JR	590
Big King, Long	620
Big King, XL	1010
Cheeseburger	300
Cheeseburger, Double	440
Cheeseburger, Kids	300
Cheeseburger. Bacon, Double	470
Chicken	390
Chicken, Kids	330
Chicken, Royale, Bacon, & Cheese	720
Chicken Royale	440
Crispy Chicken	500
Crispy Chicken, Texas BBQ	830
Crispy Chicken Bacon King	700
Halloumi	490
Halloumi, Double	680
Halloumi, Double, No Mayo	620
Halloumi, No Mayo	420
Hamburger	260
Hamburger, Kids	250
King Fish	430
Steakhouse	803
Texas BBQ, Long	540
Veggie, Kids	330
Whopper	540
Whopper, Double	870
Whopper, JR	320
BURGERS VEGETARIAN	
Veggie Bean	660
CHEESE	
Mozzarella, Sticks,3	210
Mozzarella, Sticks, 5	340
CHICKEN	
Fries	190
Nuggets, 4	190
Nuggets, 6	290
Nuggets, 9	440
Strips, Crispy	190
FRIES	
Large	400
Reg	280
Apple	30
Small	220
Super	470

BURGER KING

HASH BROWNS
	KCAL
Single	280

ICE CREAM
Oreo, Fusions	260
Cone	120

MILK SHAKE
Chocolate	430
Oreo	570
Strawberry	430
Vanilla	370

ONION RINGS
Large, 12	530
Reg, 5	230
Super, 16	710

SALAD
Chicken, Crispy	210
Garden, Side	15

SANDWICH
Bacon, Butty	240

SUNDAE
Caramel	90
Chocolate	240
Strawberry	220

CAFFE NERO

BARS
	KCAL
Apple, & Blackcurrant, Crumble	237
Oat, with Fruit Seeds & Honey	259

BISCUITS
Stem Ginger	264

BREAD
Ciabatta, Roll	180

BREAKFAST - SCRAMBLED EGG POT
with Portobello Mushroom, & Spinach	168
with Sausage, & Bacon	224

BREAKFAST CEREAL
Porridge, with Semi Skimmed Milk, no Topping	234
Porridge, with Skimmed Milk, no Topping	210
Porridge, with Soya Milk, no Topping	232

BROWNIES
Chocolate, Belgian	250
Chocolate, Belgian	241
Chocolate, Caramel & Sea Salt	257
Chocolate, GF	278

CAKE
Apricot, & Ginger, Crumble	330
Banana & Walnut Loaf	227
Banana & Walnut Loaf, Wheat Free	345
Cappuccino	553
Carrot	516
Chocolate Fudge	420
Lemon Drizzle, Organic	372
Lemon Meringue, Sicilian	498
Panettone, Classic, Mini	374
Raspberry & Amaretti, Crumble	338

CHEESECAKE
Lemon, Sicilian	343
Salted Caramel	304

CHOCOLATE
Coins	109
Dark, Venezuelan Gold, Willies Cacao, Bar	139
Milk, of the Gods, Willies Cacao, Bar	146

COFFEE - AMERICANO
Grande	23
Reg	15

COFFEE - CAPPUCCINO
Coconut Milk, Grande	88
Oat Milk, Grande	106
Semi Skimmed, Grande	107
Skimmed Milk, Grande	83
Soya Milk, Grande	97
Iced	24
Coconut Milk, Reg	50
Semi Skimmed, Reg	65
Skimmed Milk, Reg	52
Soya Milk, Reg	59
Oat Milk, Reg	64

CAFFE NERO

COFFEE - CORTADO
	KCAL
Standard	49

COFFEE - ESPRESSO
Standard	7
Con Panna	56
Tonic, Ultimate	95

COFFEE - LATTE
Coconut Milk, Grande	97
Oat Milk, Grande	134
Semi Skimmed Milk, Grande	135
Skimmed Milk, Grande	103
Soya Milk, Grande	122
Iced, Coconut	142
Iced, Semi Skimmed	155
Coconut Milk, Reg	59
Oat Milk, Reg	78
Semi Skimmed Milk, Reg	78
Skimmed Milk, Reg	62
Soya Milk, Reg	71

COFFEE - LATTE, CARAMEL
Caramelatte, Coconut Milk	380
Caramelatte, Oat Milk	417
Caramelatte, Skimmed Milk	388
Caramelatte, Soya Milk	406

COFFEE - MACCHIATTO
Standard	9

COFFEE - MOCHA
Coconut Milk, Grande	171
Oat Milk, Grande	188
Semi Skimmed Milk, Grande	363
Skimmed Milk, Grande	339
Soya Milk, Grande	179
Coconut Milk, Reg	117
Oat Milk, Reg	131
Semi Skimmed Milk, with Whipped Cream, Reg	305
Skimmed Milk, no Cream, Reg	292
Soya Milk, no Cream, Reg	126
White Chocolate, Coconut Milk	368
White Chocolate, Oat Milk	405
White Chocolate, Semi Skimmed Milk	397
White Chocolate, Skimmed milk	365
White Chocolate, Soya Milk	384

COFFEE BEANS
Chocolate Coated	133

CONSERVE
Raspberry	71
Strawberry	72

COOKIES
Caramel. Chocolate	330
Chocolate Chunk, Milk	314
Oat & Raisin	301

CREAM
Clotted	234

CAFFE NERO

CREAM
	KCAL
Whipped, for Coffee	171

CRISPS
Mature Cheddar, & Red Onion, Kettle	202
Sea Salt	205
Sea Salt & Balsamic Vinegar	201

CROISSANT
Almond	343
Apricot	260
Butter	215
Cheese Twist	333
Chocolate Twist	278
Ham & Cheddar Cheese	336
Pain au Raisin	320

DANISH PASTRY
Maple Pecan	382

DESSERT
Brownie, Chocolate, & Orange, Dolce	149
Lemon Posset, Dolce	152
Salted Caramel & Hazelnut, Dolce	137
Tiramisu, Dolce	122
White Chocolate, & Raspberry, Dolce	115

DRIED FRUIT & NUTS
Pack	236

FLATBREAD
Chicken Caesar	372
Spiced Veg, & Mango Chutney	271

FRUIT
& Seeds, Topping, for Porridge	115
Mango, & Lime	78
Topping, for Porridge	80

FRUIT SALAD
Fresh	103

GINGERBREAD
Man, Ginger Giovanni, Iced	289
Man, Gino, Christmas Special	289

HONEY
Topping, for Porridge	97

HOT CHOCOLATE
Grande, No Cream, Coconut Milk	295
Grande, No Cream, Oat Milk	340
Grande, No Cream, Semi Skimmed Milk	524
Grande, No Cream, Skimmed Milk	484
Grande, No Cream, Soya Milk	325
Milano, with Whipped Cream	458
Reg, No Cream, Coconut Milk	187
Reg, No Cream, Oat Milk	215
No Cream, Semi Skimmed Milk, Reg	398
No Cream, Skimmed Milk, Reg	374
No Cream, Soya Milk, Reg	250

JUICE
Mango & Passionfruit, Booster	196
Strawberry & Raspberry, Booster	220

CAFFE NERO

LEMONADE
	KCAL
Garden Mint	96
Raspberry	88

MARSHMALLOWS
for Hot Chocolate	20

MILK SHAKE - FRAPPE
Chocolate	215
Coffee & Caramel, Creme	503
Latte, Semi Skimmed Milk	229
Mocha Latte, Semi Skimmed Milk	265
Raspberry & White Chocolate, Creme	479
Salted Caramel & Pistachio, Creme	480
Strawberry	245
Strawberry	235
Triple Belgian Chocolate, Creme	435
Frappe, Vanilla	240
Vanilla	230

MUFFIN
Blueberry	376
Chocolate Orange, Filled	448
Cranberry & Orange, Reduced Fat	387
Lemon, with Lemon Curd Filling	398

PAIN AU CHOCOLAT
Pastry	282

PANINI
Brie, & Smoked Bacon	470
Chicken, Pesto Genovese	400
Goats Cheese, & Beetroot	414
Ham, & Mozzarella	394
Ham, & Mature Cheddar, Tostati	213
Meatball, & Mozzarella, Napoletana	583
Mozzarella, & Tomato, with Pesto	487
Mozzarella, Cheddar, & Tomato, Tostati	418
Mushroom, & Mascarpone, Tostati	395
Tuna Melt	504

PASTA SALAD
Chicken, & Bacon, Caesar	408

PIZZA
Margherita, Stonebaked, Pizzetta	419
Salami & Mozzarella, Stonebaked, Pizzetta	439

POPCORN
Sea Salt, Propercorn	87
Sea Salt & Sweet Brown Sugar, Propercorn	114

RICE CAKES
Chocolate	81

SALAD
Beetroot, Carrot, & Mixed Grain	239
Chargrilled Veg, & Mixed Grain, Pot	124
Chargrilled Vegetable, & Supergreen	120
Chicken, Butternut Squash, & Lentil, Pot	142
Chicken, Roasted Root Veg & Grain	432
Tricolore Cherry Tomato, Cucumber, & Radish	85

CAFFE NERO

SANDWICH
	KCAL
Bacon, Coffee Cured, Ciabatta, Roll	354
BLT	411
Chicken, with Rosemary Mayonnaise	309
Chicken Salad, Chargrilled	376
Cotto Ham, Salami, & Mortadella	508
Egg Mayonnaise, Free Range	433
Salmon, Smoked, & Soft Cheese	294
Sausage, Ciabatta Roll	475
Sausage, Egg, & Bacon, Ciabatta Roll	365
Tuna, Red Pepper, & Rocket	461
Vegan, Club	405
Vegan, Deli	382

SAUSAGE ROLL
Pork, & Pancetta	467

SCONE
Fruit, Sultana	287

SHORTBREAD
All Butter, Animal Bites	21
Caramel, with Belgian Chocolate	377
Bars, Crunchy, All Butter	264

SOUP
Tomato, & Mascarpone	163

SYRUP
Vanilla	97

TARTLETS
Bacon, Roasted Tomato, & Mozzarella	360
Roasted Butternut, & Red Onion	297

TEA
Black, & Peach	84
Chai Latte, Coconut Milk	188
Chai Latte, Oat Milk	230
Chai Latte, Semi Skimmed Milk	232
Chai Latte, Skimmed Milk	195
Chai Latte, Soya Milk	216
Green, & Mango	76

TEACAKES
Rich Fruit, Toasted, with Butter	286

TOASTIE
Chicken, & Bacon, Melt	412
Cotto Ham, & Cheese, Melt	434
Italian Five Cheese, Melt	450
Sundried Tomato, & Pesto	313

VEGETABLES
Crudites, & Red Pepper Houmous	129

WAFFLES
Caramel	332

YOGHURT
Berry & Granola	211
Coconut, Mango, & Passionfruit, Granola Pot	219

COSTA

BARS
Granola, Square, Traybake	329
Raspberry, & Coconut, GF	287

BISCUITS
Biscotti, Almond	155
Fruit, & Oat	228
Ginger, Stem	234
Gingerbread	176

BITES
Mallow, Millionaire	84

BREAD
Baguette, Half, SOTF	188

BREAKFAST
Bacon, Smoked, Sourdough, Roll	389
Bircher, Berry	259
Croissant, Ham, & Emmenthal	358
Granola, & Coconut, Sprinkle	85
Muffin, Scrambled Egg, & Mushroom	298
Oats, Instant, Porridge Pot	294
Porridge, Wholegrain, GF	231
Sausage, Pork, Sourdough, Roll	488
Veggie, Egg, Pot	198

BROWNIES
Chocolate, GF	309

BUNS
Brioche, Cinnamon	332
Chocolate, & Caramel, Sticky	396

CAKE
Banana, & Pecan, Loaf	325
Caramel, Crisp, Traybake	410
Carrot, Layered	576
Chocolate, Seriously	572
Chocolate, Tiffin	402
Coffee, Walnut, & Pecan	591
Iced Slice, Vegan, GF	320
Lemon, Drizzle, Loaf	365
Lemon, Drizzle, Slices, Wrapped	350
Raspberry, & Almond, Traybake	465
Raspberry & Blackcurrant Ripple	512

CHEESECAKE
New York, SOTF	564
Vanilla, Baked, Individual	384

CHOCOLATE
Coins	380
Dark, Bar	178
Flake	44
Milk, Bar	176
Truffle, Lindt	85

COFFEE - AMERICANO
Iced, Medio	57
Iced, Primo	40
No Milk, Massimo	10
No Milk, Medio	8

COSTA

COFFEE - AMERICANO
No Milk, Primo	6

COFFEE - BABYCHINO
Almond Milk	22
Coconut Milk	30
Semi Skimmed Milk	41
Semi Skimmed Milk, Lactofree	35
Skimmed Milk	29
Soya Milk	38
Whole Milk	59

COFFEE - BLACK
Cold Brew	1
Flat	4

COFFEE - CAPPUCCINO
Almond Milk, Massimo	90
Almond Milk, Massimo, Takeaway	94
Almond Milk, Medio	72
Almond Milk, Medio, Takeaway	72
Almond Milk, Primo	49
Almond Milk, Primo, Takeaway	56
Coconut Milk, Massimo	115
Coconut Milk, Massimo, Takeaway	122
Coconut Milk, Medio	92
Coconut Milk, Medio, Takeaway	92
Coconut Milk, Primo	62
Coconut Milk, Primo, Takeaway	71
Semi Skimmed Milk, Massimo	153
Semi Skimmed Milk, Massimo, Takeaway	162
Semi Skimmed Milk, Medio	122
Semi Skimmed Milk, Medio, Takeaway	122
Semi Skimmed Milk, Primo	81
Semi Skimmed Milk, Primo, Takeaway	94
Shaken, Almond Milk, Iced, Medio	65
Shaken, Almond Milk, Iced, Primo	48
Shaken, Coconut Milk, Iced, Medio	73
Shaken, Coconut Milk, Iced, Primo	56
Shaken, Semi Skimmed Milk, Iced, Medio	85
Shaken, Semi Skimmed Milk, Iced, Primo	69
Shaken, Skimmed Milk, Iced, Medio	72
Shaken, Skimmed Milk, Iced, Primo	55
Shaken, Soya Milk, Iced, Medio	82
Shaken, Soya Milk, Iced, Primo	65
Shaken, Whole Milk, Iced, Medio	104
Shaken, Whole Milk, Iced, Primo	88
Skimmed Milk, Massimo	111
Skimmed Milk, Massimo, Takeaway	120
Skimmed Milk, Medio	90
Skimmed Milk, Medio, Takeaway	90
Skimmed Milk, Primo	60
Skimmed Milk, Primo, Takeaway	70
Soya Milk, Massimo	139
Soya Milk, Massimo, Takeaway	150
Soya Milk, Medio	112

COSTA

COFFEE - CAPPUCCINO

	KCAL
Soya Milk, Medio, Takeaway	112
Soya Milk, Primo	74
Soya Milk, Primo, Takeaway	87
Whipped Milk, Almond Milk, Iced, Medio	98
Whipped Milk, Almond Milk, Iced, Primo	62
Whipped Milk, Coconut Milk, Iced, Medio	104
Whipped Milk, Coconut Milk, Iced, Primo	66
Whipped Milk, Semi Skimmed Milk, Iced, Medio	113
Whipped Milk, Semi Skimmed Milk, Iced, Primo	73
Whipped Milk, Skimmed Milk, Iced, Medio	103
Whipped Milk, Skimmed Milk, Iced, Primo	66
Ā,Â Whipped Milk, Soya Milk, Iced, Medio	110
Whipped Milk, Soya Milk, Iced, Primo	71
Whipped Milk, Whole Milk, Iced, Medio	127
Whipped Milk, Whole Milk, Iced, Primo	83
Whole Milk, Massimo	209
Whole Milk, Massimo, Takeaway	223
Whole Milk, Medio	168
Whole Milk, Medio, Takeaway	168
Whole Milk, Primo	109
Whole Milk, Primo, Takeaway	129

COFFEE - CAPPUCCINO, LACTOFREE

	KCAL
Semi Skimmed Milk, Massimo	133
Semi Skimmed Milk, Massimo, Takeaway	140
Semi Skimmed Milk, Medio	106
Semi Skimmed Milk, Medio, Takeaway	106
Semi Skimmed Milk, Primo	71
Semi Skimmed Milk, Primo, Takeaway	82
Shaken, Semi Skimmed Milk, Iced, Medio	79
Shaken, Semi Skimmed Milk, Iced, Primo	62
Whipped Milk, Semi Skimmed Milk, Iced, Medio	108
Whipped Milk, Semi Skimmed Milk, Iced, Primo	69

COFFEE - COLD BREW

	KCAL
Bonfire Spiced, Medio	88
Bonfire Spiced, Medio, Takeaway	88
Bonfire Spiced, Primo	63
Bonfire Spiced, Primo, Takeaway	63
with Whipped Milk, Semi Skimmed Milk, Medio	19
with Whipped Milk, Semi Skimmed Milk, Primo	16

COFFEE - CORTADO

	KCAL
Almond Milk, Solo	32
Almond Milk, Solo, Iced	39
Almond Milk, Solo, Takeaway	40
Coconut Milk, Solo, Iced	47
Semi Skimmed Milk, Lactofree, Solo	51
Semi Skimmed Milk, Lactofree, Solo, Iced	52
Semi Skimmed Milk, Lactofree, Solo, Takeaway	64
Semi Skimmed Milk, Solo	60
Semi Skimmed Milk, Solo, Iced	58
Semi Skimmed Milk, Solo, Takeaway	76
Skimmed Milk, Solo	42
Skimmed Milk, Solo, Iced	46

COSTA

COFFEE - CORTADO

	KCAL
Skimmed Milk, Solo, Takeaway	53
Soya Milk, Solo	55
Soya Milk, Solo, Iced	56
Soya Milk, Solo, Takeaway	69
Whole Milk, Solo	85
Whole Milk, Solo, Iced	75
Whole Milk, Solo, Takeaway	108

COFFEE - CORTADO, CARAMEL

	KCAL
Almond Milk	64
Almond Milk, Takeaway	72
Coconut Milk, Takeaway	85
Semi Skimmed Milk	89
Semi Skimmed Milk, Lactofree	81
Semi Skimmed Milk, Lactofree, Takeaway	94
Semi Skimmed Milk, Takeaway	104
Skimmed Milk	73
Skimmed Milk, Takeaway	84
Soya Milk	84
Soya Milk, Takeaway	98
Whole Milk	111
Whole Milk, Takeaway	132

COFFEE - ESPRESSO

	KCAL
Character Roast, Colombian	3
con Pana, Doppio	139
con Pana, Solo	136
Decaff, Solo	3
Doppio, Iced	39
Ristretto, Doppio	8
Ristretto, Doppio, Iced	38
Ristretto, Solo	2
Ristretto, Solo, Iced	19
Shot	3
Solo, Iced	20

COFFEE - ESPRESSO, MACCHIATO

	KCAL
Skimmed Milk, Doppio, Iced	40
Skimmed Milk, Solo, Iced	20
Whole Milk, Doppio, Iced	41
Whole Milk, Solo, Iced	21

COFFEE - ESPRESSO, MACCHIATTO

	KCAL
Almond Milk, Doppio, Iced	40
Almond Milk, Solo, Iced	20
Coconut Milk, Doppio, Iced	40
Coconut Milk, Solo, Iced	20
Semi Skimmed Milk, Doppio, Iced	41
Semi Skimmed Milk, Lactofree, Doppio, Iced	40
Semi Skimmed Milk, Lactofree, Solo, Iced	21
Semi Skimmed Milk, Solo, Iced	21
Soya Milk, Doppio, Iced	40
Soya Milk, Solo, Iced	20

COFFEE - FILTER

	KCAL
Massimo	6
Medio	4

KCAL

COSTA
COFFEE - FILTER
Primo	3

COFFEE - FLAT WHITE
Almond Milk, Primo	57
Almond Milk, Iced	57
Almond Milk, Primo, Takeaway	67
Coconut Milk, Primo	78
Coconut Milk, Iced	68
Coconut Milk, Primo, Takeaway	91
Semi Skimmed Milk, Primo	107
Semi Skimmed Milk, Iced	81
Semi Skimmed Milk, Lactofree, Primo	92
Semi Skimmed Milk, Lactofree, Iced	75
Semi Skimmed Milk, Lactofree, Primo, Takeaway	107
Semi Skimmed Milk, Primo, Takeaway	126
Skimmed Milk, Primo	75
Skimmed Milk, Iced	67
Skimmed Milk, Primo, Takeaway	89
Soya Milk, Primo	98
Soya Milk, Iced	79
Soya Milk, Primo, Takeaway	116
Whole Milk, Primo	152
Whole Milk, Iced	107
Whole Milk, Primo, Takeaway	178

COFFEE - LATTE
Latte, Almond Milk, Iced, Medio	95
Latte, Almond Milk, Iced, Primo	65
Almond Milk, Massimo	102
Almond Milk, Massimo, Takeaway	108
Almond Milk, Medio	79
Almond Milk, Medio, Takeaway	79
Almond Milk, Primo	50
Almond Milk, Primo, Takeaway	58
Coconut Milk, Massimo	137
Coconut Milk, Massimo, Takeaway	145
Coconut Milk, Medio	106
Coconut Milk, Medio, Iced	116
Coconut Milk, Medio, Takeaway	106
Coconut Milk, Primo	68
Coconut Milk, Primo, Iced	81
Coconut Milk, Primo, Takeaway	77
Semi Skimmed Milk, Iced, Medio	146
Semi Skimmed Milk, Iced, Primo	103
Semi Skimmed Milk, Lactofree, Iced, Medio	129
Semi Skimmed Milk, Lactofree, Iced, Primo	91
Semi Skimmed Milk, Lactofree, Massimo	161
Semi Skimmed Milk, Lactofree, Massimo, Takeaway	170
Semi Skimmed Milk, Lactofree, Medio	125
Semi Skimmed Milk, Lactofree, Medio, Takeaway	125
Semi Skimmed Milk, Lactofree, Primo	79
Semi Skimmed Milk, Lactofree, Primo, Takeaway	90
Semi Skimmed Milk, Massimo	188
Semi Skimmed Milk, Massimo, Takeaway	199

COSTA
COFFEE - LATTE
Semi Skimmed Milk, Medio	146
Semi Skimmed Milk, Medio, Takeaway	146
Semi Skimmed Milk, Primo	93
Semi Skimmed Milk, Primo, Takeaway	105
Skimmed Milk, Massimo	132
Skimmed Milk, Massimo, Iced	179
Skimmed Milk, Massimo, Takeaway	139
Skimmed Milk, Medio	102
Skimmed Milk, Medio, Iced	113
Skimmed Milk, Medio, Takeaway	102
Skimmed Milk, Primo	66
Skimmed Milk, Primo, Iced	79
Skimmed Milk, Primo, Takeaway	75
Soya Milk, Massimo	175
Soya Milk, Massimo, Iced	200
Soya Milk, Massimo, Takeaway	184
Soya Milk, Medio	135
Soya Milk, Medio, Iced	136
Soya Milk, Medio, Takeaway	135
Soya Milk, Primo	86
Soya Milk, Primo, Iced	96
Soya Milk, Primo, Takeaway	97
Whole Milk, Massimo	269
Whole Milk, Massimo, Takeaway	283
Whole Milk, Medio	207
Whole Milk, Medio, Iced	192
Whole Milk, Medio, Takeaway	207
Whole Milk, Primo	133
Whole Milk, Primo, Iced	138
Whole Milk, Primo, Takeaway	149

COFFEE - LATTE, BONFIRE SPICED
Almond Milk, Medio	160
Almond Milk, Primo	110
Coconut Milk, Medio	186
Coconut Milk, Primo	127
Semi Skimmed Milk, Lactofree, Medio	198
Semi Skimmed Milk, Lactofree, Primo	137
Semi Skimmed Milk, Medio	221
Semi Skimmed Milk, Primo	152
Skimmed Milk, Medio	182
Skimmed Milk, Primo	126
Soya Milk, Medio	210
Soya Milk, Primo	144
Whole Milk, Medio	277
Whole Milk, Primo	190

COFFEE - LATTE, GINGERBREAD
Almond Milk, Medio	207
Almond Milk, Medio, Takeaway	235
Almond Milk, Primo	187
Almond Milk, Primo, Takeaway	213
Coconut Milk, Medio	230
Coconut Milk, Medio, Takeaway	267

COSTA

COFFEE - LATTE, GINGERBREAD

Coconut Milk, Primo	203
Coconut Milk, Primo, Takeaway	238
Semi Skimmed Milk, Lactofree, Medio	242
Semi Skimmed Milk, Lactofree, Medio, Takeaway	285
Semi Skimmed Milk, Lactofree, Primo	212
Semi Skimmed Milk, Lactofree, Primo, Takeaway	251
Semi Skimmed Milk, Medio	262
Semi Skimmed Milk, Medio, Takeaway	315
Semi Skimmed Milk, Primo	226
Semi Skimmed Milk, Primo, Takeaway	273
Skimmed Milk, Medio	227
Skimmed Milk, Medio, Takeaway	264
Skimmed Milk, Primo	201
Skimmed Milk, Primo, Takeaway	235
Soya Milk, Medio	252
Gingerbread, Soya Milk, Medio, Takeaway	300
Soya Milk, Primo	219
Soya Milk, Primo, Takeaway	262
Whole Milk, Medio	312
Whole Milk, Medio, Takeaway	387
Whole Milk, Primo	262
Whole Milk, Primo, Takeaway	329

COFFEE - LATTE, HAZELNUT PRALINE

Almond Milk, Massimo	315
Almond Milk, Massimo, Takeaway	359
Almond Milk, Medio	284
Almond Milk, Medio, Takeaway	311
Almond Milk, Primo	250
Almond Milk, Primo, Takeaway	276
Coconut Milk, Medio	306
Coconut Milk, Medio, Takeaway	344
Coconut Milk, Primo	266
Coconut Milk, Primo, Takeaway	301
Semi Skimmed Milk, Lactofree, Medio	319
Semi Skimmed Milk, Lactofree, Medio, Takeaway	362
Semi Skimmed Milk, Lactofree, Primo	275
Semi Skimmed Milk, Lactofree, Primo, Takeaway	314
Semi Skimmed Milk, Medio	339
Semi Skimmed Milk, Medio, Takeaway	391
Semi Skimmed Milk, Primo	289
Semi Skimmed Milk, Primo, Takeaway	337
Skimmed Milk, Medio	304
Skimmed Milk, Medio, Takeaway	340
Skimmed Milk, Primo	264
Skimmed Milk, Primo, Takeaway	298
Soya Milk, Medio	329
Soya Milk, Medio, Takeaway	377
Soya Milk, Primo	282
Soya Milk, Primo, Takeaway	326
Whole Milk, Medio	389
Whole Milk, Medio, Takeaway	464
Whole Milk, Primo	325

COSTA

COFFEE - LATTE, HAZELNUT PRALINE

Whole Milk, Primo, Takeaway	392

COFFEE - MACCHIATTO

Almond Milk, Solo	8
Coconut Milk, Solo	9
Semi Skimmed Milk, Lactofree, Solo	10
Semi Skimmed Milk, Solo	11
Skimmed Milk, Solo	9
Soya Milk, Solo	10
Whole Milk, Solo	13

COFFEE - MOCHA

Almond Milk, Massimo	194
Almond Milk, Massimo, Takeaway	208
Almond Milk, Medio	155
Almond Milk, Medio, Iced	134
Almond Milk, Medio, Takeaway	160
Almond Milk, Primo	87
Almond Milk, Primo, Iced	94
Almond Milk, Primo, Takeaway	102
Coconut Milk, Massimo	219
Coconut Milk, Massimo, Takeaway	234
Coconut Milk, Medio	174
Coconut Milk, Medio, Iced	149
Coconut Milk, Medio, Takeaway	180
Coconut Milk, Primo	99
Coconut Milk, Primo, Iced	105
Mocha, Coconut Milk, Primo, Takeaway	116
Semi Skimmed Milk, Lactofree, Massimo	236
Semi Skimmed Milk, Lactofree, Massimo, Takeaway	248
Semi Skimmed Milk, Lactofree, Medio	184
Semi Skimmed Milk, Lactofree, Medio, Iced	159
Semi Skimmed Milk, Lactofree, Medio, Takeaway	190
Semi Skimmed Milk, Lactofree, Primo	105
Semi Skimmed Milk, Lactofree, Primo, Iced	113
Semi Skimmed Milk, Lactofree, Primo, Takeaway	123
Semi Skimmed Milk, Massimo	257
Semi Skimmed Milk, Massimo, Takeaway	270
Semi Skimmed Milk, Medio	200
Semi Skimmed Milk, Medio, Iced	171
Semi Skimmed Milk, Medio, Takeaway	209
Semi Skimmed Milk, Primo	115
Semi Skimmed Milk, Primo, Iced	121
Semi Skimmed Milk, Primo, Takeaway	137
Skimmed Milk, Massimo	219
Skimmed Milk, Massimo, Takeaway	230
Skimmed Milk, Medio	171
Skimmed Milk, Medio, Iced	148
Skimmed Milk, Medio, Takeaway	177
Skimmed Milk, Primo	97
Skimmed Milk, Primo, Iced	104
Skimmed Milk, Primo, Takeaway	114
Soya Milk, Massimo	245
Soya Milk, Massimo, Takeaway	261

COSTA

COFFEE - MOCHA

Soya Milk, Medio	193
Soya Milk, Medio, Iced	164
Soya Milk, Medio, Takeaway	199
Soya Milk, Primo	109
Soya Milk, Primo, Iced	116
Soya Milk, Primo, Takeaway	130
Whole Milk, Massimo	312
Whole Milk, Massimo, Takeaway	332
Whole Milk, Medio	244
Whole Milk, Iced, Primo	204
Whole Milk, Medio, Takeaway	252
Whole Milk, Primo	141
Whole Milk, Primo, Iced	146
Whole Milk, Primo, Takeaway	167

COFFEE - MOCHA CORTADO

Almond Milk	50
Almond Milk, Solo, Iced	73
Almond Milk, Takeaway	81
Coconut Milk	57
Coconut Milk, Solo, Iced	79
Coconut Milk, Takeaway	93
Skimmed Milk	56
Semi Skimmed Milk, Lactofree	61
Semi Skimmed Milk, Lactofree, Solo, Iced	83
Semi Skimmed Milk, Lactofree, Takeaway	99
Semi Skimmed Milk, Solo, Iced	65
Skimmed Milk, Takeaway	91
Skimmed Milk	67
Skimmed Milk, Solo, Iced	55
Skimmed Milk, Takeaway	109
Soya Milk, New Recipe	64
Soya Milk, Solo, Iced	85
Soya Milk, Takeaway	104
Whole Milk	83
Whole Milk, Solo, Iced	80
Whole MilkTakeaway	135

COOKIES

Chocolate, Caramel, & Hazelnut	333
Chocolate Chunk, Bake Off, SOTF	306
Chocolate Chunk	306
Toffee, & Pecan, Vegan	334

CREAM

Whipping, Extras	133

CROISSANT

Almond	321
Almond, SOTF	374
Butter	213
Butter, SOTF	267
Chocolate, & Hazelnut, SOTF	372
Cup, with Nutella	305

CUPCAKES

Banoffee	431

COSTA

CURRY

Thai, Red, Pot	275

DOUGHNUTS

Chocolatey, SOTF	309
Pineapple, & Coconut, SOTF	359

DRIED FRUIT

Mango	96

FLAPJACK

Fruity, Vegan, GF	251

FROSTINO - BELGIAN CHOCOLATE

Almond Milk, Medio	348
Almond Milk, Medio, Takeaway	348
Almond Milk, Primo	292
Almond Milk, Primo, Takeaway	292
Coconut Milk, Medio	363
Coconut Milk, Medio, Takeaway	363
Coconut Milk, Primo	303
Coconut Milk, Primo, Takeaway	303
Semi Skimmed Milk, Lactofree, Medio	374
Semi Skimmed Milk, Lactofree, Medio, Takeaway	374
Semi Skimmed Milk, Lactofree, Primo	311
Semi Skimmed Milk, Lactofree, Primo, Takeaway	311
Semi Skimmed Milk, Medio	386
Semi Skimmed Milk, Medio, Takeaway	386
Semi Skimmed Milk, Primo	320
Semi Skimmed Milk, Primo, Takeaway	320
Skimmed Milk, Medio	362
Skimmed Milk, Medio, Takeaway	362
Skimmed Milk, Primo	302
Skimmed Milk, Primo, Takeaway	302
Soya Milk, Medio	379
Soya Milk, Medio, Takeaway	379
Soya Milk, Primo	315
Soya Milk, Primo, Takeaway	315
Whole Milk, Medio	420
Whole Milk, Medio, Takeaway	420
Whole Milk, Primo	346
Whole Milk, Primo, Takeaway	346

FROSTINO - BELGIAN CHOCOLATE, COFFEE

Coffee, Almond Milk, Medio	354
Coffee, Almond Milk, Medio, Takeaway	354
Coffee, Almond Milk, Primo	295
Coffee, Almond Milk, Primo, Takeaway	295
Coffee, Coconut Milk, Medio	369
Coconut Milk, Medio, Takeaway	369
Coconut Milk, Primo	306
Coconut Milk, Primo, Takeaway	306
Semi Skimmed Milk, Lactofree, Medio	380
Semi Skimmed Milk, Lactofree, Medio, Takeaway	380
Semi Skimmed Milk, Lactofree, Primo	314
Semi Skimmed Milk, Lactofree, Primo, Takeaway	314
Semi Skimmed Milk, Medio	392
Semi Skimmed Milk, Medio, Takeaway	392

COSTA

FROSTINO - BELGIAN CHOCOLATE, COFFEE

Semi Skimmed Milk, Primo	323
Semi Skimmed Milk, Primo, Takeaway	323
Skimmed Milk, Medio	368
Skimmed Milk, Medio, Takeaway	368
Skimmed Milk, Primo	305
Skimmed Milk, Primo, Takeaway	305
Soya Milk, Medio	385
Soya Milk, Medio, Takeaway	385
Soya Milk, Primo	318
Soya Milk, Primo, Takeaway	318
Whole Milk, Medio	426
Whole Milk, Medio, Takeaway	426
Whole Milk, Primo	349
Whole Milk, Primo, Takeaway	349

FROSTINO - COFFEE

Almond Milk, Medio	101
Almond Milk, Medio, Takeaway	101
Almond Milk, Primo	70
Almond Milk, Primo, Takeaway	70
Coconut Milk, Medio	116
Coconut Milk, Medio, Takeaway	116
Coconut Milk, Primo	82
Coconut Milk, Primo, Takeaway	82
Semi Skimmed Milk, Lactofree, Medio	126
Semi Skimmed Milk, Lactofree, Medio, Takeaway	126
Semi Skimmed Milk, Lactofree, Primo	90
Semi Skimmed Milk, Lactofree, Primo, Takeaway	90
Semi Skimmed Milk, Medio	138
Semi Skimmed Milk, Medio, Takeaway	138
Semi Skimmed Milk, Primo	99
Semi Skimmed Milk, Primo, Takeaway	99
Skimmed Milk, Medio	114
Skimmed Milk, Medio, Takeaway	114
Skimmed Milk, Primo	81
Skimmed Milk, Primo, Takeaway	81
Soya Milk, Medio	131
Soya Milk, Medio, Takeaway	131
Soya Milk, Primo	94
Soya Milk, Primo, Takeaway	94
Whole Milk, Medio	172
Whole Milk, Medio, Takeaway	172
Whole Milk, Primo	125
Whole Milk, Primo, Takeaway	125

FROSTINO - MINT CHOC CHIP

Almond Milk, Medio	406
Almond Milk, Medio, Takeaway	407
Almond Milk, Primo	329
Almond Milk, Primo, Takeaway	329
Coconut Milk, Medio	421
Coconut Milk, Medio, Takeaway	422
Coconut Milk, Primo	341
Coconut Milk, Primo, Takeaway	341

COSTA

FROSTINO - MINT CHOC CHIP

Semi Skimmed Milk, Lactofree, Medio	431
Semi Skimmed Milk, Lactofree, Medio, Takeaway	432
Semi Skimmed Milk, Lactofree, Primo	349
Semi Skimmed Milk, Lactofree, Primo, Takeaway	349
Semi Skimmed Milk, Medio	442
Semi Skimmed Milk, Medio, Takeaway	444
Semi Skimmed Milk, Primo	358
Semi Skimmed Milk, Primo, Takeaway	358
Skimmed Milk, Medio	419
Skimmed Milk, Medio, Takeaway	421
Skimmed Milk, Primo	340
Skimmed Milk, Primo, Takeaway	340
Soya Milk, Medio	435
Soya Milk, Medio, Takeaway	438
Soya Milk, Primo	353
Soya Milk, Primo, Takeaway	353
Whole Milk, Medio	475
Whole Milk, Medio, Takeaway	478
Whole Milk, Primo	384
Whole Milk, Primo, Takeaway	384

FROSTINO - SALTED CARAMEL CRUNCH

Almond Milk, Medio	322
Almond Milk, Medio, Takeaway	322
Almond Milk, Primo	274
Almond Milk, Primo, Takeaway	274
Coconut Milk, Medio	337
Coconut Milk, Medio, Takeaway	337
Coconut Milk, Primo	285
Coconut Milk, Primo, Takeaway	285
Semi Skimmed Milk, Lactofree, Medio	347
Semi Skimmed Milk, Lactofree, Medio, Takeaway	347
Semi Skimmed Milk, Lactofree, Primo	293
Semi Skimmed Milk, Lactofree, Primo, Takeaway	293
Semi Skimmed Milk, Medio	359
Semi Skimmed Milk, Medio, Takeaway	359
Semi Skimmed Milk, Primo	302
Semi Skimmed Milk, Primo, Takeaway	302
Skimmed Milk, Medio	335
Skimmed Milk, Medio, Takeaway	335
Skimmed Milk, Primo	284
Skimmed Milk, Primo, Takeaway	284
Soya Milk, Medio	352
Soya Milk, Medio, Takeaway	352
Soya Milk, Primo	297
Soya Milk, Primo, Takeaway	297
Whole Milk, Medio	393
Whole Milk, Medio, Takeaway	393
Whole Milk, Primo	328
Whole Milk, Primo, Takeaway	328

FROSTINO - SALTED CARAMEL CRUNCH, COFFEE

Almond Milk, Medio	328
Almond Milk, Medio, Takeaway	328

COSTA

FROSTINO - SALTED CARAMEL CRUNCH, COFFEE

Almond Milk, Primo	277
Almond Milk, Primo, Takeaway	277
Coconut Milk, Medio	343
Coconut Milk, Medio, Takeaway	343
Coconut Milk, Primo	288
Coconut Milk, Primo, Takeaway	288
Semi Skimmed Milk, Lactofree, Medio	353
Semi Skimmed Milk, Lactofree, Medio, Takeaway	353
Semi Skimmed Milk, Lactofree, Primo	296
Semi Skimmed Milk, Lactofree, Primo, Takeaway	296
Semi Skimmed Milk, Medio	365
Semi Skimmed Milk, Medio, Takeaway	365
Semi Skimmed Milk, Primo	305
Semi Skimmed Milk, Primo, Takeaway	305
Skimmed Milk, Medio	341
Skimmed Milk, Medio, Takeaway	341
Skimmed Milk, Primo	287
Skimmed Milk, Primo, Takeaway	287
Soya Milk, Medio	358
Soya Milk, Medio, Takeaway	358
Soya Milk, Primo	300
Soya Milk, Primo, Takeaway	300
Whole Milk, Medio	399
Whole Milk, Medio, Takeaway	399
Whole Milk, Primo	331
Whole Milk, Primo, Takeaway	331

FROSTINO - STRAWBERRY

Almond Milk, Medio	384
Almond Milk, Primo	318
Coconut Milk, Medio	400
Coconut Milk, Primo	330
Semi Skimmed Milk, Lactofree, Medio	410
Semi Skimmed Milk, Lactofree, Primo	338
Semi Skimmed Milk, Medio	422
Semi Skimmed Milk, Primo	347
Skimmed Milk, Medio	398
Skimmed Milk, Primo	329
Soya Milk, Medio	415
Soya Milk, Primo	342
Whole Milk, Medio	456
Whole Milk, Primo	373

FRUIT COMPOTE

Berry, Hedgerow, SOTF	76
Mixed Berry, Topping	38

FRUIT SALAD

Breakfast	67
Snack Box, Kids	258

HOT CHOCOLATE - ALMOND MILK

Massimo	294
Massimo, Takeaway	316
Medio	207
Medio, Takeaway	226

COSTA

HOT CHOCOLATE - ALMOND MILK

Primo	118
Primo, Takeaway	152
Mini, with Flake	83
Mini, with Marshmallow	69

HOT CHOCOLATE - BLACK FOREST

Almond Milk, Medio	314
Almond Milk, Medio, Takeaway	333
Almond Milk, Primo	249
Almond Milk, Primo, Takeaway	272
Coconut Milk, Medio	333
Coconut Milk, Medio, Takeaway	355
Coconut Milk, Primo	262
Coconut Milk, Primo, Takeaway	289
Semi Skimmed Milk, Lactofree, Medio	344
Semi Skimmed Milk, Lactofree, Medio, Takeaway	367
Semi Skimmed Milk, Lactofree, Primo	269
Semi Skimmed Milk, Lactofree, Primo, Takeaway	298
Semi Skimmed Milk, Medio	361
Semi Skimmed Milk, Medio, Takeaway	387
Semi Skimmed Milk, Primo	281
Semi Skimmed Milk, Primo, Takeaway	313
Skimmed Milk, Medio	331
Skimmed Milk, Medio, Takeaway	353
Skimmed Milk, Primo	261
Skimmed Milk, Primo, Takeaway	287
Soya Milk, Medio	352
Soya Milk, Medio, Takeaway	377
Soya Milk, Primo	275
Soya Milk, Primo, Takeaway	306
Whole Milk, Medio	403
Whole Milk, Medio, Takeaway	435
Whole Milk, Primo	310
Whole Milk, Primo, Takeaway	351

HOT CHOCOLATE - BONFIRE SPICED

Almond Milk, Medio	267
Almond Milk, Medio, Takeaway	286
Almond Milk, Primo	165
Almond Milk, Primo, Takeaway	198
Coconut Milk, Medio	292
Coconut Milk, Medio, Takeaway	314
Coconut Milk, Primo	181
Coconut Milk, Primo, Takeaway	220
Semi Skimmed Milk, Lactofree, Medio	306
Semi Skimmed Milk, Lactofree, Medio, Takeaway	329
Semi Skimmed Milk, Lactofree, Primo	191
Semi Skimmed Milk, Lactofree, Primo, Takeaway	233
Semi Skimmed Milk, Medio	329
Semi Skimmed Milk, Medio, Takeaway	354
Semi Skimmed Milk, Primo	205
Semi Skimmed Milk, Primo, Takeaway	252
Skimmed Milk, Medio	289
Skimmed Milk, Medio, Takeaway	311

COSTA

HOT CHOCOLATE - BONFIRE SPICED

Skimmed Milk, Primo	180
Skimmed Milk, Primo, Takeaway	218
Soya Milk, Medio	317
Soya Milk, Medio, Takeaway	341
Soya Milk, Primo	198
Soya Milk, Primo, Takeaway	242
Whole Milk, Medio	384
Whole Milk, Medio, Takeaway	415
Whole Milk, Primo	242
Whole Milk, Primo, Takeaway	301

HOT CHOCOLATE - CARAMEL

Luxury	121
Luxury, Takeaway	159

HOT CHOCOLATE - COCONUT MILK

Massimo	331
Massimo, Takeaway	355
Medio	236
Medio, Takeaway	257
Primo	138
Primo, Takeaway	176
Mini, with Flake	97
Mini, with Marshmallow	81

HOT CHOCOLATE - GINGERBREAD & CREAM

Almond Milk, Medio	290
Almond Milk, Medio, Takeaway	309
Almond Milk, Primo	233
Coconut Milk, Medio	309
Coconut Milk, Medio, Takeaway	331
Coconut Milk, Primo	246
Coconut Milk, Primo, Takeaway	273
Semi Skimmed Milk, Lactofree, Medio	320
Semi Skimmed Milk, Lactofree, Medio, Takeaway	343
Semi Skimmed Milk, Lactofree, Primo	253
Semi Skimmed Milk, Lactofree, Primo, Takeaway	282
Semi Skimmed Milk, Medio	337
Semi Skimmed Milk, Medio, Takeaway	363
Semi Skimmed Milk, Primo	264
Semi Skimmed Milk, Primo, Takeaway	297
Skimmed Milk, Medio	307
Skimmed Milk, Medio, Takeaway	329
Skimmed Milk, Primo	244
Skimmed Milk, Primo, Takeaway	271
Soya Milk, Medio	328
Soya Milk, Medio, Takeaway	353
Soya Milk, Primo	259
Soya Milk, Primo, Takeaway	289
Whole Milk, Medio	379
Whole Milk, Medio, Takeaway	411
Whole Milk, Primo	293
Whole Milk, Primo, Takeaway	334
Almond Milk, Primo, Takeaway	256

COSTA

HOT CHOCOLATE - HAZELNUT PRALINE

Almond Milk, Medio	355
Almond Milk, Medio, Takeaway	374
Almond Milk, Primo	284
Almond Milk, Primo, Takeaway	307
Coconut Milk, Medio	374
Coconut Milk, Medio, Takeaway	396
Coconut Milk, Primo	297
Coconut Milk, Primo, Takeaway	324
Semi Skimmed Milk, Lactofree, Medio	385
Semi Skimmed Milk, Lactofree, Medio, Takeaway	408
Semi Skimmed Milk, Lactofree, Primo	304
Semi Skimmed Milk, Lactofree, Primo, Takeaway	333
Semi Skimmed Milk, Medio	402
Semi Skimmed Milk, Medio, Takeaway	428
Semi Skimmed Milk, Primo	316
Semi Skimmed Milk, Primo, Takeaway	348
Skimmed Milk, Medio	372
Skimmed Milk, Medio, Takeaway	484
Skimmed Milk, Primo	295
Skimmed Milk, Primo, Takeaway	322
Soya Milk, Medio	393
Soya Milk, Medio, Takeaway	418
Soya Milk, Primo	310
Soya Milk, Primo, Takeaway	341
Whole Milk, Medio	430
Whole Milk, Medio, Takeaway	476
Whole Milk, Primo	345
Whole Milk, Primo, Takeaway	385

HOT CHOCOLATE - LUXURY

Eat In	113
Takeaway	150

HOT CHOCOLATE - SEMI SKIMMED MILK

Mini, Lactofree, with Flake	101
Mini, Lactofree, with Marshmallow	85
Mini, with Flake	124
Mini, with Marshmallow	108
, Lactofree, Massimo	352
Lactofree, Massimo, Takeaway	377
Lactofree, Medio	252
Lactofree, Medio, Takeaway	274
Lactofree, Primo	148
Lactofree, Primo, Takeaway	190
Massimo	384
Massimo, Takeaway	413
Medio	277
Medio, Takeaway	302
Primo	165
Primo, Takeaway	212

HOT CHOCOLATE - SKIMMED MILK

Mini, with Flake	108
Mini, with Marshmallow	92
Massimo	327

COSTA

HOT CHOCOLATE - SKIMMED MILK
Massimo, Takeaway	351
Medio	232
Medio, Takeaway	254
Primo	135
Primo, Takeaway	174

HOT CHOCOLATE - SOYA MILK
Mini, with Flake	104
Mini, with Marshmallow	88
Massimo	368
Massimo, Takeaway	395
Medio	264
Ã,Â Medio, Takeaway	288
Primo	157
Primo, Takeaway	201

HOT CHOCOLATE - WHITE
Almond Milk, Massimo	276
Almond Milk, Massimo, Takeaway	300
Almond Milk, Medio	208
Almond Milk, Medio, Takeaway	234
Almond Milk, Primo	137
Almond Milk, Primo, Takeaway	164
Coconut Milk, Massimo	315
Coconut Milk, Massimo, Takeaway	348
Coconut Milk, Medio	237
Coconut Milk, Medio, Takeaway	274
Coconut Milk, Primo	156
Coconut Milk, Primo, Takeaway	194
Semi Skimmed Milk, Lactofree, Massimo	341
Semi Skimmed Milk, Lactofree, Massimo, Takeaway	380
Semi Skimmed Milk, Lactofree, Medio	256
Semi Skimmed Milk, Lactofree, Medio, Takeaway	300
Semi Skimmed Milk, Lactofree, Primo	168
Semi Skimmed Milk, Lactofree, Primo, Takeaway	213
Semi Skimmed Milk, Massimo	371
Semi Skimmed Milk, Massimo, Takeaway	417
Semi Skimmed Milk, Medio	279
Semi Skimmed Milk, Medio, Takeaway	331
Semi Skimmed Milk, Primo	183
Semi Skimmed Milk, Primo, Takeaway	236
Skimmed Milk, Massimo	310
Skimmed Milk, Massimo, Takeaway	342
Skimmed Milk, Medio	234
Skimmed Milk, Medio, Takeaway	269
Skimmed Milk, Primo	154
Skimmed Milk, Primo, Takeaway	190
Soya Milk, Massimo	353
Soya Milk, Massimo, Takeaway	395
Soya Milk, Medio	266
Soya Milk, Medio, Takeaway	313
Soya Milk, Primo	175
Soya Milk, Primo, Takeaway	223
White, Whole Milk, Massimo	457

COSTA

HOT CHOCOLATE - WHITE
Whole Milk, Massimo, Takeaway	523
Whole Milk, Medio	344
Whole Milk, Medio, Takeaway	418
Whole Milk, Primo	225
Whole Milk, Primo, Takeaway	301

HOT CHOCOLATE - WHOLE MILK
Mini, with Flake	96
Mini, with Marshmallow	80
Massimo	467
Massimo, Takeaway	501
Medio	341
Medio, Takeaway	372
Primo	208
Primo, Takeaway	267

ICE CREAM
Vanilla, Individual Tubs, SOTF	159

ICE CREAM CONE
Gingerbread	224

JUICE DRINK
Coconut, & Watermelon, Fruit Cooler, Medio	117
Coconut, & Watermelon, Fruit Cooler, Primo	88
Mango & Passionfruit, Fruit Cooler, Medio	149
Mango & Passionfruit, Fruit Cooler, Primo	112
Red Summer Berries, Fruit Cooler, Medio	198
Red Summer Berries, Fruit Cooler, Primo	150

LEMONADE
Peach	87

MACARONI CHEESE
Bolognese	481
Box	597

MARSHMALLOWS
Portion	20

MERINGUE
Pink Swirl	183
Pink Swirl, SOTF	183

MILK DRINK - CHOCOLATE
Almond Milk, Medio, Iced	200
Almond Milk, Medio, Iced, Takeaway	208
Almond Milk, Primo, Iced	143
Almond Milk, Primo, Iced, Takeaway	146
Coconut Milk, Medio, Iced	221
Coconut Milk, Medio, Iced, Takeaway	232
Coconut Milk, Primo, Iced	161
Coconut Milk, Primo, Iced, Takeaway	165
Semi Skimmed Milk, Medio, Iced	252
Semi Skimmed Milk, Medio, Iced, Takeaway	267
Semi Skimmed Milk, Primo, Iced	186
Semi Skimmed Milk, Primo, Iced, Takeaway	192
Skimmed Milk, Medio, Iced	219
Skimmed Milk, Medio, Iced, Takeaway	230
Skimmed Milk, Primo, Iced	159
Skimmed Milk, Primo, Iced, Takeaway	163

COSTA

MILK DRINK - CHOCOLATE

	KCAL
Soya Milk, Medio, Iced	242
Soya Milk, Medio, Iced, Takeaway	257
Soya Milk, Primo, Iced	178
Soya Milk, Primo, Iced, Takeaway	184
Whole Milk, Medio, Iced	299
Whole Milk, Medio, Iced, Takeaway	321
Whole Milk, Primo, Iced	226
Ã,Â Whole Milk, Primo, Iced, Takeaway	234

MILK DRINK - CHOCOLATE, LACTOFREE

Semi Skimmed Milk, Medio, Iced	235
Semi Skimmed Milk, Medio, Iced, Takeaway	249
Semi Skimmed Milk, Primo, Iced	172
Semi Skimmed Milk, Primo, Iced, Takeaway	177

MILK WHIP

Strawberry, Medio	168
Strawberry, Primo	117
Vanilla, Medio	104
Vanilla, Primo	74

MUFFIN

Banana & Pecan Breakfast Loaf	442
Blueberry	389
Caramel, Salted	391
Chocolate	485
Chocolate, with Flake	405
Lemon	399
Lotus Biscoff	467
Mini	76
Raspberry, & White Chocolate	364
Raspberry Rainbow	425

NUTS

Natural, Mixed	187

ORANGES

Easy Peeler	59

PANETTONE

Classic	377

PANINI

Brie, & Bacon	530
Goats Cheese, & Grilled Pepper, Focaccia	491
Ham, British, & Cheddar	438
Mozzarella, Tomato, & Basil	508
Tuna, Melt	471

PASTRY

Cheese, Twist	327
Chocolate, Twist	305
Pain Aux Raisins	274

POPCORN

Sweet & Salty	137

PRETZELS

Salted, Bites, Baked	97

RAISINS

Chocolate, Milk	161

COSTA

SALAD

	KCAL
Chicken, Roast	196
Cous Cous, Moroccan Styles	392
Pasta, Mozzarella, & Sun-Dried Tomato	529

SANDWICH

Chicken, Roast, & Bacon	454
Chicken, Salad, Roast	427
Egg, Free Range	342
Ham, & Cheddar Cheese, Baguette, SOTF	716
Mozzarella, & Tomato, Baguette, SOTF	670
Tuna, & Sweetcorn	395
Tuna & Cucumber, SOTF	566

SAUSAGE ROLL

Sausage Roll	400

SCONE

Cheese	391

SHORTBREAD

Bites, Mini	47
Chocolate Chunk, Milk	344
Millionaire	396

SOUP

Carrot & Coriander	167

SWEETS

Cola Bottles, Sugar Free, Vegan	87
Gummy Bears, Sugar Free, Vegan	87

SYRUP

Caramel	14
Caramel, Sugar Free	1
Cinnamon	16
Gingerbread, Sugar Free	1
Roasted Hazelnut	15
Vanilla	17

TART

Apple, Glazed, SOTF	193
Bakewell, Cherry	389
Bakewell, Mini	273
Custard, Portugese	169
Lemon	347
Mince, Vegan, GF	322

TEA - CHAI LATTE

Almond Milk, Massimo	192
Almond Milk, Massimo, Takeaway	192
Almond Milk, Medio	160
Almond Milk, Medio, Takeaway	160
Almond Milk, Primo	105
Almond Milk, Primo, Takeaway	123
Coconut Milk, Massimo	225
Coconut Milk, Massimo, Takeaway	225
Coconut Milk, Medio	190
Coconut Milk, Medio, Takeaway	190
Coconut Milk, Primo	125
Coconut Milk, Primo, Takeaway	149
Semi Skimmed Milk, Lactofree, Massimo	244

COSTA

TEA - CHAI LATTE

	KCAL
Semi Skimmed Milk, Lactofree, Massimo, Takeaway	244
Semi Skimmed Milk, Lactofree, Medio	207
Semi Skimmed Milk, Lactofree, Medio, Takeaway	207
Semi Skimmed Milk, Lactofree, Primo	135
Semi Skimmed Milk, Lactofree, Primo, Takeaway	164
Semi Skimmed Milk, Massimo	273
Semi Skimmed Milk, Massimo, Takeaway	273
Semi Skimmed Milk, Medio	234
Semi Skimmed Milk, Medio, Takeaway	234
Semi Skimmed Milk, Primo	153
Semi Skimmed Milk, Primo, Takeaway	187
Skimmed Milk, Massimo	221
Skimmed Milk, Massimo, Takeaway	221
Skimmed Milk, Medio	187
Skimmed Milk, Medio, Takeaway	187
Skimmed Milk, Primo	123
Skimmed Milk, Primo, Takeaway	147
Soya Milk, Massimo	259
Soya Milk, Massimo, Takeaway	259
Soya Milk, Medio	221
Soya Milk, Medio, Takeaway	221
Soya Milk, Primo	144
Soya Milk, Primo, Takeaway	176
Whole Milk, Massimo	348
Whole Milk, Massimo, Takeaway	348
Whole Milk, Medio	302
Whole Milk, Medio, Takeaway	302
Whole Milk, Primo	196
Whole Milk, Primo, Takeaway	245
Almond Milk, Medio, Iced	116
Almond Milk, Primo, Iced	82
Coconut Milk, Medio, Iced	132
Coconut Milk, Primo, Iced	95
Semi Skimmed Milk, Lactofree, Medio, Iced	143
Semi Skimmed Milk, Lactofree, Primo, Iced	103
Semi Skimmed Milk, Medio, Iced	156
Semi Skimmed Milk, Primo, Iced	113
Skimmed Milk, Medio, Iced	131
Skimmed Milk, Primo, Iced	93
Soya Milk, Medio, Iced	149
Soya Milk, Primo, Iced	107
Whole Milk, Medio, Iced	192
Whole Milk, Primo, Iced	141

TEA - ENGLISH

	KCAL
Breakfast	1
Breakfast, Decaff	3

TEA - FRUIT

	KCAL
Superfruity	2

TEA - GREEN

	KCAL
Jasmine	1
Simply Sencha	3

COSTA

TEA - ICED

	KCAL
Peach, Medio	95
Peach, Medio, Takeaway	97
Peach, Primo	67
Peach, Primo, Takeaway	67
Strawberry, Infusion, Medio	123
Strawberry, Infusion, Medio, Takeaway	123
Strawberry, Infusion, Primo	83
Strawberry, Infusion, Primo, Takeaway	83

TEA - MINT

	KCAL
Thoroughly Minted	3

TEACAKES

	KCAL
Fruit, No Butter, Breakfast	312
Fruit, Vegan, No Butter, Breakfast	295

TOAST

	KCAL
Brown, Seeded	382
Fruit	298
White, No Butter	275

TOASTIE

	KCAL
Cheddar, & Tomato, Slow Roasted	446
Chicken, & Bacon	418
Emmenthal, & Mushroom	436
Ham, & Cheese	307
Ham, Wiltshire, & Mature Cheddar	409
Turkey, & Trimmings	474

WAFERS

	KCAL
Cocoa, Snack	223
Vanilla, Snack	230

WAFFLES

	KCAL
Belgian, SOTF	462

WRAP

	KCAL
Chicken, & Bacon, Caesar	532
Chicken, Fajita, Roast	439
Chickpea & Mango, Spiced, Vegan, SOTF	412
Tomato, & Mozzarella	400

YOGHURT

	KCAL
Granola, Berry, Hedgerow, SOTF	299
Greek Style, 0% Fat, Organic	68

DOMINO'S PIZZA

BREAD

Garlic, Dippers	243
Garlic, Pizza	311

CHICKEN

Chick 'n' Mix	386
Kickers, Combo Box	178
Kickers	186
Strippers, Combo Box	218
Strippers	268
Wings, Combo Box	195
Wings	222
Wings, Red Hot, Franks	224
Wings, Spicy BBQ	250

COLESLAW

Portion	146

COOKIES

Portion	183

DESSERT

Cinni Dippers	200

DIP

BBQ, Big	188
BBQ	47
Garlic & Herb, Big	676
Garlic & Herb	169
Honey & Mustard	109
Red Hot, Franks, Big	23
Red Hot, Franks	6
Salsa, Tangy	43
Sweet Chilli	54

DOUGH BALLS

Twisted, with Cheese	339
Twisted, with Ham	341
Twisted, with Pepperoni	373

NACHOS

no Jalapenos	263
with Jalapenos	264

PIZZA - AMERICAN HOT

Classic Crust, Delight Mozzarella, Large	195
Classic Crust, Delight Mozzarella, Medium	174
Classic Crust, Delight Mozzarella, Personal	136
Classic Crust, Delight Mozzarella, Small	254
Classic Crust, Large	208
Classic Crust, Medium	189
Classic Crust, Personal	147
Classic Crust, Small	261
Italian Style Crust, Delight Mozzarella, Large	159
Italian Style Crust, Delight Mozzarella, Medium	140
Italian Style Crust, Delight Mozzarella, Small	209
Italian Style Crust, Large	172
Italian Style Crust, Medium	152
Italian Style Crust, Small	228
Stuffed Crust, Delight Mozzarella, Large	229
Stuffed Crust, Delight Mozzarella, Medium	207

DOMINO'S PIZZA

PIZZA - AMERICAN HOT

Stuffed Crust, Large	224
Stuffed Crust, Medium	218
Stuffed Crust, Tabasco, Delight Mozzarella, Large	229
Stuffed Crust, Tabasco, Delight Mozzarella, Medium	212
Stuffed Crust, Tabasco, Large	238
Stuffed Crust, Tabasco, Medium	221
Thin & Crispy, Delight Mozzarella, Large	143
Thin & Crispy, Delight Mozzarella, Medium	136
Thin & Crispy, Large	160
Thin & Crispy, Medium	150

PIZZA - AMERICANO

Classic Crust, Delight Mozzarella, Large	232
Classic Crust, Delight Mozzarella, Medium	206
Classic Crust, Delight Mozzarella, Personal	155
Classic Crust, Delight Mozzarella, Small	272
Classic Crust, Large	234
Classic Crust, Medium	214
Classic Crust, Small	274
Italian Style Crust, Delight Mozzarella, Large	189
Italian Style Crust, Delight Mozzarella, Medium	199
Italian Style Crust, Delight Mozzarella, Small	226
Italian Style Crust, Large	202
Italian Style Crust, Medium	219
Italian Style Crust, Small	238
Stuffed Crust, Delight Mozzarella, Large	261
Stuffed Crust, Delight Mozzarella, Medium	237
Stuffed Crust, Large	273
Stuffed Crust, Medium	251
Stuffed Crust, Tabasco, Delight Mozzarella, Large	266
Stuffed Crust, Tabasco, Delight Mozzarella, Medium	238
Stuffed Crust, Tabasco, Large	276
Stuffed Crust, Tabasco, Medium	247
Thin & Crispy, Delight Mozzarella, Large	167
Thin & Crispy, Delight Mozzarella, Medium	158
Thin & Crispy, Large	179
Thin & Crispy, Medium	247
Classic Crust, Personal	332

PIZZA - BACON DOUBLE CHEESE

Classic Crust, Delight Mozzarella, Large	201
Classic Crust, Delight Mozzarella, Medium	177
Classic Crust, Delight Mozzarella, Personal	145
Classic Crust, Delight Mozzarella, Small	254
Classic Crust, Large	219
Classic Crust, Medium	195
Classic Crust, Personal	104
Classic Crust, Small	266
Italian Style Crust, Delight Mozzarella, Large	165
Italian Style Crust, Delight Mozzarella, Medium	143
Italian Style Crust, Delight Mozzarella, Small	210
Italian Style Crust, Large	182
Ã,Â Italian Style Crust, Medium	159
Italian Style Crust, Small	233

DOMINO'S PIZZA

PIZZA - BACON DOUBLE CHEESE

Stuffed Crust, Delight Mozzarella, Large	236
Stuffed Crust, Delight Mozzarella, Medium	210
Stuffed Crust, Large	234
Stuffed Crust, Medium	224
Stuffed Crust, Tabasco, Delight Mozzarella, Large	236
Stuffed Crust, Tabasco, Delight Mozzarella, Medium	215
Stuffed Crust, Tabasco, Large	248
Stuffed Crust, Tabasco, Medium	227
Thin & Crispy, Delight Mozzarella, Large	149
Thin & Crispy, Delight Mozzarella, Medium	139
Thin & Crispy, Large	170
Thin & Crispy, Medium	157

PIZZA - BUFFALO CHICKEN

Classic Crust, Delight Mozzarella, Large	178
Classic Crust, Delight Mozzarella, Medium	155
Classic Crust, Delight Mozzarella, Personal	124
Classic Crust, Delight Mozzarella. Small	223
Classic Crust, Large	192
Classic Crust, Medium	169
Classic Crust, Personal	135
Classic Crust, Small	231
Italian Style Crust, Delight Mozzarella, Large	142
Italian Style Crust, Delight Mozzarella, Medium	121
Italian Style Crust, Delight Mozzarella, Small	179
Italian Style Crust, Large	155
Italian Style Crust, Medium	133
Italian Style Crust, Small	198
Stuffed Crust, Delight Mozzarella, Large	223
Stuffed Crust, Delight Mozzarella, Medium	188
Stuffed Crust, Large	229
Stuffed Crust, Medium	199
Stuffed Crust, Tabasco, Delight Mozzarella, Large	212
Stuffed Crust, Tabasco, Delight Mozzarella, Medium	200
Stuffed Crust, Tabasco, Large	221
Stuffed Crust, Tabasco, Medium	209
Thin & Crispy, Delight Mozzarella, Large	126
Thin & Crispy, Delight Mozzarella, Medium	200
Thin & Crispy, Large	143
Thin & Crispy, Medium	131

PIZZA - CHEESE & TOMATO

Classic Crust, Delight Mozzarella, Large	176
Classic Crust, Delight Mozzarella, Medium	153
Classic Crust, Delight Mozzarella, Personal	119
Classic Crust, Delight Mozzarella, Small	219
Classic Crust, Large	193
Classic Crust, Medium	171
Classic Crust, Personal	131
Classic Crust, Small	230
GF Crust, Delight Mozzarella, Small	188
GF Crust, Small	201
Italian Style Crust, Delight Mozzarella, Large	140
Italian Style Crust, Delight Mozzarella, Medium	120

DOMINO'S PIZZA

PIZZA - CHEESE & TOMATO

Italian Style Crust, Delight Mozzarella, Small	174
Ã,Â Italian Style Crust, Large	157
Italian Style Crust, Medium	135
Ã,Â Italian Style Crust, Small	194
Stuffed Crust, Delight Mozzarella, Large	211
Stuffed Crust, Delight Mozzarella, Medium	186
Stuffed Crust, Large	209
Stuffed Crust, Medium	201
Stuffed Crust, Tabasco, Delight Mozzarella, Large	211
Stuffed Crust, Tabasco, Delight Mozzarella, Medium	192
Stuffed Crust, Tabasco, Large	223
Stuffed Crust, Tabsaco, Medium	204
Thin & Crispy, Delight Mozzarella, Large	124
Thin & Crispy, Delight Mozzarella, Medium	115
Thin & Crispy, Large	145
Thin & Crispy, Medium	133

PIZZA - CHICKEN FEAST

Classic Crust, Delight Mozzarella, Large	184
Classic Crust, Delight Mozzarella, Medium	162
Classic Crust, Delight Mozzarella, Personal	128
Classic Crust, Delight Mozzarella, Small	231
Classic Crust, Large	198
Classic Crust, Medium	177
Classic Crust, Personal	139
Classic Crust, Small	238
Italian Style Crust, Delight Mozzarella, Lge	148
Italian Style Crust, Delight Mozzarella, Medium	128
Italian Style Crust, Delight Mozzarella, Small	186
Italian Style Crust, Lge	161
Italian Style Crust, Medium	140
Italian Style Crust, Small	206
Stuffed Crust, Delight Mozzarella, Large	219
Stuffed Crust, Delight Mozzarella, Medium	195
Stuffed Crust, Large	214
Stuffed Crust, Medium	206
Stuffed Crust, Tabasco, Delight Mozzarella, Large	219
Stuffed Crust, Tabasco, Delight Mozzarella, Medium	200
Stuffed Crust, Tabasco, Large	228
Stuffed Crust, Tabasco, Medium	209
Thin & Crispy, Delight Mozzarella, Large	132
Thin & Crispy, Delight Mozzarella, Medium	124
Thin & Crispy, Large	149
Thin & Crispy, Medium	138

PIZZA - CHOCOLATE

Lotta	211

PIZZA - DELIGHT CHICKEN

Delight Mozzarella, Large	148
Delight Mozzarella, Medium	122
Delight Mozzarella, Small	151

PIZZA - DELIGHT VEGI

Delight Mozzarella, Large	146
Delight Mozzarella, Medium	120

DOMINO'S PIZZA

PIZZA - DELIGHT VEGI

Delight Mozzarella, Small	149

PIZZA - DELUXE

Classic Crust, Delight Mozzarella, Large	193
Classic Crust, Delight Mozzarella, Medium	173
Classic Crust, Delight Mozzarella, Personal	135
Classic Crust, Delight Mozzarella, Small	251
Classic Crust, Large	207
Classic Crust, Medium	187
Classic Crust, Personal	145
Classic Crust, Small	258
Italian Style Crust, Delight Mozzarella, Large	158
Italian Style Crust, Delight Mozzarella, Medium	139
Italian Style Crust, Delight Mozzarella, Small	206
Italian Style Crust, Large	171
Italian Style Crust, Medium	151
Italian Style Crust, Small	226
Stuffed Crust, Delight Mozzarella, Large	228
Stuffed Crust, Delight Mozzarella, Medium	206
Stuffed Crust, Large	223
Stuffed Crust, Medium	217
Stuffed Crust, Tabasco, Delight Mozzarella, Large	228
Stuffed Crust, Tabasco, Delight Mozzarella, Medium	211
Stuffed Crust, Tabasco, Large	237
Stuffed Crust, Tabasco, Medium	220
Thin & Crispy, Delight Mozzarella, Large	142
Thin & Crispy, Delight Mozzarella, Medium	138
Thin & Crispy, Large	159
Thin & Crispy, Medium	153

PIZZA - FARMHOUSE

Classic Crust, Delight Mozzarella, Large	170
Classic Crust, Delight Mozzarella, Medium	149
Classic Crust, Delight Mozzarella, Personal	120
Classic Crust, Delight Mozzarella, Small	216
Classic Crust, Large	184
Classic Crust, Medium	164
Classic Crust, Personal	130
Classic Crust, Small	223
Italian Style Crust, Delight Mozzarella, Large	134
Italian Style Crust, Delight Mozzarella, Medium	115
Italian Style Crust, Delight Mozzarella, Small	171
Italian Style Crust, Large	147
Italian Style Crust, Medium	128
Italian Style Crust, Small	190
Stuffed Crust, Delight Mozzarella, Large	205
Stuffed Crust, Delight Mozzarella, Medium	182
Stuffed Crust, Large	199
Stuffed Crust, Medium	193
Stuffed Crust, Tabasco, Delight Mozzarella, Large	205
Stuffed Crust, Tabasco, Delight Mozzarella, Medium	187
Stuffed Crust, Tabasco, Large	214
Stuffed Crust, Tabasco, Medium	196
Thin & Crispy, Delight Mozzarella, Large	118

DOMINO'S PIZZA

PIZZA - FARMHOUSE

Thin & Crispy, Delight Mozzarella, Medium	111
Thin & Crispy, Large	136
Thin & Crispy, Medium	126

PIZZA - FIERY VEGI SIZZLER

Classic Crust, Delight Mozzarella, Large	160
Classic Crust, Delight Mozzarella, Medium	139
Classic Crust, Delight Mozzarella, Personal	113
Classic Crust, Delight Mozzarella, Small	202
Classic Crust, Large	174
Classic Crust, Medium	154
Classic Crust, Personal	124
Classic Crust, Small	209
Italian Style Crust, Delight Mozzarella, Large	124
Italian Style Crust, Delight Mozzarella, Medium	106
Italian Style Crust, Delight Mozzarella, Small	157
Italian Style Crust, Large	138
Italian Style Crust, Medium	118
Italian Style Crust, Small	177
Stuffed Crust, Delight Mozzarella, Large	195
Stuffed Crust, Delight Mozzarella, Medium	172
Stuffed Crust, Large	190
Stuffed Crust, Medium	184
Stuffed Crust, Tabasco, Delight Mozzarella, Large	195
Stuffed Crust, Tabasco, Delight Mozzarella, Medium	178
Stuffed Crust, Tabasco, Large	204
Stuffed Crust, Tabasco, Medium	187
Thin & Crispy, Delight Mozzarella, Large	108
Thin & Crispy, Delight Mozzarella, Medium	101
Thin & Crispy, Large	126
Thin & Crispy, Medium	116

PIZZA - FOUR VEGI

Classic Crust, Delight Mozzarella, Large	165
Classic Crust, Delight Mozzarella, Medium	145
Classic Crust, Delight Mozzarella, Personal	118
Classic Crust, Delight Mozzarella, Small	209
Classic Crust, Large	179
Classic Crust, Medium	159
Classic Crust, Personal	128
Classic Crust, Small	216
Italian Style Crust, Delight Mozzarella, Large	129
Italian Style Crust, Delight Mozzarella, Medium	111
Italian Style Crust, Delight Mozzarella, Small	164
Italian Style Crust, Large	143
Italian Style Crust, Medium	123
Italian Style Crust, Small	737
Stuffed Crust, Delight Mozzarella, Large	200
Stuffed Crust, Delight Mozzarella, Medium	178
Stuffed Crust, Large	195
Stuffed Crust, Medium	189
Stuffed Crust, Tabasco, Delight Mozzarella, Large	200
Stuffed Crust, Tabasco, Delight Mozzarella, Medium	183
Stuffed Crust, Tabasco, Large	209

DOMINO'S PIZZA

PIZZA - FOUR VEGI

Stuffed Crust, Tabasco, Medium	192
Thin & Crispy, Delight Mozzarella, Large	114
Thin & Crispy, Delight Mozzarella, Medium	107
Thin & Crispy, Large	131
Thin & Crispy, Medium	121

PIZZA - FULL HOUSE

Classic Crust, Delight Mozzarella, Large	197
Classic Crust, Delight Mozzarella, Medium	174
Classic Crust, Delight Mozzarella, Personal	145
Classic Crust, Delight Mozzarella, Small	253
Classic Crust, Large	211
Classic Crust, Medium	189
Classic Crust, Personal	155
Classic Crust, Small	260
Italian Style Crust, Delight Mozzarella, Large	161
Italian Style Crust, Delight Mozzarella, Medium	141
Italian Style Crust, Delight Mozzarella, Small	208
Italian Style Crust, Large	174
Italian Style Crust, Medium	153
Italian Style Crust, Small	228
Stuffed Crust, Delight Mozzarella, Large	228
Stuffed Crust, Delight Mozzarella, Medium	207
Stuffed Crust, Large	226
Stuffed Crust, Medium	219
Stuffed Crust, Tabasco, Delight Mozzarella, Large	231
Stuffed Crust, Tabasco, Delight Mozzarella, Medium	213
Stuffed Crust, Tabasco, Large	240
Stuffed Crust,Tabasco, Medium	221
Thin & Crispy, Delight Mozzarella, Large	145
Thin & Crispy, Delight Mozzarella, Medium	136
Thin & Crispy, Large	162
Thin & Crispy, Medium	151

PIZZA - HAM & PINEAPPLE

Classic Crust, Delight Mozzarella, Large	170
Classic Crust, Delight Mozzarella, Medium	149
Classic Crust, Delight Mozzarella, Personal	120
Classic Crust, Delight Mozzarella, Small	216
Classic Crust, Large	183
Classic Crust, Medium	164
Classic Crust, Personal	130
Classic Crust, Small	223
Italian Style Crust, Delight Mozzarella, Large	201
Italian Style Crust, Delight Mozzarella, Medium	115
Italian Style Crust, Delight Mozzarella, Small	171
Italian Style Crust, Large	147
Italian Style Crust, Medium	127
Italian Style Crust, Small	190
Stuffed Crust, Delight Mozzarella, Large	204
Stuffed Crust, Delight Mozzarella, Medium	182
Stuffed Crust, Large	199
Stuffed Crust, Medium	193
Stuffed Crust, Tabasco, Delight Mozzarella, Large	204

DOMINO'S PIZZA

PIZZA - HAM & PINEAPPLE

Stuffed Crust, Tabasco, Delight Mozzarella, Medium	187
Stuffed Crust, Tabasco, Large	213
Stuffed Crust, Tabasco, Medium	196
Thin & Crispy, Delight Mozzarella, Large	118
Thin & Crispy, Delight Mozzarella, Medium	111
Thin & Crispy, Large	135
Thin & Crispy, Medium	125

PIZZA - HOT & SPICY

Classic Crust, Delight Mozzarella, Large	171
Classic Crust, Delight Mozzarella, Medium	149
Classic Crust, Delight Mozzarella, Personal	120
Classic Crust, Delight Mozzarella, Small	215
Classic Crust, Large	185
Classic Crust, Medium	164
Classic Crust, Personal	131
Classic Crust, Small	193
Italian Style Crust, Delight Mozzarella, Large	135
Italian Style Crust, Delight Mozzarella, Medium	115
Italian Style Crust, Delight Mozzarella, Small	171
Italian Style Crust, Large	149
Italian Style Crust, Medium	128
Italian Style Crust, Small	190
Stuffed Crust, Delight Mozzarella, Large	206
Stuffed Crust, Delight Mozzarella, Medium	182
Stuffed Crust, Large	201
Stuffed Crust, Medium	193
Stuffed Crust, Tabasco, Delight Mozzarella, Large	206
Stuffed Crust, Tabasco, Delight Mozzarella, Medium	187
Stuffed Crust, Tabasco, Large	215
Stuffed Crust, Tabasco, Medium	196
Thin & Crispy, Delight Mozzarella, Large	119
Thin & Crispy, Delight Mozzarella, Medium	111
Thin & Crispy, Large	137
Thin & Crispy, Medium	126

PIZZA - HOUSE SPECIAL TANDOORI

Classic Crust, Delight Mozzarella, Large	224
Classic Crust, Delight Mozzarella, Medium	200
Classic Crust, Delight Mozzarella, Personal	167
Classic Crust, Delight Mozzarella, Small	288
Classic Crust, Large	241
Classic Crust, Medium	218
Classic Crust, Personal	180
Classic Crust, Small	300
Italian Style Crust, Delight Mozzarella, Large	188
Italian Style Crust, Delight Mozzarella, Medium	167
Italian Style Crust, Delight Mozzarella, Small	244
Italian Style Crust, Large	205
Italian Style Crust, Medium	182
Italian Style Crust, Small	267
Stuffed Crust, Delight Mozzarella, Large	259
Stuffed Crust, Delight Mozzarella, Medium	233
Stuffed Crust, Large	257

DOMINO'S PIZZA

PIZZA - HOUSE SPECIAL TANDOORI

Stuffed Crust, Medium	248
Stuffed Crust, Tabasco, Delight Mozzarella, Large	259
Stuffed Crust, Tabasco, Delight Mozzarella, Medium	239
Stuffed Crust, Tabasco, Large	271
Stuffed Crust, Tabasco, Medium	250
Thin & Crispy, Delight Mozzarella, Large	172
Thin & Crispy, Delight Mozzarella, Medium	162
Thin & Crispy, Large	257
Thin & Crispy, Medium	180

PIZZA - MEAT LOVERS

Classic Crust, Delight Mozzarella, Large	211
Classic Crust, Delight Mozzarella, Medium	189
Classic Crust, Delight Mozzarella, Personal	148
Classic Crust, Delight Mozzarella, Small	276
Classic Crust, Large	225
Classic Crust, Medium	204
Classic Crust, Personal	159
Classic Crust, Small	283
Italian Style Crust, Delight Mozzarella, Large	263
Italian Style Crust, Delight Mozzarella, Medium	155
Italian Style Crust, Delight Mozzarella, Small	231
Italian Style Crust, Large	225
Italian Style Crust, Medium	167
Italian Style Crust, Small	251
Stuffed Crust, Delight Mozzarella, Large	246
Stuffed Crust, Delight Mozzarella, Medium	222
Stuffed Crust, Large	241
Stuffed Crust, Medium	233
Stuffed Crust, Tabasco, Delight Mozzarella, Large	246
Stuffed Crust, Tabasco, Delight Mozzarella, Medium	227
Stuffed Crust, Tabasco, Large	255
Stuffed Crust, Tabasco, Medium	236
Thin & Crispy, Delight Mozzarella, Large	159
Thin & Crispy, Delight Mozzarella, Medium	151
Thin & Crispy, Large	176
Thin & Crispy, Medium	165

PIZZA - MEATEOR

Classic Crust, Delight Mozzarella, Large	246
Classic Crust, Delight Mozzarella, Medium	220
Classic Crust, Delight Mozzarella, Personal	184
Classic Crust, Delight Mozzarella, Small	294
Classic Crust, Large	249
Classic Crust, Medium	228
Classic Crust, Personal	194
Classic Crust, Small	296
Italian Style Crust, Delight Mozzarella, Large	204
Italian Style Crust, Delight Mozzarella, Medium	213
Italian Style Crust, Delight Mozzarella, Small	248
Italian Style Crust, Large	216
Italian Style Crust, Medium	233
Italian Style Crust, Small	260
Stuffed Crust, Delight Mozzarella, Large	276

DOMINO'S PIZZA

PIZZA - MEATEOR

Stuffed Crust, Delight Mozzarella, Medium	251
Stuffed Crust, Large	288
Stuffed Crust, Medium	266
Stuffed Crust, Tabasco, Delight Mozzarella, Large	280
Stuffed Crust, Tabasco, Delight Mozzarella, Medium	252
Stuffed Crust, Tabasco, Large	291
Stuffed Crust, Tabasco, Medium	261
Thin & Crispy, Delight Mozzarella, Large	182
Thin & Crispy, Delight Mozzarella, Medium	172
Thin & Crispy, Large	193
Thin & Crispy, Medium	179

PIZZA - MEATILICIOUS

Classic Crust, Delight Mozzarella, Large	202
Classic Crust, Delight Mozzarella, Medium	180
Classic Crust, Delight Mozzarella, Personal	155
Classic Crust, Delight Mozzarella, Small	263
Classic Crust, Large	216
Classic Crust, Medium	195
Classic Crust, Personal	166
Classic Crust, Small	271
Italian Style Crust, Delight Mozzarella, Large	166
Italian Style Crust, Delight Mozzarella, Medium	146
Italian Style Crust, Delight Mozzarella, Small	219
Italian Style Crust, Large	179
Italian Style Crust, Medium	158
Italian Style Crust, Small	238
Stuffed Crust, Delight Mozzarella, Large	237
Stuffed Crust, Delight Mozzarella, Medium	213
Stuffed Crust, Large	232
Stuffed Crust, Medium	224
Stuffed Crust, Delight Mozzarella, Large	237
Stuffed Crust, Tabasco, Delight Mozzarella, Medium	218
Stuffed Crust, Tabasco, Large	245
Stuffed Crust, Tabasco, Medium	227
Thin & Crispy, Delight Mozzarella, Large	150
Thin & Crispy, Delight Mozzarella, Medium	142
Thin & Crispy, Large	165
Thin & Crispy, Medium	156

PIZZA - MEATZZA

Classic Crust, Delight Mozzarella, Large	207
Classic Crust, Delight Mozzarella, Medium	185
Classic Crust, Delight Mozzarella, Personal	142
Classic Crust, Delight Mozzarella, Small	270
Classic Crust, Large	221
Classic Crust, Medium	200
Classic Crust, Personal	153
Classic Crust, Small	277
Italian Style Crust, Delight Mozzarella, Large	171
Italian Style Crust, Delight Mozzarella, Medium	151
Italian Style Crust, Delight Mozzarella, Small	225
Italian Style Crust, Large	184
Italian Style Crust, Medium	164

DOMINO'S PIZZA

PIZZA - MEATZZA

	KCAL
Italian Style Crust, Small	244
Stuffed Crust, Delight Mozzarella, Large	241
Stuffed Crust, Delight Mozzarella, Medium	218
Stuffed Crust, Large	236
Stuffed Crust, Medium	230
Stuffed Crust, Tabasco, Large	251
Stuffed Crust, Tabasco, Medium	232
Thin & Crispy, Delight Mozzarella, Large	169
Thin & Crispy, Delight Mozzarella, Medium	158
Thin & Crispy, Large	172
Thin & Crispy, Medium	162

PIZZA - MEXICAN HOT

	KCAL
Classic Crust, Delight Mozzarella, Large	202
Classic Crust, Delight Mozzarella, Medium	179
Classic Crust, Delight Mozzarella, Personal	135
Classic Crust, Delight Mozzarella, Small	257
Classic Crust, Large	219
Classic Crust, Medium	197
Classic Crust, Personal	147
Classic Crust, Small	268
Italian Style Crust, Delight Mozzarella, Large	166
Italian Style Crust, Delight Mozzarella, Medium	145
Italian Style Crust, Delight Mozzarella, Small	212
Ã,Â Italian Style Crust, Large	182
Italian Style Crust, Medium	160
Italian Style Crust, Small	236
Stuffed Crust, Delight Mozzarella, Large	236
Stuffed Crust, Delight Mozzarella, Medium	212
Stuffed Crust, Large	235
Stuffed Crust, Medium	226
Stuffed Crust, Tabasco, Delight Mozzarella, Large	236
Stuffed Crust, Tabasco, Delight Mozzarella, Medium	217
Stuffed Crust, Tabasco, Large	249
Stuffed Crust, Tabasco, Medium	229
Thin & Crispy, Delight Mozzarella, Large	150
Thin & Crispy, Delight Mozzarella, Medium	141
Thin & Crispy, Large	170
Thin & Crispy, Medium	159

PIZZA - MIGHTY MEATY

	KCAL
Classic Crust, Delight Mozzarella, Large	211
Classic Crust, Delight Mozzarella, Medium	188
Classic Crust, Delight Mozzarella, Personal	144
Classic Crust, Delight Mozzarella, Small	273
Classic Crust, Large	224
Classic Crust, Medium	203
Classic Crust, Personal	155
Classic Crust, Small	281
Italian Style Crust, Delight Mozzarella, Large	175
Italian Style Crust, Delight Mozzarella, Medium	154
Italian Style Crust, Delight Mozzarella, Small	228
Italian Style Crust, Large	188
Italian Style Crust, Medium	167

DOMINO'S PIZZA

PIZZA - MIGHTY MEATY

	KCAL
Italian Style Crust, Small	248
Stuffed Crust, Delight Mozzarella, Large	245
Stuffed Crust, Delight Mozzarella, Medium	221
Stuffed Crust, Large	240
Stuffed Crust, Medium	232
Stuffed Crust, Tabasco, Delight Mozzarella, Large	245
Stuffed Crust, Tabasco, Delight Mozzarella, Medium	226
Stuffed Crust, Tabasco, Large	254
Stuffed Crust, Tabasco, Medium	235
Thin & Crispy, Delight Mozzarella, Large	159
Thin & Crispy, Delight Mozzarella, Medium	150
Thin & Crispy, Large	176
Thin & Crispy, Medium	165

PIZZA - MIXED GRILL

	KCAL
Classic Crust, Delight Mozzarella, Large	199
Classic Crust, Delight Mozzarella, Medium	177
Classic Crust, Delight Mozzarella, Personal	145
Classic Crust, Delight Mozzarella, Small	260
Classic Crust, Large	212
Classic Crust, Medium	192
Classic Crust, Personal	156
Classic Crust, Small	267
Italian Style Crust, Delight Mozzarella, Large	163
Italian Style Crust, Delight Mozzarella, Medium	143
Italian Style Crust, Delight Mozzarella, Small	215
Italian Style Crust, Large	176
Italian Style Crust, Medium	156
Italian Style Crust, Small	235
Stuffed Crust, Delight Mozzarella, Large	233
Stuffed Crust, Delight Mozzarella, Medium	210
Stuffed Crust, Large	228
Stuffed Crust, Medium	221
Stuffed Crust, Tabasco, Delight Mozzarella, Large	234
Stuffed Crust, Tabasco, Delight Mozzarella, Medium	215
Stuffed Crust, Tabasco, Large	243
Stuffed Crust, Tabasco, Medium	224
Thin & Crispy, Delight Mozzarella, Large	147
Thin & Crispy, Delight Mozzarella, Medium	139
Thin & Crispy, Large	164
Thin & Crispy, Medium	154

PIZZA - NEW YORKER

	KCAL
Classic Crust, Delight Mozzarella, Large	200
Classic Crust, Delight Mozzarella, Medium	179
Classic Crust, Delight Mozzarella, Personal	142
Classic Crust, Delight Mozzarella, Small	263
Classic Crust, Large	214
Classic Crust, Medium	194
Classic Crust, Personal	152
Classic Crust, Small	270
GF Crust, Delight Mozzarella, Small	232
GF Crust, Small	241
Italian Style Crust, Delight Mozzarella, Large	164

DOMINO'S PIZZA
PIZZA - NEW YORKER

Italian Style Crust, Delight Mozzarella, Medium	145
Italian Style Crust, Delight Mozzarella, Small	218
Italian Style Crust, Large	178
Italian Style Crust, Medium	158
Italian Style Crust, Small	237
Stuffed Crust, Delight Mozzarella, Large	235
Stuffed Crust, Delight Mozzarella, Medium	212
Stuffed Crust, Large	230
Stuffed Crust, Medium	223
Stuffed Crust, Tabasco, Delight Mozzarella, Large	235
Stuffed Crust, Tabasco, Delight Mozzarella, Medium	217
Stuffed Crust, Tabasco, Large	244
Stuffed Crust, Tabasco, Medium	226
Thin & Crispy, Delight Mozzarella, Large	149
Thin & Crispy, Delight Mozzarella, Medium	141
Thin & Crispy, Large	166
Thin & Crispy, Medium	156

PIZZA - PEPPERONI PASSION

Classic Crust, Delight Mozzarella, Large	223
Classic Crust, Delight Mozzarella, Medium	200
Classic Crust, Delight Mozzarella, Personal	157
Classic Crust, Delight Mozzarella, Small	292
Classic Crust, Large	240
Classic Crust, Medium	218
Classic Crust, Personal	169
Classic Crust, Small	303
GF Crust, Delight Mozzarella, Small	261
Italian Style Crust, Delight Mozzarella, Large	187
Italian Style Crust, Delight Mozzarella, Medium	166
Italian Style Crust, Delight Mozzarella, Small	247
Italian Style Crust, Large	203
Italian Style Crust, Medium	182
Italian Style Crust, Small	271
Stuffed Crust, Delight Mozzarella, Large	257
Stuffed Crust, Delight Mozzarella, Medium	233
Stuffed Crust, Large	256
Stuffed Crust, Medium	247
Stuffed Crust, Tabasco, Delight Mozzarella, Large	257
Stuffed Crust, Tabasco, Delight Mozzarella, Medium	238
Stuffed Crust, Tabasco, Large	270
Stuffed Crust, Tabasco, Medium	250
Thin & Crispy, Delight Mozzarella, Large	171
Thin & Crispy, Delight Mozzarella, Medium	162
Thin & Crispy, Large	191
Thin & Crispy, Medium	180

PIZZA - RANCH BBQ

Classic Crust, Delight Mozzarella, Large	241
Classic Crust, Delight Mozzarella, Medium	212
Classic Crust, Delight Mozzarella, Personal	159
Classic Crust, Delight Mozzarella, Small	279
Classic Crust, Large	243
Classic Crust, Medium	220

DOMINO'S PIZZA
PIZZA - RANCH BBQ

Classic Crust, Personal	170
Classic Crust, Small	282
Italian Style Crust, Delight Mozzarella, Large	198
Italian Style Crust, Delight Mozzarella, Medium	205
Italian Style Crust, Delight Mozzarella, Small	233
Italian Style Crust, Large	211
Italian Style Crust, Medium	225
Italian Style Crust, Small	245
Stuffed Crust, Delight Mozzarella, Large	270
Stuffed Crust, Delight Mozzarella, Medium	243
Stuffed Crust, Large	282
Stuffed Crust, Medium	257
Stuffed Crust, Tabasco, Delight Mozzarella, Large	274
Stuffed Crust, Tabasco, Delight Mozzarella, Medium	244
Stuffed Crust, Tabasco, Large	285
Stuffed Crust, Tabasco, Medium	253
Thin & Crispy, Delight Mozzarella, Large	176
Thin & Crispy, Delight Mozzarella, Medium	164
Thin & Crispy, Large	188
Thin & Crispy, Medium	171

PIZZA - SCRUMMY

Classic Crust, Delight Mozzarella, Large	229
Classic Crust, Delight Mozzarella, Medium	205
Classic Crust, Delight Mozzarella, Personal	173
Classic Crust, Delight Mozzarella, Small	299
Classic Crust, Large	242
Classic Crust, Medium	220
Classic Crust, Personal	184
Classic Crust, Small	306
Italian Style Crust, Delight Mozzarella, Large	193
Italian Style Crust, Delight Mozzarella, Medium	172
Italian Style Crust, Delight Mozzarella, Small	254
Italian Style Crust, Large	206
Italian Style Crust, Medium	184
Italian Style Crust, Small	273
Stuffed Crust, Delight Mozzarella, Large	263
Stuffed Crust, Delight Mozzarella, Medium	238
Stuffed Crust, Large	258
Stuffed Crust, Medium	250
Stuffed Crust, Tabasco, Delight Mozzarella, Large	263
Ã,Â Stuffed Crust, Tabasco, Delight Mozzarella, Med	244
Stuffed Crust, Tabasco, Large	272
Stuffed Crust, Tabasco, Medium	252
Thin & Crispy, Delight Mozzarella, Large	177
Thin & Crispy, Delight Mozzarella, Medium	167
Thin & Crispy, Large	194
Thin & Crispy, Medium	182

PIZZA - SIZZLER

Classic Crust, Delight Mozzarella, Large	205
Classic Crust, Delight Mozzarella, Medium	183
Classic Crust, Delight Mozzarella, Personal	140
Classic Crust, Delight Mozzarella, Small	309

DOMINO'S PIZZA
PIZZA - SIZZLER

	KCAL
Classic Crust, Large	220
Classic Crust, Medium	194
Classic Crust, Personal	151
Classic Crust, Small	333
Italian Style Crust, Delight Mozzarella, Large	171
Italian Style Crust, Delight Mozzarella, Medium	153
Italian Style Crust, Delight Mozzarella, Small	211
Italian Style Crust, Large	184
Italian Style Crust, Medium	159
Italian Style Crust, Small	230
Stuffed Crust, Delight Mozzarella, Large	232
Stuffed Crust, Delight Mozzarella, Medium	224
Stuffed Crust, Large	242
Stuffed Crust, Medium	232
Stuffed Crust, Tabasco, Delight Mozzarella, Large	244
Stuffed Crust, Tabasco, Delight Mozzarella, Medium	215
Stuffed Crust, Tabasco, Large	251
Stuffed Crust, Tabasco, Medium	234
Thin & Crispy, Delight Mozzarella, Large	148
Thin & Crispy, Delight Mozzarella, Medium	146
Thin & Crispy, Large	163
Thin & Crispy, Medium	153

PIZZA - TANDOORI HOT

	KCAL
Classic Crust, Delight Mozzarella, Large	171
Classic Crust, Delight Mozzarella, Medium	149
Classic Crust, Delight Mozzarella, Personal	120
Classic Crust, Delight Mozzarella, Small	215
Classic Crust, Large	185
Classic Crust, Medium	164
Classic Crust, Personal	130
Classic Crust, Small	222
Italian Style Crust, Delight Mozzarella, Large	135
Italian Style Crust, Delight Mozzarella, Medium	115
Italian Style Crust, Delight Mozzarella, Small	170
Italian Style Crust, Large	148
Italian Style Crust, Medium	127
Italian Style Crust, Small	189
Ã,Â Stuffed Crust, Delight Mozzarella, Large	205
Stuffed Crust, Delight Mozzarella, Medium	182
Stuffed Crust, Large	200
Stuffed Crust, Medium	193
Stuffed Crust, Tabasco, Delight Mozzarella, Large	205
Stuffed Crust, Tabasco, Delight Mozzarella, Medium	188
Stuffed Crust, Tabasco, Large	214
Stuffed Crust, Tabasco, Medium	204
Thin & Crispy, Delight Mozzarella, Large	119
Thin & Crispy, Delight Mozzarella, Medium	111
Thin & Crispy, Large	136
Thin & Crispy, Medium	126

PIZZA - TANDOORI SIZZLER

	KCAL
Classic Crust, Delight Mozzarella, Large	170
Classic Crust, Delight Mozzarella, Medium	147

DOMINO'S PIZZA
PIZZA - TANDOORI SIZZLER

	KCAL
Classic Crust, Delight Mozzarella, Personal	119
Classic Crust, Delight Mozzarella, Small	213
Classic Crust, Large	183
Classic Crust, Medium	162
Classic Crust, Personal	129
Classic Crust, Small	220
Italian Style Crust, Delight Mozzarella, Large	134
Italian Style Crust, Delight Mozzarella, Medium	114
Italian Style Crust, Delight Mozzarella, Small	168
Italian Style Crust, Large	147
Italian Style Crust, Medium	126
Italian Style Crust, Small	188
Stuffed Crust, Delight Mozzarella, Large	204
Stuffed Crust, Delight Mozzarella, Medium	180
Stuffed Crust, Large	199
Stuffed Crust, Medium	192
Stuffed Crust, Tabasco, Delight Mozzarella, Large	204
Stuffed Crust, Tabasco, Delight Mozzarella, Medium	186
Stuffed Crust, Tabasco, Large	194
Stuffed Crust, Tabasco, Medium	213
Thin & Crispy, Delight Mozzarella, Large	118
Thin & Crispy, Delight Mozzarella, Medium	109
Thin & Crispy, Large	135
Thin & Crispy, Medium	124

PIZZA - TEXAS BBQ

	KCAL
Classic Crust, Delight Mozzarella, Large	208
Texas BBQ, Classic Crust, Delight Mozzarella, Medium	182
Texas BBQ, Classic Crust, Delight Mozzarella, Personal	144
Classic Crust, Delight Mozzarella, Small	236
Classic Crust, Large	211
Classic Crust, Medium	190
Classic Crust, Personal	155
Classic Crust, Small	239
GF Crust, Delight Mozzarella, Small	197
GF Crust, Small	206
Italian Style Crust, Delight Mozzarella, Large	166
Italian Style Crust, Delight Mozzarella, Medium	176
Italian Style Crust, Delight Mozzarella, Small	191
Italian Style Crust, Large	178
Italian Style Crust, Medium	195
Italian Style Crust, Small	202
Stuffed Crust, Delight Mozzarella, Large	238
Stuffed Crust, Delight Mozzarella, Medium	214
Stuffed Crust, Large	250
Stuffed Crust, Medium	228
Stuffed Crust, Tabasco, Delight Mozzarella, Large	242
Stuffed Crust, Tabasco, Delight Mozzarella, Medium	214
Stuffed Crust, Tabasco, Large	253
Stuffed Crust, Tabasco, Medium	223
Thin & Crispy, Delight Mozzarella, Large	144
Thin & Crispy, Delight Mozzarella, Medium	134
Thin & Crispy, Large	156

DOMINO'S PIZZA
PIZZA - THE CHEESEBURGER

	KCAL
Thin & Crispy, Medium	142
Classic Crust, Delight Mozzarella, Large	197
Classic Crust, Delight Mozzarella, Medium	173
Classic Crust, Delight Mozzarella, Personal	137
Classic Crust, Delight Mozzarella, Small	248
Classic Crust, Large	211
Classic Crust, Medium	188
Classic Crust, Personal	146
Classic Crust, Small	255
Italian Style Crust, Delight Mozzarella, Large	161
Italian Style Crust, Delight Mozzarella, Medium	139
Italian Style Crust, Delight Mozzarella, Small	203
Italian Style Crust, Large	175
Italian Style Crust, Medium	151
Italian Style Crust, Small	223
Stuffed Crust, Delight Mozzarella, Large	232
Stuffed Crust, Delight Mozzarella, Medium	206
Stuffed Crust, Large	227
Stuffed Crust, Medium	217
Stuffed Crust, Tabasco, Delight Mozzarella, Large	232
Stuffed Crust, Tabasco, Delight Mozzarella, Medium	211
Stuffed Crust,Tabasco, Large	241
Stuffed Crust, Tabasco, Medium	220
Thin & Crispy, Delight, Medium	134
Thin & Crispy, Delight Mozzarella, Large	146
Thin & Crispy, Large	163
Thin & Crispy, Medium	149

PIZZA - TUNA SUPREME

	KCAL
Classic Crust, Delight Mozzarella, Large	177
Classic Crust, Delight Mozzarella, Medium	152
Classic Crust, Delight Mozzarella, Personal	123
Classic Crust, Delight Mozzarella, Small	221
Classic Crust, Large	191
Classic Crust, Medium	167
Classic Crust, Personal	134
Classic Crust, Small	228
Italian Style Crust, Delight Mozzarella, Large	141
Italian Style Crust, Delight Mozzarella, Medium	119
Italian Style Crust, Delight Mozzarella, Small	176
Italian Style Crust, Large	154
Italian Style Crust, Medium	131
Stuffed Crust, Delight Mozzarella, Large	212
Stuffed Crust, Delight Mozzarella, Medium	185
Stuffed Crust, Large	206
Stuffed Crust, Medium	197
Stuffed Crust, Tabasco, Delight Mozzarella, Large	212
Stuffed Crust, Tabasco, Delight Mozzarella, Medium	191
Stuffed Crust, Tabasco, Large	220
Stuffed Crust, Tabasco, Medium	199
Thin & Crispy, Delight Mozzarella, Large	125
Thin & Crispy, Delight Mozzarella, Medium	114
Thin & Crispy, Large	142

DOMINO'S PIZZA
PIZZA - ULTIMATE BACON CHEESEBURGER

	KCAL
Thin & Crispy, Medium	129
Classic Crust, Delight Mozzarella, Large	217
Classic Crust, Delight Mozzarella, Medium	193
Classic Crust, Delight Mozzarella, Personal	156
Classic Crust, Delight Mozzarella, Small	278
Classic Crust, Large	231
Classic Crust, Medium	207
Classic Crust, Personal	167
Classic Crust, Small	285
Italian Style Crust, Delight Mozzarella, Large	181
Italian Style Crust, Delight Mozzarella, Medium	159
Italian Style Crust, Delight Mozzarella, Small	233
Italian Style Crust, Large	195
Italian Style Crust, Medium	171
Italian Style Crust, Small	253
Stuffed Crust, Delight Mozzarella, Large	262
Stuffed Crust, Delight Mozzarella, Medium	226
Stuffed Crust, Large	269
Stuffed Crust, Medium	237
Stuffed Crust, Tabasco, Delight Mozzarella, Large	252
Stuffed Crust, Tabasco, Delight Mozzarella, Medium	231
Stuffed Crust, Tabasco, Large	264
Stuffed Crust, Tabasco, Medium	240
Thin & Crispy, Delight Mozzarella, Large	165
Thin & Crispy, Delight Mozzarella, Medium	155
Thin & Crispy, Large	193
Thin & Crispy, Medium	169

PIZZA - VEG-A-ROMA

	KCAL
Classic Crust, Delight Mozzarella, Large	174
Classic Crust, Delight Mozzarella, Medium	153
Classic Crust, Delight Mozzarella, Personal	124
Classic Crust, Delight Mozzarella, Small	265
Classic Crust, Large	190
Classic Crust, Medium	164
Classic Crust, Personal	135
Classic Crust, Small	289
Italian Style Crust, Delight Mozzarella, Large	140
Italian Style Crust, Delight Mozzarella, Medium	123
Italian Style Crust, Delight Mozzarella, Small	166
Italian Style Crust, Large	153
Italian Style Crust, Medium	129
Italian Style Crust, Small	186
Stuffed Crust, Delight Mozzarella, Large	201
Stuffed Crust, Delight Mozzarella, Medium	194
Stuffed Crust, Large	211
Stuffed Crust, Medium	201
Stuffed Crust, Tabasco, Delight Mozzarella, Large	213
Stuffed Crust, Tabasco, Delight Mozzarella, Medium	185
Stuffed Crust, Tabasco, Large	220
Stuffed Crust, Tabasco, Medium	203
Thin & Crispy, Delight Mozzarella, Large	118
Thin & Crispy, Large	132

DOMINO'S PIZZA
PIZZA - VEGI CLASSIC

Thin & Crispy, Medium	123
Classic Crust, Delight Mozzarella, Large	162
Classic Crust, Delight Mozzarella, Medium	140
Classic Crust, Delight Mozzarella, Personal	114
Classic Crust, Delight Mozzarella, Small	203
Classic Crust, Large	176
Classic Crust, Medium	155
Classic Crust, Personal	124
Classic Crust, Small	210
Italian Style Crust, Delight Mozzarella, Large	126
Italian Style Crust, Delight Mozzarella, Medium	107
Italian Style Crust, Delight Mozzarella, Small	158
Italian Style Crust, Large	139
Italian Style Crust, Medium	119
Italian Style Crust, Small	178
Stuffed Crust, Delight Mozzarella, Large	196
Stuffed Crust, Delight Mozzarella, Medium	173
Stuffed Crust, Large	191
Stuffed Crust, Medium	185
Stuffed Crust, Tabasco, Delight Mozzarella, Large	205
Stuffed Crust, Tabasco, Delight Mozzarella, Medium	179
Stuffed Crust, Tabasco, Large	205
Stuffed Crust, Tabasco, Medium	187
Thin & Crispy, Delight Mozzarella, Large	110
Thin & Crispy, Delight Mozzarella, Medium	102
Thin & Crispy, Large	127
Thin & Crispy, Medium	117

PIZZA - VEGI SIZZLER

Classic Crust, Delight Mozzarella, Large	161
Classic Crust, Delight Mozzarella, Medium	140
Classic Crust, Delight Mozzarella, Personal	114
Classic Crust, Delight Mozzarella, Small	202
Classic Crust, Large	175
Classic Crust, Medium	154
Classic Crust, Personal	124
Classic Crust, Small	210
Italian Style Crust, Delight Mozzarella, Large	125
Italian Style Crust, Delight Mozzarella, Medium	106
Italian Style Crust, Delight Mozzarella, Small	158
Italian Style Crust, Large	138
Italian Style Crust, Medium	118
Stuffed Crust, Delight Mozzarella, Large	173
Stuffed Crust, Delight Mozzarella, Medium	173
Stuffed Crust, Large	190
Stuffed Crust, Medium	184
Stuffed Crust, Tabasco, Delight Mozzarella, Large	195
Stuffed Crust, Tabasco, Delight Mozzarella, Medium	178
Stuffed Crust, Tabasco, Large	204
Stuffed Crust, Tabasco, Medium	187
Thin & Crispy, Delight Mozzarella, Large	109
Thin & Crispy, Delight Mozzarella, Medium	102
Thin & Crispy, Large	126

DOMINO'S PIZZA
PIZZA - VEGI SUPEREME

Thin & Crispy, Medium	116
Thin & Crispy, Medium	122
Classic Crust, Delight Mozzarella, Large	165
Classic Crust, Delight Mozzarella, Medium	144
Classic Crust, Delight Mozzarella, Personal	116
Classic Crust, Delight Mozzarella, Small	208
Classic Crust, Large	179
Classic Crust, Medium	159
Classic Crust, Personal	127
Classic Crust, Small	215
GF Crust, Delight Mozzarella, Small	177
GF Crust, Small	186
Italian Style Crust, Delight Mozzarella, Large	129
Italian Style Crust, Delight Mozzarella, Medium	110
Italian Style Crust, Delight Mozzarella, Small	163
Italian Style Crust, Large	143
Italian Style Crust, Medium	122
Italian Style Crust, Small	183
Stuffed Crust, Delight Mozzarella, Large	200
Stuffed Crust, Delight Mozzarella, Medium	177
Stuffed Crust, Large	195
Stuffed Crust, Medium	188
Stuffed Crust, Tabasco, Delight Mozzarella, Large	200
Stuffed Crust, Tabasco, Delight Mozzarella, Medium	182
Stuffed Crust, Tabasco, Large	209
Stuffed Crust, Tabasco, Medium	191
Thin & Crispy, Delight Mozzarella, Large	114
Thin & Crispy, Delight Mozzarella, Medium	106
Thin & Crispy, Large	131

PIZZA - VEGI VOCLANO

Classic Crust, Delight Mozzarella, Medium	165
Stuffed Crust, Delight Mozzarella, Large	215
Classic Crust, Delight Mozzarella, Large	188
Classic Crust, Delight Mozzarella, Personal	130
Classic Crust, Delight Mozzarella, Small	247
Classic Crust, Large	207
Classic Crust, Medium	179
Classic Crust, Personal	143
Classic Crust, Small	307
Italian Style Crust, Delight Mozzarella, Large	154
Italian Style Crust, Delight Mozzarella, Medium	135
Italian Style Crust, Delight Mozzarella, Small	180
Italian Style Crust, Large	170
Italian Style Crust, Medium	144
Italian Style Crust, Small	203
Stuffed Crust, Delight Mozzarella, Medium	206
Stuffed Crust, Large	228
Stuffed Crust, Medium	216
Stuffed Crust, Tabasco, Delight Mozzarella, Large	214
Stuffed Crust, Tabasco, Delight Mozzarella, Medium	197
Stuffed Crust, Tabasco, Large	248
Stuffed Crust, Tabasco, Medium	218

DOMINO'S PIZZA

PIZZA - VEGI VOCLANO

	KCAL
Thin & Crispy, Delight Mozzarella, Large	131
Thin & Crispy, Delight Mozzarella, Medium	128
Thin & Crispy, Large	149
Thin & Crispy, Medium	138

POTATO WEDGES

Portion	169

WRAP

Chicken, & Bacon, Wrapzz	403
Meatball Feast, Wrapzz	526
Pepperoni Passion, Wrapzz	453
Tandoori Hot, Wrapzz	332
Texas BBQ, Wrapzz	417
Vegi Supreme, Wrapzz	301

EAT

BAGEL

	KCAL
Smoked Salmon & Cream Cheese	444

BAGUETTE

Bacon, Crispy, & Egg, Free Range	457
Brie, & Tomato	455
Cheddar, Mature, & Tomato Chutney, Malted Wheat	591
Chicken, Bacon & Avocado	504
Chicken, Herb, & Avocado, on Malted Wheat	495
Egg, Free Range, & Tomato	382
Ham, & Jarlsberg	527
Ham, & Jarlsberg, on Malted Wheat	500
Ham, Brie, & Tomato Chutney	557
Mozzarella, Pesto & Tomato	535
Salmon, Smoked, & Avocado	333
Tuna, & Cucumber	531

BARS

Fruit & Nut, Honey Toasted	195

BEANS

Edamame, Red Pepper, Spring Onion, & Coriander	8

BREAD

Banana	354

BREAKFAST

BBQ Beans, Poached Egg, & Ham Hock, Pot	414
BBQ Beans, Poached Egg, Avocado, & Feta, Pot	478
Honey, & Banana, Topping	60
Honey, Topping	43
Mango, & Coconut, Chia, Pot	188
Poached Egg, & Spinach, Omega	211

BREAKFAST CEREAL

Muesli, Apple, & Berry, Bircher	343
Porridge, Classic	180
Porridge, Quinoa, & Coconut	164

BROWNIES

Chocolate, Belgian	318

CAKE

Caramel, Carrot, & Pecan	454
Carrot	491
Chocolate, Belgian, Loaf	351
Coffee	528
Lemon, & Poppyseed, Loaf	298
Red Velvet	263

CHICKEN

Katsu, Fusion Bowl	434
Pho Ga, Fusion Bowl	423

CHOCOLATE

Caramel, Crispie	267

COFFEE

Americano	15
Americano, Iced	7
Black, Filter	1
Cappuccino	130
Chocolate Frappe, Iced	436
Cortado	88

EAT

COFFEE
Espresso	13
Flat White	122
Frappe, Iced	311
Latte	173
Latte, Iced	143
Macchiato	20
Mocha	246
Mocha Frappe, Iced	275

COOKIES
Chocolate, Triple	394
Oat, & Fruit	329

CORN
& Chickpeas, Chilli, Roasted	162

CRISPS
Cheddar & Onion	208
Sea Salt & Vinegar	209
Sea Salted	208
Thai Sweet Chilli	208

CROISSANT
All Butter	347
Almond	365
Chocolate, Almond, & Hazelnut	380
Ham, & Jarlsberg Cheese	460

DESSERT
Bakewell, Slice	466

DOUGHNUTS
Jam, Mini	170

DUMPLINGS
Gyoza, Duck, Hoisin, Fusion Bowl	682
Gyoza, Vegetable, Fusion Bowl	522

FLAPJACK
Jewelled	296

FLATBREAD
Chicken, Firecracker	436

FRUIT & NUTS
Chocolate	213

FRUIT COMPOTE
Summer Berries	14

FRUIT DRINK
Mango, & Lime, Crush, Iced	254
Summer Berry, Blitz	306

FUDGE
Scottish, Handmade	194

HOT CHOCOLATE
Portion	317

HOT POT
Beef Bourguignon	379
Chicken, Balti	383
Chicken, Panang	509
Chicken, Pulled, with Quinoa, & Lentils, Mexican	421
Chilli, Bean, Spicy & Smoky	319
Chilli, Taxan	386

EAT

HOT POT
Classic Mac	728
Mac 'N' Cheese	752
Mac 'N' Cheese, Ham Hock, & Mushroom	766
Mac 'N' Cheese, Kids	232
The Yorkie	706
Turkey, Curry	451

HOUMOUS
& Crudites, Pot	246

MANGO
Dried	82

MUFFIN
Berry, & Granola	450
Chocolate, Double	472

NUTS
Natural, Mix	222

PAIN AU RAISIN
Portion	383

PASTA
Pesto, Ultimate	958

PASTRY
Puff, Lid, for Soup	118

PEANUTS
Honey Coated, with Chilli	210

PIE
Cauliflower Cheese, & Kale, Pie Only	683
Cauliflower Cheese, & Kale, with Mash, & Gravy	932
Chicken, & Mushroom, Pie Only	598
Chicken, & Mushroom, with Mash, & Gravy	848
Steak, & Ale, Pie Only	560
Steak, & Ale, with Mash, & Gravy	811

PIZZA
Chicken, Grill	530

RAISINS
Yoghurt Coated	212

RICE CAKES
Chocolate, Dark, Belgian, Mini	120

ROLL
Bacon, British Back	390
Bacon, Poached Egg, British Back	376
Mushroom, & Poached Egg	320
Sausage, & Caramelised Onion	626

SALAD
Aubergine, Feta, & Tahini Grains	682
Chicken, & Avocado	479
Chicken, Mexican, Guacamole, & Quinoa	507
Chicken, Noodle, Spicy	399
Chicken, Satay, & Broccoli, Chargrilled, Protein Pot	298
Crayfish, Spicy, Noodles	352
Egg, Free Range, & Spinach, Protein Pot	137
Falafel, Quinoa, & Tahini, Protein Pot	346
Ham Hock, & Egg, Free Range	342
Houmous, & Falafel, Mezze	493

EAT

SALAD

Mackerel, Smoked, & Turmeric, Protein Pot	347
Salmon, Hot Smoked, Sesame	494
Salmon, Smoked, & Egg, Protein Pot	167

SANDWICH

American Melt, Grilled	586
BLT	493
Cheese, & Onion	381
Cheese, Kids	445
Cheese, Marmite, Morning Melt	424
Chicken, & Bacon, on Malted Bread	543
Chicken, Pork, Sage & Onion, Bloomer	585
Chicken, Roast, Salad, on Malted Bread	348
Chicken, Smoked, & Basil, on Stonebaked Ciabatta	458
Egg Mayonnaise, Chunky, Free Range, Malted Bread	452
Ham, & Egg, Free Range	567
Ham, & Mature Cheddar	475
Ham, & Piccalilli	560
Mushroom Melt, Grilled	500
Pastrami, New York, on Multiseed Bloomer	527
Ploughmans, Cheddar, Classic, Multiseed Bloomer	303
Prawn, Mayonnaise, & Cucumber, on Rye	447
Salmon, Smoked, & Soft Cheese, Malted Bread	352
Tuna, Mayonnaise, & Cucumber	437

SHORTBREAD

Millionaires	316

SOUP

Bean, 3, Smoked Chilli, & Tomato	183
Beef, Rendang, Malaysian	261
Broth, Shot	33
Butternut Squash, Sage, & Barley, Risotto	277
Butternut Squash, Thai	168
Chicken, & Garden Vegetable, Sm	123
Chicken, Chipotle, & Black Bean	186
Chicken, Ham, & Sweetcorn, Chowder	359
Chicken, Jerk	282
Chicken, Laksa	234
Chicken, Mushroom, & Barley	216
Chicken, Pot Pie, no Pastry	341
Chicken, Sweet Potato, & Spinach	236
Chicken, Thai Green Curry	241
Chicken Noodle, Coconut	317
Goulash, Hungarian	201
Lentil, Spiced, Spinach, & Sweet Potato	210
Meatball, Italian	232
Mushroom, Wild, & Chestnut, Sm	240
Red Pepper, & Goats Cheese, Fire Roasted	141
Sweet Potato, Chilli, & Mascarpone	261
Sweetcorn, Creamy	315
Tomato, & Basil	78
Tomato, Slow Roasted, Creamy	240
Vegetable, Moroccan, Spicy	138

EAT

TART

Pastel De Nata	220

TEA

Breakfast	2
Camomile	2
Chai Latte	243
Decaf	2
Matcha Latte	197

TOAST

Mozzarella, Tomato, & Pesto, Stonebaked Ciabatta	471
Sourdough, with Butter	180

TOASTIE

Ham, Cheese, & Dijon Mustard, Stonebaked Ciabatta	511
Tuna, & Cheddar Melt, on Ciabatta Bread	617

WRAP

Chana Gobi	574
Chicken, Satay	508
Duck, Hoisin	466
Halloumi, Chickpea, & Spinach, Spiced	535
Houmous, & Falafel	478
Sausage, & Egg, Scrambled	789

YOGHURT

Banana, Honey, & Grape Nuts	290
Skyr, with Granola, & Berry Compote	317
with Berry Compote	88

FARMHOUSE INNS

BACON
Cheese, & BBQ Sauce, Hunters, Steak Topper	440
Extra	106

BEANS
BBQ, Combo Feast	127
Extra	129

BEEF
Steak, Rib-eye, 9oz, Naked	771
Steak, Rib-eye, 9oz, with Sides	1597
Steak, Rump, 4oz, Extra	144
Steak, Rump, 8oz, Naked	415
Steak, Rump, 8oz, with Sides	1241
Steak, Sirloin, 8oz, Naked	474
Steak, Sirloin, 8oz, with Sides	1300

BHAJI
Onion, Extra	361

BREAD
Ciabatta, Garlic, Cheesy	655
Ciabatta, Garlic, Sides	450
Garlic, Combo Feast	225
Malted, & Butter, Sides	337
White, & Butter, Sides	374

BREAKFAST
All Day, with Malted Bread	1696
All Day, with White Bread	1733

BURGERS - BEEF
Patty Only, Extra	357

BURGERS - BEEF - SIGNATURE CARVERY
Double Up, with Chips, & Coleslaw	2118
with Chips, & Coleslaw	1761

BURGERS - BEEF, FARMHOUSE BBQ
Mac Stack, Double Up, with Chips, & Coleslaw	2307
Mac Stack, with Chips, & Coleslaw	1950

BURGERS - BEEF, GIANT
The Farm, with Chips, & Coleslaw	2252

BURGERS - CHEESEBURGER
Double Up, with Chips, & Coleslaw	1751
Smoked Bacon, Double Up, with Chips, & Coleslaw	1816
Smoked Bacon, with Chips, & Coleslaw	1459
with Chips, & Coleslaw	1394

BURGERS - CHICKEN
Bombay Bird, Double Up, with Chips, & Coleslaw	2481
Bombay Bird, with Chips, & Coleslaw	2121
Dirty Hunters, Double Up, with Chips, & Coleslaw	2071
Dirty Hunters, with Chips, & Coleslaw	1749
Tex Mex, Double Up, with Chips, & Coleslaw	2192
Tex Mex, with Chips, & Coleslaw	1870

BURGERS - CHICKPEA & RED PEPPER
with Chips, & Coleslaw	1366
Double Up, with Chips, & Coleslaw	1550

CHEESE
Extra	165
Parmigiana, Topper	151

FARMHOUSE INNS

CHICKEN
Breast, Curried, Skewer	1092
Breast, Extra	89
Breast, Kebab, Skewer, Combo Feast	189
Breast, Kebab, Skewer, Extra	189
Fillets, Roast, Combo Feast	179
Goujons, Southern Fried, with BBQ Dip	596
Hunters	1401
Medley, Crispy, no Sauce	1739
Smothered	1850
Southern Fried, Curried, Skewer	1325
Southern Fried, Extra	322
Southern Fried, Skewer, Combo Feast	422
Southern Fried, Skewer, Extra	422
Strips, Fully Loaded	1601
Strips, Louisiana, Combo Feast	280
Wings, Combo Feast	538
Wings, no Sauce	1015

CHIPS
Combo Feast	655
Curry Sauce, Topped, Side	796
Hunters, Topped, Side	1023
Side	655

COD
Beer Battered, with Chips, & Garden Peas, Large	1685
Beer Battered, with Chips, & Mushy Peas, Large	1736

COLESLAW
Combo Feast	306
Sides	205

CORN
Cob, Side	161

EGGS
Fried, Extra	120

FISH
Atlantic, Beer Battered, with Chips, & Mushy Peas	1817
Atlantic, Beer Battered, with Chips, & Peas	1766

FISH & CHIPS
Chip Shop Supper	2330

GAMMON
Steak, 4oz, Extra	198
Steaks, Naked	486
Steaks, Naked, with Egg, & Pineapple	672
Steaks, Naked, with Fried Egg	726
Steaks, Naked, with Pineapple	618
Steaks, with Chips, & Peas	1302

GRAVY
Extra	42

GRILLS
Mixed, Farmhouse	2202

GUACAMOLE
Portion	93

HAM
Hand Carved, & Eggs, with Chips, & Peas	1126

FARMHOUSE INNS

HASH BROWNS
Extra	78

LAMB
Shank, Minted, with Mash, & Veg	1213

LASAGNE
Beef, Naked	584
Beef, with Chips, & Garlic Bread	1381

MACARONI CHEESE
Combo Feast	232
Luxury	778

MAYONNAISE
Garlic	190

MUSHROOMS
Button, Breaded, Garlic, with Garlic Mayonnaise	655
Button, Sides	283

NACHOS
Cheesy, Big	888

ONION RINGS
Combo Feast	327
Sides	654

PATE
Chicken, Liver, with Bread, Onion Chutney, & Salad	474

PEAS
Garden, Chip Shop Supper	56
Mushy, Chip Shop Supper	107

PIE
Beef, & Ale, Slow Cooked	1184
Beef, & Ale, Slow Cooked, with Chips	1839
Beef, & Ale, Slow Cooked, with Mashed Potato	1436
Chicken, & Mushroom, No Sides	1215
Chicken, & Mushroom, with Chips	1870
Chicken, & Mushroom, with Mashes Potato	1467

PLATTER
Chicken, Sharer	2459

POTATOES
Jacket, with Baked Beans	431
Jacket, with Cheese, & Baked Beans	510
Jacket, with Mozzarella, & Cheddar Cheese	424
Jacket, with Tuna Mayonnaise	483

RIBS
Rack, Mini, Extra	204

SALAD
Chicken, & Bacon, Hot	884
Chicken, Skewer	467
Side, Combo Feast	45
Side	45

SALMON
Fillet, Scottish, Grilled	431
Fillet, Scottish, Grilled, with Hollandaise Sauce	538

SALSA
Portion	56

SANDWICH
Carvery, Bap	1149

FARMHOUSE INNS

SANDWICH
Cheese, & Chutney, Ciabatta Roll	1042
Cheese, & Chutney, Floured Bap	1027
Chicken, Bacon, & Tomato, Melt, Ciabatta Roll	1180
Chicken, Bacon, & Tomato, Melt, Floured Bap	1165
Chicken, Goujons, & Mayonnaise, Ciabatta Roll	1318
Chicken, Goujons, & Mayonnaise, Floured Bap	1303
Chicken, Hunters, Melt, Ciabatta Roll	1170
Chicken, Hunters, Melt, Floured Bap	1155
Fish Fingers, & Tartare Sauce, Ciabatta Roll	1148
Fish Fingers, & Tartare Sauce, Floured Bap	1133
Tuna Melt, Ciabatta Roll	989
Tuna Melt, Floured Bap	974

SAUCE
BBQ, Texan	144
BBQ, Texan, for Chicken Wings	72
Char Sui, Combo Feast	195
Char Sui, for Chicken Wings	130
Curry, Chip Shop Supper	141
Diane	425
Peppercorn	101
Piri Piri, Combo Feast	30
Piri Piri	40
Piri Piri, for Chicken Wings	20
Sour Cream	165
Sweet Chilli, Combo Feast	98
Sweet Chilli	131
Texan BBQ, Combo Feast	108

SAUSAGE
Extra	181
Pigs in Portionet, Extra	209

SAUSAGE & MASH
Portion	1447

SCAMPI
Wholetail, Breaded	1251
Wholetail, Breaded, Naked	550

TART
Vegetable, no Sides	483
Vegetable, with Chips	1138
Vegetable, with Mashed Potato	735

TIKKA MASALA
Chicken, no Sides	1100
Chicken, with Chips	1755
Chicken, with Pilau Rice, & Chips	1699
Chicken, with Pilau Rice	1534

YORKSHIRE PUDDING
& Pigs in Portionet, Extra	309
Extra	100
Giant, Extra	490
Wrap, All The Meats, Giant	1604
Wrap, Beef, & Horseradish, Giant	1684
Wrap, Turkey, & Cranberry, Giant	1611

GOURMET BURGER KITCHEN

BITES
Falafel	343

BURGERS
Beef, Avocado, & Bacon	2825
Beef, Cheese, & Bacon, with American Cheese	942
Beef, Classic	692
Beef, Classic, Small	533
Beef, Major Tom	922
Beef, Taxidriver	875
Californian, Vegan	503
Chicken, Chick Chick Boom, Panko	638
Chicken, Classic	445
Chicken, Classic, Panko	627
Chicken, Classic, Small	360
Chicken, Hey Pesto, Panko	1076
Chicken, Satay	552
Chicken, Satay, Panko	795
Falafel, Vegetarian	508
Lamb, Classic	578
Lamb, Lamburghini	644
Special, Jumpin Jack	642
Veggie, Classic, with Cheddar, Small	488
Veggie, Jack-in-a-Bun	465

BURGERS VEGETARIAN
Classic	513
Classic, Small	406
Classic, with American Cheese	635
Classic, with American Cheese, Small	468
Classic, with Cheddar	676
Classic, with Smoked Applewood	676
Classic, with Smoked Applewood, Small	489

CHEESE
Vegan, Extra	95

CHICKEN
Wings, Spicy	696

COFFEE
Americano	56
Cappuccino	122
Flat White	118
Latte	118

DRINK
Elderflower, Fizz	81
Ginger & Lemongrass, Fizz	82
Rhubarb & Vanilla, Fizz	83
Strawberry & Elderflower, Fizz	82

FRIES
Chunky, Small, Junior	429
Skinny, Small, Junior	454

LEMONADE
Cloudy	84

MILK SHAKE
Banana	627
Cheesecake, Strawberry & Oreo	815

GOURMET BURGER KITCHEN

PEPPERS
Jalapeno, Extras	22

SALAD
Caesar	267
Simple	83

SAUCE
Mayo, Beetroot, Vegan	146
Mayo, Harissa, Vegan	236

GREGGS
BAGUETTE
	KCAL
Bacon, & Egg, Omelette, Free Range, Hot	557
Bacon, & Sausage, Hot	600
Bacon, Hot	511
Bean, Mexican	387
Beef, & Mustard	440
Cheese, Cheddar, Mature, & Salad	482
Chicken, Mexican	529
Chicken, Peri Peri, Hot, Greggs*	514
Chicken, Roast, & Bacon, Club	501
Chicken, Southern Fried, Hot	604
Chicken, Tandoori	513
Chicken Mayonnaise, Roast	502
Ham, & Cheese	530
Ham, & Salad	442
Ham, Honey Roast, & Chicken Melt, Hot	541
Omelette, Hot	518
Sausage, & Egg, Omelette, Free Range, Hot	627
Sausage, Hot	602
Sausage, Lorne, & Bacon	647
Sausage, Lorne, & Omelette	695
Sausage, Lorne	694
Steak, Chipotle Chilli	494
Tuna, & Sweetcorn	465
Tuna, Crunch	458

BAKE
Beef, Corned	409
Cheese, & Onion	437
Chicken, & Pepperoni, Spicy	458
Chicken	422
Potato, & Meat	440
Raspberry, & Almond	70
Sausage, Bean, & Cheese	453
Steak	408
Vegetable	424

BISCUITS
Empire	280
Gingerbread, Man	173
Jammy Heart	282
Shortbread, Caramel	293
Shortbread, Chocolate, Chunks	161
Shortbread, White Chocolate, & Lemon	155

BREAD
Baguette	320
Brown, Bloomer	273
Brown, Malted	117
Rolls, Corn Topped	201
Rolls, Seeded, Oval Bite	314
Rolls, Whtite, Floured	197
Stottie, Cheese, & Onion	507
Stottie	157
Stottie, Tuna Mayonnaise	462
White, Bloomer, Loaf	122

GREGGS
BREAKFAST
	KCAL
Beans, Omelette, & Hash Browns, Veggie Box	327
Beans, Omelette, Sausages, & Hash Browns, Box	357

BREAKFAST CEREAL
Porridge, Apple, & Cinnamon, GF	232
Porridge, Creamy Oats, Simply, GF	210
Porridge, Creamy Oats, Simply	311
Porridge, Golden Syrup, GF	244
Porridge, Golden Syrup	270

BROWNIES
Chocolate, Triple, GF	97

BUNS
Belgian	393
Cinnamon	375
Iced, Finger	258
Iced, Split	367
Ring, Novelty	213

CAKE
Chocolate, Bar	359
Fondant Fancy	265
Pineapple	265
Raspberry, & Almond, Bake	63
Tottenham	346
Welsh	178

CHEESECAKE
London	449

CHERRYADE
Sparkling, No Added Sugar	20

CHICKEN
Bites, Spicy BBQ	267
Butter, Bake	316
Goujons, Southern Fried	394

COFFEE
Americano, Large	11
Americano, Reg	9
Americano, Soya Milk, Large	20
Americano, Soya Milk, Reg	19
Black, Decaf, Large	24
Black, Decaf, Reg	6
Black, Decaf, Soya Milk, Large	16
Black, Decaf, Soya Milk, Reg	16
Cappuccino, Large	111
Cappuccino, Reg	94
Espresso, Double	11
Espresso, Shot	8
Latte, Caramel, Iced, Reg	170
Latte, Caramel, Large	248
Latte, Caramel, Reg	223
Latte, Iced, Reg	111
Latte, Large	133
Latte, Pumpkin Spice, Large	253
Latte, Pumpkin Spice, Reg	228

GREGGS

COFFEE

Latte, Reg	114
Latte, Vanilla, Iced, Reg	170
Latte Vanilla, Large	248
Latte Vanilla, Reg	223
Mocha, Large	296
Mocha, Reg	233
White, Decaf, Large	24
White, Decaf, Reg	19
White, Flat	71
White, Large	45
White, Reg	34

COOKIES

Chocolate, Chunk, Triple	346
Chocolate, Milk	357
Chocolate, White	359

CRISPS

Cheese Puffs	201
Mature Cheddar & Onion	198
Salt & Vinegar, Crunchy Sticks	175
Sea Salt, & Cider Vinegar	194
Sea Salt	201
Thai Sweet Chilli	203
Tortilla, Chilli	193

CROISSANT

All Butter	306
Almond	332

DOUGHNUTS

Caramel Custard	325
Chocolate, & Vanilla, Triple	382
Chocolate, Milk, Ring	240
Chocolate, Triple	341
Coconut, Cream, Finger	390
Cream, Finger	369
Devon	239
Glazed, Ring	202
Iced, Ring	237
Jam	245
Mini	63
Pink, Jammie	323
Sugar Strand	237
Vanilla	305
Yum Yum	301
Yum Yum, Mini	131

DRINK

Mango, & Pineapple, Sparkling, No Added Sugar	15

ECLAIR

with Cream Filling	344

FRUIT

Medley	82
Tropical, Pot	72

GRAPES

Mixed	99

GREGGS

HOT CHOCOLATE

Large	281
Reg	219

JUICE

Apple, Fairtrade	70
Orange, Fairtrade	69

LEMONADE

Cloudy, Sparkling	15
Raspberry, Sparkling	10

MACARONI CHEESE

Portion	516

MUFFIN

Chocolate, Triple	462
Sticky Toffee	381

NUTS

Naked, Mixed	157

PAIN AU CHOCOLAT

Portion	312

PASTA SALAD

Chicken, & Bacon	450
Feta, & Slow Roasted Tomato	380
Tuna, Crunch	378

PASTY

Beef, & Vegetable	459
Steak, & Cheese, Roll	342

PIE

Mince, Savoury	417
Mince, Sweet	281
Scotch	367

PIZZA

Cheese, Three	552
Pepperoni, Three Cheese	617

POPCORN

Sweet & Salty, Greggs*	118

POTATO WEDGES

Southern Fried	278

PUDDING

Bread	374

RAISINS

Chocolate, & Yoghurt, Mix	128

ROLL

Bacon, & Sausage, Lorne	483
Bacon, & Egg, Omelette, Free Range, Hot	395
Bacon, & Sausage, Hot	438
Bacon, Hot	348
Cheese, & Onion, Salad, Sub	444
Cheese, Sub	216
Chicken, Roast, & Salad, Sub	351
Chicken, Tandoori, Sub	361
Ham	171
Ham, Honey Roast, & Egg Salad, Sub	338
Omelette, & Sausage, Lorne	487
Omelette, Hot	398

GREGGS

ROLL

Sausage, & Egg, Omelette, Free Range	441
Sausage, Hot	416
Sausage, Lorne	395
Tuna Mayonnaise, Sub	342

SALAD

Feta, Roast Vegetables, Mixed Grains, & Beetroot Dip	0

SANDWICH

Beef, & Tomato	334
BLT	400
Cheese, & Pickle	410
Cheese, & Tomato	395
Cheese, & Onion, Malted Brown Bread	370
Chicken, & Bacon	488
Chicken, Chargrill, Oval Bite	442
Chicken, Mexican	361
Chicken, Mexican, Oval Bite	491
Chicken, Red Thai, Bloomer	464
Chicken, Roast, & Salad	362
Egg Mayonnaise, & Tomato	387
Egg Mayonnaise, Free Range, Malted Brown Bread	371
Egg Salad, Free Range	329
Ham, Cheese, & Pickle, on Malted Bread	449
Ploughmans, Cheddar Cheese, Mature, Oval Bite	502
Tuna, & Sweetcorn	345
Tuna, Crunch, Bloomer	439
Tuna Mayonnaise, & Cucumber, Malted Brown Bread	353

SAUSAGE ROLL

Freshly Baked	328
Vegan	312

SCONE

Bran	194
Cheese	343
Fruit	297

SLICES

Bavarian	389
Custard, Vanilla	332

SNACKS

BBQ, Smoky, Crunch	104

SOUP

Chicken, & Vegetable, Creamy	129
Tomato, Cream of	213

TART

Custard	259
Custard, Portuguese	173

TEA

Green, Reg	0
Peppermint, Reg	0
Soya Milk, Large	8
Soya Milk, Reg	9
White, Large	12
White, Reg	9

GREGGS

TOASTIE

Cheese, Cheddar, & Chutney, Greggs*	460
Chicken, BBQ, & Bacon	516
Ham, & Cheddar Cheese	471

TURNOVER

Apple, Fresh Cream	461
Apple, Iced, Danish	339

WATER

Lemon, & Lime	5
Strawberry	5

WRAP

Bacon, & Cheese	385
Bean, Mexican, & Sweet Potato	457
Chicken, Chargrilled	410
Chicken, Chipotle Chilli, Mexican	470
Chicken, Peri Peri, Greggs*	484

YOGHURT

Mango, & Granola, Natural	207
Strawberry, & Granola, Natural	194

HARVESTER RESTAURANT

AVOCADO
Smashed, Build Your Own Breakfast	349

BACON
Back, Build Your Own Breakfast	83
Extra	94

BEANS
Baked, Extra	63
Baked, Heinz, Build Your Own Breakfast	63
Baked, Side, Kids Menu	51

BEEF - BRISKET
Brisket, Hickory Smoked, with Mash, & Veg	1001

BEEF - STEAK, FILLET
8oz, for Mixed Grill	287
8oz, with Fries, Mushroom, Tomato, & Onion Rings	432

BEEF - STEAK, RUMP
4oz, Build Your Own Breakfast	224
4oz, Extra, Breakfast	224
4oz, for Mixed Grill	164
4oz, Kids Menu	164
8oz, & Fries, Mushroom, Tomato, & Onion Rings	475
8oz, for Mixed Grill	329

BEEF - STEAK, SIRLOIN
10oz, Ancho Chilli	970
10oz, for Mixed Grill	521
10oz, with Fries, Mushroom, Tomato, & Onion Rings	666

BISCUITS
Oreo, Crumb, Extra	145
Oreo, Extra	93

BITES
Quorn, Southern Fried, Kids Menu	199
Quorn, Southern Fried, Starter	327

BLACK PUDDING
Build Your Own Breakfast	81
Extra	81

BREAD
Garlic, Cheesy, Side	354
Garlic, Cheesy, Tapas	633
Garlic, Side	165
Garlic, Tapas	331

BREAKFAST
Signature, Kids, No Egg	300
The Classic, No Egg	838
The Vegan	1002
The Vegan, Kids	310
The Veggie, No Egg	572
The Veggies, Kids, No Egg	378

BROCCOLI
Tenderstem, Chargrilled, Side	37
Tenderstem, Chargrilled, Side, Kids Menu	28

BROWNIES - CHOCOLATE
Belgian, with Chocolate Sauce, & Ice Cream	673
with Chocolate Sauce, Belgian, Mini	287

HARVESTER RESTAURANT

BURGERS
Bean, Beyond, Vegan	666
Bean, Patty, Extra	241
Beef, Mini, Kids Menu	330
Beef, Patty, Extra	391
Beef, The Classic	971
Chicken, Mini, Kids Menu	213
Chicken, Southern Fried, Extra	438
Chicken, The Classic	731
Plant Based, Moving Mountains, Vegan, Extra	302
The BBQ King	1117
The Big One	1808
The Cowboy	993
The Purist, Vegan	1432
The True Blue	1099

CAKE
Chocolate, Fudge, Chocolate Sauce, & Ice Cream	922

CAULIFLOWER
Buffalo, with Garlic Mayo, Starter	470

CHEESE
Halloumi, Battered, & Chips, No Peas	877
Halloumi, Extra	179
Monterey Jack, Extra	65
Stilton, Long Clawson, Extra	164

CHEESECAKE
Vanilla, Baked	622
Vanilla, Baked, Mini	260

CHICKEN - BBQ
Breast, Grilled, Kids Menu	298
BBQ	833

CHICKEN - BURGER
Breast, Extra	176

CHICKEN - BUTTERMILK
Fried, Kids Menu	253
Tenders, Fried, Starter	395

CHICKEN - CAJUN
Breast, Extra	176

CHICKEN - CAJUN, SURF & TURF
Rump Steak, Prawns, Corn, Apple & Fennel Slaw	723

CHICKEN - CARIBBEAN
with Golden Rice & Beans, Grilled Pineapple	469

CHICKEN - GRILLED
Breast, Kids Menu	176
Breast, with Jacket Potato, Simply	282

CHICKEN - ROTISSERIE
Half	510
Half, Jerk, Grilled, with Coconut Rice, & Beans	1065
Half, with Half Rack Ribs, Combo	931
Quarter, Extra	200
Quarter, Kids Menu	359
Quarter, Triple, Combo	715
Quarter, with Ribs, Original Combo	732

HARVESTER RESTAURANT

CHICKEN - SKEWERS

with Chorizo, Churrasco	964

CHICKEN - STRIPS

Kids Menu, Sm Bites	88

CHICKEN - VEGETARIAN

Quorn, Stack, BBQ	697

CHICKEN - WINGS

Sticky, Tapas	296
with BBQ, Sticky	530

CHILLI

Beef, Chipotle, Pulled	328
Non Carne, Kids Menu	545
Non Carne, Vegan, for Nachos	136
Non Carne, with Rice	542

CHIPS

Chunky, Triple Cooked, Build Your Own Breakfast	484
Chunky, Triple Cooked, Nashville Hot, Side	484
Chunky, Triple Cooked, Sage & Onion, Side	500
Chunky, Triple Cooked, Side	484
Chunky, Triple Cooked, Side, Kids Menu	218

COD

Fillet, Battered, Kids Menu	308

COD & CHIPS

with Mushy Peas	688
with Peas	675

CORN

Buttered, Side	207
Cobette, Side, Kids Menu	58

CREAM

Fluffy, Extra	103

CURRY

Vegetable, Thai Green	628

CUSTARD

Extra	90

DESSERT

Cherry Blizzard	534
Chocolate Orange, Slice	329
Cookie, Chocolate, Pizza, Build Your Own, Kids Menu	527

DESSERT - MINI COMBO

Brownie, Blackcurrant Mousse, & Cheesecake	751

EGGS - BENEDICT

Portion	668

EGGS - FRIED

Free Range, Build Your Own Breakfast	130
Free Range, Extra	85

EGGS - MEDITERRANEAN

Portion	599

EGGS - POACHED

Free Range, Build Your Own Breakfast	86

EGGS - SCRAMBLED

Free Range, Build Your Own Breakfast	108
Free Range, Build Your Own Breakfast, Kids	54
on Toast, Kids Menu, Sm Bites	265

HARVESTER RESTAURANT

FISH CAKES

Salmon, with Watercress, Melting Middle	638

FISH FINGERS

Kids Menu	220
Kids Menu, Sm Bites	166

FRIES

Halloumi, with Green Devil Sauce	427
Sweet Potato, Side	503
Sweet Potato, Side, Kids Menu	201

FRITTERS - SWEETCORN

Smoked Cheddar, & Chilli, Build Your Own Breakfast	135
Spicy, with Avocado, & Eggs	614

FRUIT SALAD

Tutti Frutti, with Strawberry Yoghurt, Kids Menu	107

GAMMON

Steak, 7oz	611
Steak, 7oz, Double Up	1076
Steak, 7oz, Double Up, with Egg, & Pineapple	1189
Steak, 7oz, Double Up, with Egg	1161
Steak, 7oz, Double Up, with Pineapple	1103
Steak, 7oz, Egg, & Pineapple	724
Steak, 7oz, for Mixed Grill	273
Steak, 7oz, with Egg	696
Steak, 7oz, with Pineapple	638

GRAVY

Chicken, Specialty, Extra	29

GRILLS

Mixed, Excludes Steak	961
Mixed, Ultimate, Excludes Steak	1999

HASH

Potato, & Spinach	334

HASH BROWNS

Build Your Own Breakfast	91

HOUMOUS

Build Your Own Breakfast	844

ICE CREAM

Extra	101
Non Dairy, Extra	223

JELLY

Peach, Fruitypot, Kids Menu	72

LAMB

Shank, Moroccan Style	1197

MACARONI CHEESE

Bites, with Smokey Ketchup	428
Cauliflower, Kids Menu	313
Extra	279
Side	279

MIXED GRILL

The Pitmaster	3389

MOUSSAKA

Feta, & Butternut Squash	654

MOUSSE

Blackcurrant	295

HARVESTER RESTAURANT

MOUSSE
Blackcurrant, Kids Menu	164
Blackcurrant, Mini	164

MUSHROOMS
Breaded, with Garlic Mayo Dip, Starter	501
Flat, Build Your Own Breakfast	12
Garlic, Oven Baked, with Garlic Bread, Starter	272

NACHOS
Starter	529
Vegan, Starter	523

ONION RINGS
Side	487

PANCAKE
Buttermilk, & Bacon, with Syrup	752
Buttermilk, with Fruit, & Syrup, Kids	192
Buttermilk, with Fruit, & Syrup	623
Side	106

PASTA
In Tomato Sauce, Kids Menu, Sm Bites	237
Spinach, & Ricotto, in Tomato & Basil Sauce	831

PEAS
Chilli & Garlic, Kickin', Side	124
Garden, Side	60
Mushy, Side	73
Side, Kids Menu	60

PIE
Cherry, Sugar Dusted	563
Cookies, & Cream	315
Fish, Cheddar Mash Topped	440

PORK - BELLY, JIM BEAM GLAZED
with Hash Potatoes, Mac & Cheese	1646

PORK - PULLED
BBQ, Extra	239
BBQ, for Nachos	239

POTATO MASH
Side, Kids Menu	94

POTATO SKINS
Cheese, & Bacon, Tapas	407
Cheese, Tapas	313

POTATOES
Jacket, Side	273
Jacket, Side, Kids Menu	273
Jacket, with Sour Cream, Side	348
Mashed, Side	212

PRAWNS
Crackerjack, with Green Devil Sauce, Starter	293

PRAWNS - GARLIC, KING
& Chilli, Extra	172
& Chilli Butter, with Garlic Bread, Starter	358

RIBS - FULL RACK, JERK BBQ
with Chicken Wings, Corn, Slaw, & Chips	1828
with Chips, Slaw, & Corn	1516

HARVESTER RESTAURANT

RIBS - FULL RACK, SLOW COOKED BBQ
in BBQ Sauce, with Chips, Slaw, & Corn	1000

RIBS - HALF RACK, BBQ
Extra	403

RIBS - HALF RACK, KIDS
Kids Menu	348

RIBS - KILO
Kiln Smoked, Bourbon Sauce	509

RICE
Chicken, Katsu, Bowl	505
Golden, & Beans, Side	229
Vegetable, Sunshine, Kids Menu	190

SALAD
Feel Good	307
Feel Good, with Cajun Chicken	503
Feel Good, with Chicken Breast	483
Feel Good, with Quorn Fillets, Cajun	850
Feel Good, with Salmon	699
Feel Good, with Steak, Rump, 8oz	644
Feel Good, with Tofu Skewers, Peri Peri	544

SALMON
Grilled, Spiked Sticky, with Golden Rice, & Beans	674
Grilled, Kids Menu	218

SANDWICH
Steak	591

SAUCE
Caribbean Curry, Steak Sauce	250
Chasseur, Steak Sauce	30
Chocolate, Belgian, Dessert	58
Chocolate, Belgian, Dessert, Kids Menu	29
Craft Ale, Bacon, & Mushroom, Steak Sauce	67
Katsu, Steak Sauce	92
Peppercorn, Steak Sauce	46
Raspberry, Dessert	57
Salted Caramel, Dessert	51
Strawberry, Dessert	57
Toffee, Fudge, Dessert	64
Toffee, Fudge, Dessert, Kids Menu	32

SAUSAGE
& Yorkie, Kids Menu	275
& Yorkie, Kids Menu, Sm Bites	192
Pork, Build Your Own Breakfast	217
Pork, Extra	217
Pork, Smoked, Cheddar, Jalapeno, with BBQ Sauce	452
Vegan	80
Vegetarian, & Yorkie, Kids Menu	265
Vegetarian, & Yorkie, Kids Menu, Sm Bites	185

SCAMPI
Extra	139
Wholetail, Whitby, Excluding Peas	425

SEA BASS
Grilled, Meal, Simply	518

HARVESTER RESTAURANT

SOUP
Tomato, & Basil	193

SPINACH
Build Your Own Breakfast	12

SPONGE PUDDING
Lemon	493
Treacle	941

SQUID
Calamari, Strips, with Garlic Mayo, Starter	278

SUNDAE
Best	255
Best, Kids Menu	239
Best, Vegan	673
Best, Vegan, Kids Menu	448
Blueberry, Eton Mess	530
Build Your Own, Kids Menu	453
Caramel, Salted, Rocky Road	618
Chocolate, Brownie, Rocky Horror	683
Chocolate, Brownie, Rocky Horror, Kids Menu	446
Passion Fruit, & White Chocolate	678
Strawberry Cheesecake	619

TAGINE
Aubergine, & Red Lentil	1077

TART
Camembert, & Cherry Tomato, Puff Pastry	635

TOFU
Skewers, Peri Peri	641

TOMATOES
Build Your Own Breakfast	6

TOPPING
Cheese, Stilton, & Bacon	352

VEGETABLES
Steamed, Side	77
Steamed, Side, Kids Menu	46
Sticks, Side, Kids Menu	44

WAFFLES - BELGIAN
Extra	390

WAFFLES - CHICKEN
Buttermilk Fried, & Bacon, with Syrup, Breakfast	1323

WRAP
Chicken, Breast, Cajun, Grilled	467
Chicken, Breast, Grilled	448
Chicken, Build Your Own, Kids Menu	415
Chicken, Buttermilk Fried	525
Halloumi	629
Quorn, Fillet, Cajun	390
Quorn, Southern Fried	475

HUNGRY HORSE

BACON
Streaky, Side, Extra	66

BAGUETTE
Cheesy Melt	755
Chicken, Club	889
Chicken, Mayo, Southern Fried	663
Fish Fingers, & Mayo	661

BEANS
Baked, Jacket Potato Topping	73
Baked, Side, Extra	73

BEEF
Steak, Rump, 12oz, Big Plate Specials	1344
Steak, Rump, 12oz, Naked, Big Plate Specials	520
Steak, Rump, 12oz, Side, Extra	435
Steak, Rump, 4oz	821
Steak, Rump, 4oz, Naked	230
Steak, Rump, 8oz	966
Steak, Rump, 8oz, Mix it Up, Big Plate Specials	289
Steak, Rump, 8oz, Naked	375
Steak, Sirloin, 9oz, Big Plate Specials	1304
Steak, Sirloin, 9oz, Naked, Big Plate Specials	480
Steak, Smothered, 8oz, Sizzler, Big Plate Specials	1364

BEEF DINNER
Roast, Sunday	967
Sunday Roast, Big Plate Specials	1597
Sunday Roasts, Kids	523

BHAJI
Onion, Extra Portion	541

BREAD
Baguette, Ā,Â½, & Butter, Extra	197
Brown, & Butter, Side	337
Garlic, Ciabatta, Cheesy	522
Garlic, Ciabatta	358
Naan, Extra	345
White, & Butter, Side	374
Wrap, Tortilla, Soft, Mix it Up, Big Plate Specials	329

BREAKFAST
All Day, Big Plate Specials	1561
Full English, Classics	845

BURGERS
Beef, & Chicken, Quadzilla	2768
Beef, Bacon, & Egg, Sunny Stacker	1308
Beef, Bacon, Chicken, & Pulled Pork, Carni-Four	2368
Beef, Classic, Double	1527
Beef, Classic	1170
Beef, Double Daddy	2219
Beef, Extra Patty	357
Beef, Sizzler, Combo, Big Plate Specials	2412
Beef, Smokin' Jack	1539
Beef, with Cheese, & Bacon, Double	1619
Beef, with Cheese, & Bacon	1262
Beef, with Cheese, Double	1553
Beef, with Cheese	1196

HUNGRY HORSE

BURGERS

Chicken, Bombay Bird	1828
Chicken, Extra Fillet	290
Chicken, Southern Fried, Double	1534
Chicken, Southern Fried, Extra Patty	360
Chicken, Southern Fried	1174
Veggie, Chinese, Double	1251
Veggie, Chinese	1021
Veggie, Hoisin, Extra Patty	185

BUTTER

Portion	29

CAKE

Chocolate, Fudge, Warm	905

CHEESE

Grated, Side, Extra	165

CHEESE - HALLOUMI

Battered, & Chips, Classics	1183
Battered, & Chips, with Baked Beans, Classics	1256
Battered, & Chips, with Garden Peas, Classics	1263
Battered, & Chips, with Mushy Peas, Classics	1303
Battered, & Chips, with Salad, Classics	1195
Battered, Mix It Up, Big Plate Specials	764
Extra	800
Fingers	886

CHEESE - POTATO TOPPING

Mozzarella, Mature Cheddar, Jacket Potato Topping	165

CHEESECAKE

Millionaires	593

CHICKEN - BREAST

Extra Portion	179

CHICKEN - CRISPY

Jumbo, with Curry Sauce, Big Plate Specials	1709

CHICKEN - FINGERS

Battered, Mix it Up, Big Plate Specials	660
Battered, Plain, Starter	607

CHICKEN - NEW YORKER

& Salad, Live Well	449
Big Plate Specials	1721
Classics	1168

CHICKEN - PARMIGIANA

Big Plate Specials	1179

CHICKEN - ROAST

Breast, Sunday, Kids Menu	508
Fillet, Sunday	864
Fillet, Sunday, Big Plate Special	1436
Half, Flattened, Mix it Up, Big Plate Specials	304

CHICKEN - SKEWER

Breast, Kebab, Mix It Up, Big Plate Specials	378
Breast, Extra	189

CHICKEN - SKEWERS

Southern Fried, Mix It Up, Big Plate Specials	844
Southern Fried, Extra	422

HUNGRY HORSE

CHICKEN - WINGS

Plain, Starter	766
with Caribbean Dressing, Starter	916
with Caribbean Dressing, Starter	757
with Char Sui Sauce, Starter	929
with Char Sui Sauce, Starter	770
with Fajita Seasoning, Starter	801
with Fajita Seasoning, Starter	642
with Garlic & Parmesan Sauce, Starter	965
with Garlic & Parmesan Sauce, Starter	806
with Hot Sauce, Starter	834
with Hot Sauce, Starter	675
with Lemon & Pepper Sauce, Starter	959
with Lemon & Pepper Sauce, Starter	800
with Piri Piri Hot Sauce, Starter	791
with Piri Piri Hot Sauce, Starter	632
with Texan BBQ Sauce, Starter	856
with Texan BBQ Sauce, Starter	697

CHILLI

Con Carne, Jacket Potato Topping	162

CHIPS

Cheesy, Side	583
Mix it Up, Big Plate Specials	574
Side	418

COD & CHIPS

Jumbo, No Sides Big Plate Specials	1605
Jumbo, with Baked Beans, Big Plate Specials	1678
Jumbo, with Garden Peas, Big Plate Specials	1665
Jumbo, with Mushy Peas, Big Plate Specials	1725
Jumbo, with Salad, Big Plate Specials	1617

COLESLAW

Jacket Potato Topping	75
Mix it Up, Big Plate Specials	100
Side	75

CORN

Cobs, Mini, Mix it Up, Big Plate Specials	39
on the Cob, Side	72

CRUMBLE

Apple	515

CURRY

Chickpea, & Sweet Potato, Big Plate Specials	2247
Chickpea, & Sweet Potato, Classics	691

CUSTARD

Extra	89

DESSERT

Piecaken, Black Forest	967
Piecaken, Black Forest, Vegan	1024

DRESSING

Caribbean, Mix It Up, Big Plate Specials	300

EGGS

Fried, Side, Extra	118

HUNGRY HORSE

FISH & CHIPS - BATTERED

	KCAL
No Sides, Classics	1337
with Baked Beans, Classics	1410
with Garden Peas, Classics	1397
with Mushy Peas, Classics	1457
with Salad, Classics	1349

FISH & CHIPS - VEGAN

Fillets, No Sides, Classics	696
Fillets, with Baked Beans, Classics	769
Fillets, with Garden Peas, Classics	756
Fillets, with Mushy Peas, Classics	816
Fillets, with Salad, Classics	708

FRIES

Dirty, Mac & Bacon, Side	910
Dirty, Mac & Cheese, Side	778
Dirty, Nacho Cheese, & Bacon, Side	760
Dirty, Pizza Topper, Side	691
Dirty, Tikka, Side	1034
Mix it Up, Big Plate Specials	546
Side	546
Sweet Potato, Mix it Up, Big Plate Specials	410
Sweet Potato, Side	410

GAMMON

15oz, Grilled, Big Plate Specials	1503
Grilled, 5oz, Classics	782
Grilled, 5oz, Mix It Up, Big Plate Specials	498

ICE CREAM

Bubblegum, Extra	120
Chocolate, Extra	99
Vanilla, Extra	97

LASAGNE

& Salad, Live Well	543
Beef, Classics	687

MACARONI CHEESE

Classics	756
Side	281

MAYONNAISE

Muddy, Extra	286

MIXED GRILL

Full Monty, Big Plate Special	1878
Mini	1308

MUSHROOMS

Breaded, Garlic	686
Side, Extra	57

NACHOS

Muchos Nachos Grande	1101

ONION RINGS

5, Side	389
Horseshoe Stacker, 20, Ã‚Â½	892
Mix it Up, Big Plate Specials	311

PASTA

Deli, Live Well	401
Deli, with Halloumi, Live Well	600

HUNGRY HORSE

PASTA

	KCAL
Deli, with Roast Chicken, Live Well	580
Deli, with Rump Steak, Live Well	545
Deli, with Salmon Fillet, Live Well	771

PEAS

Mushy, Side, Extra	120
Side, Extra	60

PIE - CHICKEN & MUSHROOM

Woodland, No Sides, Classics	1142
Woodland, with Chips, Classics	1560
Woodland, with Mash, Classics	1391

PIE - STEAK

& Ale, No Sides, Classics	1111
& Ale, with Chips, Classics	1529
& Ale, with Mash, Classics	1360

PINEAPPLE

Slice, Side, Extra	14

PIZZA

Margherita, Classics	903
Meat Feast, Classics	1229
Pepperoni, Classics	1067

PLATTER

Ultimate, Big Combo, Starter	2568

POPPADOMS

& Chutney, Extra Portion	190

POTATOES

Jacket, Mix it Up, Big Plate Specials	194
Jacket, Plain, Add Toppings Seperately	259
Jacket, Plain, Side	194
Mashed, Side, Extra	249
Roast, Extra	335

RICE

Dirty, Mix it Up, Big Plate Specials	191

ROULADE - RED CABBAGE & APPLE

Sunday Roast, Vegetarian, Big Plate Specials	1750
Sunday Roast, Vegetarian	950
Sunday Roast, Vegetarian, Kids	687

SALAD

Classic, Live Well	58
Classic, with Halloumi, Live Well	254
Classic, with Roast Chicken, Live Well	233
Classic, with Rump Steak, Live Well	198
Classic, with Salmon Fillet, Live Well	424
Dressed, Side	33
Side, Mix It Up, Big Plate Specials	49

SALMON

Fillet, Mix It Up, Big Plate Specials	370

SANDWICH

Chicken, Crispy, Big Plate Specials	2531
Chicken, Southern Fried, Steak, Big Plate Specials	2472
Halloumi, Big Plate Specials	3060

SAUCE

BBQ, Texan, Extra	90

HUNGRY HORSE

SAUCE

BBQ, Texan, Mix it Up, Big Plate Specials	180
BBQ, with Jack Daniels, Steak Sauce	146
Char Sui, Mix It Up, Big Plate Specials	325
Curry	141
Garlic, & Parmesan, Mix it Up, Big Plate Specials	199
Hot, Mix it Up, Big Plate Specials	68
Lemon, & Pepper, Mix It Up, Big Plate Specials	386
Lemon, & Garlic, Steak Sauce	160
Parmigiana, Extra	35
Peppercorn, Steak Sauce	52
Piri Piri, Extra	25
Piri Piri, Hot, Mix it Up, Big Plate Specials	50
Sour Cream	103
Sweet Chilli	82

SAUSAGE

Side, Extra	348

SAUSAGE & MASH

Vegetarian, Quorn*, Classics	541

SCAMPI

Breaded, Wholetail, & Salad, Live Well	481
Breaded, Wholetail, No Sides, Classics	939
Breaded, Wholetail, with Baked Beans, Classics	1012
Breaded, Wholetail, with Garden Peas, Classics	999
Breaded, Wholetail, with Mushy Peas, Classics	1059
Breaded, Wholetail, with Salad, Classics	951
Jumbo, No Sides, Big Plate Specials	1310
Jumbo, with Baked Beans, Big Plate Specials	1383
Jumbo, with Garden Peas, Big Plate Specials	1370
Jumbo, with Mushy Peas, Big Plate Specials	1430
Jumbo, with Salad, Big Plate Specials	1322

SOUP

Tomato, Roasted	283
Tomato, Roasted, Vegan	171

SPICES

Fajita Seasoning, Mix It Up, Big Plate Specials	52

SPONGE PUDDING

Syrup	665

SUNDAE

Candymania, Big, The Ultimate	1853
Candymania	841
Trifle-tastic	412

TIKKA MASALA

Chicken, Big Plate Specials	2366
Chicken, Classics	810

TOMATOES

Side, Extra	8

TOPPING

Hot, Steak Topper	71
New Yorker, Steak Topper	177
Sunny, Steak Topper	235
Surf, Steak Topper	172

HUNGRY HORSE

WRAP

Cheesy Melt	646
Chicken, Club	780
Chicken, Mayo, Southern Fried	554
Fish Fingers, & Mayo	552

YORKSHIRE PUDDING

Extra	100

ITSU

BARS
Brownie, Cocoa Butter	185
Chocolate, Pie, Raw	167
Coconut, Crushed, & Chocolate	293
Pecan, Cashew, & Date, Glazed	184

BEANS
Edamame, Chocolate Coated	152
Edamame	157

BEEF
Korean, Rice Bowl, No Sauce, Itsu*	445

BREAKFAST CEREAL
Porridge, Blueberry Boost	362
Porridge, Power	236
Porridge, Super Seeds	346

BROCCOLI
Tenderstem, No Dressing	29

BUNS
Bao, Avocado, & Seeds, with Egg	370
Bao, Bacon	226
Bao, Beans, & Eggs	319
Bao, Duck, Hoisin	327
Bao, Eggs Benedict	303

BURGERS
Quinoa, Rice Bowl, Veggie	826

CHICKEN
Korean, Rice Bowl, Spicy	556
Teriyaki, Rice Bowl	589
Thai, Rice Bowl	758

DRESSING
Green Herb, Large	106
Green Herb, Small	47
Sesame, Large	150
Sesame, Small	67
Teriyaki	42

DUMPLINGS
Berry, Sweet, Gyoza, Itsu*	64
Chocolate, & Banana, Gyoza, Itsu*	138
Gyoza, Chicken, & Spring Onion	251
Gyoza, Chicken, Frozen, Itsu*	157
Gyoza, Pork, & Truffle, Steamed	296
Gyoza, Pork, Itsu*	185
Gyoza, Prawn, King, Steamed	216
Gyoza, Vegetable, Fusion	240
Gyoza, Vegetable, Pot, Itsu*	5
Gyoza, Vegetable, Steamed	240
Gyoza, Vegetable, Winter Wonderland	346

FRUIT SALAD
Hawaii 5 0	113

JERKY
Beef Twerky	97

JUICE
Orange, Press	118
Veg Press	113

ITSU

JUICE DRINK
Ginger, Detox, Zinger, Super Tonic	56
Goji, Mandarin, & Lime, Super Tonic	33

KOMBUCHA
Ginger, & Lemon	18
Original	17
Passionfruit	18

MOUSSE
Chocolate	225

NOODLES
Miso, Mushroom, Kit, Itsu*	298
Ramen, Sesame, Kit, Itsu*	323
Udon, Chicken, Chargrilled	507
Udon, Chicken, Chilli	559
Udon, Curry, Kit, Itsu*	319
Udon, I'thai, Stir Fry Style	669
Udon, Satay, Itsu*	301
Chicken, Udon, Indian Inspired, Pot, Itsu*	295
Udon, with Gyoza, Veggie	455

PEAS
Dried, Wasabi	111

PRAWN CRACKERS
Peking Duck	96
Salt, & Vinegar	98
Sweet Chilli	97
Wasabi, Mild	95

PUDDING
Lemon Zinger	234
White Chocolate Dream	293

RICE CAKES
Chocolate, Dark	85
Chocolate, Milk	83
Yoghurt	80

SALAD
Chicken, Lean, Machine, No Dressing	267
Chicken, Lean, Zero Noodles, No Dressing	282
Chicken, Sesame, No Dressing	389
Chicken, Teriyaki, On a Bed, No Dressing	438
Salmon, Perfect, Bento, No Dressing	522
Salmon, Poke, On a Bed, No Dressing	494
Salmon, Poke, Zero Noodles, No Dressing	410
Salmon, Teriyaki, On a Bed, No Dressing	442
Tofu, No Meat Mondays, No Dressing	408

SEAWEED
Crispy Thins, Sea Salt Flavour	24
Crispy Thins, Sweet Soy & Sea Salt Flavour	22
Crispy Thins, Wasabi Flavour	22

SMOOTHIE
Raw Fruitifix, Beauty	216
Raw Veg Cleanse	175

SOUP
Chicken, Coconut	469
Chicken Noodle	293

	KCAL
ITSU	
SOUP	
Miso	47
Miso, Noodle, Detox	176
Miso, with Eggs, Classic, Breakfast	136
Miso, with Ham, & Eggs, Breakfast	200
Miso, with Spinach, & Eggs, Breakfast	137
Paste, Miso, Chilli, Easy , Itsu*	31
Paste, Miso, Traditional, Easy	21
Thai, Veggie	410
SUSHI	
Avocado, Baby, Rolls	266
Best of Itsu	514
Crab, & Avocado, California, Truffle	495
Crab, California Rolls	322
Crab, Prawn, & Avo, Itsu*	315
Festival	431
Health & Happiness, Box	571
Pandamania, Box	258
Salmon, & Avo, Dragon Roll	453
Salmon, Full House	584
Salmon	227
Salmon, Sashimi	162
Salmon, Super, Light	385
Salmon & Avo, Maki Rolls	309
Sharing Platter	1025
Tuna, Spicy, Dragon Roll	283
Tuna & Salmon, Sashimi Box	355
Veggie, Collection	527
Veggie, Dragon Roll	333
Veggie, Rolls, Club	180
WASABI	
Sachet, Extra	1
WATER	
Ginger, Low	65
Lemon, Low	66
Zen, Cucumber, & Mint	3
Zen, Peach, & Lychee	4
WRAP	
Chicken, Satay, Tokyo, Lean	527
Duck, Hoisin, Tokyo	508
Quinoa Burgers, Tokyo	470

	KCAL
J D WETHERSPOON	
AVOCADO	
Side or Add On	84
BACON	
Maple Cured, & American Style Cheese, Extra	168
Maple Cured, & Cheddar Cheese, Extra	170
Maple Cured, Extra	86
Rashers, Extra or Add On	103
BAGEL - AVOCADO	
Smashed	454
BAGEL - CREAM CHEESE	
Breakfast	359
BAGEL - SALMON, SMOKED	
& Cream Cheese, & Rocket, Deli Deals	430
& Cream Cheese, Breakfast	430
BANANA	
Extra or Add On	105
BEANS	
Baked, Extra or Add On	126
Baked, No Added Sugar, Kids	63
Baked, on Toast, White	551
Baked, on Toast, White, Small	244
Baked, on Toast, Wholewheat	553
Baked, on Toast, Wholewheat Small	245
BEEF - STEAK, RUMP	
10oz, & Eggs, Sunday Brunch	1225
10oz, with Peas, Tomato, & Mushrooms	635
BEEF - STEAK, SIRLOIN	
& Eggs, Brunch	1199
8oz, Skinny, with Quinoa Salad	686
8oz, Steak Club	604
BHAJI	
Onion, 2, Curry Club	331
BITES	
Macaroni Cheese, Side or Add On	278
BLACK PUDDING	
Extra or Add On	352
BLUEBERRIES	
Extra or Add On	17
BOLOGNESE	
Spaghetti, Kids	288
BREAD	
Garlic, Pizza, 11", Side	832
Garlic, Pizza, 8", Side	416
Garlic, Pizza, Large	832
Garlic, Pizza, Large, Sm Plates	832
Garlic, Pizza, Small	416
Garlic, Pizza, with Cheese, 11", Side	979
Garlic, Pizza, with Cheese, 8", Side	489
Naan, Garlic, Curry Club	291
Naan, Garlic, Extra or Add On	291
Naan, Garlic	291
Naan, Plain	224
Two Slices, & Butter, Extra or Add On	442

J D WETHERSPOON

BREAD & BUTTER PUDDING

	KCAL
Chocolate, Baileys, with Custard	478
Chocolate, Baileys, with Ice Cream	548

BREAKFAST

All Day, Brunch	1238
All Day, Brunch, Pub Classics	1238
All Day, Brunch, Small, Pub Classics	678
All Day, Brunch, Vegetarian	1175
All Day, Brunch, Vegetarian, Pub Classics	1175

BREAKFAST

All Day, Brunch, Vegetarian, Small, Pub Classics	709
American	1368
American, Small	684
Freedom	447
Large	1420
Scottish, Large	1464
Scottish, Large	1464
Scottish, Small	433
Scottish, Small	433
Scottish, Traditional	859
Scottish, Traditional	859
Small	460
Traditional	819
Vegan	879
Vegetarian	932
Vegetarian, Large	1357
Vegetarian, Small	374

BREAKFAST CEREAL

Alphabites, Multigrain	158
Porridge, Moma	250
Porridge, with Banana, & Honey MOMA!*	456
Porridge, with Blueberries, & Brown Sugar, MOMA!*	307

BROWNIES

Chocolate, with Ice Cream, Warm	800
Chocolate, with Ice Cream, Warm, Mini	425

BUNS

Chicken, Pulled	428

BURGERS - BEEF

6oz Classic	1171
BBB Burger	1720
BBQ	1679
Brie, & Bacon, Festive	1605
Caledonian	1758
Drive Thru	1796
Empire State	1949
Tennessee	1582
Ultimate	1703
with Cornish Cheese	1720

BURGERS - BEEF, STEAK

Signature, Beef Dripping Bearnaise, & Chips	1451
Signature, Beef Dripping Bearnaise, & Jacket Potato	1153
Signature, Jack Daniels Sauce, & Chips	1398
Signature, Jack Daniels Sauce, & Jacket Potato	1100

J D WETHERSPOON

BURGERS - BEEF, STEAK

	KCAL
Signature, Peppercorn Sauce, & Chips	1402
Signature, Peppercorn Sauce, & Jacket Potato	1104
Sirloin, 8oz, with Chips, Simple	1055
Sirloin, 8oz, with Jacket Potato, Simple	758
Sirloin, 8oz, with Quinoa Salad, Skinny	686
Sirloin, 8oz, with Quinoa Simple, Simple	688

BURGERS - CHICKEN

Breast, Caledonian	1618
Breast, Grilled	1031
Breast, Grilled, Skinny	453
Buttermilk, BBQ	1683
Buttermilk, Breaded, Fried	1175
Buttermilk, Drive Thru	1801
Buttermilk, Fried, & Avocado	1826
Buttermilk, Fried, & Stuffing, Festive	1641
Buttermilk, Fried, Caledonian	1763
Buttermilk, Tennessee	1587
Buttermilk, with Brie, & Smoky Chilli	1616
Grilled, & Avocado	1681
Grilled, & Stuffing, Festive	1497
Grilled, Drive Thru	1657
Grilled, with Brie, & Smoky Chilli	1472
Tennessee	1442

BURGERS - FISH

Fish	1648

BURGERS - VEGAN

Gourmet	1442
Meatless Farm	1090

BURGERS - VEGETABLE

Brie & Cranberry, with Chips, & Onion Rings, Festive	1581
Brie & Cranberry, with Chips, Festive	1275
Vegetable	1099
with Brie, & Smoky Chilli Jam	1540

CAKE

Chocolate, Fudge, with Ice Cream, Warm	897

CHEESE - AMERICAN

Burger Topping	82

CHEESE - BRIE

Extra or Add On	150

CHEESE - CHEDDAR

Burger Topping	83

CHEESE - GRATED

Extra	194

CHEESE - HALLOUMI

Extra	416
Grilled, Add on, Chicken Club	477
Grilled, Extra	416
Grilled, Extra	477
Grilled, with Rocket, & Sweet Chilli Sauce, Sm Plates	477

CHEESE - MOZZARELLA

Mozzarella, Extra	194

J D WETHERSPOON

CHICKEN - BALMORAL
Balmoral	929

CHICKEN - BITES
Breast, Battered, 10, Chicken Club	310
Breast, Battered, with Sticky Soy Sauce	411
Breast, 5, with Sticky Soy Sauce	275

CHICKEN - BUTTERMILK
Breast, Fried, Extra or Add On	350

CHICKEN - GRILLED
Breast, Chicken Club	206
Breast, Kids	206
& Ribs, Half Rack, BBQ, with Onion Rings, & Chips	1721

CHICKEN - MELT
BBQ, with Peas, Tomato, & Mushrooms	576

CHICKEN - NUGGETS
Breast, Kids	155
Quorn*, & Mini Corn Cob	431
Quorn*, Side or Add On	381
Quorn*, with Sweet Chilli	440

CHICKEN - PULLED
Extra	206

CHICKEN - QUARTER
One Leg, with BBQ Sauce, Corn, & Chips	1379
One Leg, with Sriracha Corn, & Chips	1348
Two Legs, with BBQ Sauce, Corn, & Chips	2028
Two Legs, with Sriracha, Corn, & Chips	1997

CHICKEN - STRIPS, SOUTHERN FRIED
with Smoky Chipotle Mayo, Sm Plates	653
5, Chicken Club	500
Jack Daniels Glaze, & Chips, Small	625
Jack Daniels Honey Glaze, & Chips	1166
Jack Daniels Honey Glaze, Add on, Chicken Club	370

CHICKEN - STUFFED
Bacon Wrapped, Mash, Peas, & Gravy, Pub Classics	929

CHICKEN - TRIPLE FEAST
Buttermilk Fried, Wings, & Southern Fried Strips	1838
Grilled, Wings,& Southern Fried Strips	1693

CHICKEN - WINGS, & RIBS
Half Rack, BBQ, with Onion Rings, & Chips	2020

CHICKEN - WINGS, SPICY
10, Chicken Club	1071

CHICKEN - WINGS, SRIRACHA
5, Side or Add On	588
& Blue Cheese Dip, Sm Plates	1289
Add on, Chicken Club	275

CHILLI - BEEF
Burger Topping	178
with Rice, Tortilla Chips, & Sour Cream, Pub Classics	781

CHILLI - FIVE BEAN
Burger Topping	119
with Rice, & Tortilla Chips, Pub Classics	587
with Rice, Kids	322

J D WETHERSPOON

CHIPS
Bowl, Side	955
Bowl, with Curry Sauce, Side	1071
Bowl, with Gravy	977
Extra or Add On	597
Kids	326
Side	597

CHIPS - TOPPED
BBQ Pulled Chicken, & Cheese, Sm Plates	1317
Curry Sauce, Chip Shop Style, Sm Plates	1071
Five Bean Chilli, British, Sm Plates	1074
Loaded, Cheese, Bacon, & Sour Cream, Sm Plates	1302

COD
Battered, Kids	266

CORN
Cob, Mini, Kids	226
Cobs, Mini, Side or Add on	101

CRUMBLE
Apple, Bramley, with Custard	512
Apple, Bramley, with Ice CReam	633

CURRY - CAULIFLOWER & SPIANCH
Roasted, Mangalorean, Pub Classics	883
Roasted, Mangolorean, Curry Club	883

CURRY - CHICKEN
Flaming Dragon	815

CURRY - SWEET POTATO
Chickpea, & Spinach, Curry Club	817
Spinach, & Chickpea, Pub Classics	817

DESSERT
Cookie Dough Sandwich, & Ice Cream, Warm	705
Cookie Dough Sandwich, & Ice Cream, Warm, Mini	415
Melty Mallow Stack	584
Welshcakes, Tan Y Castell	318

DIP
Garlic & Herb, Extra	177
Smoky Chilli, Extra	41

DOUGH BALLS
Sticks, with Garlic & Herb Dip	524

EGGS
Balmoral	646
Balmoral, with Haggis	619
Benedict	508
Benedict, Miners	748
Benedict, with Mushroom	472
Fried, Extra	72
Poached, Extra or Add On	63
Royale	497
Scrambled, Extra or Add On	167
Scrambled, on Toast	537
Scrambled, on Toast, Wholemeal	540

FAGGOTS
Pork, & Liver, with Chips, Mushy Peas, & Gravy	1173
Pork, & Liver, with Mash, Mushy Peas, & Gravy	844

J D WETHERSPOON

FISH & CHIPS - COD, BATTERED
& Mushy Peas	1254
& Peas	1205
Fresh, with Mushy Peas, Small, Pub Classics	717
Fresh, with Peas, Small, Pub Classics	667

FISH & CHIPS - COD, OVEN BAKED
with Mushy Peas, Pub Classics	1288
with Peas, Pub Classics	1239

FISH & CHIPS - HADDOCK, BATTERED
Fresh, with Mushy Peas, Small, Pub Classics	721
Fresh, with Peas, Small, Pub Classics	672
& Mushy Peas	1263
& Peas	1213

FISH CAKES
Haddock, & Salmon, with Side Salad	449

FRIES
Halloumi, Side or Add On	475
Halloumi, with Sweet Chilli Sauce, Sm Plates	475

FRUIT
Fresh, & Ice CReam	304
Fresh, Breakfast	178

GAMMON & EGGS - 10OZ
with Peas, Tomato, & Mushrooms, & Chips	761
with Peas, Tomato, & Mushrooms, & Jacket Potato	761

GAMMON & EGG
with Chips, 5oz	991

GRILLS
Mixed, Large, Steak Club	1416
Mixed, Steak Club	878

HADDOCK
Battered, Kids	270

HAGGIS
& Whisky Sauce, Extra	330
Extra or Add On	248
Scottish, Neeps, & Tatties	923
Scottish, Neeps, & Tatties, Small	420

HAM
Egg, & Chips, Wiltshire Cured, Kids	453
Egg, & Chips, Wiltshire Cured, Pub Classics	847
Egg, & Chips, Wiltshire Cured, Small, Pub Classics	453
Extra	56

HASH BROWNS
Two, Extra or Add On	216

HONEY
Extra or Add On	92

HOT DOG
Kids	272

ICE CREAM
Cookies & Cream, Pots	201
Eton Mess, Pots	149
Vanilla, with Raspberry Sauce, Pot, Childrens	119

JALFREZI
Chicken, Curry Club	847

J D WETHERSPOON

KORMA
Chicken, Curry Club	1004

LAMB
Cawl	480
Shank, Vegetables, Gravy, & Mash	1126

LASAGNE
Beef, British, with Dressed Side Salad	756
Vegetable, Mediterranean, with Dressed Side Salad	603

MACARONI CHEESE
Portion	584
with Chips	1181

MADRAS
Beef, Curry Club	1119

MIXED GRILL
Large, with Peas, Tomato, & Mushrooms	1416
with Peas, Tomato, & Mushrooms	878

MUFFIN
Avocado, Smashed	337
Gingerbread, Festive	449

MUSHROOMS
Extra or Add On	126

NACHOS
Sm Plates	681

ONION RINGS
Six, Side	255
Twelve, Side	510

PANCAKES - AMERICAN
Small	295
with Ice Cream, Mini	420
Maple Bacon, & Maple Flavour Syrup, Breakfast	676
Maple Flavour Syrup, & Ice Cream	715
Maple Flavour Syrup, Breakfast	590

PANINI
Brie, & Cranberry	538
Brie, Bacon, & Smoky Chilli Jam, Deli Deals	602
Cheese, & Tomato, Deli Deals	566
Chicken, Bacon, & Cheese, BBQ, Deli Deals	615
Chicken, Stuffing, Bacon, & Brie	570
Haggis, & Cheese	722
Ham, & Cheese, Wiltshire Cured, Deli Deals	530
Tuna, Cheese, & Mayo, Melt, Deli Deals	709

PASTA
Alfredo	645
Tomato, & Mascarpone	248

PASTY
Cornish, Large	1589

PEAS
Mushy, Side	248
Side	149

PIE - BEEF & DOOM BAR ALE
with Chips, & Mushy Peas	1457
with Chips, & Peas	1407
with Mash, & Mushy Peas	1128

J D WETHERSPOON

PIE - BEEF & DOOM BAR ALE

with Mash, & Peas	1078
with Chips, & Mushy Peas	1457
with Chips, & Peas	1407
with Mash, & Mushy Peas	1128
with Mash, & Peas	1078

PIE - COTTAGE

Celtic Pride, Welsh	593

PIE - MUSHROOM & VEGETABLE

No Sides	1119
with Chips	1650

PIE - STEAK & GRAVY

with Chips, Beans, & Gravy	1093
with Mash, Beans, & Gravy	764

PIZZA

BBQ Chicken & Cheese, Childrens	439
Brie, & Smoky Chilli Jam, 11", Christmas Menu	1271
Brie, & Smoky Chilli Jam, 8", Christmas Menu	636
Brie & Smoky Chilli Jam, 11"	1206
Brie & Smoky Chilli Jam, 8"	642
Carbonara, 11"	1075
Carbonara, 8"	525
Chicken, BBQ, 11"	1255
Chicken, BBQ, 8"	625
Chicken, Stuffing, Bacon, & Brie, 11"	1382
Chicken, Stuffing, Bacon, & Brie, 8"	729
Haggis, 11"	1322
Haggis, 8"	661
Ham & Mushroom, 11"	1134
Ham & Mushroom, 8"	567
Ham & Cheese, Childrens	352
Hawaiian, 11"	1165
Hawaiian, 8"	582
Hawaiian, Childrens	365
Margherita, 11"	1063
Margherita, 8"	532
Margherita, Childrens	324
Meat Feast, Spicy, 11"	1359
Meat Feast, Spicy, 8"	688
Pepperoni, 11"	1318
Pepperoni, 8"	659
Roasted Vegetable, 11"	1156
Roasted Vegetable, 8"	578
Roasted Vegetable, Childrens	364
Roasted Vegetable, Vegan, 11"	816
Roasted Vegetable, Vegan, 8"	408
Roasted Vegetable, Vegan, Childrens	291

PIZZA TOPPING

BBQ Sauce	83
Chicken, Breast	103
Chillies, Sliced	7
Mushrooms	8
Onion, Red	10

J D WETHERSPOON

PIZZA TOPPING

Pepperoni	128
Pineapple	24

POTATOES - JACKET

Grill Option	299
with Beans, & Salad, Deli Deals	483
with Beans, Kids	288
with Beef Chilli, & Sour Cream, with Salad, Deli Deals	525
with Cheese, & Salad, Deli Deals	540
with Cheese, Kids	387
with Five Bean Chilli, & Salad, Deli Deals	413
with Lurpak, Extra	299
with Roasted Vegetables, Deli Deals	374
with Roasted Vegetables, Kids	305
with Tuna, Kids	387
with Tuna Mayo, & Salad, Deli Deals	532
Mashed, Kids	134

PRAWNS

King, Spicy Coated, with Sweet Chilli Sauce	474

PUDDING - STEAK & KIDNEY

with Mash, Peas, & Gravy	951
with Chips, Peas, & Gravy, Pub Classics	1280

RIBS

Pork, BBQ, Half Rack	581
Pork, BBQ, Half Rack, Side or Add on	581
Pork, BBQ, Half Rack, with Onion Rings, Sm Plates	836
Pork, BBQ, with Coleslaw, Onions Rings, & Chips	2013

RICE

Mexican Style, Chicken Club	203

RISOTTO

Mushroom, Creamy	470

ROGAN JOSH

Lamb, Curry Club	895

ROLL

Bacon, Breakfast	287
Black Pudding, Breakfast	539
Egg, Fried, Breakfast	257
Haggis, Breakfast	311
Sausage, Breakfast	524
Sausage, Quorn*, Breakfast	436

SALAD

Ploughmans, Cheese, Plate	873

SALAD - CHICKEN

Caesar	656
Pulled, Avocado, Maple Bacon, Balsamic Vinaigrette	444

SALAD - FALAFEL

& Kale Dressing	498

SALAD - QUINOA

Side or Add on	230
with Grilled Halloumi, & Kale Dressing, Steak Club	914
with Pulled Chicken, & Kale Dressing	704

SALAD - SIDE

Side	72

J D WETHERSPOON

SALAD - SUPERFOOD

with Chicken & Balsamic Vinaigrette Dressing	444

SALMON

Smoked, Extra or Add On	100

SAMOSAS

Vegetable, 2, Curry Club	209

SANDWICH

Bacon, Butty, White	516
Bacon Butty, Wholewheat	519
Ploughmans, Cornish	654
Sausage, Butty, Quorn* White	612
Sausage, Butty, White	698
Sausage, Butty, Wholewheat	701
Sausage, Quorn*, Butty, Wholewheat	615

SAUCE

Baconnaise, Extra	191
BBQ, Burger Topping	83
BBQ, Chicken Club	83
Bearnaise, Beef Dripping	123
Cheese, & Leek, Caerphilly, Burger Topping	144
Curry, Chip Shop Style	117
Honey Glaze, Jack Daniels	70
Peppercorn, Creamy	74
Soy, Sticky, Chicken Club	101
Sriracha, Chicken Club	52
Whisky, Extra	83

SAUSAGE

Extra or Add On	168
Lincolnshire, with Chips, & Beans	1164
Pigs in Portionets, Sm Plates	497
Pork, Kids	336

SAUSAGE & MASH

Pigs in Portionets, with Beans	438
Pigs in Portionets, with Peas	449
Vegetarian, Welsh	858
Welsh, Dragon	890
Lincolnshire, with Peas, & Gravy, Pub Classics	869
Vegetarian, with Peas, & Gravy, Quorn*, Pub Classics	750

SAUSAGE - QUORN

Vegan, Extra or Add On	125
Vegan, with Chips, & Beans	1036
Vegan, with Chips, Curry Sauce, & Mushy Peas	1538
Vegan, Kids	251

SCAMPI

Breaded, Extra	232
Breaded, Kids	116
Breaded, Whitby, with Chips, & Mushy Peas	954
Breaded, Whitby, with Chips, & Mushy Peas, Small	567
Breaded, Whitby, with Chips, & Peas	907
Breaded, Whitby, with Chips, & Peas, Small	668

SQUID

Calamari, with Garlic & Herb	320

J D WETHERSPOON

STRAWBERRIES

Extra or Add On	14

SYRUP

Maple Flavoured, Extra or Add On	97

TART

Chocolate, & Salted Caramel, Dairy Free Ice Cream	855
Mince, Festive	300

TIKKA MASALA

Chicken	1105

TOAST

& Preserves, Marmalade, White	458
& Preserves, Marmalade, Wholewheat	461
& Preserves	459
& Preserves, Wholewheat Bloomer	461
Wholewheat, with Avocado, Smashed	275

TOMATOES

Halves, Grilled, Extra or Add On	16
Sliced, Extra	13

TURKEY DINNER

Breast, Stuffed, & Winter Vegetables, Festive	884

VEGETABLES

Cabbage, Leeks, Pearl Onion & Peas, Side	140
Roasted, Burger Topping	40
Roasted, Extra	80
Roasted, Kids	80
Roasted, Side	120

VINDALOO

Chicken, Curry Club	858

WRAP - BREAKFAST

Breakfast	721
Vegetarian	861

WRAP - CHICKEN

& Avocado, with Mayonnaise, Deli Deal	688
Breast, Pulled, & Sweet Chilli Sauce, Deli Deals	478
Southern Fried, Smokey Chipotle Mayo, Deli Deals	637

WRAP - HALLOUMI

Grilled, with Sweet Chilli Sauce, Deli Deals	698

WRAP - QUORN

Nuggets	498

WRAP - SALMON

Smoked, & Avocado	545

KFC

BEANS

Baked, BBQ, Large	250
Baked, BBQ, Reg	105

BURGERS

Chicken, Big Daddy, Box Meal	1355
Chicken, Big Daddy	686
Chicken, Fillet, Bacon & Cheese, Box Meal	1160
Chicken, Fillet, Bacon & Cheese	585
Chicken, Fillet, Bacon & Cheese, Meal	835
Chicken, Fillet	475
Chicken, Fillet, Meal	720
Chicken, Fillet, Mini, Streetwise	290
Chicken, Fillet, Tower	620
Chicken, Fillet, Tower, Meal	870
Chicken, Kids	265
Chicken, Meal, Kids	455
Chicken, Zinger, Box Meal	945
Chicken, Zinger	450
Chicken, Zinger, Meal	700
Chicken, Zinger, Stacker, Box Meal	1280
Chicken, Zinger, Stacker	780
Chicken, Zinger, Stacker, Meal	1030
Chicken, Zinger, Tower	595
Chicken, Zinger, Tower, Meal	845

CHICKEN

Boneless, 3 Piece, Dips Meal	765
Boneless, 4 Piece, Dips Meal	895
Boneless, Banquet, Box Meal	920
Boneless, Feast, Dipping, 12 Piece	910
Boneless, Feast, Dipping, 8 Piece	780
Bucket, Bargain, 10 Piece	850
Bucket, Bargain, 14 Piece	1090
Bucket, Bargain, 6 Piece	610
Bucket, Mighty, For One	1155
Bucket, Party, 14 Piece	1225
Bucket, Wings	1650
Drumstick, Original Recipe	170
Family Feast, 10 Piece	930
Family Feast, 6 Piece	690
Fillet, Mini	130
Fillet, Mini, Snackbox	475
Keel, Original recipe	265
Lunchbox	755
Megabox, with Gravy	930
Original Recipe, 2 Piece, Meal	730
Original Recipe, 3 Piece, Meal	970
Original Recipe, Mini Fillet, & Dip	280
Original Recipe, Mini Fillet, Meal, Kids	345
Original Recipe, Snackbox	585
Popcorn, Large	465
Popcorn, Meal	535
Popcorn, Meal, Kids	330
Popcorn, Meal, Large	710

KFC

CHICKEN

Popcorn, Reg	285
Popcorn, Small	135
Popcorn, Snackbox	480
Rib, Original Recipe	325
Thigh, Original Recipe	285
Variety, 2 Piece, Meal	1025
Variety, 3 Piece, Meal	1265
Variety, Pack, Mini	655
Wicked Variety, 10 Piece	1145
Wicked Variety, 6 Piece	905
Wing, Original Recipe	175
Wings, Hot, 6, Meal	740
Wings, Hot	85
Wings, Hot, Snackbox	510

COFFEE

Americano, Black, Reg	15
Americano, White, Reg	80
Cafe Mocha, Reg	180
Cappuccino, Reg	125
Espresso, Double	12
Espresso, Single	10
Latte, Caramel, Reg	195
Latte, Reg	140
Latte, Vanilla, Reg	195

COLA

Pepsi*, Diet or Max, Kids	2
Pepsi*, Diet or Max, Large	3
Pepsi*, Diet or Max, Reg	2
Pepsi*, Kids	100
Pepsi*, Large	180
Pepsi*, Max Cherry, Kids	5
Pepsi*, Max Cherry, Large	5
Pepsi*, Max Cherry, Reg	5
Pepsi*, Reg	130

COLESLAW

Large	320
Reg	160

COOKIES

Chocolate, Milk	375
Chocolate, White	380

CORN

Cobette	85
Cobette, Lge Portion	165

DESSERT

Kream Ball, Caramel Fudge	325
Kream Ball, Indulgent Chocolate	345
Krushems, Malteser	280
Krushems, Milky Bar	325
Krushems, Oreo	280
Krushems, Salted Caramel, Soft Serve	375
Krushems, Skittles	295
Krushems, Sour Cherry, Soft Serve	360

KFC

FRIES

	KCAL
Large	345
Reg	250

GRAVY

Large	110
Reg	45

HOT CHOCOLATE

Reg	180

JUICE

Apple, Copella*	115
Orange, Tropicana*	120

JUICE DRINK

Apple, & Blackcurrant, Robinsons*, Kids	5
Apple, & Blackcurrant, Robinsons*, Large	10
Apple, & Blackcurrant, Robinsons*, Reg	5
Blackvurrant, & Apple, Fruit Shoot	10
Orange, Fruit Shoot	10

LEMONADE

7up*, Free, Kids	5
7up*, Free, Large	10
7up*, Free, Reg	5

MUFFIN

Chocolate	555
Lemon	540

ONION RINGS

Portion	400

POTATOES

Mashed	110

RICE

Chicken, Fillet, Ricebox	490
Chicken, Fillet, Ricebox, Meal	740
Chicken, Fillet, Ricebox, with Sugar Free Drink	500
Chicken, Zinger, Ricebox	480
Chicken, Zinger, Ricebox, Meal	725
Chicken, Zinger, Ricebox, with Sugar Free Drink	480
Southern	210
Veggie, Ricebox	365
Veggie, Ricebox, Meal	615
Veggie, Ricebox, with Sugar Free Drink	365

SALAD

Chicken, Fillet	375
Chicken, Fillet, Meal	620
Chicken, Fillet, with Sugar Free Drink	375
Chicken, Zinger	350
Chicken, Zinger, Meal	600
Chicken, Zinger, with Sugar Free Drink	350
Garden, Side	75
Veggie	235
Veggie, Meal	485
Veggie, with Sugar Free Drink	235

SAUCE

BBQ, Kentucky Smoky, Dip Pot	50
Curry, Large	175

KFC

SAUCE

	KCAL
Curry, Reg	75
Hot, Original, Dip Pot	40
HP, BBQ, Heinz, Sachet	15
HP, Brown, Heinz, Sachet	15
Ketchup, Heinz, Sachet	10
Mayo, Garlic Buttermilk, Dip Pot	110
Mayonnaise, Light, Heinz, Sachet	30
Supercharger, Spicy, Dip Pot	150
Sweet Chilli, Sticky, Dip Pot	75
Tomato Sauce, Real, Dip Pot	40

SUNDAE

Berry, Mini	145
Cherry	220
Chocolate	230
Chocolate, Mini	150
Strawberry	170
Toffee	175

TANGO*

Orange, Sugar Free, Kids	3
Orange, Sugar Free, Large	5
Orange, Sugar Free, Reg	3

TEA

Black, Reg	0
Iced, Lipton*, Kids	20
Iced, Lipton*, Large	60
Iced, Lipton*, Reg	45

WRAP - BBQ

Chicken, All Stars, Streetwise, Meal	685
Chicken, Streetwise	300

WRAP - FLAMIN'

Chicken, All Stars, Streetwise, Meal	720
Chicken, Streetwise	335

WRAP - ORIGINAL RECIPE

Chicken, Twister, Kentucky Mayo, Box Meal	965
Chicken, Twister, Kentucky Mayo	500
Chicken, Twister, Kentucky Mayo, Meal	750
Chicken, Twister, Nashville Hot, Box Meal	950
Chicken, Twister, Nashville Hot	490
Chicken, Twister, Nashville Hot, Meal	735
Chicken, Twister, Smoky BBQ, Box Meal	935
Chicken, Twister, Smoky BBQ	475
Chicken, Twister, Smoky BBQ, Meal	725
Chicken, Twister, Sweet Chilli, Box Meal	945
Chicken, Twister, Sweet Chilli	485
Chicken, Twister, Sweet Chilli, Meal	735

YOGHURT

Munch Bunch	100

	KCAL			KCAL

KRISPY KREME

COFFEE
Americano, Black, 12oz	34
Americano, Black, 16oz	46
Cappuccino, 12oz	111
Cappuccino, 16oz	133
Flat White, 8oz	88
Latte, 12oz	132
Latte, 16oz	169
Mocha, 12oz	192
Mocha, 16oz	247

DOUGHNUTS
Apple Pie	296
Bites	138
Caramel, Iced, Ring	273
Chocolate, Double, Duoghnut	485
Chocolate, White, Dreamcake	405
Chocolate Dreamcake	351
Chocolate Iced, Custard Filled	289

DOUGHNUTS
Chocolate Iced, Ring, Glazed	237
Chocolate Iced, with Sprinkles	262
Chocolate Praline, Cheesecake, Duoghnut	384
Cinnamon Apple, Filled	269
Glazed, Original	200
Glazed, with a Creme Filling	371
Lemon Meringue	346
Lotus Biscoff	396
Nutty Chocolatta	379
Raspberry, Glazed	324
Reese's Peanut Butter	395
Salted Caramel, Cheesecake	367
Strawberries & Kreme	326
Strawberry Gloss	244
Vimto, Shimmer	389

HOT CHOCOLATE
12oz	234
16oz	359

ICE CREAM
Solo	240
with Caramel Sauce, & Shortbread	319
with Caramel Sauce, Shortbread, & Bites	453
with Caramel Sauce, Shortbread, & Doughnut	369
with Chocolate Sauce, & Shortbread	313
with Chocolate Sauce, Shortbread, & Bites	448
with Chocolate Sauce, Shortbread, & Doughnut	363

MILK SHAKE
Chocolate Kreme	515
Lotus Biscoff	521
Strawberries, & Kreme	515

LOCH FYNE

BEANS
Edamame, with Ginger, & Chilli	189

BEEF
Steak, Ribeye, with Chimichurri Sauce	1703

BREAD
Basket, with Balsamic Oil	797
Garlic, Starter, Kids	349

BURGERS - BEEF
Chargrilled, Pancetta, Swiss Cheese, & Burger Sauce	1669
Gruyere Cheese, No Sides, Kids	459

BUTTER
Garlic, Fish Bar	188
Garlic	188
Harissa, Fish Bar	207
Harissa	208
Lobster, Fish Bar	131
Lobster	132
Paprika, Smoked, & Sunblush Tomato, Fish Bar	192
Paprika, Smoked, & Sunblush Tomato	192
Salted	221

CABBAGE
Savoy, Shallot, & Chestnuts, Fish Bar	257
Savoy, Shallot, & Chestnuts	257
Savoy, Shallot, & Chestnuts, Side, Kids	128

CARROTS
Rainbow, with Harissa Butter, Fish Bar	109
Rainbow, with Harissa Butter	126

CHEESE
Plate, Scottish	595

CHIPS
Twice Cooked, Fish Bar	526
Twice Cooked	526

COD
Fillet, Panko Crusted, No Sides, Kids	380
Fillet, Roasted, Pancetta, & Red Wine Lentils	883
Grilled, Line Caught, Fish Bar	325
Pan Fried, Line Caught, Fish Bar	399
Steamed, Line Caught, Fish Bar	319

CREME BRULEE
Portion	621

CRUDITES
Starter, Kids	166

CRUMBLE
Plum, Granola, Baked	691

CURRY
Cauliflower, & Squash, Goan, Spiced	460
Malabar, King Prawn, Kids	303
Seafood, Goan	565

DESSERT
Chocolate, Fondant	568

DUCK
Smoked, Gressingham, Fig, & Goats Cheese	241

LOCH FYNE

FISH

Megrim, Whole, Grilled, Fish Bar	415
Megrim, Whole, Pan Fried, Fish Bar	490
Megrim, Whole, Steamed, Fish Bar	415

FISH & CHIPS

Cod, Battered	1620
Haddock, Battered	1373
Haddock, Takeaway	1437
Portion	1624

FISH CAKES

Haddock, No Sides, Kids	407
Haddock, Smoked, with Mustard Leeks	733

FRIES

French, Fish Bar	616
French	560
French, Side, Kids	420
Halloumi, with Chimichurri	743

FRUIT

Plate, Kids	34

GNOCCHI

Spinach, Mushroom, Blue Cheese, Leek, & Artichoke	1114

HADDOCK

Smoked, Poached	643

ICE CREAM

Amaretti Amaretto, Luxury	136
Chocolate Split, Luxury	129
Mint Chocolate, Luxury	122
Strawberry, Luxury	82
Vanilla, 3 Scoops, Luxury	305
Vanilla, Luxury	110
Vanilla, Vegan, Luxury	102
Walnut, Luxury	130

ICE LOLLY

Apple, Organic, Kids	17
Rainbow, Organic, Kids	18
Tropical, Organic, Kids	20

KETCHUP

Portion	20

LANGOUSTINE

Grilled, with Romesco Sauce, Premium	823

LINGUINE

Pomodoro, Kids	234
Prawn, & Chilli	729

LOBSTER

Thermidor, Whole, with Basmiti Rice	688
Thermidor, Whole, with French Fries	1211

MACKEREL - FILLET, CURED

Red Cabbage, & Apple, with Honey Mustard, Main	474
Red Cabbage, & Apple, with Honey Mustard, Starter	346

MACKEREL - WHOLE

Grilled, Fish Bar	849
Pan Fried, Fish Bar	923
Steamed, Fish Bar	849

LOCH FYNE

MAYONNAISE

Portion	113

MONKFISH

Roast, Smoked Pancetta, & Red Wine Lentils	1033

MUSSELS

Scottish, Rope Grown, Main	1186
Scottish, Rope Grown, Starter	375

OIL

& Balsamic Vinegar	323
Chilli, Roasted, Fish Bar	114
Chilli, Roasted	152

OLIVES

Nocellara	186

OYSTERS

Fyne Vinegar, 1	62
Fyne Vinegar, 12	674
Fyne Vinegar, 3	173
Fyne Vinegar, 6	339
My First Oyster	61
Soy & Ginger, 1	68
Soy & Ginger, 12	680
Soy & Ginger, 3	179
Soy & Ginger, 6	345
Wasabi & Cucumber, 1	71
Wasabi & Cucumber, 12	683
Wasabi & Cucumber, 3	182
Wasabi & Cucumber, 6	348

PAKORA

Samphire, & Sweet Potato, with Date Chutney	404

PEAS

Mushy	68

PEPPERS

Padron, with Smoked Sea Salt	199

PETIT POIS

Side, Kids	29

PIE

Apple, No Ice Cream	314

PLATTER

Shellfish, with Lobster, & Crab	1420

PORK

Belly, Black Pudding Mash, Spinach, & Apple Puree	748

POTATOES

Dauphinoise, Fish Bar	615
Dauphinoise	615
Mashed, Creamed, with Chives, Fish Bar	248
Mashed, Creamed, with Chives	248
Mashed, Side, Kids	74
New, Sauteed, Fish Bar	191
New, Sauteed	191
New, with Butter, Fish Bar	238
New, with Butter	239
New. with Butter. Side. Kids	119

LOCH FYNE

PRAWNS
Karagee, with Soy & Ginger Sauce	325
King, Chilli & Garlic, Pan Fried	857

PUDDING
Sticky Toffee, with Tablet Ice Cream	1194

SALAD - GREEN
Fish Bar	126
Side	126

SALAD - WARM WINTER
Puy Lentil & Red Pepper Dressing, Main	603
Puy Lentil & Red Pepper Dressing, Starter	311

SALMON
Fillet, No Sides, Kids	199
Grilled, Scottish, Fish Bar	536
Pan Fried, Scottish, Fish Bar	611
Smoked, Plate, Classic	337
Steamed, Scottish, Fish Bar	536

SALSA
Verde	176

SAMPHIRE
with Lemon	11

SAUCE
Chimichurri, Fish Bar	114
Chimichurri	114
Cream Anglaise	62
Pesto, Wild Garlic	54
Pesto, Wild Garlic	54
Soy, & Ginger, Fish Bar	23
Soy, & Ginger	23

SAUSAGE
Chorizo, in Parsley & White Wine	393

SAUSAGE ROLL
Mini	244

SCALLOPS
with Chickpea, & Nduja Stew	311

SCOTCH EGG
Haggis, Curried Potato Cream, & Turnip	773

SEA BASS
Fillet, No Sides, Kids	250
Whole, Grilled, Fish Bar	596
Whole, Pan Fried, Fish Bar	670
Whole, Steamed, Fish Bar	593

SEA BREAM
Gilt Head, Grilled, Fish Bar	274
Gilt Head, Pan Fried, Fish Bar	311
Gilt Head, Steamed, Fish Bar	274

SEAFOOD
Clams, Cockles, & Chorizo, on Sourdough	353
Grill	1003

SORBET
Lemon, Luxury	62
Pear, Luxury	63
Raspberry, Luxury	65

LOCH FYNE

SOUP
Fish	468

SPINACH
Buttered, Fish Bar	50
Buttered	50

SQUID
Salt & Pepper	490

SUNDAE
Popcorn	564

SWEET POTATO
Wedges, Side, Kids	283

TART
Squash. & Ricotta, with Beetroot	140

TORTELLONI
Beetroot, & Ricotta, Goats Cheese Cream, Main	566
Beetroot, & Ricotta, Goats Cheese Cream, Starter	321
Crab, Devonshire, with Lemon Oil	731
Crab, Devonshire, with Lemon Oil, Premium	712

TRIFLE
Black Forest	788

TUNA
Chargrilled, Fish Bar	396
Grilled, Fish Bar	392
Pan Fried, Fish Bar	433

TURBOT
Whole, Grilled, Fish Bar	604
Whole, Pan Fried, Fish Bar	589
Whole, Steamed, Fish Bar	604

VEGETABLES
Sticks, Side, Kids	166

MCDONALD'S

BREAKFAST CEREAL

Porridge, Oat So Simple, & Syrup	326
Porridge, Oat So Simple, & Jam	233
Porridge, Oat So Simple, & Sugar	206
Porridge, Oat So Simple, Apple & Cherry	228
Porridge, Oat So Simple, Plain	194

BROWNIES

Chocolate	273

BURGERS

Beef, The Canadian Stack	686
Beef, The French Stack	714
Beef, The Italian Stack	647
Beef, The Swiss Stack	721
Big Mac	508
Cheeseburger, Bacon, Double	495
Cheeseburger, Double	445
Cheeseburger	301
Chicken, Indian	590
Chicken, Jamaican	644
Chicken Legend, with BBQ Sauce	484
Chicken Legend, with Cool Mayo	529
Chicken Legend, with Hot & Spicy Mayo	519
Filet-O-Fish	329
Hamburger	250
Mayo Chicken	319
McChicken Sandwich	388
Quarter Pounder, Double, with Cheese	750
Quarter Pounder, with Cheese	518
Vegetable, Deluxe	380

CARROTS

Sticks	34

CHEESE

Melt, Dippers	255
Melt, Dippers, Shareboc	765

CHICKEN

McNuggets, 6 Pieces	259
McNuggets, 9 Pieces	388
Nuggets, Sharebox, 20	863
Selects, 3 Pieces	359
Selects, 5 Pieces	599

COFFEE

Black, Large	8
Black, Medium	6
Cappuccino, Large	124
Cappuccino, Medium	94
Caramel Frappe, Iced	313
Espresso, Double Shot	1
Espresso, Single Shot	1
Flat White, Semi Skimmed Milk	86
Latte, Large	192
Latte, Medium	142
Latte, Millionaires	198
Latte, Toffee, Large	227

MCDONALD'S

COFFEE

Latte, Toffee	183
Latte. Iced	94
White, Large	40
White, Medium	30

COLA

Coca-Cola, Diet	1
Coca-Cola	170
Coke, Zero	1

COOKIES

Triple Chocolate	321

DOUGHNUTS

Millionaires	250
Sugared Donut	189

FANTA

Orange	76

FLATBREAD

Cheesy, Bacon	298

FRIES

French, Large	444
French, Medium	337
French, Small	237

FRUIT

Bag, Apple & Grape	46

FRUIT SHOOT

Apple & Blackcurrant, Robinsons	10

HAPPY MEAL

Carrot Sticks	34
Cheeseburger, No Sides	301
Chicken Nuggets, 4, No Sides	173
Fish Fingers, No Sides	194
Fries, Small	237
Hamburger, No Sides	250
Wrap, Chicken, Crispy, No Sides	248
Wrap, Chicken, Grilled, No Sides	181
Wrap, Veggie, No Sides	209

HASH BROWNS

Single	136

HOT CHOCOLATE

Medium	173

ICE CREAM CONE

Portion	145
with Flake	190

IRN BRU

Portion	80

JUICE

Orange, Tropicana	108

JUICE DRINK

Oasis	67

LEMONADE

Sprite, Zero	4
Strawberry, Frozen	207

MCDONALD'S

MCFLURRY
Maltesers	283
Oreo	267
Smarties	280

MCMUFFIN
Bacon, & Egg, Double	401
Bacon, & Egg	348
Egg, & Cheese	295
Sausage, & Egg, Double	565
Sausage, & Egg	430

MILK
Organic	125

MILK SHAKE
Banana, Large	495
Banana, Medium	386
Banana, Small	203
Chocolate, Large	488
Chocolate, Medium	380
Chocolate, Small	200
Strawberry, Large	488
Strawberry, Medium	379
Strawberry, Small	200
Vanilla, Large	483
Vanilla, Medium	377
Vanilla, Small	198

MUFFIN
Mixed Berry	298

PANCAKE
& Syrup	477
& Sausage, with Syrup	612

PIE
Apple, Hot	250

ROLL
Bacon, with Tomato Ketchup	351

SALAD
Chicken, No Bacon, Grilled	133
Chicken, with Bacon, Grilled	183
Crispy Chicken, No Bacon	265
Crispy Chicken, with Bacon	315
Side, Shaker	18

SMOOTHIE
Mango & Pineapple, Iced, Large	236
Mango & Pineapple, Iced, Medium	187

TEA
with Milk	6

WRAP
Breakfast, Sausage, & Egg, with Brown Sauce	609
Breakfast, Sausage, & Egg, with Ketchup	605
Chicken, Grilled	181
Chicken, Spicy, Snack	322
Chicken & Bacon One, Crispy, BBQ	500
Chicken & Bacon One, Grilled, BBQ	366
Chicken One, Crispy, Garlic Mayo	479

MCDONALD'S

WRAP
Chicken One, Crispy, Hot Cajun	503
Chicken One, Crispy, Sweet Chilli	474
Chicken One, Grilled, Garlic Mayo	345
Chicken One, Grilled, Hot Cajun	369
Chicken One, Grilled, Sweet Chilli	340
Veggie One, Spicy	364

NANDO'S

AVOCADO

	KCAL
Extra	85
Salad Extra	170

BREAD

Garlic, Kids Menu	218
Garlic, Large, Side	698
Garlic, Reg, Side	349
Pitta, Toasted, with Butter, Extra	246

BROCCOLI

Long Stem, Large, Side	48
Long Stem, Reg, Side	24
Long Stem, Side, Kids Menu	12

BROWNIES

Salted Caramel	389

BURGERS

Beanie, Peri Peri, Extra Hot	593
Beanie, Peri Peri, Hot	552
Beanie, Peri Peri, Lemon & Herb	521
Beanie, Peri Peri, Mango & Lime	534
Beanie, Peri Peri, Medium	531
Beanie, Plain	511
Chicken, Breast, Peri-Peri, Extra Hot	469
Chicken, Breast, Peri-Peri, Hot	428
Chicken, Breast, Peri-Peri, Lemon & Herb	397
Chicken, Breast, Peri-Peri, Mango & Lime	410
Chicken, Breast, Peri-Peri, Medium	407
Chicken, Breast, Plain, Kids Menu	296
Chicken, Breast, Plain	387
Chicken, Butterfly Burger, Peri Peri, Extra Hot	663
Chicken, Butterfly Burger, Peri Peri, Hot	622
Chicken, Butterfly Burger, Peri Peri, Lemon & Herb	591
Chicken, Butterfly Burger, Peri Peri, Mango & Lime	604
Chicken, Butterfly Burger, Peri Peri, Medium	601
Chicken, Butterfly Burger, Plain	581
Chicken, Double, Peri Peri, Extra Hot	607
Chicken, Double, Peri Peri, Hot	566
Chicken, Double, Peri Peri, Lemon & Herb	535
Chicken, Double, Peri Peri, Mango & Lime	548
Chicken, Double, Peri Peri, Medium	545
Chicken, Double, Plain	525
Chicken, Sunset Burger, Peri Peri, Extra Hot	680
Chicken, Sunset Burger, Peri Peri, Hot	639
Chicken, Sunset Burger, Peri Peri, Lemon & Herb	608
Chicken, Sunset Burger, Peri Peri, Mango & Lime	621
Chicken, Sunset Burger, Peri Peri, Medium	618
Chicken, Sunset Burger, Plain	598
Mushroom, & Halloumi, Peri Peri, Extra Hot	743
Mushroom, & Halloumi, Peri Peri, Hot	702
Mushroom, & Halloumi, Peri Peri, Lemon & Herb	671
Mushroom, & Halloumi, Peri Peri, Mango & Lime	684
Mushroom, & Halloumi, Peri Peri, Medium	681
Mushroom, & Halloumi, Plain	661
Supergreen, Peri Peri, Extra Hot	487

NANDO'S

BURGERS

	KCAL
Supergreen, Peri Peri, Hot	446
Supergreen, Peri Peri, Lemon & Herb	415
Supergreen, Peri Peri, Mango & Lime	428
Supergreen, Peri Peri, Medium	425
Supergreen, Plain	405
Sweet Potato, & Butternut, Kids Menu	333
Sweet Potato, & Butternut, Pattie Only, Kids Menu	219
Sweet Potato, & Butternut, Peri Peri, Extra Hot	511
Sweet Potato, & Butternut, Peri Peri, Hot	470
Sweet Potato, & Butternut, Peri Peri, Lemon & Herb	439
Sweet Potato, & Butternut, Peri Peri, Mango & Lime	452
Sweet Potato, & Butternut, Peri Peri, Medium	449
Sweet Potato, & Butternut, Plain	429

CAKE

Carrot	737
Choc-A-Lot	582

CHEESE

Feta, Extra	138
Halloumi, Grilled, Extra	177
Halloumi, Sticks, & Dip	441

CHEESECAKE

Caramel, Gooey	415
White Chocolate, & Raspberrry	446

CHICKEN

Breast, Fillet, Grilled, Peri-Peri, Extra Hot	220
Breast, Fillet, Grilled, Peri-Peri, Hot	179
Breast, Fillet, Grilled, Peri-Peri, Lemon & Herb	148
Breast, Fillet, Grilled, Peri-Peri, Mango & Lime	161
Breast, Fillet, Grilled, Peri-Peri, Med	158
Breast, Fillet, Grilled, Plain, Salad Extra	138
Breast, Fillet Plain, Kids Menu	138
Butterfly, Crispy, Peri Peri, Extra Hot	414
Butterfly, Crispy, Peri Peri, Hot	373
Butterfly, Crispy, Peri Peri, Lemon & Herb	342
Butterfly, Crispy, Peri Peri, Mango & Lime	355
Butterfly, Crispy, Peri Peri, Medium	352
Butterfly, Crispy, Plain	332
Half, Peri-Peri, Extra Hot	650
Half, Peri-Peri, Hot	609
Half, Peri-Peri, Lemon & Herb	578
Half, Peri-Peri, Mango & Lime	591
Half, Peri-Peri, Med	588
Half, Plain	568
Quarter, Breast, Peri-Peri, Extra Hot	405
Quarter, Breast, Peri-Peri, Hot	364
Quarter, Breast, Peri-Peri, Lemon & Herb	333
Quarter, Breast, Peri-Peri, Mango & Lime	346
Quarter, Breast, Peri-Peri, Medium	343
Quarter, Breast, Plain	323
Quarter, Leg, & Peri-Peri, Extra Hot	327
Quarter, Leg, Peri-Peri, Hot	286
Quarter, Leg, Peri-Peri, Lemon & Herb	255

NANDO'S

CHICKEN

Quarter, Leg, Peri-Peri, Mango & Lime	268
Quarter, Leg, Peri-Peri, Medium	265
Quarter, Leg, Plain	245
Thighs, Deboned, Peri-Peri, Extra Hot	637
Thighs, Deboned, Peri-Peri, Hot	596
Thighs, Deboned, Peri-Peri, Lemon & Herb	565
Thighs, Deboned, Peri-Peri, Mango & Lime	578
Thighs, Deboned, Peri-Peri, Medium	575
Thighs, Deboned, Plain	555
Thighs 2, Salad Extra, Peri Peri, Extra Hot	359
Thighs 2, Salad Extra, Peri Peri, Hot	318
Thighs 2, Salad Extra, Peri Peri, Lemon & Herb	287
Thighs 2, Salad Extra, Peri Peri, Mango & Lime	300
Thighs 2, Salad Extra, Peri Peri, Medium	297
Thighs 2, Salad Extra, Plain	277
Whole, Peri-Peri, Extra Hot	1218
Whole, Peri-Peri, Hot	1177
Whole, Peri-Peri, Lemon & Herb	1146
Whole, Peri-Peri, Mango & Lime	1159
Whole, Peri-Peri, Medium	1156
Whole, Plain	1136
Wings, Peri-Peri, Extra Hot, 10	868
Wings, Peri-Peri, Extra Hot, 3	318
Wings, Peri-Peri, Extra Hot, 5	475
Wings, Peri-Peri, Hot, 10	827
Wings, Peri-Peri, Hot, 3	277
Wings, Peri-Peri, Hot, 5	434
Wings, Peri-Peri, Lemon & Herb, 10	796
Wings, Peri-Peri, Lemon & Herb, 3	246
Wings, Peri-Peri, Lemon & Herb, 5	403
Wings, Peri-Peri, Mango & Lime, 10	809
Wings, Peri-Peri, Mango & Lime, 3	259
Wings, Peri-Peri, Mango & Lime, 5	416
Wings, Peri-Peri, Medium, 10	806
Wings, Peri-Peri, Medium, 3	256
Wings, Peri-Peri, Medium, 5	413
Wings, Plain, 10	786
Wings, Plain, 3, Kids Menu	236
Wings, Plain, 3	236
Wings, Plain, 5	393

CHIPS

Kids Menu	336
Large, Side	1256
Peri Salted, Large, Side	1260
Peri Salted, Reg, Side	467
Reg, Side	465

COFFEE

Americano	0
Cappuccino	73
Espresso	0
Latte	63

NANDO'S

COLESLAW

Large, Side	526
Reg, Side	263

CORDIAL

Green, Kids Menu	26

CORN

Cob, Kids Menu	72
Cob, Large, Side	288
Cob, Reg, Side	144

DIP

Red Pepper, & Chilli, with Pitta	464

FROZEN YOGHURT

Chocolate	79
Mango	71
Strawberry	70

HOT CHOCOLATE

Portion	291

HOUMOUS

Peri Drizzle, & Pitta	819
Salad Extra	204

ICE CREAM

Chocolate	145
Coconut	157
Mango	99
Vanilla, Kids Menu	158
Vanilla	161

ICE LOLLY

Chilly Billy	30

JUICE

Apple, Pressed	134
Orange	118

JUICE DRINK

Mango Quencher	120

LEMONADE

Cloudy	143

MASH

Creamy, Large, Side	496
Creamy, Reg, Side	248

MILK

Organic, Kids Menu	113

MUSHROOMS

Portabello, Extra	105

NUTS

Peri-Peri	793

OLIVES

Mixed, Spicy	138

PEAS

Macho, Large, Side	283
Macho, Reg, Side	141

PEPPER

Chargrilled, Extra	39

PINEAPPLE

Slice, Grilled, Extra	37

NANDO'S

RELISH
Chilli, Jam, Extra	149

RICE
Spicy, Large, Side	492
Spicy, Reg, Side	246

ROLL - CHICKEN, LIVERS
Portuguese, Peri Peri, Extra Hot	622
Portuguese, Peri Peri, Hot	581
Portuguese, Peri Peri, Lemon & Herb	550
Portuguese, Peri Peri, Mango & Lime	563
Portuguese, Peri Peri, Medium	560
Portuguese, Plain	540

ROLL - STEAK, FILLET
Prego, Peri Peri, Extra Hot	487
Prego, Peri Peri, Hot	446
Prego, Peri Peri, Mango & Lime	428
Prego, Peri Peri, Medium	425
Prego, Plain	405

ROLL - STEAK, FILLETS
Prego, Peri Peri, Lemon & Herb	415

SALAD - CAESAR
Side	285
with Chicken Breast, Peri Peri, Extra Hot	504
with Chicken Breast, Peri Peri, Hot	463
with Chicken Breast, Peri Peri, Lemon & Herb	432
with Chicken Breast, Peri Peri, Mango & Lime	445
with Chicken Breast, Peri Peri, Med	442
with Chicken Breast, Plain	422

SALAD - GRAINS N GREENS
Side, Kids Menu	104
Large, Side	356
Side	189
with Chicken Breast, Peri Peri, Extra Hot	409
with Chicken Breast, Peri Peri, Hot	368
with Chicken Breast, Peri Peri, Lemon & Herb	337
with Chicken Breast, Peri Peri, Mango & Lime	350
with Chicken Breast, Peri Peri, Medium	347
with Chicken Breast, Plain	327

SALAD - HOUSE
Side	126
with Chicken Breast, Peri Peri, Extra Hot	345
with Chicken Breast, Peri Peri, Hot	304
with Chicken Breast, Peri Peri, Lemon & Herb	273
with Chicken Breast, Peri Peri, Mango & Lime	286
with Chicken Breast, Peri Peri, Medium	283
with Chicken Breast, Plain	263

SALAD - MIXED LEAF
Large, Side	25
Reg, Side	13
with Chicken Breast, Peri Peri, Extra Hot	244
with Chicken Breast, Peri Peri, Hot	203
with Chicken Breast, Peri Peri, Lemon & Herb	172
with Chicken Breast, Peri Peri, Mango & Lime	185

NANDO'S

SALAD - MIXED LEAF
with Chicken Breast, Peri Peri, Medium	182
with Chicken Breast, Plain	162

SANDWICH
Beanie, Pitta, Peri Peri, Extra Hot	602
Beanie, Pitta, Peri Peri, Hot	561
Beanie, Pitta, Peri Peri, Lemon & Herb	530
Beanie, Pitta, Peri Peri, Mango & Lime	543
Beanie, Pitta, Peri Peri, Medium	540
Beanie, Pitta, Plain	520
Chicken, Breast, Peri-Peri, Extra Hot, Pitta	478
Chicken, Breast, Peri-Peri, Hot, Pitta	437
Chicken, Breast, Peri-Peri, Lemon & Herb, Pitta	406
Chicken, Breast, Peri-Peri, Mango & Lime, Pitta	419
Chicken, Breast, Peri-Peri, Medium, Pitta	416
Chicken, Breast, Plain, Pitta	396
Chicken, Double, Pitta, Peri Peri, Extra Hot	616
Chicken, Double, Pitta, Peri Peri, Hot	575
Chicken, Double, Pitta, Peri Peri, Lemon & Herb	544
Chicken, Double, Pitta, Peri Peri, Mango & Lime	557
Chicken, Double, Pitta, Peri Peri, Medium	554
Chicken, Double, Pitta, Plain	534
Chicken, Thigh, Fino Pitta, Peri Peri, Extra Hot	838
Chicken, Thigh, Fino Pitta, Peri Peri, Hot	797
Chicken, Thigh, Fino Pitta, Peri Peri, Lemon & Herb	766
Chicken, Thigh, Fino Pitta, Peri Peri, Mango & Lime	779
Chicken, Thigh, Fino Pitta, Peri Peri, Medium	776
Chicken, Thigh, Fino Pitta, Plain	756
Mushroom, Halloumi, Peri Peri, Pitta, Extra Hot	727
Mushroom, Halloumi, Peri Peri, Pitta, Hot	686
Mushroom, Halloumi, Peri Peri, Pitta, Lemon & Herb	655
Mushroom, Halloumi, Peri Peri, Pitta, Mango & Lime	668
Mushroom, Halloumi, Peri Peri, Pitta, Medium	665
Mushroom, Halloumi, Pitta, Plain	645
Steak, Fillet, & Veg, Peri Peri, Extra Hot	531
Steak, Fillet, & Veg, Peri Peri, Hot	490
Steak, Fillet, & Veg, Peri Peri, Lemon & Herb	459
Steak, Fillet, & Veg, Peri Peri, Mango & Lime	472
Steak, Fillet, & Veg, Peri Peri, Medium	469
Steak, Fillet, & Veg, Plain	449
Supergreen, Peri Peri, Pitta, Extra Hot	536
Supergreen, Peri Peri, Pitta, Hot	495
Supergreen, Peri Peri, Pitta, Lemon & Herb	464
Supergreen, Peri Peri, Pitta, Mango & Lime	477
Supergreen, Peri Peri, Pitta, Medium	474
Supergreen, Pitta, Plain	454
Sweet Potato, Butternut, Pitta, Peri Peri, Extra Hot	560
Sweet Potato, Butternut, Pitta, Peri Peri, Hot	519
Sweet Potato, Butternut, Pitta, Peri Peri, Lemon Herb	488
Sweet Potato, Butternut, Pitta, Peri Peri, Mango Lime	501
Sweet Potato, Butternut, Pitta, Peri Peri, Medium	498
Sweet Potato, Butternut, Pitta, Plain	478

NANDO'S

SAUCE

Peri Peri Drizzle, Side	97
Perinaise, Condiments	159

SPINACH

Saucy, Large, Side	195
Saucy, Reg, Side	98

STEW

Cataplana, Veggie	515

SWEET POTATO

& Butternut Squash, Fino Side	174
& Butternut Squash, Side, Kids Menu	71
Mash, Fino Side	97
Mash, Kids Menu	48

TART

Custard, Naughty Natas	169

TEA

Infusions, All Flavours	0
Organic, Everyday	23
Rubro, Iced	57

TOMATOES

Kids Menu	13

VEGETABLES

Chargrilled, Fino Side	93

WRAP

Beanie, Peri Peri, Extra Hot	736
Beanie, Peri Peri, Hot	695
Beanie, Peri Peri, Lemon & Herb	664
Beanie, Peri Peri, Mango & Lime	677
Beanie, Peri Peri, Medium	674
Beanie, Plain	654
Chicken, Breast, Peri-Peri, Extra Hot	613
Chicken, Breast, Peri-Peri, Hot	572
Chicken, Breast, Peri-Peri, Lemon & Herb	541
Chicken, Breast, Peri-Peri, Mango & Lime	554
Chicken, Breast, Peri-Peri, Medium	551
Chicken, Breast, Plain	531
Chicken, Double, Peri Peri, Extra Hot	750
Chicken, Double, Peri Peri, Hot	709
Chicken, Double, Peri Peri, Lemon & Herb	678
Chicken, Double, Peri Peri, Mango & Lime	691
Chicken, Double, Peri Peri, Medium	688
Chicken, Double, Plain	668
Chicken, Grilled, Mozam, Peri Peri, Extra Hot	546
Chicken, Grilled, Mozam, Peri Peri, Hot	505
Chicken, Grilled, Mozam, Peri Peri, Lemon & Herb	474
Chicken, Grilled, Mozam, Peri Peri, Mango & Lime	487
Chicken, Grilled, Mozam, Peri Peri, Medium	484
Chicken, Grilled, Mozam, Plain	464
Mushroom, & Halloumi, Peri-Peri, Extra Hot	802
Mushroom, & Halloumi, Peri-Peri, Hot	761
Mushroom, & Halloumi, Peri-Peri, Lemon & Herb	730
Mushroom, & Halloumi, Peri-Peri, Mango & Lime	743
Mushroom, & Halloumi, Peri-Peri, Medium	740

NANDO'S

WRAP

Mushroom, & Halloumi, Plain	720
Steak, Fillet, & Veg, Peri Peri, Extra Hot	623
Steak, Fillet, & Veg, Peri Peri, Hot	582
Steak, Fillet, & Veg, Peri Peri, Lemon & Herb	551
Steak, Fillet, & Veg, Peri Peri, Mango & Lime	564
Steak, Fillet, & Veg, Peri Peri, Medium	561
Steak, Fillet, & Veg, Plain	541
Supergreen, Peri Peri, Extra Hot	670
Supergreen, Peri Peri, Hot	629
Supergreen, Peri Peri, Lemon & Herb	598
Supergreen, Peri Peri, Mango & Lime	611
Supergreen, Peri Peri, Medium	608
Supergreen, Plain	588
Sweet Potato, & Butternut, Peri Peri, Extra Hot	694
Sweet Potato, & Butternut, Peri Peri, Hot	653
Sweet Potato, & Butternut, Peri Peri, Lemon & Herb	622
Sweet Potato, & Butternut, Peri Peri, Mango & Lime	635
Sweet Potato, & Butternut, Peri Peri, Medium	632
Sweet Potato, & Butternut, Plain	612

PIZZA EXPRESS

BOLOGNESE
Penne, Al Forno	674

BREAD
Garlic, with Mozzarella	356

CALZONE
'Nduja, Restaurant	1196
Verdure, Restaurant	906

CANNELLONI
Spinach, & Ricotta, Al Forno	705

DESSERT
Chocolate Fondant, with Vanilla Ice Cream	918
Parfait, Chocolate, & Amaretto	275

DOUGH BALLS
Doppio	828
GF, with Garlic Butter	370
Plain	396
Vegan	336
without Butter	230

DRESSING
House, Light	135

ICE CREAM
Chocolate, & Chocolate Straw, Coppa Gelato	246
Strawberry, & Chocolate Straw, Coppa Gelato	211
Vanilla, Gelato, Side	114

LASAGNE
Classica, Al Forno	712

MUSHROOMS
Garlic, Baked	329

OLIVES
Marinate	137

PENNE
Pepperonata, Al Forno	542

PIZZA
American, Classic	1019
American, Hot, Romana	1010
American Hot, Leggera, Wholemeal	548
Barbacoa, Romana	1118
Calabrese	1275
Carbonara, Romana	1486
Diavlo, Leggera, Wholemeal	556
Diavlo, Romana	1167
Fiorentina, Classic	942
Funghi di Bosco, Romana	1096
Giardiniera, Classic, Vegan	843
Giardiniera, Leggera, Wholemeal, Vegan	556
Giardiniera, Romana, Vegan	970
La Reine, Classic	898
La Reine, Leggera, Wholemeal	498
La Rosie, Piccolo, Restaurant	455
Margherita, Bufala, Romana	1152
Margherita, Classic	834
Margherita, Classic, Vegan	711
Padana, Leggera, Wholemeal	587

PIZZA EXPRESS

PIZZA
Padana, Leggera, Wholemeal, Vegan	560
Padana, Romana, Vegan	911
Pollo, ad Astra, Leggera	599
Pollo, ad Astra, Romana	1145
Pollo, Forza, Leggera, Wholemeal	578
Pollo, Forza, Romana	1253
Sloppy Giuseppe, Classic	897
Veneziana, Classic	938
Veneziana, Classic, Vegan	815

PRAWNS
King, with Spicy 'Nduja	326

RISOTTO
con Funghi	668

SALAD
Pollo, no Dressing	502
Pollo, with Dough Balls, Piccolo	283
Pollo, with Dressing, & Dough Sticks	954
Pollo, with Polenta Chips, Piccolo	265

SUNDAE
Ic Cream, with Chocolate Sauce, Piccolo	149
Ice Cream, with Fruit Sauce, Piccolo	131

TOMATOES
Roasted	67

PIZZA HUT

	KCAL
APPLES	
Salad Station	10
BACON	
Bits, Salad Station	104
BEETROOT	
Diced, Salad Station	10
BITES	
Cheesy	469
Cinnamon, Hot	472
Cinnamon, Kids	248
Hot Dog	404
BOLOGNESE	
Spaghetti, Little Boss	198
BREAD	
Garlic	511
Garlic, with Mozzarella	689
BREADSTICKS	
Salad Station	245
BROWNIES	
Chocolate, Hot	600
BROWNIES	
Chocolate, Kids	394
CARROTS	
Shredded, Salad Station	10
CHEESE TRIANGLES	
Fried	425
Oven Baked	396
CHEESECAKE	
Chocolate, Honeycomb	639
I Can't Believe It's Not	513
Strawberries, & Cream	537
CHICKEN	
Bites	397
Breaded, & Fries, Fried, Big Boss	619
Breaded, & Fries, Fried, Little Boss	548
Breaded, & Fries, Oven Baked, Big Boss	472
Breaded, & Fries, Oven Baked, Little Boss	400
Breaded, & Seasoned Fries, Fried, Big Boss	704
Breaded, & Seasoned Fries, Fried, Little Boss	563
Breaded, & Seasoned Fries, Oven Baked, Big Boss	533
Breaded, & Seasoned Fries, Oven Baked, Little Boss	421
Melt, BBQ Americano	396
Melt, Garlic Mushroom	447
Melt, Naked	246
Melt, Pepperoni	423
Nuggets, Southern Fried	248
Wings	379
CHOCOLATE	
Beans, Ice Cream Factory	460
Chips, Ice Cream Factory	516
Toffee, Crunch, Ice Cream Factory	465
Tricolor, Pieces, Ice Cream Factory	542

PIZZA HUT

	KCAL
COLESLAW	
Salad Station	38
COOKIES	
Dough, Chocolate Chip, Hot	651
Dough, S'mores, Hot	691
Dough, Salted Caramel, Hot	631
CORN	
Cob, 3, Side	203
Cob, 5, Side	328
Cob, Mini, Side	328
CROUTONS	
Salad Station	85
CUCUMBER	
Salad Station	2
DIP	
BBQ	35
Blue Cheese, Salad Station	75
Garlic Sauce	89
Sour Cream, & Chive, Dressing	102
DRESSING	
French, Low Fat, Salad Station	15
DRESSING	
Olive Oil, & Balsamic Vinegar, Salad Station	124
Ranch, Salad Station	79
Thousand Island, Salad Station	54
FLATBREAD	
BBQ Steak, & Chicken	535
Chicken Delight	440
Ham, & Garlic Mushroom	459
Tuna, & Sweetcorn	457
Virtuous Veg	375
Virtuous Veg, Vegan	332
FRIES	
Cheesy, Fried, Side	854
Cheesy, Oven Baked, Side	680
Fried, Side	673
Oven Baked, Side	355
Seasoned, Fried, Side	702
Seasoned, Oven Baked, Side	384
Sweet Potato, Side	772
ICE CREAM	
Vanilla, Ice Cream Factory, Kids	192
Vanilla, Ice Cream Factory	329
ICE CREAM FLOAT	
Cream Soda, Black Cherry	300
Cream Soda	300
ICE LOLLY	
Orange	69
KETCHUP	
BLANK	99
LASAGNE	
Beef	790
Beef, with Garlic Bread, Big Boss	523

PIZZA HUT

LETTUCE

	KCAL
Mix, Salad Station	2

MACARONI CHEESE

Big Boss	412
BLANK	824
with Chicken, Pulled	867
with Garlic Mushrooms	894

MAYONNAISE

Garlic, Salad Station	92
Light, Salad Station	77

MILK SHAKE

Chocoholic, Kids	273
Chocoholic	622
Oreo, Kids	309
Oreo	775
Salted Caramel, Kids	328
Salted Caramel	679
Strawberry, Kids	287
Strawberry	698
Vanilla, Kids	263
Vanilla	581

OIL

Garlic, & Chilli, Salad Station	180

ONION RINGS

Fried, Side	236
Oven Baked, Side	154

ONIONS

Crispy, Salad Station	125
Red, Salad Station	7

PASTA

Cheesy, Little Boss	385

PASTA BAKE

Cheese, 4, & Spinach, Buffet	245
Marinara, Buffet	273

PASTA SAUCE

Cheese, Buffet	128
Marinara, Buffet	87

PENNE

Buffet	265

PEPPERS

Jalapeno, Poppers, Fried	438
Jalapeno, Poppers, Oven Baked	354
Jalapeno, Salad Station	2
Mixed, Salad Station	3

PIZZA

All About Mushrooms, Cheesy Bites Crust	2224
All About Mushrooms, Deep Pan, Large	2072
All About Mushrooms, Deep Pan, Reg	1014
All About Mushrooms, GF	918
All About Mushrooms, Stuffed Crust, Individual	1224
All About Mushrooms, Stuffed Crust, Large	2224
All About Mushrooms, Thin Crust, Individual	894
All About Mushrooms, Thin Crust, Large	1472

PIZZA HUT

PIZZA

	KCAL
All About Mushrooms, Vegan, Deep Pan, Large	1979
All About Mushrooms, Vegan, Deep Pan, Reg	964
All About Mushrooms, Vegan, GF	959
All About Mushrooms, Vegan, Thin Crust, Individual	827
All About Mushrooms, Vegan, Thin Crust, Large	1378
BBQ Americano, Cheesy Bites Crust	2584
BBQ Americano, Deep Pan, Large	2432
BBQ Americano, Deep Pan, Reg	1158
BBQ Americano, GF	1068
BBQ Americano, Stuffed Crust, Individual	1374
BBQ Americano, Stuffed Crust, Large	2584
BBQ Americano, Thin Crust, Individual	1038
BBQ Americano, Thin Crust, Large	1840
BBQ Jack 'N' Cheese, Cheesy Bites Crust	2296
BBQ Jack 'N' Cheese, Deep Pan, Large	2144
BBQ Jack 'N' Cheese, Deep Pan, Reg	1038
BBQ Jack 'N' Cheese, GF	942
BBQ Jack 'N' Cheese, Stuffed Crust, Individual	1248
BBQ Jack 'N' Cheese, Stuffed Crust, Large	2296
BBQ Jack 'N' Cheese, Thin Crust, Individual	912
BBQ Jack 'N' Cheese, Thin Crust, Large	1536
Chicken Supreme, Cheesy Bites Crust	2344
Chicken Supreme, Deep Pan, Large	2192
Chicken Supreme, Deep Pan, Reg	1050
Chicken Supreme, GF	954
Chicken Supreme, Stuffed Crust, Individual	1260
Chicken Supreme, Stuffed Crust, Large	2344
Chicken Supreme, Thin Crust, Individual	930
Chicken Supreme, Thin Crust, Large	1592
Hawaiian, Cheesy Bites Crust	2216
Hawaiian, Deep Pan, Large	2072
Hawaiian, Deep Pan, Reg	1008
Hawaiian, GF	912
Hawaiian, Stuffed Crust, Individual	1212
Hawaiian, Stuffed Crust, Large	2216
Hawaiian, Thin Crust, Individual	888
Hawaiian, Thin Crust, Large	1472
Hot 'N' Spicy, Vegan, Deep Pan, Large	1976
Hot 'N' Spicy, Vegan, Deep Pan, Reg	966
Hot 'N' Spicy, Vegan, GF	870
Hot 'N' Spicy, Vegan, Thin Crust, Individual	840
Hot 'N' Spicy, Vegan, Thin Crust, Large	1368
Hot 'N' Spicy Chicken, Cheesy Bites Crust	2408
Hot 'N' Spicy Chicken, Deep Pan, Large	2256
Hot 'N' Spicy Chicken, Deep Pan, Reg	1092
Hot 'N' Spicy Chicken, GF	996
Hot 'N' Spicy Chicken, Stuffed Crust, Individual	1302
Hot 'N' Spicy Chicken, Stuffed Crust, Large	2408
Hot 'N' Spicy Chicken, Thin Crust, Individual	972
Hot 'N' Spicy Chicken, Thin Crust, Large	1656
Hot 'N' Spicy Veg, Cheesy Bites Crust	2296
Hot 'N' Spicy Veg, Deep Pan, Large	2152

PIZZA HUT
PIZZA

	KCAL
Hot 'N' Spicy Veg, Deep Pan, Reg	1050
Hot 'N' Spicy Veg, GF	954
Hot 'N' Spicy Veg, Stuffed Crust, Individual	1260
Hot 'N' Spicy Veg, Stuffed Crust, Large	2296
Hot 'N' Spicy Veg, Thin Crust, Individual	924
Hot 'N' Spicy Veg, Thin Crust, Large	1536
Jack N Ch**se, Vegan, Deep Pan, Large	2058
Jack N Ch**se, Vegan, Deep Pan, Reg	994
Jack N Ch**se, Vegan, GF	984
Jack N Ch**se, Vegan, Thin Crust, Individual	873
Jack N Ch**se, Vegan, Thin Crust, Large	1457
Margherita, Cheesy Bites Crust	2280
Margherita, Deep Pan, Big Boss	453
Margherita, Deep Pan, Large	2128
Margherita, Deep Pan, Little Boss	423
Margherita, Deep Pan, Reg	1038
Margherita, GF, Big Boss	433
Margherita, GF, Little Boss	412
Margherita, GF	942
Margherita, Stuffed Crust, Individual	1248
Margherita, Stuffed Crust, Large	2280
Margherita, Thin Crust, Big Boss	374
Margherita, Thin Crust, Individual	918
Margherita, Thin Crust, Large	1528
Margherita, Thin Crust, Little Boss	327
Margherita, Vegan, Deep Pan, Large	2163
Margherita, Vegan, Deep Pan, Reg	1056
Margherita, Vegan, GF	958
Margherita, Vegan, Thin Crust, Individual	935
Margherita, Vegan, Thin Crust, Large	1563
Meat Feast, Cheesy Bites Crust	2528
Meat Feast, Deep Pan, Large	2376
Meat Feast, Deep Pan, Reg	1140
Meat Feast, Epic, Cheesy Bites Crust	2592
Meat Feast, Epic, Deep Pan, Large	2448
Meat Feast, Epic, Deep Pan, Reg	1188
Meat Feast, Epic, Stuffed Crust, Individual	1398
Meat Feast, Epic, Stuffed Crust, Large	2592
Meat Feast, Epic, Thin Crust, Individual	1068
Meat Feast, Epic, Thin Crust, Large	1848
Meat Feast, GF	1044
Meat Feast, Stuffed Crust, Individual	1350
Meat Feast, Stuffed Crust, Large	2528
Meat Feast, Thin Crust, Individual	1020
Meat Feast, Thin Crust, Large	1776
New York Hot Dog, Cheesy Bites Crust	2720
New York Hot Dog, Deep Pan, Large	2568
New York Hot Dog, Deep Pan, Reg	1248
New York Hot Dog, GF	1152
New York Hot Dog, Stuffed Crust, Individual	1458
New York Hot Dog, Stuffed Crust, Large	2720

PIZZA HUT
PIZZA

	KCAL
New York Hot Dog, Thin Crust, Individual	1128
New York Hot Dog, Thin Crust, Large	1968
Pepperoni, Cheesy Bites Crust	2384
Pepperoni, Deep Pan, Large	2232
Pepperoni, Deep Pan, Reg	1092
Pepperoni, Epic, Cheesy Bites Crust	2760
Pepperoni, Epic, Deep Pan, Large	2616
Pepperoni, Epic, Deep Pan, Reg	1266
Pepperoni, Epic, GF	1170
Pepperoni, Epic, Stuffed Crust, Individual	1476
Pepperoni, Epic, Stuffed Crust, Large	2760
Pepperoni, Epic, Thin Crust, Individual	1146
Pepperoni, Epic, Thin Crust, Large	2008
Pepperoni, GF	996
Pepperoni, Stuffed Crust, Individual	1296
Pepperoni, Stuffed Crust, Large	2384
Pepperoni, Thin Crust, Individual	972
Pepperoni, Thin Crust, Large	1632
Philly Cheese Steak, Cheesy Bites Crust	3000
Philly Cheese Steak, Deep Pan, Large	2848
Philly Cheese Steak, Deep Pan, Reg	1392
Philly Cheese Steak, GF	1302
Philly Cheese Steak, Stuffed Crust, Individual	1602
Philly Cheese Steak, Stuffed Crust, Large	3000
Philly Cheese Steak, Thin Crust, Individual	1278
Philly Cheese Steak, Thin Crust, Large	2248
Supreme, Cheesy Bites Crust	2600
Supreme, Deep Pan, Large	2440
Supreme, Deep Pan, Reg	1158
Supreme, GF	1068
Supreme, Stuffed Crust, Individual	1368
Supreme, Stuffed Crust, Large	2600
Supreme, Thin Crust, Individual	1038
Supreme, Thin Crust, Large	1840
Texas Meat Meltdown, Cheesy Bites Crust	2880
Texas Meat Meltdown, Deep Pan, Large	2728
Texas Meat Meltdown, Deep Pan, Reg	1308
Texas Meat Meltdown, GF	1014
Texas Meat Meltdown, Stuffed Crust, Individual	1524
Texas Meat Meltdown, Stuffed Crust, Large	2880
Texas Meat Meltdown, Thin Crust, Individual	1188
Texas Meat Meltdown, Thin Crust, Large	2256
The G.O.A.T, Cheesy Bites Crust	2456
The G.O.A.T, Deep Pan, Large	2312
The G.O.A.T, Deep Pan, Reg	1134
The G.O.A.T, GF	1032
The G.O.A.T, Stuffed Crust, Individual	1338
The G.O.A.T, Stuffed Crust, Large	2456
The G.O.A.T, Thin Crust, Individual	1002
The G.O.A.T, Thin Crust, Large	1696
Veggie, Cheesy Bites Crust	2184
Veggie, Deep Pan, Large	2032

PIZZA HUT
PIZZA
Veggie, Deep Pan, Reg	984
Veggie, Epic, Cheesy Bites Crust	2320
Veggie, Epic, Deep Pan, Large	2176
Veggie, Epic, Deep Pan, Reg	1062
Veggie, Epic, GF	966
Veggie, Epic, Stuffed Crust, Individual	1272
Veggie, Epic, Stuffed Crust, Large	2320
Veggie, Epic, Thin Crust, Individual	942
Veggie, Epic, Thin Crust, Large	1568
Veggie, GF	888
Veggie, Stuffed Crust, Individual	1194
Veggie, Stuffed Crust, Large	2184
Veggie, Thin Crust, Individual	864
Veggie, Thin Crust, Large	1432
Veggie, Vegan, Deep Pan, Large	1932
Veggie, Vegan, Deep Pan, Reg	933
Veggie, Vegan, GF	929
Veggie, Vegan, Thin Crust, Individual	812
Veggie, Vegan, Thin Crust, Large	1332

PIZZA TOPPING
Chicken	20
Ham	13
Pepperoni	34
Peppers	2
Pineapple	21
Sweetcorn	15
Tuna	14

POTATO SALAD
Salad Station	27

RIBS
Pork, BBQ	582
Pork, Rack, All American	787

ROLLS
Jack 'N' Roll, Vegan	305

SALSA
Salad Station	12

SAUCE
BBQ	119
Chocolate, Ice Cream Factory, Kids	32
Chocolate, Ice Cream Factory	59
Hot & Spicy	65
Hut House Seasoning	322
Raspberry, Ice Cream Factory	263
Sweet Chilli	175

SULTANAS
Salad Station	55

SWEETCORN
Salad Station	15

TOMATOES
Cherry, Salad Station	3

TOPPING
Gold Crunch, Ice Cream Factory	681

PIZZA HUT
TOPPING
Lemon Crunch, Ice Cream Factory	382
Sprinkles, Ice Cream Factory	421
Strawberry Crunch, Ice Cream Factory	382

TORTILLA CHIPS
Salad Station	96

VINEGAR
Sarsons	21

WRAP
Chicken, & Cheese, Little Boss	535
Chicken, & Sweetcorn, Little Boss	426
Chicken, Big Boss	396
Tuna, & Cheese	350
Tuna, & Sweetcorn	245
Tuna	210

PRET A MANGER

ALMONDS
Chocolate, Dark	235

AVOCADO
Smashed, on Bread, GF	293

BAGUETTE
Artichoke, Olives, & Tapenade, Vegan	454
Avocado, Olives, & Tomato, with Rocket	529
Beetroot, Smashed, Pistachios, & Feta	531
Brie, Tomato, & Basil, White	431
Cheddar, & Pickle, Posh	620
Cheddar, & Pickle, Posh, Veggie Pret	615
Chicken, & Bacon, Caesar, White	595
Chuna Mayo, Vegan	491
Egg Mayo, & Tomatoes, Breakfast	309
Egg Mayonnaise, & Bacon, Breakfast	326
Egg Mayonnaise, & Avocado	533
Egg Mayonnaise, & Bacon	494
Egg Mayonnaise, & Roasted Tomatoes	447
Egg Mayonnaise, & Salmon, Smoked	503
Egg Mayonnaise, Free Range, & Avocado, Breakfast	335
Eggless Mayo, & Cress, Vegan	602
Ham, & Pickles, Jambon Beurre, White	355
Ham, Pulled, Egg, & Pickles, White	624
Mozzarella, & Pesto, Italian	549
Mozzarella, & Pesto, Italian, with Vegan Mayo	523
Mozzarella, Chipotle, Hot	422
Prosciutto, Italian	536
Prosciutto, Posh	518
Salmon, Smoked, Soft Cheese, & Dill	453
Salmon, Smoked, with Egg Mayo, Breakfast	339
Tuna Mayo, & Cucumber, Pole & Line Caught, White	540
Veggie, Italian	517
Veggie, Italian, with Vegan Mayo	510

BANANA
Portion	62

BARS
Choc	348
Chocolate, Milk	145
Chocolate Brownie	291
Dairy Free, Chocolatey, Coconut Bite	208
Love Bar	325
Nut	248
Popcorn	171
Pret Bar	279

BISCUITS
Ginger Snap	240
Gingerbread	197

BITES
Almond Butter	142

BREAD
Baguette, Losange, for Soup	214
Focaccia, Brie, & Bacon	687
Focaccia, Mozzarella, Pesto, & Roasted Tomatoes	465

PRET A MANGER

BREAD
Focaccia, Mushroom, Creamy, Toasted	370
Focaccia, Salt Beef, & Pickles	616
GF, for Soup	132

BREAKFAST
Acai, & Almond Butter, Bowl	371
Bacon, Brioche	420
Bacon & Egg Brioche	490
Fruit, Yoghurt, & Granola, Bowl	263
Ham, & Egg, Brioche	408
Mango, & Banana, Sunshine, Bowl	253
Poached Egg, & Beans, Power Pot	238
Sausage, & Egg, Brioche	585
Veggie Brioche	346

BREAKFAST CEREAL
Bircher Muesli, Bowl	299
Honey, Granola, Pot	272
Porridge, Coconut	218
Porridge, No Topping	242

BUTTER
Almond, Easy Peasy Almond Squeezy	191

CAKE
Banana, Slice	223
Carrot, Slice	309
Lemon Drizzle, GF, Slice	409
Pecan Slice	467
Victoria Sponge	464

CHEESECAKE
Lemon, Pot	321

CHOCOLATE
Dark, with Sea Salt	136

COFFEE
American, Black, Iced	1
Americano, Black	3
Americano, White, Iced	35
Cappuccino	92
Cappuccino, Soya	92
Cappucino, Oat Milk	116
Filter Coffee	3
Flat White	80
Flat White, Rice-Coconut	102
Flat White, Soya	77
Frappe, Chocolate	439
Frappe, Classic	251
Latte, Iced	120
Latte, Pumpkin Spice	167
Latte, Rice-Coconut, Iced	151
Latte, Rice-Coconut	150
Latte, Skimmed Milk	118
Latte, Soya, Iced	113
Latte, Soya	113
Latte, Soya, Pumpkin Spice	162
Macchiato	5

PRET A MANGER

COFFEE

Mocha, Coconut, Iced	190
Mocha, Iced	185
Mocha, Rice-Coconut	216
Mocha, Semi Skimmed Milk	185
Mocha, Skimmed, Iced	143
Mocha, Soya, Iced	160
Mocha, Soya	181

COOKIES

Chocolate, Chunk	370
Chocolate, Dark, & Almond Butter	377
Fruit, Oat & Spelt	347
Pecan, & Caramel	391

CORN CAKES

Chocolate Covered, Dark	239

CRANBERRIES

& Seeds, Topping, for Breakfast	122
in Coats, Yoghurt Coating	234

CRISPS

Mature Cheddar, & Red Onion	200
Sea Salt, & Organic Cider Vinegar	196
Sea Salt	203
Smokey Chipotle	203
Vegetable, Carrot, Beetroot, & Parsnip	202

CROISSANT

Almond	374
Butter, French	291
Ham, Cheese, Tomato & Bacon	338
Jam	335
Mozzarella & Tomato	322

DANISH PASTRY

Cinnamon	489

DHAL

Butternut, & Lentil	246

DRESSING

Chilli, Ancho	46
Feta	132
Green, Zingy	52

DRIED FRUIT

Mango	119

FLATBREAD

Artichokes, Olive Tapenade, Rocket, & Basil	421
Avocado, Mexican	485
Chicken, Pesto, & Rocket	567
Falafel, Avocado, & Chipotle	470
Greek, Green	402
Salmon, & Avocado	592
Summer, Italian	431

FRUIT

Fruit Salad	111
Mango & Lime	92
Melon, & Blueberry	38
Superfruit Salad, Pot	61

PRET A MANGER

FRUIT & NUT MIX

with Chocolate Covered Raisins	177

FRUIT COMPOTE

Topping, for Breakfast	24

GINGER BEER

Pure Pret	129

GRATIN

Butternut Squash, & Cauliflor	514

HONEY

Breakfast Topping	107

HOT CHOCOLATE

Coconut, Iced	260
Iced	256
Portion	256
Rice-Coconut	288
Skimmed, Iced	213
Soya, Iced	230
Soya	251

JUICE

Apple	120
Carrot	50
Daily Greens	144
Ginger & Apple, Shot	55
Hot Shot	47
Orange, Freshly Squeezed, Natural, Super	105
Orange, Large	168

JUICE DRINK

Apple, Fizz, Sparkling, Pure	112
Cranberry & Raspberry, Still	175
Grape & Elderflower, Sparkling, Pure Pret	109
Green Tea, Yoga Bunny, Sparkling, Pure	116
Orange, & Passion Fruit, Still	135

KOMBUCHA

Ginger	43

LEMONADE

Rhubarb, Pure	118
Still, Lemon & Ginger, Pure	153

MACARONI CHEESE

& Greens, Vegan	560
Kale, & Cauliflower	549
Lasagne	572
Prosciutto	586

MILK

Babyccino, with Chocolate Sprinkles	14
Cold, for Kids	94
Rice-Coconut	150

MOUSSE

Chocolate	306

MUFFIN

Double Berry	441

NUTS

Naked	254

PRET A MANGER
OMELETTE
Bacon, & Spinach	199
Egg, & Chorizo, Spicy	196
Eggs, & Corn, Spicy	223
Feta, & Red Pepper	167
Mushroom, & Spinach	182
Squash, Soft Cheese, & Feta	201

PAIN AU RAISIN
Portion	394

POPCORN
Rock Salt	143
Sweet, & Salt	163

SALAD
Asian, Style, Veggie Pot	202
Chicken, & Avocado, Smashed	346
Chicken, Bang Bang	378
Chicken, Italian, Chef's	635
Chicken, Italian, Chef's, without Dressing	401
Egg, & Avocado, Smashed	315
Egg, & Spinach, Protein Pot	104
Falafel, Mezze	337
Greek, Pret's	358
Protein Box	321
Roast Beets, Squash, & Feta, Veggie Box	357
Salmon, & Avocado, Smashed	315
Salmon, & Egg, Smoked, Protein Pot	134
Salmon, Cali-Style	489
Squash, Roast, Pecans, & Feta Dressing	225
Sweet Potato Falafel, & Smashed Beets, Veggie Box	407
Tuna, Nicoise	469

SALMON
Smoked, Protein Box	409

SANDWICH
Avocado, Smashed, Carrots, & Dill, GF	313
BLT, Best Ever	525
Cheddar, Mature, & Pret Pickle	517
Cheddar, Mature, & Pret Pickle, Veggie Pret	512
Cheese, Kids	422
Chicken, Avocado, & Basil	482
Chicken, Caesar, & Smashed Avo, GF	452
Club, Carrot, & Houmous, Smoky	411
Club, Classic Super	526
Egg, Free Range, & Tomato, on Rye	429
Egg Mayo, Free Range, Kids	315
Egg Mayo, Free-Range	367
Falafel, Halloumi, & Pickles, Brioche, Hot	520
Falafel, Halloumi, & Pickles, Brioche	482
Ham, & Cheese	531
Ham, Kids	300
Houmous, & Red Peppers, GF	426
New Yorker, on Rye, Veggie	571
Salmon, Scottish, Smoked	421
Salmon, Smoked, & Soft Cheese, GF	297

PRET A MANGER
SANDWICH
Super Greens, & Reds	447
The VLT	345
Tuna, & Cucumber	447

SMOOTHIE
Almond, Protein Power	639
Almond Butter, & Berries	534
Avocado	272
Berry Blast	239
Coco-Berry, Bircher	265
Mango, & Pineapple	209
Mango	143
Strawberry, & Banana	211
Super Greens	265
Vitamin Volcano	130

SOUP
Broth, Chicken, Shiitake, & Miso	127
Broth, Chicken, Shiitake, & Miso, Side	79
Chicken, & Butternut, Risotto	208
Chicken, & Butternut, Risotto, Side	123
Chicken, Broccoli, & Brown Rice	85
Chicken, Curry, Coconut	217
Chicken, Fajita	194
Chicken, Fajita, Side	115
Chicken, Katsu	237
Chicken, Katsu, Side	141
Chicken, Roast, & Root Veg	196
Chicken, Roast, & Root Veg, Side	116
Chowder, Sweetcorn, Smoky	217
Chowder, Sweetcorn, Smoky, Side	129
Miso	38
Mushroom, Risotto	203
Mushroom, Risotto, Side	121
Pea, & Mint	183
Pea, & Mint, Side	108
Tomato, Souper, Side	123
Vegetable, Red Thai	184
Vegetable, Red Thai, Side	110

TART
Bakewell, Slice	467

TEA
Black, Iced	0
Ceylon, Breakfast	14
Chamomile	0
Earl Grey, Black	14
Fennel, & Mint	0
Green, & Peach	88
Green, Iced	0
Green, Iced, with Blood Orange, & Pomegranate	50
Green, Tropical	0
Green, White Matcha, Oolong	0
Latta, Matcha, Semi-Skimmed, Iced	136
Latta, Matcha, Skimmed, Iced	113

PRET A MANGER

TEA

Latte, Chai, Coconut, Iced	262
Latte, Chai, Iced	218
Latte, Chai, Organic	218
Latte, Chai, Skimmed, Iced	218
Latte, Chai, Soya, Iced	288
Latte, Matcha, Iced	150
Latte, Matcha	205
Latte, Matcha, Soya, Iced	130
Latte, Turmeric, Iced	141
Latte, Turmeric	198
Latte, Turmeric, Semi-Skimmed, Iced	134
Latte, Turmeric, Soya, Iced	128
Latte, Turmeric Skimmed, Iced	1107
Lemon, & Ginger, Infusion	100
Peppermint, Peace	0
Peppermint	0
Raspberry, & Pomegranate, Infusion	98
Rooibos Cacao	0
Turmeric Tonic	0

TOASTIE

Brie, Avocado & Tomato	562
Cheese, Classic	599
Halloumi, & Red Pepper	556
Ham, Cheese, & Mustard	561
Tuna Melt	537

WATER

Spring, Sparkling	0

WRAP

Avocado, & Herb Salad	509
Avocado, & Herb Salad, Veggie Pret	512
Chicken, Bang Bang	433
Chicken, Spicy, Hot	495
Duck, Hoisin, Salad	459
Falafel, & Halloumi, Hot	624
Houmous, & Chipotle	412
Mushroom, Hoisin, Vegan	377
Ragu, & Red Pepper, Vegan, Hot	420
Swedish Meatball, Hot	663
Sweet Potato, Mexican	339

YOGHURT

Coconut, & Mango, Bowl	287
Mango, Chia, Pot	116

PREZZO

ANTIPASTI

Meats, Cured, Sharers	979

BITES

Pizza, Sharers	860
Pizza, Spicy, Sharers	860

BITES

Pizza, Spicy, Starter	356
Pizza, Starter	356

BOLOGNESE

Spaghetti	589
Spaghetti, with King Prawns	564

BREAD

Garlic, Pizza, Large, Sharers	892
Garlic, Starter	271
Garlic, with Balsamic Onions, & Mozzarella, Starter	520
Garlic, with Mozzarella, Starter	386

BROCCOLI

Tenderstem, & Cauliflower	88

BROWNIE

Chocolate, Dome	467

BRUSCHETTA

Tomato, Starter	415

BURGER

Calabrese, with Fries	1382

CALZONE

Spicy Carne	898
Tre Carni	930

CARBONARA

Spaghetti, Chicken, Al Forno	1033
Spaghetti	662

CHEESE

Mozzarella, Breaded, Starter	561

CHEESECAKE

Honeycomb Smash, Mini	219
Honeycomb Smash	500
Vanilla, with Caramel Sauce, Mini	203
Vanilla, with Raspberries, Mini	242

CHICKEN

Breast, Chargrilled, with Mushrooms	384

DESSERT

Affogato	320

FLATBREAD

Sharers	849

FRIES

House, Side	582
Truffle Oil Infused, Side	671

HOUMOUS

Italian, Starter	667

ICE CREAM

Chocolate	194
Strawberry	171
Vanilla	171

	KCAL		KCAL
PREZZO		**PREZZO**	
LASAGNE		**RISOTTO**	
Traditional, Al Forno	687	Prawn, King, & Salmon	471
MEATBALLS		**SALAD**	
Giant, Starter	453	Caesar, Chicken, no Garlic Bread	737
MUSHROOMS		Caprese, Starter	241
Stuffed, Baked, Starter	395	Chicken, Bacon & Avocado, no Garlic Bread	512
OLIVES		Lentil, Beetroot, & Butternut, no Garlic Bread	321
Marinated	102	Mix, Side	103
PANNA COTTA		Rocket, with Italian Cheese, Side	93
with Fruit Compote, Mini	126	**SALMON**	
with Fruit Compote	375	Fillet, Roast, with Vegetables	483
PASTA		**SEA BASS**	
Penne, Alla Rusticana	756	with Vegetables, & Pesto	506
Penne, Arrabbiata	501	**SORBET**	
Penne, Aubergine	554	Raspberry	13
Penne, Goats Cheese, Al Forno	1033	**SPAGHETTI & MEATBALLS**	
Penne, Gorgonzola	633	Al Forno	903
Penne, Pancetta, Pea, & Mushroom, Light	492	**SQUID**	
Penne, Pesto & Pea	681	Calamari, Starter	702
Penne, Prawn, Spicy, & Basil Pesto, Light	506	**TART**	
Penne, Salmon, Oak Smoked	840	Chocolate, Salted Caramel	599
PASTRY		**TIRAMISU**	
Cannoli, Mini	282	Portion	323
PIZZA			
Chicken & Roasted Pepper, Large	1111		
Chicken & Roasted Pepper, Reg	923		
Chicken Primavera, Light	524		
Fiorentina, Large	1016		
Fiorentina, Reg	699		
Goats Cheese, & Aubergine, Light	554		
Goats Cheese, & Red Pepper, Large	1053		
Goats Cheese, & Red Pepper, Reg	910		
Margherita, Large	837		
Margherita, Reg	705		
Margherita Royale, Premium	979		
Mushroom, Garlic, Large	725		
Mushroom, Garlic, Reg	595		
Pepperoni, Posh, Premium	1242		
Tre Gusti, Large	1339		
Tre Gusti, Reg	929		
Tropicana, Large	1018		
Tropicana, Reg	783		
Vesuvio, Large	1052		
Vesuvio, Reg	872		
PRAWNS			
King, Starter	406		
PUDDING			
Sticky Toffee	631		
RAVIOLI			
Lobster, & Crab	510		
RISOTTO			
Chicken, & Asparagus	787		
Mushroom	725		

STARBUCKS

BANANA
Fairtrade	108

BARS
Caramel, Stick, Crispy	185
Granola	326
Pistachio, Vegan	326
Raspberry, Stick, Crispy	181
Rocky Road	333

BREAD
Banana	381
Ciabatta, Cheese, & Marmite, Mini	355
Focaccia, Brie, & Cran-Merry	384

BREAKFAST
Eggs, Scrambled, Tomato, & Spinach, Hot Box	262

BREAKFAST CEREAL
Berry Good Bircher	286
Porridge, 5 Grain	285
Porridge, Oatmeal, Classic	303

BROWNIES
Chocolate, Christmas Tree	372

BURRITO
Breakfast, All Day, Vegan	388

CAKE
Carrot, Loaf	323
Chocolate, Christmas Bauble, Loaf	392
Lemon, Loaf	352

COFFEE - AMERICANO
Grande	16
Short	5
Tall	11
Venti	22

COFFEE - AMERICANO, ICED
Grande	16
Tall	11
Venti	22

COFFEE - CAPPUCCINO
Almond Milk, Grande	74
Almond Milk, Short	35
Almond Milk, Tall	67
Almond Milk, Venti	104
Coconut Milk, Grande	120
Coconut Milk, Short	57
Coconut Milk, Tall	108
Coconut Milk, Venti	168
Oat Milk, Grande	213
Oat Milk, Short	100
Oat Milk, Tall	191
Oat Milk, Venti	297
Semi Skimmed Milk, Grande	143
Semi Skimmed Milk, Short	68
Semi Skimmed Milk, Tall	129
Semi Skimmed Milk, Venti	201
Skimmed Milk, Grande	103

STARBUCKS

COFFEE - CAPPUCCINO
Skimmed Milk, Short	49
Skimmed Milk, Tall	93
Skimmed Milk, Venti	144
Soy, Grande	119
Soy, Short	56
Soy, Tall	107
Soy, Venti	167
Whole Milk, Grande	181
Whole Milk, Short	85
Whole Milk, Tall	163
Whole Milk, Venti	253

COFFEE - CAPPUCCINO, ICED
Almond Milk, Grande	70
Almond Milk, Tall	58
Almond Milk, Venti	83
Coconut Milk, Grande	113
Coconut Milk, Tall	92
Coconut Milk, Venti	131
Oat Milk, Grande	201
Oat Milk, Tall	162
Oat Milk, Venti	230
Semi Skimmed Milk, Grande	136
Semi Skimmed Milk, Tall	110
Semi Skimmed Milk, Venti	156
Skimmed Milk, Grande	97
Skimmed Milk, Tall	80
Skimmed Milk, Venti	113
Soy, Grande	113
Soy, Tall	92
Soy, Venti	131
Whole Milk, Grande	171
Whole Milk, Tall	138
Whole Milk, Venti	196
with Cold Foam, Skimmed Milk, Grande	69
with Cold Foam, Skimmed Milk, Tall	57
with Cold Foam, Skimmed Milk, Venti	93

COFFEE - COLD BREW
Grande	1
Short	0
Tall	1
Venti	1

COFFEE - COLD BREW, LATTE
Almond Milk, Grande	53
Almond Milk, Tall	40
Almond Milk, Venti	63
Coconut Milk, Grande	91
Coconut Milk, Tall	69
Coconut Milk, Venti	108
Oat Milk, Grande	169
Oat Milk, Tall	127
Oat Milk, Venti	199
Semi Skimmed Milk, Grande	110

STARBUCKS

COFFEE - COLD BREW, LATTE

Semi Skimmed Milk, Tall	83
Semi Skimmed Milk, Venti	130
Skimmed Milk, Grande	77
Skimmed Milk, Tall	58
Skimmed Milk, Venti	91
Soy, Grande	91
Soy, Tall	69
Soy, Venti	107
Whole Milk, Grande	142
Whole Milk, Tall	108
Whole Milk, Venti	168

COFFEE - COLD BREW, NITRO

10oz	4
Tall	4
with Caramel Cold Foam, Skimmed Milk, 10oz	23
with Caramel Cold Foam, Skimmed Milk, Tall	28
with Cold Foam, Skimmed Milk, 10oz	21
with Cold Foam, Skimmed Milk, Tall	26

COFFEE - CORTADO

Almond Milk	34
Coconut Milk	50
Oat Milk	84
Semi Skimmed Milk	59
Skimmed Milk	44
Soy	50
Whole Milk	72

COFFEE - ESPRESSO

Con Panna, Doppio	80
Con Panna, Solo	64
Doppio	11
Solo	6
Macchiato, Almond Milk, Doppio	15
Macchiato, Almond Milk, Solo	7
Macchiato, Coconut Milk, Doppio	17
Macchiato, Coconut Milk, Solo	8
Oat Milk, Doppio	23
Oat Milk, Solo	9
Macchiato, Semi Skimmed Milk, Doppio	19
Macchiato, Semi Skimmed Milk, Solo	7
Macchiato, Skimmed Milk, Doppio	16
Macchiato, Skimmed Milk, Solo	7
Macchiato, Soy, Doppio	17
Macchiato, Soy, Solo	8
Macchiato, Whole Milk, Doppio	21
Macchiato, Whole Milk, Solo	9

COFFEE - FILTER

Grande	3
Short	2
Tall	2
Venti	4

COFFEE - FLAT WHITE

Almond Milk, Short	47

STARBUCKS

COFFEE - FLAT WHITE

Coconut Milk, Short	73
Oat Milk, Short	126
Semi Skimmed Milk, Short	87
Ã‚Â Skimmed Milk, Short	63
Soy, Short	73
Whole Milk, Short	108

COFFEE - LATTE

Almond Milk, Grande	92
Almond Milk, Short	43
Almond Milk, Tall	74
Almond Milk, Venti	121
Coconut Milk, Grande	164
Coconut Milk, Short	77
Coconut Milk, Tall	130
Coconut Milk, Venti	214
Oat Milk, Grande	269
Oat Milk, Short	127
Oat Milk, Tall	212
Oat Milk, Venti	350
Semi Skimmed Milk, Grande	180
Semi Skimmed Milk, Short	85
Semi Skimmed Milk, Tall	143
Semi Skimmed Milk, Venti	235
Skimmed Milk, Grande	128
Skimmed Milk, Short	60
Skimmed Milk, Tall	102
Skimmed Milk, Venti	168
Soy, Grande	149
Soy, Short	70
Soy, Tall	119
Soy, Venti	195
Whole Milk, Grande	228
Whole Milk, Short	108
Whole Milk, Tall	181
Whole Milk, Venti	298
Cardamon Vanilla, Coconut Milk, Grande	148
Cardamon Vanilla, Coconut Milk, Short	77
Cardamon Vanilla, Coconut Milk, Tall	118
Cardamon Vanilla, Coconut Milk, Venti	207
Cardamon Vanilla, Oat Milk, Grande	269
Cardamon Vanilla, Oat Milk, Short	137
Cardamon Vanilla, Oat Milk, Tall	213
Cardamon Vanilla, Oat Milk, Venti	366
Cardamon Vanilla, Semi Skimmed Milk, Grande	179
Cardamon Vanilla, Semi Skimmed Milk, Short	93
Cardamon Vanilla, Semi Skimmed Milk, Tall	143
Cardamon Vanilla, Semi Skimmed Milk, Venti	248
Cardamon Vanilla, Skimmed Milk, Grande	127
Cardamon Vanilla, Skimmed Milk, Short	67
Cardamon Vanilla, Skimmed Milk, Tall	101
Cardamon Vanilla, Skimmed Milk, Venti	180
Cardamon Vanilla, Soy, Grande	148

STARBUCKS
COFFEE - LATTE

Cardamon Vanilla, Soy, Short	77
Cardamon Vanilla, Soy, Tall	118
Cardamon Vanilla, Soy, Venti	207
Cardamon Vanilla, Whole Milk, Grande	228
Cardamon Vanilla, Whole Milk, Short	117
Cardamon Vanilla, Whole Milk, Tall	181
Cardamon Vanilla, Whole Milk, Venti	312
Eggnog, Grande	344
Eggnog, Short	170
Eggnog, Tall	272
Eggnog, Venti	366
Gingerbread, Almond Milk, Grande	254
Gingerbread, Almond Milk, Short	143
Gingerbread, Almond Milk, Tall	197
Gingerbread, Almond Milk, Venti	300
Gingerbread, Coconut Milk, Grande	327
Gingerbread, Coconut Milk, Short	177
Gingerbread, Coconut Milk, Tall	247
Gingerbread, Coconut Milk, Venti	392
Gingerbread, Oat Milk, Grande	432
Gingerbread, Oat Milk, Short	225
Gingerbread, Oat Milk, Tall	318
Gingerbread, Oat Milk, Venti	523
Gingerbread, Semi Skimmed Milk, Grande	343
Gingerbread, Semi Skimmed Milk, Short	184
Gingerbread, Semi Skimmed Milk, Tall	258
Gingerbread, Semi Skimmed Milk, Venti	412
Gingerbread, Skimmed Milk, Grande	290
Gingerbread, Skimmed Milk, Short	160
Gingerbread, Skimmed Milk, Tall	222
Gingerbread, Skimmed Milk, Venti	346
Gingerbread, Soy, Grande	312
Gingerbread, Soy, Short	170
Gingerbread, Soy, Tall	236
Gingerbread, Soy, Venti	373
Gingerbread, Whole Milk, Grande	391
Gingerbread, Whole Milk, Short	207
Gingerbread, Whole Milk, Tall	291
Gingerbread, Whole Milk, Venti	472
Toffee Nut, Almond Milk, Grande	256
Toffee Nut, Almond Milk, Short	146
Toffee Nut, Almond Milk, Tall	200
Toffee Nut, Almond Milk, Venti	302
Toffee Nut, Coconut Milk, Grande	314
Toffee Nut, Coconut Milk, Short	172
Toffee Nut, Coconut Milk, Tall	239
Toffee Nut, Coconut Milk, Venti	374
Toffee Nut, Oat Milk, Grande	434
Toffee Nut, Oat Milk, Short	228
Toffee Nut, Oat Milk, Tall	321
Toffee Nut, Oat Milk, Venti	524
Toffee Nut, Semi Skimmed Milk, Grande	345

STARBUCKS
COFFEE - LATTE

Toffee Nut, Semi Skimmed Milk, Short	187
Toffee Nut, Semi Skimmed Milk, Tall	260
Toffee Nut, Semi Skimmed Milk, Venti	413
Toffee Nut, Skimmed Milk, Grande	293
Toffee Nut, Skimmed Milk, Short	163
Toffee Nut, Skimmed Milk, Tall	224
Toffee Nut, Skimmed Milk, Venti	347
Toffee Nut, Soy, Grande	314
Toffee Nut, Soy, Short	173
Toffee Nut, Soy, Tall	239
Toffee Nut, Soy, Venti	374
Toffee Nut, Whole Milk, Grande	393
Toffee Nut, Whole Milk, Short	209
Toffee Nut, Whole Milk, Tall	293
Toffee Nut, Whole Milk, Venti	473
Vanilla, Almond Milk, Grande	164
Vanilla, Almond Milk, Short	79
Vanilla, Almond Milk, Tall	127
Vanilla, Almond Milk, Venti	210
Vanilla, Coconut Milk, Grande	222
Vanilla, Coconut Milk, Short	107
Vanilla, Coconut Milk, Tall	172
Vanilla, Coconut Milk, Venti	285
Vanilla, Oat Milk, Grande	342
Vanilla, Oat Milk, Short	162
Vanilla, Oat Milk, Tall	265
Vanilla, Oat Milk, Venti	438
Vanilla, Semi Skimmed Milk, Grande	253
Vanilla, Semi Skimmed Milk, Short	121
Vanilla, Semi Skimmed Milk, Tall	196
Vanilla, Semi Skimmed Milk, Venti	324
Vanilla, Skimmed Milk, Grande	201
Vanilla, Skimmed Milk, Short	96
Vanilla, Skimmed Milk, Tall	155
Vanilla, Skimmed Milk, Venti	257
Vanilla, Soy Milk, Grande	222
Vanilla, Soy Milk, Short	106
Vanilla, Soy Milk, Tall	172
Vanilla, Soy Milk, Venti	284
Vanilla, Whole Milk, Grande	301
Vanilla, Whole Milk, Short	143
Vanilla, Whole Milk, Tall	233
Vanilla, Whole Milk, Venti	386

COFFEE - LATTE, ICED

Almond Milk, Grande	65
Almond Milk, Tall	54
Almond Milk, Venti	78
Coconut Milk, Grande	105
Coconut Milk, Tall	85
Coconut Milk, Venti	123
Oat Milk, Grande	185
Oat Milk, Tall	149

STARBUCKS

COFFEE - LATTE, ICED

	KCAL
Oat Milk, Venti	214
Semi Skimmed Milk, Grande	125
Semi Skimmed Milk, Tall	102
Semi Skimmed Milk, Venti	146
Skimmed Milk, Grande	90
Skimmed Milk, Tall	74
Skimmed Milk, Venti	106
Soy, Grande	104
Soy, Tall	85
Soy, Venti	122
Whole Milk, Grande	158
Whole Milk, Tall	128
Whole Milk, Venti	183
Eggnog, Grande	237
Eggnog, Tall	191
Eggnog, Venti	332
Gingerbread, Almond Milk, Grande	227
Gingerbread, Almond Milk, Tall	185
Gingerbread, Almond Milk, Venti	261
Gingerbread, Coconut Milk, Grande	276
Gingerbread, Coconut Milk, Tall	224
Gingerbread, Coconut Milk, Venti	316
Gingerbread, Oat Milk, Grande	347
Gingerbread, Oat Milk, Tall	280
Gingerbread, Oat Milk, Venti	397
Gingerbread, Semi Skimmed Milk, Grande	287
Gingerbread, Semi Skimmed Milk, Tall	233
Gingerbread, Semi Skimmed Milk, Venti	329
Gingerbread, Skimmed Milk, Grande	252
Gingerbread, Skimmed Milk, Tall	205
Gingerbread, Skimmed Milk, Venti	289
Gingerbread, Soy, Grande	266
Gingerbread, Soy, Tall	216
Gingerbread, Soy, Venti	305
Gingerbread, Whole Milk, Grande	320
Gingerbread, Whole Milk, Tall	259
Gingerbread, Whole Milk, Venti	366
Toffee Nut, Almond Milk, Grande	230
Toffee Nut, Almond Milk, Tall	188
Toffee Nut, Almond Milk, Venti	262
Toffee Nut, Coconut Milk, Grande	278
Toffee Nut, Coconut Milk, Tall	227
Toffee Nut, Coconut Milk, Venti	317
Toffee Nut, Oat Milk, Grande	349
Toffee Nut, Oat Milk, Tall	283
Toffee Nut, Oat Milk, Venti	398
Toffee Nut, Semi Skimmed Milk, Grande	289
Toffee Nut, Semi Skimmed Milk, Tall	235
Toffee Nut, Semi Skimmed Milk, Venti	330
Toffee Nut, Skimmed Milk, Grande	254
Toffee Nut, Skimmed Milk, Tall	207
Toffee Nut, Skimmed Milk, Venti	290

	KCAL
Toffee Nut, Soy, Grande	268
Toffee Nut, Soy, Tall	219
Toffee Nut, Soy, Venti	306
Toffee Nut, Whole Milk, Grande	322
Toffee Nut, Whole Milk, Tall	261
Toffee Nut, Whole Milk, Venti	367

COFFEE - LATTE, MACCHIATO

	KCAL
Almond Milk, Grande	78
Almond Milk, Short	34
Almond Milk, Tall	78
Almond Milk, Venti	102
Coconut Milk, Grande	119
Coconut Milk, Short	54
Coconut Milk, Tall	89
Coconut Milk, Venti	163
Oat Milk, Grande	195
Oat Milk, Short	97
Oat Milk, Tall	162
Oat Milk, Venti	272
Semi Skimmed Milk, Grande	132
Semi Skimmed Milk, Short	66
Semi Skimmed Milk, Tall	110
Semi Skimmed Milk, Venti	184
Skimmed Milk, Grande	94
Skimmed Milk, Short	47
Skimmed Milk, Tall	79
Skimmed Milk, Venti	133
Soy, Grande	110
Soy, Short	55
Soy, Tall	92
Soy, Venti	154
Whole Milk, Grande	166
Whole Milk, Short	83
Whole Milk, Tall	138
Whole Milk, Venti	232

COFFEE - MACCHIATO

	KCAL
Caramel, Almond Milk, Grande	155
Caramel, Almond Milk, Short	74
Caramel, Almond Milk, Tall	122
Caramel, Almond Milk, Venti	193
Caramel, Coconut Milk, Grande	205
Caramel, Coconut Milk, Short	98
Caramel, Coconut Milk, Tall	161
Caramel, Coconut Milk, Venti	253
Caramel, Semi Skimmed Milk, Grande	229
Caramel, Semi Skimmed Milk, Short	109
Caramel, Semi Skimmed Milk, Tall	180
Caramel, Semi Skimmed Milk, Venti	281
Caramel, Skimmed Milk, Grande	187
Caramel, Skimmed Milk, Short	89
Caramel, Skimmed Milk, Tall	146
Caramel, Skimmed Milk, Venti	231
Caramel, Soy, Grande	205
Caramel, Soy, Short	97

STARBUCKS

COFFEE - MACCHIATO

Caramel, Soy, Tall	161
Caramel, Soy, Venti	253
Caramel, Whole Milk, Grande	273
Caramel, Whole Milk, Short	129
Caramel, Whole Milk, Tall	215
Caramel, Whole Milk, Venti	335

COFFEE - MACCHIATO, CARAMEL

Oat Milk, Grande	308
Oat Milk, Short	145
Oat Milk, Tall	243
Oat Milk, Venti	377

COFFEE - MACCHIATO, ICED

Caramel, Almond Milk, Grande	140
Caramel, Almond Milk, Tall	110
Caramel, Almond Milk, Venti	171
Caramel, Coconut Milk, Grande	179
Caramel, Coconut Milk, Tall	141
Caramel, Coconut Milk, Venti	216
Caramel, Oat Milk, Grande	259
Caramel, Oat Milk, Tall	205
Caramel, Oat Milk, Venti	307
Caramel, Semi Skimmed Milk, Grande	199
Caramel, Semi Skimmed Milk, Tall	157
Caramel, Semi Skimmed Milk, Venti	239
Caramel, Skimmed Milk, Grande	164
Caramel, Skimmed Milk, Tall	129
Caramel, Skimmed Milk, Venti	199
Caramel, Soy, Grande	178
Caramel, Soy, Tall	141
Caramel, Soy, Venti	215
Caramel, Whole Milk, Grande	232
Caramel, Whole Milk, Tall	183
Caramel, Whole Milk, Venti	276

COFFEE - MISTO

Almond Milk, Grande	48
Almond Milk, Short	24
Almond Milk, Tall	33
Almond Milk, Venti	64
Coconut Milk, Grande	81
Coconut Milk, Short	41
Coconut Milk, Tall	56
Coconut Milk, Venti	109
Oat Milk, Grande	149
Oat Milk, Short	76
Oat Milk, Tall	102
Oat Milk, Venti	200
Semi Skimmed Milk, Grande	98
Semi Skimmed Milk, Short	50
Semi Skimmed Milk, Tall	67
Semi Skimmed Milk, Venti	132
Skimmed Milk, Grande	69
Skimmed Milk, Short	35

STARBUCKS

COFFEE - MISTO

Skimmed Milk, Tall	47
Skimmed Milk, Venti	92
Soy, Grande	81
Soy, Short	41
Soy, Tall	55
Soy, Venti	108
Whole Milk, Grande	126
Whole Milk, Short	64
Whole Milk, Tall	86
Whole Milk, Venti	169

COFFEE - MOCHA

Almond Milk, Grande	225
Almond Milk, Short	128
Almond Milk, Tall	179
Almond Milk, Venti	256
Coconut Milk, Grande	263
Coconut Milk, Short	143
Coconut Milk, Tall	206
Coconut Milk, Venti	300
Oat Milk, Grande	342
Oat Milk, Short	174
Oat Milk, Tall	261
Oat Milk, Venti	389
Semi Skimmed Milk, Grande	283
Semi Skimmed Milk, Short	151
Semi Skimmed Milk, Tall	220
Semi Skimmed Milk, Venti	322
Skimmed Milk, Grande	249
Skimmed Milk, Short	137
Skimmed Milk, Tall	196
Skimmed Milk, Venti	283
Soy, Grande	263
Soy, Short	143
Soy, Tall	205
Soy, Venti	299
Whole Milk, Grande	315
Whole Milk, Short	163
Whole Milk, Tall	242
Whole Milk, Venti	359
White Choc, Almond Milk, Grande	350
White Choc, Almond Milk, Short	188
White Choc, Almond Milk, Tall	276
White Choc, Almond Milk, Venti	426
White Choc, Coconut Milk, Grande	388
White Choc, Coconut Milk, Short	204
White Choc, Coconut Milk, Tall	306
White Choc, Coconut Milk, Venti	479
White Choc, Oat Milk, Grande	466
White Choc, Oat Milk, Short	235
White Choc, Oat Milk, Tall	369
White Choc, Oat Milk, Venti	588
White Choc, Semi Skimmed Milk, Grande	408

STARBUCKS

COFFEE - MOCHA

White Choc, Semi Skimmed Milk, Short	212
White Choc, Semi Skimmed Milk, Tall	322
White Choc, Semi Skimmed Milk, Venti	507
White Choc, Skimmed Milk, Grande	374
White Choc, Skimmed Milk, Short	198
White Choc, Skimmed Milk, Tall	295
White Choc, Skimmed Milk, Venti	459
White Choc, Soy, Grande	387
White Choc, Soy, Short	203
White Choc, Soy, Tall	306
White Choc, Soy, Venti	478
White Choc, Whole Milk, Grande	440
White Choc, Whole Milk, Short	225
White Choc, Whole Milk, Tall	347
White Choc, Whole Milk, Venti	551

COFFEE - MOCHA, ICED

with Whipped Cream, Almond Milk, Grande	277
with Whipped Cream, Almond Milk, Tall	210
with Whipped Cream, Almond Milk, Venti	310
Ã,Â with Whipped Cream, Coconut Milk, Grande	317
with Whipped Cream, Coconut Milk, Tall	241
with Whipped Cream, Coconut Milk, Venti	354
with Whipped Cream, Oat Milk, Grande	397
I with Whipped Cream, Oat Milk, Tall	305
with Whipped Cream, Oat Milk, Venti	446
with Whipped Cream, Semi Skimmed Milk, Grande	337
with Whipped Cream, Semi Skimmed Milk, Tall	257
with Whipped Cream, Semi Skimmed Milk, Venti	378
with Whipped Cream, Skimmed Milk, Grande	302
with Whipped Cream, Skimmed Milk, Tall	229
with Whipped Cream, Skimmed Milk, Venti	338
with Whipped Cream, Soy, Grande	316
with Whipped Cream, Soy, Tall	241
with Whipped Cream, Soy, Venti	354
with Whipped Cream, Whole Milk, Grande	370
with Whipped Cream, Whole Milk, Tall	283
with Whipped Cream, Whole Milk, Venti	415

COFFEE - MOCHA, ICED, WHITE

with Whipped Cream, Almond Milk, Grande	387
with Whipped Cream, Almond Milk, Tall	290
with Whipped Cream, Almond Milk, Venti	458
with Whipped Cream, Coconut Milk, Grande	415
with Whipped Cream, Coconut Milk, Tall	314
with Whipped Cream, Coconut Milk, Venti	497
with Whipped Cream, Oat Milk, Grande	474
with Whipped Cream, Oat Milk, Tall	361
with Whipped Cream, Oat Milk, Venti	577
with Whipped Cream, Semi Skimmed Milk, Grande	430
with Whipped Cream, Semi Skimmed Milk, Tall	326
with Whipped Cream, Semi Skimmed Milk, Venti	517
with Whipped Cream, Skimmed Milk, Grande	405
with Whipped Cream, Skimmed Milk, Tall	305

STARBUCKS

COFFEE - MOCHA, ICED, WHITE

with Whipped Cream, Skimmed Milk, Venti	483
with Whipped Cream, Soy, Grande	415
with Whipped Cream, Soy, Tall	313
with Whipped Cream, Soy, Venti	497
with Whipped Cream, Whole Milk, Grande	454
with Whipped Cream, Whole Milk, Tall	345
with Whipped Cream, Whole Milk, Venti	550

COOKIES

Chocolate, Milk, Chunk	363
Chocolate, Triple	372
Oat, & Raisin	321

CROISSANT

Almond	339
Butter	255

CUPCAKES

Salted Caramel, Twinkle & Sprinkle	437

FRAPPUCCINO - CARAMEL

with Whipped Cream, Almond Milk, Grande	363
with Whipped Cream, Almond Milk, Mini	191
with Whipped Cream, Almond Milk, Tall	264
with Whipped Cream, Almond Milk, Venti	420
with Whipped Cream, Coconut Milk, Grande	379
with Whipped Cream, Coconut Milk, Mini	200
with Whipped Cream, Coconut Milk, Tall	277
with Whipped Cream, Coconut Milk, Venti	438
with Whipped Cream, Oat Milk, Grande	413
with Whipped Cream, Oat Milk, Mini	218
with Whipped Cream, Oat Milk, Tall	305
with Whipped Cream, Oat Milk, Venti	475
with Whipped Cream, Semi Skimmed Milk, Grande	388
with Whipped Cream, Semi Skimmed Milk, Mini	205
with Whipped Cream, Semi Skimmed Milk, Tall	284
with Whipped Cream, Semi Skimmed Milk, Venti	431
with Whipped Cream, Skimmed Milk, Grande	373
with Whipped Cream, Skimmed Milk, Mini	197
with Whipped Cream, Skimmed Milk, Tall	272
with Whipped Cream, Skimmed Milk, Venti	431
with Whipped Cream, Soy, Grande	379
with Whipped Cream, Soy, Mini	200
with Whipped Cream, Soy, Tall	277
with Whipped Cream, Soy, Venti	438
with Whipped Cream, Whole Milk, Grande	402
with Whipped Cream, Whole Milk, Mini	212
with Whipped Cream, Whole Milk, Tall	296
with Whipped Cream, Whole Milk, Venti	463
Light, No Whip, Skimmed Milk, Grande	127
Light, No Whip, Skimmed Milk, Mini	72
Light, No Whip, Skimmed Milk, Tall	93
Light, No Whip, Skimmed Milk, Venti	156

FRAPPUCCINO - CARAMEL CREAM

with Whipped Cream, Almond Milk, Grande	305
with Whipped Cream, Almond Milk, Mini	167

STARBUCKS
FRAPPUCCINO - CARAMEL CREAM

with Whipped Cream, Almond Milk, Tall	227
with Whipped Cream, Almond Milk, Venti	358
with Whipped Cream, Coconut Milk, Grande	327
with Whipped Cream, Coconut Milk, Mini	178
with Whipped Cream, Coconut Milk, Tall	245
with Whipped Cream, Coconut Milk, Venti	385
with Whipped Cream, Oat Milk, Grande	373
with Whipped Cream, Oat Milk, Mini	202
with Whipped Cream, Oat Milk, Tall	283
with Whipped Cream, Oat Milk, Venti	441
with Whipped Cream, Semi Skimmed Milk, Grande	339
with Whipped Cream, Semi Skimmed Milk, Mini	185
with Whipped Cream, Semi Skimmed Milk, Tall	319
with Whipped Cream, Semi Skimmed Milk, Venti	399
with Whipped Cream, Skimmed Milk, Grande	319
with Whipped Cream, Skimmed Milk, Mini	174
with Whipped Cream, Skimmed Milk, Tall	239
with Whipped Cream, Skimmed Milk, Venti	375
with Whipped Cream, Soy, Grande	327
with Whipped Cream, Soy, Mini	178
with Whipped Cream, Soy, Tall	245
with Whipped Cream, Soy, Venti	385
with Whipped Cream, Whole Milk, Grande	358
with Whipped Cream, Whole Milk, Mini	194
with Whipped Cream, Whole Milk, Tall	270
with Whipped Cream, Whole Milk, Venti	422

FRAPPUCCINO - CHAI TEA

with Whipped Cream, Almond Milk, Grande	313
with Whipped Cream, Almond Milk, Mini	159
with Whipped Cream, Almond Milk, Tall	215
with Whipped Cream, Almond Milk, Venti	354
with Whipped Cream, Coconut Milk, Grande	334
with Whipped Cream, Coconut Milk, Mini	171
with Whipped Cream, Coconut Milk, Tall	232
with Whipped Cream, Coconut Milk, Venti	380
with Whipped Cream, Oat Milk, Grande	377
with Whipped Cream, Oat Milk, Mini	195
with Whipped Cream, Oat Milk, Tall	267
with Whipped Cream, Oat Milk, Venti	433
with Whipped Cream, Semi Skimmed Milk, Grande	345
with Whipped Cream, Semi Skimmed Milk, Mini	177
with Whipped Cream, Semi Skimmed Milk, Tall	241
with Whipped Cream, Semi Skimmed Milk, Venti	393
with Whipped Cream, Skimmed Milk, Grande	326
with Whipped Cream, Skimmed Milk, Mini	166
with Whipped Cream, Skimmed Milk, Tall	226
with Whipped Cream, Skimmed Milk, Venti	370
with Whipped Cream, Soy, Grande	334
with Whipped Cream, Soy, Mini	170
with Whipped Cream, Soy, Tall	232
with Whipped Cream, Soy, Venti	379
with Whipped Cream, Whole Milk, Grande	363

STARBUCKS
FRAPPUCCINO - CHAI TEA

with Whipped Cream, Whole Milk, Mini	186
with Whipped Cream, Whole Milk, Tall	255
with Whipped Cream, Whole Milk, Venti	415

FRAPPUCCINO - CHOCOLATE CREAM

with Whipped Cream, Almond Milk, Grande	293
with Whipped Cream, Almond Milk, Mini	154
with Whipped Cream, Almond Milk, Tall	210
with Whipped Cream, Almond Milk, Venti	340
with Whipped Cream, Coconut Milk, Grande	316
with Whipped Cream, Coconut Milk, Mini	166
with Whipped Cream, Coconut Milk, Tall	228
with Whipped Cream, Coconut Milk, Venti	367
with Whipped Cream, Oat Milk, Grande	362
with Whipped Cream, Oat Milk, Mini	190
with Whipped Cream, Oat Milk, Tall	263
with Whipped Cream, Oat Milk, Venti	421
with Whipped Cream, Semi Skimmed Milk, Grande	327
with Whipped Cream, Semi Skimmed Milk, Mini	172
with Whipped Cream, Semi Skimmed Milk, Tall	237
with Whipped Cream, Semi Skimmed Milk, Venti	381
with Whipped Cream, Skimmed Milk, Grande	307
with Whipped Cream, Skimmed Milk, Mini	162
with Whipped Cream, Skimmed Milk, Tall	221
with Whipped Cream, Skimmed Milk, Venti	357
with Whipped Cream, Soy, Grande	315
with Whipped Cream, Soy, Mini	166
with Whipped Cream, Soy, Tall	227
with Whipped Cream, Soy, Venti	366
with Whipped Cream, Whole Milk, Grande	327
with Whipped Cream, Whole Milk, Mini	182
with Whipped Cream, Whole Milk, Tall	251
with Whipped Cream, Whole Milk, Venti	403

FRAPPUCCINO - COFFEE

No Whip, Almond Milk, Grande	192
No Whip, Almond Milk, Mini	89
No Whip, Almond Milk, Tall	138
No Whip, Almond Milk, Venti	239
No Whip, Coconut Milk, Grande	208
No Whip, Coconut Milk, Mini	98
No Whip, Coconut Milk, Tall	152
No Whip, Coconut Milk, Venti	257
No Whip, Oat Milk, Grande	242
No Whip, Oat Milk, Mini	116
No Whip, Oat Milk, Tall	180
No Whip, Oat Milk, Venti	294
No Whip, Semi Skimmed Milk, Grande	217
No Whip, Semi Skimmed Milk, Mini	103
No Whip, Semi Skimmed Milk, Tall	159
No Whip, Semi Skimmed Milk, Venti	217
No Whip, Skimmed Milk, Grande	202
No Whip, Skimmed Milk, Mini	95
No Whip, Skimmed Milk, Tall	147

STARBUCKS
FRAPPUCCINO - COFFEE

No Whip, Skimmed Milk, Venti	250
No Whip, Soy, Grande	208
No Whip, Soy, Mini	98
No Whip, Soy, Tall	152
No Whip, Soy, Venti	257
No Whip, Whole Milk, Grande	231
No Whip, Whole Milk, Mini	110
No Whip, Whole Milk, Tall	170
No Whip, Whole Milk, Venti	282
Coffee Light, No Whip, Skimmed Milk, Grande	118
Coffee Light, No Whip, Skimmed Milk, Mini	59
Coffee Light, No Whip, Skimmed Milk, Tall	83
Coffee Light, No Whip, Skimmed Milk, Venti	129

FRAPPUCCINO - COOKIE & CREAM

with Whipped Cream, Almond Milk, Grande	368
with Whipped Cream, Almond Milk, Mini	179
with Whipped Cream, Almond Milk, Tall	266
with Whipped Cream, Almond Milk, Venti	429
with Whipped Cream, Coconut Milk, Grande	397
with Whipped Cream, Coconut Milk, Mini	193
with Whipped Cream, Coconut Milk, Tall	288
with Whipped Cream, Coconut Milk, Venti	463
with Whipped Cream, Oat Milk, Grande	439
with Whipped Cream, Oat Milk, Mini	214
with Whipped Cream, Oat Milk, Tall	320
with Whipped Cream, Oat Milk, Venti	512
with Whipped Cream, Semi Skimmed Milk, Grande	404
with Whipped Cream, Semi Skimmed Milk, Mini	196
with Whipped Cream, Semi Skimmed Milk, Tall	293
with Whipped Cream, Semi Skimmed Milk, Venti	470
with Whipped Cream, Skimmed Milk, Grande	383
with Whipped Cream, Skimmed Milk, Mini	186
with Whipped Cream, Skimmed Milk, Tall	277
with Whipped Cream, Skimmed Milk, Venti	446
with Whipped Cream, Soy, Grande	391
with Whipped Cream, Soy, Mini	190
with Whipped Cream, Soy, Tall	284
with Whipped Cream, Soy, Venti	456
with Whipped Cream, Whole Milk, Grande	423
with Whipped Cream, Whole Milk, Mini	206
with Whipped Cream, Whole Milk, Tall	308
with Whipped Cream, Whole Milk, Venti	493

FRAPPUCCINO - DOUBLE CHOC CHIP CREAM

with Whipped Cream, Almond Milk, Grande	365
with Whipped Cream, Almond Milk, Mini	187
with Whipped Cream, Almond Milk, Tall	263
with Whipped Cream, Almond Milk, Venti	444
with Whipped Cream, Coconut Milk, Grande	394
with Whipped Cream, Coconut Milk, Mini	201
with Whipped Cream, Coconut Milk, Tall	286
with Whipped Cream, Coconut Milk, Venti	478
with Whipped Cream, Oat Milk, Grande	435

STARBUCKS
FRAPPUCCINO - DOUBLE CHOC CHIP CREAM

with Whipped Cream, Oat Milk, Mini	222
with Whipped Cream, Oat Milk, Tall	318
with Whipped Cream, Oat Milk, Venti	528
with Whipped Cream, Semi Skimmed Milk, Grande	400
with Whipped Cream, Semi Skimmed Milk, Mini	204
with Whipped Cream, Semi Skimmed Milk, Tall	291
with Whipped Cream, Semi Skimmed Milk, Venti	486
with Whipped Cream, Skimmed Milk, Grande	379
with Whipped Cream, Skimmed Milk, Mini	194
with Whipped Cream, Skimmed Milk, Tall	275
with Whipped Cream, Skimmed Milk, Venti	461
with Whipped Cream, Soy, Grande	388
with Whipped Cream, Soy, Mini	198
with Whipped Cream, Soy, Tall	281
with Whipped Cream, Soy, Venti	471
with Whipped Cream, Whole Milk, Grande	419
with Whipped Cream, Whole Milk, Mini	214
with Whipped Cream, Whole Milk, Tall	306
with Whipped Cream, Whole Milk, Venti	509

FRAPPUCCINO - ESPRESSO

No Whip, Almond Milk, Grande	185
No Whip, Almond Milk, Mini	93
No Whip, Almond Milk, Tall	128
No Whip, Almond Milk, Venti	230
No Whip, Coconut Milk, Grande	201
No Whip, Coconut Milk, Mini	101
No Whip, Coconut Milk, Tall	140
No Whip, Coconut Milk, Venti	247
No Whip, Oat Milk, Grande	233
No Whip, Oat Milk, Mini	119
No Whip, Oat Milk, Tall	165
No Whip, Oat Milk, Venti	282
No Whip, Semi Skimmed Milk, Grande	209
No Whip, Semi Skimmed Milk, Mini	106
No Whip, Semi Skimmed Milk, Tall	146
No Whip, Semi Skimmed Milk, Venti	256
No Whip, Skimmed Milk, Grande	195
No Whip, Skimmed Milk, Mini	98
No Whip, Skimmed Milk, Tall	135
No Whip, Skimmed Milk, Venti	241
No Whip, Soy, Grande	200
No Whip, Soy, Mini	101
No Whip, Soy, Tall	140
No Whip, Soy, Venti	247
No Whip, Whole Milk, Grande	222
No Whip, Whole Milk, Mini	113
No Whip, Whole Milk, Tall	157
No Whip, Whole Milk, Venti	270
Light, No Whip, Skimmed Milk, Grande	112
Light, No Whip, Skimmed Milk, Mini	63
Light, No Whip, Skimmed Milk, Tall	79
Light, No Whip, Skimmed Milk, Venti	128

STARBUCKS
FRAPPUCCINO - GINGERBREAD

with Whipped Cream, Almond Milk, Grande	342
with Whipped Cream, Almond Milk, Mini	175
with Whipped Cream, Almond Milk, Tall	246
with Whipped Cream, Almond Milk, Venti	399
with Whipped Cream, Coconut Milk, Grande	363
with Whipped Cream, Coconut Milk, Mini	186
with Whipped Cream, Coconut Milk, Tall	262
with Whipped Cream, Coconut Milk, Venti	421
with Whipped Cream, Oat Milk, Grande	392
with Whipped Cream, Oat Milk, Mini	201
with Whipped Cream, Oat Milk, Tall	287
with Whipped Cream, Oat Milk, Venti	454
with Whipped Cream, Semi Skimmed Milk, Grande	367
with Whipped Cream, Semi Skimmed Milk, Mini	188
with Whipped Cream, Semi Skimmed Milk, Tall	266
with Whipped Cream, Semi Skimmed Milk, Venti	426
with Whipped Cream, Skimmed Milk, Grande	352
with Whipped Cream, Skimmed Milk, Mini	180
with Whipped Cream, Skimmed Milk, Tall	254
with Whipped Cream, Skimmed Milk, Venti	410
with Whipped Cream, Soy, Grande	358
with Whipped Cream, Soy, Mini	183
with Whipped Cream, Soy, Tall	259
with Whipped Cream, Soy, Venti	417
with Whipped Cream, Whole Milk, Grande	381
with Whipped Cream, Whole Milk, Mini	195
with Whipped Cream, Whole Milk, Tall	277
with Whipped Cream, Whole Milk, Venti	441
Light, No Whip, Skimmed Milk, Grande	155
Light, No Whip, Skimmed Milk, Mini	76
Light, No Whip, Skimmed Milk, Tall	114
Light, No Whip, Skimmed Milk, Venti	191

FRAPPUCCINO - GINGERBREAD CREME

with Whipped Cream, Almond Milk, Grande	288
with Whipped Cream, Almond Milk, Mini	150
with Whipped Cream, Almond Milk, Tall	208
with Whipped Cream, Almond Milk, Venti	330
with Whipped Cream, Coconut Milk, Grande	317
with Whipped Cream, Coconut Milk, Mini	164
with Whipped Cream, Coconut Milk, Tall	230
with Whipped Cream, Coconut Milk, Venti	363
with Whipped Cream, Oat Milk, Grande	358
with Whipped Cream, Oat Milk, Mini	186
with Whipped Cream, Oat Milk, Tall	262
with Whipped Cream, Oat Milk, Venti	410
with Whipped Cream, Semi Skimmed Milk, Grande	323
with Whipped Cream, Semi Skimmed Milk, Mini	168
with Whipped Cream, Semi Skimmed Milk, Tall	235
with Whipped Cream, Semi Skimmed Milk, Venti	370
with Whipped Cream, Skimmed Milk, Grande	302
with Whipped Cream, Skimmed Milk, Mini	157
with Whipped Cream, Skimmed Milk, Tall	219

STARBUCKS
FRAPPUCCINO - GINGERBREAD CREME

with Whipped Cream, Skimmed Milk, Venti	346
with Whipped Cream, Soy, Grande	311
with Whipped Cream, Soy, Mini	161
with Whipped Cream, Soy, Tall	226
with Whipped Cream, Soy, Venti	356
with Whipped Cream, Whole Milk, Grande	342
with Whipped Cream, Whole Milk, Mini	177
with Whipped Cream, Whole Milk, Tall	250
with Whipped Cream, Whole Milk, Venti	392

FRAPPUCCINO - JAVA CHIP

with Whipped Cream, Almond Milk, Grande	433
with Whipped Cream, Almond Milk, Mini	222
with Whipped Cream, Almond Milk, Tall	311
with Whipped Cream, Almond Milk, Venti	509
with Whipped Cream, Coconut Milk, Grande	413
with Whipped Cream, Coconut Milk, Mini	211
with Whipped Cream, Coconut Milk, Tall	295
with Whipped Cream, Coconut Milk, Venti	487
with Whipped Cream, Oat Milk, Grande	462
with Whipped Cream, Oat Milk, Mini	238
with Whipped Cream, Oat Milk, Tall	335
with Whipped Cream, Oat Milk, Venti	541
with Whipped Cream, Semi Skimmed Milk, Grande	438
with Whipped Cream, Semi Skimmed Milk, Mini	225
with Whipped Cream, Semi Skimmed Milk, Tall	315
with Whipped Cream, Semi Skimmed Milk, Venti	514
with Whipped Cream, Skimmed Milk, Grande	423
with Whipped Cream, Skimmed Milk, Mini	217
with Whipped Cream, Skimmed Milk, Tall	303
with Whipped Cream, Skimmed Milk, Venti	498
with Whipped Cream, Soy, Grande	429
with Whipped Cream, Soy, Mini	220
with Whipped Cream, Soy, Tall	308
with Whipped Cream, Soy, Venti	504
with Whipped Cream, Whole Milk, Grande	451
with Whipped Cream, Whole Milk, Mini	232
with Whipped Cream, Whole Milk, Tall	326
with Whipped Cream, Whole Milk, Venti	528
Light, No Whip, Skimmed Milk, Grande	192
Light, No Whip, Skimmed Milk, Mini	104
Light, No Whip, Skimmed Milk, Tall	137
Light, No Whip, Skimmed Milk, Venti	228

FRAPPUCCINO - MARSHMALLOW

with Whipped Cream, Almond Milk, Grande	307
with Whipped Cream, Almond Milk, Mini	162
Ã,Â with Whipped Cream, Almond Milk, Tall	220
with Whipped Cream, Almond Milk, Venti	357
with Whipped Cream, Coconut Milk, Grande	336
with Whipped Cream, Coconut Milk, Mini	177
with Whipped Cream, Coconut Milk, Tall	242
with Whipped Cream, Coconut Milk, Venti	389
with Whipped Cream, Oat Milk, Grande	377

STARBUCKS
FRAPPUCCINO - MARSHMALLOW

with Whipped Cream, Oat Milk, Mini	198
with Whipped Cream, Oat Milk, Tall	274
with Whipped Cream, Oat Milk, Venti	437
with Whipped Cream, Semi Skimmed Milk, Grande	342
with Whipped Cream, Semi Skimmed Milk, Mini	180
with Whipped Cream, Semi Skimmed Milk, Tall	247
with Whipped Cream, Semi Skimmed Milk, Venti	397
with Whipped Cream, Skimmed Milk, Grande	321
with Whipped Cream, Skimmed Milk, Mini	169
with Whipped Cream, Skimmed Milk, Tall	231
with Whipped Cream, Skimmed Milk, Venti	373
with Whipped Cream, Soy, Grande	330
with Whipped Cream, Soy, Mini	174
with Whipped Cream, Soy, Tall	237
with Whipped Cream, Soy, Venti	383
with Whipped Cream, Whole Milk, Grande	361
with Whipped Cream, Whole Milk, Mini	190
with Whipped Cream, Whole Milk, Tall	262
with Whipped Cream, Whole Milk, Venti	419

FRAPPUCCINO - MATCHA TEA

with Whipped Cream, Almond Milk, Grande	323
with Whipped Cream, Almond Milk, Mini	160
with Whipped Cream, Almond Milk, Tall	228
with Whipped Cream, Almond Milk, Venti	365
with Whipped Cream, Coconut Milk, Grande	347
with Whipped Cream, Coconut Milk, Mini	172
with Whipped Cream, Coconut Milk, Tall	247
with Whipped Cream, Coconut Milk, Venti	392
with Whipped Cream, Oat Milk, Grande	396
with Whipped Cream, Oat Milk, Mini	196
with Whipped Cream, Oat Milk, Tall	284
with Whipped Cream, Oat Milk, Venti	447
with Whipped Cream, Semi Skimmed Milk, Grande	359
with Whipped Cream, Semi Skimmed Milk, Mini	178
with Whipped Cream, Semi Skimmed Milk, Tall	256
with Whipped Cream, Semi Skimmed Milk, Venti	406
with Whipped Cream, Skimmed Milk, Grande	338
with Whipped Cream, Skimmed Milk, Mini	167
with Whipped Cream, Skimmed Milk, Tall	240
with Whipped Cream, Skimmed Milk, Venti	382
with Whipped Cream, Soy, Grande	346
with Whipped Cream, Soy, Mini	172
with Whipped Cream, Soy, Tall	246
with Whipped Cream, Soy, Venti	392
with Whipped Cream, Whole Milk, Grande	379
with Whipped Cream, Whole Milk, Mini	188
with Whipped Cream, Whole Milk, Tall	272
with Whipped Cream, Whole Milk, Venti	428

FRAPPUCCINO - MOCHA

with Whipped Cream, Almond Milk, Grande	330
with Whipped Cream, Almond Milk, Mini	174
with Whipped Cream, Almond Milk, Tall	240

STARBUCKS
FRAPPUCCINO - MOCHA

with Whipped Cream, Almond Milk, Venti	394
with Whipped Cream, Coconut Milk, Grande	345
with Whipped Cream, Coconut Milk, Mini	183
with Whipped Cream, Coconut Milk, Tall	253
with Whipped Cream, Coconut Milk, Venti	412
with Whipped Cream, Oat Milk, Grande	376
with Whipped Cream, Oat Milk, Mini	201
with Whipped Cream, Oat Milk, Tall	280
with Whipped Cream, Oat Milk, Venti	449
with Whipped Cream, Semi Skimmed Milk, Grande	353
with Whipped Cream, Semi Skimmed Milk, Mini	188
with Whipped Cream, Semi Skimmed Milk, Tall	260
with Whipped Cream, Semi Skimmed Milk, Venti	421
with Whipped Cream, Skimmed Milk, Grande	339
with Whipped Cream, Skimmed Milk, Mini	180
with Whipped Cream, Skimmed Milk, Tall	249
with Whipped Cream, Skimmed Milk, Venti	405
with Whipped Cream, Soy, Grande	345
with Whipped Cream, Soy, Mini	183
with Whipped Cream, Soy, Tall	253
with Whipped Cream, Soy, Venti	412
with Whipped Cream, Whole Milk, Grande	366
with Whipped Cream, Whole Milk, Mini	195
with Whipped Cream, Whole Milk, Tall	271
with Whipped Cream, Whole Milk, Venti	436
Light, No Whip, Skimmed Milk, Grande	135
Light, No Whip, Skimmed Milk, Mini	72
Light, No Whip, Skimmed Milk, Tall	91
Light, No Whip, Skimmed Milk, Venti	159

FRAPPUCCINO - MOCHA, WHITE CHOC

with Whipped Cream, Almond Milk, Grande	358
with Whipped Cream, Almond Milk, Mini	181
with Whipped Cream, Almond Milk, Tall	252
with Whipped Cream, Almond Milk, Venti	424
with Whipped Cream, Coconut Milk, Grande	374
with Whipped Cream, Coconut Milk, Mini	190
with Whipped Cream, Coconut Milk, Tall	265
with Whipped Cream, Coconut Milk, Venti	424
with Whipped Cream, Oat Milk, Grande	406
with Whipped Cream, Oat Milk, Mini	208
with Whipped Cream, Oat Milk, Tall	292
with Whipped Cream, Oat Milk, Venti	460
with Whipped Cream, Semi Skimmed Milk, Grande	382
with Whipped Cream, Semi Skimmed Milk, Mini	194
with Whipped Cream, Semi Skimmed Milk, Tall	272
with Whipped Cream, Semi Skimmed Milk, Venti	433
with Whipped Cream, Skimmed Milk, Grande	368
with Whipped Cream, Skimmed Milk, Mini	187
with Whipped Cream, Skimmed Milk, Tall	260
with Whipped Cream, Skimmed Milk, Venti	418
with Whipped Cream, Soy, Grande	374
with Whipped Cream, Soy, Mini	190

STARBUCKS
FRAPPUCCINO - MOCHA, WHITE CHOC

	KCAL
with Whipped Cream, Soy, Tall	265
with Whipped Cream, Soy, Venti	424
with Whipped Cream, Whole Milk, Grande	395
with Whipped Cream, Whole Milk, Mini	202
with Whipped Cream, Whole Milk, Tall	283
with Whipped Cream, Whole Milk, Venti	448
Light, White Choc, No Whip, Skimmed Milk, Grande	155
Light, White Choc, No Whip, Skimmed Milk, Mini	78
Light, White Choc, No Whip, Skimmed Milk, Tall	99
Light, White Choc, No Whip, Skimmed Milk, Venti	166

FRAPPUCCINO - ROOBIOS TEA

	KCAL
with Whipped Cream, Almond Milk, Grande	305
with Whipped Cream, Almond Milk, Mini	152
with Whipped Cream, Almond Milk, Tall	216
with Whipped Cream, Almond Milk, Venti	343
with Whipped Cream, Coconut Milk, Grande	329
with Whipped Cream, Coconut Milk, Mini	164
with Whipped Cream, Coconut Milk, Tall	235
with Whipped Cream, Coconut Milk, Venti	370
with Whipped Cream, Oat Milk, Grande	378
with Whipped Cream, Oat Milk, Mini	188
with Whipped Cream, Oat Milk, Tall	272
with Whipped Cream, Oat Milk, Venti	425
with Whipped Cream, Semi Skimmed Milk, Grande	341
with Whipped Cream, Semi Skimmed Milk, Mini	170
with Whipped Cream, Semi Skimmed Milk, Tall	244
with Whipped Cream, Semi Skimmed Milk, Venti	384
with Whipped Cream, Skimmed Milk, Grande	320
with Whipped Cream, Skimmed Milk, Mini	160
with Whipped Cream, Skimmed Milk, Tall	228
with Whipped Cream, Skimmed Milk, Venti	360
with Whipped Cream, Soy, Grande	329
with Whipped Cream, Soy, Mini	164
with Whipped Cream, Soy, Tall	234
with Whipped Cream, Soy, Venti	370
with Whipped Cream, Whole Milk, Grande	361
with Whipped Cream, Whole Milk, Mini	180
with Whipped Cream, Whole Milk, Tall	259
with Whipped Cream, Whole Milk, Venti	406

FRAPPUCCINO - STARWBERRIES & CREAM

	KCAL
with Whipped Cream, Soy, Venti	402
with Whipped Cream, Almond Milk, Grande	402
with Whipped Cream, Almond Milk, Mini	173
with Whipped Cream, Almond Milk, Tall	235
with Whipped Cream, Almond Milk, Venti	378
with Whipped Cream, Coconut Milk, Grande	344
with Whipped Cream, Coconut Milk, Mini	185
with Whipped Cream, Coconut Milk, Tall	252
with Whipped Cream, Coconut Milk, Venti	402
with Whipped Cream, Oat Milk, Grande	387
with Whipped Cream, Oat Milk, Mini	209
with Whipped Cream, Oat Milk, Tall	287

STARBUCKS
FRAPPUCCINO - STRAWBERRIES & CREAM

	KCAL
with Whipped Cream, Oat Milk, Venti	452
with Whipped Cream, Semi Skimmed Milk, Grande	355
with Whipped Cream, Semi Skimmed Milk, Mini	191
with Whipped Cream, Semi Skimmed Milk, Tall	261
with Whipped Cream, Semi Skimmed Milk, Venti	415
with Whipped Cream, Skimmed Milk, Grande	337
with Whipped Cream, Skimmed Milk, Mini	181
with Whipped Cream, Skimmed Milk, Tall	246
with Whipped Cream, Skimmed Milk, Venti	393
with Whipped Cream, Soy, Grande	344
with Whipped Cream, Soy, Mini	185
with Whipped Cream, Soy, Tall	252
with Whipped Cream, Whole Milk, Grande	373
with Whipped Cream, Whole Milk, Mini	201
with Whipped Cream, Whole Milk, Tall	275
with Whipped Cream, Whole Milk, Venti	435

FRAPPUCCINO - TOFFEE NUT

	KCAL
with Whipped Cream, Almond Milk, Grande	350
with Whipped Cream, Almond Milk, Mini	180
with Whipped Cream, Almond Milk, Tall	252
with Whipped Cream, Almond Milk, Venti	406
with Whipped Cream, Coconut Milk, Grande	371
with Whipped Cream, Coconut Milk, Mini	191
with Whipped Cream, Coconut Milk, Tall	268
with Whipped Cream, Coconut Milk, Venti	429
with Whipped Cream, Oat Milk, Grande	350
with Whipped Cream, Oat Milk, Mini	207
with Whipped Cream, Oat Milk, Tall	293
with Whipped Cream, Oat Milk, Venti	462
with Whipped Cream, Semi Skimmed Milk, Grande	375
with Whipped Cream, Semi Skimmed Milk, Mini	193
with Whipped Cream, Semi Skimmed Milk, Tall	272
with Whipped Cream, Semi Skimmed Milk, Venti	434
with Whipped Cream, Skimmed Milk, Grande	360
with Whipped Cream, Skimmed Milk, Mini	185
with Whipped Cream, Skimmed Milk, Tall	260
with Whipped Cream, Skimmed Milk, Venti	418
with Whipped Cream, Soy, Grande	366
with Whipped Cream, Soy, Mini	188
with Whipped Cream, Soy, Tall	265
with Whipped Cream, Soy, Venti	424
with Whipped Cream, Whole Milk, Grande	389
with Whipped Cream, Whole Milk, Mini	200
with Whipped Cream, Whole Milk, Tall	283
No Whip, Skimmed Milk, Grande	155
No Whip, Skimmed Milk, Mini	76
No Whip, Skimmed Milk, Tall	114
No Whip, Skimmed Milk, Venti	191

FRAPPUCCINO - TOFFEE NUT CREME

	KCAL
with Whipped Cream, Almond Milk, Grande	296
with Whipped Cream, Almond Milk, Mini	155
with Whipped Cream, Almond Milk, Tall	214

STARBUCKS

FRAPPUCCINO - TOFFEE NUT CREME

	KCAL
with Whipped Cream, Almond Milk, Venti	337
with Whipped Cream, Coconut Milk, Grande	325
with Whipped Cream, Coconut Milk, Mini	170
with Whipped Cream, Coconut Milk, Tall	236
with Whipped Cream, Coconut Milk, Venti	370
with Whipped Cream, Oat Milk, Grande	366
with Whipped Cream, Oat Milk, Mini	191
with Whipped Cream, Oat Milk, Tall	268
with Whipped Cream, Oat Milk, Venti	418
with Whipped Cream, Semi Skimmed Milk, Grande	331
with Whipped Cream, Semi Skimmed Milk, Mini	173
with Whipped Cream, Semi Skimmed Milk, Tall	241
with Whipped Cream, Semi Skimmed Milk, Venti	377
with Whipped Cream, Skimmed Milk, Grande	310
with Whipped Cream, Skimmed Milk, Mini	162
with Whipped Cream, Skimmed Milk, Tall	225
with Whipped Cream, Skimmed Milk, Venti	354
with Whipped Cream, Soy, Grande	319
with Whipped Cream, Soy, Mini	167
with Whipped Cream, Soy, Tall	232
with Whipped Cream, Soy, Venti	363
with Whipped Cream, Whole Milk, Grande	350
with Whipped Cream, Whole Milk, Mini	183
with Whipped Cream, Whole Milk, Tall	256
with Whipped Cream, Whole Milk, Venti	399

FRAPPUCCINO - VANILLA CREAM

	KCAL
with Whipped Cream, Almond Milk, Grande	291
with Whipped Cream, Almond Milk, Mini	149
with Whipped Cream, Almond Milk, Tall	206
with Whipped Cream, Almond Milk, Venti	336
with Whipped Cream, Coconut Milk, Grande	315
with Whipped Cream, Coconut Milk, Mini	160
with Whipped Cream, Coconut Milk, Tall	224
with Whipped Cream, Coconut Milk, Venti	363
with Whipped Cream, Oat Milk, Grande	362
with Whipped Cream, Oat Milk, Mini	184
with Whipped Cream, Oat Milk, Tall	260
with Whipped Cream, Oat Milk, Venti	419
with Whipped Cream, Semi Skimmed Milk, Grande	327
with Whipped Cream, Semi Skimmed Milk, Mini	166
with Whipped Cream, Semi Skimmed Milk, Tall	233
with Whipped Cream, Semi Skimmed Milk, Venti	377
with Whipped Cream, Skimmed Milk , Tall	217
with Whipped Cream, Skimmed Milk, Grande	306
with Whipped Cream, Skimmed Milk, Mini	156
with Whipped Cream, Skimmed Milk, Venti	353
with Whipped Cream, Soy, Grande	314
with Whipped Cream, Soy, Mini	160
with Whipped Cream, Soy, Tall	215
with Whipped Cream, Soy, Tall	223
with Whipped Cream, Soy, Venti	363
with Whipped Cream, Whole Milk, Grande	346

STARBUCKS

FRAPPUCCINO - VANILLA CREAM

	KCAL
with Whipped Cream, Whole Milk, Mini	176
with Whipped Cream, Whole Milk, Tall	248
with Whipped Cream, Whole Milk, Venti	400

FRAPPUCCINO - WHITE CHOC CREAM

	KCAL
with Whipped Cream, Almond Milk, Grande	313
with Whipped Cream, Almond Milk, Mini	156
with Whipped Cream, Almond Milk, Tall	218
with Whipped Cream, Almond Milk, Venti	352
with Whipped Cream, Coconut Milk, Grande	335
with Whipped Cream, Coconut Milk, Mini	168
with Whipped Cream, Coconut Milk, Tall	236
with Whipped Cream, Coconut Milk, Venti	378
with Whipped Cream, Oat Milk, Grande	380
with Whipped Cream, Oat Milk, Mini	192
with Whipped Cream, Oat Milk, Tall	273
with Whipped Cream, Oat Milk, Venti	432
with Whipped Cream, Semi Skimmed Milk, Grande	346
with Whipped Cream, Semi Skimmed Milk, Mini	174
with Whipped Cream, Semi Skimmed Milk, Tall	246
with Whipped Cream, Semi Skimmed Milk, Venti	392
with Whipped Cream, Skimmed Milk, Grande	326
with Whipped Cream, Skimmed Milk, Mini	164
with Whipped Cream, Skimmed Milk, Tall	230
with Whipped Cream, Skimmed Milk, Venti	368
with Whipped Cream, Soy, Grande	334
with Whipped Cream, Soy, Mini	168
with Whipped Cream, Soy, Tall	236
with Whipped Cream, Soy, Venti	378
with Whipped Cream, Whole Milk, Grande	365
with Whipped Cream, Whole Milk, Mini	184
with Whipped Cream, Whole Milk, Tall	261
with Whipped Cream, Whole Milk, Venti	414

FRUIT SALAD

	KCAL
Pot	72

HOT CHOCOLATE - CARAMEL

	KCAL
with Whipped Cream, Almond Milk, Grande	486
with Whipped Cream, Almond Milk, Short	302
with Whipped Cream, Almond Milk, Tall	361
with Whipped Cream, Almond Milk, Venti	633
with Whipped Cream, Coconut Milk, Grande	517
with Whipped Cream, Coconut Milk, Short	319
with Whipped Cream, Coconut Milk, Tall	381
with Whipped Cream, Coconut Milk, Venti	674
with Whipped Cream, Oat Milk, Grande	582
with Whipped Cream, Oat Milk, Short	355
with Whipped Cream, Oat Milk, Tall	422
with Whipped Cream, Oat Milk, Venti	758
with Whipped Cream, Semi Skimmed Milk, Grande	534
with Whipped Cream, Semi Skimmed Milk, Short	328
with Whipped Cream, Semi Skimmed Milk, Tall	392
with Whipped Cream, Semi Skimmed Milk, Venti	695
with Whipped Cream, Skimmed Milk, Grande	506

STARBUCKS
HOT CHOCOLATE - CARAMEL

with Whipped Cream, Skimmed Milk, Short	313
with Whipped Cream, Skimmed Milk, Tall	374
with Whipped Cream, Skimmed Milk, Venti	659
with Whipped Cream, Soy, Grande	517
with Whipped Cream, Soy, Short	319
with Whipped Cream, Soy, Tall	381
with Whipped Cream, Soy, Venti	674
with Whipped Cream, Whole Milk, Grande	560
with Whipped Cream, Whole Milk, Short	343
with Whipped Cream, Whole Milk, Tall	408
with Whipped Cream, Whole Milk, Venti	729

HOT CHOCOLATE - CLASSIC

with Whipped Cream, Almond Milk, Grande	221
with Whipped Cream, Almond Milk, Tall	181
with Whipped Cream, Almond Milk, Venti	263
with Whipped Cream, Coconut Milk, Grande	263
with Whipped Cream, Coconut Milk, Short	144
with Whipped Cream, Coconut Milk, Tall	216
with Whipped Cream, Coconut Milk, Venti	320
with Whipped Cream, Oat Milk, Grande	347
with Whipped Cream, Oat Milk, Short	178
with Whipped Cream, Oat Milk, Tall	286
with Whipped Cream, Oat Milk, Venti	436
with Whipped Cream, Semi Skimmed Milk, Grande	284
with Whipped Cream, Semi Skimmed Milk, Short	152
with Whipped Cream, Semi Skimmed Milk, Tall	234
with Whipped Cream, Semi Skimmed Milk, Venti	350
with Whipped Cream, Skimmed Milk, Grande	247
with Whipped Cream, Skimmed Milk, Short	137
with Whipped Cream, Skimmed Milk, Tall	203
with Whipped Cream, Skimmed Milk, Venti	299
with Whipped Cream, Soy, Grande	262
with Whipped Cream, Soy, Short	143
with Whipped Cream, Soy, Tall	215
with Whipped Cream, Soy, Venti	319
with Whipped Cream, Whole Milk, Grande	318
with Whipped Cream, Whole Milk, Short	167
with Whipped Cream, Whole Milk, Tall	262
with Whipped Cream, Whole Milk, Venti	397
with Whipped Cream, Almond Milk, Short	127

HOT CHOCOLATE - HAZELNUT

with Whipped Cream, Almond Milk, Grande	464
with Whipped Cream, Almond Milk, Short	285
with Whipped Cream, Almond Milk, Tall	341
with Whipped Cream, Almond Milk, Venti	609
with Whipped Cream, Coconut Milk, Grande	495
with Whipped Cream, Coconut Milk, Short	302
with Whipped Cream, Coconut Milk, Tall	362
with Whipped Cream, Coconut Milk, Venti	650
with Whipped Cream, Oat Milk, Grande	560
with Whipped Cream, Oat Milk, Short	337
with Whipped Cream, Oat Milk, Tall	403

STARBUCKS
HOT CHOCOLATE - HAZLENUT

with Whipped Cream, Oat Milk, Venti	733
with Whipped Cream, Semi Skimmed Milk, Short	311
with Whipped Cream, Whole Milk, Tall	389
with Whipped Cream, Whole Milk, Venti	705
with Whipped Cream, Semi Skimmed Milk, Grande	512
with Whipped Cream, Semi Skimmed Milk, Tall	372
with Whipped Cream, Semi Skimmed Milk, Venti	671
with Whipped Cream, Skimmed Milk, Grande	484
with Whipped Cream, Skimmed Milk, Short	295
with Whipped Cream, Skimmed Milk, Tall	354
with Whipped Cream, Skimmed Milk, Venti	634
with Whipped Cream, Soy, Grande	495
with Whipped Cream, Soy, Short	302
with Whipped Cream, Soy, Venti	649
with Whipped Cream, Whole Milk, Grande	538
with Whipped Cream, Whole Milk, Short	325

HOT CHOCOLATE - MARSHMALLOW

with Whipped Cream, Almond Milk, Grande	302
with Whipped Cream, Almond Milk, Short	168
with Whipped Cream, Almond Milk, Tall	238
with Whipped Cream, Almond Milk, Venti	363
with Whipped Cream, Coconut Milk, Grande	375
with Whipped Cream, Coconut Milk, Short	204
with Whipped Cream, Coconut Milk, Tall	296
with Whipped Cream, Coconut Milk, Venti	459
with Whipped Cream, Oat Milk, Grande	482
with Whipped Cream, Oat Milk, Short	257
with Whipped Cream, Oat Milk, Tall	379
with Whipped Cream, Oat Milk, Venti	597
with Whipped Cream, Semi Skimmed Milk, Grande	392
with Whipped Cream, Semi Skimmed Milk, Short	212
with Whipped Cream, Semi Skimmed Milk, Tall	308
with Whipped Cream, Semi Skimmed Milk, Venti	480
with Whipped Cream, Skimmed Milk, Grande	339
with Whipped Cream, Skimmed Milk, Short	186
with Whipped Cream, Skimmed Milk, Tall	267
with Whipped Cream, Skimmed Milk, Venti	411
with Whipped Cream, Soy, Grande	360
with Whipped Cream, Soy, Short	197
with Whipped Cream, Soy, Tall	284
with Whipped Cream, Soy, Venti	439
with Whipped Cream, Whole Milk, Grande	441
with Whipped Cream, Whole Milk, Short	237
with Whipped Cream, Whole Milk, Tall	347
with Whipped Cream, Whole Milk, Venti	544

HOT CHOCOLATE - SIGNATURE

with Whipped Cream, Almond Milk, Grande	383
with Whipped Cream, Almond Milk, Short	242
with Whipped Cream, Almond Milk, Tall	280
with Whipped Cream, Almond Milk, Venti	509
with Whipped Cream, Coconut Milk, Grande	415
with Whipped Cream, Coconut Milk, Short	259

STARBUCKS

HOT CHOCOLATE - SIGNATURE

with Whipped Cream, Coconut Milk, Tall	300
with Whipped Cream, Coconut Milk, Venti	550
with Whipped Cream, Oat Milk, Grande	479
with Whipped Cream, Oat Milk, Short	294
with Whipped Cream, Oat Milk, Tall	341
with Whipped Cream, Oat Milk, Venti	634
with Whipped Cream, Semi Skimmed Milk, Grande	431
with Whipped Cream, Semi Skimmed Milk, Short	268
with Whipped Cream, Semi Skimmed Milk, Tall	310
with Whipped Cream, Semi Skimmed Milk, Venti	571
with Whipped Cream, Skimmed Milk, Grande	403
with Whipped Cream, Skimmed Milk, Short	253
with Whipped Cream, Skimmed Milk, Tall	292
with Whipped Cream, Skimmed Milk, Venti	535
with Whipped Cream, Soy, Grande	414
with Whipped Cream, Soy, Short	259
with Whipped Cream, Soy, Tall	299
with Whipped Cream, Soy, Venti	550
with Whipped Cream, Whole Milk, Grande	457
with Whipped Cream, Whole Milk, Short	282
with Whipped Cream, Whole Milk, Tall	327
with Whipped Cream, Whole Milk, Venti	605

HOT CHOCOLATE - WHITE

with Whipped Cream, Almond Milk, Grande	348
with Whipped Cream, Almond Milk, Short	185
with Whipped Cream, Almond Milk, Tall	273
with Whipped Cream, Almond Milk, Venti	422
with Whipped Cream, Coconut Milk, Grande	391
with Whipped Cream, Coconut Milk, Short	201
with Whipped Cream, Coconut Milk, Tall	307
with Whipped Cream, Coconut Milk, Venti	481
with Whipped Cream, Oat Milk, Grande	480
with Whipped Cream, Oat Milk, Short	235
with Whipped Cream, Oat Milk, Tall	378
with Whipped Cream, Oat Milk, Venti	601
with Whipped Cream, Semi Skimmed Milk, Grande	414
with Whipped Cream, Semi Skimmed Milk, Short	210
with Whipped Cream, Semi Skimmed Milk, Tall	325
with Whipped Cream, Semi Skimmed Milk, Venti	511
with Whipped Cream, Skimmed Milk, Grande	375
with Whipped Cream, Skimmed Milk, Short	195
with Whipped Cream, Skimmed Milk, Tall	295
with Whipped Cream, Skimmed Milk, Venti	459
with Whipped Cream, Soy, Grande	391
with Whipped Cream, Soy, Short	201
with Whipped Cream, Soy, Tall	307
with Whipped Cream, Soy, Venti	480
with Whipped Cream, Whole Milk, Grande	450
with Whipped Cream, Whole Milk, Short	223
with Whipped Cream, Whole Milk, Tall	354
with Whipped Cream, Whole Milk, Venti	560

STARBUCKS

MACARONI CHEESE

Vegan, Hot Box	470

MUFFIN

Bacon, & Egg	394
Blueberry	409
Chocolate, Triple	470
Cran-Merry Cheesecake	438
Halloumi, & Avocado	436
Lemon	424

PAIN AU CHOCOLAT

Portion	258

PAIN AU RAISIN

Portion	293

PANINI

Festive Feast	534
Ham, & Cheese, GF	341
Ham, & Cheese	424
Tomato, & Mozzarella	409
Tuna Melt	414

PASTRY

Cinnamon Swirl	482
Twist, Chocolate	275

PIE

Mince	403

ROLL

Bacon, Smoked	334
Breakfast, All Day	463

SALAD

Chicken	269
Vegetables, Roasted, Vegan	270

SANDWICH

Chicken, & Hickory Bacon	380
Egg Mayonnaise, Free Range	492

STARBUCKS

SANDWICH

Sausage	478
Turkey, Tis' the Season	534

SHORTBREAD

Chocolate Caramel	368
Chocolate Chunk, Fairtrade	493

SLICE

Caramel, Nut	383

SUB

Turkey, & Swiss Style Cheese, Pretzel	382

TEA

Chai, Grande	0
Chai, Latte, Almond Milk, Grande	186
Chai, Latte, Almond Milk, Short	92
Chai, Latte, Almond Milk, Tall	143
Chai, Latte, Almond Milk, Venti	241
Chai, Latte, Coconut Milk, Grande	221
Chai, Latte, Coconut Milk, Short	109
Chai, Latte, Coconut Milk, Tall	170

STARBUCKS
TEA

	KCAL
Chai, Latte, Coconut Milk, Venti	289
Chai, Latte, Oat Milk, Grande	292
Chai, Latte, Oat Milk, Short	143
Chai, Latte, Oat Milk, Tall	227
Chai, Latte, Oat Milk, Venti	389
Chai, Latte, Semi Skimmed Milk, Grande	239
Chai, Latte, Semi Skimmed Milk, Short	117
Chai, Latte, Semi Skimmed Milk, Tall	185
Chai, Latte, Semi Skimmed Milk, Venti	315
Chai, Latte, Skimmed Milk, Grande	208
Chai, Latte, Skimmed Milk, Short	103
Chai, Latte, Skimmed Milk, Tall	160
Chai, Latte, Skimmed Milk, Venti	271
Chai, Latte, Soy, Grande	220
Chai, Latte, Soy, Short	109
Chai, Latte, Soy, Tall	170
Chai, Latte, Soy, Venti	289
Chai, Latte, Whole Milk, Grande	268
Chai, Latte, Whole Milk, Short	131
Chai, Latte, Whole Milk, Tall	208
Chai, Latte, Whole Milk, Venti	355
Chai, Short	0
Chai, Tall	0
Chai, Venti	0
Chamomile, Grande	0
Chamomile, Short	0
Chamomile, Tall	0
Chamomile, Venti	0
Earl Grey, Grande	0
Earl Grey, Short	0
Earl Grey, Tall	0
Earl Grey, Venti	0
Emperor's Cloud & Mist, Short	0
Emperor's Clouds & Mist, Grande	0
Emperor's Clouds & Mist, Tall	0
Emperor's Clouds & Mist, Venti	0
English Breakfast, Grande	0
English Breakfast, Short	0
English Breakfast, Tall	0
English Breakfast, Venti	0
Hibiscus, Grande	0
Hibiscus, Short	0
Hibiscus, Tall	0
Hibiscus, Venti	0
Iced, Hibiscus, Shaken, Grande	0
Iced, Hibiscus, Shaken, Tall	0
Iced, Hibiscus, Shaken, Venti	0
Iced, Lemonade, Black Tea, Shaken, Grande	46
Iced, Lemonade, Black Tea, Shaken, Tall	35
Iced, Lemonade, Black Tea, Shaken, Venti	56
Iced, Lemonade, Blackberry Mojito, Shaken, Grande	89
Iced, Lemonade, Blackberry Mojito, Shaken, Tall	67

STARBUCKS
TEA

	KCAL
Iced, Lemonade, Blackberry Mojito, Shaken, Venti	110
Iced, Lemonade, Green Tea, Shaken, Grande	46
Iced, Lemonade, Green Tea, Shaken, Tall	35
Iced, Lemonade, Green Tea, Shaken, Venti	56
Iced, Lemonade, Hibiscus, Shaken, Grande	46
Iced, Lemonade, Hibiscus, Shaken, Tall	35
Iced, Lemonade, Hibiscus, Shaken, Venti	56
Iced, Lemonade, Mango, Black Tea, Shaken, Grande	110
Iced, Lemonade, Mango, Black Tea, Shaken, Tall	83
Iced, Lemonade, Mango, Black Tea, Shaken, Venti	137
Iced, Mango, Tropical, Grande	135
Iced, Mango, Tropical, Tall	104
Iced, Mango, Tropical, Venti	170
Iced, Matcha, Almond Milk, Grande	68
Iced, Matcha, Almond Milk, Tall	53
Iced, Matcha, Almond Milk, Venti	80
Iced, Matcha, Coconut Milk, Grande	117
Iced, Matcha, Coconut Milk, Tall	91
Iced, Matcha, Coconut Milk, Venti	136
Iced, Matcha, Oat Milk, Grande	188
Iced, Matcha, Oat Milk, Tall	148
Iced, Matcha, Oat Milk, Venti	216
Iced, Matcha, Semi Skimmed Milk, Grande	128
Iced, Matcha, Semi Skimmed Milk, Tall	100
Iced, Matcha, Semi Skimmed Milk, Venti	148
Iced, Matcha, Skimmed Milk, Grande	93
Iced, Matcha, Skimmed Milk, Tall	72
Iced, Matcha, Skimmed Milk, Venti	108
Iced, Matcha, Soy, Grande	107
Iced, Matcha, Soy, Tall	83
Iced, Matcha, Soy, Venti	124
Iced, Matcha, Whole Milk, Grande	161
Iced, Matcha, Whole Milk, Tall	126
Iced, Matcha, Whole Milk, Venti	185
Iced, Peach Citrus, Grande	64
Iced, Peach Citrus, Tall	48
Iced, Peach Citrus, Unsweetened, Grande	0
Iced, Peach Citrus, Unsweetened, Tall	0
Iced, Peach Citrus, Unsweetened, Venti	0
Iced, Peach Citrus, Venti	80
Iced, Rooibos, Latte, Almond Milk, Grande	59
Iced, Rooibos, Latte, Almond Milk, Tall	46
Iced, Rooibos, Latte, Almond Milk, Venti	67
Iced, Rooibos, Latte, Coconut Milk, Grande	108
Iced, Rooibos, Latte, Coconut Milk, Tall	85
Iced, Rooibos, Latte, Coconut Milk, Venti	123
Iced, Rooibos, Latte, Oat Milk, Grande	178
Iced, Rooibos, Latte, Oat Milk, Tall	141
Iced, Rooibos, Latte, Oat Milk, Venti	203
Iced, Rooibos, Latte, Semi Skimmed Milk, Grande	118
Iced, Rooibos, Latte, Semi Skimmed Milk, Tall	94
Iced, Rooibos, Latte, Semi Skimmed Milk, Venti	135

STARBUCKS
TEA

	KCAL
Iced, Rooibos, Latte, Skimmed Milk, Grande	83
Iced, Rooibos, Latte, Skimmed Milk, Tall	66
Iced, Rooibos, Latte, Skimmed Milk, Venti	95
Iced, Rooibos, Latte, Soy, Grande	97
Iced, Rooibos, Latte, Soy, Tall	77
Iced, Rooibos, Latte, Soy, Venti	111
Iced, Rooibos, Latte, Whole Milk, Grande	151
Iced, Rooibos, Latte, Whole Milk, Tall	119
Iced, Rooibos, Latte, Whole Milk, Venti	172
Jasmine Pearls, Grande	0
Jasmine Pearls, Short	0
Jasmine Pearls, Tall	0
Jasmine Pearls, Venti	0
Matcha, Latte, Almond Milk, Grande	276
Matcha, Latte, Almond Milk, Short	45
Matcha, Latte, Almond Milk, Tall	73
Matcha, Latte, Almond Milk, Venti	125
Matcha, Latte, Coconut Milk, Grande	155
Matcha, Latte, Coconut Milk, Short	74
Matcha, Latte, Coconut Milk, Tall	120
Matcha, Latte, Coconut Milk, Venti	202
Matcha, Latte, Oat Milk, Grande	276
Matcha, Latte, Oat Milk, Short	134
Matcha, Latte, Oat Milk, Tall	214
Matcha, Latte, Oat Milk, Venti	360
Matcha, Latte, Semi Skimmed Milk, Grande	186
Matcha, Latte, Semi Skimmed Milk, Short	89
Matcha, Latte, Semi Skimmed Milk, Tall	144
Matcha, Latte, Semi Skimmed Milk, Venti	242
Matcha, Latte, Skimmed Milk, Grande	133
Matcha, Latte, Skimmed Milk, Short	63
Matcha, Latte, Skimmed Milk, Tall	102
Matcha, Latte, Skimmed Milk, Venti	174
Matcha, Latte, Soy, Grande	154
Matcha, Latte, Soy, Short	74
Matcha, Latte, Soy, Tall	119
Matcha, Latte, Soy, Venti	201
Matcha, Latte, Whole Milk, Grande	235
Matcha, Latte, Whole Milk, Short	113
Matcha, Latte, Whole Milk, Tall	182
Matcha, Latte, Whole Milk, Venti	306
Mint Blend, Grande	0
Mint Blend, Short	0
Mint Blend, Tall	0
Mint Blend, Venti	0
Mint Citrus, Green Tea, Grande	0
Mint Citrus, Green Tea, Short	0
Mint Citrus, Green Tea, Tall	0
Mint Citrus, Green Tea, Venti	0
Pineapple, Green, Grande	64
Pineapple, Green, Tall	48
Pineapple, Green, Unsweetened, Grande	0

STARBUCKS
TEA

	KCAL
Pineapple, Green, Unsweetened, Tall	0
Pineapple, Green, Unsweetened, Venti	0
Pineapple, Green, Venti	80
Rooibos, Latte, Almond Milk, Grande	86
Rooibos, Latte, Almond Milk, Short	42
Rooibos, Latte, Almond Milk, Tall	67
Rooibos, Latte, Almond Milk, Venti	112
Rooibos, Latte, Coconut Milk, Grande	145
Rooibos, Latte, Coconut Milk, Short	71
Rooibos, Latte, Coconut Milk, Tall	113
Rooibos, Latte, Coconut Milk, Venti	189
Rooibos, Latte, Oat Milk, Grande	266
Rooibos, Latte, Oat Milk, Short	130
Rooibos, Latte, Oat Milk, Tall	208
Rooibos, Latte, Oat Milk, Venti	347
Rooibos, Latte, Semi Skimmed Milk, Grande	176
Rooibos, Latte, Semi Skimmed Milk, Short	86
Rooibos, Latte, Semi Skimmed Milk, Tall	137
Rooibos, Latte, Semi Skimmed Milk, Venti	229
Rooibos, Latte, Skimmed Milk, Grande	123
Rooibos, Latte, Skimmed Milk, Short	60
Rooibos, Latte, Skimmed Milk, Tall	96
Rooibos, Latte, Skimmed Milk, Venti	161
Rooibos, Latte, Soy, Grande	144
Rooibos, Latte, Soy, Short	71
Rooibos, Latte, Soy, Tall	113
Rooibos, Latte, Soy, Venti	188
Rooibos, Latte, Whole Milk, Grande	225
Rooibos, Latte, Whole Milk, Short	110
Rooibos, Latte, Whole Milk, Tall	175
Rooibos, Latte, Whole Milk, Venti	293
Strawberry, Black, Grande	64
Strawberry, Black, Tall	48
Strawberry, Black, Unsweetened, Grande	0
Strawberry, Black, Unsweetened, Tall	0
Strawberry, Black, Unsweetened, Venti	0
Strawberry, Black, Venti	80
Youthberry, Grande	0
Youthberry, Short	0
Youthberry, Tall	0
Youthberry, Venti	0

TOAST

	KCAL
Fruit, Luxury	455

TOASTIE

	KCAL
Cheese, Five	482
Chicken, & Bacon, BBQ	480
Ham, Hickory, & Cheese	479

WRAP

	KCAL
Chicken, & Avocado	390
Vegan, Very Merry	543

YOGHURT

	KCAL
Berry Crunch, Pot	250

SUBWAY

BACON
2 Strips, Portion	40

BEEF
Patty, Big, Portion	142
Steak, Portion	94

BREAD
Garlic, Cheesy, Savers Menu	275

CHEESE
Cheddar, Peppered	39
Cheddar, Processed	40
Monterey Cheddar	57

CHICKEN
Breast, Portion	85
Strips, Teriyaki Glazed, Portion	101
Tikka, Portion	89

COOKIES
Chocolate Chip Candy	211
Chocolate Chunk	216
Double Choc Chip	215
Oatmeal Raisin	195
Raspberry Cheesecake	207
White Chip Macadamia Nut	213

DANISH PASTRY
Apricot Crown	419
Cinnamon Swirl	207
Vanilla Crown	329

DOUGHNUTS
Chocolate	351
Sugared	352

EGGS
Patty, Portion	55

FLATBREAD
Bacon, Egg, & Cheese, with Salad, Breakfast	296
Bacon, with Salad, Breakfast	293
Chicken, & Bacon, Ranch Melt, with Salad	515
Chicken, BBQ, Pizza, with Salad	366
Chicken, Breast, with Salad	321
Chicken, Pizziola, with Salad	457
Chicken, Teriyaki, with Salad	321
Chicken, Tikka, with Salad	325
Egg, & Cheese, with Salad, Breakfast	260
Ham, with Salad	307
Italian BMT, with Salad	428
Meatball Marinara, with Salad	454
Mega Melt, with Salad, Breakfast	473
Pepperoni, Spicy, Pizza, with Salad	359
Sausage, Egg, & Cheese, with Salad, Breakfast	436
Sausage, with Salad, Breakfast	396
Spicy Italian, with Salad	497
Steak, & Cheese, with Salad	369
Subway Melt, with Cheese, & Salad	386
Tuna, with Salad	371
Turkey, & Ham, with Salad	309

SUBWAY

FLATBREAD
Turkey, Breast, with Salad	292
Vegan, with Salad	236
Veggie Delite, with Salad	236
Veggie Supreme, Pizza Sub, with Salad	253

GARLIC BREAD
Cheesy, with Steak, Ultimate, 6"	527

HASH BROWNS
Savers Menu	169

MEATBALLS
Marinara, Portion	218

MUFFIN
Blueberry	394
Chocolate Chunk	243
Double Chocolate Chip	351
Raspberry, & White Chocolate	389

NACHOS
with Salsa, Cheese, & Jalapenos, Savers Menu	347

PEPPERONI
Salami, & Cheese, Spicy Italian, Portion	262
Salami, & Ham, Italian BMT, Portion	192

SALAD
Chicken, & Bacon, Ranch Melt, without Dressing	334
Chicken, Breast, without Dressing	138
Chicken, Chipotle Melt, without Dressing	268
Chicken, Pizziola, without Dressing	274
Chicken, Rotisserie-Style, without Dressing	160
Chicken, Teriyaki, without Dressing	153
Chicken, Thai, without Salad	218
Chicken Tikka, without Dressing	142
Ham, without Dressing	124
Italian BMT, without Dressing	246
Meatball, Marinara, without Dressing	270
Spicy Italian, without Dressing	314
Steak, & Cheese, without Dressing	186
Subway Melt, with Cheese, without Dressing	205
Tuna, without Dressing	188
Tuna Nicoise, without Dressing	347
Turkey, & Ham, without Dressing	126
Turkey, Breast, without Dressing	109
Vegan, without Dressing	205
Veggie Delite, without Dressing	52
Veggie Patty, without Dressing	212

SAUCE
Barbecue	39
Chilli, Hot	48
Chilli, Sweet	46
Chipotle Southwest	90
Deli Mustard	23
Honey Mustard	32
Ketchup	22
Mayonnaise, Lite	50
Ranch	43

SUBWAY

SAUCE

	KCAL
Sriracha	27
Sweet Onion	34

SAUSAGE

Portion	176

SUBS - BACON

9 Grain Honey Oat Bread, Breakfast, 6"	291
9 Grain Wheat Bread, Breakfast, 6"	277
Hearty Italian Bread, Breakfast, 6"	278
Italian Herb & Cheese Bread, Breakfast, 6"	310
Italian White Bread, Breakfast, 6"	265

SUBS - BACON, EGG & CHEESE

9 Grain Honey Oat Bread, Breakfast, 6"	294
9 Grain Wheat Bread, Breakfast, 6"	336
Hearty Italian Bread, Breakfast, 6"	282
Italian Herb & Cheese Bread, Breakfast, 6"	313
Italian White Bread, Breakfast, 6"	269

SUBS - CHICKEN & BACON, RANCH MELT

with Salad, 9 Grain Honey Oat Bread, 6"	513
with Salad, 9 Grain Wheat Bread, 6"	499
with Salad, Hearty Italian Bread, 6"	500
with Salad, Italian Herb & Cheese Bread, 6"	532
with Salad, Italian White Bread, 6"	487

SUBS - CHICKEN BREAST

9 Grain Honey Oat Bread, 6"	319
9 Grain Wheat Bread, 6"	304
with Salad, Hearty Italian Bread, 6"	306
with Salad, Italian Herb & Cheese Bread, 6"	338
with Salad, Italian White Bread, 6"	293

SUBS - CHICKEN PIZZIOLA

with Salad, 9 Grain Honey Oat Bread, 6"	455
with Salad, 9 Grain Wheat Bread, 6"	440
with Salad, Hearty Italian Bread, 6"	442
with Salad, Italian Herb & Cheese Bread, 6"	474
with Salad, Italian White Bread, 6"	429

SUBS - CHICKEN TERIYAKI

with Salad, 9 Grain Honey Oat Bread, 6"	319
with Salad, 9 Grain Wheat Bread, 6"	320
with Salad, Hearty Italian Bread, 6"	306
with Salad, Italian Herb & Cheese Bread, 6"	338
with Salad, Italian White Bread, 6"	293

SUBS - CHICKEN TIKKA

with Salad, 9 Grain Honey Oat Bread, 6"	323
with Salad, 9 Grain Wheat Bread, 6"	309
with Salad, Hearty Italian Bread, 6"	310
with Salad, Italian Herb & Cheese Bread, 6"	342
with Salad, Italian White Bread, 6"	297

SUBS - CHICKEN, BBQ, PIZZA

with Salad, 9 Grain Honey Oat Bread, 6"	364
with Salad, 9 Grain Wheat Bread, 6"	349
with Salad, Hearty Italian Bread, 6"	351
with Salad, Italian Herb & Cheese Bread, 6"	382
with Salad, Italian White Bread, 6"	338

SUBWAY

SUBS - CHICKEN, CHIPOTLE MELT

	KCAL
with Salad, 9 Grain Wheat Bread, 6"	436
with Salad, Italian White Bread, 6"	429

SUBS - CHICKEN, NACHO SALSA

Hearty Italian Bread, Savers Menu, 6"	503

SUBS - EGG & CHEESE

9 Grain Honey Oat Bread, Breakfast, 6"	258
9 Grain Wheat Bread, Breakfast, 6"	299
Hearty Italian Bread, Breakfast, 6"	245
Italian Herb & Cheese Bread, Breakfast, 6"	277
Italian White Bread, Breakfast, 6"	232

SUBS - HAM SALAD

9 Grain Honey Oat Bread, 6"	305
9 Grain Wheat Bread, 6"	291
9 Grain Wheat Bread, Kids Pak, 4"	182
Hearty Italian Bread, 6"	292
Italian Herb & Cheese Bread, 6"	324
Italian White Bread, 6"	279
Italian White Bread, Kids Pak, 4"	182

SUBS - ITALIAN BMT

Ultimate Cheesy Garlic Bread, 6"	720
with Salad, 9 Grain Honey Oat Bread, 6"	426
with Salad, 9 Grain Wheat Bread, 6"	412
with Salad, Hearty Italian Bread, 6"	414
with Salad, Italian Herb & Cheese Bread, 6"	445
with Salad, Italian White Bread, 6"	401

SUBS - ITALIAN, SPICY

with Salad, 9 Grain Honey Oat Bread, 6"	495
with Salad, 9 Grain Wheat Bread, 6"	481
with Salad, Hearty Italian Bread, 6"	483
with Salad, Italian Herb & Cheese Bread, 6"	514
with Salad, Italian White Bread, 6"	470

SUBS - MARGHERITA PIZZA

Hearty Italian, Savers Menu	359

SUBS - MEAT FEAST

Italian Herbs & Cheese Bread, Savers Menu, 6"	450

SUBS - MEATBALL MARINARA

with Salad, 9 Grain Honey Oat Bread, 6"	452
with Salad, 9 Grain Wheat Bread, 6"	438
with Salad, Hearty Italian Bread, 6"	439
with Salad, Italian Herb & Cheese Bread, 6"	471
with Salad, Italian White Bread, 6"	426
with Salad, Ultimate Cheesy Garlic Bread, 6"	799

SUBS - MEGA MELT

9 Grain Honey Oat Bread, Breakfast, 6"	471
9 Grain Wheat Bread, Breakfast, 6"	512
Hearty Italian Bread, Breakfast, 6"	458
Italian Herb & Cheese Bread, Breakfast, 6"	490
Italian White Bread, Breakfast, 6"	445

SUBS - PEPPERONI PIZZA, SPICY

with Salad, 9 Grain Honey Oat Bread, 6"	357
with Salad, 9 Grain Wheat Bread, 6"	343
with Salad, Hearty Italian Bread, 6"	344

SUBWAY

SUBS - PEPPERONI PIZZA, SPICY

with Salad, Italian Herb & Cheese Bread, 6"	376
with Salad, Italian White Bread, 6"	331

SUBS - SAUSAGE

9 Grain Honey Oat Bread, Breakfast, 6"	394
9 Grain Wheat Bread, Breakfast, 6"	380
Hearty Italian Bread, Breakfast, 6"	382
Italian Herb & Cheese Bread, Breakfast, 6"	413
Italian White Bread, Breakfast, 6"	369

SUBS - SAUSAGE, EGG & CHEESE

9 Grain Honey Oat Bread, Breakfast, 6"	434
9 Grain Wheat Bread, Breakfast, 6"	475
Hearty Italian Bread, Breakfast, 6"	422
Italian Herb & Cheese Bread, Breakfast, 6"	453
Italian White Bread, Breakfast, 6"	409

SUBS - STEAK & CHEESE

with Salad, 9 Grain Honey Oat Bread, 6"	367
with Salad, 9 Grain Wheat Bread, 6"	353
with Salad, Hearty Italian Bread, 6"	354
with Salad, Italian Herb & Cheese Bread, 6"	386
Ã,Â with Salad, Italian White Bread, 6"	341

SUBS - SUBWAY MELT WITH CHEESE

& Salad, 9 Grain Honey Oat Bread, 6"	384
& Salad, 9 Grain Wheat Bread, 6"	369
& Salad, Hearty Italian Bread, 6"	371
& Salad, Italian Herb & Cheese Bread, 6"	402
& Salad, Italian White Bread, 6"	358

SUBS - TUNA

with Salad, 9 Grain Honey Oat Bread, 6"	369
with Salad, 9 Grain Wheat Bread, 6"	355
with Salad, Hearty Italian Bread, 6"	356
with Salad, Italian Herb & Cheese Bread, 6"	388
with Salad, Italian White Bread, 6"	343

SUBS - TURKEY & HAM

with Salad, 9 Grain Honey Oat Bread, 6"	307
with Salad, 9 Grain Wheat Bread, 6"	293
with Salad, Hearty Italian Bread, 6"	294
with Salad, Italian Herb & Cheese Bread, 6"	326
with Salad, Italian White Bread, 6"	281

SUBS - TURKEY BREAST

with Salad, 9 Grain Honey Oat Bread, 6"	290
with Salad, 9 Grain Wheat Bread, 6"	276
with Salad, 9 Grain Wheat Bread, Kids Pak, 4"	184
with Salad, Hearty Italian Bread, 6"	277
with Salad, Italian Herb & Cheese Bread, 6"	309
with Salad, Italian White Bread, 6"	264
with Salad, Italian White Bread, Kids Pak, 4"	180

SUBS - VEGAN

with Salad, 9 Grain Honey Oat Bread, 6"	234
with Salad, 9 Grain Wheat Bread, 6"	371
with Salad, Hearty Italian Bread, 6"	221
with Salad, Italian Herb & Cheese Bread, 6"	252
with Salad, Italian White Bread, 6"	208

SUBWAY

SUBS - VEGGIE DELITE

with Salad, 9 Grain Honey Oat Bread, 6"	234
with Salad, 9 Grain Wheat Bread, 6"	219
with Salad, 9 Grain Wheat Bread, Kids Pak, 4"	147
with Salad, Hearty Italian Bread, 6"	221
with Salad, Italian Herb & Cheese Bread, 6"	252
with Salad, Italian White Bread, 6"	208
with Salad, Italian White Bread, Kids Pak, 4"	142

SUBS - VEGGIE PATTY

with Salad, 9 Grain Wheat Bread, 6"	381
with Salad, Italian White Bread, 6"	373

SUBS - VEGGIE SUPREME PIZZA

with Salad, 9 Grain Honey Oat Bread, 6"	251
with Salad, 9 Grain Wheat Bread, 6"	237
with Salad, Hearty Italian Bread, 6"	239
with Salad, Italian Herb & Cheese Bread, 6"	270
with Salad, Italian White Bread, 6"	226

TUNA

Portion	135

TURKEY

Breast, & Ham, Portion	72
Breast, Portion	56

VEGETARIAN

Veggie Patty, Portion	160

WRAP - CHICKEN BBQ

& Bacon, Tomato Basil Wrap, Signature	553

WRAP - CHICKEN CAESAR

Rotisserie-Style, Signature	596

WRAP - STEAK

Chipotle, & Cheese, Tomato Basil Wrap, Signature	660

WRAP - TURKEY & BACON

& Guacamole, Signature	554

WRAP - VEGAN

& Garlic Aioli, Tomato Basil Wrap, Signature	729

TABLE TABLE

BACON

Back, Cooked, Breakfast	49

BAGEL

Cinnamon, & Raisin, Breakfast	293

BEANS

Baked, in Tomato Sauce, Breakfast	91

BEEF - ROAST

Dinner, Kids Menu	671
Topside, Dinner	1398

BEEF - STEAK

Rib-eye, 10oz	1033
Rump, 8oz, with Chips	835
Rump, 8oz, with Salad	550
Rump, 8oz, with Skinny Fries, Value Menu	675
Sirloin, 8oz, & Prawns, King, Surf & Turf Combo	1108
Sirloin, 8oz, with Chips	847
Sirloin, 8oz, with Salad	563

BLACK PUDDING

Slice, Breakfast	122

BREAD

Garlic, Flatbread, Side	306
Garlic, Flatbread, with BBQ Dip	492
Garlic, Flatbread, with Cheese, Side	456
Garlic, Flatbread, with Tomato Dip	496
Garlic, Side, Kids Menu	109
Garlic, Starter, Kids Menu	112

BROCCOLI

Tenderstem, Side	139

BROWNIES

Chocolate, Triple	666
Chocolate, Warm, Value Menu	523

BUBBLE & SQUEAK

Breakfast	169

BURGERS

Beef, with Chips, Kids Menu	619
Chicken, & Avocado	1121
Chicken, with Jacket Potato, & Beans	453
Lamb, & Feta	1015
Mac & Cheese	1380
Mac & Cheese, Value Menu	822
Sloppy Joe	1073
Steak, with Cheese, & Bacon, Double Stack	1308
Steak, with Cheese, Double Stack	1245
Steak, with Cheese, Value Menu	952
Surf & Turf	1471

BUTTER

Salted, Portion, Breakfast	48

CAKE

Chocolate, Fudge, Sensation	810
Lemon, Drizzle	144

CAULIFLOWER CHEESE

Sunday Roast	283

TABLE TABLE

CHEESE

Camembert, Baked, Starter	622

CHEESECAKE

Baked	551
Strawberry, Mini	223

CHICKEN

Breast, Pancetta, Wrapped, & Mozzarella Stuffed	947
Breast, Topped, Bacon & Cheese, with Chips	747
Breast, Topped, Bacon & Cheese, with Jacket Potato	760
Escalope	1357
Forestiere	713
Goujons, Buttermilk, & Rosemary, Starter	407
Paprika, Value Menu	525
Poppin, with Chips, & Beans, Kids Menu	394
Roast, Kids Menu	581
Wings, BBQ, Starter	304

CHICKEN DINNER

Half, Roast	1458

CHIPS

Side, Kids Menu	181
Side	363

COD

Bites, Breaded, Kids Menu	507

CORN

Cob, Side, Kids Menu	79

CROISSANT

Breakfast	161

CRUMBLE

Apple, Bramley, & Blackberry	633

CRUMPETS

Sourdough, Breakfast	91

CURRY

Chicken, Kids Menu	444
Chicken, Makhani	934

DOUGHNUTS

Mini, Kids Menu	203

DRIED FRUIT MIX

Breakfast	308

EGGS

Boiled, Single, Breakfast	82
Fried, Single, Breakfast	108
Poached, Single, Breakfast	79
Scrambled, Breakfast	269

FISH & CHIPS

Battered, with Peas, Value Menu	909
Haddock, Hand Battered, with Peas, Value Menu	1087

FRIES

Dirty, Side	516
Halloumi, Side	586
Skinny Cut, Side	328
Sweet Potato, Side	290
Tiger, Side	353

TABLE TABLE

FRUIT MIX

Berry, Breakfast	23

FRUIT SALAD

Breakfast	49
Kids Menu	49

GAMMON

Steak, with Chips, & Egg, Value Menu	769
Steak, with Chips, & Eggs	877
Steak, with Chips, & Pineapple	953
Steak, with Chips, & Pineapple, Value Menu	699
Steak, with Chips, Egg, & Pineapple	807
Steak, with Jacket Potato, & Eggs	890
Steak, with Jacket Potato, & Pineapple	751
Steak, with Jacket Potato, Egg, & Pineapple	820

HADDOCK

Beer Battered, & Chips, with Mushy Peas	1125
Beer Battered, & Chips, with Peas	1087

HAM

Egg, & Chips, Dayime Value Menu	857

HASH BROWNS

Single, Breakfast	94

HONEY

Breakfast	65

ICE CREAM

Dairy, with Caramel Sauce	277
Dairy, with Chocolate Sauce	276
Dairy, with Raspberry Sauce	273
Vanilla, with Caramel Sauce, Kids Menu	199
Vanilla, with Chocolate Sauce, Kids Menu	199
Vanilla, with Raspberry Sauce, Kids Menu	197

JAM

Strawberry, Breakfast	33

LAMB

Rump	631

LASAGNE

Beef, & Pork, Value Menu	577
Beef, Luxury	949
Sweet Potato, & Feta	704
Sweet Potato, & Feta, Value Menu	608

MEATBALLS

Chicken, Kids Menu	177

MIXED GRILL

Table Table	1205
Table Table, with Rump Steak, 8oz	1355

MUFFIN

Blueberry, Breakfast	114

MUSHROOMS

Breaded, Garlic & Herb	314
with Butter, Breakfast	161

NACHOS

Loaded, Sharing	1175

TABLE TABLE

SALAD

Bacon, & Blue Cheese	387
Chicken, Grilled	233
Halloumi, Grilled	360
Mixed, Side, Kids Menu	23
Mixed, Side	39

SANDWICH

Chicken, & Bacon, Club, Open, Value Menu	835

SAUCE

Bearnaise	122
Diane	73
Peppercorn, Creamy	29

SAUSAGE

Breakfast	114
Quorn*, Breakfast	78

SAUSAGE & MASH

Bangers, Kids Menu	402
Vegetarian, Bangers, Kids Menu	354

SCAMPI

Breaded, & Chips, with Mushy Peas	828
Breaded, & Chips, with Peas	790

SORBET

Coconut	233

SOUP

Broccoli	255
Carrot, & Coriander	261
Leek, & Potato	312
Mushroom, Cream Of	291

SPAGHETTI BOLOGNAISE

Kids Menu	322

SPREAD

Sunflower, Portion, Breakfast	43

SQUID

Calamari, with Sweet Chilli, Starter	438

SUNDAE

Chocolate, Churros	748
Chocolate, with Kit Kat	526
Chocolate Browne, Mini, Value Menu	277
Funny Face, Kids Menu	196

SYRUP

Maple, Breakfastr	62

TART

Lemon	450

TOAST

GF, Breakfast	84
Malted, Breakfast	92
White, Breakfast	92

TOMATOES

Half, Breakfast	9

TORTE

Chocolate, Greek Yoghurt, Mini	295

TABLE TABLE
VEGETABLES
Sticks, Side, Kids Menu	26
Sticks, Starter, Kids Menu	48

VEGETABLES MIXED
Green, Side	112

YOGHURT
Greek Style	87
Strawberry, Frozen, Kids Menu	142
Strawberry, Kids Menu	115
Strawberry	115
Vanilla	96

THE REAL GREEK FOOD COMPANY LTD
ASPARAGUS
Grilled, Hot Meze	140

CHEESE
Halloumi, Grilled, Hot Meze	151
Halloumi, Skewers, Hot Meze	118
Halloumi, Skewers, Kids Menu	118

CHICK PEAS
Revithia, Cold Meze	286

CHICKEN
Skewers, Hot Meze	177
Skewers, Kids Menu	88

CHIPS
Side	528

COD
Salt, Hot Meze	346

CRUDITES
Cold Meze	37

DESSERT
Watermelon, Sweet & Salty	124
Yoghurt, Greek with Raspberries	223

DIP
Aioli, Parsley	176
Dip, Selection	589
Mayonnaise, Lemon, Preserved	279
Melitzanasalata, Cold Meze	236
Relish, Chilli, Smoked	42
Relish, Sun-Dried Tomato & Roast Red Pepper	92

DOLMADES
Cold Meze	254

FLATBREAD
Greek, Cold Meze	615
Greek, with Olive & Dukkah, Nibbles	538

HOUMOUS
Cold Meze	298

LAMB
Cutlets, Hot Meze	881
Kefte, Hot Meze	344
Skewers, Hot Meze	255

NUTS
Mixed, Athenian, Nibbles	479

OCTOPUS
Grilled, Hot Meze	447

OLIVES
Nibbles	317

PARCELS
Tiropitakia, Filo Pastry, Hot Meze	416

PORK
Skewers, Hot Meze	281

POTATOES
New, in Olive Oil & Lemon Juice, Hot Meze	293

RICE
Saffron, Hot Meze	406

THE REAL GREEK FOOD COMPANY LTD

SALAD

Cos	42
Tabouleh, Cold Meze	117
Watermelon, Mint & Feta, Cold Meze	102

SARDINES

Grilled, Hot Meze	619

SOUVLAKI

Lamb, Kefte	730
Lamb	607
Pork	633
Souvlaki, Halloumi & Vegetable	451

SQUID

Kalamari, Grilled, Hot Meze	286

TARAMASALATA

Cold Meze	913

TZATZIKI

Cold Meze	163

TOBY CARVERY

AUBERGINE

Stack, Grilled	150

BACON

Back, Breakfast, All You Can Eat	188

BAKE

Leek, Crumble, Carvery	103
Potato, & Carrot, Carvery	121
Potato, & Leek, Carvery	120
Potato, & Parsnip, Carvery	145
Potato, & Squash, Carvery	123
Tomato, Crumble, Carvery	112

BEANS

Baked, Breakfast, All You Can Eat	76
Baked, Side, Kids Menu	76
Green, Carvery	44
Romano, Carvery	59

BEEF

Roast, Carvery	274

BISCUITS

Oreo, Crumb, Sundae Topping	97

BITES

Onion	61

BOLOGNESE

Spaghetti, Kids Menu	233

BREAD

Brown, Sandwich Choice	387
Ciabatta, Sanwich Choice	293
Ciabatta, with Lurpak	337
Garlic, Ciabatta	364
Garlic, Ciabatta, with Cheese	529
Garlic, Kids Menu	182
White, Bap, Sandwich Choice	324
White, Sandwich Choice	420
Wholemeal, Bap, Sandwich Choice	246

BREAKFAST CEREAL

Porridge, Breakfast, All You Can Eat	243

BROCCOLI

Carvery	39

BROWNIES

Chocolate, Millionaires	896
Chocolate, Pieces, Mini	259

BUBBLE & SQUEAK

Carvery	85

BURGERS

Beef, Roast, with Roast Potatoes	1320
Chicken, Kids Menu	370
Very Vegan, with Roast Potatoes	960

BUTTERNUT SQUASH

Carvery	467

CABBAGE

Red, with Cranberry, & Orange, Carvery	79
Seasonal, Carvery	196

TOBY CARVERY

CAKE
Chocolate, & Raspberry, Fondant	584
Chocolate, Fudge	574
Mousse, Chocolate, & Orange	319

CARROTS
Carvery	31

CAULIFLOWER CHEESE
Carvery	37
Portion	59

CHEESECAKE
Vanilla, Baked	782

CHICKEN
Nuggets, Kids Menu	190
Strips, Southern Fried, Spicy, with BBQ Sauce	302
Wings, BBQ Sauce	387

CHICKEN DINNER
Baby's	123

CHILLI
Non Carne, with Basmati Rice	442

CHOCOLATE
Flake, Extra	44

COOKIES
Chocolate Chip, Sundae Topping	256

CORN
Cob, Mini, Carvery	49
Cob, Mini, Side, Kids Menu	58
Cob, Mini, Side	133

COURGETTE
Lemon & Thyme, Roasted, Carvery	35

CREAM
Whipped, for Desserts	148

CRUMBLE
Apple, Blackberry, & Redcurrant, Kids Menu	379
Apple, Blackberry, & Redcurrant, Mini	299
Apple, Blackberry, & Redcurrant	423
Apple, Bramley, & Cinnamon, Mini	279
Apple & Cinnamon, with Custard, Kids Menu	359

CUSTARD
for Desserts	135
Soya, Vegan, for Desserts	80

DESSERT
Knickerbocker Glory	543

DUMPLINGS
in Onion Gravy, Carvery	469

EGGS
Fried, Free Range, Breakfast, All You Can Eat	143
Scrambled, Breakfast, All You Can Eat	108

FRUIT COMPOTE
Apple, Blackberry, & Redcurrant, Porridge Topping	42
Apple, with Cinnamon, Porridge Topping	67
Toffee, Apple, & Banana, Porridge Topping	82

TOBY CARVERY

GAMMON
Pomegranate Glaze, Carvery	196

GRAVY
Breakfast, All You Can Eat	54
Classic, Carvery	23
Cranberry, Carvery	208

HASH
Potato, Cheese, & Onion, Breakfast, All You Can Eat	97

HONEYCOMB
Pieces, Sundae Topping	78

HOUMOUS
with Veg, & Bread	474

ICE CREAM
for Desserts	115
Kids Menu	179
No Sauce	213

ICE LOLLY
Pip Organic, Kids Menu	20

LAMB
Roast, Carvery	214

LASAGNE
Lentil, & Sage	427

LEEKS
Carvery	30

MACARONI CHEESE
Carvery	100
Kids Menu	150

MARSHMALLOWS
Sundae Topping	50

MUSHROOMS
Garlic	228
Roasted, Breakfast, All You Can Eat	425

MUSTARD
English, Carvery	194
Wholegrain, Carvery	213

NACHOS
in a Yorkie, Sharing	1358

ONIONS
in Gravy, Carvery	61

PARCELS
Broccoli, & Brie	492
Chilli Cheese	376

PARSNIP
Honey Roast, Carvery	163
with Marmalade Glaze	125

PEAS
Carvery	80

PIE
Allotment	352
Apple	246
Mushroom, & Ale, Roast	761

TOBY CARVERY

PLATTER
Taster	1867

PORK
Roast, No Crackling, Carvery	135

POTATO
Carvery	669

POTATOES
Diced, Breakfast, All You Can Eat	91
Mashed, Carvery	99
Roast, Beef Dripping, Carvery	111
Roast, Bowl, Side	229
Roast, Carvery	94
Roast, Loaded	321

PRAWN COCKTAIL
King, with Bread	417
King, with Wholemeal Bread, Mini, Kids Menu	300

PROFITEROLES
Baileys	490

PUDDING
Arctic Roll, with Whipped Cream	418
Summer	331
Three Little	1145

SALAD
Caesar, Side	191
Caesar	334
Super Green, no Cheese, Side	64
Super Green, no Cheese	127
Super Green, with Cheese, Side	83
Super Green, with Cheese, Small, Side	73
Super Green, with Cheese	145
Turkey, Avocado, & Bacon	497

SALMON
En Pappillote	368

SANDWICH FILLING
Beef, Roast, Mushroom, & Chutney, Add Bread	641
Cheese, & Chutney, Add Bread	266
Hunters Gammon, Add Bread	501
Pork, Roast, Add Bread	521
Prawn, King, Add Bread	332
Turkey, Roast, Club, Add Bread	530

SAUCE
Apple, Carvery	103
Bread, Carvery	443
Chocolate, Belgian	58
Cranberry, Carvery	210
Horseradish, Carvery	178
Lemon, Sicillian	55
Mint, Carvery	45
Parsley, Carvery	467
Strawberry	57
Toffee, Devon Cream	64

TOBY CARVERY

SAUSAGE
& Giant Yorkshire Pudding, Kids Menu	327
Pigs, In Portionets, Mini	531
Pork, British, Breakfast, All You Can Eat	217
Quorn, Breakfast, All You Can Eat	128
Quorn*, & Giant Yorkshire Pudding, Kids Menu	292

SORBET
Trio	453

SOUP
Small, Side	58
Tomato, with Wholemeal Bread, Kids Menu	226

SPINACH
Creamed, Carvery	41

SPONGE
Apricot, with Custard	406
Cherry, with Custard	399
Rhubarb, with Custard	410
Rolo Toffee, with Custard	509
Strawberry, with Custard	407
Treacle	526

SPROUTS
Carvery	64
with Bacon, Maple, Carvery	76

STRAWBERRIES
& Cream	200
& Ice Cream	167

STUFFING
Sage, & Cranberry, Carvery	340
Sage, & Onion, Carvery	204

SUNDAE
Best of British	588
Chocolate, & Toffee	454
Chocolate, Heaven, Kids Menu	362
Cookie Dough	503
Honeycomb Dream	423
Make Your Own, Kids Menu	281
Mango, & Passion Fruit, Blizzard	385

SWEDE
Carvery	7

SWEET POTATO
Carvery	146

TART
Lemon, Creamy, with Raspberries, & Whipped Cream	628

TOAD IN THE HOLE
Veggie	1073

TOAST
White, Breakfast, All You Can Eat	478

TOMATOES
Plum, Breakfast, All You Can Eat	15

TURKEY
Roast, Carvery	118

TOBY CARVERY
VEGETABLES
Leeks, Cabbage, & Peas, Carvery	59
Mediterranean Style, Roasted, Carvery	397
Roast, with Gravy, Carvery	317
Root, Roast	347
Sticks, & Cheesy, BBQ, Dip, Kids Menu	106
Sticks, Side, Kids Menu	31

WAFERS
Extra	8

YORKSHIRE PUDDING
& Gravy, Side	168
& Gravy, Vegetarian, Side	215
Breakfast, All You Can Eat	381
Carvery	626
Sandwich Choice	328
Stuffed, Beef	313

VINTAGE INNS
BAKE - SLOW ROASTED TOMATO
& Almond, with Roast Potatoes, & Veg	1170

BEANS
Baked, Side, Childrens	80

BEEF - STEAK SIRLOIN, 8OZ
Triple Cooked Chips, Onions Rings, Roasted Tomato	966

BEEF - STEAK, FILLET, 7OZ
Triple Cooked Chips, Onion Rings, Roasted Tomato	798

BEEF - STEAK, RIBEYE, 10OZ
Triple Cooked Chips, Onion Rings, Roasted Tomato	963

BEEF - STEAK, RUMP, 8OZ
Triple Cooked Chips, Onion Rings, Roasted Tomato	927

BEEF BOURGUIGNON
Porcini, Slow Cooked, with Mash, Carrots, & Dumplings	432

BEEF DINNER, SIRLOIN
Yorkshire Pudding, Roast Potatoes, Veg, & Gravy	1598

BEEF DINNER, TRIO
Turkey, & Pork, Roast Potatoes, Veg, & Gravy	1379

BITES
Black Pudding	417
Black Pudding, Yorkshire	367
Yorkshire Pudding	299

BREAD
Garlic, Side, Childrens	373

BREAD & BUTTER PUDDING
Marmalade, with Custard	642

BROWNIES - CHOCOLATE
Belgian, Chocolate Sauce, & Irish Liqueur Ice Cream	832
with Vanilla Ice Cream, Childrens	553

BURGERS
Beef, Chargrilled, Dirty	1324
Beef, Chargrilled, with Mayo, Relish, & Onion Rings	734
Beef, no Sides, Children's	173
Beef, Prime, Dirty	933
Beef, Prime, with Mayo, Relish, & Onion Rings	343
Beef, Wagyu, with Salsa, Mayo, & Onion Rings	1460
Chicken, no Sides, Childrens	328
Chickpea, & Aubergine, Spiced	447
Plant Based, Moving Mountanis, with Side Salad	601

CAULIFLOWER
Roasted, Spiced, with Couscous, & Coconut Sauce	1104

CAULIFLOWER CHEESE
Portion	222

CHEESE
Camembert, Garlic & Rosemary, Baked	1035
Cheeseboard, with Biscuits, Grapes, & Chutney	1122

CHEESECAKE
Blackcurrant, & Prosecco	471
Caramel, Biscuit, Vegan, with Banana	777
Vanilla, Baked	414

VINTAGE INNS

CHICKEN
Hunters, with Bacon, & Tomato Sauce, & Chips	1478
Hunters, with Gammon, Chips, & BBq Sauce	1430
Wings, Southern Fried	599

CHIPS
Side, Childrens	698
Triple Cooked	499

COD
Battered, Fillet, no Sides, Childrens	290
Loin, & Chorizo Roasted Potatoes	572
Loin, & Tomatoes, Heirloom	330

CREME BRULEE
Apricot, with Biscuits	416

CRUMBLE
Winter Fruit, Spiced, with Custard	557
Winter Fruit, Spiced, with Soya Custard	572

DESSERT
Eton Mess	372

FISH & CHIPS - COD, BATTERED
Chips, Mushy Peas, & Tartare Sauce, Lunch Bites	963
Chips, Mushy Peas, & Tartare Sauce	1330

FISH CAKES - LOBSTER
with Bouillabaisse, Broccoli, & Potatoes, Lunch Bites	441
with Bouillabaisse, Broccoli, & Potatoes	602

FLATBREAD - GARLIC BUTTER
with Cheese, Stonebaked, Sharers & Grazing	864

FRIES
Skin On, Side, Childrens	539
Sweet Potato, Side, Childrens	293
Sweet Potato	377

GAMMON
Steak, 4oz, with Eggs, & Chips, Lunch Bites	765
Steak, 8oz, with Eggs, & Chips	1262

ICE CREAM
Chocolate, Childrens	355
Chocolate, Double	315
Irish Cream Liqueur	255
Vanilla, Childrens	278
Vanilla Pod	122

ICE LOLLY
Tropical Fruit, Childrens	20

JELLY
Peach, Childrens	144

KEBAB
Lamb Kofta, with Tzatziki, & Dressed Slaw, Starter	340

LAMB - DINNER, RUMP
Yorkshire Pudding, Roast Potatoes, Veg, & Gravy	1758

LAMB - DUO
Rump, & Shepherd's Pie, Veg, & Red Wine Jus, Main	1204

LAMB - RACK
Roasted, with Veg, & Spiced Potatoes	1142

VINTAGE INNS

LASAGNE
Beef, & Red Wine	583
Beef, no Sides, Children's	349

MUSHROOMS - GARLIC, BAKED
& Chees, Steak Add On	109
& Cheddar Sauce, with Rustic Bread, Starter	296

OLIVES
Mixed, Marinated in Garlic & Red Pepper	184

ONION RINGS
Homemade	86

PASTA
Tomato, Childrens	238

PATE
Duo, with Rustic Bread, Starter	432

PEAS
Side, Childrens	45

PIE - APPLE, BRAMLEY
with Custard, & Vanilla Pod Ice Cream	754

PIE - CHICKEN & MUSHROOM
with Mash, Roasted Carrots, & Veg	942

PIE - LEMON MERINGUE
Portion	393

PIE - STEAK & ALE
with Mash, Seasonal Veg, & a Jug of Gravy	1004

PIZZA
Chicken, Spicy Cajun, Stonebaked	1288
Four Cheese, Stonebaked	1209
Margherita, Childrens	577
Margherita, Stonebaked	963
Meat Feast, Stonebaked	1404
Vegetable, Roasted, with Pesto, Stonebaked	1134

PLATTER
Mezze, Sharers & Grazing	1293
Pudding, Tasting	2391
Sticky, Sharers & Grazing	2200

PORK - BELLY, ROAST
Yorkshire Pudding, Roast Potatoes, Veg, & Gravy	1703

PORK - BELLY, SLOW COOKED
with Mash, Crackling & Veg	1365

POTATOES
Baby, Side, Childrens	77
Mashed, Side, Children's	141
Roast	482

PRAWN COCKTAIL
with Lobster, with Rustic Bread, Starter	751

PRAWNS
Garlic, Steak Add On	209
Tempura, with Rice Cracker, & Soy, Lime & Chilli Dip	475

PUDDING
Sticky Toffee, with Butterscotch Sauce, & Custard	356

RIBS
Pork, Caramelised Sticky, with Mango Salsa	466

VINTAGE INNS

RICE
Sunshine, Side, Childrens	190

RISOTTO
Mushroom, Wild	1045
Mushroom, Wild, with Chicken	1243
Mushroom, Wild, with Halloumi	1443
Mushroom, Wild, with Salmon	1871
Seafood, with Roasted Tomatoes	1097

SALAD - CAESAR
with Chicken, & Garlic Flatbread	1201
with Garlic Flatbread	710
with Halloumi, & Garlic Flatbread	1050
with Salmon, & Garlic Flatbread	1141

SALAD - DUCK
Aromatic	337

SALAD - SIDE
Childrens	46

SALAD - WHEATBERRY
Apple, & Cranberry	1223
Apple, & Cranberry, with Chicken, Lunch Bites	1212
Apple, & Cranberry, with Chicken	1459
Apple, & Cranberry, with Halloumi, Lunch Bites	1064
Apple, & Cranberry, with Halloumi	1311
Apple, & Cranberry, with Lamb Koftas, Lunch Bites	890
Apple, & Cranberry, with Lamb Koftas	1137
Apple, & Cranberry, with Salmon, Lunch Bites	1078
Apple, & Cranberry, with Salmon	1753

SALMON
Pesto Crusted, & Mascarpone, Broccoli, Butter Sauce	1107

SANDWICH
Beef, Brisket, on Sourdough, no Chips	729
Beef, Roast, on a Rustic Roll, no Chips	1086
Chicken, & Camembert, Hot, on Foccacia, no Chips	769
Fish Finger, Cod, on a Rustic Roll, no Chips	578
Ham, & Cheddar, Melt, on Sourdough, no Chips	733

SAUCE
Bearnaise, Steak Sauce	210
Beef Dripping, Steak Sauce	162
Peppercorn, Steak Sauce	46

SAUSAGE
Pork, with Gravy, no Sides, Childrens	278

SCALLOPS
Extra	47
Black Pudding, Minted Pea Puree, Bacon, Starter	731

SEA BASS
with Pancetta Veloute, Broccoli, & Mash	754

SOUP
Broccoli, & Stilton	213
Pea, Mint, & Ham	302
Pea & Mint	204

SQUID - CALAMARI
Salt, Pepper, Chorizo, & Chipotle Chilli Mayo, Starter	476

VINTAGE INNS

STUFFING
Lemon & Thyme, Bacon Wrapped, Extra	385

TART
Carrot, & Apricot Chutney, & Salad, & Baby Potatoes	1078

TURKEY DINNER
Yorkshire Pudding, Roast Potatoes, Veg, & Gravy	1408

VEGETABLES
Skewer, no Sides, Childrens	83
Sticks, Side, Childrens	38

WRAP
Jackfruit, Smoky, with Side Salad, Vegan	233
Jackfruit, Smoky, without Chips	215

YORKSHIRE PUDDING
Extra	99
Roast Potatoes, Veg, & Gravy, No Meat, Childrens	660
Roast Potatoes, Veg, & Gravy, No Meat	660

WAGAMAMA

BANANA
Panko, Salted Caramel Ice Cream, Katsu	275

BEANS
Edamame, with Chilli	255
Edamame, with Salt	247

BEEF
Teriyaki, & Rice, Donburi	935

BROCCOLI
& Bok Choi, Wok-Fried, Greens	182

BUNS
Beef, Korean BBQ, & Red Onion, Steamed, Hirata	332
Mushroom, & Panko Aubergine, Steamed, Hirata	352
Pork, Belly, & Panko Apple, Steamed, Hirata	562

CAKE
Chocolate, Caramel, Smoked	519
Mango, & Matcha, Layer	258

CAULIFLOWER
Bang Bang	474

CHEESECAKE
Salted Caramel	383
White Chocolate, & Matcha	514
White Chocolate, & Ginger	454

CHICKEN
Crispy, with Sesame, & Soy Sauce, Tori Kara Age	441
Grilled, & Soba Noodles, Kids Menu	458
Grilled, Katsu, Naked	607
Grilled, Katsu, with Amai Sauce, Mini, Kids Menu	412
Grilled, Katsu, with Curry Sauce, Mini, Kids Menu	434
Panko, Katsu, Amai Sauce, Mini, Kids Menu	463
Panko, Katsu, Curry Sauce, Mini, Kids Menu	486
Rice, Egg, Stir Fry, Cha Han, Mini, Kids Menu	406
Skewers, Teriyaki, Yakitori	267
Teriyaki, & Rice, Donburi	787

CHILLI
Side	2

CURRY - CHICKEN
& Sticky Rice, Katsu	1127
& White Rice, Nikko	948
& White Rice, Raisukaree	1161

CURRY - FISH
Sea Bream, & White Rice, Nikko	939

CURRY - PRAWN
& White, Rice, Firecracker	1083
& White Rice, Raisukaree	1072

CURRY - SEITAN
Panko Crusted, with Sticky Rice, Vegatsu	1160

CURRY - VEGETABLE YASAI
& Sticky Rice, Katsu, Amai Sauce, Mini, Kids Menu	384
& Sticky Rice, Katsu, Curry Sauce, Mini, Kids Menu	407
& Sticky Rice, Katsu	1161
& White Rice, Nikko	798

WAGAMAMA

DUCK
Grilled, Teriyaki, with Rice, Donburi	1407
Lettuce, Wraps	336
Wrap, with Cucumber, & Hoisin Sauce	441

DUMPLINGS
Chicken, Steamed, Gyoza	224
Duck, Fried, Gyoza	373
Pork, Pulled, Steamed, Gyoza	231
Prawn, Fried, Gyoza	235
Yasai, Steamed, Gyoza	210

EGGS
Tea Stained, Side	94

FISH
Bites, Crispy, with Amai Sauce, Mini, Kids Menu	579
Bites, Crispy, with Curry Sauce, Mini, Kids Menu	579
White, Grilled, with Soba Noodles, Kids Menu	388

ICE CREAM
Caramel, Salted	496
Chocolate, & Orange Blossom	299
Coconut, Reika	449
Coffee, Vietnamese	471
Guava, Pink, & Passion Fruit	163
Strawberry, & Yuzu	319
Vanilla, Pod, Kids Menu	137
Vanilla, Pod	459

ICE LOLLY
Blackcurrant, & Apple, Little Ko Pop	32
Mango, & Apple, Little Ko Pop	38

JUICE
Apple, & Orange, Mini, Kids Menu	87
Apple, Mini, Kids Menu	68
Blueberry, Spice	191
Carrot	72
Fruit	146
Orange	110
Positive	159
Power	158
Raw	97
Tropical	172

KIMCHI
Side	16

NOODLES
Plain, Side	321

NOODLES - BEEF
Brisket, Tantanmen, Ramen	669
Steak, Sirloin, Chilli, Ramen	730
Steak, Sirloin, Teriyaki, Soba, Teppanyaki	909
Bulgogi, Soba, Teppanyaki	877

NOODLES - CHICKEN
Ginger, Udon, Teppanyaki	691
Grilled, Chilli, Ramen	617
Grilled, Ramen, Mini, Kids Menu	409

WAGAMAMA

NOODLES - CHICKEN
Grilled, Ramen	500
Yaki Soba, Mini, Kids Menu	374

NOODLES - CHICKEN & PRAWN
Pad-Thai, Teppanyaki	809
Yaki Soba, Teppanyaki	717
Yaki Udon, Teppanyaki	664

NOODLES - CHICKEN, PRAWN, PORK, MUSSELS
Wagamama, Ramen	708

NOODLES - COD
Miso Glazed, Ramen	659
Mokutan Soba, Teppanyaki	831

NOODLES - LAMB
Teriyaki, Soba, Teppanyaki	942

NOODLES - PORK
Belly, Shirodashi, Ramen	971

NOODLES - PRAWN
Chilli,& Kimchee, Ramen	543

NOODLES - SALMON
Teriyaki, Soba, Teppanyaki	892

NOODLES - TOFU
& Vegetable, Yasai, Pad-Thai, Teppanyaki	809
& Veg, Yasai, Rice Noodles, Ramen, Mini, Kids Menu	275
& Veg, Yasai, Thin Noodles, Ramen, Mini, Kids Menu	297
& Vegetable, Yasai Yaki Soba, Mini, Kids Menu	364
Kare Burosu, Ramen	615

NOODLES - VEGETABLE
Yasai Yaki Soba, Teppanyaki	764

PICKLE
Japanese, Side	4

PRAWNS
in Breadcrumbs, Crispy, Chilli Sauce, Ebi Katsu	282
Skewers, Lollipop, Kushiyaki	142

RICE
Brown, Side	395
Steamed, Side	543
Sticky, Side	498

SALAD
Beef, Sirloin, & Shiitake Mushrooms	463
Chicken, & Prawn, Pad Thai	315
Chicken, Harusame, Glass Noodle	441
Raw	335
Tofu, Harusame, Glass Noodle	438

SOUP
Miso, & Japanese Pickles, Side	41

SQUID
Balls, Tama	357
Chilli, Crispy, Side	503

STIR FRY
Avant Gard'n, Vegan	567

TART
Yuzu, & Lemon	306

WAGAMAMA

TOFU
Rice, Egg, Stir Fry, Cha Han, Mini, Kids Menu	359

TUNA
Steak,Nuoc Cham, Seared	468

VEGETABLES
Tempura	385

WIMPY

BACON
Slice	65

BEANS
Baked, Heinz, Extra	69

BREAKFAST
All Day	832
Country	359
Hashbrown	396
Sunrise	340
The Great Wimpy	758

BROWNIES
Chocolate	639

BURGERS
Bean, Spicy, & Slaw, Stack, Vegetarian	673
Bean, Spicy, Vegetarian	557
Bender, in a Bun, with Cheese	527
Cheese Burger, Double	647
Cheese Burger	433
Cheeseburger, Junior, with Beans, Kids	477
Cheeseburger, Junior, with Chips, Kids	601
Cheeseburger, Junior, with Salad, Kids	422
Chicken, Fillet, Firecracker Sauce	498
Chicken, Fillet, with BBQ Sauce	503
Chicken, Fillet, with Wimpy Mayo	527
Chicken, Gourmet	510
Fish Finger	577
Halfpounder, Original	876
Halfpounder with Bacon & Cheese	861
Hamburger	392
Junior, with Beans, Kids	436
Junior, with Chips, Kids	560
Junior, with Salad, Kids	381
Kingsize	823
Mega	789
Quarterpounder, Club	736
Quarterpounder, Patty Only	264
QuarterPounder, Smoky BBQ	693
QuarterPounder, with Cheese, Original	613
QuarterPounder, with Mushroom	646
Quarterpounder with Bacon & Cheese	597
Quorn, Southern Fried, Spicy, Vegetarian	506

CHEESE
Mozzarella, Melts, 6	390
Slices, Extras	41

CHICKEN
Platter, Gourmet	645
Strips, & Chips	685
Strips, with Beans, Kids	310
Strips, with Chips, Kids	433
Strips, with Salad, Kids	254
Wings, Coated, with BBQ Sauce	477
Wings, Coated, with Firecracker Sauce	466

WIMPY

CHIPS
Large	333
Reg	267
Sweet Potato, Large	340
Sweet Potato, Reg	269

CHOCOLATE
Flake, for Sundae	45

COFFEE
Americano, Black, Large	5
Americano, Black, Reg	3
Americano, with Milk, Large	26
Americano, with Milk, Reg	16
Cappuccino, Large	109
Cappuccino, Reg	81
Esspresso, Large	5
Esspresso, Reg	3
Latte, Large	139
Latte, Reg	111
Mocha, Large	248
Mocha, Reg	183
Shot, Extra	3

COLA
Pepsi, Diet, Kids	2
Pepsi, Diet, Large	3
Pepsi, Diet, Reg	2
Pepsi, Large	181
Pepsi, Max, Kids	1
Pepsi, Max, Large	2
Pepsi, Max, Reg	2
Pepsi, Reg	143

COLESLAW
Extra	171

CREAM
Extra, for Desserts	70
Extra, for Drinks	39

DESSERT
Brown Derby with Dairy Ice Cream	436

DRESSING
Caesar	219
French	60
Wimpy Mayo	199

EGGS
Fried, Extra	90
Fried, on Toast, White	458
Scrambled, Extra	65
Scrambled, on Toast, White	409

FISH
Bites, with Beans, Kids	255
Bites, with Chips, Kids	379
Bites, with Salad, Kids	200

FISH & CHIPS
Cod	705

WIMPY

GRILLS
International	1024
Wimpy	803

HASH BROWNS
Extra	98

HOT CHOCOLATE
without Cream, Large	281
without Cream, Reg	224

ICE CREAM
Extra	95

ICE CREAM FLOAT
7 Up	99
Pepsi, Diet	96
Pepsi	183
Pepsi Max	96
Tango Orange	97

JAM
Extra	48

JELLY
Orange, Pot, Kids	3
Strawberry, Pot, Kids	5

JUICE
Apple, Kids	122
Apple, Large	206
Apple, Reg	163
Orange, Kids	120
Orange, Large	202
Orange, Reg	160

LEMONADE
7 Up, Free, Kids	5
7 Up, Free, Large	9
7 Up, Free, Reg	7

MARMALADE
Extra	49

MILK
Kids	125
Large	211
Reg	167

MILK SHAKE
Banana, Thick, Kids	187
Banana, Thick, Large	300
Banana, Thick, Reg	244
Choco Toffee Popcorn, Thick, Reg	425
Chocolate, Peppermint, Thick, Reg	365
Chocolate, Thick, Kids	189
Chocolate, Thick, Large	303
Chocolate, Thick, Reg	246
Lime, Thick, Kids	152
Lime, Thick, Large	243
Lime, Thick, Reg	197
Strawberry, Thick, Kids	187

WIMPY

MILK SHAKE
Strawberry, Thick, Large	299
Strawberry, Thick, Reg	243
Vanilla, Thick, Kids	151
Vanilla, Thick, Large	241
Vanilla, Thick, Reg	196

MUFFIN
Bacon, & Egg	347
Bacon, & Hasbrown	445
Hashbrown	380
Sausage, & Egg	380
Sausage, & Hashbrown	478

MUSHROOMS
Extra	110

ONION RINGS
8	317
CheesO, 4	481

PANCAKE
& Ice Cream, no Toppings, Kids	178
& Ice Cream, no Toppings	344

PEAS
Extras	86

PEPPER
Jalapeno, Burger Extras	1

POTATO FILLING
Bacon	65
Beans, Baked, Heinz	79
Cheese, Grated	189
Coleslaw	194
Mushrooms	137

POTATOES
Baked, Jacket, Half, with Beans, Kids	297
Baked, Jacket, Half, with Cheese, Kids	347
Baked, Jacket, Half, with Chips, Kids	421
Baked, Jacket, Half, with Salad, Kids	241
Baked, Jacket, Plain, with Butter	516
Jacket, with Butter, & Salad, add Fillings Seperately	523

SALAD
Chicken, Breaded, no Dressing	360
Chicken, Gourmet, no Dressing	317
Junior, Side, Kids	8
Mixed, Side	67
Quorn, Southern Fried, Spicy, no Dressing	320

SAUCE
BBQ	41
Chocolate, for Sundae	81
Firecracker	29
Ketchup	29
Mango, for Sundae	25
Maple Flavoured, for Sundae	86
Special	114
Strawberry, for Sundae	80

WIMPY
SAUCE
Summer Fruits, for Sundae	38
Toffee Fudge, for Sundae	91
Wimpy Mayo	100

SAUSAGE
Bender, with Egg & Chips, Grill	628
Patty, Extra	98
Pork, Bender	271
Pork, Breakfast	130
with Beans, Kids	322
with Chips, Kids	446
with Egg & Chips, Grill	615
with Salad, Kids	267

SMOOTHIE
Mango, Iced	181
Summer Fruits, Iced	274

SQUASH
Apple, & Blackcurrant, Kids	4
Orange, Kids	3

SUNDAE
Brownie	591
Ice Cream, No Toppings, Kids	95
Ice Cream, No Toppings	159
Knickerbocker Glory	372

TANGO*
Orange, Free, Kids	3
Orange, Free, Large	4
Orange, Free, Reg	3

TEA
Black, Large	1
Black, Reg	1
Herbal, Large	3
Herbal, Reg	2
with Milk, Large	22
with Milk, Reg	14

TEACAKES
Toasted, with Butter	295

TOAST
White, with Butter	279

TOASTIE
Cheese, & Red Onion, White	391
Cheese, & Tomato, White	386
Cheese, with Beans, White, Kids	400
Cheese, with Chips, White, Kids	521
Cheese, with Salad, White, Kids	345
Chicken, BBQ, White	523
Ham, & Cheese, White	436

TOPPING
Flake, Crushed, for Drinks	45
Fruit Cocktail, for Sundae	18
Fudge, Pieces, Mini	40
Marshmallows, Mini, for Drinks	32

WIMPY
TOPPING
Marshmallows, Mini, for Sundae	32
Strawberries, for Sundae	10

TORTE
Apple, no Toppings	245

VEGETABLES
Sticks, Carrot, & Cucumber, Kids	24

WAFFLES
Eskimo, no Toppings	663

Useful Resources

Weight Loss
Weight Loss Resources is home to the UK's largest calorie and nutrition database along with diaries, tools and expert advice for weight loss and health.
Tel: 01733 345592   Email: helpteam@weightlossresources.co.uk
Website: www.weightlossresources.co.uk

Products to Help You Keep Track
From food diaries to weight graphs and calorie counted recipe books visit the wlr shop.
Tel: 01733 345592   Email: helpteam@weightlossresources.co.uk
Website: www.weightlossresources.co.uk/shop

Dietary Advice
The British Dietetic Association has helpful food fact leaflets and information on how to contact a registered dietitian.
Tel: 0121 200 8080 Email: info@bda.uk.com
Website: www.bda.uk.com

Healthy Eating
The British Nutrition Foundation has lots of in depth scientifically based nutritional information, knowledge and advice on healthy eating for all ages.
Tel: 0207 7557 7930 Email: postbox@nutrition.org.uk
Website: www.nutrition.org.uk

Healthy Heart
The British Heart Foundation provides advice and information for all on all heart aspects from being healthy, to living with heart conditions, research and fundraising.
Tel: 0207 554 000 Email: via their website
Website: www.bhf.org.uk

Cancer Research
Cancer Research UK is the leading UK charity dedicated to research, education and fundraising for all forms of cancer.
Tel: 0300 123 1022 Email: via their website
Website: www.cancerresearchuk.org

Diabetes Advice

Diabetes UK is the leading charity working for people with diabetes. Their mission is to improve the lives of people with diabetes and to work towards a future without diabetes
Tel : 0345 123 2399 Email: info@diabetes.org.uk
Website: www.diabetes.org.uk

Beating Bowel Cancer

Beating Bowel Cancer is a leading UK charity for bowel cancer patients, working to raise awareness of symptoms, promote early diagnosis and encourage open access to treatment choice for those affected by bowel cancer.Tel: 08450 719301 Email: nurse@beatingbowelcancer.org
Website: www.beatingbowelcancer.org

Safety and Standards

The Food Standards Agency is an independent watchdog, set up to protect the public's health and consumer interests in relation to food.
Tel: 0207 276 8829 Email: helpline@foodstandards.gsi.gov.uk
Website: www.food.gov.uk

Feedback

If you have any comments or suggestions about The Calorie, Carb & Fat Bible, or would like further information on Weight Loss Resources, please call, email, or write to us:

Tel:	01733 345592
Email:	helpteam@weightlossresources.co.uk
Address:	Rebecca Walton,
	Weight Loss Resources Ltd,
	2C Flag Business Exchange,
	Vicarage Farm Road,
	Peterborough,
	PE1 5TX.

Reviews for The Calorie Carb & Fat Bible

'What a brilliant book. I know I'll be sinking my teeth into it.'
GMTV Nutritionist Amanda Ursell, BSc RD

'To help you make low-cal choices everyday, invest in a copy.'
ZEST magazine

'There is no doubt that the food listings are extremely helpful
for anyone wishing to control their calorie intake in order to lose
pounds or maintain a healthy weight.'
Women's Fitness magazine

'Useful if you don't want to exclude any overall food groups.'
Easy Living magazine

'Quite simply an astonishing achievement by the authors.'
Evening Post, Nottingham

'The book gives you all the basic information so you can work out
your daily calorie needs.'
Woman magazine

'This is a welcome resource in view of the 'national epidemic of obesity.'

Bryony Philip, Bowel Cancer UK

'The authors seem to understand the problems of slimming.'

Dr John Campion

'Jam-packed with info on dieting, and full to bursting point with the calorie, carbohydrate and fat values of thousands of different foods, it's the perfect weight loss tool.'

Evening Express, Aberdeen

'Excellent resource tool - used by myself in my role as a Practice Nurse.'

Pam Boal, Sunderland

'I recently bought your book called the Calorie, Carb & Fat Bible and would love to tell you what a brilliant book it is. I have recently started a weight management programme and I honestly don't know where I'd be without your book. It has helped me a lot and given me some really good advice.'

Rachel Mitchell

About Weight Loss Resources

If you want to lose weight in a healthy, sustainable way, you'll find all the tools and support you need at wlr. Available on your phone, tablet, or PC.

HERE'S THE HIGHLIGHTS:

- Track calories: how many you need, how many you've consumed and burned, and how many you have left

- New Visual Food Diary, a more relaxed way to track. Enables you to reflect on choices and gain insights about your relationship with food

- The best kept online UK food database

- 1000s of recipes and meal ideas that you can add to your online diary and adapt to suit yourself

- Create and calorie count your own recipes and diet plans

- Set a weight loss goal, see how many calories you need to get there, and the date you can expect to reach it

- Fantastic support from our knowledgeable Helpteam, available 7 days a week

You can take a free trial at www.weightlossresources.co.uk or give us a call on 01733 345592